Lymphatic Tissues and In Vivo Immune Responses

edited by

Beat A. Imhof
Basel Institute for Immunology
Basel, Switzerland

Sonia Berrih-Aknin
CCML,CNRS URA-1159
Le Plessis-Robinson, France

Sophie Ezine
INSERM U-345,Hôspital Necker
Paris, France

Marcel Dekker, Inc. New York • Basel • Hong Kong

Library of Congress Cataloging-in-Publication Data

Lymphatic tissues and in vivo immune responses / edited by Beat Imhof,
S. Berrih-Aknin, S. Ezine.
p. cm.
Proceedings of the Tenth International Conference on Lymphatic Tissues and Germinal Centres in Immune Reactions, held in Compiégne, France, July 1-5, 1990.
Includes bibliographical references and index.
ISBN 0-8247-8528-2 (alk. paper)
1. Immune response--Congresses. 2. Lymphatics--Congresses.
I. Imhof, Beat. II. Berrih-Aknin, S. (Sonia). III. Ezine, S. (Sophie).
IV. International Conference on Lymphatic Tissues and Germinal Centres in Immune Reactions (10th: 1990: Compiégne, France)
[DNLM: 1. Cell Movement--physiology--congresses. 2. Immunity, Cellular--congresses. 3. Lymphocytes--physiology--congresses.
4. Lymphoid Tissue--physiology--congresses. QW 568 L9854 1990]
QR186.L9 1991
599'.029--dc20
DNLM/DLC
for Library of Congress 91-24647
CIP

This book is printed on acid free paper.

Marcel Dekker, Inc.
270 Madison Avenue, New York 10016

Current printing (last digit):
10 9 8 7 6 5 4 3 2 1

PRINTED IN THE UNITED STATES OF AMERICA

Preface

This book contains the proceedings of the Tenth International Conference on Lymphatic Tissues and Germinal Centres in Immune Reactions, called the 10th Germinal Centre Conference (GCC), held in Compiègne, France, July 1–5, 1990.

Over the last few years knowledge of functional molecules has increased dramatically. Genes of many reagents (cytokines, growth factors, and regulatory proteins) are now cloned, and pure recombinant products are available. However, most of these substances were found by well-defined assays in vitro. The aim of these conferences, organized about every 3 years, is to stimulate research on the function of molecules in vivo. This book explains many details—on the molecular level—of what has been described as immunological phenomenology. In an attempt to clarify a subject as complex as in vivo immunology, it has been divided into separate components.

One section is devoted to the detailed characterization of T lymphocytes and the differentiation from their progenitors. A new facet is the finding that the earliest T-cell progenitors bear low levels of the CD4 molecule before they become the so called $CD4^-8^-$ double-negative cells. Production of transgenic mice has allowed conclusions to be made on positive and negative selection during T-cell maturation. The differentiating cells always interact with accessory cells. The 20 chapters on thymic epithelial cells describe their characteristics and function and their probable accessory role. The various phenotypes can now be defined by monoclonal marker antibodies.

Corresponding to T cells is the immunology of B lymphocytes, their differentiation and interaction with follicular dendritic cells. The latter are described extensively in the section on accessory cells. Highlights are the presentation of a germinal center culture system allowing the interaction of B cells, follicular dendritic cells, and T cells in a controlled microenvironment. A further new, and certainly important, finding is that follicular dendritic cells can be infected by human immunodeficiency virus.

Much effort has been spent on the question of how lymphocytes migrate from the location of emergence to their site of action. The section on lymphocyte migration and homing includes chapters describing the phenotype of migrating cells, their regulation, and the adhesion molecules involved in homing. Tissue-specific vascular adhesion appears to be regulated by the local microenvironment. To deal with the peripheral response of mature lymphocytes, special attention is given to the mucosal immune system. Large numbers of lymphocytes can be found in the gut of adult animals permanently infected by its feces. A further problem arises if the peripheral immune system erroneously reacts against self-antigens, and the section on animal models for autoimmune diseases, i.e., diabetes or myasthenia gravis, may help to unravel this question.

We are grateful to the Commission of the European Communities, the Association Française contre les Myopathies, the Ministère des Affaires Etrangères, the Basel Institute for Immunology, and many private companies for support of the conference.

Our heartful thanks go to Paul Nieuwenhuis, who stood by us with much helpful advice during the preparations of the meeting; to Sigbjørn Fossum, whose experience organizing the 9th GCC saved us from many pitfalls; and to the other members of the scientific committee, Jean-François Bach, Dennis G. Osmond, Jean Paul Thiery, and G. Jeanette Thorbecke, whose many suggestions helped us establish the scientific program. Finally, we thank Jacques F. A. P. Miller, who gave the honorary lecture to celebrate the 10th GCC, and Jean-François Bach, Richard L. Boyd, Eugene Butcher, B. J. Fowlkes, Delphine Guy Grand, Marion D. Kendall, H. Robson MacDonald, Polly Matzinger, Thomas T. McDonald, Joost J. Oppenheim, Dennis G. Osmond, Martine Papiernik, Klaus Rajewsky, Jean Paul Thiery, G. Jeanette Thorbecke, Willem van Ewijk, Hartmut Wekerle, and Rolf Zinkernagel, all experts in their fields, who chaired the sessions and wrote the corresponding introductions to the sections in this book.

Beat A. Imhof
Sonia Berrih-Aknin
Sophie Ezine

Contents

ACCESSORY CELLS

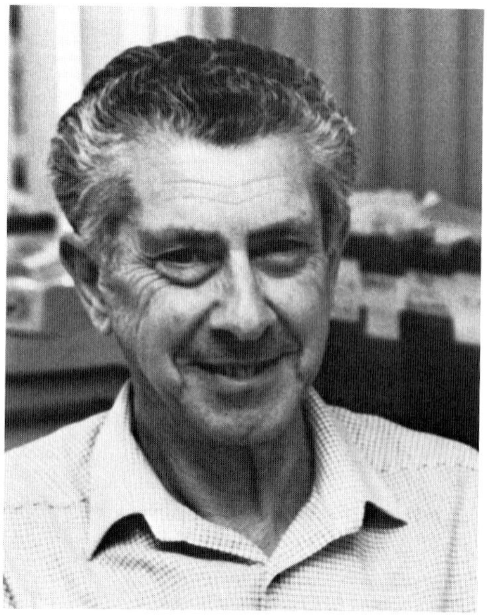

J. F. A. P. Miller

Do Self-Tolerant T Cells Exist In Vivo?

J. F. A. P. Miller
The Walter and Eliza Hall Institute of Medical Research, Royal Melbourne Hospital, Victoria, Australia

I am very grateful to the Organizers of the 10th International Conference on Lymphatic Tissues and Germinal Centres in Immune Reactions who have invited me to give this honorary lecture. This series of conferences has been very successful in bringing together numerous investigators, thus enabling them to present their most interesting results and create lively discussions. I was fortunate to participate in some of the early Conferences, notably the one held in Padova in 1968 (1), where I had the opportunity to show our evidence for T- and B-cell cooperation in antibody responses. This was an entirely new line of work, but the exact mechanism of the interaction was not clear. Several possibilities were envisaged at the next Conference, held in Uppsala in 1970 (2), including one in which "T cells might interact with antigen to produce factors [that] might facilitate the differentiation of B cells in response to certain antigens." We now, of course, know that the T-cell interleukins, IL-2 and IL-4, are involved in helping B cells produce antibody.

As a topic for this Honorary Lecture, I have chosen to examine a question raised 30 years ago by Sir Michael Woodruff: "Has anybody ever demonstrated that there are such things as tolerant cells?" (3) (T cells were unknown in those days). I presume tolerant T cells may be defined as cells able to produce specific antigen receptors, potentially able to perceive and bind to antigen-presenting cells, but unable to be switched on for reasons that have not been clarified. Clearly Sir Michael's question is an important one for if, for example, T cells tolerant to self-components do exist, it is incumbent upon us to determine whether some autoimmune reactions may result from their reactivation and how this may occur and be prevented. Moreover, if there are T cells tolerant to oncogene products, their reactivation may help limit tumor growth. But if self-tolerant T cells do exist and circulate around aimlessly, the question arises as to what could possibly be their role. Why should they not cease to exist? In the case of B cells, the work of Goodnow and colleagues has clearly demonstrated the existence of functionally silenced B cells in which surface immunoglobulin M (IgM) was downregulated (4). Such B cells are apparently not deleted and could still have some useful function; e.g., in antigen processing. T cells on the other hand do not possess such a processing function, so that the persistence of any functionally silenced T cells, if it occurs, certainly poses an enigma.

Whether T cells tolerant to self-components exist may now again be asked primarily because of the clear-cut demonstration of intrathymic clonal elimination of self-reactive T cells (5–8). If, however, the induction of self-tolerance is limited to antigens synthesized by thymic stromal cells during T-cell maturation, a major dilemma has to be faced. Must the entire array of the body's self-antigens be exhibited in the thymus? Otherwise, how could T cells capable of recognizing self-components unique to extrathymic tissues be negatively selected? Some autoantigens could of course be shed in the circulation and taken up by certain cells, such as dendritic cells or macrophages, which could reach the thymus where they would impose tolerance (9). If, however, as has been documented (10), major histocompatibility complex (MHC) class I molecules present peptides from endogenously synthesized proteins, such as self-components, and class II from exogenously synthesized proteins, such as shed antigens, how could differentiating class I reactive $CD8^+$ T cells be negatively selected within the thymus by shed antigens? Among the universe of peptides derived from self-constituents, some at least are unlikely to be represented within thymus tissue. It is therefore reasonable to ask whether T cells reactive to such peptides in the context of class I molecules do become tolerant and, if so, by what mechanism? Are they eliminated peripherally or functionally silenced? It is this question that we hope to solve, and I will not consider here the artificial situation in which tolerance is induced following exposure to *exogenous* antigens (e.g., see refs. 11 and 12), as this may not mimic the natural situation involving self-components synthesized from within cells. I will therefore limit this discussion to tolerance to bona fide self-constituents *synthesized* by body cells.

Transgenic technology has been used to introduce a gene whose product should potentially be able to be recognized by T lymphocytes. For example, several investigators microinjected particular MHC class II genes into fertilized eggs and analyzed transgenic offspring for tolerance to the transgene. In transgenic mice in which potentially responding T cells utilized a particular Vβ gene whose product could be detected by a monoclonal antibody, evidenced for the existence of tolerant (anergized) T lymphocytes was claimed. Thus, transgenic mice expressing I-E on β cells, but not in the thymus, were tolerant of I-E but had not deleted anti-Vβ17a-bearing T cells. These could not be stimulated in vitro with anti-Vβ17 monoclonal antibody in contrast to the Vβ17a-bearing T cells of SJL mice which lack I-E (13). Conceivably, therefore, I-E in the transgenic mice had not eliminated but functionally silenced potentially I-E reactive, Vβ17a-bearing T cells, which may thus be regarded as tolerant cells. A similar situation has been claimed to occur in other experiments in which Mls antigens or I-E was expressed on thymus cortical epithelial cells or in nude mice. In these models, T cells bearing particular Vβ genes were not deleted and were unable to respond in vitro in mixed lymphocyte reaction (MLR) to stimulation with appropriate anti-Vβ monoclonal antibodies except when supplemented with IL-2 (14–16). Such T cells were said to be anergic, anergy being defined as unresponsiveness in MLR with no apparent clonal deletion and unresponsiveness to anti–T-cell receptor (anti-TCR) or anti-CD3 monoclonal antibodies in the absence of added IL-2.

These data do not, however, exclude deletion as the tolerogenic mechanism. $V\beta17^+$ and $V\beta11^+$ T cells, for example, make only a minor contribution to MLR directed to I-E antigens in vitro, which implies that other cells, presumably of higher affinity, account for the bulk of the response (17). In peripheral tolerance to class II or Mls antigens, therefore, only the high-affinity T cells may have been deleted (possibly intrathymically on cortical epithelium or extrathymically in other cases). The $V\beta17^+$ T cells, being of lower affinity, would behave as virgin cells, which have been shown not to respond to anti-CD3 or anti-TCR monoclonal antibodies except in the presence of IL-2 (18). In other words, deletion of high-affinity clones and insufficient priming of low-affinity clones could explain all the results. If so, the evidence for the existence of tolerant, or anergic, cells remains questionable.

To determine what the situation might be in mice expressing unique class I molecules extrathymically, my colleagues and I microinjected into fertilized mouse eggs a class I gene (H-$2K^b$) linked to various tissue-specific promoters, such as the rat insulin promoter (RIP) and the sheep metallothionein promoter (MT). Tolerance to the transgene product was tested in transgenic offspring both in vivo and in vitro. Briefly, a search was made for lymphocytic infiltration in the transgene-producing tissues, the mice were grafted with skin from appropriate donors, and spleen cells were tested in vitro for cytotoxic activity against various targets. The results have been published (19–22) and only a brief summary is given here. No lymphocytic infiltration was ever seen at any stage in transgene-expressing tissues, even if the mice were given normal syngeneic (nontransgenic) spleen cells intravenously or stimulated with spleen cells from donors expressing H-$2K^b$. Infiltration was seen in transgenic recipients of H-$2K^b$ immune spleen cells, particularly in thymectomized irradiated hosts (21). This florid infiltrate did, however, subside with time, raising the possibility that peripheral tolerance may even have been induced in immune cells (21). H-$2K^b$-bearing skin was not rejected in older mice who had lost more than 75% of their β cells that were overexpressing H-$2K^b$ (19,22). This loss of tolerance thus appeared to occur when the concentration of the tolerated H-$2K^b$ fell below some critical threshold.

In vitro, spleen cells from young RIP mice could not kill the specific target, EL4, but did kill the third-party target, P815. Thymus cells, on the other hand, could kill both targets, clearly suggesting that tolerance was not imposed intrathymically. Spleen cells from older RIP mice (those that had lost most of their β cells) killed both targets, which agrees with the in vivo data. Most interestingly, reactivity to EL4 was restored to young spleen cells by providing them with IL-2 (20). Conceivably, therefore, cytolytic T cell precursors (CTL_p) specific for H-$2K^b$ were neither eliminated nor permanently silenced. Indeed, there may be no need to impose tolerance on these cells: withholding "help" would ensure an effective state of tolerance in vivo. Silencing or elimination of the "helper" cells would be sufficient to maintain tolerance. The potentially reactive CTL would persist and be activated only when the concentration of tolerogen fell below some threshold (e.g., in the older RIP mice), or upon delivery of both antigen and "help" (e.g., in the IL-2–supplemented CTL assays). The target cell for tolerance may thus be the IL-2–producing $CD8^+$ T cell that helps class I alloresponses (23). Tolerance would not be imposed upon these cells within the thymus, since $CD8^+$ T cells do not "see" shed antigens. Hence, these cells could help the alloresponse of thymus lymphocytes. By contrast, tolerance would be imposed on these cells in the periphery where antigen (shed or otherwise) is available, and the specific delivery of IL-2 would thus be limited in the spleen but not in the thymus. Alternatively, the target cells for tolerance in this transgenic model could be high-affinity anti-H-$2K^b$ T cells, which would either have been eliminated peripherally or functionally silenced. The low-affinity cells would have escaped but would be poorly equipped to deal with the rejection of skin grafts in vivo, or the killing of specific targets in vitro unless given help in the form of additional IL-2.

It has been repeatedly asked whether the thymus in our transgenic mice might not express a few molecules of transgene product, albeit too low to be detected by the immunoperoxidase technique. Could not such few molecules be involved in deleting clones of transgene reactive T cells? This is unlikely for several reasons: (1) In the RIP mice, tolerance waned as β-cell loss progressed; it is unlikely that intrathymic synthesis of a few transgene molecules should cease at the time of β-cell loss. (2) In the MT mice, tolerance persisted for life even following adult thymectomy, irradiation and injection of marrow, and grafting of thymus from syngeneic nontransgenic donors. Such a thymus graft would of course be unable to synthesize transgenic molecules. (3) It can always be argued that shed antigen reached the thymus where it would eliminate transgene reactive T cells. This is unlikely to be the case for $CD8^+$ T cells, which do not "see" exogenous antigen (10). It is also an unlikely possibility, since thymus cells in the RIP mice were reactive in vitro at the stage when spleen cells were specifically tolerant.

The question of how all potentially T cells could be tolerized by a few β cells has often been raised. Since the frequency of alloreactive T cells is of the order of 10%, a large pool of potentially reactive cells must have been eliminated or silenced by a rather small pool of β cells expressing the transgene in our RIP mice. Presumably, new T cells, recently emigrated from the thymus, would have had ample opportunity to circulate through the islets to perceive the antigen. The sensitivity of some T-cell subsets to a negative signal may perhaps continue for a short time after leaving the thymus; thus, antigen encounter during this critical period would lead to inactivation. Evidence in favor of this comes from studies showing that the same signal could tolerize thymocytes, but activate splenic T cells (24). Alternatively, the newly derived T cells may have encountered shed antigen, not in the islets, but at some other peripheral site where they would be eliminated or functionally silenced.

To examine the fate of anti–H-$2k^b$ CTLp in transgenic mice expressing H-$2K^b$ in an extrathymic site, we mated RIP-K^b transgenic mice to mice transgenic for an anti–H-$2K^b$ TCR. In single TCR transgenic mice, >95% of the T cells were $CD8^+$ and their TCR had

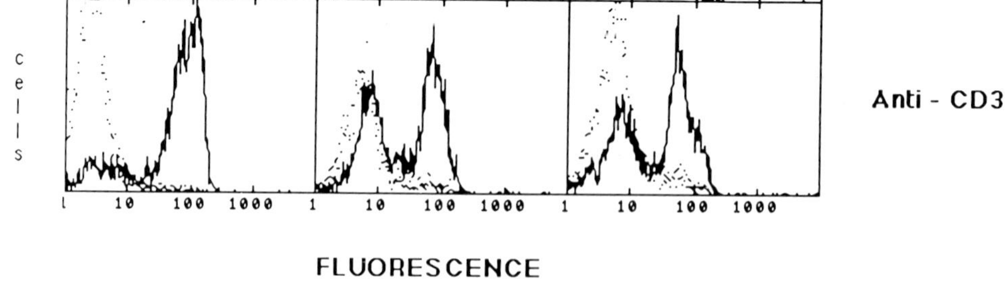

Figure 1 Flow cytometry of peripheral blood lymphocytes from mice of the following transgenic mouse lines: RIP-K^b (RIP), anti-K^b TCR (TCR) and double transgenics (RIP × TCR). The cells were stained with monoclonal antibodies against the Vβ11 transgene product or against the T-cell receptor complex, CD3. Negative controls for each mouse are indicated by the dotted line. Note the prevalence of Vβ11-positive cells in the TCR transgenics; these cells are not deleted in the double transgenic mice, which produce extra-thymic H-$2K^b$. (From unpublished data of G. Morahan and J. F. A. P. Miller.)

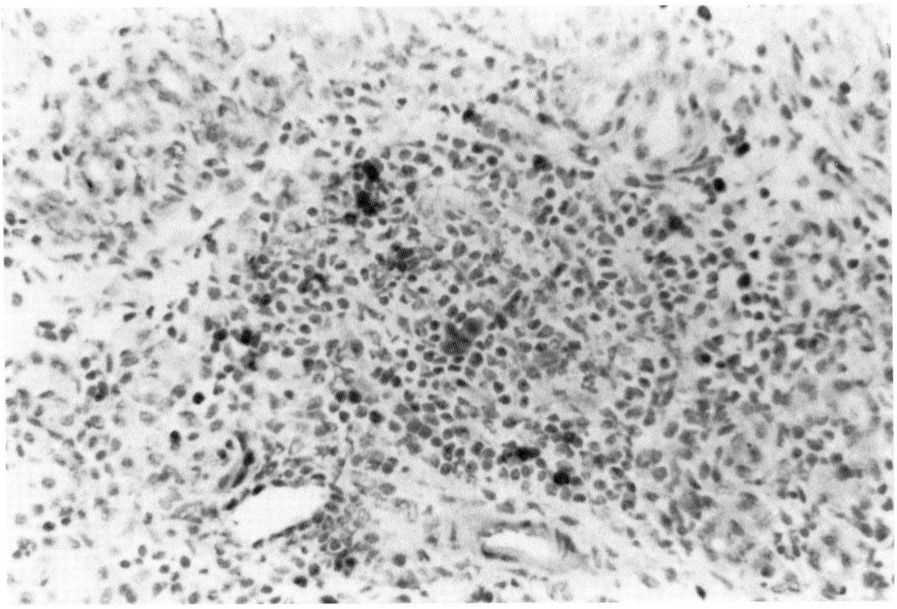

(a)

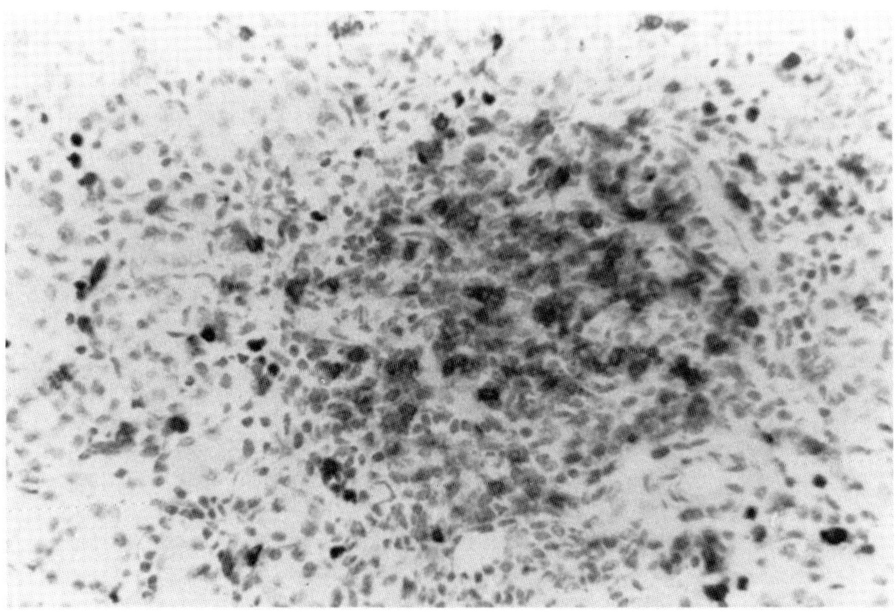

(b)

Figure 2 Lymphocytic infiltrate in pancreatic islets of double transgenic offspring of matings between RIP-K^b and anti–H-$2K^b$ transgenic mice. Immunoperoxidase sections stained with (a) anti-insulin antibody, and (b) anti-Vβ11. (From unpublished data of G. Morahan and J. F. A. P. Miller.)

the Vβ11 marker of the cytotoxic T lymphocyte (CTL) clone from which the TCR α and β genes were isolated. The double transgenic offspring showed no difference in the proportion of Vβ11-positive CD8$^+$ cells in peripheral blood, spleen, or lymph nodes (Fig. 1). In striking contrast to single transgenic RIP-K^b mice, variable lymphocytic infiltration was evident at different stages in some of the pancreatic islets (Fig. 2). The infiltrating cells were mostly CD8$^+$ and had the Vβ11 marker of the transgene. They did, however, lack IL-2 receptors, as determined by immunoperoxidase staining with an anti–IL-2R monoclonal antibody and they were small lymphocytes that appeared inactive. This contrasts with the situation in the diabetes-prone NOD mice in which up to 10% of the cells in the islet infiltrates were reported to be IL-2R$^+$ (25). In vitro, spleen cells from double transgenic mice showed little cytolytic activity toward EL4 and none toward P815. When IL-2 was supplied, the P815 targets were not killed but the EL4 targets were killed even at a very low effector: target cell ratio. Clearly the CD8$^+$ anti-H-2K^b CTLp were present in vivo but were unable to react against the β cells, either because of a defect in IL-2 delivery, or because the T cells bearing the transgene TCR had too low an affinity for H-2K^b. Whatever the case may be, these observations do suggest the existence of tolerant T cells, although we do not know how long these may last.

Intrathymic clonal deletion does not therefore appear to be the tolerogenic mechanism in our transgenic systems. Tolerance seems to have been induced at a peripheral level, possibly by targeting some high-affinity effector cell and disturbing IL-2 production. We have attempted to determine whether peripheral tolerance in our transgenic models eventually eliminates T cells, which as suggested above might be functionally silenced, at least for a period of time. Spleen cells from tolerant transgenic mice bearing skin grafts were injected intravenously into thymectomized irradiated syngeneic nontransgenic recipients which were later grafted with tail skin from appropriate donors. In preliminary experiments, third-party grafts were rejected within 15 days but most of the recipient mice failed to reject the grafts which has been tolerated in the original donors (Table 1). This suggested either that the specific T cells in the tolerant transgenic mice had been deleted, or that they had been permanently functionally silenced. The situation should become clearer when clonotype-identifiable T cells from TCR-RIP-K^b double transgenic mice are parked in appropriately skin grafted immunoincompetent hosts.

Tentatively, it may be concluded that self-tolerant T cells may exist in vivo, at least for an undefined period of time. It remains to be seen whether they can be specifically reactivated, and if so by what mechanisms. The implications of this work for autoimmune reactivity and stimulation of tumor immunity are clear.

Table 1 Survival of C57BL/10 Skin Grafts on Adult Thymectomized Irradiated bml Mice Receiving Spleen Cells from Young Transgenic RIP-K^b Mice Tolerant of C57BL/10 Tail Skin

	No. of mice showing graft survival (days)		
Skin graft donor	<15	38	>70
C57BL/10	0	1	4
BALB/c	5	0	0

Another experiment gave similar results. Unpublished data of J. F. A. P. Miller.

ACKNOWLEDGMENTS

The investigations performed in the author's laboratory were supported by grants from the National Health and Medical Research Council of Australia, the Buckland Foundation, and the Multiple Sclerosis Society of Australia.

REFERENCES

1. Miller JFAP, Mitchell GF. Interaction between two distinct cell lineages in an immune response. In: *Lymphatic Tissue and Germinal Centres in Immune Response*. L Fiore-Donati and MG Hanna Jr., eds. Plenum, New York. *Adv. Exp. Med. Biol.* 1969; 5:455–463.
2. Miller JFAP. Interaction between T cells and B cells in humoral antibody responses. In: *Morphological and Functional Aspects of Immunity*, Proceedings of the IIIrd International Conference of Lymphatic Tissues and Germinal Centres in Immune Reaction, Uppsala, 1970. K Lindahl-Kiessing, G Alm, and MG Hanna, Jr, eds. Plenum, New York, 1971, pp. 93–102.
3. Woodruff MFA. In Discussion after Mitchison NA. Blood transfusion in fowl: An example of immunological tolerance requiring the persistence of antigen. In: *Biological Problems of Grafting*. Blackwell, Oxford, England, 1959, p. 258.
4. Goodnow CC, Crosbie J, Adelstein S, Lavoie TB, Smith-Gill SJ, Brink RA, Pritchard-Briscoe H, Wotherspoon JS, Loblay RH, Raphael K, Trent RJ, Basten A. Altered immunoglobulin expression and functional silencing of self-reactive B lymphocytes in transgenic mice. *Nature* 1988; 334: 676–682.
5. Kappler JW, Roehm M, Marrack P. T cell tolerance by clonal elimination in the thymus. *Cell* 1987; 49:273–280.
6. Kisielow P, Blüthmann H, Staerz UD, Steinmetz M, von Boehmer H. Tolerance in T-cell-receptor transgenic mice involves deletion of nonmature $CD4^+8^+$ thymocytes. *Nature* 1988; 333: 742–746.
7. MacDonald HR, Sneider R, Lees RK, Howe RC, Acha-Orbea H, Fetenstein H, Zinkernagel RM, Hengartner H. T cell receptor V_β use predicts reactivity and tolerance to Mls^a-encoded antigens. *Nature* 1988; 332:40–45.
8. Sha WC, Nelson CA, Newberry RD, Kranz DM, Russell JH, Loh D. Positive and negative selection of an antigen receptor on T cells in transgenic mice. *Nature* 1988; 336:73–76.
9. Nieuwenhuis P, Stet RJM, Wagenaar JPA, Wubbena AS, Kampinga J, Karrenbeld A. The transcapsular route: a new way for (self-) antigens to by-pass the blood-thymus barrier? *Immunol. Today* 1988; 9:372–376.
10. Braciale TJ, Morrison LA, Sweetser MT, Sambrook J, Gething M-J, Braciale VL. Antigen presentation pathways to class I and class II MHC-restricted T lymphocytes. *Immunol. Rev.* 1987; 98:85–114.
11. Rammensee H-G, Kroschewski R, Frangoulis B. Clonal anergy induced in mature $V\beta6^+$ T lymphocytes on immunizing $Mls\text{-}1^b$ mice with $Mls\text{-}1^a$ expressing cells. *Nature* 1989; 339: 541–544.
12. Waldmann H, Cobbold SP, Qin S. Tolerance induction using CD4 and CD8 monoclonal antibodies. *Prog. Immunol.* 1989; 7:147–155.
13. Burkly LC, Lo D, Kanagawa O, Brinster RL, Flavell RA. T-cell tolerance by clonal anergy in transgenic mice with nonlymphoid expression of MHC class II I-E. *Nature* 1989; 342:564–566.
14. Ramsdell F, Lantz T, Fowlkes BJ. A nondeletional mechanism of thymic self tolerance. *Science* 1989; 246:1038–1041.
15. Hodes RJ, Sharrow SO, Solomon A. Failure of T cell receptor Vβ negative selection in an athymic environment. *Science* 1989; 246:1041–1044.
16. Fry AM, Jones LA, Kruisbeek AM, Matis LA. Thymic requirement for clonal deletion during T cell development. *Science* 1989; 246:1044–1046.

17. Gao E-K, Kanagawa O, Sprent J. Capacity of unprimed $CD4^+$ and $CD8^+$ T cells expressing Vβ11 receptors to respond to I-E alloantigens in vivo. *J. Exp. Med.* 1989; 170:1947–1957.
18. Byrne JA, Butler JL, Cooper MD. Differential activation requirements for virgin and memory T cells. *J. Immunol.* 1988; 141:3249–3257.
19. Allison J, Campbell IL, Morahan G, Mandel TE, Harrison L, Miller JFAP. Diabetes in transgenic mice resulting from over-expression of class I histocompatibility molecules in pancreatic β cells. *Nature* 1988; *333*:529–533.
20. Morahan G, Allison J, Miller JFAP. Tolerance of class I histocompatibility antigen expressed extra-thymically. *Nature* 1989; *339*:622–624.
21. Morahan G, Brennan F, Bhathal PS, Allison J, Cox KO, Miller JFAP. Expression in transgenic mice of class I histocompatibility antigens controlled by the metallothionein promoter. *Proc. Natl. Acad. Sci. U.S.A.* 1989; *86*:3782–3786.
22. Miller JFAP, Morahan G, Allison J. Extra-thymic acquisition of tolerance by T lymphocytes. *Cold Spring Harbor Symp. Quant. Biol.* 1990; *54*:807-813.
23. Singer A, Munitz TI, Golding H, Rosenberg AS, Mizuochi T. Recognition requirement for the activation, differentiation and function of T-helper cells specific for class I MHC alloantigens. *Immunol. Rev.* 1987; 98:143–170.
24. Matzinger P, Guerder S. Does T-cell tolerance require a dedicated antigen-presenting cell? *Nature* 1989; 338:74–76.
25. Signore A, Pozzilli P, Gale EAM, Andreani D, Beverley PCL. The natural history of lymphocyte subsets infiltrating the pancreas of NOD mice. *Diabetologia* 1989; 32:282–289.

THYMIC EPITHELIAL CELLS

1
The Diversity of Thymic Epithelial Cells

Marion D. Kendall[1] **and Richard Boyd**[2]
[1]*Cell Biology Unit and Thymus Research Laboratory, United Medical and Dental Schools of Guy's and St. Thomas's Hospitals, London, England;*
[2]*Monash University, Melbourne, Australia*

Heterogeneity of epithelial cells of the thymus is a fundamental component of the formation and function of thymic microenvironments. Not only are there functionally different regions in the gland, but the close apposition of bone marrow-derived cells, nerves, and their products with epithelial cells could influence the maturation or differentiation of a particular cell or group of cells. Thus, either positive or negative selection could be achieved locally, perhaps before clonal expansion, to form the final T-cell repertoire. Also, recently the importance of the thymus in the neuroendocrinimmune axis has become widely accepted and factors controlling the microenvironment are important research topics.

Using the descriptions of human epithelial cells by van de Wijngaert et al. (1), the epithelial cells of all vertebrates can be classified into six or more types.

The type 1 cell (subcapsular/perivascular), characterized by the presence of a basal lamina (and in man, curious tubular inclusions), is positive to antibodies belonging to group II (2). These cells have keratins similar to those of the basal layer of skin epidermis. They totally surround the cortex, isolating cortical blood vessels from cortical parenchyma and extend to the corticomedullary junction. Many are positive with the antibody A2B5 to a neuronal ganglioside (3), are positive with antibodies to all known thymic hormones (especially well illustrated by thymopsin alpha$_1$ and thymulin antibodies), and to oxytocin, neurophysin, and to a lesser extent vasopressin. They are generally, except occasionally on the cortical side, class II major histocompatibility (MHC) negative. Being part of the subcapsular cortex, they form the region where double-negative CD4/CD8 thymocytes are mainly located, and where there is a plexus of nerves containing NA, VIP, CGRP, NP-Y and TK neuropeptides (4,5).

These cells, joined to type 2 epithelial cells by desmosomes, form the cortical microenvironment with types 3 and 4 (of the deep cortex), and can be identified by their positive reaction to antibodies in group III (2). They are MHC class II positive (more so, the deeper into the cortex). The ultrastructure of types 2 and 3 cells indicate very active cells, and it is thought that they almost certainly produce most of the cytokines known to be secreted by the thymus and also perhaps some hormones. Probably a specialized form of these cells are thymic nurse cells (TNCs), which have been known to hold, by emperiopoleisis, hundreds of thymocytes. Thymic nurse cells have the same antigens as other cortical epithelial cells except Thy-1 (6), and in addition they are positive to A2B5, oxytocin, neurophysin, and vasopressin (7). The deep cortical type 4 cell is, by ultrastructural features, a dying cell often conspicuous after manipulations of the thymus when regrowth appears in the cortex. Most of the thymus cortex has a few nerve fibers ramifying through, and these may contain any of the neuropeptides above.

The medulla is typified by types 5 (relatively undifferentiated cells sharing many features, except a basal lamina, with type 1 cells) and type 6 epithelial cells (associated with Hassall's corpuscles). Antibodies of group IV (2) react with some or all of the cells. However, this area of van de Winjgaert et al.'s description needs extending, as both ultrastructural studies of rodents and immunohistochemistry indicate a greater degree of diversity of epithelial forms. In addition the strongly MHC class II–positive macrophages and interdigitating cells of this region confuse the issue at the light microscopic level. For example, there is a novel medullary MHC class II epitope but it could be on bone marrow–derived cells or epithelial cells (8). In general, medullary epithelial cells are well keratinized, although some have a distinctive keratin complement (9). Many secrete hormones, and in old age these cells may be the dominant medullary epithelial component. Some are positive with antibodies to oxytocin and vasopressin. Some are strongly MHC positive, whereas others are MHC class II negative. Rodent thymuses often also have greatly hypertrophied slightly keratinized, often MHC class II–positive epithelial cells.

The epithelial cell secretion of thymulin is circadian, reaching a peak in man about 8 a.m. (10), and is under the influence of central nervous system hormones such as growth hormone, prolactin (11), and adrenocorticotropin (12), thus confirming the thymus as part of the neuro-endocrine-immune axis.

Hassall's corpuscles are still largely inexplicable but they have their own unique array of antigens (group V) and share some with other medullary epithelial cells (2). They show variations in number and size with age and increase after manipulations of the thymus.

Thymic medullary epithelial cells could be innervated as there is a plexus of acetylcholinesterase-positive fibers and cells (13), although the presence of cholinergic innervation is disputed (13,14). Very recently, however, choline acetyltransferase activity has been demonstrated in the thymus (15), and the medulla would be the most likely candidate for this activity. Enolase-positive and CGRP-positive cells have also been observed in the medulla, and occasionally in the cortex close to septa.

Thus, the major regions of the thymus each have their own complement of epithelial cells, each creating microenvironments that could favor either the first steps in maturation and differentiation (subcapsular/perivascular regions), thymocyte maturation and selection (cortex), or the final selection and development of mature T cells in the medulla.

REFERENCES

1. van de Wijngaert FP, Kendall MD, Schuurman HJ, Rademakers LHMP, and Kater L. Heterogeneity of human thymus epithelial cells at the ultrastructural level. Cell Tiss Res 1984, 237:227–237.
2. Kampinga J, Berges S, Boyd R, Brekelmans P, Colic M, Ewijk W van, Kendall MD, Ladyman H, Nieuwenhuis P, Ritter M, Schuurman H-J, Tournefier A. Thymic epithelial antibodies: Immunohistological analysis and introduction of nomenclature. Summary of the Epithelium

Workshop held at the 2nd Workshop *The Thymus. Histophysiology and Dynamics in the Immune System*. Thymus 1989, 13:165–173.
3. Haynes BF. The human thymic microenvironment. Adv Immunol 1984; 36:87–142.
4. Weihe E, Muller S, Fink T, Zentel HJ. Tachykinins, calcitonin gene-related peptide and neuropeptide Y in nerves of the mammalian thymus: interactions with mast cells in autoimmune and sensory neuroimmunomodulation? Neurosci Lett 1989, 100:77–82.
5. Al-Shawaf A, Cowen T, and Kendall MD. Identification of neural profiles containing vasoactive intestinal polypeptide, acetylcholinesterase, and catecholamines in the rat thymus. J Anat in press.
6. Lampert IA, Ritter MA. The origin of the diverse epithelial cells of the thymus: Is there a common stem cell? Thymus Update 1988, 1:5–25.
7. Geenen V, Defresne MP, Robert F, Legros JJ, Franchimont P, Boniver J. The neurohormonal thymic microenvironment: immunocytochemical evidence that thymic nurse cells are neuroendocrine cells. Neuroendocrinology 1988, 47:365–8.
8. Murphy DB, Lo D, Rath S, Brinster RL, Flavell RA, Slanetz A, Janeway CA. A novel MHC class II epitope expressed in thymic medulla but not in cortex. Nature 1989, 338:765–8.
9. Nicolas JF, Savino W, Reano A, Viac J, Brochier J, Dardenne M. Heterogeneity of thymic epithelial cell (TEC) keratins—immunohistochemical and biochemical evidence for a subset of highly differentiated TEC in the mouse. J Histochem Cytochem 1985, 33:687–694.
10. Safieh B, Kendall MD, personal observations.
11. Dardenne M, Savino W. Neuroendocrine control of the thymic epithelium: modulation of thymic endocrine function, cytokeratin expression and cell proliferation by hormones and neuropeptides. Prog Neurobiol Immunol 1990, 3:18–25.
12. Buckingham J, Safieh B, Kendall MD, personal observations.
13. Kendall MD, Al-Shawaf A, Zaidi SAA. The cholinergic and adrenergic innervation of the rat thymus. Adv Exp Med Biol 1988, 237:255–261.
14. Nance DM, Hopkins DA, Beigler D. Re-investigation of the innervation of the thymus gland in mice and rats. Brain Behav Immunol 1987, 1:134–147.
15. Tria MA, Vantini G, Fiori M, Rossi A. Choline acetyltransferase activity in the murine thymus. Ist International Conference International Society for Neuroimmuno-modulation, Florence, Italy, May 23–26, 1990.

2
Monoclonal Antiepithelial Antibody Workshop II
Flow Cytometric and Biochemical Analysis of Thymic Epithelial Cell Heterogeneity

Heather Ladyman,[1] Richard Boyd,[2] Pieter Brekelmans,[3] Miodrag Čolić,[4] Willem van Ewijk,[3] Brita von Gaudecker,[5] Jaap Kampinga,[6] Marion Kendall,[7] Paul Nieuwenhuis,[8] Henk-Jan Schuurman,[9] Annick Tournefier,[10] and Mary Ritter[1]

[1]Hammersmith Hospital, London, England; [2]Monash Medical School, Melbourne, Australia; [3]Erasmus University, Rotterdam, The Netherlands; [4]Institute for Experimental Medicine, Military Medical Academy, Belgrade, Yugoslavia; [5]Anatomisches Institut, Christian Albrechts Universitat zu Kiel, Kiel, Federal Republic of Germany; [6]Quadrant Research Foundation, Cambridge Research Laboratories, Cambridge, England; [7]Unit of Cell Biology, United Medical and Dental Schools, St. Thomas's Campus, London, England; [8]University of Groningen, Groningen, The Netherlands; [9]University Hospital, Utrecht, The Netherlands; [10]Université Pierre et Marie Curie, Paris, France

INTRODUCTION

T cells are known to mature and to be selected within the thymic microenvironment. In order to analyze the cellular and molecular interactions that take place during this process several monoclonal antibodies (MAbs) have been raised to molecules present on/in thymic epithelial cells. In order to compare and analyze MAbs from different laboratories and to improve the efficiency of research in this field a series of workshops have been organized. Workshop I concentrated on immunohistochemical analysis, and resulted in the classification of MAbs according to their staining patterns (CTES; clusters of thymic epithelial staining), as reported at Rolduc, April 1989 (1). Workshop II was designed to give additional information on the reactivity of the MAbs (electron microscopic localization, nonepithelial reactivity), and also some biochemical analysis of the antigens that they recognize. Results from this second workshop are reported in this chapter (the MAbs included are given in Table 1).

Table 1 Monoclonal Antibodies Included in the Workshop

MAb no.	Clone	Isotype	CTES group	Staining pattern
H1	MR19	IgM	II	s/c, pv, med ep.
H2	MR10	IgM	II	s/c, pv, med ep.
H3	MR6	IgG1	IIIB	cort, subpop. med et.
H4	8.18	IgM	VA	HC
H5	N8.2	IgM	VD	HC, ass. med ep., subpop. lys.
H6	HTS1	IgM	XXb	s/c, cort, subpop. med ep.
H7	HTS6	IgM	I	all TEC
H8	HTS8	IgM	II	s/c, pv. med ep.
M1	ER-TR5	IgM	II	s/c, pv, med ep.
M2	IVC4	IgM	II	s/c, pv, med ep.
M3	M-15F7		III	cort ep.
M4	MTS9	IgG	IIIB	cort, subpop. med ep.
M5	ER-TR4	IgM	IIIB	cort, subpop. med ep.
M6	4F1E4	IgM	IIIB	cort, subpop. med ep.
M7	M-14F10		IV	med, HC ep.
M8	MTS39	IgM	I	all TEC
M9	MTS1	IgM	I	all TEC
M10	MTS10	IgM	II	s/c, pv, med ep.
M11	MTS5			
M12	MTS44	IgG	IIIB	cort, subpop, med ep.
M13	MTS38	IgG	IIIC2	cort, ep., thys
M14	MTS32	IgG	IIIC2	cort ep., thys
M15	MTS20	IgM	IVA	med ep.
M16	MTS7	IgM	XXc	subpop. cort, med ep.
M17	MTS37	IgG	XXc	subpop. cort, med ep.
M18	MTS33	IgG	XXd	subpop. med ep., cort thys
R1	HIS39	IgM	II	s/c, pv, med ep.
R2	R-MC-18		II	s/c, pv, med ep.
R3	HIS38	IgM	IIIA	cort ep.
R4	R-MC-13		IIIA	cort ep.
R5	HIS37	IgM	IIIB	cort, subpop. med ep.
R6	R-MC-14		IIIB	cort, subpop. med ep.
R7	R-MC-17		IIIC	cort ep, subpop. leuc.
R8	R-MC-20		VE	HC, assoc. med, s/c ep.
R9	HIS46	IgM	XXa	maj. cort, med, min. s/c ep.

Abbreviations: s/c = subcapsule, pv = perivascular, med = medulla, cort = cortical, ep = epithelium, TNC = thymic nurse cell, thys = thymocytes, mac = macrophage, IDC = interdigitating cell, c/m junct = corticomedullary junction.

Table 2 Electron Microscopy

MAb no.	Cells recognized	Localization
H1	s/c, pv, med ep.	cytoplasmic
H2	s/c, pv, med ep.	cytoplasmic
H3	cort ep, TNC, thys, med mac/IDC.	cell membrane
H4	HC, assoc med ep.	cell membrane
M3	cort, c/m junct ep.	cell membrane
M6	cort ep, thys.	cytoplasmic, cell membrane

Abbreviations: s/c = subcapsule, pv = perivascular, med = medulla, cort = cortical, ep = epithelium, TNC = thymic nurse cell, thys = thymocytes, mac = macrophage, IDC = interdigitating cell, c/m junct = corticomedullary junction.

ELECTRON MICROSCOPY (EM): METHOD

Murine and pediatric human thymus samples were processed for immuno-EM using gold-coupled secondary reagents with subsequent silver enhancement (2).

Results and Discussion

The aim of the EM was to clarify the thymic cells recognized by the MAbs and to assess whether their antigens are intracellular or localized on the cell membrane. Results have so far been obtained for six MAbs (Table 2). However, not all reagents worked well in this technique, and the method is very time consuming.

COMPARISON WITH CYTOKERATINS: METHOD

All MAbs were tested in double immunostaining experiments with polyclonal guinea pig anticytokeratin, using species-specific secondary antibodies on cryostat sections of human, rat, or mouse thymus (3). This protocol was repeated using the polyclonal antikeratin as the first antibody to test for blocking of MAb labeling by the anticytokeratin antibody.

Results and Discussion

Seven antimouse (M1, M2, M3, M5, M7, M10, M15) but none of the antihuman or antirat TEC MAbs were blocked by preincubation with polyclonal anticytokeratin antibody. The seven blocked MAbs are therefore probably antikeratin in nature. Monoclonal antibodies M3 and M5 were chosen for further double-labeling studies with MAbs specific for either cytokeratin 8 (CK8) or 18 (CK18), since their staining patterns were similar to the CK8/CK18 distribution. This revealed only double-positive cells, indicating that M3 and M5 may recognize epitopes present on CK8 and/or CK18.

IMMUNOSTAINING ON SINGLE CELL SUSPENSIONS: METHOD

Suspensions of thymocytes, peripheral blood mononuclear cells (PBMCs), and splenic lymphocytes were prepared, separated over ficoll when necessary, from the mouse, rat, and human. The MAb panel was screened against each cell type by indirect immunofluorescence using FITC-conjugated rabbit antimouse immunoglobulin (Ig) or rabbit antirat Ig antibody as secondary reagents. Cells were analyzed by flow cytometry.

Results and Discussion

The four antihuman TEC MAbs tested for reactivity with pediatric human thymocytes (PHTs) were all found to be positive, although they differed in the number of cells stained and the intensity of staining (Table 3). All nine of the antirat TEC panel were screened against adult rat thymocytes (ARTs), but only two were positive (see Table 3). In contrast, 12 of the 18 antimouse TEC panel MAbs stained varying percentages of adult mouse thymocytes (AMTs), ranging from 43 to 98%, and showing a broad range of staining intensity (see Table 3). Five of these MAbs gave varying results from the different participating laboratories, and must therefore be retested for clarification. Those antimouse TEC MAbs that were positive on AMTs were tested against fetal mouse thymocytes (FMTs), and most were positive; the percentage of positive cells and the intensity of staining showed some differences (Table 4). Only three of the antimouse TEC MAbs were positive on adult mouse spleen lymphocytes (AMSLs) (see Table 4). Compilation of these antimouse TEC MAbs data gives interesting profiles for the cell surface ligands recognized by these MAbs (see Table 4), with what appear to be developmentally associated changes in the intensity of cell surface expression and the percentage of positive cells.

Table 3 Flow Cytometry on Thymocytes

MAb no.	% positive	Staining intensity
H1	4.7	hi
H2	5.3	mod
H3	28.2	low
H4	12.4	low
R4	19	low
R7	41	low
M7	43[a]	low
M8	64	low
M9	98[a]	low/mod
M10	85[a]	low
M11	94[a]	low/mod
M12	66[a]	mod
M13	62	low/mod/hi
M14	96	hi
M15	56	low
M16	80	mod
M17	90	mod/hi
M18	84	low/mod/hi

M6 = Usually negative but occasionally gave high-intensity staining. MAbs H5 to H8 were not tested. Other MAbs not shown were negative. All MAbs tested on thymocytes of the appropriate species.

[a]Results inconsistent between different laboratories.

Table 4 Antimouse Antibody Panel

	Compilation of flow cytometry results					
	FMT		AMT		AMSL	
MAb no.	%	intensity	%	intensity	%	intensity
M8	10	low	64	low	negative	
M10	9	low	85	low	negative	
M11	10	low	94	low	negative	
M13	20	low	62	low/mod/hi	negative	
M14	41	low/mod	96	hi	17	low
M15	18	low	56	low	negative	
M17	96	mod/hi	90	mod/hi	42	low/mod
M18	19	low	84	low/mod/hi	45	low/mod/hi

FMT = fetal mouse thymocytes. AMSL = adult mouse spleen lymphocytes. AMT = adult mouse thymocytes.

RELATIVE MOLECULAR MASS OF ANTIGENS DETECTED BY MABS: METHOD

Cell lysates were prepared using detergent buffers containing proteolytic inhibitors at 4°C from either pediatric human thymic stromal cells or thymocytes, adult mouse thymic stromal cells or thymocytes, or axolotl thymic epithelial cells. Lysates were run on SDS-PAGE electrophoresis, transferred electrophoretically onto either nitrocellulose or nylon membranes (4), and analyzed by immunoblotting with the MAbs.

Table 5 Relative Molecular Mass of Antigens Detected by the MAbs

Antibody no.	Relative mol. mass (kD)
H1	51, 39.5, 14.2
H2	51, 39.5, 14.2
H3	200
H6	47, 44, 43, 40
H7	58, 50, 47, 43
M2	38
M6	108, 95
M8	43
M9	58, 47, 43, 40
M11	58, 47, 43, 40
M12	43
M16	43
R5	43

For MAbs not included in this table the relative molecular mass of their antigen is not known.

Results and Discussion

Results were obtained for 13 of the 35 MAbs in the workshop (Table 5); some MAbs revealed several bands on the western blots, whereas others only gave single bands. For MAb M6, the structure (glycosylation, PI linkage) and function (adhesion and proliferation assays) of the antigen recognized have been studied in detail (Chapter 12). Clearly much more work needs to be done in order to further analyze the many molecules recognized by the workshop antibodies.

REFERENCES

1. Kampinga J , Berges S, Boyd R, Brekelmans P , Colic M, van Ewijk W, Kendall MD, Ladyman H, Nieuwenhuis P, Ritter MA, Schuurman H-J, Tournefier A. Thymic epithelial antibodies: Immunohistological analysis and introduction of nomenclature. Summary of the Epithelium Workshop held at the 2nd Workshop *The Thymus. Histophysiology and Dynamics in the Immune System.* Thymus 1989; 13:165–73.
2. von Gaudecker B, Larche M, Schuurmann H-J, Ritter M. Analysis of the fine distribution of thymic epithelial microenvironmental molecules by immuno-electron microscopy. Thymus 1989; 13:187–194.
3. Kanariou M, Huby R, Ladyman H, Colic M, Sivolapenko G, Lampert I, Ritter M. Immunosuppression with cyclosporin A alters the thymic microenvironment. Clin. Exp. Immunol. 1989; 78:263–270.
4. Laemmli UK. Cleavage of structural proteins during the assembly of the head of bacteriophage T4. Nature 1970; 227:680–85.

3

Molecular Heterogeneity Within the Subcapsular Medullary (CTES II) Subpopulation of Thymic Epithelium

Mary A. Ritter, Jantien Zijlstra, Ania Kaminski, Aruna Sareen, and Heather Ladyman
Royal Postgraduate Medical School, London, England

INTRODUCTION

The thymus provides a milieu that is critical to the development of a fully functional T-cell repertoire that is major histocompatibility complex (MHC) restricted and tolerant to self. This thymic influence is thought to be mediated by stromal cells (epithelium, dendritic cells, and macrophages) that together constitute the thymic microenvironment. We and others have used monoclonal antibodies (MAbs) to identify heterogeneity within the epithelial component of the thymic microenvironment (1–3). These reagents have now been grouped according to the intrathymic location of the antigens to which they bind: panepithelial (CTES I); subcapsular, perivascular, and medullary epithelium (CTES II); cortical epithelium (CTES III); medullary epithelium (CTES IV); and Hassall's corpuscles (CTES V) (3). These data raise the possibility that discrete microenvironments may exist for different stages of intrathymic T-cell differentiation.

In this study, we have analyzed our CTES II group of MAbs in further detail to determine the molecular nature and nonepithelial distribution of the antigens to which these reagents bind. Our data demonstrate that there is considerable molecular heterogeneity within the subcapsular/perivascular/medullary subpopulation of epithelial cells.

MATERIALS AND METHODS

Monoclonal Antibodies

Six CTES II MAbs were included in this study. Rat MAb IVC4 was raised to mouse thymic epithelium (2), but also labels human thymus (3). Mouse MAbs MR10, MR14, and MR19 were all raised to human tissue and do not react with other species tested (1). Mouse MAbs 3A and 4B were raised to BSA-coupled thymulin (Sigma, U.K.) and screened by both immunohistochemistry of frozen thymic sections and by ELISA; both MAbs react with human, mouse, and rat thymic tissue. The binding of the MAbs 3A and 4B is inhibited by

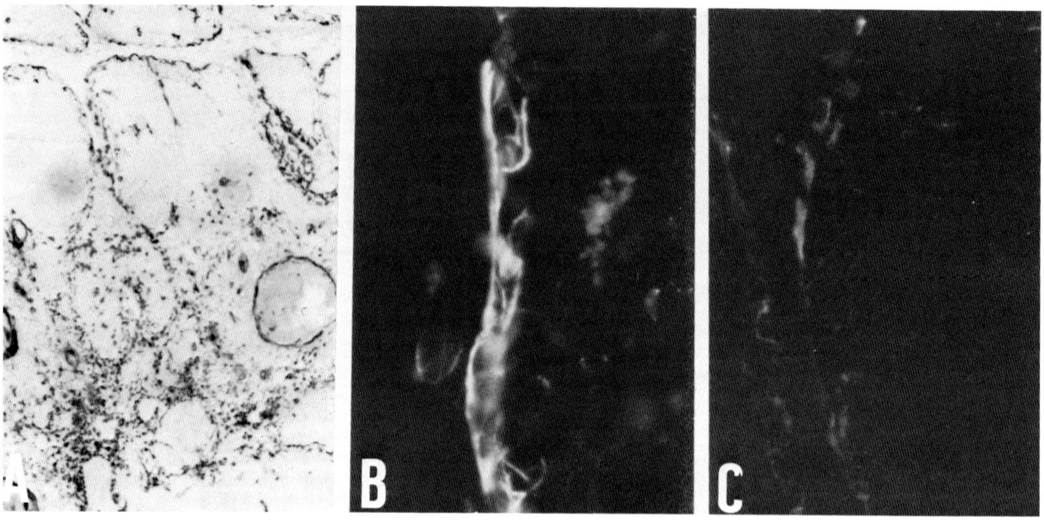

Figure 1 (A) Human pediatric thymus stained with CTES II MAb MR19 by indirect immunoperoxidase (no histological counterstain), showing labeling of subcapsular and medullary epithelium. (B) Subcapsular region of human pediatric thymus stained in indirect immunofluorescence with MAb MR19 to show "thick" subcapsular labeling (CTES IIA). (C) Subcapsular region of human pediatric thymus stained in indirect immunofluorescence with MAb MR10 to show "thin" subcapsular labeling (CTES IIB).

preincubation of the MAbs with pure thymulin. All MAbs are of immunoglobulin M (IgM) isotype. By immunohistochemistry, all MAbs showed typical CTES labeling of subcapsular, perivascular, and medullary (a major subpopulation) epithelium. However, MAb MR19 revealed a thicker layer of subcapsular epithelium (CTES IIA) than that seen with the MAbs MR10 and MR14 (CTES IIB) (Fig. 1).

Flow Cytometry

Fresh cell suspensions of pediatric thymocytes and peripheral blood leukocytes (dextran separation) were stained by indirect immunofluorescence using either FITC-rabbit antimouse Ig or FITC-rabbit antirat Ig (Dakopatts, Denmark) as appropriate. Cells were analyzed immediately after staining by flow cytometry (EPICS Profile, Coulter, U.S.A.).

Western Blotting

The molecular weights of the molecules detected by CTES II MAb were determined by Western blotting. Fresh thymic tissue (mouse or human) was teased to remove the majority of thymocytes, and the resultant stromal preparation lysed in buffer containing 0.5% NP40 and 1mM PMSF (4). Lysates were separated by SDS-PAGE (10, 12.5, and 15%) under both reducing and nonreducing conditions prior to transfer to a nylon membrane. Membranes with incubated with MAbs using a multichannel system (Immunetics, U.S.A.), and antibody binding was visualized using peroxidase-conjugated second layer reagents (Dakopatts).

RESULTS

Flow Cytometry

Mouse antihuman MAbs MR10, MR14, and MR19 all gave strong labeling (mean windows: MR10/MR14, 53; MR19, 59) of between 5.3 and 8.2% of thymocytes (Fig. 2) and 10.1 to 11.5% of peripheral blood leukocytes. Mouse antithymulin MAbs 3A and 4B gave strong staining (mean windows: 3A, 44; 4B, 108) of between 6.4 and 10.1% of thymocytes. Rat antimouse MAb IVC4 labelled no cells of hemopoietic origin.

Western Blotting

Monoclonal antibody MR10, MR14, and MR19 all gave the same three bands of 51.0, 39.5, and 14.2 kD under both reducing and nonreducing conditions (Fig. 3). Monoclonal antibody IVC4 detected a single molecule of 38 kD. Monoclonal antibody 3A revealed a band of approximately 100 kD, whereas MAb 4B identified no molecule in this system.

DISCUSSION

We have raised monoclonal antibodies to thymic epithelial cells in order to dissect the molecules that may be involved in T-lymphocyte differentiation (1,2). Several groups have now produced MAbs that label the subcapsular, perivascular, and medullary epithelium of the thymus (3); however, whether all these CTES II reagents detect the same molecule or whether there are many different molecules that characterize this subpopulation of epithelial cells is not known. In this study, we have analyzed the molecular weight of the antigens detected by our panel of CTES II MAbs. We have also studied the presence of these antigens on nonepithelial cell types, since we have found that some molecules are shared between thymic epithelium and lymphocytes (4).

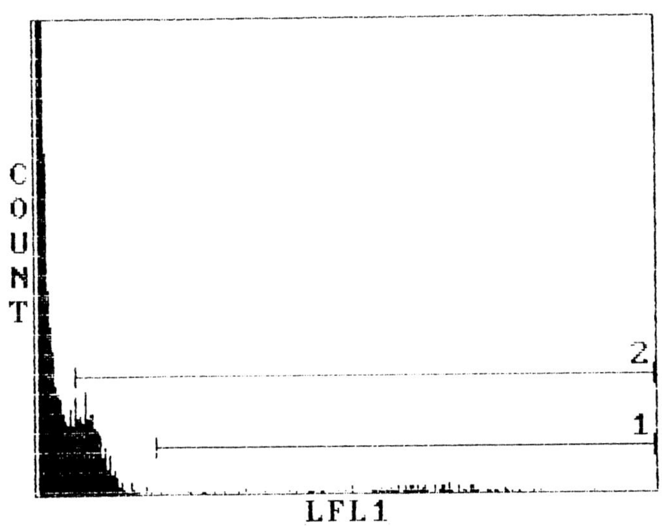

Figure 2 Flow cytometric analysis (fluorescence histogram) of human pediatric thymocytes labeled in indirect immunofluorescence with MAb MR19. Window 1 (excludes background staining with isotype matched negative control antibody) shows 5.3% of thymocytes are strongly MR19 positive.

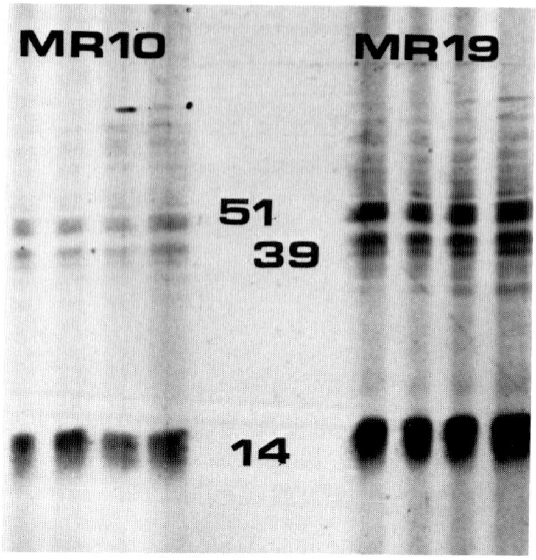

Figure 3 Western blotting analysis of human pediatric thymic stroma using MAbs MR10 (left hand panels) and MR19 (right hand panels), showing three bands of 51.0, 39.5, and 14.2 kD. 15% SDS-PAGE, nonreducing conditions.

Our data indicate that there is considerable molecular heterogeneity within the subcapsular, perivascular, medullary epithelial subpulation. Monoclonal antibody IVC4 binds to an epithelial-specific 38-kD molecule. Since binding of this MAb to thymus sections is blocked by preincubation with a polyclonal antikeratin antibody, the target antigen for MAb IVC4 is likely to be a keratin. Antithymulin MAb 3A and 4B recognize the same epithelium. This is consistent with other studies which have shown that it is the CTES II epithelial cells that are responsible for the secretion of thymic hormones (5). Interestingly a small number of lymphocytes were also positive with the antithymulin antibodies. This has also been observed in immuno–electron microscopic studies of the thymus (Kendall, personal communication), and may represent thymulin binding to its receptor in situ. It is not surprising that MAb 4B gave no band by Western blotting, since the molecular w eight of the thymulin nonapeptide is approximately 800 D. The 100-kD protein detected by MAb 3A may be a thymulin precursor rather than the hormone itself, although this MAb must also recognize mature thymulin, since its binding is blocked by the synthetic thymulin nonapeptide.

Monoclonal antibodies MR10 and MR14 were thought to be of different specificity from MR19, based on differences in the degree of labeling of the subcapsular epithelium ("thin" vs "thick") (3). However, the fact that the antigen to which they bind is indistinguishable by Western blotting suggests that the differences observed may perhaps be due differences of affinity rather than of specificity. In addition, all three MAbs give strong labeling of a small subpopulation of thymocytes. The relationship between the three separate bands detected by the MAbs and the function of these "shared" epithelial-lymphocyte molecules is currently under investigation.

REFERENCES

1. De Maagd RA, MacKenzie WA, Schuurman HJ, Ritter MA, Price KM, Broekhuizen R, Kater L. The human thymus microenvironment: Heterogeneity detected by monoclonal anti-epithelial cell antibodies. Immunology 1985; 54:745–54.
2. Kanariou M, Huby R, Ladyman HM, Colic M, Sivolapenko G, Lampert I, Ritter MA. Immunosuppression with cyclosporin A alters the thymic microenvironment. Clin. Exp. Immunol. 1989; 78:263–70.
3. Kampinga J, Berges S, Boyd R, Brekelmans P, Colic M, van Ewijk W, Kendall MD, Ladyman HM, Nieuwenhuis P, Ritter MA, Schuurman HJ, Tournifier A. Thymus 1989; 13:165–73.
4. Larche M, Lamb JR, Ritter MA. A novel T lymphocyte molecule that may function in the induction of self-tolerance and MHC-restriction within the human thymic microenvironment. Immunology 1988; 64:101–5.
5. Dardenne M, Bach JF. Functional biology of thymic hormones. In: Kendall MK and Ritter MA (eds.). *Thymus Update*. Vol. 1. London, Harwood Academic, 1988, pp. 101–116.

4
Epithelial Cell Expression of Interleukin-4 Receptor Complex

Ishak Mat,[1] David Melcher,[2] and Mary A. Ritter[1]
[1]*Royal Postgraduate Medical School, Hammersmith Hospital, London, England;*
[2]*Royal Sussex County Hospital, Brighton, England*

INTRODUCTION

Monoclonal antibody (MAb) MR6 was raised to epithelial cells of the human thymic cortex as part of a study designed to analyze the inductive and proliferative stimuli provided by the thymic microenvironment for the developing T cells (1). The molecule recognized by MAb MR6 was later found to be present at low levels on the surface of lymphocytes, macrophages, and dendritic cells (2,3). However, of all normal tissues studied, only thymic epithelium showed strong expression. The molecule detected by MAb MR6 (MR6-Ag) has an apparent molecular weight of 200 kD, but is highly sensitive to proteolysis, yielding a molecule of 145 kD (4). The distribution and density of the MAb MR6-Ag appeared to be similar to that of the human interleukin-4 (IL-4) receptor (IL-4R) (5). Subsequently, MAb MR6 was found to block IL-4–induced immune responses (6), providing functional evidence for the view that MAb MR6 may be recognizing part of the human IL-4R complex. The strong expression of MAb MR6-Ag on cortical thymic epithelial cells (TECs) led us to investigate whether exogenously added IL-4 will bind to these cells. We now present a preliminary immunohistochemical analysis on the distribution of IL-4-binding cells in human thymus using biotinylated IL-4. Additionally, we have also examined the expression of the MAb MR6-Ag/IL-4R complex in other epithelia. In a previous study (7), it was found that the expression of the complex was upregulated in a number of epithelial tumors. In this study, we have examined a larger number of breast tumors using MAb MR6.

METHODS

Immunohistochemical Analysis of Human Thymus Using Biotinylated IL-4 (IL-4B)

Surface-bound IL-4 can be eluted from lymphocytes by exposure to low pH (8). We have adapted this technique to investigate the possibility that thymic epithelium carries surface-bound IL-4. Fresh frozen sections of pediatric human thymus (5 μ) were washed for 5 min in 0.1% acetic acid, 150 mM NaCl, pH 2.9. The sections were then transferred to 0.01M Tris-HCl, 0.5M NaCl, pH 2.9 for 2 min, fixed in ice-cold methanol:acetone (1:1) mixture for 10 min, and transferred to pH 7.6 Tris buffer. Unwashed sections were processed similarly but using pH 7.4 instead of pH 2.9 solution. Interleukin-4B (F4000 Fluorokine IL-4 kit, R & D Systems, British Biotechnology, U.K.) was added to the washed and unwashed sections using a modification of the manufacturer's protocol. Briefly, 50μl of a 1/5 dilution of the reconstituted IL-4B was added to the sections and incubated for 60 min at 4°C. The sections were washed with RDF1 buffer (provided in the kit) to remove unbound cytokine reagent and were then incubated with the avidin-FITC for 30 min at 4°C in the dark. Sections were mounted in Citifluor (Citifluor Ltd, U.K.) and examined using an Olympus HD-2 UV microscope. As controls, sections were incubated with (a) avidin-FITC alone, (b) MAb MR6, (c) anti-CD1, and (d) anticytokeratin mouse MAb. Monoclonal antibody MR6 was used as neat supernatant, anti-CD1 and anti-CK MAbs were used at 1/100 dilution. Mouse MAb were followed by FITC conjugated rabbit antimouse immunoglobulin (Ig) (Dakopatts, Denmark). The intensity of staining was estimated by noting the time required to expose the section using the automatic exposure meter of the UV microscope.

Immunohistochemical Analysis of Breast Tissues

Frozen sections (5 μ) were analyzed by indirect immunoperoxidase using mouse MAb MR6 or an isotype-matched (IgG_1) negative control followed by HRP conjugated rabbit antimouse Ig (Dakopatts, Denmark) as described previously (7).

RESULTS

Acid-Washing of the Thymus Sections Increased the Intensity of Labeling with IL-4B but Not MAb MR6, Anti-CD1, or Anticytokeratin

The intensity of staining is expressed as mean fluorescent index, an inverse of the mean from eight determinations of exposure time (Table 1). Washing of thymus sections with pH 2.9 buffer significantly increased the intensity of labeling by IL-4B ($p \leq 0.02$) but not for MAb MR6 ($p \leq 0.4$), anti-CD1 ($p \leq 0.66$), or anti-CK ($p \leq 0.65$). Histological examination revealed that cells labeled with IL-4B were found in the cortex of the thymus (Fig. 1a) with weak labeling of cells in the medulla. The morphology and cellular distribution of the positive cells suggested that they were epithelial in nature and dual immunofluorescent analysis to confirm this is now in progress.

Table 1 Effect of Acid Washing of Thymus Sections on the Intensity of Labeling with IL-4B, MAb MR6, anti-CD1, and anti-CK Antibodies

	Mean fluorescent index[a]	
Reagents	Not acid washed	Acid washed
Biotinylated IL-4	0.198 ± 0.01[b]	0.267 ± 0.02[b]
MAb MR6	0.588 ± 0.03	0.555 ± 0.04
anti-CD1	0.238 ± 0.04	0.205 ± 0.05
anti-CK	0.038 ± 0.05	0.040 ± 0.06

[a]Mean fluorescent index = 1/mean exposure time from eight determinations. Statistical analysis was performed using Student's t-test.
[b]$p \leq 0.02$ for IL-4B on washed vs not washed sections. No other comparison was statistically significant.

Immunohistochemical Analysis of MAb MR6-Ag/IL-4R Expression in Breast Tissues

Immunoperoxidase labeling was scored by eye for the intensity and approximate percentage of positive cells in each tissue sample. The frequency of MAb MR6+ samples is represented in Table 2. Two-thirds of normal breast samples showed weak to moderate staining with MAb MR6. In these samples, approximately 30% of the cells were MAb MR6+. Approximately 50% of breast tumors were MAb MR6+, and in these samples 50–80% of the cells were positive. Dual immunofluorescence analysis showed that greater than 80% of the MAb MR6+ cells were also keratin+ (4). All benign proliferation tissues examined were strongly MAb MR6+ (Fig. 2a). In low-grade tumors, approximately 54% were MAb MR6+, with most showing moderate to strong expression. However, in high-grade tumors, only 31% were MAb MR6+, with all showing only weak staining.

DISCUSSION

Monoclonal antibody MR6 gives strong staining of cortical epithelial cells of the thymus and functional analysis has suggested that the MAb MR6 antigen may be associated with the IL-4 receptor (6). In this study, the results of immunohistochemical analysis of human thymus sections using IL-4B provide evidence that some cortical TEC express IL-4 receptors. While MAb MR6 was found not to inhibit the binding of IL-4 (data not shown), inhibition of IL-4–induced immune responses suggested that the MAb MR6 antigen may be associated with the IL-4 receptor signal transduction pathway. However, cortical TECs are a relatively quiescent population of cells, and are generally not known to proliferate rapidly in the normal postnatal and adult situation. This raises the questions as to the possible role of the IL-4R expressed on these cells. There have been a number of explanations, including prevention of functional maturation of self-reactive thymocytes by sequestration of available IL-4, leading to negative selection (9), or presentation of IL-4 to the actively growing immature thymocytes, perhaps contributing to positive selection (3). The observation that acid washing increases the intensity of labeling with IL-4B suggests that cortical TECs may serve as a reservoir for IL-4. This observation, in addition to the finding that IL-4 did not modify TEC proliferation in vitro (10), favors the hypothesis that cortical TECs present IL-4 to the immature cortical thymocytes, probably influencing the

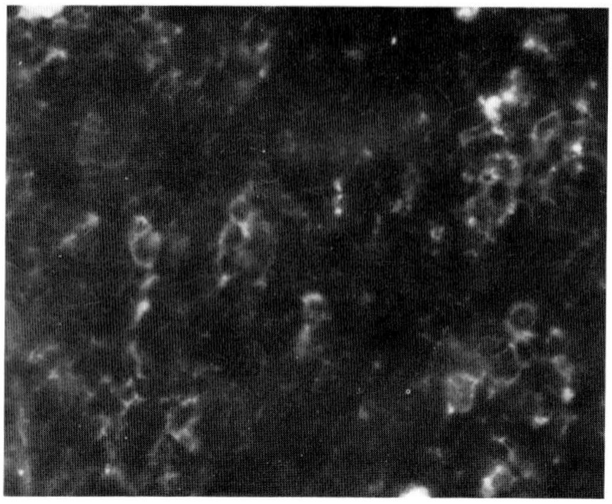

(a)

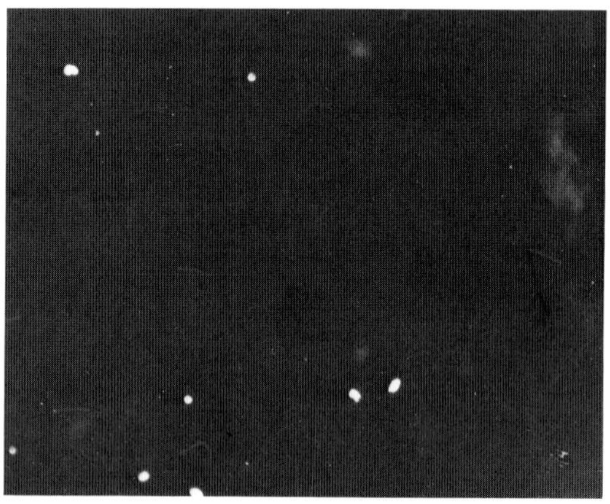

(b)

Figure 1 Labeling of thymic cortical epithelial cells with (a) biotinylated IL-4 (x425), and (b) negative control (x425). IL-4B labeled epitheliallike cells in the cortex. Some thymocytes appear to be weakly stained.

Table 2 Expression of MAb MR6-Ag/IL-4R Complex in Normal Tissues and Tumors of the Breast

	Labeling with MR6	
Type of tissues	% positive	Intensity of staining[a]
Normal	66 (6/9)	+/++
Benign proliferation	100 (6/6)	++/+++
Grades I & II	54 (13/24)	+/++/+++
Grade III	31 (5/16)	+

[a]Intensity of staining: weak = +, moderate = ++ and strong = +++.

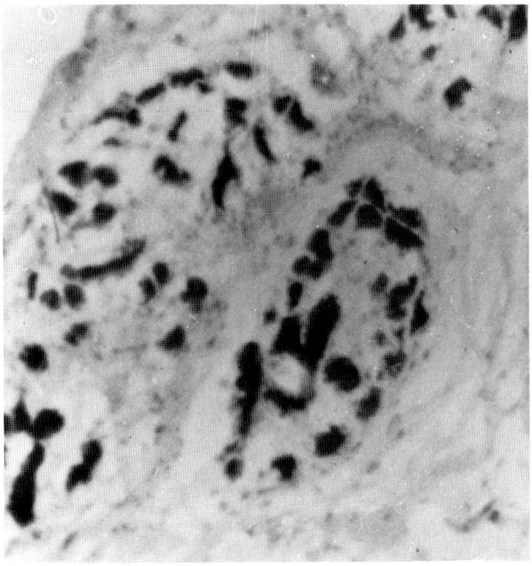

(a)

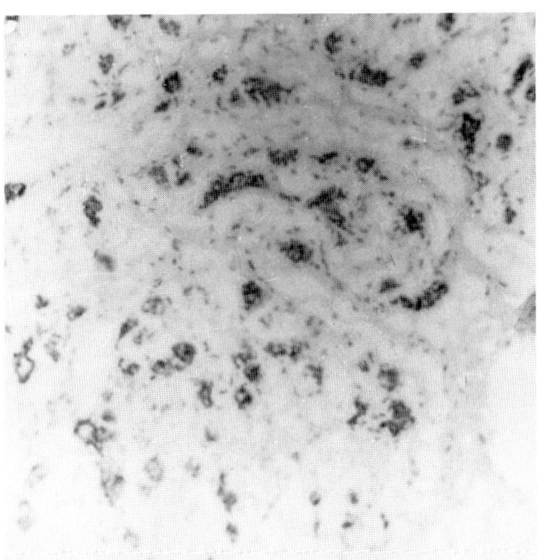

(b)

Figure 2 Upregulation of the MAb MR6-Ag/IL-4R complex expression in benign proliferation of breast. Sections were analyzed by indirect immunoperoxidase using (a) MAb MR6, and (b) isotype-matched irrelevant monoclonal antibody (x225). Sections were counterstained with hematoxylin. Isotype-matched antibody did not yield any reaction product. (Staining seen is hematoxylin only.)

maturation and expansion of the double-positive population. However, exactly why benign proliferation and low-grade tumors of the breast showed upregulation in the expression of the Mab MR6-Ag/IL-4R complex is much less clear, although it is possible that IL-4 may act as either a growth or maturation factor for epithelium depending on the state of maturity of the target cell, as is the case for T and B lymphocytes. The finding that the expression of the complex was downregulated in high-grade tumors suggests that the MAb MR6-Ag/IL4R complex may be involved early in the process of epithelial tumorigenisis.

REFERENCES

1. De Maagd, R. A., Mackenzie, W. A., Schuurman, H.-J., Ritter, M. A., Price, K. M., Broekhuizen, R., and Kater, L. The human thymus microenvironment: Heterogeneity detected by monoclonal anti-epithelial cell antibodies. Immunology 1985; 54:745–754.
2. Larche, M., Lamb, J. R., and Ritter, M. A. A novel T lymphocyte molecule that may function in the induction of self-tolerance and MHC-restriction within the human thymic microenvironment. Immunology 1988; 64:101–105.
3. von Gaudecker, B., Larche, M., Schuurman, H.-J., and Ritter, M. A. Analysis of the fine distribution of thymic epithelial microenvironment molecules by immunoelectron microscopy. Thymus 1989; 13:187.
4. Mat, I., Larche, M., Melcher, D., and Ritter, M. A. Br. J. Cancer 1990 (in press).
5. Park, L. S., Friend, D., Sassenfeld, H. M., and Urdal, D. L. Characterization of the human B cell stimulatory factor-1 receptor. J. Exp. Med. 1987; 166:476.
6. Larche, M., Lamb, J. R., O'Hehir, R. E., Imami-Shita, N., Zanders, E. D., Quint, D. E., Moqbel, R., and Ritter, M. A. Functional evidence for a monoclonal antibody that binds to the human interleukin 4 receptor. Immunology 1988; 65:617.
7. Al Jabaari, B., Ladyman, H. M., Larche, M., Sivolapenko, G. B., Epenetos, A. A., and Ritter, M. A. Elevated expression of the interleukin 4 receptor in carcinoma—a target for immunotherapy? Br. J. Cancer 1989; 59:910.
8. Zubet, C. E., Galizzi, J.-P., Valle, A., et al. Interleukin 4 receptors on normal B lymphocytes: Characterization and regulation. Eur. J. Immunol. 1990; 20:551.
9. Larche, M., and Ritter, M. A. IL-4, oncogenesis, and the thymus. In: M. K. Kendall and M. A. Ritter (eds.). *Thymus Update*. Vol. 2. London, Harwood Academic, 1989, pp. 59–72.
10. Saly, A. H., Hadden, E. M., Touraine, J. L., and Hadden, J. M. Effects of cytokines on human thymic epithelial cells in culture: IL-1 induces thymic epithelial cell proliferation and change in morphology. Cell. Immunol. 1989; 1214(1):13.

5

In Situ Hybridization Studies on the TNF-α in the Mouse Thymus

Role of Tumor Necrosing Factor α in the Prevention of Radiation-Induced Thymic Lymphomas

Philippe Delvenne, Marie-Paule Defresne, Chantal Humblet, Marie-Therese Martin, Anne Michel Rongy, Robert Courtoy, Roland Greimers, Catherine Delvenne, Jean Michel Paulus, Jean Claude Grosdent, and Jacques Boniver

University Hospital of Liège, Liège, Belgium

INTRODUCTION

In C57BL/Ka mice, a split-dose whole body irradiation regimen induces thymic lymphoblastic lymphomas (1). During the latency period preceding the onset of lymphomas, preneoplastic cells are detected in the thymus (2,3). Simultaneously deep alterations to marrow prothymocytes (3,4) and thymocyte subpopulations occur (5), together with a deep disturbance in the function of thymic epithelium (6). Interestingly, lymphoma development can be inhibited if a graft of normal bone marrow cells is given early after the split-dose irradiation (1). To explain the mechanism of lymphoma prevention, we proposed the hypothesis that grafted marrow cells provide the thymus with precursors of thymocytes and of nonepithelial stroma cells; consequently cytokine production may be restored in the thymus, leading to reconstitution of thymic epithelium (7). Gamma interferon, which is known to act on epithelial cells of various origins (8), and particularly on thymic epithelium by inducing class II molecule expression and even thymic hormone production (9,10), is one of the candidate cytokines. Our strategy to test this hypothesis was at three levels: (a) Is it possible to prevent radiation-induced thymic lymphomas by injecting exogenous cytokines instead of bone marrow cells? (b) What are the effects of exogenous cytokines on thymic epithelial cells in vitro? (c) Is there any evidence of increased

Table 1 Thymic Cells with TNF-α Transcripts[a]

Days after last irradiation	Controls	4.0 × 1.75 Gy	4.0 × 75 Gy + BM graft
15	17	15	7
30	13	3	73
45	4	14	26
80	12	14	3

[a]Number of cells with TNF-α transcripts per thymic section examined at magnification 400x.

cytokine production within the thymus in bone-marrow–grafted irradiated mice. In this chapter, we will show the preliminary results of experiments, which are now in progress to answer this third question.

EXPERIMENTAL DATA

We compared cytokine production in situ within the thymus of mice which are submitted to a leukemogenic split-dose irradiation, or which are grafted with normal bone marrow cells after such irradiations. Presently, the in situ hybridization methodology for tumor necrotizing factor α (TNF-α) transcripts is available in our laboratory. The molecular probe is a cyclic deoxyribonucleic acid fragment of a 1644 base pair (bp) inserted into the polylinker site of the pGEM-I plasmid (Promega). Sense or antisense ribonucleic acid probes were prepared and in situ hybridization performed (11,12).

Table 1 shows the results of a first experiment. The data are the average numbers of cells with TNF-α transcripts per thymic section in each experimental group. In the thymus of normal adult mice, very few cells showed autoradiographic signals for TNF-α transcripts. After a split-dose leukemogenic irradiation, the number of cells with TNF-α transcripts was quite similar to controls; by contrast, in marrow-grafted and irradiated animals, there was a striking increase of the number of TNF-α–positive cells between the fifteenth and forty-fifth days after treatment.

DISCUSSION

The data reported here yield new insight for the mechanism of lymphoma prevention by bone marrow grafting after a split-dose irradiation of 4.0 × 1.75 Gy: We demonstrate the transient accumulation of cells with TNF-α transcripts in the thymus of marrow-grafted irradiated animals. Interestingly, this occurs when several effects of bone marrow grafting are apparent: restoration of thymic epithelial cell capacities as well as of thymic histiocytic and dendritic cell numbers, and disappearance of preneoplastic cells (13). These data, together with the observed effects of exogenous TNF-α on thymic lymphoma development (7) and on the in vitro functional activities of thymic epithelial cells (10) suggest that the transient increase of TNF-α production in the thymus might be related to the mechanism of lymphoma prevention. Indeed, the produced TNF-α in marrow-grafted irradiated animals might contribute to the elimination of preleukemic cells either directly by a cytotoxic effect or indirectly by restoring thymic epithelium and hence signals for normal thymocyte differentiation perhaps incompatible with the progression of preneoplastic cells toward lymphoma growth.

ACKNOWLEDGMENTS

The studies mentioned in this chapter were financially supported by the Fund of Scientific Medical Research (Belgium), the Research Fund of the Faculty of Medicine of Liège University (Belgium), the Centre Anticancéreus près l'Université) de Liège, the Bekales Foundation, and Boehringer Ingelheim International.

The authors are grateful to Professor W. Fiers of the University of Ghent, Belgium, for providing the TNF-α molecular probe.

REFERENCES

1. Kaplan HS. On the natural history of the murine leukemias. Presidential address. Cancer Res. 1967; 1325–1340.
2. Haran-Ghera N. Dependent and autonomous phases during leukemogenesis. Leukemia Res. 1978; 2:11–21.
3. Boniver J, Decleve A, Lieberman M, Honsik C, Travis M, Kaplan HS. Marrow thymus interaction during radiation leukemogenesis in C57Bl/Ka mice. Cancer Res. 1981; 41:390–392.
4. Pazmino NH, Mc Ewan R, Ihle JN. Radiation leukemia in C57Bl/6 mice. III—Correlation of altered expression of terminal deoxynucleotidyl-transferase to induction of leukemia. J. Exp. Med. 1978; 148:1338–1350.
5. Rongy AM, Humblet C, Lelievre P, Greimers R, Defresne MP, Boniver J. Abnormal thymocyte subpopulations in split dose irradiated C57Bl/Ka mice before the onset of lymphomas. Effects of bone marrow grafting. Thymus (in press).
6. Defresne MP, Greimers R, Lenaerts P, Boniver J. Effects of marrow grafting on preleukemic cells and thymic nurse cells in C57Bl/Ka mice after a leukemogenic split dose irradiation. JNCI 1986; 77:1079–1085.
7. Boniver J, Humblet C, Defresne MP. Tumor Necrosis Factor and Interferon Y inhibit the development of radiation-induced thymic lymphomas in C57Bl/Ka mice. Leukemia 1989; 8: 611–613.
8. Papiernik M, Dombret H, Stefanos S, Wretzerbin J. Control of Ia antigen expression on phagocytic cells of the thymic reticulum by Interferon-gamma and prostaglandins. Eur. J. Immunol. 1986; (16):296–300.
9. Berry SF, Arenzana-Seisdebos F, Cohen S, Devos R, Charron D, Virelizier JL. Interferon modulates HLA class II antigen expression on cultured human thymic epithelial cells. J. Immunol. 1985; 135:1165–1171.
10. Defresne MP, Humblet C, Rongy AM, Greimers R, Boniver J. Effect of interferon-gamma and tumor necrosis factor-alpha on lymphoepithelial interactions within nurse cells. Eur. J. Immunol. 1990; 20:429–432.
11. Beissert S, Bergholz M, Waase I, Lepsien G, Schauer A, Pfizenmaier K, Krönke M. Regulation of tumor necrosis factor gene expression in colorectal adenocarcinoma: In vivo analysis by in situ hybridization. Proc. Natl. Acad. Sci. U.S.A. 1989; 86:5064–5068.
12. Hogan B, Constantini F, Lacy E. *Manipulating the Mouse Embryo*. Cold Spring Harbor Laboratories, Cold Spring Harbor, New York. 1986, pp. 228–235.
13. Sprecher E, Giloh H, Rahamin E, Yefenof E, Becker Y. Cytofluorometric analysis of thymic interdigitating cells from C57Bl/6 mice prior and after leukemogenic X irradiation. Leukemia Res. 1989; 13:799–809.

6
Human Thymic Stromal Cells Produce Interleukin-1, Interleukin-3, and Soluble CD23

Ali H. Dalloul, Patrice Debré, Fateh Ouaaz, Michel Arock, and M. Djavad Mossalayi
Laboratoire d'Immunologie Cellulaire, Hôpital Pitié-Salpêtrière, Paris, France

INTRODUCTION

The thymic microenvironment is a complex specialized tissue made of epithelial components, mesenchymal cells forming the thymic capsule and septae, and cells originating from bone marrow: monocytes and interdigitating cells (1). The passage of T-cell precursors through the thymus is an obligatory step for the generation of competent T lymphocytes (1). Earliest identifiable human thymocytes are $CD7^+2^-3^-4^-8^-$ (2). Factors involved in the differentiation of these precursors remained poorly understood. Recently, we have shown that, in contrast to interleukins (IL) 1–4, a sequential incubation with IL-1 and soluble CD23 (sCD23) could induce pre–T-cell maturation (3,4). However, proliferation of these precursors was observed with IL-3 (5). To study relevance of these data to T-cell ontogeny, we investigated the production of these cytokines by thymic stromal cells. Our results point to the ability of various thymic stroma cells to secrete above factors.

MATERIALS AND METHODS

Monoclonal Antibodies (MAbs)

Monomorphic anti–HLA DR (Beckton Dickinson, Mountain View, California); pananti-cytokeratin (Boehringer. Mannheim, Meylan, France); anti-vimentin (Amersham, U.K.); OKM1 (CD11b, Ortho clone, Raritan, New Jersey), IoM2, anti-CD14 (Immunotech, Marseille, France), fluorescein-anti-mouse immunoglobulins (Ig) (Beckton dickinson), and Avidin-Biotin peroxidase complex (Vector, Burlingame, California), and anti–IL-3 MAb (Genzyme, Boston, Massachusetts).

Obtaining and Culture of Stromal Cells

Adherent cells were obtained by adherence on plastic flasks. Epithelial cells were grown from thymic explants as described (6), using McCoy's medium containing 10% FCS, 100 IU/ml penicillin, 100 μg/ml streptomycin, 2.5 μg/ml amphotericin B, 0.4 μg/ml hydrocortisone, 10^{-7} M choleratoxin, and 20 ng/ml epidermal growth factor (all from Sigma). Fibroblasts were grown either from thymic explants, or from E^- thymic cells after adherence, in the presence of medium containing 10% FCS and above antibiotics.

Cytokine Assays

Cell supernatants were collected 48 hr after medium change. Soluble CD23 was assayed by RIA as described (7). Interleukin-1β was assayed by ELISA (Roussel Uclaf). Interleukin-3 was assayed by the ability to promote basophil-containing myeloid colonies from human bone marrow (8) as compared to rIL-3.

RESULTS

Separation and Identification of Thymic Stromal Cells

Thymic adherent cells (TADs), fibroblasts (TFs), and epithelial cells (TECs) have distinct morphology. In addition, they differ in their phenotype, as shown on Table 1. Thymic epithelial cells were strongly cytokeratin positive and vimentin negative, whereas fibroblasts were only vimentin positive. Thymic fibroblasts were pure, whereas TECs contained 5% contaminating fibroblasts, but no T cells or monocytes. Thymic adherent cells were mostly monocytic (>90% CD11b, CD14) and contained <5% cytokeratin-positive and/or vimentin-positive cells.

Only TECs Produce IL-3

Forty-eight-hour thymic stromal cell supernatants were added to bone marrow cell cultures at 20% final dilution, in methylcellulose cultures. Myeloid colonies were scored at day 10, and individual colonies picked up and stained with Giemsa. Only TEC supernatant promoted the proliferation of marrow precursors, with a significant percentage of basophil-containing colonies. Thymic epithelial cells produced high amounts of IL-3 when compared to activated T cells. However, this property seems to be dependent on activation fate of these cells. Indeed, continuous growth of TECs in the presence of EGF is needed for this production. Finally, IL-3 activity was abolished following addition of anti–IL-3 MAbs to the cultures (Table 2).

Table 1 Surface Marker Analysis of Thymic Stromal Cells

Cells	HLA-c1.I	HLA-DR	Keratin	Vimentin	CD11b	CD14
TEc	+	+	++	–	–	–
TF	+	+	–	++	–	–
TAD	+	+[a]	–[b]	–[b]	++	++

Results shown as negative, weakly (+) or strongly positive (++).
[a]10% (++).
[b]2% (++) cells.

Table 2 TECs Produce Interleukin-3

Medium colonies	Total colonies[a]	% Basophil-containing
Control	1 ± 1	ND
TEC-sup[b]	64 ± 35	21 ± 4
"+ anti IL-3 (100ng)	28 ± 2	0
r IL-3 (20ng)	53 ± 3	26 ± 6
"+ anti IL-3 (100ng)	21 ± 3	0
TEC-sup (–HC)[c]	67 ± 28	23 ± 5
TEC-sup (–EGF)	3 ± 2	ND
TF-sup	2 ± 1	ND
TAD-sup	1 ± 1	ND

[a]Colony formation: 5 ± 10^5 bone marrow cells incubated with supernatants from epithelial (TEC), fibroblast (TF), and adherent cells (TAD)
[b]Supernatant at 20% final dilution, mean + SD from 4 experiments done in triplicate.
[c]Supernatant from cells cultured for 7 days without hydrocortisone (HC) or epidermal growth factor (EGF).

IL-1 Is Secreted by Thymic Stromal Cells

Without stimulation, supernatants from TADs and TFs did not contain any IL-1 activity (Table 3), whereas low IL-1 levels were observed in some TEC supernatants. Following stimulation with LPS or TPA, all cells studies secreted IL-1. However, TAD produced highest IL-1 levels in these conditions (Table 3).

TECs Produce sCD23

We failed to detect any soluble CD23 (tested by RIA) in supernatants from above stromal cells. Meanwhile, when stimulated with IL-4, TADs produced significant levels of sCD23, whereas very low levels was found in TEC-derived supernatants. Since hydrocortisone (necessary for optimal TEC growth) inhibits CD23 expression on B lymphocytes, we assayed to whether the same effect was responsible for TECs' failure to secrete sCD23. Indeed, Table 4 shows that TECs grown with hydrocortisone-free medium secreted sCD23. This production was enhanced by IL-4.

DISCUSSION

Our results show that epithelial cells and monocytes from thymic stroma produce cytokines with a possible role in T-cell ontogeny. Interleukin-1 is produced by stimulated TADs, TFs,

Table 3 Interleukin-1 Production by Thymic Stromal Cells

Stimulation	TECs	TADs	TFs
No	30 ± 20[a]	0	0
LPS (10 μg/ml)	50 ± 15	400 ± 25	100 ± 25
PMA (100 ng/ml)	100 ± 20	120 ± 10	120 ± 10

[a]pg per 10^6 cells/ml.

Table 4 Thymic Stromal Cells Produce sCD23

Stimulation	TECs	TADs	TFs
Medium	0	0	0
Medium + IL-4 (200 μ)	0	24 ± 7[a]	0
Medium (–HC)[b]	8.5 ± 2.5	ND	ND
Medium (–HC) + IL-4	81 ± 15	ND	ND

[a]ng x 10^6 cells/ml.
[b]TEC cultured in medium without hydrocortisone.

and TECs, which correlate previous finding (6). Of interest, we have recently shown that IL-1 acts in synergy with sCD23 for the maturation of prothymocytes. CD23 was also secreted by TECs, and this activity is inhibited by hydrocortisone and enhanced by IL-4. In addition, we recently found CD23-mRNA (messenger ribonucleic acid) in cultured TECs as well as thymic sections. Of interest, it was mainly localized in the subcapsular area and deep cortex (data not shown).

Interleukin-3 is another cytokine exclusively produced by TECs. These cells secrete very high amounts of IL-3 when continuously grow with EGF. We also detected IL-3–specific mRNA in these cells (C. Fourcade, unpublished data). This finding is interesting in the light of IL-3's potential role in supporting autorenewal of prothymocytes.

Finally, although monocytes may play a role in T-cell proliferation and differentiation, the major role seems to be devoted to TECs as regards their intrathymic localization.

REFERENCES

1. Barton F. Haynes: The human thymic microenvironment. Adv. Immunol. 1984; 36:87.
2. Bertho J.M, Mossalayi M.D, Dalloul A.H, Mouterde G, Debré P: Isolation of an early T-cell precursor (CFU-TL) from Human bone marrow. Blood 1990; 75:1064.
3. Mossalayi M.D, Dalloul A.H, Bertho, J.M, Lecron J.C, Goube de Laforest P, Debré P: In vitro differentiation and proliferation of purified human thymic and bone marrow CD7+2-T cell precursors. Exp. Hematol. 1990; 18:326.
4. Dalloul A.H, Mossalayi M.D, Dellagi K, Bertho J.M, Debré P: Factor requirements for activation and proliferation steps of human cD2+3,4,8- early thymocytes. Eur. J. Immunol. 1989; 19:1985.
5. Mossalayi M.D, Lecron J.C, Dalloul A.H, Sarfati M, Bertho J.M, Hofstetter H, Delespesse G, Debré P: Soluble CD23 and Interleukin 1 synergistically induce early human thymocyte maturation. J. Exp. Med. 1990; 171:959.
6. Le P.T, Tuck, D.T, Dinarello C.A, Haynes B.F, Singer KH: Human thymic epithelial cells produce interleukin 1. J. Immunol. 1987; 1 38:2520.
7. Delespesse G, Sarfati M, Peleman R: Influence of recombinant IL4, IFN alpha and IFN gamma on the production of human IgG binding factor (soluble CD23). J. Immunol. 1989; 142:132.
8. Lanotte M, Arock M, Lacaze N, Guy Grand D: Murine basophil mast cell differentiation, toward optimal conditions for selective growth and maturation of basophil and allied cells. J. Cell Physiol. 1986; 129:199.

7
Thymulin-Secreting Cells in Humans
Distribution, Light Microscope Histochemistry, and Plasma Thymulin Levels

Marion D. Kendall,[1] Bared Safieh,[1] Aruna Sareen,[2] Graham Venn,[3] Lorna Matheson,[1] and Mary Ritter[2]
[1]*Thymus Research Laboratory and Cell Biology, United Medical and Dental Schools of Guy's and St. Thomas's Hospitals, London, England;* [2]*RPMS, London, England;* [3]*United Medical and Dental Schools of Guy's and St. Thomas's Hospitals, London, England*

INTRODUCTION

The thymic hormone, thymulin, is secreted by a subset of medullary epithelial cells (1) and by cells of the subcapsular cortex. In humans, the thymus atrophies with age and loses much of the cortex but a large medullary component remains (2), and no studies have been undertaken to establish that the medulla in old age still secretes thymulin.

Thus, this study was initiated for the dual purposes of examining thymulin secretion in old age and to seek correlations between peripheral blood (PB) subsets, thymocyte phenotype, function, and plasma thymulin levels.

The study was commenced comparatively recently, and the results must be regarded as preliminary. Despite this, there are many facts that have already emerged, and these are briefly reported here and will be documented in full later.

MATERIALS AND METHODS

Blood was taken, with ethical permission, from normal young adults (n = 13), from 60 patients undergoing open heart surgery, and from 17 age-matched controls. All samples were taken 8–9 a.m., kept on ice, and centrifuged at 4°C before storing the plasma at –70°C for the estimation of thymulin by radioimmunoassay (RIA) (3). Values below 150 fg/ml were regarded as not determined (ND), as this was below the detection limit of the assay. In four cardiac cases, blood samples were also taken at 0.5- or 1.0-hr intervals through surgery and afterwards. Whole blood was used for flow cytometry with monoclonal antibodies (MAbs) directed to CD4 and CD8 antigens. Small portions of thymus gland, normally discarded at surgery, were prepared for flow cytometry using the same MAbs, and other portions frozen by conventional methods for immunocytochemistry using an antikeratin MAb (LP34, Dakopatts High Wycanbe, England), and immunoglobulin M (IgM) MAb raised in mouse against synthetic thymulin (4β, our unpublished data), and appropriate negative and positive controls. The specificity of 4β had previously been tested by ELISA and by preabsorption of the MAb with pure thymulin prior to immunohistochemistry.

RESULTS

Mean patient age was 65+/–7 years. Thymic tissue of all patients was fatty but contained patches of medulla (0.5–0.1 mm diameter), often with Hassall's corpuscles. Small patches of cortex were generally associated with the medulla or with blood vessels.

The medullary tissue in all samples contained numerous cells positive with LP34 and many, but not all, of these were positive with 4β. Other epithelial cells positive to 4β were found around cortical blood vessels and in some patients around patches of cortex.

The mean plasma thymulin level for cardiac patients (364+/–245 fg/ml, 7 ND) was not significantly different from healthy adults of a similar age range (350+/–120 fg/ml, 2 ND). There was, however, a much greater variation among cardiac patients, with 25% having very high plasma thymulin levels (up to 1428 fg/ml).

The percentage of $CD4^+$ or $CD8^+$ cells in the peripheral blood (PB) of cardiac patients was slightly lower but similar to the normal ranges for adults >20 years.

Considering only patients with high plasma thymulin levels: these had highly significantly lower (P = <0.001, d.f. = 20) percentages of PB $CD4^+$ cells (27.5+/–11%) compared with normal adults (48+/–11%) and, of PB $CD8^+$ cells (18+/–5% against 38+/–9% in normal adults).

When thymulin levels for all patients were plotted against the percentage of $CD8^+$ thymocytes, a bell-shaped distribution was found with normal thymulin plasma values generally coinciding with the highest percentage of $CD8^+$ thymocytes. Thus, the percentage of $CD8^+$ thymocytes was low (<35% of total mononuclear cells) in patients with either low or high plasma thymulin levels.

The mean CD4:CD8 ratio for cardiac patients was 1.5+/–0.7 compared to 1.4 for young adults. The ratio of CD4:CD8 thymocytes in the cardiac patients (1.2+/–0.8, n = 31) was not significantly different from PB ratios.

When four patients were serially sampled throughout surgery and afterwards, thymulin levels dropped in all patients (ND in three patients) and remained low until 3–4 hr postoperatively when they were elevated above the original (8 a.m.) values.

DISCUSSION

The thymus gland of these elderly cardiac patients was fully functional with regard to the production of thymulin. This was evidenced by the presence of thymulin-containing cells in all the thymus glands examined (even when greatly atrophied), and also, plasma thymulin levels were similar to those of normal age-matched adults.

However, thymulin levels in 25% of the patients were very high; far higher than those recorded in normal adults (3). This could result from the immediate stress of the operation, or alternatively may represent a group predisposed to stress. This aspect of the study needs further investigation.

The changes in thymulin values throughout surgery and recovery are very interesting. Similar earlier studies designed to examine the possibility of hypofunctioning of the pituitary and adrenals in cardiac surgery (4) found no evidence for that, but did document rises in adrenocorticotropin (ACTH) and later rises in cortisol that occur postoperatively. In our study, the rise in thymulin occurred in all four cases just after the rise in ACTH and before the rise in cortisol. This provides further evidence that control of plasma thymulin is part of the hypothalamic-pituitary axis. In this context its release has been shown to be affected by other pituitary hormones (5). Work is currently underway to further examine these neuroimmune interactions.

REFERENCES

1. Savino W, Dardenne M, Bach JF. Thymic hormone containing cells. II Evolution of cells containing the serum thymic factor (FTS or thymulin) in normal and autoimmune mice, as revealed by anti-FTS monoclonal antibodies. Relationship with Ia bearing cells. Clin Exp Immunol 1983; 51:1–6.
2. Steinmann GG. Changes in the human thymus during ageing. In: *The Human Thymus Histophysiology and Pathology*. HK Muller-Hermelink (ed.). Curr Top Pathol 1986; 75:43–88.
3. Safieh B, Kendall MD, Norman JC, Metreau E, Dardenne M, Bach JF, Pleau JM. A new radioimmunoassay for the thymic peptide thymulin, and its application for measuring thymulin in blood samples. J Immunol Methods 1990; 127:255–265.
4. Chambers DJ, Karimanzandi N, Braimbridge MV, Dunham J, Brooks F, Quiney J, Slavin B. Hormonal and electrolyte responses during and after open heart surgery. Thor Cardiovasc Surg 1984; 32:358–364.
5. Dardenne M, Wilson S. Neuroendocrine control of the thymic epithelium: Modulation of thymic endocrine function, cytokeratin expression and cell proliferation by hormones and neuropeptides. PNEI 1990; 3:18–25.

8

Differentiation of Epithelial Stroma During Ontogenesis of the Thymus

Comparison of Antigen Expression Within the Developing Thymus Anlage and in the Pharyngeal Region

Klaus-Ulrich Hartmann and Eryati Darwin
Institute for Experimental Immunology, Philipps-University, Marburg, Federal Republic of Germany

MATERIALS AND METHODS

BDF1 mice were bred in our colony; the day when a vaginal plug was observed was considered as gestational day 0 (GD). The thymus of seven embryos (GD 17) were minced, freed of the majority of thymocytes, and incubated for 1 hr with collagenase. 5×10^6 cells were given three times i.p. to LOU rats; 4 days following the last (intracardial) injection, the spleen cells were prepared and fused with myeloma cells (Sp2/F0) following standard procedures. The growing hybridomas were then screened for antibody binding to cryosections of fetal (GD 17) thymus. Selected hybridomas were cloned twice.

Antibody binding was investigated on 5-μm cryostat sections of whole embryos or of isolated organs. After fixation with acetone the sections were incubated with hybridoma supernatant (resp. purified immunoglobulins) 60 min, followed by incubations with biotinylated goat-antirat immunoglobulin (Ig) (Sigma Bioch.), with streptavidin-biotin-peroxidase complex (Amersham), and with diaminobenzidine/H2O2 in TRIS buffer; most sections were weakly counterstained with hematoxylin before embedding in glycerol gelatine.

CRYOSECTION OF WHOLE MOUSE EMBRYOS

Two rat monoclonal antibodies reacting with epithelial stroma cells of embryonic mouse thymus have been selected: MAb Th1-115/7 stained mainly the epithelial stroma cells of the thymus cortex. In cryosections already GD 11 a fine reticular staining in the center of the thymus anlage could be seen. Following GD 13, the monoclonal antibody (MAb) 115–positive cells were located predominantly within the cortical regions of the thymus. Staining—and probably antigen expression—of the thymus cortex was most intensive between GD 14 and GD 18 (Fig. 1), but somewhat reduced staining of cortical epithelial cells could be observed in thymus of newborn and adult animals.

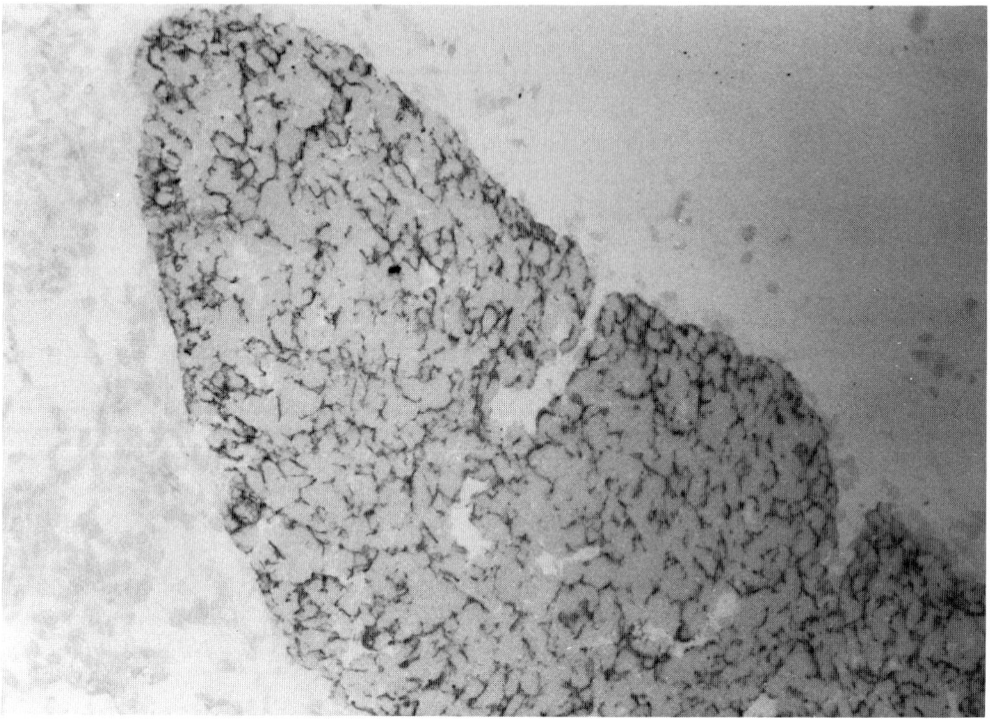

Figure 1 MAb Th1-115/7. Thymus GD 17.

MAb 115 also stains the mucosal epithelial of the pharynx and of the developing cavum nasi and canalis tympanopharyngis (Fig. 2), and distinct patches of cells occur in the esophagus, the collecting tubes of the kidney, and the epithelium of the gallbladder.

MAb Th-101/7 bound to epithelial stroma cells within the thymus medulla. MAb 101–positive cells could be observed in the center of the thymus anlage already at GD 11. Following GD 13, the MAb 101–positive cells form clusters, most intensively stained between GD 15 and birth (Fig. 3). MAb 101–positive cell clusters are present in the medulla of adult thymus.

In addition, MAb 101 bound to distinct areas of submucosa cells of the pharynx, of the cavum nasi (Fig. 4), and of the trachea. The papillae filiformes of the tongue were MAb 101 positive (GD 15), as were the epithelial cells around the hair follicle. (These extrathymic staining patterns could also be observed in embryos of congenital thymus-deficient nu/nu mice.)

HYPOTHESIS

The roles of the surface molecules recognized by MAb 115 and MAb 101 are not yet known. The expression of these antigens along the pharynx might be explained by a common ontogenic development of pharyngeal epithelium and thymus anlage. It seems that these antigens are expressed in epithelial layers of areas of differentiation, of folding (formation of the cavum nasi), or invagination, and of intensive interactions between endodermal and ectodermal tissues.

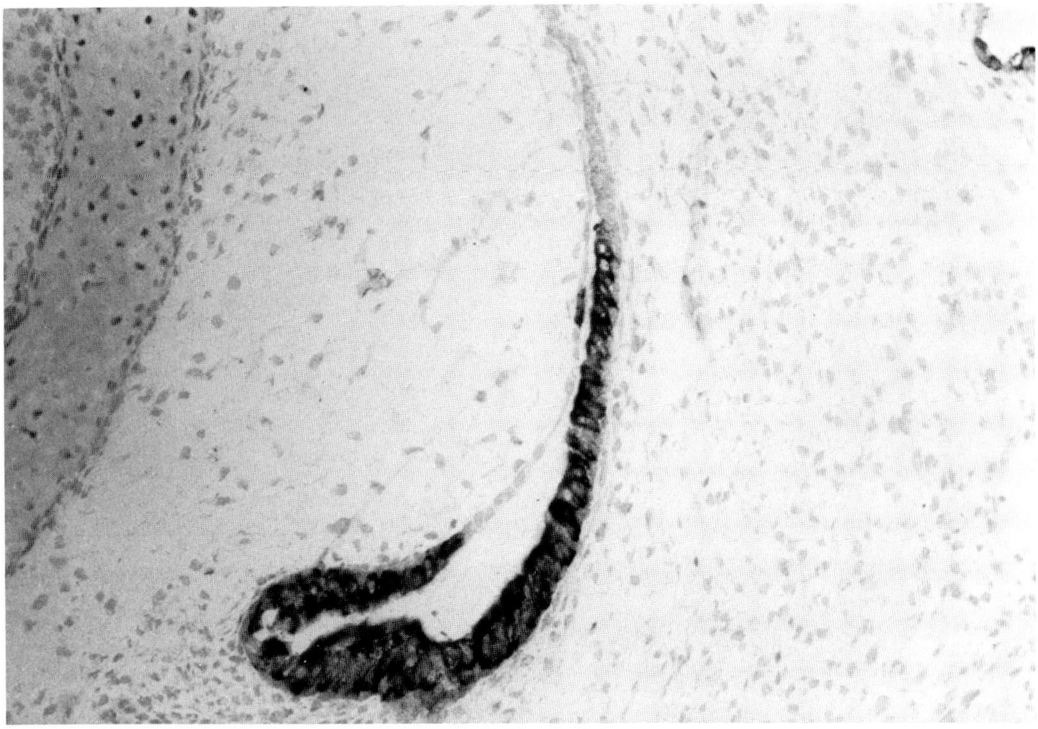

Figure 2 MAb Th1-115/7. Pharynx.

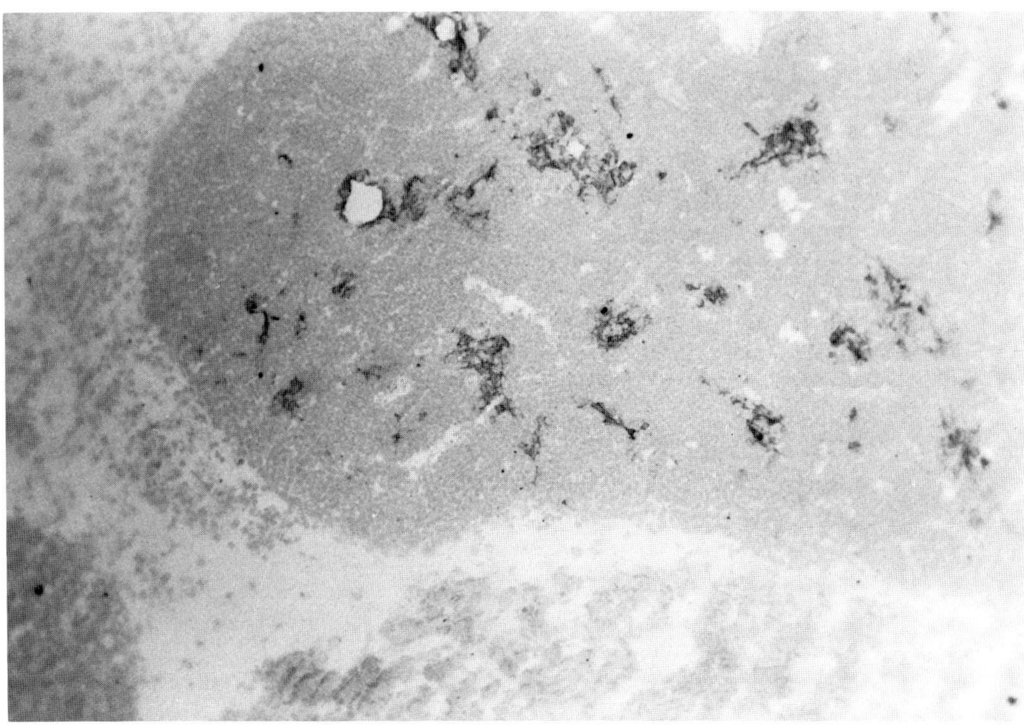

Figure 3 MAb Th2-101/5. Thymus GD 17.

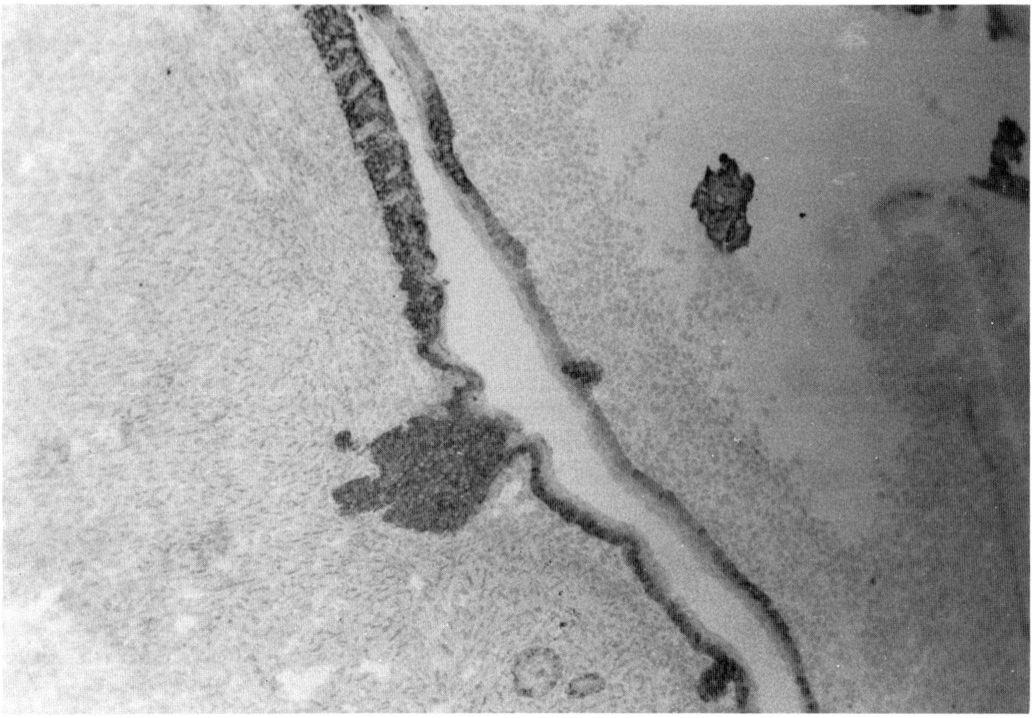

Figure 4 MAb Th2-101/5. Pharynx.

Monoclonal 115 and also MAb 101 stain epithelial layers in areas where sensory functions develop, i.e., tasting, smelling, and feeling, especially at the entrance of the pharynx. Thus, the simultaneous antigen expression in areas of the development of sensory regions and on thymus epithelial cells might suggest or at least (together with other observations) would be compatible with the hypothesis that the thymus anlage originated from a "sensory organ" located at the pharynx during evolution.

In addition, if cryosections of early embryos are stained with monoclonal antibodies directed against the major histocompatibility complex (MHC) class 1 structures (MAb R 1.9.6), the thymus anlage expresses MHC class 1 molecules earlier than other organs. If the sequence of antigen expression during ontogenesis follows phylogenesis, then this observation could suggest that MHC-like molecules had served as receptors in the primordial thymus anlage before descendence into the mediastinum.

9
Ontogenetic Development of the Thymic Stroma of Wistar Rats

Angeles Vicente and Agustin G. Zapata
Complutense University, Madrid, Spain

INTRODUCTION

The thymus is a central lymphoid organ in which T-cell precursors mature and differentiate governed partially by the nonlymphoid components of the thymic stroma, consisting of epithelial cells, macrophages, and interdigitating/dendritic cells. Whereas T-cell subset differentiation is well evidenced, relatively little is known of the origin and development of the thymus microenvironment. In rats, classic studies reported the histogenesis of the thymus (1) and recently, the development of some nonlymphoid cell populations has been described (2–5), but a systematic ontogenic study correlating structure and specific cell marker expression is lacking. In this regard, the present study analyzes by in situ immunohistochemistry, histoenzymology, and electron microscopy the appearance and development of the nonlymphoid components of Wistar rat thymus during both embryonic and postnatal life.

MATERIALS AND METHODS

Wistar rat thymus glands were sampled from day 13 of fetal life to day 11 after birth. Thymuses were removed aseptically from both neonatal rats and 17- to 20-days old fetuses. Fetuses from earlier embryonic stage were fixed in toto. Thymic samples were processed routinely for light and transmission electron microscopy. For immunohistochemistry, the samples were fixed either in lysine periodate–paraformaldehyde–glutaraldehyde or Bouin's fixative and embedded in paraffin wax. Cell marker characterization was achieved by an indirect immunoperoxidase-labeling assay on 6-uμ thick sections using the listed mouse monoclonal antibodies (MAb), antisera, or lectins in Table 1, and developing routinely the peroxidase reaction with 0.05% 3,3-diaminobenzidine (Sigma, St. Louis, Missouri). Enzymatic activities were determined on 7-μm thick frozen sections using the indicated substrates in Table 1.

Table 1

MAb	Dilution	Specificity
OX-18 (Serotec)	1/200	MHC class I antigens
OX-6 (Serotec)	1/200	MHC class II antigens
HIS-19 (Histology Dept. Groningen Univ)	1/50	MHC class II antigens
ED 1 (Free University Amsterdam)	1/1000	Medullary macrophages
ED 2 (Free University Amsterdam)	1/1000	Cortical and cortico-medullary macrophages
OX-42 (Serotec)	1/100	Macrophages
Cytokeratin polyclonal antibody (BioGenes, Dublin, CA)	1 mg/ml	56Kd and 64Kd Keratins
RMC-20 (courtesy of Dr. Colic, Belgrade)	1 mg/ml	Medullary epithelial cells
Lectins	**Dilution**	**Specificity**
Ulex phosphatase	20 mg/ml	Medullary epithelial cells
Tetragonolobus purpureas (Sigma)	20 mg/ml	Medullary epithelial cells
Enzymes		**Substrates**
Acid phosphatase		Naphthyl AS biphosphate
Non-spescific esterase		α-Naphthyl acetate
5′-nucleotidase		Adenosin-5′-mono-phosphate
ATPase		Adenosin-5′-tri-phosphate

RESULTS AND DISCUSSION

Histology

The thymus of earlier stages (d 13) consists of two separated homogeneous epithelial lobes isolated from the pharyngeal epithelium. At days 14–15, the thymic primordium, which has descended ventrocaudally, is a single organ with an incipient cortex-medulla differentiation. From this stage, the thymus gland grows and clearly defined cortex and medulla become evident. These results agree with the reported histogenesis of mammalian thymus (6–8), although some authors report that the cortex-medulla differentiation occurs late (d 21) in rat fetuses (9).

Epithelial Cells

The thymic primordium of 13-day-old fetuses contains a homogeneous population of epithelial cells showing few filaments and desmosomes, which in the following stages (d 14–15), differentiates into several epithelial cell types. An epithelial cell type forms a subcapsular continuous layer which remains in the adult thymus. A second cell population constitutes the cortical stroma-supporting elements in later embryonic stages and adult rats. Apparently related to it, after birth, there appear cortical lymphoepithelial clusters which resemble of in vitro nurse cells. In the medullary area, there occur diverse epithelial cells, characterized mainly by the presence of thick bundles of filaments and electron-dense granules, which in further stages constitute three main epithelial cell types. One, relatively similar to the cortical stroma-supporting elements exhibits short cell processes and few filaments and desmosomes. Most of the medullary epithelial cells increase the cytokeratin content and eventually associated to form Hassall's bodies. In this regard, nonspecific esterase and acid phosphatase activities closely associated with Hassall's bodies after birth occur earlier in isolated medullary epithelial cells. A third type of medullary epithelial cell evident from day 18 of gestation corresponds to secretory, hypertrophied cells containing electron-dense granules and small vesicles which converge to form large vacuoles. These results confirm the heterogeneity of the epithelial components of embryonic thymus. In mice and humans, MAbs specific to thymic stroma demonstrate such a heterogeneity from the first stages of embryonic life (7,10). TGP, Ulex, and RCM-20-positive cells are restricted to a few medullary epithelial elements which appear on day 19/20 and persist after birth. Cytokeratin-positive cells appear in 17-day-old fetal thymuses, increasingly rapidly in later stages to constitute an extensive network in both cortex and medulla after birth. This late expression of cytokeratin could be accounted to the used antiserum which recognizes exclusively large molecular weight keratins (56–64 kD). Colic et al. (6) point out that fetal thymus expresses only some low molecular weight polypeptides, confirming indirectly our results.

Medullary epithelial cells express surface major histocompatibility (MHC) class II and more weakly class I molecules from day 15 of embryonic life. At day 16–18 there is an increase of MHC class I molecule expression on medullary epithelial cells, and on days 19–20 cortical epithelial cells express for the first time MHC class II antigens (Fig. 1). After birth cortical epithelial cells show surface MHC class I molecules. Both in situ and in vitro reports evidence the expression of MHC molecules on the epithelial cells of thymic cortex and medulla, although medullary cells exhibit a higher expression than cortical epithelium (7,10,12). Other authors agree, in concordance with our results, on the time of the appearance of these molecules and the earlier expression of class II and of class I antigens (13). Ultrastructural results in mouse indicate that the first thymic cells showing MHC class II correspond to medullary stroma-supporting cells and secretory, hypertrophied elements (11).

Development of Thymic Macrophages and IDCs/DCs

Although phagocytic cells are identified in 15-day-old fetal thymus, cells expressing macrophage cell markers appear on days 19–20. In addition, nonspecific esterase and acid phosphatase activities become evident on day 17/18 of gestation. At birth, however, there

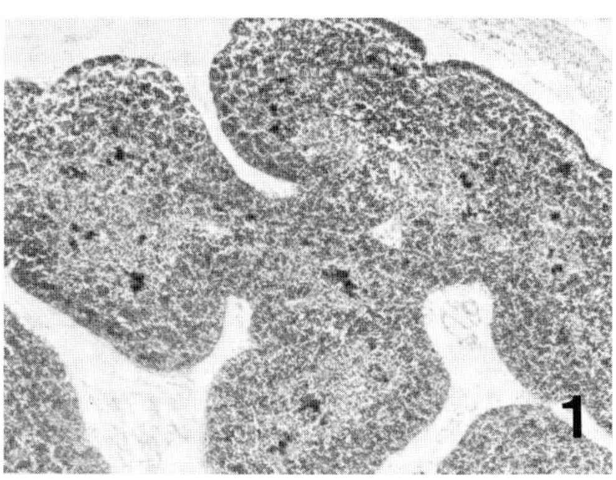

Figure 1 Expression of MHC class II molecules on the cortical epithelial cells of 19–20-day embryonic rats.

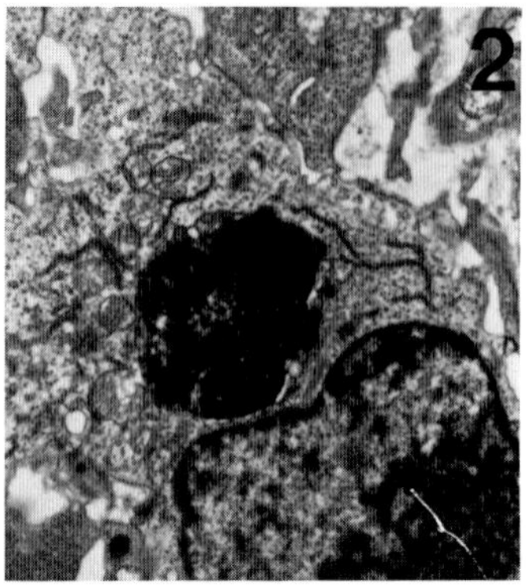

Figure 2 Macrophages in the embryonic thymus of Wistar rats.

is an important increase in these activities as well as in the number of $ED1^+$ cells and, in lesser amount, of $ED2^+$ cells. Duijvestijn et al. (2) observed macrophages in 17-days-old rat fetuses, and Sminia et al. (4) agree with our results on the appearance and further development of both ED1 and ED2 macrophage populations in the last days of rat gestation. Thus, it is difficult to correlate the ultrastructural results with the pattern of expression of $ED1^+$ and $ED2^+$ cells. Macrophages observed during embryonic life (Fig. 2) could represent two subtypes of the same cell population equivalent to that described by Milicavic et al. (14) in adult rat thymus. In addition, they could be $ED1^+$ cells, the only cell macrophage population described in rat embryonic thymus (4). On the other hand, $ED2^+$ cells which appear around birth correspond principally to the population of cortical macrophages containing engulfed lymphocytes. Expression of MHC class II molecules on medullar dendritic cells has been reported in adult thymus (12), although a weak Ia reactivity has been described on medullary macrophages (11). According to our results, isolated Ia^+ dendritic cells occur in the thymic medulla of 20-day-old fetuses (see Fig. 1), and after birth, they increase considerably (Fig. 3). Other authors (3) have related this postnatal increase to a continuous migration of bone marrow–derived precursors. Typical interdigitating cells are, however, observed in the medulla of 17-day-old fetuses in agreement with previous reports (8),

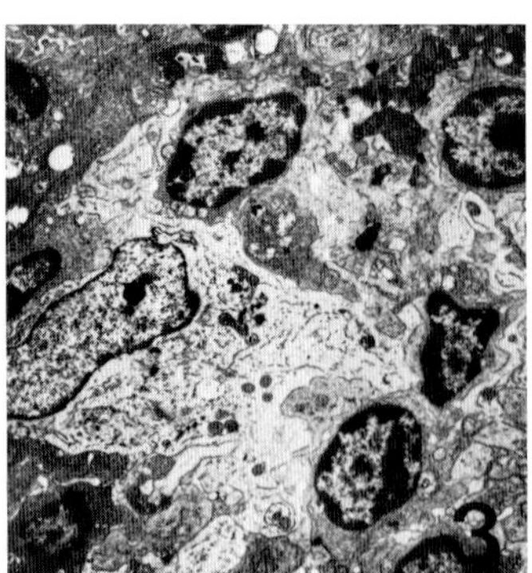

Figure 3 Presence of isolated Ia+ dendritic cells in the thymic medulla of neonatal Wistar rats.

although Duijvestijn et al. (2) find them only from day 19 of gestation. Remarkably, these IDCs exhibit cored tubules which in skin Langerhans cells have been related to receptor internalization and membrane recycling (15).

CONCLUSIONS

Our results suggest a gradual morphofunctional maturation of thymic nonlymphoid components with an early diversification of epithelial cell populations and later appearance of IDCs/DCs and macrophages. Likewise, the expression of MHC molecules occurs earlier in the epithelial component than in dendritic cells, although the highest expression is raised around birth in both cell populations. Remarkably, although lymphocytes maturate rapidly in the thymus, mature thymocytes only migrate to peripheral lymphoid organs at birth or in the first days of postnatal life (16) when, according to the present results, the nonlymphoid components of thymus are fully functional. Thus, as recently pointed out by Marrack et al. (17), our results suggest a correlation between the maturation of thymic stromal components and the acquisition of functional competence by T cells.

REFERENCES

1. Harland M. Early histogenesis of the thymus in the white rat. Anat Rec 1940;77:247–271.
2. Duijvestijn AM, Sminia T, Köhler YG, Janse EM, Hoefsmit ECM. Ontogeny of the rat thymus microenvironment: Development of the interdigitating cell and macrophage populations. Dev Comp Immunol 1984;8:947–956.
3. Higley HR, O'Morchoe CCC. Morphometric analysis of thymic medullary non-lymphoid cell changes during postnatal development. Dev Comp Immunol 1984;8:711–719.
4. Sminia T, van Asselt AA, van de Ende MB, Dijkstsra CD. Rat thymus macrophages: An immunohistochemical study on fetal, neonatal and adult thymus. Thymus 1986;8:141–150.
5. Colic M, Jovanovic S, Mitrovic S, Dujic A. Immunohistochemical identification of six cytokeratin-defined subsets of the rat thymic epithelial cells. Thymus 1989;13:175–185.
6. von Gaudecker B, Müller-Hermelink HK. Ontogeny and organization of the stationary non-lymphoid cells in the human thymus. Cell Tissue Res 1980;207:287–306.
7. van Vliet E, Jenkinson EJ, Kingston R, Owen JJT, van Ewijk W. Stromal cell types in the developing thymus of the normal and nude mouse embryo. Eur J Immunol 1985; 15:675–681.
8. Moraux-Moyson A, Scheiff JM, Haumont S. Thymus histogenesis in C3H mice. Thymus 1988;12:89–109.
9. Aboussaouira T, Moustafa Y, Idelman S. Image analysis of cell proliferation in rat thymus throughout development. Thymus 1988;12:167–186.
10. Haynes BF, Scearce RM, Lobach DF, Hensley LL. Phenotypic characterization and ontogeny of mesodermal-derived and endocrine epithelial components of the human thymic microenvironment. J Exp Med 1984;159:1149–1168.
11. Van Ewijk W, Rouse RV, Weissman IL. Immunoelectron microscopic identification of I-A and H-2K bearing cells. J Histochem Cytochem 1980;28:1089–1099.
12. Barclay AN, Mayrhofer G. Bone marrow origin of Ia-positive cells in the medulla of rat thymus. J Exp Med 1981;153:1666–1671.
13. Jenkinson E, van Ewijk W, Owen JJT. Major histocompatibility complex antigen expression on the epithelium of the developing thymus in normal and nude mice. J Exp Med 1981;153: 280–293.
14. Milicevic NM, Milicevic Z, Colic M, Mujovic S. Ultrastructural study of macrophages in the rat thymus, with special reference to the cortico-medullary zone. J Anat 1987;150:89–998.

15. Hanau D, Fabre M, Schmitt DA, Garaud JC, Pauly G, Cazenave JP. Appearance of Birbeck granule-like structures in anti-T6 antibody-treated human epidermal Langerhans cells. J Invest Dermatol 1988;90:298–304.
16. Ceredig R, MacDonald HR, Jenkinson EJ. Flow microfluorometric analysis of mouse thymus development in vivo and in vitro. Eur J Immunol 1983;13:185–190.
17. Marrack P, Kushnir E, Born W, McDuffie M, Kappler J. The development of helper T cell precursors in mouse thymus. J Immunol 1988;140:2508–2514.

10

Analysis of Molecules Shared by Rat T Cells and Their Thymic Epithelial Microenvironment

Russell Hargreaves, Ann McCormack, and Mary A. Ritter
Royal Postgraduate Medical School, London, England

INTRODUCTION

Epithelial cells within the thymus are thought to play an important role in the proliferation and maturation of T lymphocytes via cell-cell contact and secretion of soluble molecules. We and colleagues have raised monoclonal antibodies (MAbs) to identify the epithelial molecules involved in these processes (1–4). However, we have recently found that some MAbs which detect heterogeneity within the epithelial component of the thymic microenvironment recognize molecules that are also present on T-lymphocyte subpopulations (1,2,3). We have now further investigated the phenomenon of shared lymphocyte-epithelial molecules by raising MAbs in a system where mice were immunized with activated rat T lymphocytes and the resulting supernatant MAbs screened for epithelial reactivity on sections of rat thymus. Our data indicate that many molecules are shared between T cells and thymic epithelium, suggesting that the interaction between the epithelial microenvironment and the developing lymphocytes is a synergistic one.

MATERIALS AND METHODS

Fusion

Six-week-old female (CBA × Balb/c) F_1 mice were immunized intraperitoneally with a mixture of Complete Freunds Adjuvant and approximately 10^7 cells generated from a mixed lymphocyte reaction (MLR) using AS rat T cells stimulated with AUGUST adherent spleen cells. Two subsequent immunizations followed at 2-week intervals with a mixture of Incomplete Freunds Adjuvant and AS anti-AUGUST MLR cells. Three days after the last immunization, spleen cells were fused with myeloma line NSO using standard fusion protocol (4). Hybridomas were cloned by limiting dilution.

Screening

Immunohistology

Hybridoma supernatants were screened by indirect immunofluorescence on 5-μm frozen tissue sections of rat thymus using a rabbit antimouse immunoglobulin (Ig) FITC (Dakopatts, Denmark) second layer. Additional screening was done on human thymus.

Flow Cytometric Analysis

Fresh thymocyte and spleen cell suspensions were prepared from 6- to 8-week-old female AS rats. The panel of monoclonals was then incubated at saturating concentrations with the cells for 45 min, washed twice with HEPES buffered medium, and then incubated for 45 min with rabbit antimouse Ig FITC second layer. Finally, the cells were washed three times with medium and analyzed immediately (EPICS Profile, Coulter, U.S.A.).

T-Cell Separation

The spleen of an 8-week-old rat was teased and the cells resuspended in 1 ml of prewarmed RPMI medium containing 10% FCS. This suspension was then layered on to 1 g of prewet nylon wool, and the nylon wool column incubated at 37°C for 45 min. Ten milliliters of warm medium was then passed through the column and the eluted cells collected. These cells were processed for FACS analysis using the above method.

RESULTS

MAb Panel

Two fusions were carried out, both producing a similar panel of antibodies. Immunohistology revealed MAbs that labeled each of the major subsets of thymic epithelium: panepithelium (CTES I); subcapsular, perivascular, and medullary epithelium (CTES II); cortical epithelium (CTES III); and medullary epithelium only (CTES IV) (full CTES classification in ref. 3). For initial studies three of these (SB1, SB3, and XA5) were selected for more detailed analysis (see following two sections).

Tissue Distribution

Monoclonal antibody SB3 gave high-intensity staining of both medullary, perivascular, and subcapsular epithelium in rat and human thymus (Fig. 1), typical of the CTES II pattern. Monoclonal antibody SB1 was positive on both cortical epithelium, and a small amount of medullary epithelium (Fig. 2), typical of a CTES IIIB reagent. Monoclonal antibody XA5–positive epithelial cells reside only in the medulla of rat and human thymus (Fig. 3).

FACS Analysis

Indirect immunofluorescence analysis with antibody SB3 revealed surface labeling of 11% of rat splenocytes and approximately 5% of rat thymocytes. Neither MAbs XA5 nor SB1 displayed any surface positivity on either thymus or spleen cells. These data suggest the presence of intracellular molecules.

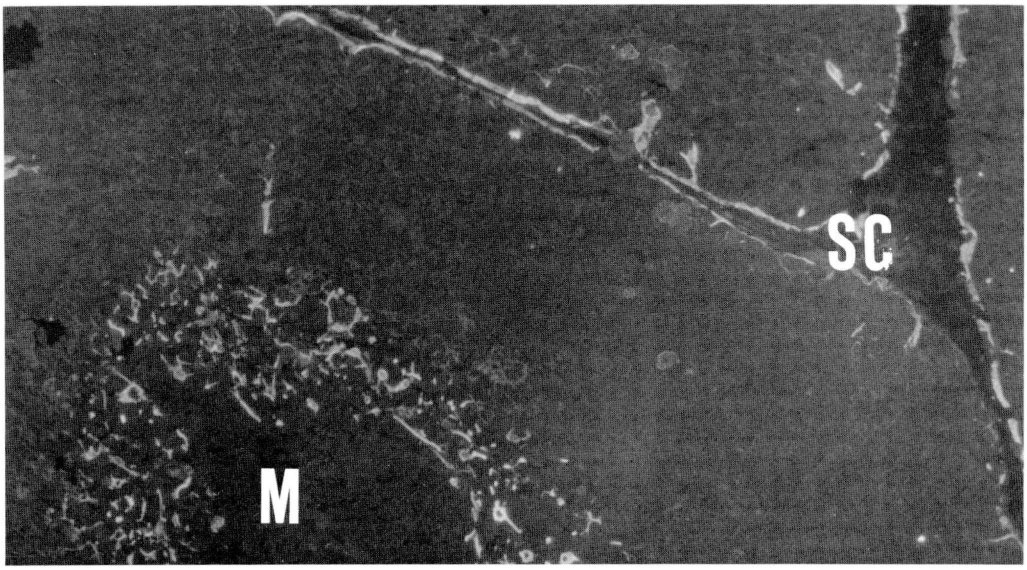

Figure 1 Rat thymus tissue sections stained with MAb SB3 by indirect immunofluorescence showing labeling of both medullary (M) and subcapsular (S) epithelium. (Magnified 187.5×)

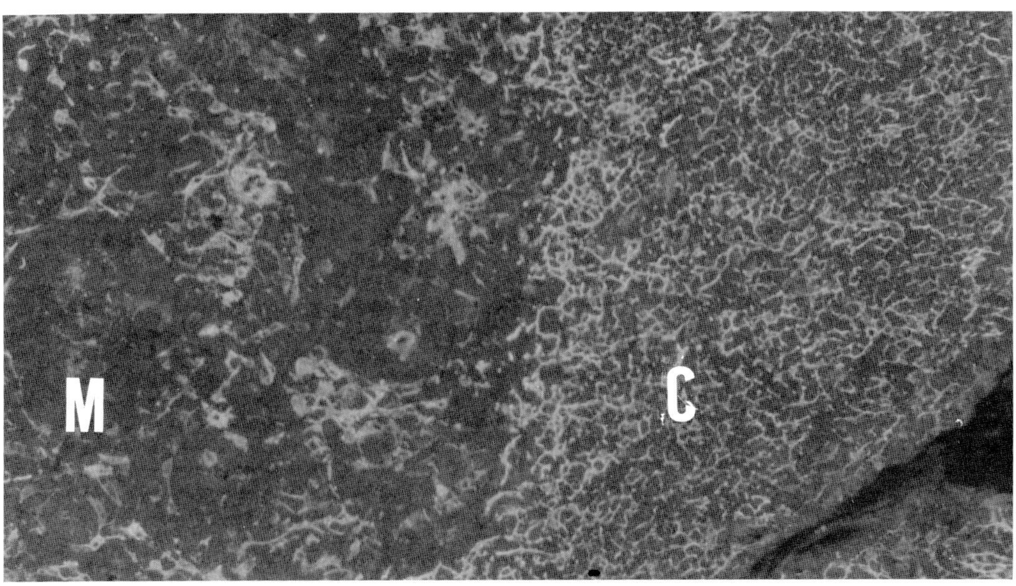

Figure 2 MAb SB1 labeling cortical (C) and some medullary (M) epithelia in rat thymus. (Magnified 187.5×)

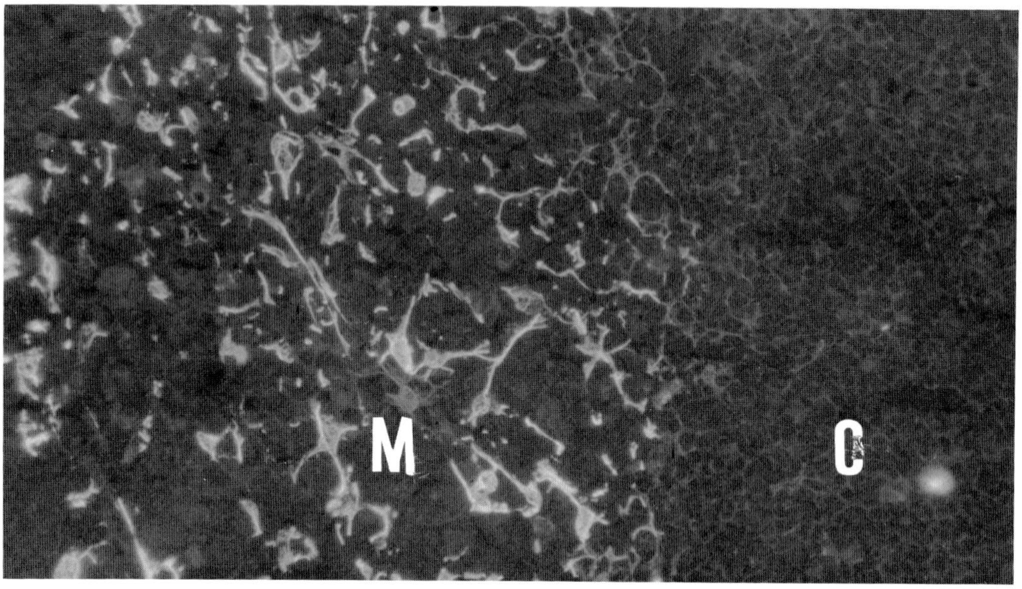

Figure 3 Rat thymus stained by immunofluorescence with MAb XA5 showing labeling only within the medulla (M). (Magnified 375×)

Cytospins

Cytospin preparations of B-depleted splenocytes were fixed and analyzed by indirect immunofluorescence. Monoclonal antibodies SB1 and XA5 gave intracellular labeling, localized predominantly to the nucleus. No intracellular staining was seen with MAb SB3.

DISCUSSION

Previous studies in which MAbs have been raised to thymic epithelium have revealed that some of these reagents detect molecules that are also present on T lymphocytes (1–3). In this study, we have investigated the extent of this phenomenon in a system where MAbs were generated against activated T cells and then screened on thymic epithelium. Two panels of MAbs were produced in this way, each containing a wide range of thymic epithelial staining patterns comparable to those generated after immunization with thymic stromal cells. Thus "shared antigens" were found to characterize each of the following epithelial subpopulations: all epithelial cells (CTES I); subcapsular, perivascular, and medullary epithelium (CTES II); cortical epithelium (CTES III); and medullary epithelium (CTES IV). In more detailed studies one of these reagents (SB3) has been shown to recognize a cell surface molecule while two others (MAbs SB1 and XA5) bind to intracellular antigens. Similar studies are in progress with the other reagents in our MAb panel.

Clearly the next stage in the investigation will be to analyze the molecular nature of these shared antigens by immunoprecipitation and Western blotting techniques to determine whether it is the same molecule that is present on/in the two cell types, as is the case for the human and murine shared antigens that we have studied (2). The function of such molecules will then be investigated to determine their role in T-cell differentiation. These studies should also shed light on what appears to be a two-way synergistic interaction between developing T cells and their thymic microenvironment.

REFERENCES

1. Ritter MA, and Haynes BF. Summary of thymic epithelium workshop. In: *Leucocyte Typing III*. A. McMichael, PCL Beverley, S Cobbold, MJ Crumpton, W Gilks, FM Gotch, N Hogg, M Horton, N Ling, ICM MacLennan, DY Mason, C Milstein, D Speigelhalter and H Waldmann (eds.). Oxford University Press, 1987, p. 247.
2. Larche M, Lamb JR, Ritter MA. A novel T lymphocyte molecule that may function in the induction of self-tolerance and MHC-restriction within the human thymic microenvironment. Immunology 1988;64:101–5.
3. Kampinga J, Berges S, Boyd RL, Brekelmans P, Colic M, van Ewijk W, Kendall MD, Ladyman H, Niewenhuis P, Ritter MA, Schuurman H-J, Tournifier A. Thymic epithelial antibodies: Immunohistological analysis and introduction of nomenclature. Thymus 1989; 14:165–73.
4. De Maagd RA, MacKenzie WA, Schuurman H-J, Ritter MA, Price KM, Broekhuizen R, Kater L. The human thymus microenvironment: heterogeneity detected by monoclonal anti-epithelial cell antibodies. Immunology 1985; 54:745–54.

11

Identification of Molecules Shared Between Subcapsular/Medullary Epithelium, Granulocytes, and a Subset of Macrophages in Rat Thymus

Miodrag Colić, Sonja Gašić, Ljiljana Popović, and Aleksandar Dujić
Military Medical Academy, Belgrade, Yugoslavia

INTRODUCTION

The thymic microenvironment plays a very important role in positioning, differentiation, and maturation of T cells, acting by direct contact with thymocytes or by soluble products (1). However, very little is known regarding individual molecules involved in these processes. Hybridoma technology enables identification of new antigens on thymic non-lymphoid cells and their subsequent functional analysis. The first interlaboratory workshop and systematization of a large panel of monoclonal antibodies (MAbs) predominantly recognizing the antigens of thymic epithelial cells resulted in their preliminary clustering and nomenclature (2). We present here the immunoreactivity of two new MAbs produced in our laboratory which recognize molecules shared between subcapsular/medullary epithelium, granulocytes, and a subset of macrophages in rat thymus and discuss their relationship with other MAbs reactive with the thymic microenvironment.

MATERIALS AND METHODS

Animals

AO rats, 6–8 weeks old, both sexes and BALB/c mice, female, 8 weeks old, bred at the Farm for Experimental Animals, MMA, Belgrade, were used.

Immunization and Fusion

BALB/c mice were immunized i.p. with 0.4 ml homogenized rat thymus with complete Freund's adjuvant (FA) (Torlak, Belgrade, YU) in physiological saline. Thymic homogenate, which contained enriched nonlymphoid cells, was prepared after excess thymocytes had been removed by i.p. injection of hydrocortisone (Galenika, Belgrade, Yu) (150 mg/kg b.w.) 2 days before the experiment. The procedure was repeated with incomplete FA and without FA, respectively, at 2-week intervals. Fusion was performed 3 days after the last immunization, as previously described (3). Briefly, spleen cells from immunized mice were fused with P 3x63-Ag8.653 myeloma cells using PEG 1500 and plated out into 96-well plates (Flow Laboratories, Irving, Scotland). Hybridomas were selected for in HAT medium (Serva, Heidelberg, FRG) and screened by immunoperoxidase staining on cryostat thymic sections, as described below. Positive clones were cloned by limiting dilution.

Immunohistochemistry

Cryostat sections of the thymus or cytospins of cultured thymic macrophages were fixed in acetone, incubated with supernatants of MAbs for 60 min, followed by blocking of endogenous peroxidase activity in methanol containing 0.3% H_2O_2. After that, sections were incubated with $F(ab')_2$ preparation of sheep antimouse immunoglobulin (Ig) coupled with peroxidase or isotype specific goat antimouse Ig biotinylated antibodies (Amersham International, Amersham Bucks, UK) and subsequent streptavidin-peroxidase. Revelation of the peroxidase activity was performed using 0.06% diaminobenzidine (DAB) and 0.10% H_2O_2.

Double immunostaining was used to compare immunoreactivity of produced MAbs with other MAbs (for details, see Results). In all combinations MAbs mutually differed in isotype specificity. Four double immunofluorescence staining the sequence of incubations was as follows: first MAb, goat antimouse Ig isotype-specific biotinylated antibody, streptavidin Texas Red; seemed MAb, sheep antimouse Ig isotype-specific FITC-conjugated antibody. The dual combination of streptavidin-biotin immunoperoxidase and immunoalkaline phosphatase was also used. Sections/cytospins were incubated with the first MAb and subsequent isotype-specific secondary coupled with alkaline phosphatase, then with secondary MAb and corresponding isotype-specific antibody coupled with peroxidase. Alkaline phosphatase (AP) reaction (red color) was visualized using naphthol AS-MX phosphate, fast red, and 1 M levamisole (to block endogenous AP activity). Peroxidase reactions activity (brown color) was demonstrated using DAB and H_2O_2 as described. All controls in which one of the MAbs was replaced by an irrelevant mouse MAb of the same isotype gave negative results.

Other Antibodies

K 8.13 MAb reactive with various cytokeratin polypeptides was purchased from ICN, Farmakos-ICN, Belgrade.

ED1 MAb was a generous gift of Dr. C. Dijkstra (Free University, Amsterdam), whereas R-MC series of MAbs (23, 42, and 45) were produced in our laboratory (3,4).

Cultivation of Thymic Macrophages

Small fragments of thymic tissues were cultivated onto glass Petri dishes using serum-free medium (Biorich 2, Flow) and 30% L conditioned medium (supernatant of L 929 fibroblast cell line) as a source of macrophage colony-stimulating factor. This medium inhibited the proliferation of fibroblasts and epithelial cells and favored the growth of macrophage colonies. Macrophages were identified by their morphology, presence of nonspecific esterase activity, and reactivity with ED1 MAb (specific for rat cells belonging to the monocyte/macrophage lineage) (5).

Macrophage–Thymocyte Rosettes

Adherent macrophages grown in culture were detached using PBS containing 0.02% EDTA. Rosettes were performed by mixing macrophages with syngeneic thymocytes in ration 1:100 and 3 hr incubation at +4°C.

Flow Cytometry

Cell suspension of thymocytes and peripheral blood cells were stained by MAbs and subsequent antimouse Ig-FITC antibody (Amersham International, UK). Red blood cells were lysed using ammonium-sulfate before fixation with 0.4% formaldehyde. The percentage of labeled cells was evaluated on an EPICS-CS cytofluorimeter (Coulter, FRG). Lymphocytes, monocytes or granulocytes in peripheral blood were identified according to the forward light scatter.

RESULTS

Two monoclonal antibodies (R-MC 46 and 47) from the fusion, reactive with thymic nonlymphoid cells, were cloned. They differed in isotype specificity (IgG_1 and IgM, respectively) but showed a very similar staining pattern in the thymus. Both Abs bound to subcapsular/medullary epithelium and isolated cells throughout the cortex and septa morphologically resembled granulocytes and macrophages (Fig. 1a). Labeling in the cortex was very characteristic with clusterlike appearance. The clusters were different in size, staining or a very large with heavily stained central cell and surrounding positive thymocyte in a rosettelike form (Fig. 1b).

The identification of each cell type recognized by these two MAbs was performed using double immunostaining and flow cytometry.

Dual immunostaining with R-MC 46/47 MAbs and K 8.13 MAb recognizing all epithelial cells in the rat thymus (6) showed that R-MC antibodies stained keratin-positive cells in the subcapsule (Fig. 2a,b.) and most cells in the medulla. However, R-MC 46.47 MAbs showed more confluent staining, also seen outside epithelium in a granular form.

A subset of R-MC $46/47^+$ cortical macrophages was identified using double staining with R-MC 42 MAb specific for cortical macrophages (4). These dual combinations demonstrated that more than 50% cells in clusters were double positive. We further tested thymic macrophages in culture 2 weeks after cultivation and found that 20–50% adherent macrophages are R-MC $46/47^+$ (Fig. 3). Staining was present both in cytoplasm (small or large granular content) and on membranes of some cells. Some macrophages forming rosettes with thymocyte (25–40%) were also positive (Fig. 4). Thymocyte in rosettes were slightly positive or negative.

To study whether R-MC 46 and 47 MAbs stain granulocytes we used flow cytometric analysis of peripheral blood cells. Figure 5 shows that most granulocytes identified by forward light scatter were positive with both antibodies (85–95% and 90–97%, respectively). The analysis of monocyte bitmap showed that 30–45% monocytes were also positive. No positivity was detected on the lymphocyte population. Flow cytometry of thymocytes in suspension showed that less than 2% cells were R-MC $46/47^+$. R-MC $46/47^+$ granulocytes were identified on thymic sections using double staining with R-MC 45 MAb (4). These cells were frequently associated with some R-MC 23^+ blood vessels (3) which were also weakly R-MC $46/47^+$ (not shown).

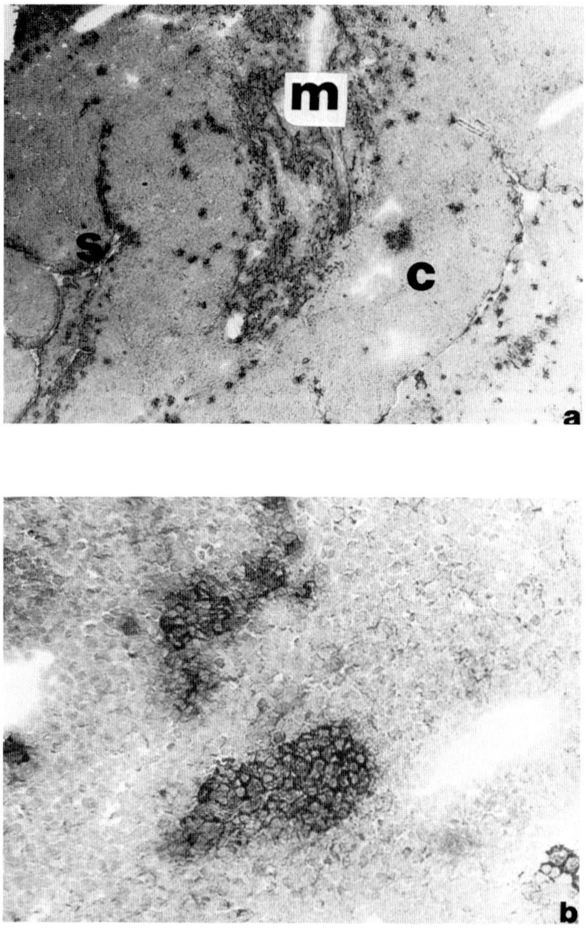

Figure 1 Streptavidin-biotin immunoperoxidase staining of the rat thymus with R-MC 46 MAb. Note staining of the subcapsular/medullary epithelium and isolated cells throughout the cortex (a). Staining of the cortical cells in a cluster-like appearance (b). S = subcapsula; C = cortex; M = medulla. (Magnifications: [a] ×40 [b] ×100)

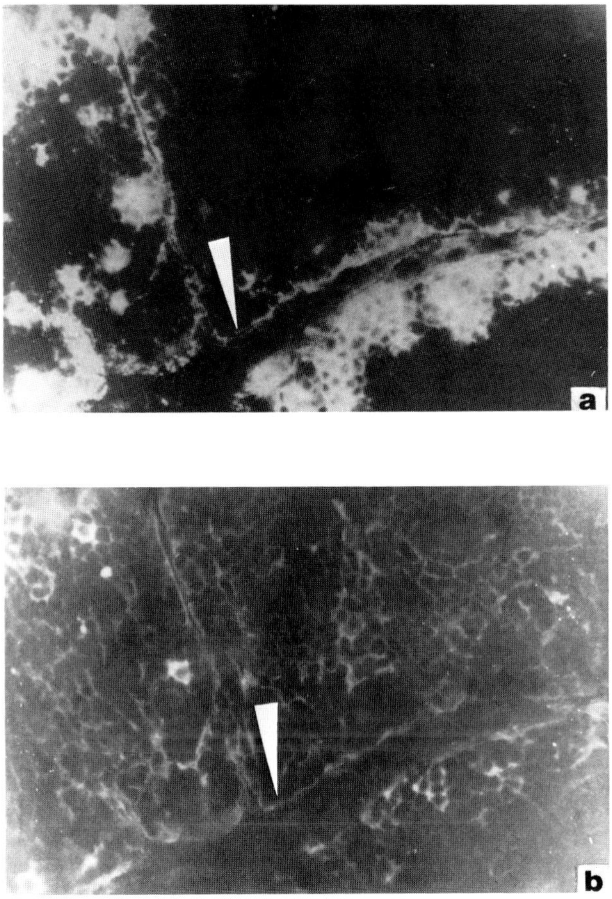

Figure 2 Double immunofluorescence of the rat thymus with R-MC 47 MAb (a) and K.8.13 MAb (b). Note that R-MC 47 stains the subcapsular (keratin-positive) epithelium (arrows) and clusters of keratin-negative cells. (Magnification: ×450)

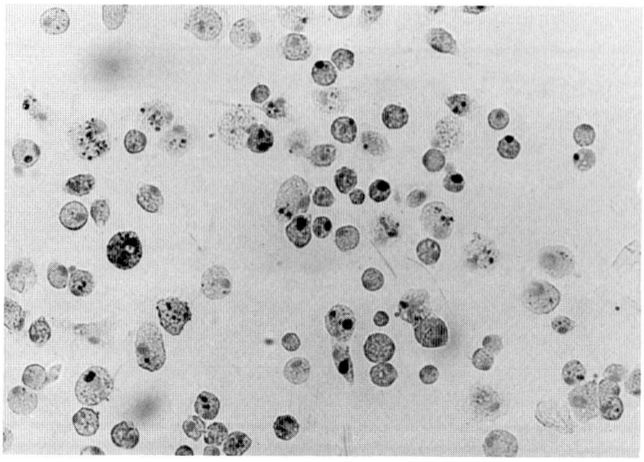

Figure 3 A monolayer of thymic macrophages in culture stained with R-MC 46 MAb. Note that the manority of cells show predominant intracytoplasmic granular staining. (Magnification: ×100)

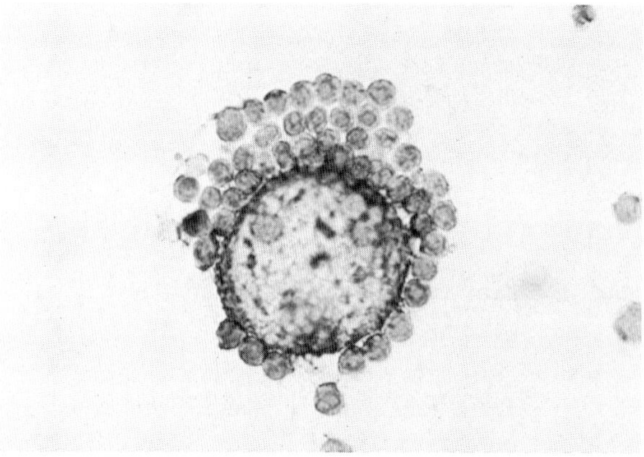

Figure 4 An adherent macrophage from thymic culture forming rosettes with syngeneic thymocytes is R-MC 47^{+}.

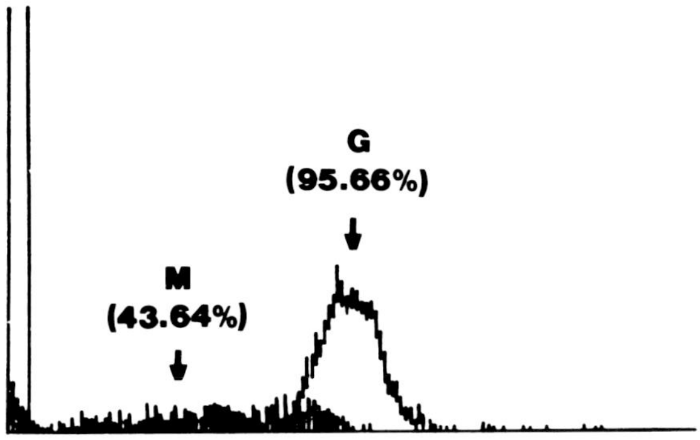

Figure 5 Fluorescence profile of granulocytes (G) and monocytes (M) stained with R-MC 47 MAb.

DISCUSSION

Based on the immunoreactivity of R-MC 46 and 47 MAbs presented in this work, it can be concluded that they recognize antigen(s) shared between granulocytes/macrophages and thymic epithelial cells. The characteristic staining pattern of these reagents in the thymus delineates them from other MAbs against the thymic microenvironmental components already produced in our laboratory (3,4).

Certain MAbs raised to thymic epithelium in humans also stain isolated macrophages/granulocytes and a subset of thymic epithelial cells (7) but their restriction in binding only to Hassall's corpuscles and different staining pattern indicate that R-MC 46/47 and these MAbs probably do not detect the same antigens.

We carefully examined the re activity of a large panel of MAbs produced to myeloid antigens in humans recently presented at the 4th International Conference of Leucocyte Differentiation Antigens and found that MAbs clustered into CD13 and CD15 bind granulocytes/monocytes and some epithelial cells (8). However, no data regarding staining of thymic epithelium with these reagents were given.

Two MAbs (R2-1A6 and R2-2B1) produced by Ishii et al. (9) stain macrophages, granulocytes, and some reticular elements in the rat, including thymic epithelium. These MAbs probably differ from R-MC 46 and 47 MAbs in that they have different staining pattern and recognize high molecular mass (220 kD) proteins, whereas both our MAbs immunoprecipitate small 3.5-kD polypeptide from rat granulocytes (manuscript in preparation). Polypeptides with a similar mol mass (4 kD) possessing chemotactic activity for hemopoietic T lymphocyte precursors have been isolated from culture supernatant of a rat thymic epithelial cell line (IT-45) (10). The small mol mass of antigens recognized by R-MC 46 and 47 MAbs and characteristic staining pattern of granulocytes associated with some tissue blood vessels (not shown) indicate their similarity to p.8.14 antigens recognized by 5.5 MAb in humans (11), for which it is suggested to have a role in homing of granulocytes and monocytes into inflamed tissues. All these data are attractive for further functional characterization of R-MC 46/47 antigens, especially their possible roles in T-cell development.

REFERENCES

1. Lobach DF, Haynes BF. Ontogeny of the human thymus during fetal development. J Clin Immunol 1987; 7:81–97.
2. Kampinga J, Berges S, Boyd RL, Brekelmans P, Colic M, Ewijk van W et al. Thymic epithelial antibodies: Immunohistological analysis and introduction of nomenclature. Thymus 1989; 13:165–73.
3. Colic M, Matanovic D, Hegedis Lj, Dujic A. Immunohistochemical characterization of rat thymic non-lymphoid cells. I. Epithelial and mesenchimal components defined by monoclonal antibodies. Immunology 1988; 67:277–84.
4. Colic M, Popovic Lj, Gasic S, Dragojevic-Simic V, Milicevic NM, Matanovic D. et al. Immunohistochemical characterization of rat thymic non-lymphoid cells. II. Macrophages and granulocytes defined by monoclonal antibodies. Immunology 1990; 69:416–22.
5. Dijkstra CD, Dopp EA, Joling P, Kraal G. The heterogeneity of mononuclear phagocytes in lymphoid organs: distinct macrophage populations in the rat recognized by monoclonal antibodies ED1, ED2 and ED3. Immunology 1985; 54:589–99.
6. Colic M, Jovanovic S, Mitrovic S, Dujic A. Immunohistochemical identification of six cytokeratin-defined subsets of the rat thymic epithelial cells. Thymus 1989; 13:175–85.
7. Ritter MA, Haynes BF. Summary of thymic epithelium workshop. In: McMichael A, Beverley P, Hagg N, Horton M. (eds.). *Leucocyte Typing III. White Cell Differentiation Antigens.* Oxford, England, Oxford University Press, 1987, p. 247–8.
8. Knapp W. Myeloid section report. In: Knapp W. et al. (ed.). *Leucocyte Typing IV. White Cell Differentiation Antigens.* Oxford, England, Oxford University Press 1989, p. 747–80.
9. Ishii Y, Matsuura A, Iwaki H, Takami T, Kikuchi K. Two closely related expressed on granulocytes, macrophages and some reticular elements in rat lymphoid tissues: characterization by monoclonal antibodies. Immunology 1984; 51:477–87.
10. Imhof BA, Deugnier MA, Itoh T, Theiry JP. T lymphocyte precursors migrate towards chemotactic peptides secreted by embryonic or juvenile thymus. Adv Exp Biol Med 1988; 237:565–70.
11. Hogg N, Allen C, Edgeworth J. Monoclonal antibody 5.5 reacts with p8,14, a myeloid molecule associated with some vascular endothelium. Eur J Immunol 1989; 19:1053–61.

12
A Novel Adhesion Molecule on Mouse Thymic Epithelium and T Lymphocytes

Nesrina Imami, Heather Ladyman, and Mary A. Ritter
Royal Postgraduate Medical School, Hammersmith Hospital, London, England

INTRODUCTION

Thymic epithelial cells play an important role in the differentiation and selection of developing T lymphocytes. In a previous study, we raised monoclonal antibodies (MAbs) to thymic epithelium in order to identify cell surface molecules that may be involved in these developmental processes (1). One such reagent, the rat MAb 4F1, recognizes cortical epithelium in tissue sections of mouse thymus. In this chapter, we describe the structural and functional analysis of the molecule to which 4F1 binds (4F1-antigen). Our data indicate that the 4F1-antigen may be a novel adhesion molecule composed of both PI-linked and transmembrane forms which is found not only on some epithelial cells, but also on the surface of certain T lymphocytes. In addition, 4F1-antibody blocks lymphocyte-epithelial adhesion and T-cell proliferation in a mixed lymphocyte reaction (MLR). Thus, the 4F1-antigen may be involved in both intrathymic T-lymphocyte differentiation and peripheral T-cell function.

MATERIALS AND METHODS

Expression of the 4Fl-antigen was analyzed by immunofluorescence and/or immunoperoxidase techniques on: thymus tissue sections, monolayer cultures of thymoma cell lines (TM25*114,103 and 120; containing both epithelial and lymphoid cells) (2), and suspensions of thymocytes and thymoma lymphocytes (TM25*114,103, 120 and BW5147; 10^6) using flow cytofluorimetry (EPICS) (3). To assess the function of this antigen MLR were performed using BALB/c (H-2^d) spleen cells as responders and T_4 (H-$2^{k/b}$)–irradiated spleen cells as stimulators.

The biochemical nature of the 4F1-antigen was assayed by: Western blotting, using the modified system of Laemmli (4); surface iodination of cells and immunoprecipitation (5); inhibition of glycosylation by tunicamycin and enzyme digestion with endoglycosidase F (5); and finally, phospholipase C treatment to remove PI-linked surface molecules (6).

RESULTS AND DISCUSSION

Distribution and Expression of the 4F1-Antigen

The 4F1 gives strong labeling of cortical epithelium, and also weakly stains small patches of epithelium in the medulla of the mouse thymus (Fig. 1). The 4F1-antigen is highly conserved, since the antibody also stains thymuses of other species; for example, 26-week fetal human thymus (all thymic epithelial cells [TEC]), chicken thymus (perivascular TECs), goat thymus (medullary TECs), and axolotol thymus (7) as well as epithelial cells within other mouse organs (kidney tubules and gut). This molecule appears early during thymus ontogeny (day 11; the earliest stage analyzed); thus, it is present at the time of colonization by the first stem cells.

Staining of the thymoma cell lines confirmed the reactivity of 4F1 with epithelial cells but showed that transformed lymphoid cells were also strongly positive (Fig. 2). Flow cytometric analysis showed high expression of 4F1-antigen on the surface of these thymoma lymphocytes. The molecule is also sometimes present on normal Balb/c thymocytes, and on the BW 5147 lymphoid cell line, indicating that the 4F1-antigen is not acquired passively from the epithelial cells but is synthesized by the thymocytes

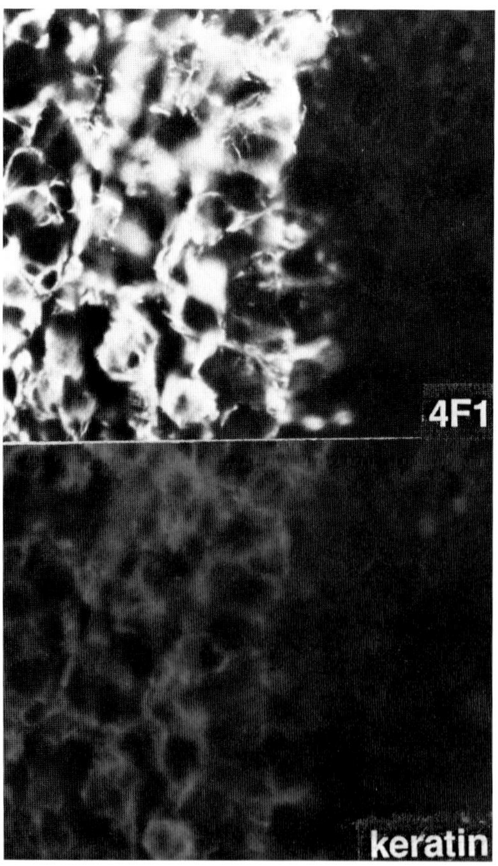

Figure 1 Dual immunofluorescence staining of normal mouse thymus.

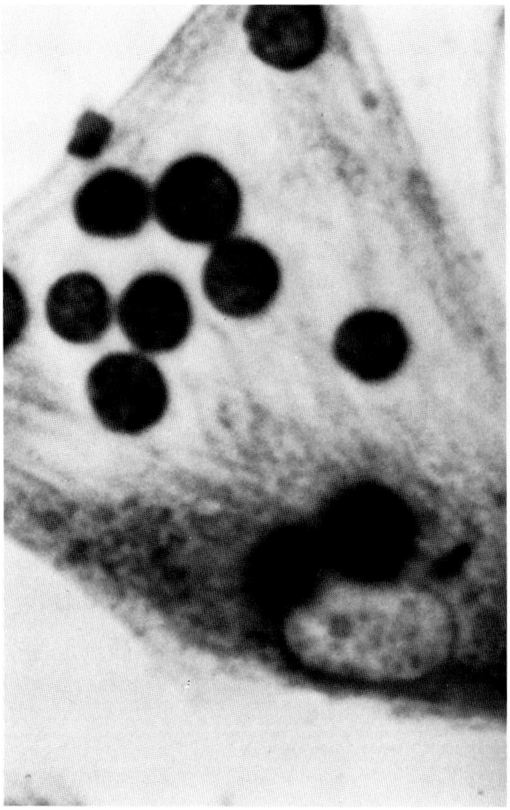

Figure 2 Immunoperoxidase staining of thymoma line.

themselves. Similarly, epithelial thymoma cells grown in isolation from any lymphocytes show strong 4F1-antigen expression. Thus, both lymphoid and epithelial cells must be capable of synthesizing the molecule. Electron microscopy also shows the presence of the molecule on both cell types. However, since not all normal thymocyte samples bear 4F1-antigen the molecule may be upregulated under certain conditions such as infection/activation and transformation.

Functional Analysis of the 4F1-Antigen

Addition of 4F1 to mixed cultures of thymoma lymphocytes and epithelial cells almost completely inhibited the adhesion that normally occurs between the two cell types; an isotype-matched control MAb had no effect. Thus, that the 4F1-antigen may be important in the interaction of developing thymocytes and their epithelial microenvironment. In the MLR MAb 4F1, but not the isotype matched control antibody, totally inhibited the proliferative response of mature peripheral T cells in a dose-dependent manner (Table 1). The 4F1 MAb therefore appears to recognize a molecule that is important in T-cell adhesion and activation.

Table 1 Inhibition of Proliferation by MAb 4F1

	3H-TdR cpm +/−%SE	
Antibody dilution	4F1	IVC4
1 : 2	230 +/− 15	6542 +/− 9
1 : 4	125 +/− 15	6357 +/− 10
1 : 8	1498 +/− 13	6138 +/− 11
1 : 16	3770 +/− 9	7168 +/− 12

Biochemical Analysis of the 4F1-Antigen

The following cell types were analyzed by Western blotting and immunoprecipitation: epithelial thymoma cells (line TM25*F1), normal thymic epithelium, lymphoid thymoma lines TM25*114 and BW 5147, and normal thymocytes. The molecule to which 4F1 binds was found to have the following properties (Fig. 3): (a) There are always two bands of approximately 108+/−5 kD and 95+/−5 kD. (b) The same two bands are present under both reducing and nonreducing conditions. (c) The same two bands are seen for both lymphoid and epithelial cells.

Glycosylation of the 4F1-antigen was analyzed using either tunicamycin in culture or by treating immunoprecipitates with endoglycosidase F (Endo F). When cells were grown in the presence of tunicamycin there was a slight reduction in the intensity of the two bands, but since tunicamycin partially inhibits total protein synthesis as well as the fact that even at 2 μg/ml of tunicamycin the cells stopped adhering to each other and to tissue culture flasks, further studies of glycosylation were performed using Endo F. With this enzyme there was a significant reduction in the intensity of both bands, but neither reduction in weight nor disappearance of the band as expected. Therefore, further studies will

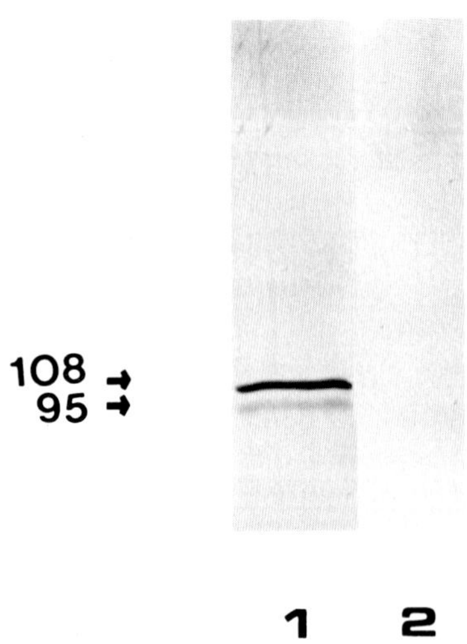

Figure 3 Western blotting analysis of the 4F1-antigen.

concentrate on digestion of O-linked and other sugars. Analysis of membrane insertion using PI-PLC showed that there was a considerable reduction of the lower, 95-kD, band after PI-PLC treatment. In addition, PI-PLC treatment of thymic tissue sections showed a significant reduction in the fluorescence intensity of 4F1 staining, but again this was never complete.

There therefore appear to be two distinct cell surface forms of the 4F1 molecule, a 95-kD lower molecular weight form that has a PI linkage and a 108-kD form that is probably anchored to the cell via a transmembrane segment. Whether the molecule is glycosylated remains yet to be resolved. The cellular distribution of the 4F1-antigen together with its biochemical characteristics suggest that this is a novel molecule, previously unidentified. Other molecules with a similar molecular mass (e.g., HERMES molecules) are not expressed in two forms on the cell surface, and those that are known to be expressed in two forms (e.g., CD58, Leu 8) have a lower molecular weight and different tissue distribution. Future studies are planned to identify the human homologue of the murine 4F1-antigen using gene cloning technologies.

REFERENCES

1. Kanariou M, Huby R, Ladyman H, Colic M, Sivolapenko G, Lampert I, Ritter M. Immunosuppression with cyclosporin A alters the thymic microenvironment. Clin Exp Immunol 1989; 78:263–70.
2. Spanopoulou E, Early A, Elliot J, Crispe N, Ladyman H, Ritter MA, Watt S, Grosveld F, Kioussis D. Complex lymphoid and epithelial thymic tumours in Thy 1-myc transgenic mice. Nature 1989; 342:185–9.
3. Larche M, Lamb JR, O'Hehir RE, Imami N, Zanders ED, Quint DE, Moqbel R, Ritter MA. Functional evidence for a monoclonal antibody that binds to the human IL-4 receptor. Immunology 1988; 65:617–22.
4. Laemmli UK. Cleavage of structural proteins during the assembly of the head of bacteriophage T4. Nature 1970; 227:680–5.
5. Newman RA, Sutherland R, Greaves MF. The biochemical characterisation of a cell surface antigen associated with lymphoblastic leukemia and lymphocyte precursors. J Immunol 1981; 126:2024–30.
6. Pierres M, Naquet P, Barbet J, Marchetto S, Marics I, Devaux C, Barad M, Hyman R, Rougon G. Evidence that murine hematopoietic cell subset marker J11d is attached to a glycosylphosphatidylinositol membrane anchor. Eur J Immunol 1987; 17:1781–5.
7. Kampinga J, Berges S, Boyd R, Brekelmans P, Colic M, van Ewijk W, Kendall MD, Ladyman H, Nieuwenhuis P, Ritter MA, Schuurman H-J, Tournefier A. Thymic epithelial antibodies: Immunohistological analysis and introduction of nomenclature. Summary of the Epithelium Workshop held at the 2nd Workshop. *The Thymus. Histophysiology and Dynamics in the Immune System.* Thymus 1989; 13:165–73.

13

Characterization of Murine Thymic Nonlymphoid Cell Subpopulations and Their Secretory Products In Vitro

Jacob Shoham
Bar-Ilan University, Ramat-Gan, Israel

INTRODUCTION

The thymus is a most complex organ that ontogenically develops first as a structured blend of cells of epithelial and mesenchymal origin, each differentiating ultimately to several subpopulations (1,2), which presumably have different growth requirements and different functional activities. This composite structure, which forms the thymic stroma, directs the crucial maturational events of progenitor T cells, which migrate into the thymus. The thymic stromal cells perform this function by both direct contact with the lymphoid cells and by the secretion of several soluble factors (3,4). The analysis of this interaction can be done at different levels. In vivo studies were employed (5) but they cannot provide answers at the cellular and molecular levels. The use of thymic organ cultures (6) helps in this analysis, but is insufficient for fine dissection of the phenomena involved. Thymic stromal cell lines (7,8) have major advantages in terms of cell definition and reproducibility of activities. However, they may not faithfully represent in vivo activities. Cultivation of stromal cells as primary cultures was attempted by several investigators (9,10). However, the difficulties in obtaining homogeneous thymic stromal cell subpopulations in primary cultures were repeatedly noticed. This is particularly true for murine stromal cells. Moreover, preservation of cell characteristics is known to be poor when cells are grown on plastic surface in the presence of serum.

CONDITIONS FOR CULTIVATION OF THYMIC NONLYMPHOID CELL SUBPOPULATIONS

In choosing our approach to the study of thymic stromal cell function, we directed our efforts toward identifying those variables which will permit the cells to maintain their respective gene set as committed differentiated cells at levels approximating those in vivo. These variables are of three categories: (a) Nutrients included in the medium which should be serum free and contain, beside basic constituents, a set of trace elements, hormones, and growth factors, the type and concentration of which are specifically tailored for each cell type. (b) Extracellular matric (ECM) which contains a mixture of proteins (e.g. collagens, glycoproteins, such as fibronectin and laminin, proteoglycans), which are largely insoluble because of extensive crosslinking. (c) Tissue specific factors which represent localized signals between neighboring cells in the same tissue.

With these considerations in mind, we decided to use primary cultures in order to increase the chance of preserving the true functional nature of the cells. We established conditions which allowed us to grow selectively and reproducibly three nonlymphoid subpopulations of the thymus—epithelial cells, mesenchymal cells, and thymic macrophages—in primary cultures. These cells were grown on ECM in defined medium (a defined medium was not yet established for thymic macrophages). Some details about growth requirements, structural characteristics, and functional activities are presented in Tables 1–3, respectively. We have evidence that by adopting this approach we preserved better cell functions (11,12). The following is a short discussion of the conditions which enabled us to establish these cultures.

Cell Dissociation

Each cell type needs different treatment. The epithelial cell cultures develop from partially digested tiny pieces of thymus, using a selected batch of collagenase. The mesenchymal cells can be grown only after dissociation of the tissue to single cell level, using a different selected batch of collagenase. The macrophages are preferentially separated by teasing through a wire mesh, without enzymatic treatment. The need for different collagenase batches for each cell type is not surprising; each cell type has different attachments to the various collagens in the tissue ECM.

Extracellular Matrix

There is a sound basis, theoretical and practical, for the importance of ECM for cell growth and differentiation in culture. Theoretically, ECM represents a major manifestation of

Table 1 Essential Growth Requirements of Three Murine Thymic Nonlymphoid Cell Subpopulations in Culture

	Epithelial cells	Mesenchymal cells	Thymic macrophages
Method of Cell preparation	Selected collagenase[a] small pieces	Selected collagenase single cells	Teasing on wire mesh
Growth requirements			
1. Need for ECM	+++	++++	++++
2. Essential soluble factors	Insulin EGF Hydrocortisone	Transferrin HDL Selenium Hydrocortisone	Serum CSF

[a]A different collagenase batch had to be selected for each cell subpopulation.

Abbreviations: EGF, epidermal growth factor; HDL, high density lipoprotein; CSF, colony-stimulating factor.

mesenchymal-epithelial cell interaction, which is a basic feature of all metazoan organisms (13). It serves for cell support and orientation and is a source of growth and differentiation stimuli in both embryonal and adult life. Experimentally, many recent studies have demonstrated the advantages of using ECM as a substrate for cell growth and differentiation in culture. Several methods of preparing ECM-coated plates for cell culture were described (14). We chose to use the method of Gospodarowicz et al. (15), which is based on the preparation of matrix from endothelial cells of bovine cornea. Monolayers of such cells are grown in tissue culture dishes and then removed by dilute detergent treatment. Extracellular matrix secreted by the monolayer cells remain attached to the dish and on top of it cells can be cultivated. This method results in homogeneous ECM coating of plates and the ECM components are in correct stoichiometry and chemical relationships.

The use of ECM in our cultures dramatically improved attachment, plating efficiency, and response to growth factors. It was absolutely necessary for mesenchymal cells and macrophages, which could not survive without it. Epithelial cells were somewhat less dependent on ECM, but also could not proliferate in its absence.

Nutrients and Soluble Factors

The analysis of growth requirements of cultured cells in serum-free medium was pioneered by several groups (16). It was shown that each cell type needs a specific set of nutrients and growth factors, in addition to the common ones, in order to proliferate and function optimally. Indeed, we found that the epithelial and mesenchymal cells have specific growth requirement (see Table 1) (11). In spite of considerable efforts, we could not yet determine the specific, serum-free medium conditions for thymic macrophages.

STRUCTURAL CHARACTERISTICS

Table 2 summarizes some of the structural characteristics of the three populations. The definition of the epithelial cells relies on the presence of desmosones and tonofilaments, the positive staining for keratin, and the negative one for vimentin. The mesenchymal cells and macrophages are negative for the first three criteria and positive for vimentin. Further characterization of the cells suggest that the epithelial cells are probably of medullary origin as judged by their staining with *Ulex europaeus* agglutinin, ER-TR5 antibodies, and the ability to form Hassel's corpuscles. The mesenchymal cells may be actually endothelial cells—They have typical morphology as a monolayer and are dependent on high density lipoprotein and selenium, which are known growth-promoting factors of endothelial cells. The macrophages were positively identified by phagocytosis of latex particles and by nonspecific esterase staining.

ACTIVITIES OF MEDIUM CONDITIONED BY THYMIC NONLYMPHOID CELLS

Some activities of culture supernatants (CS) of these cell cultures were determined already (Table 3). We first looked for the presence of known cytokines in the CS. Three cytokine activities were identified in the epithelial CS: IL-6, and two colony-stimulating factors (CSF)—G-CSF and M-CSF. The determination of the molecular basis for these activities is under current investigation as well as the search for other known cytokine activities. In addition, we tested CS effect on thymocyte function. Spontaneous thymocyte proliferation was strongly supported by epithelial and mesenchymal, but not macrophage CS. The

Table 2 Structural Characteristics of the Three Cultured Thymic Nonlymphoid Cell Subpopulations

	Epithelial cells	Mesenchymal cells	Thymic macrophages
Morphology			
SEM Shape	Flat	Round	ND
Surface	Homogeneous	Mixed texture	
MV	Small	Large + blebs	
TEM Mitochrondria	+++	+++	ND
RER	+++	+++	
Desmosomes	+++	–	
Tonofilaments	+++	–	
Immunocytochemistry[a]			
Vimentin (VIM 13.2)[b]	–	+++	++
Keratin (A-1)[c]	+++	–	–
MHC class I (20-8-4)[d]	++	+	+
MHC class II (25-9-17)[d]	+	–	++
Thymic cortical epithelium (ER-TR4)[e]	–	–	–
Thymic medullary epithelium (ER-TR5)[e]	+	–	–
Thymic macrophages (ER-TR6)[e]	–	–	+
Cytochemistry and other			
Phagocytosis (latex)	–	–	+++
UEA	+++	ND	ND
NSE	–	–	+++
Sudan red	–	+++[f]	ND
PAS	–	+++[f]	ND

[a]Parentheses designate the monoclonal antibody used for the respective marker. Staining by immunofluorescence.
[b–e]The antibodies were donated by Drs. Geiger, Sun, Sachs, and van Ewijk, respectively.
[f]In aging culture (<20 days).
Abbreviations: SEM, Scanning electron microscopy; MV, microvilli; TEM, transmission electron microscopy; ND, not done; RER, rough endoplasmic reticulum; UEA, *Ulex europaeus* agglutinin; NSE, nonspecific esterase; PAS, periodic acid Schiff.

epithelial cells could be further distinguished by the ability of their CS to enhance concanavalin A–induced proliferation and IL-2 production in thymocytes. The responsive thymocyte subpopulation was the one that *does not* bind peanut agglutinin. The CS of an established thymic epithelial cell line displayed only part of these activities at a considerably lower level. The CS from primary kidney cell culture was completely devoid of activity.

The results suggest that primary thymic stromal cell cultures, cultivated under the defined conditions described here, may better preserve physiological secretory activities, and probably also other cell functions, compared with established cell lines. Furthermore,

Table 3 Activities of Medium Conditioned by the Three B Thymic Nonlymphoid Cells in Culture

	Epithelial cells	Mesenchymal cells	Thymic macrophages (unstimulated)
Known cytokines[a]			
IL-1 (D10)	–	–	–
IL-2 (CTLL)	–	–	–
IL-3 (AC2)	–	–	–
IL-4 (CTLS)	–	–	ND
IL-6 (B9)[b]	++	++	ND
CSF (BM colonies)	++	++	NA
G-CSF (32D)[b]	++	ND	ND
M-CSF (14D14)[b]	++	ND	ND
IFN (L_{929}^{+VSV})	–	–	–
Effect on thymocytes			
PR-spontaneous	+++	+++	–
Con A induced	+++	+	+
IL-2 production	+++	–	–
IL-3 production	+++	++	–

[a]The name of the line (or method) used for determination of the respective lymphokine is in parentheses.
[b]Activity neutralized by respective antibodies. The activity on 32D cells was originally ascribed by us to IL-3 (12). We now have evidence that it is related to the presence of G-CSF, and no IL-3 is present in the CS.
Abbreviations: PR, proliferative response; NA, not applicable (the growth medium contains CSF); MB, bone marrow; VSV, vesicular stomatitis virus.

the results are compatible with the hypothesis that the soluble factors, secreted by thymic stromal cells, are active on either very early or late stages of thymic differentiation, whereas the main intrathymic stages of differentiation are conceivably dependent primarily on direct contact with stromal cells.

REFERENCES

1. Le Dourain NM, Jotereau FV. The ontogeny of the thymus. In: Kendall MD (ed). *The Thymus Gland.* London, Academic Press, 1981, pp. 37–62.
2. Kendall MD. The cells of the thymus. In: Kendall MD (ed). *The Thymus Gland.* London, Academic Press, 1981, pp. 63–84.
3. Haynes BF. The role of thymic microenvironment in promotion of early stages of human T cell maturation. Clin. Res. 1986; 34:422–430.
4. Shoham J. The role of thymic hormones in regulating T-cell activity and lymphokine production In: Aiuti F, Rosen F. and Cooper MD (eds). *Recent Advance in Primary and Acquired Immunodeficiencies.* New York, Raven Press, 1986, pp. 101–118.
5. Stutman O. Ontogeny of T cells. Clin Immunol Allergy 1985; 5:191–263.
6. Jenkins J, Franchi L, Kingstone R, Owen JJT. Effect of deoxyguanosine on lymphoporesis in the developing thymus rudiment in vitro application in the production of chimric thymus rudiments. Eur. J. Immunol. 1982; 1 2:583–587.
7. Itoh T. Establishment of an epithelial cell line from rat thymus. Am. J. Anat. 1979; 156:99–105.

8. Glimcher LH, Kruisbeek AM, Paul WE, Green I. Functional activity of a transformed thymic epithelial cell line. Scand. J. Immunol 1983; 17:1–9.
9. Jason JM, Janeway CA. *In vitro* cultivation of non-lymphoid thymic cells: morphological and immunological characterization. Clin. Immunol. Immunopathol. 1984; 30:214–221.
10. Sunn TT, Bonitz P, Burnes EH. Cell culture of mammalian thymic epithelial cells: Growth, structural and antigenic properties. Cell. Immunol. 1984; 83:1–12.
11. Eshel I, Savion N, Shoham J. Analysis of thymic stromal cell subpopulations grown in vitro on extracellular matrix in defined medium. I. Growth conditions and morphology of murine thymic epithelial and mesenchymal cells. J. Immunol. 1990; 144:1554–1562.
12. Eshel I, Savion N, Shoham J. Analysis of thymic stromal cell subpopulations grown in vitro on extracellular matrix in defined medium. II. Cytokine activities in murine thymic epithelial and mesenchymal cell culture supernatants. J. Immunol. 1990; 144:1563–1570.
13. Yamada KM, ed. *Cell Interactions and Development.* New York, Wiley Intersciences, 1983.
14. Reid LCM. Regulation of growth and differentiation of mammalian cells by hormones and extracellular matrix. In: Ahmed F. Schulz J. Smith EE. Whelan WJ. (eds). *From Gene to Protein: Translation into Biotechnology.* New York, Academic Press, 1982, pp. 53–74.
15. Gospodarowicz D, Delgado D, Vlodavsky I. Permissive effect of extracellular matrix on cell proliferation *in vitro.* Proc. Natl. Acad. Sci. 1980; 77:4094–4099.
16. Barnes O. Sato J. Serum free cell culture: A unifying approach. Cell 1980; 22:649–656.

14
In Situ Effects of Estrogens on the Stroma of Rat Thymus

Ana M. Moreno and Agustin G. Zapata
Complutense University, Madrid, Spain

INTRODUCTION

There is a compelling body of evidence indicating that sex steroids induce profound changes in the histology and function of the mammalian thymus gland. Despite the fact that most authors agree on the induced histological changes, involved mechanisms and affected cell populations are little known. Some authors have pointed out that helper T cells are especially affected by sex steroids (1), whereas others claim an increased number of thymic single positive cell populations, mainly $CD4^{+}CD8^{-}$ after 17-β-estradiol treatment (2). On the other hand, it is not clearly established if sex steroids directly affect the thymocytes, or if their effects are mediated throughout the nonlymphoid components of thymic stroma. Estrogen receptors are located particularly in epithelial cells (2), which could be involved in thymic hormone production (3), but some reports identify binding sites for estrogens on thymic lymphoblasts or proliferating thymocytes (4). In any case, a systematic analysis of the changes affecting the nonlymphoid components of thymic stroma is lacking, and the present study analyzes the effects along the time of two different doses of estradiol benzoate (EB) on the structure, vascular permeability, and nonlymphoid cell populations of adult rat thymus.

MATERIALS AND METHODS

Three-month-old female Wistar rats were injected subcutaneously with either 100 or 500 μg of EB dissolved in 0.1 ml of corn oil. Controls received the oil injection only. At 2, 7, 15, and 21 days after treatment, rats were sacrificed by decapitation, body weights determined, and the thymus removed, weighed, and processed for routine light and transmission electron microscopy, while blood samples were collected and plasma used to determine estradiol concentration by radioimmunoassay.

Histological and Histometrical Studies

On 10 different sections by lobe and rat routinely processed for light microscopy the following parameters were determined: (a) relative areas occupied either by cortex or medulla; (b) thymic cortex and medulla weight; (c) frequency of cortical and medullary lymphocytes; (d) percentage of cortical and medullary pycnotic cells; (e) cortical and medullary mitotic index. The results, expressed as the mean ±SEM, were compared by Student's "t" test.

Immunohistochemistry and Histoenzymatic Studies

Cell marker characterization was achieved on 7-μm thick cryosections by an indirect immunoperoxidase labeling assay using monoclonal antibodies (MAbs) and lectins listed in Table 1. The peroxidase reaction was developed routinely with 0.05%, 3,3diaminobenzidine (Sigma, St. Louis, Missouri). Enzymatic activities were determined on 7-μm thick frozen sections using the indicated substrates in Table 1.

Vascular Permeability

Thymic vascular permeability was studied at the same days (2, 7, 15, and 21 days) in control and 500-μg EB-injected rats. Both groups of animals were injected with a single dose (8 mg/ml) of MAb His-17 (pan T, Histology Dept., Groningen Univ.), the intrathymic presence of which was detected by indirect immunoperoxidase labeling assay 2 hr after injection.

Table 1

Polyclonal antibodies	Dilution	Specificity
Anti-Cytokeratin (BioGenes, Dublin, CA)	1 mg/ml	56-64 Kd.
Anti-thymosin β_4 (George Washington Univ.)	1:2500	Thymosin β_4
Monoclonal antibodies		
His-19 (Histology Dept., Groningen Univ.)	1:200	MHC Cl II antigens
OX-18 (Serotec)	1:100	MHC Cl I antigens
His-37 (Histology Dept., Groningen Univ.)	1:1	Cortical epithelial cells
His-38 (Histology Dept., Groningen Univ.)	1:1	Cortical epithelial cells
His-39 (Histology Dept., Groningen Univ.)	1:9	Medullary epithelial cells
ED1 (Free University, Amsterdam)	1:1000	Macrophages
ED2 (Free University, Amsterdam)	1:2000	Macrophages
Lectins		
Ulex europaeus (Sigma)	1 mg/ml	Medullary epithelial cells
Enzymes		Substrates
Acid phosphatase		Naphthyl AS biphosphate
Nonspecific esterase		α-Naphthyl acetate

RESULTS AND DISCUSSION

Plasma Estradiol Levels

Two days after treatment, rats injected with 100 μg/ml of EB increase approximately by three the plasma estradiol levels, whereas in the case of rats injected with 500 μg of EB the increase is 30 times. Nevertheless, in both cases, the values almost reach control levels on day 7.

Histological and Morphometrical Results

A decrease in the relative weight of both total thymus and cortex occurs from day 2 in rats treated with both doses of estradiol (Figs. 1 and 2). The higher dose induces the lowest values on day 7. Moreover, on day 21 the organ had not recovered the relative weight of control rats (Figs. 1 and 2). In the case of medulla, only the high dose produces a fast decrease of the relative weight. Low doses induce certain decrease only on last days. A significant decrease in thymus weight, affecting principally the cortical area, as well as a considerably delay in the recovery after sex steroid treatment has been reported by numerous authors (5,6).

In both cortex and medulla of EB-treated rats, the number of lymphocytes decreases significantly in all the days studied (Fig. 3). Again, the high dose induced the lowest values on day 7, the number of lymphocytes does not reach control values on day 21 and the decrease in the number of medullary lymphocytes is specially evident on day 21. A progressive loss of cortical thymic lymphocytes has been noted by most authors in estrogen-treated mammals (6), whereas medullary lymphoid cell populations have been pointed out to be affected or only depleted after severe treatment (5). Besides, a selective effect of the estrogens on lymphocyte populations of the outer cortex has been reported by Gulino et al. (4). In agreement, our results demonstrate "empty" subcapsular areas in the treated rats and lymphoblast degeneration has been ultrastructurally observed in these areas.

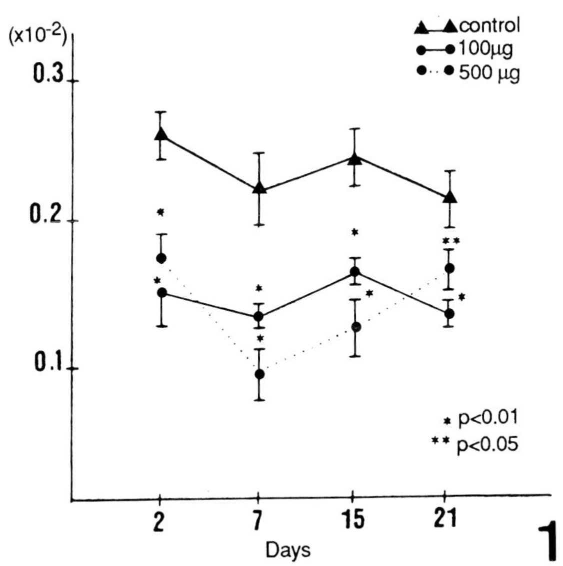

Figure 1 Relative weight of the thymus in control and EB-treated rats.

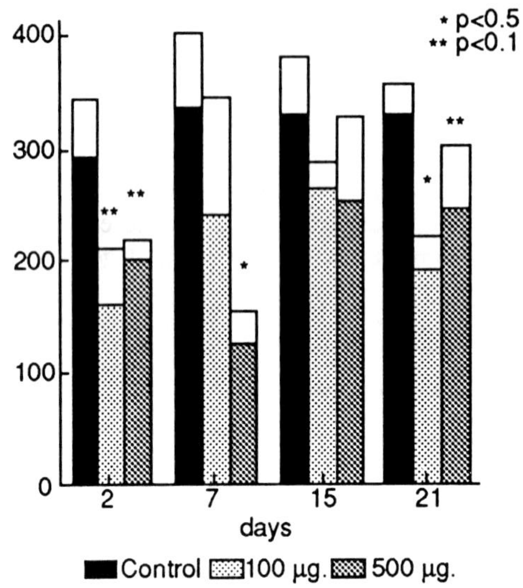

Figure 2 Relative weight of thymic cortex in control and EB-treated rats..

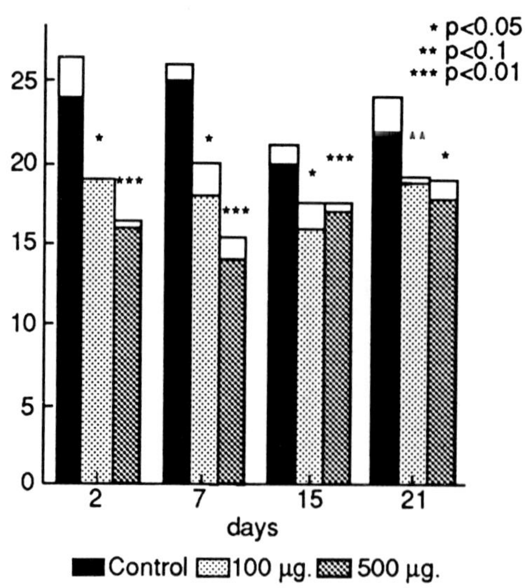

Figure 3 Frequency (number of cortical lymphocytes/μm^2) in control and EB-treated rats..

An intense cortical erythropoiesis is observed a few days after EB treatment, probably associated with degeneration of epithelial cells. A relationship between intrathymic erythropoiesis, degeneration of both cortical lymphocytes and epithelial-reticular cells, increased macrophage activity, and high levels of circulating sex hormones has been pointed out in *Sturnus unicolor* (7). Other authors have reported, however, no effects of estrogens on thymic epithelial-reticular cells, although the assumption is difficult of supporting because of the known presence of estrogen receptors on the thymic epithelial component (3). On the other hand, it is unclear from our own results if the degenerated epithelial cells come from hyperplastic epithelial elements which contain enlarged cytoplasmic vacuoles, or if these last elements represent thymic hormones–producing cells negatively regulated by EB.

The decreased number of cortical lymphocytes in treated animals could be related to both an increase in the number of cortical pyknotic cells on day 7 and a decreased mitotic index in the cortex on days 2 and 7. The decreased mitotic index in the cortex could be in turn related to the degeneration of subcapsular lymphoblasts. In the medulla the lower mitotic index observed in treated rats can contribute also the decrease in the number of medullary lymphocytes, but a lower number of cortical-differentiating lymphocytes can account also for the medulla condition. In this regard, a decrease of double positive $CD4^+8^+$ T cells has been recently reported in mice treated with 17-β-estradiol (2). A similar explanation could be given to the observed decrease of medullary pyknotic cells.

Changes in Specific Nonlymphoid Cell Populations

Observed changes after EB treatment affected principally epithelial cells and macrophages. No remarkable differences were found either in the number of cell marker expression of dendritic cells.

Epithelial Cells

Two days after EB treatment, the number of subcapsular epithelial cells demonstrated by their reactivity both with cytokeratin and MAb His-19 increases considerably. His-39^+ medullary cells show certain decreases on day 7. On days 2, 7, and 15, the staining both for His-37 and His-38 disappears on some cortical areas. The reactivity reappears on day 21. In the corticomedullary area, there is a decrease in the number of Ulex-positive epithelial cells on days 2, 7, and 15.

Thymosin β4-Containing Cells

In controls, thymosin β4-containing cells occur principally at the cortico–medullary border and in low numbers in the medulla. After treatment, most cells disappear completely throughout the thymus gland, reappearing on day 21 at the corticomedullary border but not in the medulla.

MHC Class II Antigen Expression

There is a decreased expression of MHC class II antigens on day 7 in epithelial cells, and an altered pattern in the cortex where the MHC class II antigen expression disappears in some areas.

Macrophages

After sex steroid treatment there is a general increase in the number of macrophages. Increased $ED1^+$ cells occur throughout the thymus and remain on day 21. $ED2^+$ cells, in correlation with the activity of both nonspecific esterase and acid phosphatase, increase in all regions except in the medulla, but exclusively on days 2 and 7.

Vascular Permeability

Antigens can bypass the blood-thymus barrier and reach the thymic parenchyma throughout a transcapsular route (8). Thus, 2 hr after intravenous injection of control rats with a MAb His-17, raised against T cells, numerous thymocytes appear stained principally in the subcapsular subtrabecular zones and in lesser amount in the medulla and around the cortical and medullary blood vessels. On the contrary, in EB-treated rats injected with MAb His-17, there is a striking decrease in the number of positively stained thymocytes of both subcapsular and subtrabecular zones and an increase in the medulla and around blood vessels of the cortex and medulla. These results indicate that the sex hormone increase notably the vascular permeability of the thymus gland favoring the entry of molecules throughout the thymic-blood barrier rather than by a transcapsular route.

CONCLUSIONS

Our results confirm profound alterations in both lymphoid and nonlymphoid cell populations after estrogen treatment. Important modifications in specific epithelial cell populations of the thymic cortex, principally, but also of the medulla, the almost disappearance of thymosin β_4-producing cells, probably associated with the ultrastructurally observed degeneration of epithelial cells, the altered pattern of MHC class II antigen expression in epithelial cells, as well as the demonstrated modifications in vascular permeability suggest indirectly a role of thymic epithelial cells in immunological changes induced by sex hormones. Nevertheless, the elimination of subcapsular large lymphoid cells, corroborated by light and electron microscopy, demonstrates also a direct effect of estradiol on thymic lymphoid cell populations. Further research could be focused on the phenotypic characterization of such a large lymphocyte population and on the analysis of the effects induced by its elimination in intrathymic T-cell differentiation.

REFERENCES

1. Barr IG, Kardir Khalid BA, Pearce P, Toh B-H, Bartlett PF, Scollay RG, Funder JW. Dihydrostestosterone and estradiol deplete corticosensitive thymocytes lacking in receptors for these hormones. J Immunol 1982; 128:2825–2828.
2. Screpanti I, Morone S, Meco D, Santoni A, Gulino A, Paolino R, Crisanti A, Mathieson BJ, Franti L. Steroid sensitivity of thymocyte subpopulations during intrathymic differentiation. Effects of 17β-estradiol and dexamethasone on subsets expressing T cell antigen receptor or IL-2 receptor. J Immunol 1989; 142:3378–3383.
3. Stimson WH, Crylly PJ. Effects of steroids on the secretion of immunoregulatory factors by thymic epithelial cell cultures. Immunology 1981; 44:401–407.
4. Gulino A, Screpanti I, Torrisi MR, Frati L. Estrogen receptors and estrogen sensitivity of fetal thymocytes are restricted to blast lymphoid cells. Endocrinology 1985; 117:47–54.
5. Sobhon P, Jirasattham C. Effect of sex hormones on the thymus and lymphoid tissue of ovariectomized rats. Acta Anat 1974; 89:211–225.
6. Sfikakis A, Sfikakis P, Varonas D. Oestradiol induced interaction between adrenals and thymus in the female rats. Acta Endocrinol 1981; Suppl. 244:41–42.

7. Fonfria J, Barrutia MG, Garrido E, Ardavin CF, Zapata A. Erythropoiesis in the thymus of the spotless starling, *Sturnus unicolor*. Cell Tissue Res 1983; 232:445–455.
8. Nieuwenhuis P, Stet RJN, Wagenaar JPA, Wubbena AS, Kampinga J, Karrenbeld. The transcapsular route: a new way for (self-)antigens to by-pass the blood-thymus barrier? Immunol Today 1988; 9:372–375.

15

Chicken Fetal Thymus Organ Culture

A Model for T-Cell Development Within the Thymic Microenvironment

Natalie J. Davidson, Andrew G. Bean, and Richard L. Boyd
Monash University Medical School, Prahran, Australia

INTRODUCTION

A marked degree of conservation in both thymic microanatomy and thymocyte ontogeny between the avian and mammalian classes has been demonstrated by the development of monoclonal antibodies (MAbs) directed against lymphoid and nonlymphoid components of the avian thymus (1,2). Examination of chicken thymic development in a fetal thymus organ culture (FTOC) system will provide further insight into the mechanisms of thymopoiesis in avian, and therefore, higher species. A similar culture system has been successfully utilized to investigate early events in murine thymocyte development (3,4), and provides a unique model in which to monitor and manipulate thymic cellular interactions in an isolated environment.

This chapter summarizes the development of both lymphoid and stromal components of the chicken thymus in FTOC, establishing a system in which to further examine the nature of the thymic microenvironment and the mechanisms of its influence upon lymphopoiesis.

MATERIALS AND METHODS

Fetal Thymus Organ Culture

Thymic lobes were isolated from 10-day-old Australorp/White Leghorn F_1 hybrid embryos and cultured (5).

Antibodies

The MAb CT3, CT4, CT8, and TCR-1 (avian homologues of CD3, CD4, CD8, and γδ TCR (T-cell receptor), respectively (6–8) were gratefully received from Drs. C. H. Chen and M. D. Cooper. MUI-83 (thymocytes and subpopulation of peripheral T cells) and a large panel of stromal cell–reactive MAbs, produced in this laboratory, have been described elsewhere (5,9).

Flow Cytometry

Suspensions of cultured and embryonic thymus were prepared and labeled using an indirect immunofluorescence technique for flow cytometry. Flow cytometric analysis was performed using FACScan instrumentation (Becton Dickinson, Mountainview, CA, U.S.A.) (5).

Indirect Immunofluorescence of Frozen Tissue Sections

Air-dried tissue sections (4–6 μm), of cultured and uncultured thymus, were stained with rabbit anti-keratin (Dakopatts, Carpinteria, CA, U.S.A.) (revealed by TRITC-conjugated anti-rabbit immunoglobulin; Silenus, Melbourne, Australia) and MAb supernatant (revealed with FITC-conjugated sheep (F(ab)′2) anti-mouse; Silenus) (5).

RESULTS AND DISCUSSION

This study was aimed at addressing chicken FTOC as a valid system in which to examine early events in thymocyte differentiation and to identify and functionally assess the microenvironmental components directing this process. The integrity of thymic function in vitro was assessed by a detailed examination of thymocyte subset ontogenesis in comparison to that of age-matched control embryos by employing flow cytometric analysis (data from selected time points presented in Table 1). The stromal composition of cultured thymus was examined by indirect immunofluorescence of frozen tissue sections and again compared to that of control embryos (summary presented in Table 2).

Table 1 Thymocyte Development in Chicken Fetal Thymus Organ Culture

	% Positive cells				
Phenotype	0-day FTOC	6-day FTOC	16-day-old embryos	10-day FTOC	20-day-old embryos
$CD4^-CD8^-$	94.0 ± 2.5	31.0 ± 7.3	7.8 ± 1.9	10.0 ± 3.5	7.4 ± 3.4
$CD4^+CD8^+$	0	25.3 ± 10.4	87.4 ± 4.1	37.4 ± 9.9	91.8 ± 2.4
$CD4^+CD8^-$	2.6 ± 1.9	5.5 ± 2.0	0.7 ± 0.7	2.7 ± 2.3	<1
$CD4^-CD8^+$	4.3 ± 1.7	38.1 ± 6.1	4.2 ± 2.5	50.1 ± 4.1	1.2 ± 0.4
$CD3^+$	1.0 ± 0.3	51.6 ± 17.0	53.2 ± 2.7	58.0 ± 12.7	73.2 ± 10.9
$\gamma\delta TCR^+$	2.0 ± 1.4	38.3 ± 2.7	5.9 ± 2.4	16.1 ± 2.7	3.2 ± 1.1
$MUI\text{-}83^+$	15.5 ± 8.7	81.0 ± 8.9	95.6 ± 3.2	51.2 ± 15.7	91.9 ± 4.9
$MUI\text{-}36^+$	2.2 ± 0.6	53.1 ± 10.9	18.8 ± 9.9	33.9 ± 10.1	11.4 ± 8.6
$MUI\text{-}78^+$	9.3 ± 4.0	15.9 ± 8.4	3.1 ± 1.8	16.5 ± 2.9	8.7 ± 5.9

Development of thymocyte subpopulations in FTOC, assessed by flow cytometry at 0, 6, and 10 days of culture. Data for age-matched controls (16 & 20 de) is presented for comparison.

Table 2 Stromal Population Development in Chicken Fetal Thymus Organ Culture

Cell type	MAb	Adult	0-day FTOC	8-day FTOC	18-day-old embryos
Ep	MUI-54	C & M Ep subpop ST/SC Ep	pan Ep	normal	pan Ep
	MUI-52	isol C Ep	isol + cells (mid-lobe)	increased	isol C Ep
	MUI-62	M Ep clust	rare, isol Ep	normal	M Ep clust
	MUI-70	ST/SC Ep, M PV Ep	isol Ep	irregular	isol ST, M PV Ep
Ep and Non-ep	MUI-78 (Class II)	isol C Ep conf M Ep & non-ep	isol EP & non-ep	increased	adult reactivity
	MUI-66	M Ep clust, isol K+/– C, PVC, KNA	pan Ep	increased	adult reactivity
Non-ep	MUI-79	MØ (M>C)	rare MØ	increased	adult reactivity
	MUI-82	M blood vessels	negative	negative	adult reactivity

The development of MAb-defined thymic stromal subpopulations at 0 (10-day-old embryos) and 8 days of FTOC assessed by indirect immunofluorescence of frozen tissue sections. Data for age-matched control (18 day-old embryos) and adult thymus MAb reactivity are presented for comparison. Thymic MAb reactivity from 6–10 days FTOC was found to be similar and can therefore be related to Table 1.

Abbreviations: C=cortex, clust=clusters, conf=confluent, d=day, Ep=epithelium, FTOC=fetal thymus organ culture, isol=isolated, k=keratin, M=medulla, MØ=macrophage, OC=organ culture, PV=perivascular, SC=subcapsular, ST=subtrabecular.

Ontogenesis of Thymocyte Subpopulations in FTOC

Results provided herein demonstrate that FTOC provides an environment supporting TCR (γδ) gene rearrangement and TCR/CD3 expression (Table 1). An increase in the proportion of $\gamma\delta TCR^+$ thymocytes noted in FTOC may reflect favorable in vitro conditions for the development of this population and/or a lack of cellular migration to peripheral tissues normally occurring in 15-day-old embryos (1). All CD4/CD8-defined thymocyte subpopulations developed in FTOC arising from an initial 10-day-old embryo population of primarily double negative (DN) thymocytes (Table 1), although developmental trends differed somewhat to that in the embryo. A low representation of $CD4^+CD8^+$ (double positive) thymocytes was readily observed. A block in development of double positives (DP) may result from the lack of maintenance of a required stromal environment, or alternatively, the supply of thymocyte precursors, with limited capacity for self-renewal (10), may be exhausted. A progressive, though somewhat slowed, decrease in the proportion of double negative thymocytes suggests that this population has the capacity to differentiate in FTOC, but development was partially blocked prior to the double positive stage. This may be accounted for by the high levels of $CD4^-CD8^+$ thymocytes present in

FTOC, possibly containing a DN→DP intermediary subset, as described in the murine thymus (11). This $CD4^-CD8^+$ population may also contain $\gamma\delta TcR^+$ thymocytes, shown to be present in embryonic thymus by Bucy et al. (12). A predominance of $CD8^+$ to $CD4^+$ thymocytes has also been demonstrated in murine FTOC and may be attributed to the differential maintenance of the stromal environment required by these subpopulations, as suggested by Ceredig (3).

MUI-83 defines an antigen (Mr 60/85 kDa) present on the majority of thymocytes from 12 days old and a subpopulation of peripheral T cells (13). Slightly decreased levels at 6 days FTOC (Table 1) may reflect a decreased capacity for thymocyte development in FTOC, which further decreased with time in culture. The antigen defined by MUI-36 (Mr 90 kD) is present on B cells and a subpopulation of thymic macrophages and thymocytes. Expression of this antigen was greatly enhanced on thymocytes in culture, the significance of which is yet to be determined. Thymocyte expression of MUI-78 (avian class II reagent, B-L) was enhanced in FTOC and was probably passively acquired from $B\text{-}L^+$ thymic stromal elements (14), also demonstrating increased expression on tissue sections.

Thymic Stromal Composition of Cultured Fetal Thymus

In an examination of the degree of conformity between the stromal composition of FTOC thymus and embryonic thymus, it was found that most MAb-defined stromal populations were present in vitro, although in some cases the degree of representation or distribution/organization was altered. Stromal populations have been classed into three major categories on the basis of MAb reactivity, including: (a) epithelial, (b) epithelial and nonepithelial, and (c) nonepithelial cells. Stromal composition, represented by a small group of antibodies, of the thymus at 0 (10-day-old embryos) and 8 days FTOC with 18-day-old embryos and adult reactivity provided for comparison, is presented in Table 2.

The MAb-defined epithelial stroma, including cortical, medullary, and type I (subcapsule, subtrabeculae, perivascular), was represented in FTOC. MUI-54 and MUI-62 (Fig. 1a) showed normal reactivity, while the cortical epithelial reactivity of MUI-52 was enhanced and may represent an antigen activated in vitro (2,9). The MAbs reactive with type 1 epithelium (e.g., MUI-70) displayed irregular reactivity, staining groups of reticular cells with limited resemblance to formal type 1 structures. This has also been noted in murine FTOC (D. Godfrey, personal communication), and may result from removal of the thymus from its native environment and the lack of an operative vascular system.

The category of epithelium and nonepithelium is represented by two MAbs, the first being a class II reagent (MUI-78) showing increased expression in FTOC (Fig. 1b); the second, MUI-66, shows reactivity with a variety of cell types, but of particular interest are medullary epithelial clusters of a morphologically less differentiated type (2). Enhanced reactivity with this reagent was observed in FTOC and may reflect a slowed epithelial maturation in vitro.

The third category, nonepithelial stroma, includes MUI-79, reacting with a subpopulation of thymic macrophages, showing enhanced reactivity in FTOC. This may be a result of increased activity due to the phagocytosis of dead/dying thymocytes (15), the proportions of which increase with time in culture. MUI-82 reacts with endothelium of medullary blood vessels and was negative at the onset of culture (10-day-old embryos), as blood vessels do not form until after this age (16), and thus not unexpectedly on cultured thymus.

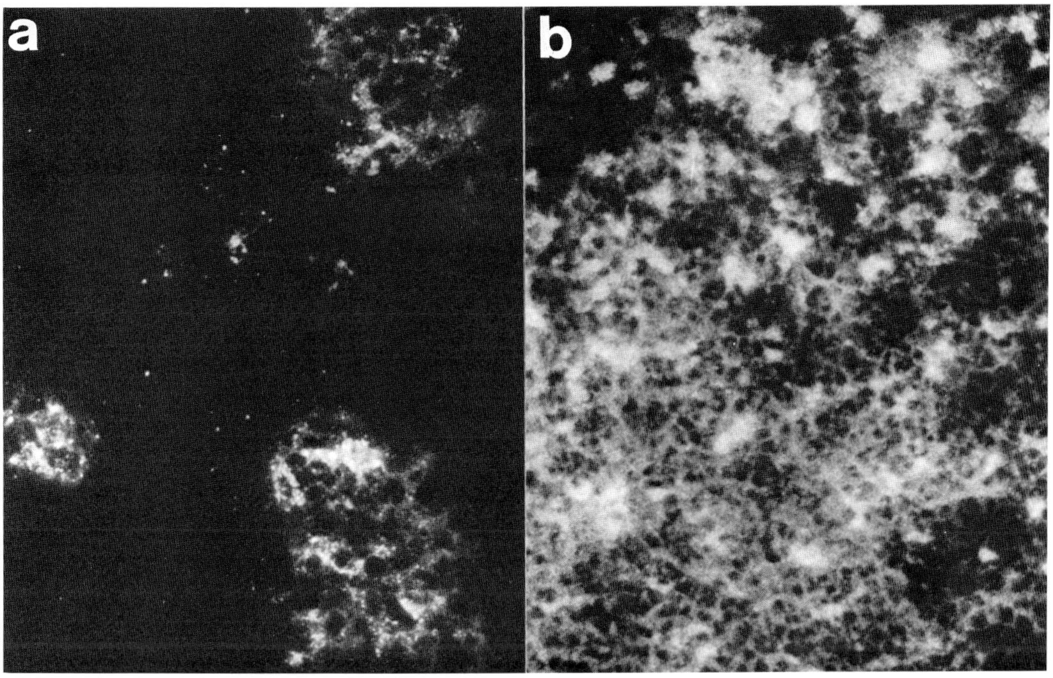

Figure 1 Expression of (a) MUI-62 (medullary epithelial clusters and secreted glycoprotein, Mr 60/200 kD), and (b) MUI-78 (chicken class II, B-L) on 10-day-old-embryo thymus cultured for 8 days, as determined by indirect immunofluorescence of frozen tissue sections. Extensive reactivity was observed with MUI-78, whereas MUI-62 appeared identical to that of age-matched 18-day-old-embryo thymus (refer Table 2).

Summary and Conclusions

The data presented herein demonstrate that stromal populations present in the normal embryonic thymus are represented in FTOC. In some cases, deviation is noted, although this is not unexpected considering the constraints of an in vitro system. Thymocyte differentiation, involving TCR gene rearrangement and TCR/CD3 expression has been demonstrated in chicken FTOC. This indicates that FTOC is sufficient for thymocyte development and further implies that the essential components of the microenvironment must be present in vitro. Having established the validity of this system, the possibility that some of the antigens/stromal cells recognized by our panel of MAbs are involved in thymocyte differentiation may be examined by masking these epitopes using the MAbs and assessing the effect of this treatment upon thymocyte development. Experiments to address this hypothesis are underway. It is expected that this system of FTOC will yield valuable insight into the nature of thymic function in the avian system.

ACKNOWLEDGMENTS

This work was supported by grants from the National Health and Medical Research Council (860396), the Anti-Cancer Council of Victoria (131658) and the Monash University Special Research Grant Scheme.

REFERENCES

1. Cooper MD, Bucy RP and Chen CH. T cell development in birds. In: *The Avian Model in Developmental Biology: From Organism to Genes*. Editions du CRNS-1990, EMBO Symposium, Dec. 13–15, 1989.
2. Boyd RL, Wilson TJ, van de Water J, Haapanen LA, and Gershwin ME. Selective abnormalities in the thymic microenvironment associated with avian scleroderma, an inherited fibrotic disease of L200 chickens. J Autoimmun (in press).
3. Ceredig R. Differentiation potential of 14-day fetal mouse thymocytes in organ culture. Analysis of CD4/CD8-defined single-positive and double-negative cells. J Immunol 1988; 141:355–362.
4. Born W, McDuffie M, Roehm N, Kushnir E, White J, Thorpe D, Stefano J, Kappler J and Marrack P. Expression and role of the T cell receptor in early thymocyte differentiation in vitro. J Immunol 1987; 138:999–1008.
5. Davidson NJ and Boyd RL. Avian fetal thymus organ culture: Thymocyte kinetics and development. (in preparation).
6. Chen CH, Ager LL, Gartland GL and Cooper MD. Identification of a T3/T cell receptor complex in chicken. J Exp Med 1986; 164:375–389.
7. Chan MM, Chen CH, Ager LL and Cooper MD. Identification of the avian homologues of mammalian CD4 and CD8 antigens. J Immunol 1988; 140:2133–2138.
8. Sowder JT, Chen CH, Ager LL, Chang MM and Cooper MD. A large subpopulation of avian T cells express a homologue of the mammalian Tγδ receptor. J Exp Med 1988; 167:315–322.
9. Wilson WJ, Davidson NJ and Boyd RL. Phenotypic analysis of the chicken thymic microenvironment during ontogenic development. (in preparation).
10. Penit C, Vasseur F and Papiernik M. In vivo dynamics of $CD4^-CD8^-$ thymocytes. Proliferation, renewal and differentiation of different cell subsets studied by DNA biosynthetic labelling and surface detection. Eur J Immunol 1988; 18:1343–1350.
11. MacDonald HR, Budd RC and Howe RC. A $CD3^-$ subset of $CD4^-CD8^+$ thymocytes: A rapidly cycling intermediate in the generation of $CD4^+CD8^+$. Eur J Immunol 1988; 18:519–523.
12. Bucy RP, Chen CH and Cooper MD. Ontogeny of T cell receptors in the chicken thymus. J Immunol 1990; 144:1161–1168.
13. Bean AG, Davidson NJ, Wilson TJ, Ward HA and Boyd RL. CTCA-1: A novel chicken thymocyte antigen. 1990 (in preparation).
14. Sharrow SO, Ozato K and Sachs DH. Phenotypic expression of I-A and I-E/C subregion determinants on murine thymocytes. J Immunol 1980; 125:2263–2268.
15. Izon DJ, Boyd RL, Waanders GA and Kelso A. The myelopoietic inducing potential of mouse thymic stromal cells. Cell Immunol 1989; 124:264–277.
16. Kendall MD. Avian thymus glands: A review. Dev Comp Immunol 1980; 4:191–210.

16

An Immuno–Electron Microscopic Study of Epithelial Cells, Macrophages, and Phagocytosis of Thymocytes in the Mouse Thymus

Marion D. Kendall,[1] Geoff Morgan,[1] Susan A. Billingsley,[2] and Ann G. Clarke[2]
[1]*Cell Biology and Thymus Laboratory, United Medical and Dental Schools of Guy's and St. Thomas's Hospitals, London, England;*
[2]*Institute of Animal Physiology and Genetic Research, AFRC, Babraham, England*

INTRODUCTION

The cells of the thymic microenvironment that influence the maturation and differentiation of thymocytes are mainly epithelial cells and bone marrow–derived cells. However, it is still not clear precisely which cells enact negative and positive selection and where it occurs. For example, chimera studies suggest that for T cells recognizing major histocompatibility complex (MHC) class II, positive selection occurs by interaction with thymic cortical epithelial cells, and medullary bone marrow–derived cells enact negative selection. However, cortical epithelium can present self-hemoglobin in vivo and could enact negative selection (1).

This study, to be reported in full elsewhere, was therefore initiated to examine, at the electron microscopic (EM) level, the relationships between MHC class II on cells of the microenvironment, and dying apoptotic cells.

MATERIALS AND METHODS

C57BL male and female mice were sacrificed before mating (virgin controls), after mating to CBA males (pregnant females) on various days of pregnancy (day 1 = day of vaginal plug) or in old age (14 months).

After Sagatal anesthetization and fixation (0.1% glutaraldehyde and 3% paraformaldehyde in 0.1 M cacodylate buffer) by slow perfusion (over 5–10 min) through the heart, the thymus was excised and further immersion fixed for 1 hr. After an overnight wash in cacodylate buffer and infiltration with 2.3 M sucrose in PBS/BSA (with 0.05% thimerosal as a preservative), tissues were frozen in liquid N_2 and ultrathin frozen sections cut at –110–120°C on a Reichert. Sections were processed as previously detailed (2) using 10 nm immunogold (Biocell Research Laboratories, Cardiff, England) to visualize epitopes labeled with rat antimouse M5/114. This IgG2b monoclonal antibody (MAb) only reacts with class II (Ia) cell surface components (3). Appropriate immunoreactivity was controlled by using rat antimouse immunoglobulin Ig_{2b} (IgG_{2b}) antibodies, YTS 191 raised to CD4; YTS 169 to CD8 as positive controls, or replacing the second layer with the carrier as a negative control, or by using an inappropriate MAb (Mac 58 raised to a potato virus).

RESULTS (Figs. 1–3)

Morphological preservation was good, allowing epithelial cells to be distinguished by identification of desmosomes and tonofilament bundles. A few blocks showed some degree of shrinkage. There were some gold particles over the sections with Mac 58, and virtually no gold when the MAbs were omitted. Endothelial cells and eosinophils were all negative. YTS 191 and YTS 169 labeled almost all thymocytes of the cortex and some in the medulla.

Gold particles were not observed on all epithelial cells with MAb M5/114, but the pattern was consistent throughout pregnancy. Type 1 cells (subcapsular/perivascular) were generally negative on the capsular surface but occasionally expressed a very low level of mainly surface labeling where they touched adjacent type 2 cells. Types 2, 3, and 4 cortical epithelial cells in control and old animals were strongly labeled on their surfaces, and in addition in pregnancy, when these cells became phagocytic, gold particles were found internally around the edges of electron-lucent vacuoles and scattered within the cytoplasm. Type 4 cells of the deep cortex were variable but negative in the medulla around developing Hassall's corpuscles.

Type 5 epithelial medullary cells were generally class II negative, or only weakly positive on the surface. Other, hypertrophic medullary epithelial cells were strongly positive, and had many gold particles on the membranes of their vacuoles.

In virgin female mice, the majority of cortical and corticomedullary macrophages (containing electron-lucent "lipidic" inclusions but no obvious remnants of thymocytes) were class II negative. During pregnancy and in old age, class II–positive macrophages appeared in the cortex in rosettes. They had few if any of the above lipidic inclusions and contained degrading apoptotic thymocytes. Interdigitating cells of the medulla were all class II positive.

DISCUSSION

Changes in the pregnant mouse thymus were similar to those found previously (4). The distribution of class II products in this study differed form previous work (5,6) with respect to macrophages and type 1 and medullary epithelial cells. Like Nabarra et al. (7), we found great variability in class II expression on macrophages. They estimated about 50% of macrophages are class II positive, but it has been shown elsewhere (8) that after dissociating the cells of the thymus, Ia-positive macrophages augment thymocyte proliferation but Ia-negative cells decrease viability and proliferation by forming rosettes. In this study, expression of class II antigens occurred on cells actively engulfing apoptotic thymocytes and rosette-forming cells were class II positive. Since Ia expression in phagocytic cells of the thymic reticulum (9) and cultured epithelial cells (10) is upregulated by locally secreted cytokines (interferon-γ and prostaglandins), the microenvironment might be modified at different physiological times (pregnancy and old age).

We found type 1 and medullary epithelial cells were generally class II negative. These cells also share other antigenic determinants; e.g., group II cluster antigens, A2B5

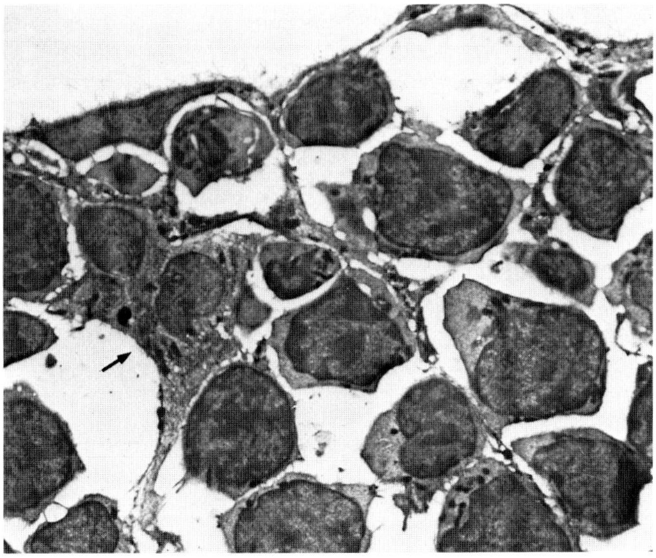

Figure 1 Low-power EM to show position of subcapsular epithelial cells, which are MHC class II negative, and adjacent type 2 cells, which are positive (<–). 12-day pregnant mouse. (Magnification: ×3000)

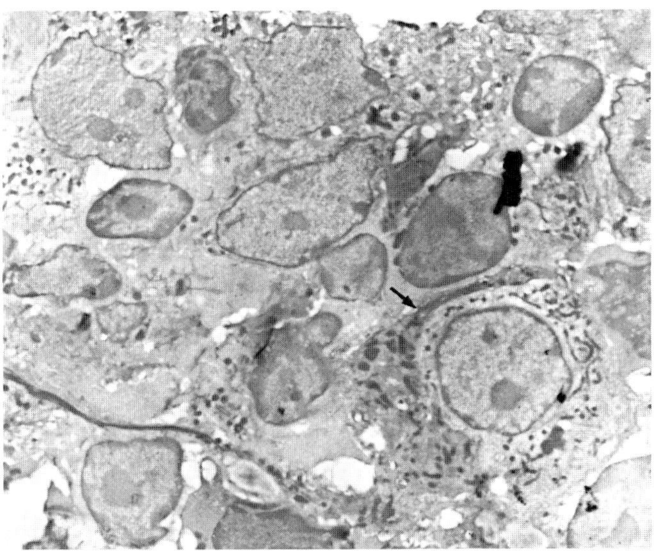

Figure 2 Low-power EM to show a group of MHC class II–negative medullary cells and a small Hassall's corpuscle and surrounding type 4 cell (<–) both of which are MHC class II negative. Young virgin female mouse. (Magnification: ×3000)

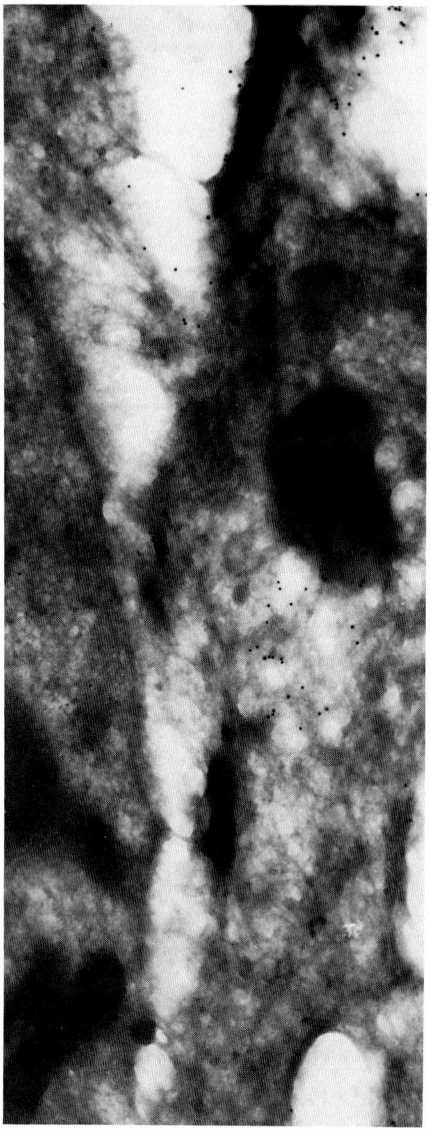

Figure 3 Immunogold particles demonstrating MHC class II antigens on the surface and in vacuoles of a type 3 cortical epithelial cell. The thymocyte on the left is unlabeled. 12-day pregnant mouse. (Magnification: ×30,000)

positivity and contain thymic hormone peptides. Since they are situated at the points of entry and exit to the thymus, these cells may not be involved in thymocyte "education" and may not need therefore to express class II.

ACKNOWLEDGMENTS

This work was supported by a grant from the Nuffield Foundation (AGC). Thanks are due to Professor H. Waldman for the YTS monoclonal antibodies and to Dr. J. Butcher for the Mac 58 monoclonal antibody.

REFERENCES

1. Lorenz RG, Allen PM. Thymic cortical epithelial cells can present self-antigens in vivo. Nature 1989; 337:560–562.
2. Morgan G, Wooding FBP, Beckeers JF, Freisen HG. An immunological cryo-ultrastructural study of a sequential appearance of proteins in placental binucleate cells in early pregnancy in the cow. J Reprod Fertil 1989; 86:745–52.
3. Battacharya A, Dorf ME, Springer TA. A shared alloantigenic determination on Ia antigens encoded by the I-A and I-E subregions: evidence for I region gene duplication. J Immunol 1981; 127:2488–2495.
4. Clarke AG, Kendall MD. Histological changes in the thymus during mouse pregnancy. Thymus 1989; 14:65–78.
5. van Ewijk W, Rouse RV, Weissman IL. Distribution of H-2 microenvironments in the mouse thymus. J Histochem Cytochem 1980; 28:1089–99.
6. Farr AG, Nakane PK. Cells bearing Ia antigens in the murine thymus. An ultrastructural study. Am J Pathol 1983; 111:88–97.
7. Nabarra B, Papiernik M. Phenotype of thymic stromal cells. An immunoelectron microscopic study with anti-IA, anti-MAC-1, and anti-MAC-2 antibodies. Lab Invest 1988; 58:524–31.
8. Zepp F, Schulte-Wissermann H, Mannhardt W. Macrophage subpopulations regulate intrathymic T-cell development. Thymus 1984; 6:279–93, 295–308.
9. Papiernik M, Dombret H, Stephanos S, Weitzerbin J. Control of Ia antigen expression on phagocytic cells of the thymic reticulum by interferon-gamma and prostaglandins. Eur J Immunol 1986; 16:296–300.
10. Berrih S, Arenzana-Seisdedos F, Cohen S, Devos R, Charron D, Virelizier J-L. Interferon-gamma modulates HLA class II antigen expression on cultured human thymic epithelial cells. J Immunol 1985; 135:1165–1171.

17

Involvement of Class II Major Histocompatibility Complex Molecules and CD3 in a Step of Intrathymic Lymphopoiesis Controlled by Thymic Nurse Cells

Marie Paule Defresne, Chantal Humblet, Anne-Michel Rongy, Roland Greimers, and Jacques Boniver
Laboratory of Pathological Anatomy and Cytopathology, University Hospital of Liège, Liège, Belgium

INTRODUCTION

Thymic nurse cells (TNCs) are multicellular complexes (1) which represent a microenvironment in vivo where thymocytes establish interactions with subcapsular epithelial cells (2,3), expressing class II major histocompatibility complex (MHC) molecules: they have been suspected to be responsible for positive selection of self-MHC–restricted T cells (4) and/or for negative selection (5). The nature of the recognition molecules responsible for the cell-cell interactions observed within TNCs is not yet known. However, the role of the T-cell receptor (TCR) and of MHC class II antigens has been suspected from two sets of experiments. First, postnatal treatment of mice with anti-CD3 antibodies inhibits the interactions of immature thymocytes with class II–positive cortical epithelial cells (6). Second, we recently demonstrated that interferon-γ (IFN-γ) stimulates epithelial cells isolated from TNCs to establish interactions with thymocytes in vitro. This stimulation correlates with an increase in the expression of MHC class II antigens at the surface of epithelial cells (7).

In order to study the involvement of these molecules in the formation of TNCs, we analyzed the effects of anti-Ia and anti-CD3 MAbs on the formation of TNCs in vitro, when epithelial cells isolated from TNCs are incubated with immature fetal thymocytes.

EXPERIMENTAL DATA: INHIBITION OF IN VITRO TNC FORMATION WITH ANTI-Ia OR ANTI-CD3 MAb

In all the experiments, C57BL/Ka mice were used. The TNCs were isolated by enzymatic digestion of thymuses and repeated sedimentations (8). The epithelial cells isolated from these complexes were incubated with 16- to 17-day-old fetal thymocytes in hanging-drop culture and tested for their capacity to form new lymphoepithelial complexes (7,9).

As shown earlier (7), 25+/–5% of the epithelial cells isolated from TNCs formed lymphoepithelial complexes in these conditions. This percentage strikingly increased to 54+/–11% when the epithelial cells had been cultured for 3–4 days in the presence of rmIFN-γ (7). Simultaneously, an increase in the expression of Ia antigens at the surface of epithelial cells was observed (7).

Epithelial cells isolated from TNCs and cultured with or without rmIFN-γ were tested for their capacity to form in vitro complexes in the presence of anti-Ia MAb (200 μg/ml) in the hanging-drop culture (rat IgG antimouse Ia antigens, clone M5/114, Hybritech, San Diego, California, and mouse IgM anti–I-A, clones B17-263.R1 and B17-123-R2, Serotec, Wiesbaden, West Germany). As shown in Table 1, these antibodies partially inhibited the capacity of TNC-derived epithelial cells to form in vitro complexes: The values observed were 10+/–6% for epithelial cells cultured in medium alone and 18+/–6% for rmIFN-γ–stimulated epithelial cells.

The 16- to 17-day-old fetal thymocytes were incubated with anti-CD3 MAb during 30 min at 37°C (hamster anti-CD3, clone 145-2C11, generously given by Dr. O. Leo) (9), and after washing, tested for their capacity to form in vitro complexes with epithelial cells isolated from TNCs. In other experiments, the same MAb was added to the hanging-drop culture. In both cases, the anti-CD3 MAb partially inhibited the formation of lymphoepithelial complexes (Table 2). The values observed were indeed 12+/–2% as compared to 25+/–5% and 24+/–2% in the absence of MAb or after the addition of an irrelevant hamster antimouse MAb (anti–Qa 2) used as control.

DISCUSSION

This study demonstrates that anti-Ia as well as anti-CD3 MAb partially inhibit the in vitro lymphoepithelial complexes formation between epithelial cells isolated from TNCs and immature thymocytes.

Freshly isolated TNCs as well as TNC-derived epithelial cells cultured for 5 days express class II MHC molecules (1,7). rmIFN-γ increased this expression and simultaneously stimulated their capacity to establish interactions with thymocytes (7). Here again, anti-Ia MAb partially inhibited the in vitro complex formation. The Ia molecules might thus facilitate cell-cell interactions within TNCs.

Anti-CD3 MAb also inhibited the formation of lymphoepithelial complexes. It has been previously shown that subpopulations of cortical thymocytes express TCR: This

Table 1 Effect of Anti-Ia MAb on the Capacity of Epithelial Cells Isolated from TNCs to Form Lymphoepithelial Complexes in Vitro

	% of epithelial cells forming complexes[a]			
	After culture in medium		After incubation with rmIFN-γ	
MAb added	none	Anti-Ia	None	Anti-Ia
	25+/–5	7+/–3	54+/–11	18+/–6

[a]The data represent the mean values and SD obtained from three separate experiments each involving three to five assays.

Table 2 Effect of Anti-CD3 MAb on the Capacity of Epithelial Cells Isolated from TNCs to Form Lymphoepithelial Complexes in Vitro

	% of epithelial cells forming complexes[a]		
MAb added	none	Anti-CD3	Anti-Qa 2
	25+/−5	12+/−2	24+/−2

[a]The data represent the mean values and SD obtained from three separate experiments each involving three to five assays.

expression is restricted to areas of thymocyte membrane in contact with processes of epithelial cells expressing Ia antigens (10). Moreover, injections of MAb against TCR B chain or CD3 lead to an arrest of intrathymic differentiation at the transition for immature CD4CD8 double positive to single positive mature thymocytes: This maturation arrest correlates with a nearly complete abrogation of thymocyte-epithelial interactions within TNCs (6). These findings support the hypothesis that TNCs control a maturation step of cortical thymocytes via TCR/MHC interactions.

Such interactions have been proposed to play a role in the selection of MHC-restricted receptor repertoire (11). Whether they are involved in the positive and/or in the negative selection has still to be determined. Observations made in TCR transgenic mice suggest that thymic stromal cells expressing MHC molecules play a role in positive selection (12). On the other hand, the findings that thymocytes within TNCs are at a pretolerant stage (13), and that TNC-derived epithelial cells can present self-antigens in vivo (5) imply that they could be involved in negative selection.

ACKNOWLEDGMENTS

This work was supported by the Fund for Medical Scientific Research, the Centre Anticancéreux près l'Université de Liège, the Research Fund of the Faculty of Medicine at Liège University, and Boehringer Ingelheim International.

REFERENCES

1. Wekerle H. Ketelsen U.P. Thymic nurse cells. Ia-bearing epithelium involved in T lymphocyte differentiation? Nature 1980; 283:402–4.
2. Defresne M.P. Goffinet G. Boniver J. In situ characterization in freeze-fractured mouse thymuses of lymphoepithelial complexes ultrastructurally similar to isolated thymic nurse cells. Tissue Cell 1986; 18:321–30.
3. Van Ewijk W. Cell surface topography of thymic microenvironments. Lab. Invest. 1988; 59: 579–90.
4. Kyewski B.A. Thymic nurse cells: possible sites of T-cell selection. Immunol. Today 1986; 7:374–9.
5. Lorenz R.G. Allen P.M. Thymic cortical epithelial cells can present self-antigens in vivo. Nature 1989; 337:560–2.
6. Kyewski B.A. Schirrmacher V. Allison J.P. Antibodies against the T cell receptor/CD3 complex interfere with distinct intra-thymic cell-cell interactions in vivo: correlation with arrest of T cell differentiation. Eur. J. Immunol. 1989; 19:857–63.

7. Defresne M.P. Humblet C. Rongy A.M. Greimers R. Boniver J. Effect of interferon-gamma and tumor necrosis factor alpha on lymphoepithelial interactions within thymic nurse cells. Eur. J. Immunol. 1990; 20:429–32.
8. Defresne M.P. Rongy A.M. Greimers R. Boniver J. Cellular aspects of radiation leukemogenesis in C57BL/Ka mice. II. Thymic microenvironment and nurse cells. Leukemia Res. 1986; 10:783–9.
9. Leo O. Foo D. Sachs D.H. Samelson L.E. Bluestone J.A. Identification of a monoclonal antibody specific for a murine T3 polypeptide. Proc. Natl. Acad. Sci. U.S.A. 1987; 34:1374–8.
10. Farr A.G. Anderson S.K. Marrack P. Kappler J. Expression of antigen-specific, major histocompatibility complex-restricted receptors by cortical and medullary thymocytes in situ. Cell 1985; 43:543–50.
11. Emmrich F. Cross-linking of CD4 and CD8 with the T-cell receptor complex: Quaternary complex formation and T-cell repertoire selection. Immunol. Today 1988; 9:296–9.
12. Von Boehmer H. Teh H.S. Kisielow P. The thymus selects the useful, neglects the useless and destroys the harmful. Immunol. Today 1989; 10:57–61.
13. Penninger J. Klima J. Kroemer G. Dietrich H. Hala K. Wick G. Intra-thymic nurse cell lymphocytes can induce a graft-versus-host reaction with high efficiency. Dev. Comp. Immunol. 1989; 13:313–27.19.

18

Unique Thymic Microenvironment for T-Cell Development in Spontaneous Thymoma BUF/Mna Rats

Taichi Ezaki, Kenjiro Matsuno, and Masahiko Kotani
Kumamoto University Medical School, Kumamoto, Japan

INTRODUCTION

BUF/Mna rats develop spontaneous benign thymomas of epithelial origin with nearly 100% incidence at 9–15 months of age in an autosomal dominant manner (1). In a previous study, we have demonstrated that there is a unique differentiation pathway at intrathymic and postthymic stages of T-cell development in this rat strain (2). It has been assumed that the thymic microenvironment play some role in the unusual cortical differentiation pathway for T-cell development. Very recently, we have recognized numerous lymphoepithelial cell complexes, so called thymic nurse cells (TNCs) increasing in situ in ordinary paraffin sections of the thymomas in BUF/Mna rats. In this report, we will focus on the TNCs by separating them from thymuses at various ages and investigating some of their immunological characteristics.

MATERIALS AND METHODS

Rats

Male inbred BUF/Mna (RT-I^{u}) rats and DA (RT-1^{a}) rats were obtained from our rat colonies at the Laboratory Animal Center for Experimental Research, Kumamoto University Medical School. More than three animals per assay were examined.

Separation of TNCs

Thymuses were minced into small pieces and placed into dissociation bottles containing 20 ml of 0.25% trypsin (Wako Pure Chemical Industries, Osaka, Japan) in Ca^{2+}- and Mg^{2+}-free phosphate-buffered saline (PBS) with collagenase (1 mg/ml; Wako) and deoxyribonuclease (25 μg/ml; Sigma, St. Louis, Missouri). The dissociation was achieved by stirring at about 200 rpm for 20 min at room temperature. The cell suspensions were washed once, resuspended in PBS, and then fetal calf serum (FCS) was carefully underlaid at the bottom of the tubes. The TNCs were isolated by four or five runs of sedimentation at 1g according to the method of Wekerle et al. (3).

Tissue Preparation for Histology and Immunochemistry

Thymuses were fixed in Carnoy's fixative, dehydrated in ethanol, and embedded in paraffin for methylgreen-pyronin (MGP) staining and hematoxylin-eosin (H&E) staining. For enzyme-histochemistry and immunohistochemistry, thymuses were fresh frozen in liquid nitrogen and 6-μm-thick cryosections were made. Smears of isolated TNCs were also made. The indirect immunoenzymatic method was employed for the immunostaining as described previously (2).

RESULTS AND DISCUSSION

Histological Changes in the Thymus with Age and Identification of TNCs In Situ

No noticeable structural changes were seen until 3 months of age. As previously reported (2), the thymic weight reached its first peak around 2–3 months of age and began to reincrease from 8–9 months (start of tumorigenesis) after a period of slight decrease for about 6 months. Then, with age, the cortical areas showing a remarkable increment of lymphocytes and starry neoplastic epithelial cells gradually occupied most parts of the thymus, whereas the medullary areas became narrower and segmented like islets in the enlarged cortical areas. At 9 months after birth, numerous TNCs were readily found in ordinary paraffin sections of the thymus (Fig. 1a,b). Since it is difficult to identify TNCs in situ in the normal thymus because of their small population size, there has been a repeated argument concerning their reality in situ (4,5). However, this thymoma model provides a clear evidence for the existence of TNCs in situ. Some pyroninophilic cells enclosed in TNCs were often found by the MGP staining (Fig. 1a), indicating their high content of ribonucleic acid. This agrees with the fact of frequent mitotic figures within TNCs (3). These structures were found to be cytokeratin positive (Fig. 1c) and class II antigen positive (Fig. 1d) by the immunostaining.

Characterization and Quantification of Isolated TNCs

The TNCs were isolated from thymuses at various ages. Most of the TNCs from thymomas usually enclosed 10–100 viable lymphoid cells (Fig. 2). They were class I positive, class II positive, and cytokeratin positive but acid phosphatase negative and nonspecific esterase negative, indicating their epithelial origin but not phagocytic origin (data not shown). There was no distinct difference in their morphology between thymomas and normal control thymuses. In BUF/Mna rats, the absolute numbers of TNCs per whole thymus were higher than those of control DA rats at all ages examined (Fig. 3a), but TNCs per gram of thymus were almost similar to those of DA rats till 2 months of age (Fig. 3b). These two values burst out increasing at 8 months of age, which was immediately before or in good accordance with the onset of thymomas. Furthermore, in order to examine the proportion of TNCs that contained proliferative cells, 5-bromo-2′-deoxyuridine (BrdU 4 mg/100g body weight; Sigma) was injected intraperitoneally 1 hr before TNC separation. More than 300 TNCs were examined for the presence of BrdU-positive cells within the TNCs. In

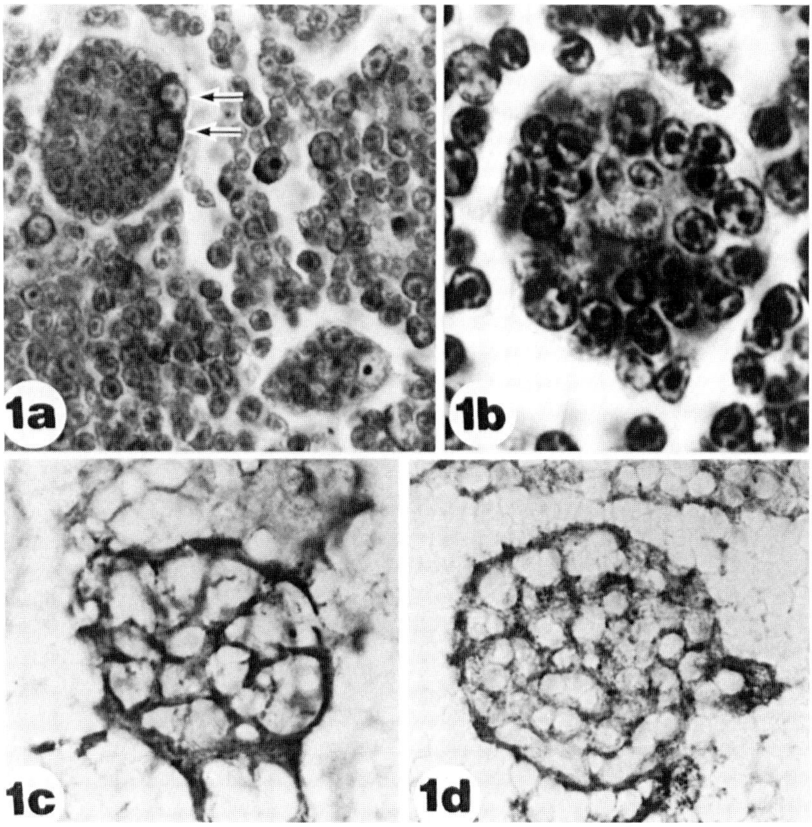

Figure 1 Identification of TNC in situ in the thymomas of BUF/Mna rats. (a) Two TNCs in the cortical area. Pyroninophilic cells (arrows) were seen within the TNCs. MGP staining. (Magnification: ×800). (b) Higher magnification of a TNC. H&E. (Magnification: ×1600). (c) Immunoperoxidase staining with rabbit antibovine keratin antibody (DAKO Corp., California). (Magnification: ×800). (d) Immunoperoxidase staining of class II antigen with OX6 (Sera-Lab Ltd., Sussex, England). (Magnification: ×800).

23-month-old thymoma BUF/Mna rats, 35 ± 4% of TNCs contained BrdU-positive cells, whereas TNCs from 6-week-old DA and BUF/Mna rats showed only 16 ± 6% and 24 ± 6% positivities, respectively. This indicates that TNCs in the thymoma rats have higher capability of supporting cell proliferation within them. Our preliminary immunohistochemical analysis has revealed that many of the TNCs can actually produce demonstrable level of FTS (Facteur thymique serique) (6). All these data strongly suggest that the increase of TNCs in BUF/Mna rats may be responsible for the increment of thymocytes in the thymus. It seems less likely that macrophages are actually involved in the cause of the unique T-cell development, since there was no significant difference between thymomas and control thymuses in histological distribution of macrophage populations as revealed by the immunostaining with ED1, ED2, and ED3 (7) (data not shown).

In conclusion, we have clearly demonstrated TNCs in situ in the thymoma of BUF/Mna rats. These TNCs seem to play the primary role in the unusual increment of

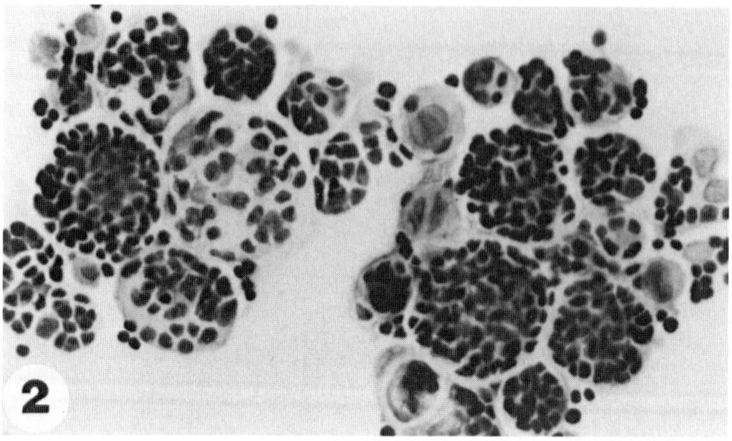

Figure 2 A smear of isolated TNCs. Hematoxylin staining. (Magnification: ×500)

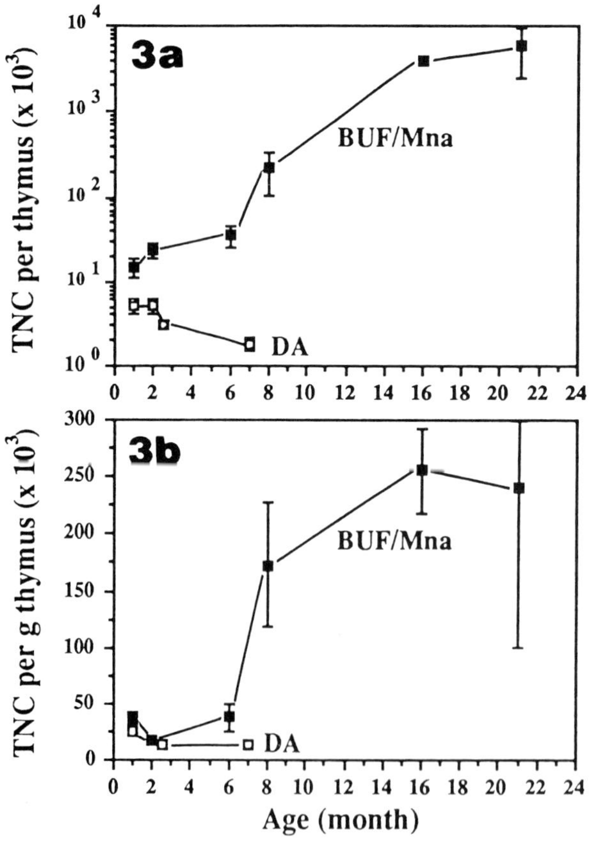

Figure 3 Quantification of TNCs isolated from thymuses of various ages. (a) Number of TNCs in the thymus of various ages. (b) Number of TNCs/g thymus.

thymocytes and their unique development in the thymus. The results and our previous results (2) suggest that TNCs in BUF/Mna rats are at least morphologically normal but functionally hyperactive in producing thymocytes. BUF/Mna rats may thus provide a useful model to study the regulatory roles of thymic microenvironment, especially TNCs, for T-cell development.

REFERENCES

1. Matsuyama M, Yamada C, Hiai H. A single dominant susceptible gene determines spontaneous development of thymoma in BUF/Mna rat. Jpn J Cancer Res (Gann) 1986; 77:1066–8.
2. Ezaki T, Kawatsu R, Matsuno K, Kotani M. Characterization of intrathymic and extrathymic T cell development in spontaneous thymoma Buffalo/Mna rats. Thymus 1990; 16:67-87.
3. Wekerle H, Ketelsen U-P, Ernst M. Thymic nurse cells. Lymphoepithelial cell complexes in murine thymuses: morphological and serological characterization. J Exp Med 1980; 151:925–44.
4. Kyewski BA, Kaplan HS. Lymphoepithelial interactions in the mouse thymus: phenotypic and kinetic studies on thymic nurse cells. J Immunol 1982; 128:2287–94.
5. van de Wijngaert FP, Rademakers LHPM, Schuurman H-J, de Weger RA, Kater L. Identification and *in situ* localization of the "thymic nurse cell" in man. J Immunol 1983; 130:2348–51.
6. Bach J-F, Dardenne M, Pleau J-M. Biochemical characterization of a serum thymic factor. Nature 1977; 266:55–7.
7. Sminia T, van Asselt AA, van de Ende MB, Dijkstra CD. Rat thymus macrophages: an immunohistochemical study on fetal, neonatal and adult thymus. Thymus 1986; 8:141–50.

19
Viral Infection of the Thymus

Jan Gossmann, Jürgen Löhler, Thomas Kratzberg, and Fritz Lehmann-Grube
Heinrich-Pette-Institut für Experimentelle Virologie und Immunologie an der Universität Hamburg, Federal Republic of Germany

INTRODUCTION

Because of the central role the thymus plays in the functioning of the immune system we wanted to know the histopathological consequences of a viral infection for this organ. Our model was the adult mouse acutely infected with the lymphocytic choriomeningitis (LCM) virus, which is well suited because the agent multiplies to high concentrations in parenchymal as well as lymphoid tissues, including the thymus (1,2). For the experiments we employed the WE strain of LCM virus and C57BL/6J (B6) mice, which were raised and maintained under specific pathogen–free conditions.

REPLICATION OF LCM VIRUS IN AND ELIMINATION FROM THE THYMUS

After intraperitoneal (i.p.) inoculation of 10^6 mouse infectious units (IU), the virus multiplied in the thymus attaining infectious virus concentrations as high as 10^8 IU/g on day 7; subsequently the titers declined to essentially undetectable levels by day 12. Immunohistochemically, viral antigen was found predominantly in foci of epithelial/reticular cells in the medulla (Fig. 1a) and occasionally in macrophages.

PATHOLOGY OF THE THYMUS IN THE LCM VIRUS-INFECTED MOUSE

At intervals after i.p. inoculation, thymuses were weighed and subsequently analyzed histologically and immunohistochemically. Beginning on day 5 and extending to day 12 after infection, rapid involution was observed, as evidenced by a more than 50% reduction

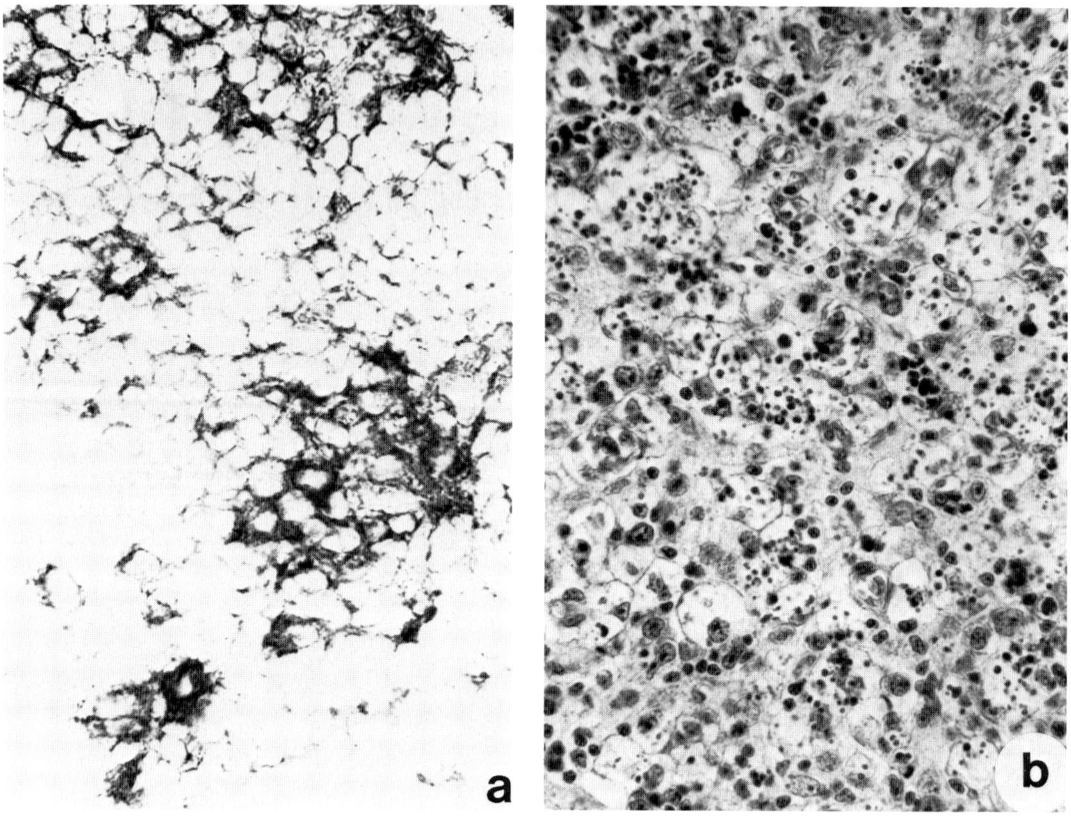

Figure 1 (a) LCM viral antigen in medullary epithelial/reticular cells of the thymus. Eight days after i.p. infection with 10^6 IU of LCM virus. Frozen section, indirect immunoalkaline phosphatase method. (Magnification ×360) (b) Apoptosis of cortical thymocytes. Eight days after i.p. infection with 10^6 IU of LCM virus. H&E. (Magnification ×460).

of weight. Histological inspection revealed nearly complete apoptosis of cortical thymocytes (Fig. 1b) and necrotizing changes of the medullary stroma with swollen and vacuolated cytoplasm, disappearance of immunoreactivity of intracellular keratin, and deposition of fibrinoid. Multinucleated reticular cells became visible, and activation of macrophages was prominent. These alterations were maximal around day 9 after infection. On day 12, signs of repair were obvious.

For a more detailed inspection, sections of frozen and paraffin-embedded specimens were stained by the use of monoclonal antibodies (MAbs) and various immunohistochemical methods for the cellular expression of CD8, CD4, major histocompatibility complex (MHC) classes I and II antigens, MAC 1, F4/80, B 220 and interleukin-2 receptor (IL-2R) p55 α chain. Furthermore, the peanut agglutinin (PNA) lectin binding of the cells was examined. Loss of CD4 and CD8 cell surface antigens on one hand and of PNA-binding ability on the other revealed a precipitous drop in the numbers of cortical

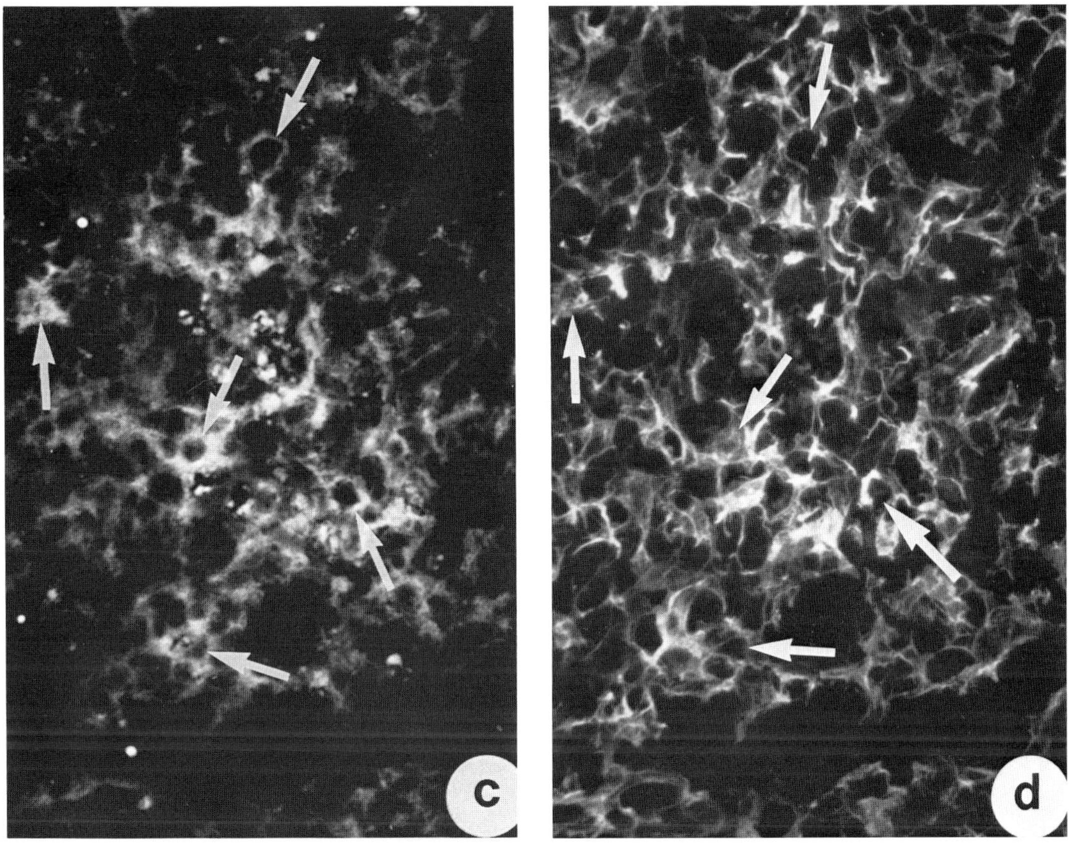

Figure 1 (Continued)
(c and d) IL-2R α chains on keratin-positive cells of the thymic medulla. Nine days after infection with 10^6 IU of LCM virus, frozen sections of the thymus were double stained with rat anti–IL-2R MAb 7D4 (c) and a rabbit keratin-specific antiserum (d), followed by anti-rat-IgG and anti-rabbit-IgG antibodies conjugated with FITC and Texas Red, respectively. Arrows point to double-positive cells. (Magnification ×460).

thymocytes with a close to total absence of PNA-positive lymphocytes on day 9. The number of double positive, double negative, and CD4-positive cells was more drastically reduced than the number of CD8-positive cells, a visual impression that was confirmed by FACS data (Table 1). Presumably, as a consequence of this lymphocytolysis, the normally fine reticular MHC class II immunostaining was obscured by a more compact appearance of the now broadened and roundish reticulum cells. The MHC class I immunolabeling was strongly positive throughout the cortex, the cells of which are normally essentially free of this antigen. While thymocytes vanished during the infectious process, the number of MAC 1–positive cells was greatly enlarged. B cells also showed an abnormal distribution, and increased numbers were located in the cortex instead of the corticomedullary junction.

Table 1 Numbers of Subset Thymocytes During Viral Infection

	Number of cells per thymus[b]			
Day after infection[a]	$CD4^+$	$CD8^+$	$CD4^+CD8^+$	$CD4^-CD8^-$
Uninfected	5.3×10^6[c]	2.8×10^6	1.3×10^8	7.7×10^6
9	6.2×10^5	1.1×10^6	3.3×10^6	5.7×10^5

[a]C57BL/6J mice were infected by intraperitoneal injection of 10^6 infectious units of LCM virus on day 0 or left uninfected.

[b]Thymocyte cell suspensions from individual mice were double labeled with biotinylated CD4 and FITC-coupled CD8 monoclonal antibodies followed by streptavidin-PE. 5000 cells were analyzed on a FACScan, dead cells being excluded on the basis of forward and side scatter.

[c]Calculated from the numbers of cells recovered per thymus and the percentages of the respective subset thymocytes.

IL-2R EXPRESSION IN THE THYMUS OF LCM VIRUS-INFECTED MICE

Having found that the LCM virus infection led to the predominant lysis of PNA-positive cortical thymocytes, we wanted to know whether thymic cells bearing the IL-2R were also affected. Staining of frozen sections with antibodies specific for the p55 α chain revealed diminished numbers of IL-2R–positive thymocytes in infected mice, with a total loss on day 9; subsequently, such cells reappeared attaining sizeable numbers on day 12, when regeneration was also evident histologically. Surprisingly, at the same time we found IL-2R on epithelial/reticular cells in the medulla, especially in areas which were positive for LCM virus antigen. Immunofluorescence double-labeling experiments with three different MAbs directed against p55 α chain, namely, 7D4 (3), AMT 13 (4), and PC 61 (5), and polyclonal antibodies against keratin on one hand and the same antibodies and antiserum against LCM virus on the other disclosed that a considerable portion of the non–T cells expressing IL-2R were indeed epithelial/reticular cells and that some of them (although not all) were LCM virus-positive (see Fig. 1c and 1d). We also found weak expression of IL-2R on an occasional epithelial/reticular cell in the medulla of uninfected mice.

PARTICIPATION OF T-CELL SUBSETS IN THYMIC PATHOLOGY

It is well established that the pathological lesions of the central nervous system and liver in LCM virus–infected mice are mediated by virus-specific T cells (6,7), and the same is true for the peripheral lymphoid organs (our unpublished observations), which led to the question of whether the observed thymus changes were likewise of an immunopathological nature. Injection into mice of anti–Thy-1.2 MAb C depletes them of their peripheral T lymphocytes but leaves thymocytes intact (8). In infected mice thus treated, thymic alterations did not occur.

To further elucidate the contribution of T lymphocytes to both elimination of the virus and pathological changes, mice were treated with the CD4-specific MAb YTS 191.1 or the CD8-specific MAb YTS 169.4 (9), which depletes them of peripheral CD4 (leaving behind the CD8) T lymphocytes and of peripheral CD8 (leaving behind the CD4) T lymphocytes, respectively. As had been found for other organs (9) the CD8 cell-free mice were unable to

Table 2 Virus Titers in the Thymus of LCM Virus–Infected Mice Depleted of T-Lymphocyte Subsets by Treatment with MAbs

	Day after infection[b]	
Treatment[a]	9	12
No antibody	$6.3 \pm 2.2 \times 10^{7}$[c]	$8.1 \pm 0.5 \times 10^{3}$
α CD4	$7.1 \pm 4.2 \times 10^{7}$	$1.5 \pm 0.8 \times 10^{5}$
α CD8	$5.5 \pm 1.4 \times 10^{8}$	$1.1 \pm 0.2 \times 10^{8}$
α CD4 + α CD8	$1.4 \pm 0.9 \times 10^{9}$	$2.8 \pm 0.5 \times 10^{8}$

[a]C57BL/6J mice were injected once intravenously on day 5 after infection with 100 μg of either CD4 or CD8 MAb (9) or a combination of both.
[b]Mice were infected by intraperitoneal inoculation of 10^6 infectious units of LCM virus on day 0.
[c]Infectious units per g thymus ± SEM in three mice.

clear the virus from the thymus, whereas the antiviral potential of mice devoid of CD4 cells was not greatly affected (Table 2), which confirms our previous conclusion that elimination of LCM virus from murine tissues depends principally on CD8 cytotoxic T lymphocytes (CTLs) (10). Surprisingly, in infected CD4 lymphocyte–depleted mice the thymic cortex was found to be largely intact and other alterations associated with thymic involution were all but absent. In contrast, in CD8 cell–depleted mice, the pathological alterations of the thymic cortex were as marked as in infected but not antibody-treated mice. Treatment with MAbs directed against Thy-1, CD8, or CD4 did not measurably affect the high expression of IL-2R on epithelial/reticular cells in LCM virus-infected mice.

CONCLUSIONS

We interpret our findings to mean that most of the alterations in the thymus of LCM virus-infected mice are not caused directly by the virus or by its elimination, which is mediated by CD8-positive T cells but rather result from an immunopathological process with CD4-positive T lymphocytes playing the essential part.

Our search of the literature has revealed just one previous publication in which the presence of IL-2R on nonhematopoietic cells in vivo has been mentioned (11). We found it on the epithelial/reticular cells of the thymic medulla, where it might facilitate the communication with IL-2–producing thymocytes. This, of course, is speculation as is our explanation for the upregulation of the IL-2R during infection with LCM virus. Expression of this receptor was greatly augmented even after elimination of all circulating T lymphocytes or of T-cell subsets, and was clearly related both qualitatively and quantitatively with the presence of the virus. Perhaps its increased appearance on epithelial/reticular cells is directly caused by the virus or, more likely, by mediators (cytokines or other inflammatory products) that are locally released from macrophages or thymic stroma cells during the infection. As to the relatively high number of CD8-positive T lymphocytes in the thymus of LCM virus-infected mice, this possibly results from the influx of antivirally active mature CD8-positive CTLs, which we have shown to enter the organ from the circulation (12).

ACKNOWLEDGMENTS

This work was aided by a research grant from the Wilhelm Sander-Stiftung, Neustadt an der Donau. The Heinrich-Pette-Institut is financially supported by Freie und Hansestadt Hamburg and Bundesministerium für Jugend, Familie, Frauen und Gesundheit.

REFERENCES

1. Löhler J, Lehmann-Grube F. Immunopathologic alterations of lymphatic tissues of mice infected with lymphocytic choriomeningitis virus. I. Histopathologic findings. Lab. Invest. 1981; 44: 193–204.
2. Moskophidis D, Lehmann-Grube F. The immune response of the mouse to lymphocytic choriomeningitis virus. III. Differences of numbers of cytotoxic T lymphocytes in spleens of mice of different strains. Cell. Immunol. 1983; 77:279–89.
3. Malek TR, Robb RJ, Shevach EM. Identification and initial characterization of a rat monoclonal antibody reactive with the murine interleukin 2 receptor-ligand complex. Proc. Natl. Acad. Sci. U.S.A. 1983; 80:5694–8.
4. Osawa H, Diamantstein T. A rat monoclonal antibody that binds specifically to mouse T lymphoblasts and inhibits IL 2 receptor functions: A putative anti-IL 2 receptor antibody. J. Immunol. 1984; 132:2445–50.
5. Lowenthal JW, Corthesy P, Tougne C, Lees R, MacDonald HR, Nabholz M. High and low affinity IL 2 receptors: Analysis by IL 2 dissociation rate and reactivity with monoclonal antireceptor antibody PC 61. J. Immunol 1985; 135:3988–94.
6. Cole GA, Nathanson N, Prendergast RA. Requirement for theta-bearing cells in lymphocytic choriomeningitis virus-induced central nervous system disease. Nature 1972; 238:335–7.
7. Zinkernagel RM, Haenseler E, Leist T, Cerny A, Hengartner H, Althage A. T cell-mediated hepatitis in mice infected with lymphocytic choriomeningitis virus. Liver cell destruction by H-2 class I-restricted virus-specific cytotoxic T cells as a physiological correlate of the ^{51}Cr-release assay? J. Exp. Med. 1986; 164:1075–92.
8. Opitz HG, Opitz U, Hewlett G, Schlumberger HD. A new model for investigations of T-cell functions in mice: Differential immunosuppressive effects of two monoclonal anti-Thy-1.2 antibodies. Immunobiology 1982; 160:438–53.
9. Moskophidis D, Cobbold SP, Waldmann H, Lehmann-Grube F. Mechanisms of recovery from acute virus infection: Treatment of lymphocytic choriomeningitis virus-infected mice with monoclonal antibodies reveals that Lyt-2^+ T lymphocytes mediate clearance of virus and regulate the antiviral antibody response. J. Virol. 1987; 61:1867–74.
10. Lehmann-Grube F, Moskophidis D, Löhler J. Recovery from acute virus infection. Role of cytotoxic T lymphocytes in the elimination of lymphocytic choriomeningitis virus from spleens of mice. Ann. N.Y. Acad. Sci. 1988; 532:238–56.
11. Hofman FM, von Hanwehr RI, Dinarello CA, Mizel SB, Hinton D, Merill JE. Immunoregulatory molecules and IL 2 receptors identified in multiple sclerosis brain. J. Immunol. 1986; 136: 3239–45.
12. Gossmann J, Löhler J, Lehmann-Grube F. Entry of antivirally active T lymphocytes into the thymus of virus-infected mice. J Immunol (in press).

20
Atrophy of the Rat Thymus
Effects of 2,3,7,8-Tetrachlorodibenzo-*p*-dioxin on the Epithelial Microenvironment Assessed at the Ultrastructural Level: A Comparison with *bis*(tri-*n*-butyltin)oxide

Eric J. De Waal,[1] Louk H. P. M. Rademakers,[2] Henk-Jan Schuurman,[1,2] Henk Van Loveren,[1] and Joseph G. Vos[1]
[1]*National Institute of Public Health and Environmental Protection, Bilthoven, The Netherlands;* [2]*University Hospital, Utrecht, The Netherlands*

INTRODUCTION

2,3,7,8-Tetrachlorodibenzo-*p*-dioxin (TCDD) induces lymphocyte depletion in the rat thymic cortex (1). The mechanism of action has not yet been elucidated. In vitro studies point to a direct action of TCDD on thymic epithelial cells (2–4). It has been suggested that TCDD enhances terminal differentiation of thymic epithelial cells to a state in which they loose the ability to support thymocyte maturation (3). On the other hand, both a direct cytotoxic effect of TCDD on thymocytes and a TCDD-induced change in T-lymphocyte stem cells in the bone marrow have been claimed (5,6). In order to test the hypothesis that TCDD affects the cortical epithelium of the rat thymus in vivo, we studied TCDD-induced epithelial cell changes at the ultrastructural level. *Bis*(tri-*n*-butyltin)oxide (TBTO) was used a reference, as this compound is known for its direct toxic action on thymocytes (7).

EXPERIMENTAL DESIGN

In two separate experiments, juvenile male Wistar rats (8 animals/compound/dose; 12 control animals) were intubated once orally with either TCDD (50 or 150 μg/kg body-weight) or TBTO (30 or 90 mg/kg) and sacrificed at 4 or 10 days thereafter. The thymus was weighed and subsequently fixed by immersion for conventional electron microscopy. Cortical regions were selected from two tissue blocks of each thymus.

The epithelial cells were studied on electron micrographs. For each epithelial cell type ultrastructural features were semiquantitatively assessed and statistically analyzed by a two-way ANOVA (analysis of variance) (day, treatment), with the level of statistical significance at $p < 0.05$.

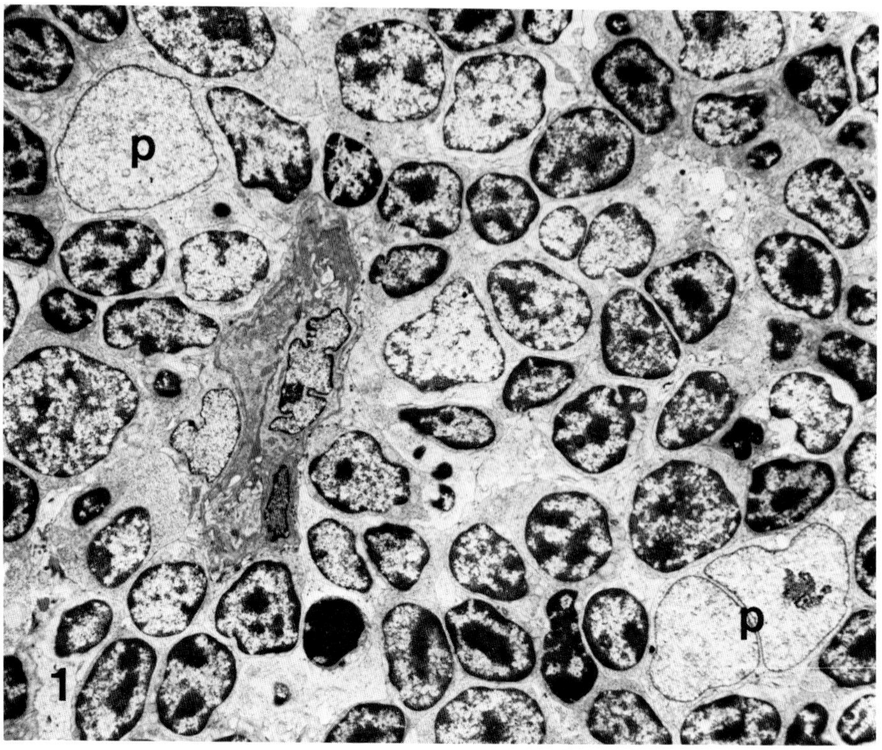

Figure 1 Two pale epithelial cells (P) in the thymic cortex of a control animal. (Magnification: ×2500).

RESULTS AND DISCUSSION

The thymic weight was diminished in a dose-dependent manner both at 4 and 10 days after exposure to TCDD (45–50% and 66–85% reduction, respectively) and at 4 days after administration of TBTO (23–38% reduction). At 10 days after administration of TBTO, this change was significant at the 90 mg/kg level only (34% reduction).

In the normal rat thymus the cortical epithelium showed heterogeneity at the ultrastructural level. Judged by their nuclear and cytoplasmic electron density, three different types of epithelial cells were recognized in the cortex, designated as pale, intermediate, and dark cells (8). The pale cells (Fig. 1) predominated, whereas the intermediate and dark cells occurred at much lower numbers. Similar cell types have been described in the human thymus (9). The spectrum in morphology is thought to reflect a differentiation process within the thymic epithelium, progressing from pale to dark cells (9).

At 10 days after administration of 50 μg/kg TCDD, focally aggregates of epithelial cells were observed. This change was far more marked after exposure to 150 μg/kg TCDD, especially at 10 days after exposure (Table 1, Fig. 2). Epithelial cell aggregates were not found after treatment with TBTO.

Another TCDD-induced change was a relative shift from pale to intermediate epithelial cell types. This effect was most prominent after administration of 150 μg/kg TCDD (Table 1; Figs. 2 and 3). The dark epithelial cells remained few in numbers. A less

Table 1 Principal Ultrastructural Changes in the Cortical Epithelium

	Controls	TCDD 50 μg/kg 4 days	TCDD 50 μg/kg 10 days	TCDD 150 μg/kg 4 days	TCDD 150 μg/kg 10 days
Formation of cell aggregates	–	–	↑	↑↑	↑↑↑
Frequency of					
pale cells	–	↓	↓	↓↓	↓↓
intermediate cells	–	↑	↑	↑↑	↑↑

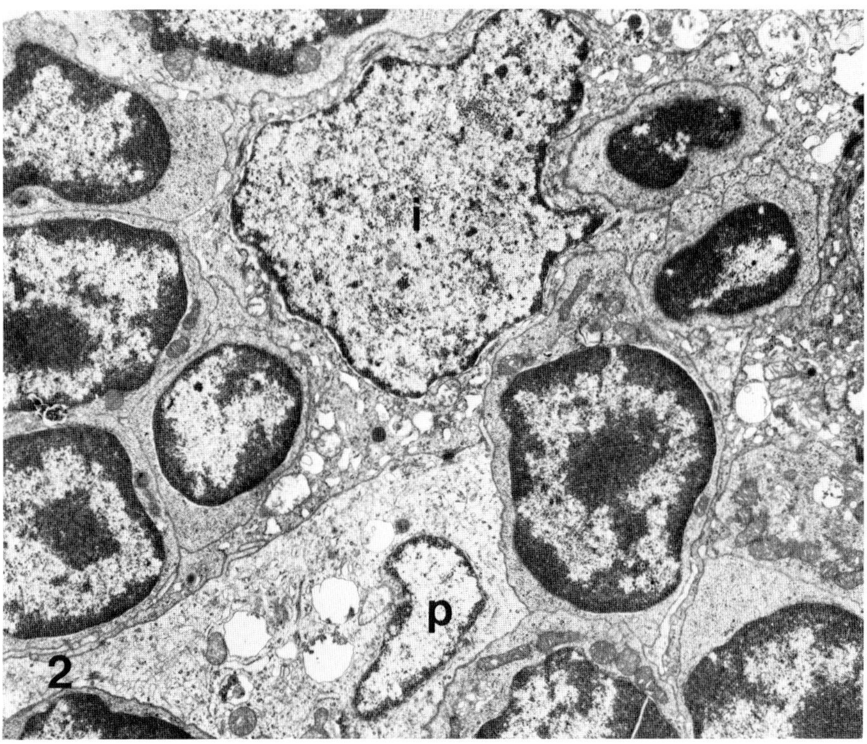

Figure 2 Ten days after administration of 150 μg/kg TCDD. An intermediate (I) and a pale cell (P) are shown forming part of an epithelial cell aggregate. (Magnification: ×7500).

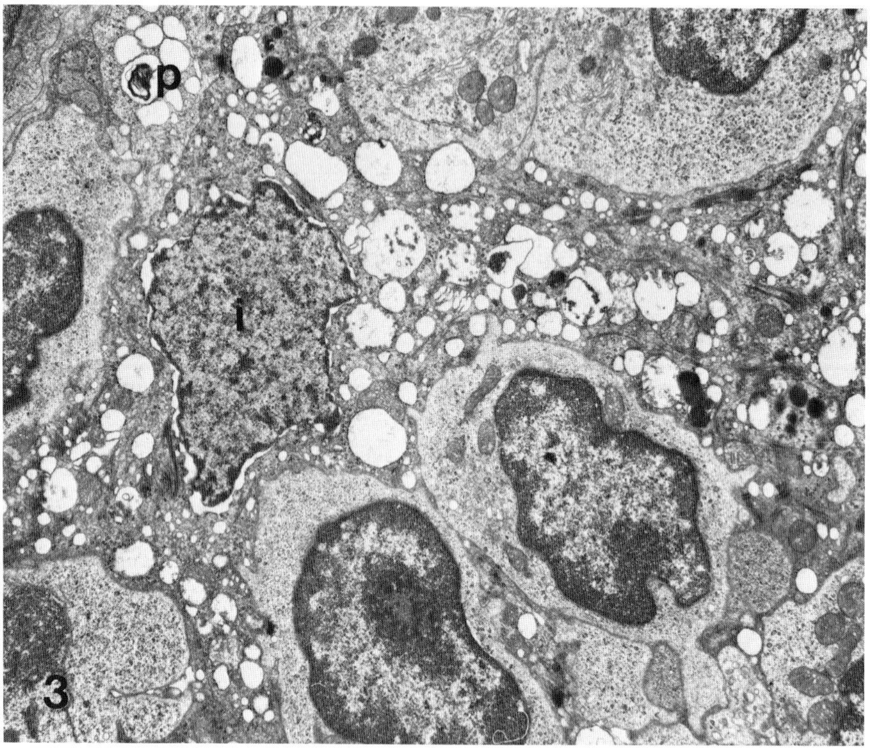

Figure 3 A vacuolated intermediate epithelial cell (I) seen at 10 days after exposure to 150 μg/kg TCDD. A small piece of a vacuolated pale cell (P) is shown also. (Magnification: ×8000).

pronounced shift of epithelial cell types was found after exposure to TBTO at the 30 mg/kg dose level only.

Following administration of 150 μg/kg TCDD, an increased vacuolation of pale and dark epithelial cells was seen. A similar trend occurred in the intermediate cells (Fig. 3). The subcapsular epithelium was also affected. Following exposure to TBTO, vacuolation was less prominent as compared with the TCDD-induced effect. The increased vacuolation indicates an altered secretory state of the epithelium owing to the depletion of thymocytes.

We conclude from these results that TCDD affects the epithelial microenvironment in the thymic cortex in vivo. At the ultrastructural level this phenomenon is reflected by the formation of epithelial cell aggregates and a more differentiated state of the cortical epithelium. In contrast, there is no evidence that TBTO specifically acts on cortical epithelial cells.

REFERENCES

1. Vos JG, Luster MI. Immune alterations. In: Kimbrough, RD, Jensen AA (eds.). *Halogenated Biphenyls, Terphenyls, Naphthalenes, Dibenzodioxins and Related Products*. Amsterdam, Elsevier Science Publishers, 1989; pp. 295–322.
2. Cook JC, Greenlee WF. Characterization of a specific binding protein for 2,3,7,8-tetrachlorodibenzo-*p*-dioxin in human thymic epithelial cells. Mol Pharmacol 1989; 35:713–719.

3. Greenlee WF, Dold KM, Irons RD, Osborne R. Evidence for direct action of 2,3,7,8-tetrachlorodibenzo-*p*-dioxin (TCDD) on thymic epithelium. Toxicol Appl Pharmacol 1985; 79:112–120.
4. Cook JC, Dold KM, Greenlee WF. An in vitro model for studying the toxicity of 2,3,7,8-tetrachlorodibenzo-*p*-dioxin to human thymus. Toxicol Appl Pharmacol 1987; 89:256–268.
5. McConkey DJ, Hartzell P, Duddy SK, Håkansson H, Orrenius S. 2,3,7,8-Tetrachlorodibenzo-*p*-dioxin kills immature thymocytes by Ca^{2+}-mediated endonuclease activation. Science 1988; 242:256–259.
6. Fine JS, Silverstone AE, Gasiewicz TA. Impairment of prothymocyte activity by 2,3,7,8-tetrachlorodibenzo-*p*-dioxin. J Immunol 1990; 144:1169–1176.
7. Vos JG, de Klerk A, Krajnc EI, Kruizinga W, van Ommen B, Rozing J. Toxicity of bis(tri-*n*-butyl-tin)oxide in the rat. II. Suppression of thymus-dependent immune responses and of parameters of nonspecific resistance after short-term exposure. Toxicol Appl Pharmacol 1984; 75:387–408.
8. Kendall MD, Schuurman HJ, Fenton J, Broekhuizen R, Kampinga J. Implantation of cultured thymic fragments in congenitally athymic (nude) rats. Ultrastructural characteristics of the developing microenvironment. Cell Tissue Res 1988; 254:283–294.
9. Van de Wijngaert FP, Kendall MD, Schuurman HJ, Rademakers LHPM, Kater L. Heterogeneity of epithelial cells in the human thymus. An ultrastructural study. Cell Tissue Res 1984; 237: 227–237.

T CELLS

21
The Development and Selection of T Lymphocytes

B. J. Fowlkes
Laboratory of Cellular and Molecular Immunology, National Institute of Allergy and Infectious Diseases, National Institutes of Health, Bethesda, Maryland

EARLY EVENTS IN T-CELL DIFFERENTIATION

Mature T cells use a surface receptor (TCR) which allows them to respond to a diverse array of foreign antigens. At the heart of this receptor is an αβ (or γδ) heterodimer which is noncovalently linked to five invariant chains (CD3 and ζ (1,2). Accessory molecules (CD4 or CD8) may participate as an intimate part of the receptor complex, either serving a signaling function, enhancing affinity for the ligand, or both (3). If the αβ heterodimer engages an antigenic peptide embedded in a molecule encoded by the major histocompatibility complex (MHC) of an antigen-presenting cell, this specific interaction induces a series of intracellular events which results in the activation of the cell.

Mature T cells develop in the thymus from stem cells originating from the fetal liver or, in the adult, from the bone marrow. These stem cells undergo a number of differentiative and selective events in order to generate the mature T cells which migrate to the peripheral lymphoid organs (1,4). As Roland Scollay relates in this session, the earliest precursor cells to arrive in the thymus express low levels of CD4, no CD8, and bear no TCR (Abstract 1.42). These cells rapidly undergo rearrangement of all the TCR genes (α, β, γ, and δ) (4). The inductive signals that initiate rearrangement are not known.

The first cells to appear during fetal development bearing TCR are those with γδ receptors (2). In the mouse, cells bearing TCRαβ are not detected for another three days (day 16 of gestation). While there is no evidence that TCR$\gamma\delta^+$ cells can give rise to the TCR$\alpha\beta^+$ cells, it appears that both lineages do arise from a common precursor. The mechanism responsible for this lineage diversification has not been resolved (3).

As these cells rearrange their TCR genes, they lose surface CD4, becoming CD4^-8^-, and subsequently pass through a period in which they transiently express interleukin-2 receptors (IL-2R) prior to a CD4^+8^+ (double positive) stage (4,5). Whether the IL-2R detected on these cells serves a function in growth and/or differentiation is still a matter of controversy. In mature T cells, the IL-2R is expressed as a result of TCR stimulation. It is not obvious what could be the inductive signal responsible for expression of IL-2R by $CD4^-8^-TCR^-$ immature thymocytes.

Prior to expression of the CD4 and CD8 accessory molecules, the IL-2R is lost. This stage of T-cell development is phenotypically distinguishable from the pre–$IL\text{-}2R^+$ stage (Pgp^-, HSA^+) and appears to be the major proliferative phase of thymocyte development (4,5). As maturation proceeds, the accessory molecules, CD4 and CD8, appear on the surface of these still-blasting cells. The mechanism promoting this event is not known but, interestingly, the transition to the $CD4^+8^+$ stage does not occur in *scid* mice, that are unable to rearrange their TCR genes. The expression of CD4 and CD8 does not occur simultaneously; instead, one precedes the other by a few hours in fetal development (4). In most strains of mice, CD8 appears before CD4.

Whether TRCαβ is expressed on the surface at the early $CD4^-8^+$ stage is a matter of controversy. Most reports from the murine system show that TCRαβ is expressed later in the $CD4^+8^+$ stage, when the majority of the cells become smaller in size. The bulk of $CD4^+8^+$ cells with TCR express low levels of receptor and do not exhibit the immune functions of mature peripheral T cells (4).

While fully functional γδ cells, with Vγ3Vδ1 receptors, are present by day 13 of murine fetal development, thymocytes bearing other specific γδ receptors arise in the days of gestation that follow (2). These subsets of $TCR\gamma\delta^+$ cells appear in an ordered sequence that correlates with the proximity of each V region to the Cγ locus. Interestingly, these different subsets of $TCR\gamma\delta^+$ cells are destined for export, each to a specific epithelial tissue in the periphery. Since $\gamma\delta^+$ thymocytes appear so early and prior to the appearance of the $\alpha\beta^+$ cells, it is reasonable to speculate that these cells may be required for the differentiation of the $\alpha\beta^+$ cells. The fact that thymocytes in *scid* mice never mature to the $CD4^+8^+$ stage and have no TCR-positive cells should be considered in this regard.

REQUIREMENT FOR POSITIVE SELECTION IN T-CELL MATURATION

As will be discussed in this session, further development of the αβ lineage to full functional maturity is a result of interactions between the TCR on the T cell and MHC molecules expressed by thymic stromal cells, an event termed positive selection (6). Prior to this event, a diverse array of clonotypic TCRs is generated by the rearrangement of random contributions of germline-encoded elements, V,Jα and V,D,Jβ. This diversity is increased by the imprecision in recombinational joining and the nonencoded nucleotides added at the junctions. Diversity is reduced, however, by selective mechanisms operating at the cellular level in the thymus. As a result of positive selection, the peripheral T-cell repertoire is biased toward recognition of foreign antigen presented by MHC molecules of the type expressed on thymic epithelial cells. This phenomenon was first demonstrated in experiments using hematopoietic chimeras and thymus-transplanted mice (4,6). The existence of positive selection is supported also by experiments in which antibodies to MHC and the CD4 or CD8 coreceptors were found to block T-cell development (7).

More recently, it became possible to follow the fate of individual TCR-bearing cells, either with antibodies directed at TCRs (of defined specificities), or through the use of TCR transgenic mice (6,8). In the transgenic mice, the introduction of already-rearranged TCR genes into the germ line suppressed the rearrangement of the endogenous TCR genes such that the majority of T cells express the transgenic TCR. With these mice, positive selection could be clearly demonstrated, since mature T cells with transgenic TCR developed *only* if the thymic epithelium expressed the appropriate allelic form of MHC. These systems had an advantage in that the fate of individual TCR-bearing thymocytes could be assessed directly without the added complications of priming by immunization or reading out reactivity by functional assays.

T-cell receptor transgenic mice also were used to show that the MHC class specificity of the TCR determines the commitment to the CD4 or CD8 lineage (8). These experimental results suggested a role for the CD4 and CD8 molecules in positive selection. Even more convincing were the experiments showing that in vivo treatment with antibodies to the accessory molecules blocks development of the appropriate MHC class–specific subset (anti-CD8 of class I and anti-CD4 of class II). These latter results strongly support the concept that the CD4 and CD8 molecules serve as coreceptors in the interaction that promotes selective maturation (3,7).

Although these various experimental approaches establish that T-cell maturation and MHC restriction are the result of positive selection in the thymus, there are many aspects of this process that are not, as yet, understood. We do not know what effect positive selection has on rearrangement of the TCR genes. While productive rearrangement and expression of TCRβ appears to suppress further rearrangement at the β locus, this does not appear to be the case for α. Could the positive selection event then serve as the signal to terminate TCR α gene rearrangement? Mature T cells recognize antigen as a processed peptide embedded in the MHC molecule of an antigen-presenting cell. Similarly, self-peptides may occupy the binding site of MHC on thymic epithelial cells. If so, non–MHC genes should affect selection. In this regard, we do not know the actual ligand on the epithelial cell and whether accessory and/or adherence molecules are involved in this process, or whether there are requirements for second signals. It is important also to understand if positive selection is a stage-specific event and, if so, the stage of T maturation at which this event occurs. Relevant to this issue is the actual mechanism by which the TCR specificity determines the selective expression of CD4 or CD8 (3).

To address these latter questions, our laboratory has produced transgenic mice which constitutively express CD8 on their T cells throughout development. By mating the CD8 transgenic to class I–specific TCRαβ transgenic mice, we have been able to examine the effect of ecotopic CD8 expression on the selection of the TCR. The results indicate that the class I–specific TCR is not expressed on mature CD4 cells (which bear also the transgenic CD8); moreover, positive selection of the receptor is substantially improved in the CD8 subset. These findings are consistent with a model for positive selection in which selection occurs at a stage in which both CD4 and CD8 are expressed. The data are consistent also with a model in which positive selection by class I MHC generates an instructive signal which directs the differentiation to the CD8 lineage.

That positive selection occurs at a double positive stage is supported by studies presented in this session. Patrice Hugo has examined the level of TCR αβ in the fetus and finds that low levels of TCRαβ first appear on day 16.5 on some $CD4^+8^+$ thymocytes (Abstract 1.39). By days 17–18, high levels of TCRαβ are expressed on a few of the $CD4^+8^+$ cells. Interestingly, this subset of $CD4^+8^+$ thymocytes with high levels of TCR expresses lower levels of either CD4 or CD8 compared to the TCR^{low} double positives. This conversion occurs without an increase in cell size. Most likely, this transitional population represents cells which have upregulated TCR as a result of positive selection. The associated downregulation of one or the other accessory molecule converts these cells to the $CD4^+8^-$ or $CD4^-8^+$ phenotype. It is these latter populations that develop immunocompetence and are exported to the periphery (5).

A transitional subpopulation is also demonstrated by Pamela Ohashi using class I (H-$2D^b$)–specific TCRαβ transgenic mice (Abstract 1.55). She observes a subset of

$CD4^+8^+$ thymocytes with intermediate levels of transgenic TCR in H-2^{bd} mice (which are able to select the transgenic receptor), but not in H-2^{dd} mice, the nonselecting haplotype. Taken together, these studies strongly support the concept that positive selection occurs at the $CD4^+8^+$ stage.

Interestingly, neither Hugo nor Ohashi and their collaborators find a change in cell size of the $CD4^+8^+$ cells which upregulate TCR. This observation is consistent with previous results showing that cell division occurs predominantly at the late $CD4^-8^-$ (IL-$2R^-$) and early $CD4^+8^+TCR^-$ stages (4,5). Thus, it would appear that positive selection is a signal for differentiation and further maturation without a requirement for cell division. The in vivo labeling studies carried out by Claude Penit indicate that incorporation of label occurs during the transitional $CD4^-8^-$ to $CD4^+8^+$ proliferative stage, and that the TCR^{high} cells persist longer in the labeled state (~3 days) than the TCR^{low} $CD4^+8^+$ thymocytes (Abstract 1.40). These data are consistent with a model in which positive selection rescues cells from a genetically programmed death. In nontransgenic mice, very few of the maturing cells should have the appropriate specificity to be rescued by this selective mechanism. Thus, in addition to the nonproductive TCR gene rearrangements and the effect of clonal deletion (discussed below), the failure to positively select many of the immature T cells could account for the inordinate amount of cell death which occurs in the thymus.

SELECTIVE MECHANISMS THAT PREVENT SELF-REACTIVITY

The early studies using chimeric mice, in which the fate of lymphocytes developing in an MHC-incompatible environment was assessed, demonstrated that tolerance to self-antigens could be acquired in the thymus (9–11). Once individual TCR could be followed directly using either anti-TCR antibodies or TCR transgenic mice, it was shown that T cells bearing self-reactive TCR are eliminated during development in the thymus (6). Moreover, the injection of neonates or fetal organ cultures with certain toxins or the appropriate cells could induce the deletion of specific T cells. These data established clonal deletion as a major mechanisms for inducing self-tolerance in the thymus. Other experiments suggested that clonal deletion can occur at the $CD4^+8^+$ stage and that the CD4/CD8 coreceptors are used in the interaction that induces deletion (4). This conclusion is supported also in Penit's and Hugo's presentations showing that $V\beta6^{high}$ ($CD4^+8^+$) cells are absent in Mls-1^a-bearing mice ($V\beta6^+$ cells are Mls-1^a reactive) (Abstracts 1.40 and 1.39).

It has been known for quite some time that self-tolerance can occur as a result of an interaction of a developing T cell with a bone marrow–derived hematopoietic cell. Results from our laboratory and others demonstrated that tolerance induction by clonal deletion is very efficiently mediated by bone marrow–derived cells. The question arises as to whether the epithelium can also induce deletion. The evidence on this question comes from either chimeric or transgenic mice with allo-MHC expressed only on the thymic epithelium and shows that clonal deletion by epithelial cells is quite poor (7). In a few cases, however, a reduction of the relevant receptor-bearing cells is observed. It has been suggested that this reduction may represent the deletion of only those clones with TCR of high affinity for epithelial antigens. Hopefully, the use of $TCR\alpha\beta$ transgenic mice may help to clarify these issues. What is important, nevertheless, is that even when clonal deletion fails to occur, T cells can be tolerized by another mechanism which induces clonal anergy. That is, those clones with specificity only for the epithelial-type antigens are not clonally deleted, but can be functionally inactivated. Thus, self-tolerance can be induced in the thymus by both clonal deletion and clonal anergy. While it is clear that bone marrow–derived hematopoietic cells can induce clonal deletion, the role of the thymic epithelium in tolerance induction by either clonal deletion or anergy needs further and more direct experimentation.

A number of critical questions remain unanswered on the subject of self-tolerance. Although it is well established that clonal deletion can occur in $CD4^+8^+$ thymocytes, it is possible that this event may operate also at a later stage. The stage at which clonal anergy occurs has not been determined (7). It is of interest to know whether other tolerance mechanisms operate in the thymus. With regard to the last issue, the downregulation of TCR and/or accessory molecules has been proposed as an additional mechanism for inducing tolerance (4).

DIFFERENTIAL SIGNALING AND DEVELOPMENTAL FATES

It is obvious from the previous discussion that two opposing forces are operating in the thymus. An interaction of a developing T cell with a bone marrow–derived hematopoietic cell induces clonal deletion, while an interaction with thymic epithelium leads to functional maturity (positive selection). Since both of the events can involve the same TCR and MHC, what are the variables that determine these two developmental fates? A number of possibilities exist. T-cell signaling may vary during the different stages as a result of changes in TCR density, the association of TCR-associated signaling components, participation of the coreceptor molecules (CD4 and CD8), etc. Therefore, if positive and negative selection are distinct stage-specific events, the quantity or quality of the signals delivered to the T cell may change.

Another consideration is that two cell types are inducing these different selection events. T-cell interaction with ligands on different stromal cells may involve unique accessory/adherence molecules, second signals, and/or presentation of tissue-specific peptides by MHC. Since distinct tissues are responsible for these selective events, and since T cells migrate through the thymus as they mature, the anatomical distribution of tissues (and peptides) could also be important in differential signaling.

As to whether positive and negative selection are ordered events, Ohashi's results show that in a TCRαβ transgenic mouse with specificity for either $Mls\text{-}1^a$ or LCMV, clonal deletion mediated by the two antigens occurs at different stages, one before and one after the upregulation of TCR density (Abstract 1.55). Although this difference in the stage of deletion could occur as a result of the differential affinity of the transgenic TCR for the two ligands, certainly the density of TCR, the stage at which the T cells encounter the antigen, the anatomical distribution of the antigen, or properties related to antigen processing and/or presentation may bear on these interactions.

From our knowledge of T-cell development, it is apparent that any T-cell precursor entering the thymus has a relatively low probability of differentiating to maturity. Only those clones that productively rearrange their TCR genes, fail to be clonally deleted, and have sufficiently reactivity to undergo positive selection will survive. Thus, the peripheral T-cell repertoire is dependent not only upon the production of a diverse set of T-cell receptors, but also on the successful interaction of these receptors with specific components of the thymic microenvironment.

ACKNOWLEDGMENTS

The author gratefully acknowledges the editorial assistance of Brenda Rae Marshall.

REFERENCES

1. Marrack P, Kappler J. The T cell receptor. Science 1987; 238:1073–9.
2. Raulet DH. The structure, function, and molecular genetics of the γ/δ T cell receptor. Ann Rev Immunol 1989; 7:175–207.
3. Robey EA, Fowlkes BJ, Pardoll DM. Molecular mechanisms for lineage commitment in T cell development. Semin Immunol 1990; 2:24–34.
4. Fowlkes BJ, Pardoll DM. Molecular and cellular events of T cell development. Adv Immunol 1989; 44:207–64.
5. Scollay R, Wilson A, D'Amico A, Kelly K, Egerton M, Pearse M, Wu L, Shortman K. Developmental status and reconstitution potential of subpopulations of murine thymocytes. Immunol Rev 1988; 104:81–120.
6. Blackman M, Kappler J, Marrack P. The role of the T cell receptor in positive and negative selection of developing T cells. Science 1990; 248:1335–41.
7. Ramsdell F, Fowlkes BJ. Clonal deletion versus clonal anergy: the role of the thymus in inducing self tolerance. Science 1990; 248:1342–8.
8. von Boehmer H, Kisielow P. Self-nonself discrimination by T cells. Science 1990; 248:1369–73.
9. Schwartz RH. The role of gene products of the major histocompatibility complex in T cell activation and cellular interactions. In: Paul WE (ed). *Fundamental Immunology*. New York, Raven Press, 1984, pp. 379–438.
10. Sprent J, Lo D, Gao E-K, Ron Y. T cell selection in the thymus. Immunol Rev 1988; 101:171–90.
11. Schwartz RH. Acquisition of immunologic self-tolerance. Cell 1989; 57:1073–81.

22
Growth and Maturation Requirements for CD7⁺ Early Human Thymocytes

M. Djavad Mossalayi, Christine Fourcade, Ali H. Dalloul, and Patrice Debré
Laboratoire d'Immunologie, Hôpital Pitié-Salpêtrière, Paris, France

INTRODUCTION

$CD7^+2^-3^-4^-8^-$ cells are known to be earliest identifiable T-cell precursors (1–3). We recently isolated these precursors with more than 90% purity from both human thymic and bone marrow cells (3). Of interest, they are able to acquire mature T-cell antigen expression following appropriate in vitro culturing (1–4). Meanwhile, factors necessary for their autorenewal and/or differentiation remained ill defined. In the present study, we attempted to assay effect of interleukins (IL) 1, 2,3, and 4 and recombinant soluble CD23 (rsCD23) (5) on early T-cell development. Purified $CD7^+$ precursors were thus incubated with one or a combination of these molecules. Mitogenic effect was studied by thymidine uptake and cell differentiation was quantified by surface markers as well as sensitivity to the mitogenic effect of CD3 or CD2 monoclonal antibodies (MAbs). Our data present evidence of distinguished effects of these cytokine on $CD7^+$ precursors.

MATERIALS AND METHODS

Monoclonal Antibodies

Monoclonal antibodies to the following antigens were used: CD3, CD4, CD8, CD25, CD7, CD3/TCR αβ (WT31) (Ortho Pharmaceutical, Raritan, New Jersey); CD23 (Immunotech, Marseille, France); TCR αβ, TCR δ, and comitogenic CD_{I+III} (2). Cell markers are evaluated by the indirect immunofluorescence method using a FACStar (Becton Dickinson, Grenoble, France).

Cell Cultures

Purified $CD7^+2^-$ precursors were obtained from neonatal thymic fragments as detailed elsewhere (3). They were then incubated in MacCoy's 5A medium containing 20% human

Table 1 Effect of Various Cytokines on CD7⁺ Prothymocyte Proliferation

Cytokines	—	rIL-1	rIL-2	rIL-3	rIL-4	rsCD23
CPM × 10^3	1.7*	2.1	2.0	5.9	1.9	1.7

Thymidine uptake by 4.10^4 purified $CD7^+2^-$ cells following 4-day incubation with various cytokines. Mean of 8 experiments (SE<10%).

AB serum and one or a combination of rsCD23 (25 ng/ml) (5), rIL-1β (50 U/ml), rIL-2 (100 U/ml), rIL-3 (10 U/ml), rIL-4 (100 U/ml) (Glaxo, Geneva, Switzerland), IOB8 (CD23, μg/ml), IOT14 (CD25, 25 μg/ml). The cells were then tested for their surface markers. For direct effect of above cytokines on $CD7^+$ cell proliferation, ^{3}HTdr was added at day 3 and radioactivity measured 24 hr later. Treated cells were also assayed for their ability to proliferate in response to rIL-2 and CD3 (25 μg/ml) or $CD2_{I+III}$ (1/400 ascite) MAbs (2).

RESULTS

IL-3 Significantly Induces $CD7^+$ Cell Proliferation

Purified $CD7^+$ cells were incubated for 72 hr in presence of various cytokines. ^{3}HTdr was then added and thymidine uptake measured 24 hr later. As shown in Table 1, only cells incubated with IL-3 showed significant mitogenesis ($p < 0.005$) as compared to other culture conditions.

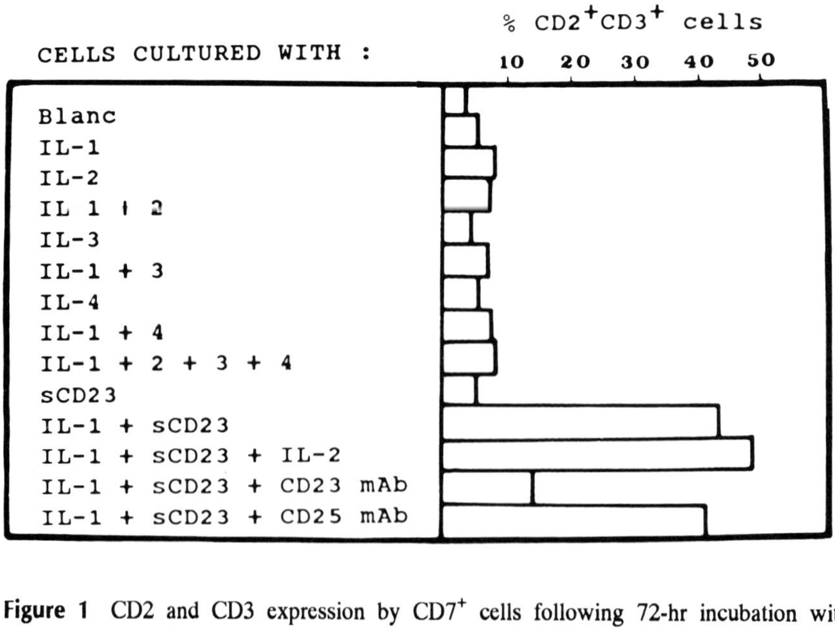

Figure 1 CD2 and CD3 expression by $CD7^+$ cells following 72-hr incubation with various cytokines (see methods).

Table 2 Effect of IL-1 + sCD23 Treatment on Cell Responses to Various T-Cell Mitogens

Cells pretreated with	Postincubation factors						
	—	IL-2	IL-4	CD2	CD2 + IL-2	CD3	CD3 + IL-2
Non	1.6*	1.9	1.8	2.0	2.2	1.9	1.9
IL-1 + sCD3	1.4	3.1	4.2	3.1	10.5	2.2	7.8

$CD7^+$ cells were incubated 24 hr with/without IL-1 + sCD23, washed thereafter, and postincubated 48 hr in the presence of various T-cell mitogens. CPM $\times$ $10^3/4.10^4$ cells.

IL-1 + sCD23 Induced Surface Mature T-Cell Antigen Acquirement by $CD7^+$ Cells

Prothymocytes were incubated 48 hr with various cytokines as above and their surface markers assayed thereafter. As shown on Figure 1, only cells incubated with Il-1 + sCD23 showed significant acquisition of CD2 and CD3 expression ($p < 0.001$). $CD2^+3^+$ progeny were TCR $\alpha\beta^+$, $HNK1^-$, expressed CD8 (55%) or CD4 (37%), and only 4% were $CD4^+8^+$. Sequential studies indicate that IL-1 induces $CD7^+$ cell responsiveness to rsCD23 (data not shown).

Acquisition of Mature T-cell Functions by $CD7^+$ Precursors

As IL-1 + sCD23 induced CD2 and CD3 expression by $CD7^+$ cells, we subsequently investigated whether this antigen expression is functional. IL-1 + sCD23 treated cells were thus washed and incubated with mitogenic CD2 and CD3 MAbs, IL-2, and/or IL-4. ^{3}HTdr was added 48 hr later and thymidine uptake measured the day after. As shown in Table 2, by contrast to untreated precursors, cells incubated with IL-1 + sCD23 could respond to CD2 and CD3 triggering in presence of IL-2. IL-4 have low but significant mitogenic effect.

DISCUSSION

The above data indicate that IL-3 can induce proliferation of human $CD7^+2^-$ prothymocytes. Of interest, surface phenotype of prothymocytes was not altered following this treatment. Such an IL-3 effect was previously reported in an early human T-cell leukemia (6). Together, these findings suggest that IL-3 is an autorenewal factor for $CD7^+$ precursors. Interleukins -2 and -4 only promoted the proliferation of more mature $CD2^+$ cells. Our results also confirmed the ability of sCD23 to induce differentiation of IL-1–treated $CD7^+$ precursors (2). CD23 is the low-affinity receptor for immunoglobulin E (IgE) ($IgER_{II}$) (7). It is expressed on B cells, monocytes/macrophages, eosinophils, platelets, and epidermal Langerhans cells (7). Surface CD23 is cleaved into soluble fragments (sCD23) following an autoproteolytic process (7). This sCD23 has various biological activities such as the control of IgE synthesis, induction of B- and T-cell proliferation, and the differentiation of B and T cell precursors (7,8). We have recently shown that rsCD23 also promotes myeloid colony generation by early $CD34^+$ precursors (9). Together, these data suggest that sCD23 has high differentiating activity on various, IL-1–induced early hematopoietic stem cells. The physiological significance of these data remains to be investigated. Recent data from our group (see A. H. Dalloul et al., p. 37, this volume) showed that cultured epithelial cells derived from human thymus are able to secrete IL-1, IL-3, and sCD23. Direct evidence of the in situ presence of these cytokines and TCR specificity of in vitro matured thymocytes need more studies. However, these data suggest a direct role of soluble factors in the differentiation and/or proliferation of early thymocytes.

REFERENCES

1. Haynes BF, Martin ME, Key H, Kurtzberg J. Early events in human T cell ontogeny: phenotypic characterization and immunohistological localization of T cell precursors in early human fetal tissues. J Exp Med 1988; 168:1061–1080.
2. Mossalayi MD, Lecron JC, Dalloul AH, Sarfati M, Bertho JM, Hofstetter H, Delespesse G, Debré P. Soluble CD23 (FcERII) and interleukin 1 synergistically induce early human thymocyte maturation. J Exp Med 1990; 171:959–964.
3. Mossalayi MD, Dalloul AH, Bertho JM, Lecron JC, Goube de Laforest P, Debré P. In vitro differentiation and proliferation of purified human thymic and bone marrow $CD7^+$ $CD2^-$ T-cell precursors. Exp Hematol 1990; 18:326–331.
4. Bertho JM, Mossalayi MD, Dalloul AH, Mouterde G, Debré P. Isolation of an early T-cell precursors (CFU-TL) from human bone marrow. Blood 1990; 75:1064–1068.
5. Ludin C, Hofstetter H, Sarfati M, Levy CA, Suter U, Alaimo D, Kilcherr G, Frost H, Delespesse G. Cloning and expression of the cDNA coding for a human lymphocyte IgE receptor. EMBO J 1987; 6:109–114.
6. Schneider EM, Lorentz I, Leoppold S, Zischer H, Clark SC. Generation of mature $CD3^+$ and T cell receptor $(TCR)^+$ T cells from a leukemic analogue of the putative human stem cell by T cell conditioned medium containing IL-3, IL-2 and GM-CSF. Leukemia 1988; 2:282–289.
7. Delespesse G, Sarfati M, Hofstetter H. Human IgE-binding factors. Immunol Today 1989; 10:159–164.
8. Armitage RJ, Goff LK, Beverley PCL. Expression and functional role of CD23 on T cells. Eur J Immunol 1989; 19:31–35.
9. Mossalayi MD, Arock M, Bertho JM, Blanc C, Dalloul AH, Hofstetter H, Sarfati M, Delespesse G, Debré P. Proliferation of early human myeloid precursors induced by interleukin-1 and recombinant soluble CD23. Blood 1990; 75:1924–1927.

23

Evidence of In Vitro Maturation of Murine Single Positive Thymocytes from Double Negative Precursors with Interleukin-2 Receptors

Myra Small[1] and Rochelle A. Diamond[2]
[1]*Sackler School of Medicine, Tel Aviv University, Ramat Aviv, Israel;*
[2]*California Institute of Technology, Pasadena, California*

INTRODUCTION

Study of in vitro maturation of thymocyte precursors on thymic stromal monolayers has long been the hope of immunologists wishing to unravel some of the complexities of intrathymic events and lineage relationships. In organ cultures, where all the components are supplied in the correct locations, such maturation has been shown to occur (1). We wished to add exogenous precursors to primary heterogeneous stromal cell cultures (2,3). As a source of precursors we have investigated thymocytes with interleukin-2 (IL-2) receptors since evidence has suggested that they give rise to at least some mature T cells (4–6). Although one-step panning on 7D4 antibody allowed us to isolate a 90% double negative (DN) population, we aimed at better purification. This was achieved by complement elimination that was followed by antibody panning (>97% DN). The precursor cells were then added to primary cultures of thymic stromal cells in order to determine whether antigens characteristic of mature T cells could develop in culture.

MATERIALS AND METHODS

C57Bl mice were used at 4–12 weeks of age. The antibodies used were: RL 172.4, antimouse CD4 (cells from ATCC); 3.155, antimouse CD8 (cells from ATCC); PE-L3T4, antimouse CD4 (Becton Dickinson); FITC-Ly2, antimouse CD8 (Becton Dickinson); 500A2, antimouse CD3, (a hamster IgG from Dr. J. Allison); FITC-goat antihamster Ig (a purified goat IgG from Oganon Tecknika); 7D4, antimouse IL-2Rα (cells from ATCC).

Cultures of thymic stromal cells were pregrown for 2 weeks, essentially as described previously (2,3), but in D-valine MEM (Sigma) with considerably lower levels of amino acids than the DMEM used before, and perhaps this underlies the poorer than usual epithelial cell growth and more abundant macrophages. In an attempt to limit the growth of bone marrow–derived stromal cells as well as any residual monolayer-derived thymocytes,

2-deoxyguanosine at 1.35 mM was added to the medium (7), either after a week or from time zero. The medium was deoxyguanosine-free for the last 1–3 days. Indomethacin at 2×10^{-5} M was added 1 day before the thymocyte inoculum. Cultures were grown in 5% CO_2. Control 3T3 fibroblasts were obtained from Dr. B. Wold, California Institute of Technology, Pasadena. Panning dishes (Falcon 1008) were prepared with 7D4 ascites fluid at 1:1000 in phosphate-buffered saline (PBS) for 2 hr at room temperature. Free antibody was decanted, 0.25% BSA in PBS left overnight at 4°, and dishes were washed before use with panning medium (PM=calcium- and magnesium-free HBSS + 0.25% BSA + 5 mM sodium azide). Double negative thymocytes were prepared from thymuses carefully cleaned of lymph nodes and blood, essentially as described previously (6). Two or three rounds of complement lysis were performed with optimal concentrations of RL 172.4, 3.155, and baby rabbit C′ (Pel Freeze) for 45 min at 37°. Viable cells were recovered on gradients of Ficoll-metrizoate and washed. Double negative cells in 1 ml PM were panned for 1 hr at 4° with rocking. Unattached cells were removed by 10 washes with PM. 0.04% EDTA in PBS was added for 15 min at 37°, the cells were detached by vigorous pipetting, spun and resuspended in RPMI + 5% FCS. Aliquots were saved for antibody staining and the rest added (with indomethacin) to thymic stromal cultures or control dishes, usually at 2×10^{6} cells/culture (<1% of original cell numbers). Within 4 hr most thymocytes adhered to stromal cells with epithelial morphology. They were harvested from the upper surface at specified times by swirling and decanting of the plates followed by addition of calcium and magnesium-free PBS for 30 min and additional swirling. Antibody staining was performed on about 10^{5} cells in 50 μl essentially as described (8). For two-color staining of CD4/CD8, directly conjugated antibodies were used. $1–2\times10^{4}$ formalin-fixed cells were analyzed on an Ortho System 50H cell sorter with a 5W argon laser exciting at 488 nm. Cell populations to be analyzed were selected in terms of forward scatter vs 90° scatter. The boundaries for cells expressing CD4 (PE), CD8 (FITC) or CD3 (+2nd antibody-FITC) were set according to the fluorescence of control samples from the same day.

RESULTS AND DISCUSSION

The population of precursor cells generated in this study can be seen in Figs. 1 and 2 to be $CD4^-$, $CD8^-$, $CD3^-$. The cells adhering to 7D4-coated dishes were >90% IL-2R^+, >90% Thy-1^+, and within 20 hr virtually all of the cells incorporated [^{3}H]thymidine when checked by autoradiography. By isolating the IL-2R^+ subset of DN thymocytes we sought to obtain early thymocytes (4–6) without contamination by mast cells, macrophages, etc., and without the DN subset that has been found to acquire antigens overnight in the absence of a thymic environment (9). Although the significance of constitutively expressed IL-2 receptors is not clear at present, scattered positive cells are fund in the adult thymus (10).

As can be seen in Fig. 1, development in terms of high levels of CD3 expression was detected when the precursors were cocultivated with primary cultures of thymic stromal cells. High levels of CD3 were not seen when the cells were cultured on a 3T3 monolayer. Since cells also burrow under the monolayer or remain bound we cannot attach quantitative significance to the percentage of cells that expressed this receptor-related antigen. In initial experiments precursor cells attached mainly to large stromal cells at the periphery of the cultures. After addition of indomethacin, however, precursors were bound throughout the culture, suggesting interference by prostaglandins in the vicinity of macrophages. Morphologically the stromal cells that bound the precursors resembled those identified elsewhere as cortical epithelial cells (3).

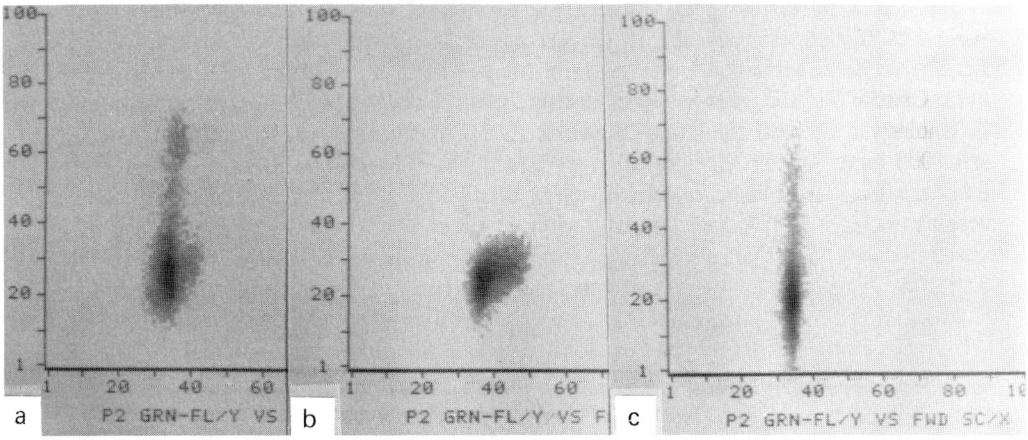

Figure 1 CD3 antigen in (a) normal thymocytes (b) 7D4$^+$DN precursors and (c) precursors cocultured 3 days with thymic stromal cultures.

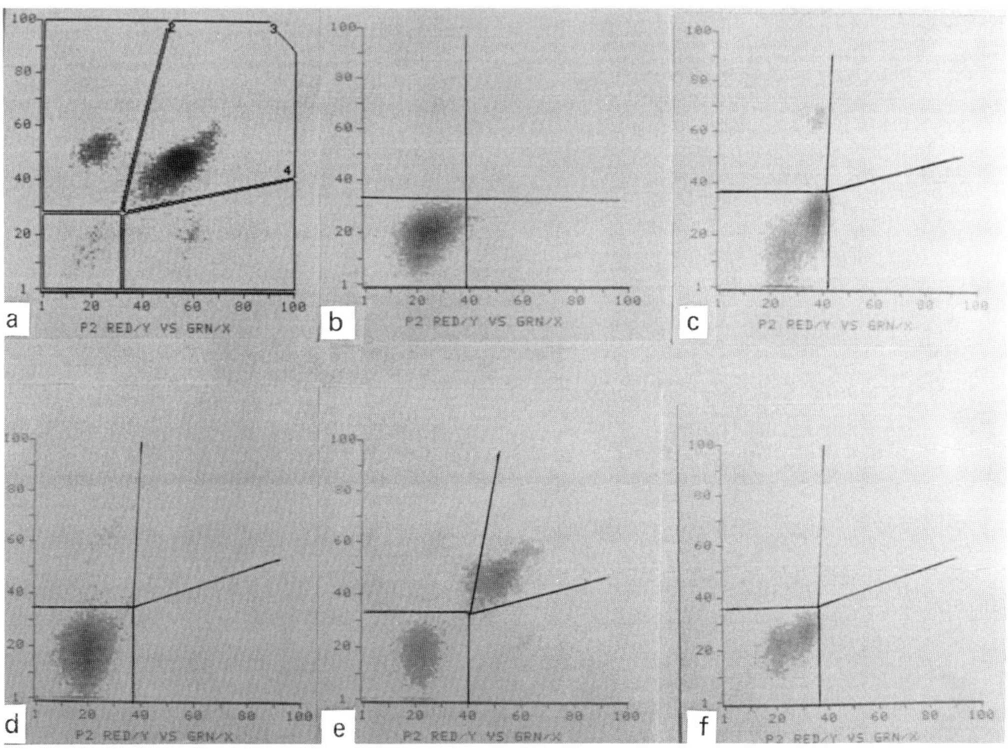

Figure 2 CD4 and CD8 antigens in (a) normal thymocytes, (b) 7D4$^+$DN precursors, (c, d, and e) precursors cocultured 3 days with thymic stromal cultures, or (f) precursors cocultured 3 days with 3T3 cells.

In Fig. 2, we see that cells with a $CD4^+$ SP phenotype developed when the precursors were cocultivated with primary thymic stromal cultures. This was apparent at 1 or 3 days but not when the same cells were cultured 1 day without a monolayer or 3 days with 3T3 cells. Double positive cells were also detected but surprisingly the SP population appeared to be derived directly from the DN cells. Thus, in spite of many results interpreted as evidence for DN→DP→SP (9), it seems that a DN→$SPCD4^+$ pathway is also possible. This idea has recently been taken one step further in an elegant communication by Palacios et al. (12). Using a line of thymic precursor cells, these authors found that the cells could mature to $CD4^+$SP upon a stromal epithelial line, whereas they became DP, $CD4^+$, and $CD8^+$ in heterogeneous stromal cultures, thus pointing to the importance of the stromal microenvironment in determining the outcome. While some $CD8^+$ SP cells have been found by several groups to be immature (9), this has not been reported for $CD4^+$SP, although heterogeneity of this population has been suggested (9). In a continuation of our approach (M. Small and I. L. Weissman, unpublished results) it has been possible to check two additional important points by using three-color FACS analysis of live cells. By propidium iodide exclusion, viable cells appear to be gaining mature phenotype in culture. These cells of mature phenotype have also been shown to be derived from the immature precursors by use of congenic mice with the Thy-1 locus differing from that of the strain used in the stromal cultures. We should also mention recent reports of others describing stages of T-cell development in vitro from bone marrow precursors (13), and also the importance of bone marrow–derived stromal cells in T-cell development (14).

We consider the present experiments as preliminary. They suggest that IL-$2R^+$, $CD4^-$, $CD8^-$, $CD3^-$ thymocytes can become $CD3^+$Hi and $CD4^+$SP within a thymic microenvironment in culture. In addition it appears that $CD4^+$SP can be derived directly from DN precursors.

NOTE ADDED IN PROOF

Patrice Hugo et al. (this volume) have detected $CD4^+CD8^-CD3^-$ intermediate thymocytes in vivo. Thus the $CD4^+$SP cells obtained here could be either $CD4^+CD8^-CD3^+$ or $CD4^+CD8^-CD3^-$ together with $CD4^+CD8^+CD3^+$ or $CD4^-CD8^-CD3^+$ cells. Current experiments (M. Small and I. L. Weissman, unpublished results) indicate that cells with all four of these phenotypes can develop in the thymic stromal cultures.

REFERENCES

1. Ceredig R. Differentiation potential of 14-day fetal mouse thymocytes in organ cultures. J. Immunol. 1988; 141:355–362.
2. Small M., Barr-Nea L., Aronson M. Culture of thymic epithelial cells from mice and age-related studies on the growing cells. Eur. J. Immunol. 1984; 14:936–942.
3. Small M., Van Ewijk W., Gown A.M., Rouse R.V. Identification of subpopulations of mouse thymic epithelial cells in culture. Immunology 1989; 68:371–377.
4. Shimonkevitz R., Husmann, L., Bevan M., Crispe I. Transient expression of IL-2 receptor precedes the differentiation of immature thymocytes. Nature 1987; 329:157–159.
5. Jenkinson E.J., Kingston R., Owen J.J.T. Importance of IL-2 receptors in intra-thymic generation of cells expressing T-cell receptors. Nature 1987; 329:160–162.
6. Boyer P.D., Diamond R.A., Rothenberg E.V. Changes in inducibility of IL-2 receptor α chain and T cell receptor expression during thymocyte differentiation in the mouse. J. Immunol. 1989; 142:4121–4130.

7. Jenkinson E.J., Franchi L.F., Kingston R., Owen J.J.T. Effect of deoxyguanosine on lymphopoiesis in developing thymus rudiments in vitro. Eur. J. Immunol. 1982; 12:583–587.
8. Boyer P .D., Rothenberg E.V. IL-2 Receptor inducibility is blocked in cortical-type thymocytes. J. Immunol. 1988; 140:2886–2892.
9. Fowlkes B.J., Pardoll D.M. Molecular and cellular events of T-cell development. Adv. Immunol. 1989; 44:207–264.
10. Ceredig R., Lowenthal J.W., Nabholtz M., MacDonald H.R. Expression of interleukin-2 receptors as a differentiation marker on intrathymic stem cells. Nature 1985; 314:98–100.
11. Havran W., Poenie M., Kimura J., Tsien R., Weiss A., Allison J. Expression and function of the CD3-antigen receptor on murine $CD4^{+}8^{+}$ thymocytes. Nature 1987; 330:170–173.
12. Palacios R., Studer S., Samaridis J., Pelkonen J. Thymic epithelial cells induce in vitro differentiation of PRO-T lymphocyte clones into TCRαβ/T3+ and TCRγδ/T3+ cells. EMBO J. 1989; 8:4053–4063.
13. Deugnier M-A., Imhof B.A., Bauvois B., Dunon D., Denoyelle M., Thiery J-P. Characterization of rat T cell precursors sorted by chemotactic migration toward thymotaxin. Cell 1989; 56:1073–1083.
14. Papiernik M., Penit C., El Rouby S. Control of prothymocyte proliferation by thymic accessory cells. Eur. J. Immunol. 1987; 17:1303–1310.

24

$CD4^+CD8^-CD3^-$ Thymocytes

An Alternative Route to Generate Double-Positive, $CD4^+CD8^+$ Thymocytes

P. Hugo,[1,2] G. A. Waanders,[1] R. Scollay,[2] K. Shortman,[2] and R. L. Boyd[1]

[1]*Monash Medical School, Prahran, Victoria, Australia;*
[2]*The Walter and Eliza Hall Institute of Medical Research, Parkville, Victoria, Australia*

INTRODUCTION

Careful analysis of T-cell differentiation events with multiple markers has allowed the identification of some small but distinct thymocyte subsets, such as $CD4^-CD8^+$ cells which are CD3 negative (1–3). This established that the CD4/CD8 markers alone were insufficient to define mature T cells. This $CD4^-CD8^+$ subset was shown to give rise, both in vitro (2,4) and in vivo (5,6), to $CD4^+CD8^+$ cells, and led investigators to seek a $CD4^+CD8^-CD3^-$ subset. However, this population was missed (1,2,4,6–8) or not clearly delineated (3). In this report, we readdress the existence of such a $CD4^+CD8^-CD3^-$subset.

MATERIALS AND METHODS

Mice

Female mice 4–8 weeks of age were used. Embryos were aged by a vaginal plug assessment.

Multicolor Flow Cytometric Analysis

Cells were stained and analyzed by a protocol described elsewhere (9,10).

Labeling of Outer Cortical Thymocytes

Thymuses were dipped into RPMI-1640, 10% FCS, 200 μg/ml Hoechst 33342 (Calbiochem-Behring, USA) for 30 min at 23°C and then washed (3). Cells were then stained with antibodies and analyzed with a FACS II (B.D.). Outer cortical cells were detected as bright blue-fluorescent cells.

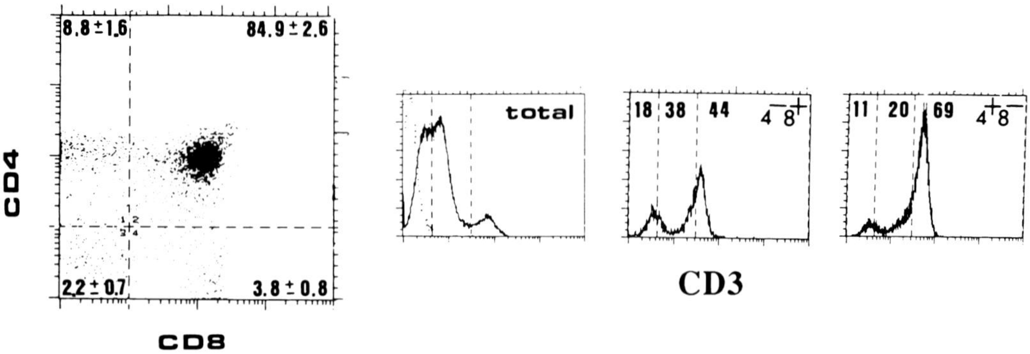

Figure 1 Existence of $CD4^+CD8^-CD3^-$ thymocytes. Adult CBA thymocytes were stained with αCD3, αCD4, and αCD8 antibodies. The plots show CD4 vs CD8 expression (left box) and CD3 expression on gated $CD4^-CD8^+$ or $CD4^+CD8^-$ subsets. Profiles of total cells labeled with FITC-conjugated alone (.......) or anti-CD3 + conjugate (———). The data are from 12 experiments.

RESULTS AND DISCUSSION

$CD4^+CD8^-CD3^-$ Thymocytes in Adult CBA Mice

Staining for CD4, CD8, and CD3 allowed us to visualize a proportion (18.4% ± 5.6) of immature (CD3-negative) cells in the $CD4^-CD8^+$ subset. A significant, although lower, proportion (10.9% ± 2.7) of CD3-negative cells was also found among the $CD4^+CD8^-$ subset (Fig. 1), but the $CD4^+CD8^-CD3^-$ were more numerous than the $CD4^-CD8^+CD3^-$ cells (1 vs 0.7% of the total thymocytes) in the CBA thymus.

Strain Variation of $CD4^+CD8^-CD3^-$ Cells

It was proposed that the $CD4^+CD8^-CD3^-$ subset varies from strain-to-strain (14). We found indeed a marked variation of the $CD4^+CD8^-CD3^-/CD4^-CD8^+CD3^-$ ratio being 0.2±0.1, 0.4±0.2, 0.3±0.1, and 1.6±0.6 in C57BL/10, Balb/c, DBA-2, and CBA/H, respectively, explaining the difficulty in seeing such a subset in some strains (1,2,4,6–8).

$CD4^+CD8^-CD3^-$ Thymocytes Are Blastic Outer Cortical Cells

It is tempting to ascribe the same precursor status to this novel $CD4^+CD8^-CD3^-$ subset as the $CD4^-CD8^+CD3^-$ cells. As such, we would expect the immature $CD4^+$ cells to be blastic and outer cortical (3,6,11). our results fulfill this expectation, since they were found be blastic and clearly distinguishable from their mature (CD3-positive) counterpart (Fig. 2). They were also found to be highly concentrated in the outer cortex (Fig. 3).

Phenotype of $CD4^+CD8^-CD3^-$ Thymocytes

The global phenotype of immature $CD4^+$ cells was shown to be different from $CD4^-CD8^-$ CD3-negative (Table 1), showing that CD4 expression is not the only distinguishing marker between these two subsets. The immature CD4-positive cells were identical to the immature CD8-positive cells for several markers tested.

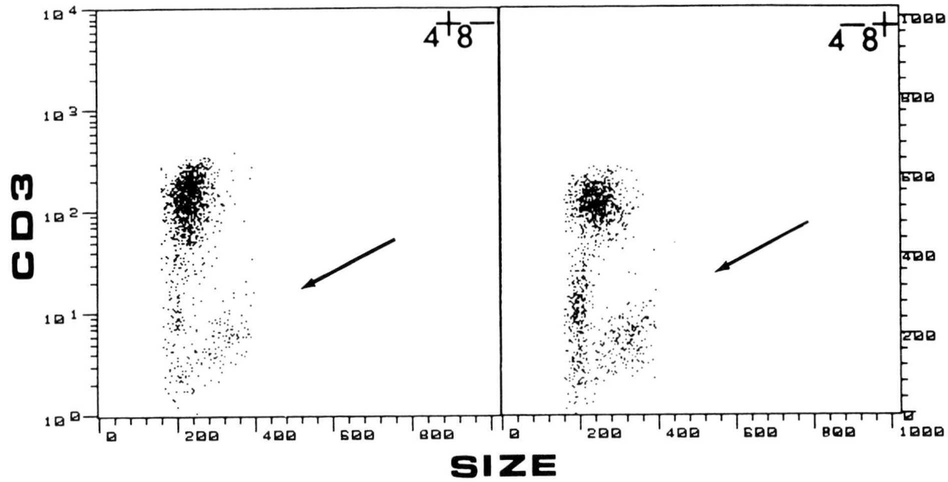

Figure 2 Cell size of the $CD4^+CD8^-CD3^-$ thymocytes. Forward light scatter, related to cell size, was determined for $CD4^+CD8^-$ and $CD4^-CD8^+$ subsets and plotted versus their CD3 expression. Arrows indicate the $CD3^-$ immature cells.

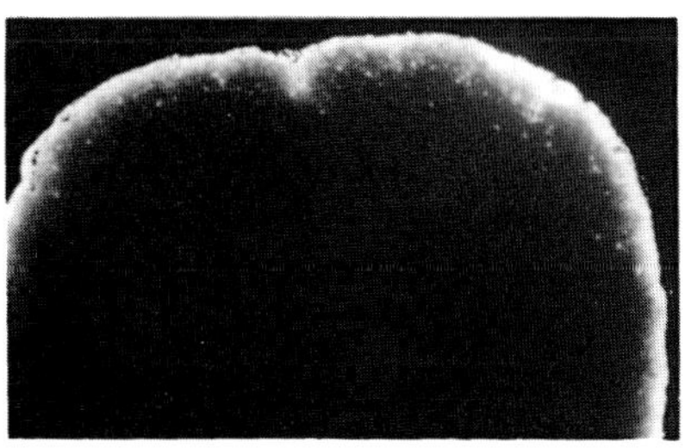

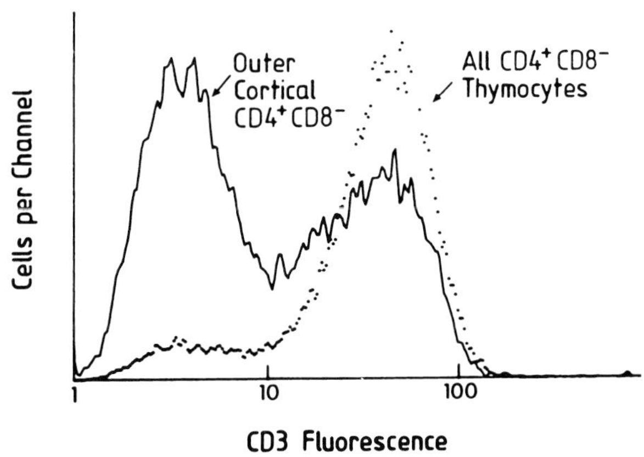

Figure 3 In situ localization of the $CD4^+CD8^-CD3^-$ cells. Thymic lobes were immersed in Hoechst 33342 (left panel), and $CD8^-$ cells were isolated and labeled for CD4 and CD3. CD3 profiles of gated Hoechst 33342^+ outer cortical (———) and total $CD4^+CD8^-$ cells (.......) are presented.

Table 1 Phenotype of $CD4^+CD8^-CD3^-$ Cells

Marker	$CD4^-CD8^-CD3^-$	$CD4^+CD8^-CD3^-$	$CD4^-CD8^+CD3^-$
Thy-1	low to high	high	high
HSA	low to high	high	high
CD5	– to low	low	low
LFA-1	– to high	high	high
IL-2Rα	– or +	–	–
Pgp-1	– or high	–	–
MEL-14	–	– to low	– to low
H-2K	low or high	– to low	– to low
MTS-35[a]	high	high	high

Adult CBA thymocytes were assessed for the expression of several markers by five-colour analysis. (a) Marker for immature thymocytes (Godfrey et al., in preparation).

Ontogeny of $CD4^+CD8^-CD3^-$ Cells

The putative precursor activity of the $CD4^+CD8^-CD3^-$ cells predicts that they appear before $CD4^+CD8^+$ cells during fetal life, as do the $CD4^-CD8^+CD3^-$ cells (12). Indeed, the $CD4^+CD8^-CD3^-$ cells were detected before the $CD4^+CD8^+CD3^-$ cells (days 15 and 16, respectively) (Table 2), as were the $CD4^-CD8^+CD3^-$ cells, although with slightly different kinetics.

Kinetics of $CD4^+CD8^-CD3^-$ Cells After Cortisone Treatment

The $CD4^-CD8^+CD3^-$ cells are cortisone-sensitive (3), and we noted here that the $CD4^+CD8^-CD3^-$ subset also disappeared after cortisone treatment (Table 3). Appreciable numbers of immature $CD4^+$ and $CD8^+$ cells were seen at days 5–6 posttreatment, and at days 6–7 for the $CD4^+CD8^+CD3^-$ cells. Thus, the kinetics of both immature ($CD4^+$/$CD8^+$) subsets correlated well with the subsequent production of $CD4^+CD8^+CD3^-$ cells, as recently reported during thymic reconstitution after irradiation (13).

Table 2 Ontogeny of Immature $CD4^+$ Cells

	Days of Fetal Life				
	15	16	16.5	17	18
$CD4^-8^-3^-$	92.8[a]	73.5	35.3	21.3	8.4
$CD4^-8^+3^-$	0.3	9.6	23.9	7.6	3.3
$CD4^+8^-3^-$	4.0	4.9	4.0	6.0	2.3
$CD4^+8^+3^-$	0	8.0	31.1	55.3	36.3

[a]%; values are the mean of three experiments.

Table 3 Appearance of Immature CD4$^+$ Thymocytes After Cortisone Treatment

	Day post-treatment								
	2	4	5	6	7	8	9	10	14
CD4$^-$8$^-$3$^-$	0.8[a]	0.3	0.1	17	11	14	3.5	4.6	28.2
CD4$^-$8$^+$3$^-$	0.2	0	0.5	8.7	4.9	4.0	6.3	5.5	7.5
CD4$^+$8$^-$3$^-$	0	0	0.3	6.5	6.2	9.1	15	6.4	11.3
CD4$^+$8$^+$3$^-$	0	0	1.4	4.5	7.2	112	196	360	693

Mice received i.p. 125 mg of dexamethasone per kg body weight.
[a]Cells ($\times 10^{-5}$)/thymus obtained from two experiments.

CONCLUSIONS

We have demonstrated the existence of CD4$^+$CD8$^-$CD3$^-$ cells in the murine thymus. Since they were outer cortical blastic cells, and their phenotype and kinetics during ontogeny were similar to that of CD4$^-$CD8$^+$CD3$^-$ cells, they could be considered as a transient precursor. This is supported by the recent demonstration that both subsets give rise to CD4$^+$CD8$^+$ cells in culture (13,14). Therefore, it appears that not only the CD4$^-$CD8$^+$CD3$^-$ route, but also the CD4$^+$CD8$^-$CD3$^-$ route can be taken by the CD4$^-$CD8$^-$CD3$^-$ cells to generate CD4$^+$CD8$^+$ cells, while we and others (13) have shown strong strain preferences toward one or the other pathways.

ACKNOWLEDGMENTS

We thank Becton Dickinson who sponsored the presentation of these results. P. Hugo is supported by a postdoctoral fellowship from the MRC of Canada. This work was supported by the NH and MRC Australia (No. 860396), NIH USA (No. AI17310) and Anti-Cancer Council of Victoria (No. 131658).

REFERENCES

1. Paterson DJ, Williams AF. An intermediate cell in thymocyte differentiation that expresses CD8 but not CD4 antigen. J Exp Med 1987; 166:1603–8.
2. MacDonald HR, Budd RC, Howe RC, A CD3$^-$ subset of CD4$^-$8$^+$ thymocytes: A rapidly cycling intermediate in the generation of CD4$^+$8$^+$. Eur J Immunol 1988; 18:519–23.
3. Shortman K, Wilson A, Egerton M, Pearse M, Scollay R. Immature CD4$^-$CD8$^+$ murine thymocytes. Cell Immunol 1988; 113:462–77.
4. Nikolic-Zugic J, Moore MW, Bevan MJ. Characterization of the subset of immature thymocytes which can undergo rapid in vitro differentiation. Eur J Immunol 1989; 19:649–53.
5. Nikolic-Zugic J, Bevan MJ. Thymocytes expressing CD8 differentiate into CD4$^+$ cells following intrathymic injection. PNAS 1988; 85:8633–37.
6. Guidos CJ, Weissman IL, Adkins B. Intrathymic maturation of murine T lymphocytes from CD8$^+$ precursors. PNAS 1989; 86:7542–46.
7. Boyer PD, Diamond RA, Rothenberg EV. Changes in inducibility of IL-2 receptor α-chain and T cell-receptor expression during thymocyte differentiation in the mouse. J Immunol 1989; 142:4121–30.

8. Pénit C, Vasseur F. Sequential events in thymocyte differentiation and thymus regeneration revealed by a combination of bromodeoxyuridine DNA labeling and anti-mitotic drug treatment. J Immunol 1988; 140:3315–23.
9. Hugo P, Waanders GA, Scollay R, Shortman K, Boyd RL. Ontogeny of a novel $CD4^+CD8^-CD3^-$ thymocyte subpopulation; a comparison with $CD4^-CD8^+CD3^-$ thymocytes. Int Immunol 1990; 2:209–18.
10. Hugo P, Waanders GA, Boyd RL, Scollay R. The $CD4^+CD8^+CD3^{high}$ thymocytes represent a cortisone-resistant subset differentiating converting into mature T-cells. In: *Lymphatic Tissues and In Vivo Immune Responses*. Ezine S., Berrih-Aknin S., Imhof B. (eds.). Plenum Press, New York, 1991, pp. 155–9.
11. Pénit C, Vasseur F. Cell proliferation and differentiation in the fetal and early postnatal mouse thymus. J Immunol 1989; 142:3369–77.
12. Kisielow P, Leiserson W, von Boehmer H. Differentiation of thymocytes in fetal organ culture: Analysis of phenotypic changes accompanying the appearance of cytolytic and interleukin 2-producing cells. J Immunol 1984; 133:1117–23.
13. Matsumoto K, Yoshikai Y, Matsuzaki G, Asano T, Nomoto K. A novel $CD3^-J11d^+$ subset of $CD4^+CD8^-$ cells repopulating thymus in radiation bone marrow chimeras. Eur J Immunol 1989; 19:1203–07.
14. Wilson A, Petri HT, Scollay R, Shortman K. The acquisition of CD4 and CD8 during the differentiation of early thymocytes in short-term culture. Int Immunol 1989; 1:605–12.

25

Interleukin-7 Induces Proliferation and Maturation of Human Thymocyte Subsets

Leanne W. Vollger and Christel H. Uittenbogaart
University of California at Los Angeles School of Medicine, Los Angeles, California

INTRODUCTION

Intrathymic stimuli which promote T-cell differentiation include cell surface interaction molecules and soluble mediators such as thymic hormones and cytokines. One cytokine which is likely to play an important role in the thymus is interleukin-7 (IL-7). It was originally described as a growth factor for pre–B cells (1). More recently, IL-7 has been reported to induce proliferation of human and murine thymocytes (2–6) and peripheral blood T cells (7,8). While IL-7 was isolated as a product of bone marrow stromal cells (1,9), IL-7 ribonucleic acid has been identified in human and in murine thymus tissue (9,10). Therefore, it is likely that IL-7 is produced by stromal cells in the thymus as well as in the bone marrow, and that IL-7 may play a role in thymocyte development.

MATERIALS AND METHODS

Reagents

Human rIL-7 was a gift from Immunex, Seattle, Washington. Monoclonal antibodies (MAbs) Leu-2 (anti-CD8), Leu-3 (anti-CD4), Leu-4 (anti-CD3), and Leu-18 (anti-CD45RA) conjugated with fluorescein (FITC) or phycoerythrin (PE) were obtained from Becton-Dickinson (Mountain View, California). FITC-conjugated goat antimouse immunoglobulin (Ig), PE-conjugated 2H4 (anti-CD45RA) and unconjugated 2H4 were obtained from Coulter (Hialeah, Florida).

Thymocyte Preparation and Culture

Normal thymus specimens were obtained in the course of corrective cardiac surgery for children. Thymocyte suspensions were prepared as described previously (11). Thymocytes were passed over a nylon wool column to remove non–T cells and debris. Thymocytes were cultured in serum-free medium (AT-IMDM) as described (12).

Evaluation of Proliferation and Inhibition of Proliferation

Thymocyte proliferation was estimated in [^{3}H]thymidine ([^{3}H]TdR) uptake assays (11). Mitomycin C (Sigma, St. Louis, MO) and hydroxyurea (Sigma) were used to inhibit thymocyte proliferation. Thymocytes were incubated with mitomycin C (25 μg/ml) for 30 min at 37°C and then washed three times. Alternatively, hydroxyurea was added to thymocytes and maintained throughout the culture period.

Immunofluorescence

Thymocytes were stained as described (11). Samples were analyzed on a FACScan flow cytometer (Becton Dickinson Immunocytometry Systems, San Jose, California).

Isolation of CD45RA$^-$ Thymocytes

Magnetic beads covalently attached to goat antimouse IgG/IgM (Kirkegaard and Perry, Gaithersburg, MD) were incubated in AT-IMDM containing 2% BSA for 24 hr. Then, magnetic beads were incubated with 2H4 antibody (1.25 tests of 2H4 as defined by the manufacturer/10^8 beads/ml) in AT-IMDM for 8 hr at 4°C before use. Beads were washed to remove excess 2H4. Thymocytes and 2H4-coated beads were combined at 5×10^6 beads/1×10^7 thymocytes/ml and incubated at 4°C on a rotator for 1 hr. Beads, with CD45RA$^+$ cells bound, were removed with a magnet, and CD45RA depleted cells were recovered. CD45RA-depleted thymocytes were exposed a second time to 2H4-coated beads for 12 hr. Following separation, thymocytes were phenotyped and analyzed using FITC-conjugated Leu-18 and PE-conjugated 2H4 to detect CD45RA and FITC-conjugated goat anti-mouse to detect any 2H4 antibody bound to cells during separation.

RESULTS

IL-7 Promotes the Appearance of a Population of Large Cells Expressing a Mature Phenotype

Human thymocytes were cultured in serum-free medium with or without 200 U/ml IL-7. After 10–14 days in culture with IL-7, a population of large cells appeared (Fig. 1, top right). Phenotypic analysis of the whole cell population revealed an increase in cells of a mature phenotype compared to day 0 and compared to cells cultured in medium alone. Specifically, there was an increase in the percentage of cells expressing CD45RA antigen. In IL-7, 38% of cells expressed CD45RA on day 11 compared to 7% on day 0. In medium alone, 13% of thymocytes expressed CD45RA on day 11 compared to 7% on day 0. The density of CD45RA expression was also increased after 11 days of culture in the presence of IL-7: mean fluorescence channel (MFC) of 574 in IL-7, compared to MFC of 475 in medium alone. In addition, the density of CD3 was increased after 11 days in culture with IL-7 (MFC 553 in IL-7, and MFC 469 in medium alone). The percentages of CD4 and CD8 single positive cells increased in IL-7 and in medium alone (Fig. 1). However, CD4 and CD8 were expressed at very low density on cells cultured in medium alone compared to cells cultured in IL-7 (Fig. 1).

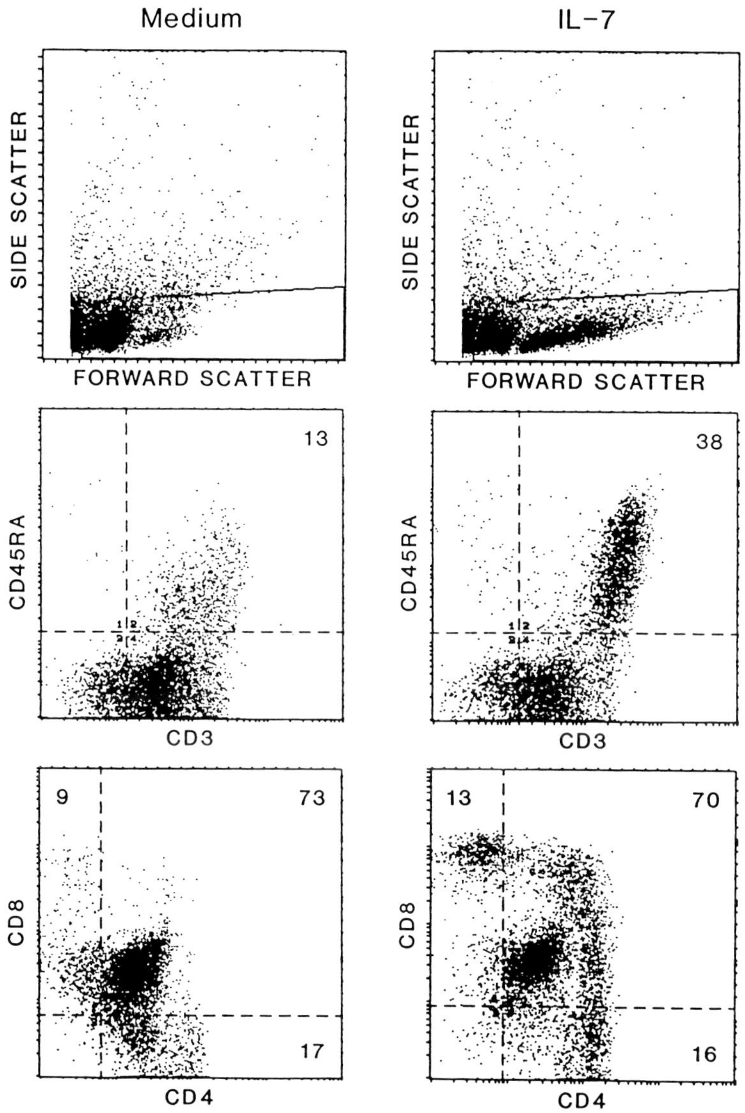

Figure 1 IL-7 induces thymocyte maturation. Thymocytes were cultured in medium alone or with 200 U/ml IL-7. Fluorescence histograms show cell size (forward scatter), granularity (side scatter), and surface expression of CD3, CD45RA, CD4, and CD8. Numbers show the percentage of cells present in the quadrants indicated. Thymocyte phenotypes after 11 days in culture in medium alone (left panels) or with 200 U/ML IL-7 (right panels) are shown. Representative results are shown for one of 10 experiments performed.

Changes in Phenotype Do Not Represent a Transient State of Activation

Thymocytes were cultured with IL-7, and on day 13 an aliquot of cells was phenotyped, and cultures were continued with or without IL-7. Twelve days after removal of IL-7, thymocytes maintained the same phenotype as those cultured continuously in IL-7 (data not shown).

IL-7 Induces Thymocyte Proliferation

Using serum-free culture conditions, we found that IL-7 consistently induced a low level of thymocyte proliferation (Table 1). Proliferation was detectable at 200 U/ml IL-7 and was maximal at 1000 U/ml. The observed changes in the number of CD45RA-positive cells might be accounted for by proliferation of a small population of CD45RA-positive cells, or by de novo CD45RA expression. To investigate these possibilities, two approaches were taken. First, the ability of IL-7 to induce differentiation of CD45RA-negative thymocytes was tested. Second, the proliferation requirement for phenotypic changes was tested.

IL-7 Induces CD45RA Expression on CD45RA-Negative Precursors

After CD45RA-positive cells were removed, the resulting CD45RA-depleted thymocytes were greater than 99.5% CD45RA-negative (Fig. 2). CD45RA-depleted thymocytes were cultured in medium alone or with 200 U/ml IL-7. After 14 days of culture in IL-7, 14.6% of these thymocytes expressed CD45RA. In contrast, CD45RA-depleted thymocytes cultured in medium alone contained no CD45RA-positive cells (Fig. 2). Therefore, CD45RA-negative thymocytes differentiated into CD45RA-positive thymocytes only when cultured in the presence of IL-7.

IL-7 Induces Differentiation in the Absence of Proliferation

To determine if proliferation was required for the appearance of mature CD45RA-positive, bright CD3-positive cells, thymocytes were either cultured in the presence of 10 mM

Table 1 IL-7 Induces Proliferation of Human Thymocytes

U/ml IL-7	CPM + SD
0	333 ± 268
20	422 ± 97
200	1,404 ± 294
500	1,625 ± 240
1000	2,280 ± 284
2000	1,491 ± 259

Data are expressed as mean cpm per 10^5 cells ± standard deviation (SD). Thymocytes were cultured in serum-free medium with IL-7 (20-2000 U/ml) and pulsed with [^{3}H]thymidine on the fifth day of culture.

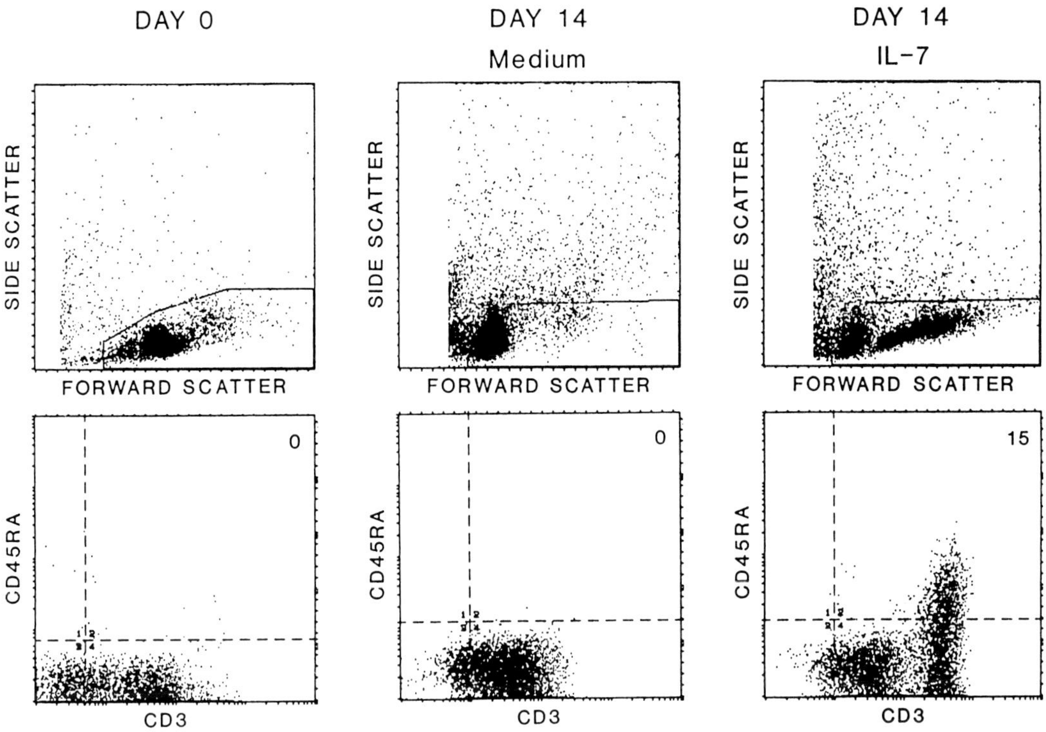

Figure 2 IL-7 induces CD45RA expression on $CD45RA^-$ thymocytes. The phenotype of $CD45RA^-$ thymocytes on day 0 of culture is shown in the left panels. $CD45RA^-$ thymocytes were phenotyped again after 14 days of culture in medium alone (middle panels) or with 200 U/ml IL-7 (right panels).

hydroxyurea or else pretreated with mitomycin C to inhibit proliferation. Similar results were obtained with both procedures. Results of one representative experiment are shown in Figure 3 and Table 2. Hydroxyurea, 10 mM, was added to thymocyte cultures either on day 0 or on day 5 and maintained throughout the culture period. By day 5, a significant amount of cell death had occurred, and the number of CD45RA-positive cells decreased in all culture conditions from 6.8×10^5 CD45RA-positive cells on day 0 to 1.4×10^5 CD45RA-positive cells on day 5 (Table 2). On day 5, very little difference was observed between the phenotypes of thymocytes cultured in IL-7 or medium alone. However, on day 11, cells cultured in IL-7 showed increased expression of CD45RA and increased CD3 density, in the presence (Fig. 3) and in the absence of hydroxyurea. In medium alone, with or without hydroxyurea, the CD3/CD45RA immunofluorescence pattern remained similar to that seen on day 0 and on day 5 (Fig. 3). Between days 5 and 11, IL-7 caused a large increase in the number of CD45RA-positive cells: a 13.6-fold increase in the absence of hydroxyurea, and a 10.7-fold increase in the presence of hydroxyurea (Table 2). Similar changes in phenotype and in numbers of CD45RA-positive cells were observed whether hydroxyurea was added on day 0 or on day 5. These data indicate that IL-7 does induce phenotypic changes indicating differentiation in the absence of proliferation.

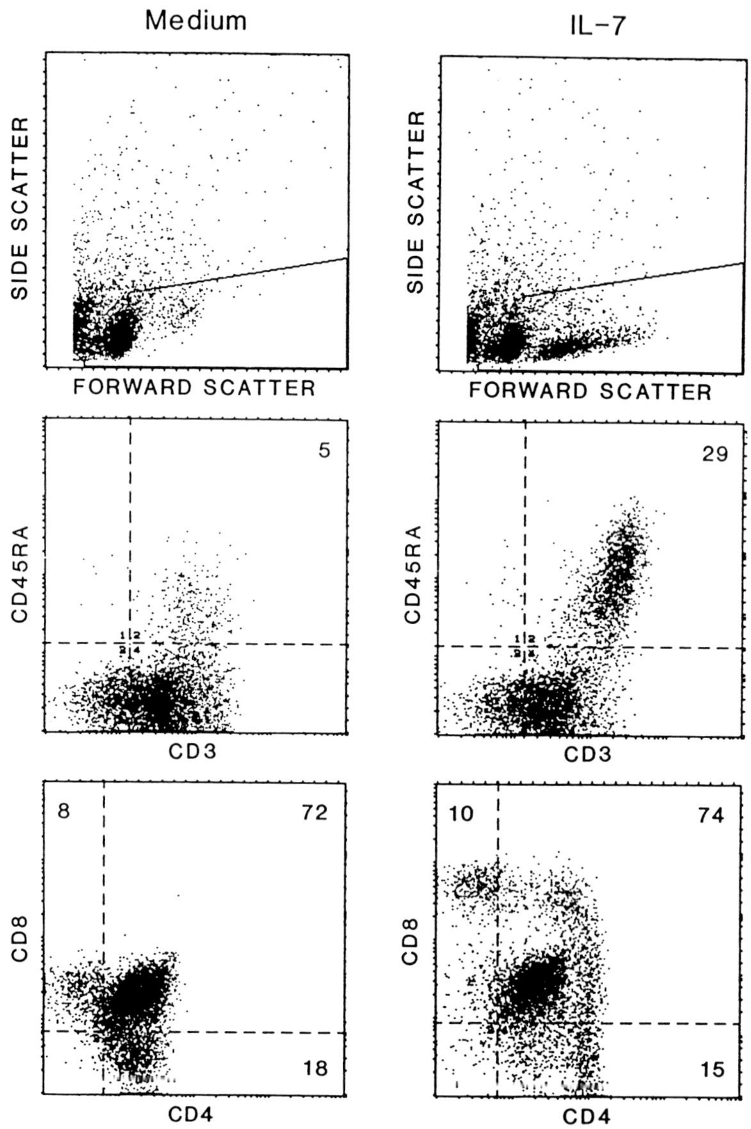

Figure 3 Thymocytes cultured in the presence of hydroxyurea. Thymocytes were cultured in the presence of 10 mM hydroxyurea either in medium (left panels) or with 200 U/ml IL-7 (right panels). Expression of CD3, CD45RA, CD4, and CD8 on the eleventh day in culture is shown.

Table 2 Absolute Numbers of CD45RA⁺ Thymocytes During Culture in the Presence or Absence of Hydroxyurea

Culture conditions	Day 0	Day 5	Day 11
Control			
medium	6.8 ± 10^5	1.4 ± 10^5	2.7 ± 10^5
IL-7	6.8 ± 10^5	1.4 ± 10^5	1.9 ± 10^6
Hydroxyurea (day 0)			
medium	6.8 ± 10^5	ND	1.7 ± 10^5
IL-7	6.8 ± 10^5	ND	1.5 ± 10^6
Hydroxyurea (day 5)			
medium	6.8 ± 10^5	1.4 ± 10^5	1.5 ± 10^5
IL-7	6.8 ± 10^5	1.4 ± 10^5	1.5 ± 10^6

Thymocytes were cultured in medium or in medium plus IL-7 (200 U/ml) either with or without hydroxyurea for 11 days. Hydroxyurea was added on day 0 or on day 5 as indicated. Total cell numbers were counted under a microscope, and cell phenotype was analyzed by immunofluorescence and flow cytometry. The absolute number of $CD45RA^+$ cells was calculated from these measurements. ND, not done.

DISCUSSION

Previous reports have shown that IL-7 induces the proliferation of several lymphocyte populations. Here we present the first evidence that IL-7 can also induce thymocyte differentiation. Interleukin-7 promoted the generation of a population of large, mature thymocytes which expressed high-density CD3 and CD45RA in vitro. We found that phenotypic changes induced by IL-7 (a) do not represent a transient state of activation, (b) may partly result from low level proliferation of mature thymocytes, and (c) do result from differentiation of CD45RA-negative precursors to CD45RA-positive thymocytes.

Induction of CD45RA expression is not unique to IL-7. We have reported similar phenotypic changes induced by IL-4 (12), and we have observed CD45RA-positive thymocytes after culture with IL-2 plus PHA-P (unpublished observations). The mechanism of IL-7 action, however, appears to be different from that of IL-4 or IL-2. Anti–IL-4 antibodies did not inhibit phenotypic changes by IL-7, indicating that IL-7 actions were not mediated by IL-4 (unpublished observations). Interleukin-2 receptor p55 (CD25) expression was not detected on thymocytes before or after culture with IL-7, suggesting that IL-2 may not be involved in IL-7–induced changes. Also, the increased CD45RA expression by IL-2 plus PHA-P is dependent on proliferation, and probably represents expansion of CD45RA-positive cells (unpublished observations).

The functional significance of CD45RA expression on thymocytes is not known. However, the pattern of CD45RA expression has raised some intriguing hypotheses. While CD45RA is expressed on only a small population of thymocytes, it is present on virtually all cord blood T cells (13). Therefore, it has been proposed that thymocyte acquisition of CD45RA is a required step for export to the periphery (13). Pilarski et al. have suggested that expression of CD45RA allows thymocyte survival (14). Our data indicate that IL-7 may be an important regulator of de novo CD45RA expression in the thymus.

ACKNOWLEDGMENTS

This work was supported by grant CH-439 from the American Cancer Society, grants CA42735 and CA09120 from the National Institutes of Health and by the Concern Foundation. We thank Dr. Steven Gillis for providing us with human interleukin-7.

REFERENCES

1. Namen AE, Schmierer AE, March CJ, Overell RW, Park LS, Urdal DL, Mochizuki DY. B-cell precursor growth promoting activity: purification and characterization of a growth factor active on lymphocyte precursors. J Exp Med 1988; 167:988.
2. Varma C, Chantry D, Brennan F, Turner M, Katz F, Feldmann M. Interleukin 7 and interleukin 4 stimulate human thymocyte growth through distinct mechanisms. Cytokine 1990; 2:55.
3. Conlon PJ, Morrissey PJ, Nordan RP, Grabstein KH, Prickett KS, Reed SG, Goodwin R, Cosman D, Namen AE. Murine thymocytes proliferate in direct response to interleukin-7. Blood 1989; 74:1368.
4. Watson JD, Morrissey PJ, Namen AE, Conlon PJ, Widmer MB. Effect of IL-7 on the growth of fetal thymocytes in culture. J Immunol 1989; 143:1215.
5. Chantry D, Turner M, Feldmann M. Interleukin 7 (murine pre-B cell growth factor/ lymphopoietin 1) stimulates thymocyte growth: regulation by transforming growth factor beta. Eur J Immunol 1989; 19:783.
6. Okazaki H, Ito M, Sudo T, Hattori M, Kano S, Katsura Y, Minato N. IL-7 promotes thymocyte proliferation and maintains immunocompetent thymocytes bearing alpha/beta or gamma/delta T-cell receptors in vitro: synergism with IL-2. J Immunol 1989; 143:2917.
7. Welch PA, Namen AE, Goodwin RG, Armitage R, Cooper MD. Human IL-7: a novel T cell growth factor. J Immunol 1989; 143:3562.
8. Armitage RJ, Namen AE, Sassenfeld HM, Grabstein KH. Regulation of human T cell proliferation by IL-7. J Immunol 1990; 144:938.
9. Namen AE, Lupton S, Hjerrild K, Wignall J, Mochizuki DY, Schmierer A, Mosley B, March CJ, Urdal D, Gillis S, Cosman D, Goodwin RG. Stimulation of B-cell progenitors by cloned murine interleukin-7. Nature 1988; 333:571.
10. Goodwin RG, Lupton S, Schmierer A, Hjerrild KJ, Jerzy R, Clevenger W, Gillis S, Cosman D, Namen AE. Human interleukin 7: molecular cloning and growth factor activity on human and murine B lineage cells. Proc Natl Aced Sci U.S.A. 1989; 86:302.
11. Uittenbogaart CH, Higashitani S, Schmid I, Vollger LW, Boone T, Clement LT. Interleukin-4 induces expression of CD45RA antigen on human thymocyte subpopulations. Int Immun 1990 (in press)
12. Uittenbogaart CH, Cantor Y, Fahey JL. Growth of human malignant lymphoid cell lines in serum free medium. In Vitro 1983; 19:67.
13. Tedder TF, Clement LT, Cooper MD. Human lymphocyte differentiation antigens HB-10 and HB-11. I. Ontogeny of antigen expression. J Immunol 1985; 134:2983.
14. Pilarski LM, Deans JP. Selective expression of CD45R isoforms and of maturation antigens during human thymocyte differentiation: observations and a hypothesis. Immunol Letters 1989; 21:187.

26

CD4$^+$CD8$^+$CD3^{high} Thymocytes Represent a Cortisone-Resistant Subset Differentiating into Mature T Cells

P. Hugo,[1,2] G. A. Waanders,[1] R. L. Boyd,[1] and R. Scollay[2]
[1]*Monash Medical School, Prahran, Victoria, Australia;*
[2]*The Walter and Eliza Hall Institute of Medical Research, Parkville, Victoria, Australia*

INTRODUCTION

Only 2–4% of CD4$^+$CD8$^+$ thymocytes are expected to convert into mature T cells (1), by differentiation events not yet well defined (2). A clear understanding of these could help in deciphering the exact target of negative selection for instance, since it is controversial at what stage deletion occurs (3,4). It has been proposed that the density of (TCR) T-cell receptor/CD3 complex could play a role in negative selection (5). In this regard, the identification of a CD4$^+$CD8$^+$ subset expressing high level of CD3 (CD3^{high}), presumed to represent the immediate precursor of mature T cells, is noteworthy (2). Here we have characterized and positioned this subset within the T-cell differentiation pathway.

MATERIALS AND METHODS

Mice

All mice were used at 4–8 weeks of age. Embryos were aged by a vaginal plug assessment.

Fetal Thymic Organ Cultures (FTOC)

FTOC were prepared with day 14 thymic lobes as described elsewhere (6).

Multicolor Flow Cytometric Analysis

Cells were stained for three-color analysis by a protocol extensively described elsewhere (7). Staining for five-color analysis was done in the following stages: (a) one of the antibodies, Thy-1 (30-H12), MEL-14, HSA(M1/69), H-2K^k (11-4.1), IL-2R (PC.61), CD5 (53-7.3), LFA-1 (I21/7.7), or CD44 (Pgp-1) (IM7.81); (b) allophycocyanin (APC)-conjugated goat anti-immunoglobulin (anti-Ig) (Caltag Lab, USA); (c) normal Ig;

(d) phycoerythrin PE–conjugated anti-CD4 (GK-1.5, B.D.)/biotin-conjugated rat anti-CD8 (53.6.7, B.D.)/FITC-conjugated anti-CD3ε (145-2C11); (e) streptavidin-conjugated Texas red (TRIC, Caltag). Dead cells were excluded by propidium iodide uptake. In some cases APC-conjugated anti-CD4 and TRIC-conjugated sheep anti-Ig were used when TCR αβ (H57-597), Vβ8.2 TCR (F23.2), Vβ6 (44-22-1), or MTS 35 biotin-conjugated antibodies (a marker for immature thymocytes; Godfrey et al., in preparation) were revealed by streptavidin-conjugated PE (Caltag). Controls consisted of either unstained cells or thymocytes incubated with the second stage reagents alone. Stained cells, 1-1.5 × 10^5, cells were analyzed with a FACScan or FACStar^{plus} (B.D.).

RESULTS AND DISCUSSION

CD4$^+$CD8$^+$ Expressing Intermediate or High Levels of CD3

CD4$^+$CD8$^+$ cells are mainly CD3-negative or CD3^{low}, but ~ 2-4% expressed intermediate/high levels of CD3 (CD3$^{int/high}$) (Fig. 1). While CD4$^+$CD8$^+$CD3^{lo} cells bore typical levels of CD4 and CD8, we found here that the CD4$^+$CD8$^+$CD3$^{int/high}$ cells expressed lower level of either CD4 or CD8 (8). When analyzed closely down-regulation of CD4/CD8 was shown to occur at the CD4$^+$CD8$^+$CD3^{high} stage (8).

Phenotype of CD4$^+$CD8$^+$CD3$^{int/high}$ Cells

CD4$^+$CD8$^+$CD3$^{int/high}$ cells were shown to have a phenotype intermediate between typical CD4$^+$CD8$^+$ cells and mature thymocytes (Table 1). Interestingly, they displayed a transitional expression for some markers, as shown by the intensity of H-2K and MTS 35 which identifies immature thymocytes (Godfrey et al., in preparation).

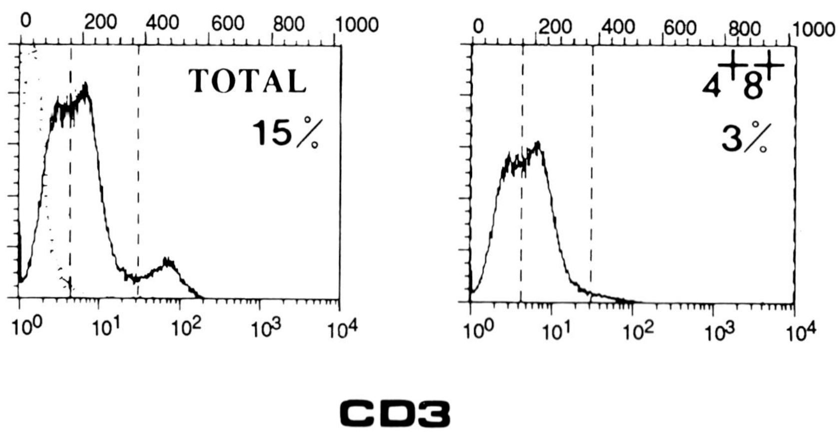

Figure 1 CD4$^+$CD8$^+$ expressing high-level CD3. Adult CBA thymocytes were stained for CD4, CD8, and CD3. The profiles of total thymocytes labeled with the conjugate alone (......) or the anti-CD3 + conjugate (———) are compared to the one of gated CD4$^+$CD8$^+$ cells. These results are representative of 12 independent experiments.

Table 1 Phenotype of $CD4^+CD8^+CD3^{high}$ Cells

Marker	$CD4^+CD8^+$	$CD4^+CD8^+CD3^{int/high}$	Mature thymocytes[a]
Thy-1	high	high	low
HSA	high	high	–/int
CD5	low	high	high
LFA-1	high	high	high
IL-2Rα	–	–	–
Pgp-1	–	–	–/+
MEL-14	–/low	–/high	–/high
H-2K	low	low/high	high
αβTcR	low	int/high	high
MTS-35[b]	high	–/high	–

Adult CBA thymocytes were analyzed by five-color analysis.
[a]$CD4^+CD8^-CD3^+/CD4^-CD8^+CD3^+$.
[b]Marker for immature thymocytes (Godfrey et al., in preparation).

Ontogeny of $CD4^+CD8^+CD3^{high}$ Cells

If $CD4^+CD8^+CD3^{high}$ cells are the immediate precursors of mature T cells they should appear before the latter during ontogeny but after the $CD4^+CD8^+CD3^{-/low}$ cells. We thus monitored this in the FTOC, embryo, and during reconstitution following cortisone treatment. $CD4^+CD8^+CD3^{high}$ cells appeared after $CD4^+CD8^+CD3^{-/low}$ and before the burst of mature T cells in all models (Tables 2 and 3). The few mature $CD4^+/CD8^+$ cells in the early embryo are misleading having been shown to be TCR δ–positive cells (7,9). In this experiment we noted that >99.5% of $CD4^+CD8^+CD3^{-/low}$ cells were wiped out 12 hr after cortisone treatment, while as much as 16% of the $CD4^+CD8^+CD3^{hi}$ cells remained (~40% for mature thymocytes; data not shown) indicating that cortisone-resistance being acquired place at this stage.

Negative Selection Occurs After Upregulation of TCR/CD3 Complex on $CD4^+CD8^+CD3^{low}$ Cells

Using the model where TCR Vβ6 epitope is deleted in Mls-1[a] but not Mls-1[b] mice (3), we have identified the target of negative selection by comparing the Vβ6 expression among different subsets in DBA-2 (H-2[d], Mls-1[a]) and Balb/c (H-2[d], Mls-1[b]) mice. No difference was noted between the two strains for $CD4^+CD8^+CD3^{low}$ cells (Table 4). However, $V\beta6^+$ cells were significantly lower in the Mls-1[a] strain among the $CD4^+CD8^+CD3^{int}$ subset, and were deleted in the $CD4^+CD8^+CD3^{high}$ subset as for the mature T cells, whereas no significant changes were noted for the TCR Vβ8.2 epitope (nondeleted) in all these subsets (data not shown). Negative selection has therefore begun at the $CD4^+CD8^+CD3^{int}$ stage, and was complete at the $CD4^+CD8^+CD3^{high}$ stage, confirming the proposal that density of TCR/CD3 complex is important for this process (5).

CONCLUSION

In this report, we have characterized the previously ill-defined $CD4^+CD8^+CD3^{high}$ cells. Their kinetics during thymic development and their phenotype suggest that they represent

Table 2 Ontogeny of $CD4^+CD8^+CD3^{high}$ Cells

	Subsets (% of total thymocytes)				
Ontogenic stage	$CD4^+8^+3^-$	$CD4^+8^+3^{low}$	$CD4^+8^+3^{high}$	$CD4^+8^-3^{high}$	$CD4^-8^+3^{high}$
d 3	26.0	6.0	0	0.2	1.3
d 6	37.0	19.4	0.6	0.7	1.4
d 12	25.0	27.0	2.5	2.2	5.3
E16	5.5	2.0	0.1	0.6	1.3
E16.5	25.7	6.5	0.3	0.8	0.8
E17	59.1	3.5	0.3	0.8	1.4
E18	57.0	18.3	0.7	4.9	1.2
E19	39.5	37.4	1.4	4.9	1.0
Neo	41.1	42.0	2.6	7.5	1.0
Adult	39.2	45.6	1.0	7.2	3.1

Thymocytes from CBA fetal thymic lobes cultured for 3, 6, or 12 days (d), or embryos of different days (E), neonatal (Neo) or adult mice were triple-labeled and the proportion of various subsets determined.

the immediate precursor of the TCR $\alpha\beta^+$ mature thymocytes. Supporting this, is the observation that $CD4^+CD8^+CD3^{high}$ cells do mature into single positives when injected intrathymically (unpublished observation). Overall, the following sequence can be mapped: $CD4^+CD8^+CD3^{low}$ cells upregulate their TCR/CD3 complex, becoming $CD4^+CD8^+CD3^{int}$, at which point negative selection is operative, and when they reach the stage of $CD4^+CD8^+CD3^{high}$ they downregulate either CD4 or CD8, acquire cortisone-resistance, and modulate the expression of various surface markers to convert into mature T cells.

Table 3 Appearance of $CD4^+CD8^+CD3^{high}$ Cell After Cortisone Treatment

Days	Subsets (cells $\times 10^{-6}$)/thymus				
post-treatment	$CD4^+8^+3^-$	$CD4^+8^+3^{low}$	$CD4^+8^+3^{high}$	$CD4^+8^-3^{high}$	$CD4^-8^+3^{high}$
6	4.5	1.6	0.02	0.9	0.9
7	7.2	2.6	0.04	0.6	0.4
8	11.3	4.1	0.06	0.4	0.2
9	9.7	11.3	0.3	1.0	0.4
10	36.0	48.9	1.0	2.9	1.1
14	69.4	97.7	2.1	9.6	3.0

Mice received i.p. 125 mg of dexamethasone per kg body weight. Results obtained from two experiments.

Table 4 Deletion of TCR $V\beta6^+$ Cells at $CD4^+CD8^+CD3^{int}$ Stage

Subsets		DBA-2 (Mls-1^a, H-2^b)	Balb/c^d (Mls-1^b, H-2^d)
$CD4^+8^+3^{low}$	$V\beta6^{low}$	4.4 ± 0.1[1,2]	5.2 ± 0.5
$CD4^+8^+3^{int}$	$V\beta6^{int}$	4.0 ± 0.8[3]	6.2 ± 0.6
$CD4^+8^+3^{high}$	$V\beta6^{high}$	0.7 ± 0.2[4]	8.3 ± 1.0
$CD4^+8^-3^{high}$	$V\beta6^{high}$	0.2 ± 0.1[4]	6.5 ± 0.9
$CD4^-8^+3^{high}$	$V\beta6^{high}$	0.2 ± 0.1[4]	5.9 ± 0.5

[1]Mean % ± SD from at least 4 individual mice.
[2]$p > 0.05$ by Student "t" test.
[3]$p \leq 0.01$ by Student "t" test.
[4]$p \leq 0.001$ by Student "t" test.

ACKNOWLEDGMENT

We thank Becton Dickinson who sponsored the presentation of these results. P. Hugo is supported by a postdoctoral fellowship from the MRC of Canada. This work was supported by the NH and MRC Australia (No. 860396), NIH USA (No. AI17310) and Anti-Cancer Council of Victoria (No. 131658).

REFERENCES

1. von Boehmer H. The developmental biology of T lymphocytes. Ann Rev Immunol 1988; 6: 309–26.
2. Fowlkes BJ, Pardoll DM. Molecular and cellular events of T cell development. Adv Immunol 1989; 44:207–64.
3. Kisielow P, Bluthmann H, Staerz UD, Steinmetz M, von Boehmer H. Tolerance in T-cell-receptor transgenic mice involved deletion of nonmature $CD4^+CD8^+$ thymocytes. Nature 1988; 333: 742–46.
4. Kappler JW, Roehm N, Marrak P. T cell tolerance by clonal elimination in the thymus. Cell 1987; 49:273–80.
5. MacDonald HR. T cell repertoire selection during development. Curr Opin Immunol 1989; 2:199–203.
6. Waanders GA, Boyd RL. The effects of interleukin 2 on early and late thymocyte differentiation in fetal thymus organ culture. Int Immunol 1990; 2:461–468.
7. Hugo P, Waanders GA, Scollay R, Shortman K, Boyd RL. Ontogeny of a novel $CD4^+CD8^-CD3^-$ thymocyte subpopulation: a comparison with $CD4^-CD8^+CD3^-$ thymocytes. Int Immunol 1990; 2:209–18.
8. Hugo P, Boyd RL, Waanders GA, Petrie HT, Scollay R. Timing of deletion of autoreactive $V\beta6^+$ cells and down-modulation of either CD4 or CD8 on phenotypically distinct $CD4^+8^+$ subsets of thymocytes expressing intermediate or high levels of T cell receptor. Int Immunol (in press).
9. Itohara S, Nakanishi N, Kanagawa O, Kubo R, Tonegawa S. Monoclonal antibodies specific to native murine T-cell receptor $\tau\delta$: Analysis of $\tau\delta$ T cells during thymic ontogeny and in peripheral lymphoid organs. PNAS 1989; 86:5094–98.

27
Emigration of Atypical Subpopulations from the Murine Thymus

Katherine A. Kelly and Roland Scollay
The Walter and Eliza Hall Institute of Medical Research, Melbourne, Australia

INTRODUCTION

The thymus is responsible for the production of T cells. Approximately 1% of thymocytes emigrate to seed the peripheral lymphoid organs per day (1). Previous studies have shown that the majority of these cells are the typical $CD3^+4^+8^-$ and $CD3^+4^-8^+$ mature T cells. In this chapter, we investigate the emigration of minor populations of $CD4^+8^+$ and $CD4^-8^-$ cells from the thymus of adult mice.

METHODS

In order to trace recent thymic emigrants we used the technique of intrathymic injection of fluorescein isothiocyanate, followed by flow cytometric analysis of FITC-positive cells appearing in the lymph nodes and spleen 16 hr later (1). For analysis of the $CD4^-8^-$ population, CD4-positive, CD8-positive and immunoglobulin–positive cells were depleted prior to flow cytometric analysis using a combination of complement mediated cytotoxicity and magnetic bead (Amerlex M, Amersham) depletion (2). Five- to six-week-old CBA/CaH mice were used throughout.

RESULTS AND DISCUSSION

Emigration of $CD4^+8^+$ Cells

Figure 1 shows that while the majority of cells emigrating from the thymus express either CD4 or CD8, a small proportion (approximately 2%) of cells express both CD4 and CD8. Further examination of these cells indicates they express CD3 (Fig. 2), indicating that they come from a small selected subset of relatively mature thymic $CD4^+8^+$ cells and are not a

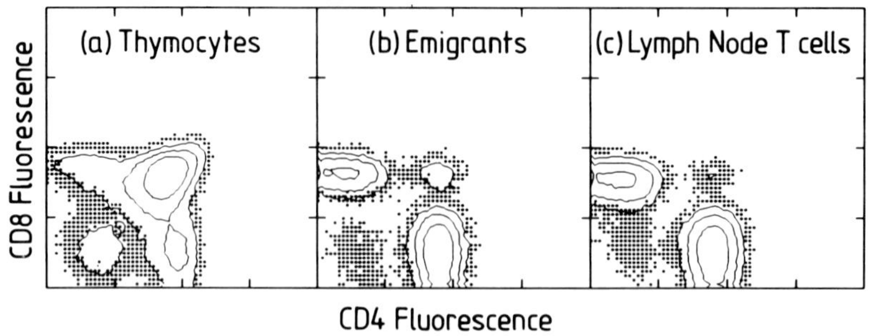

Figure 1 Two-color plots of CD4 vs CD8 on (a) thymocytes, (b) recent thymic emigrants, and (c) lymph node T cells. Data are represented over a 4-decade log scale.

random sample. They have a forward light scatter profile similar to $CD3^+4^+8^+$ thymocytes but different from the $CD3^+4^+8^+$ cells detected in lymph nodes (Fig. 3). This suggests that they are "real" $CD4^+8^+$ cells rather than doublets of $CD4^+8^-$ and $CD4^-8^+$ cells we have shown to constitute the majority of apparently $CD4^+8^+$ events in lymph nodes (3). While $CD4^+8^+$ T cells are rare in murine lymph nodes and spleen (3), it has been reported that they are more common among populations of intestinal intraepithelial lymphocytes (4). One possible explanation for this finding is selective migration of $CD4^+8^+$ cells to this site.

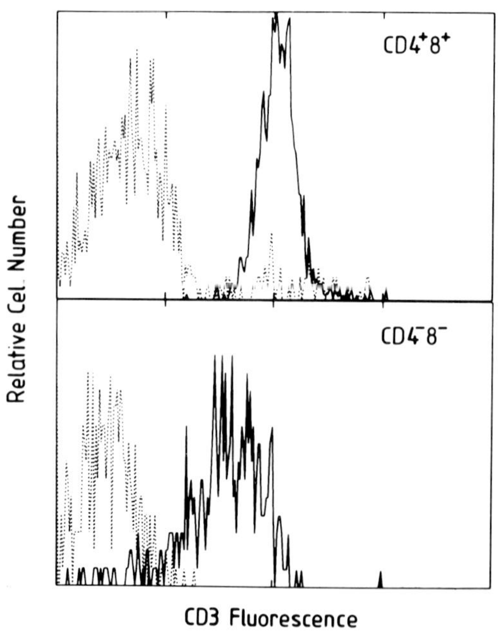

Figure 2 Log fluorescence staining of CD3 on $CD4^+8^+$ (top) and $CD4^-8^-$ emigrants (bottom). Broken lines indicate control staining on the same selected subpopulations.

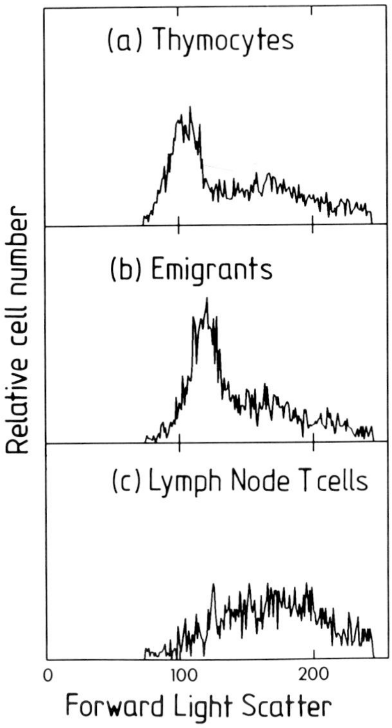

Figure 3 Forward light scatter profiles of $CD3^+4^+8^+$ thymocytes, recent thymic emigrants, and lymph node T cells, respectively.

Emigration of $CD4^-8^-$ Cells

The possibility of emigration of $CD3^+4^-8^-$ cells from the thymus is of interest as a small ~1%) population of these cells exists in the thymus as well as in lymph nodes and spleen, but little is known of their origin. In addition, TCR γδ-positive cells are known to be enriched in this population (5,8). Approximately 1% of recent thymic emigrants express neither CD4 nor CD8 (see Fig. 1), and the vast majority of these express CD3 (see Fig. 2). Figure 4 shows a further subdivision among $CD4^-8^-$ thymic emigrants located in the spleen, based on TCR αβ and TCR γδ expression, and the data indicate that the majority of $CD4^-8^-$ emigrants express TCR γδ.

Within the $CD4^-8^-$TCR $\alpha\beta^+$ thymic subpopulation, an unusually high proportion of cells expresses products of the Vβ8 gene family (6). These cells are known to increase in number with age (7). The data in Table 1 compare the proportion of Vβ8-positive cells among $CD4^-8^-$TCR$\alpha\beta^+$ thymocytes, splenic emigrants and splenocytes. It is evident that splenic $CD4^-8^-$TCR αβ cells and the splenic migrants have a similar high proportion of Vβ8-positive cells, but this proportion is significantly lower than among the equivalent intrathymic population. This indicates a selective emigration pattern for $CD4^-8^-$TCR $\alpha\beta^+$ subsets.

Overall our data show that some rare intrathymic subpopulations are represented among the cells leaving the thymus. Their significance to peripheral immune responses remains to be determined.

Table 1 TCR Vβ8 Expression Among $CD4^{-}8^{-}TCR\alpha\beta^{+}$ Thymocytes, Recent Thymic Emigrants, and Splenic T Cells as Determined by Flow Cytometery Using Monoclonal Antibody F23.1

Cell origin	% TCR $V\beta8^{+}$
Thymocytes	81 ± 2
Emigrants	48 ± 7
Spleen	53 ± 7

Standard deviations are based on determination in three to six different experiments.

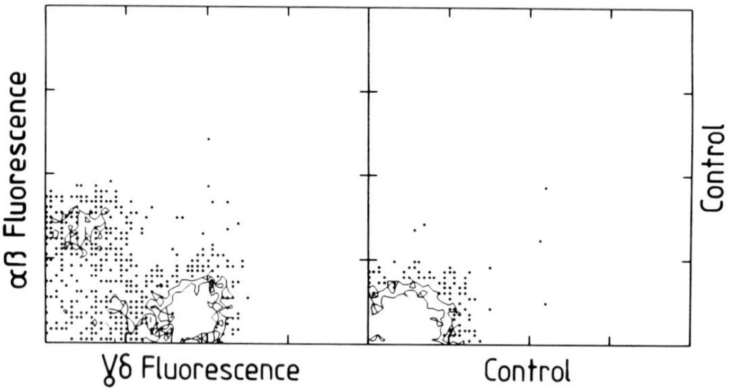

Figure 4 Two-color plot of TCR αβ and TCR γδ expression on $CD3^{+}4^{-}8^{-}$ thymic emigrants. Data are represented over a 4-decade log scale.

REFERENCES

1. Scollay R, Butcher E, Weissman I. Thymus cell migration: Quantitative studies on the rate of migration of cells from the thymus to the periphery in mice. Eur J Immunol 1980; 10:210–8.
2. Kelly K, Shortman K, Scollay R. The surface phenotype of activated T lymphocytes. Immunol Cell Biol 1988; 66:297–306.
3. Kelly K, Pilarski L, Shortman K, Scollay R. $CD4^{+}CD8^{+}$ cells are rare among *in vitro* activated mouse or human T lymphocytes. Cell Immunol 1988; 117:414–24.
4. Mosley RL, Styre D, Klein JR. $CD4^{+}CD8^{+}$ murine intestinal intraepithelial lymphocytes. Int mmunol 1990; 2:361–5.
5. Itohara S, Nakanishi N, Kanagawa O, Kubo R, Tonegawa S. Monoclonal antibodies specific to native murine T cell receptor γδ: Analysis of T cells during thymic ontogeny and peripheral lymphoid organs. Proc Natl Acad Sci USA 1989; 86:5094–8.
6. Wilson A, Ewing T, Owens T, Scollay R, Shortman K. T cell antigen receptor expression by subsets of Ly-2⁻L3T4⁻ ($CD4^{-}CD8^{-}$) thymocytes. J Immunol 1988; 140:1470–6.

7. Egerton M, Scollay R. Intrathymic selection of murine TCR$\alpha\beta^+$ CD4$^-$CD8$^-$ thymocytes. Int Immunol 1990; 2:157–63.
8. Wu L, Pearce M, Egerton M, Petrie H, Scollay R. CD4$^-$8$^-$ thymocytes that express the T cell receptor may have previously expressed CD8. Int Immunol 1990; 2:51–6.

28
Abnormal Increase of $CD4^-CD8^-$ and $CD4^-CD8^+$ Thymocytes in C57BL/Ka Split-Dose Irradiated Mice

A.-M. Rongy,[1] R. Greimers,[1] C. Humblet,[1] M. P. Defresne,[1] M. Papiernik,[2] and J. Boniver[1]
[1]*Laboratory of Pathological Anatomy and Cytopathology, University Hospital at Liège, Liège, Belgium;*
[2]*Necker Hospital, Paris, France*

INTRODUCTION

Fractionated whole-body x-irradiation (4×1.75 Gy at weekly intervals) induces a high percentage of thymic lymphomas in C57BL/Ka mice (1). During the latency period preceding lymphoma development, potential neoplastic (preleukemic) cells appear in the thymus (2,3). Simultaneously, the pool of marrow prothymocytes is reduced (2,4,5), the stromal cells are damaged (3,6), and deep alterations of the thymocyte subpopulations occur. Previous data showed a drop of the percentage of $CD4^+CD8^+$ thymocytes together with an increase of $CD4^-CD8^-$ and $CD4^-CD8^+$ cells (7).

These thymocytes subpopulations are known to be heterogeneous, as defined by the expression of CD3 molecules and the rearrangement and expression of the T-cell receptor (TCR) complex. The lack of CD3 expression is a characteristic feature of very early thymocytes (8); the early $CD4^-CD8^-CD3^-$ cells were shown to convert into $CD4^-CD8^+CD3^-$ precursors (9–12). Recent data suggest that $CD4^-CD8^+CD3^-$ (10,11,13,14) and probably $CD4^+CD8^-CD3^-$ (15) represent a transient differentiation step between $CD4^-CD8^-$ and $CD4^+CD8^+$. By contrast, the $CD4^-CD8^-CD3^+$ cells do not seem to have precursor activity in transfer experiments (16,17); they are not the precursor of the $CD4^+CD8^+CD3^+$ cells. They may derive from a different lineage but recent studies suggest that they may derive from $CD4^+CD8^+$ cells which have downregulated CD4 and CD8 after simultaneous interactions with both classes I and II major histocompatibility complex (MHC) antigens (18,19); they seem to be mature cells which have undergone partial selection (20–22).

In the present report, we show data on the expression of CD3 molecules on the increased $CD4^-CD8^-$ and $CD4^-CD8^+$ subsets in the thymus of preleukemic irradiated mice.

EXPERIMENTAL DATA

Expression of CD4, CD8, and CD3

The following antibodies were used for labeling: anti-CD4 (clone GK 1.5), anti-CD8 (clone 53-6.7), and anti-CD3 (clone 145-2C11); this latter antibody labels mostly the highly CD3-expressing cells. Using appropriate fluorochromes, three-color analysis was performed with a FACScan flow cytometer. In the normal thymus, eight major subsets have been described suing the CD4, CD8, and CD3 markers (23,24), as shown in Figure 1A:

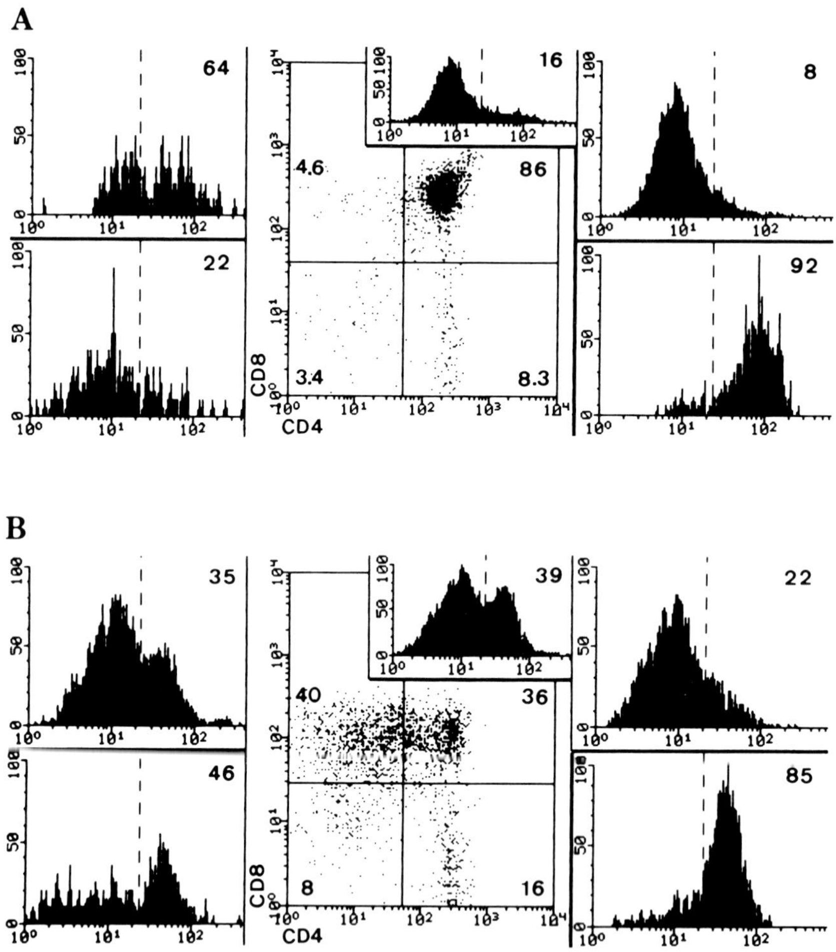

Figure 1 Three-color analysis of C57BL/Ka thymocytes using anti-CD8 biotin detected by Duochrome (a streptavidin conjugated with a tandem PE-Texas Red), anti-CD4-PE and anti-CD3-FITC. (A) Normal mouse, and (B) a mouse which had received a split-dose irradiation 45 days before. Thymocytes were analyzed on the basis of CD4 vs CD8 expression (central panel), the whole population (central histogram) and all four subpopulations were assessed for the CD3 expression (peripheral panels: upper left $CD4^-CD8^+CD3^+$, bottom left $CD4^-CD8^-CD3^+$, upper right $CD4^+CD8^+CD3^+$, bottom right $CD4^+CD8^-CD3^+$). Two × 10^4 per mouse were analyzed on a FACScan flow cytometer (Becton Dickinson).

Unselected thymocytes and all four subpopulations defined by the CD4 and CD8 expression were assessed for the high-level CD3 expression. Most $CD4^+CD8^-$ (90%) and 55–70% of $CD4^-CD8^+$ cells were CD3 positive. Less than 10% of the $CD4^+CD8^+$ subset showed a high level of CD3 expression. The CD3 antigen is also expressed on the surface of 20–30% of the $CD4^-CD8^-$ cells.

Table 1 shows the results of a representative experiment in which C57BL/Ka mice were sacrificed at different time intervals after a split-dose irradiation regimen. At some time intervals, important individual variations were noted. The significant phenotypic alterations can be summarized as follows:

1. The $CD4^+CD8^+$ population was reduced at 15, 30, and 45 days after the treatment, whereas the percentage of the $CD3^+$ cells among them was increased (Fig. 1B).
2. At the same time intervals, the percentage of $CD4^-CD8^+$ subset was higher than in controls, while the ratio of $CD3^+$ vs $CD3^-$ cells was generally unchanged. Sixty and 75 days after the completion of the irradiation, the percentage of $CD4^-CD8^+$ thymocytes was normalized but the CD3-positive fraction was increased compared to controls (up to 90% of the $CD4^-CD8^+$ subset).
3. The $CD4^+CD8^-$ subset was not modified, neither its $CD3^+$ fraction (Fig. 1B).
4. The most striking alterations occurred in the $CD4^-CD8^-$ population, which increased 30 and 45 days after the split-dose irradiation. Moreover, during the whole preleukemic period an average of 40–60% of the $CD4^-CD8^-$ cells expressed CD3; in some individual cases 85% of $CD4^-CD8^-$ were positive with the anti-CD3 antibody (Fig. 1B).

Expression of TCR αβ

Table 2 shows the expression of CD3 and TCR αβ (as defined by anti-CD3, clone 145-2C11 and anti-TCR αβ, clone H57-597 monoclonal antibodies) after a leukemogenic irradiation, in the whole thymus and in the $CD4^-CD8^-$ subset. The increase of $CD3^+$ in the

Table 1 Percentage of Thymic Subpopulations in C57BL/Ka Mice After a Leukemogenic Split-Dose Irradiation

		Days postirradiation				
Subsets	Control	15	30	45	60	75
$CD4^+CD8^+$	86.6 ± 3.4	79.1 ± 6.1	68.0 ± 12.9	72.2 ± 13.0	87.1 ± 2.7	80.2 ± 7.5
$CD3^+$ fraction	6.5 ± 2.0	11.9 ± 6.0	17.4 ± 4.1	12.7 ± 4.9	9.0 ± 5.3	8.8 ± 3.7
$CD4^-CD8^-$	2.5 ± 0.9	1.6 ± 0.7	6.0 ± 3.1	8.2 ± 4.0	1.5 ± 0.6	3.7 ± 2.6
$CD3^+$ fraction	24.1 ± 5.4	20.5 ± 3.8	60.1 ± 9.6	55.0 ± 19.3	44.8 ± 19.4	60.2 ± 24.1
$CD4^+CD8^-$	7.9 ± 1.3	10.9 ± 2.0	9.8 ± 4.0	9.6 ± 4.4	6.3 ± 1.9	10.0 ± 0.9
$CD3^+$ fraction	86.2 ± 5.3	80.9 ± 5.5	89.7 ± 4.8	81.2 ± 10.1	92.9 ± 2.8	87.0 ± 5.2
$CD4^-CD8^+$	3.1 ± 0.9	8.5 ± 4.1	15.2 ± 8.9	8.6 ± 5.1	4.1 ± 1.9	5.5 ± 3.8
$CD3^+$ fraction	58.7 ± 8.7	57.5 ± 18.3	57.1 ± 13.2	66.7 ± 7.7	76.9 ± 6.7	84.3 ± 3.1

Expression of CD3 was analyzed for each subset defined by the expression of CD4 and CD8 (mean of 4 mice ± SE).

Table 2 Expression of CD3 and TCR αβ in Total Population (T) and in Freshly Isolated $CD4^-CD8^-$ (DN) from Individual Normal Thymus and from Individual Mice Irradiated 50 Days Before

			4 × 1.75 Gy									
	Control		Mouse 1		Mouse 2		Mouse 3		Mouse 4		Mouse 5	
	T	DN	T	DN	T	DN	T	DN	T	DN	T	DN
$CD3^+$	14.5 ± 1.5	23.0 ± 0.7	25.2	53.0	16.3	38.0	32.0	69.5	17.1	58.2	17.1	28.6
TCR αβ	13.8 ± 1.3	19.2 ± 0.9	21.1	50.0	15.5	35.1	29.0	65.6	14.3	47.9	15.5	28.0

DN were isolated using complement-dependent lysis prior to magnetic cell separation.

whole population as in the freshly isolated $CD4^-CD8^-$ thymocytes was correlated with the expression of the heterodimer αβ of the antigenic receptor.

DISCUSSION

Two successive phases were defined during the preleukemic period. (a) During the first 2 months, we observed an increased of $CD4^-CD8^+$ cells without alteration of the balance of "mature" CD3-positive vs "immature" CD3-negative subset, a relative enrichment for $CD4^-CD8^-$, particularly of the CD3-positive subset and a drop of the $CD4^+CD8^+$ subpopulation. (b) Later on, no significant alterations of the percentages of the different subsets defined by CD4 and CD8 expression were seen; however, there was an increase of the cells which express CD3 and the TCR αβ, especially in the $CD4^-CD8^-$ subset.

These increased $CD4^-CD8^-CD3^+$ cells belong most probably to the TCR αβ–positive subset (Table 2). This phenotypic alteration is difficult to explain as the differentiation step of these cells remains unclear. They might derive from $CD4^-CD8^-CD3^-$ and constitute a distinct lineage, as the $CD4^-CD8^-CD3^+$ TCR νδ or they could derive from $CD4^+CD8^+$ cells which have lost both CD4 and CD8 (21,22). We have no experimental data to conclude but anyway an alteration of the differentiation pathway is observed. Further studies are under investigation to analyze the relationship of this increased population and the preleukemic cells found in the thymus of irradiated mice (2,3). On the other hand, previous studies have shown that preleukemic thymuses contain an abnormal subpopulation with precursor activity in transfer experiments, which is distinct from the preleukemic cells (7). Whether this abnormal subpopulation might be related to the $CD4^-CD8^-$ $CD3^+$ TCR αβ cells remains to be determined.

REFERENCES

1. Kaplan H.S. Brown M.B. J. Natl. Cancer Inst. 1952; 13:185–208.
2. Boniver J, Decleve A, Lieberman M, Honsik C, Travis M, Kaplan H.S. Cancer Res 1981; 41:390–92.
3. Defresne MP, Greimers R, Lenaerts P, Boniver J. J Natl Cancer Inst 1986; 77:1079–85.
4. Pazmino NH, Mc Ewans R, Ihle JN. J Exp Med 1978; 148:1338–50.
5. Van Bekkum DW, Boersma WJA, Eliason JL, Knaan S. Leukemia Res 1984; 8:461–71.
6. Defresne MP, Rongy AM, Greimers R, Boniver J. Leukemia Res 1986; 10:783–89.
7. Rongy AM, Greimers R, Humblet C, Defresne MP, Boniver J. Thymus 1990; 16:7–27.

8. Fowkles BJ, Pardoll D. Adv Immunol 1989; 44:207–64.
9. Penit C, Vasseur F. J Immunol 1988; 140:3315–23.
10. Penit C, Vasseur F. J Immunol 1989; 142:3369–77.
11. Shortman K, Wilson A, Egerton M, Pearse M, Scollay R. Cell Immunol 1988; 113:462–79.
12. Nikolic-Zugic J, Bevan MJ. Proc Natl Acad Sci USA 1988; 85:8633–37.
13. Guidos CJ, Weissman IL, Adkins B. Proc Natl Acad Sci USA 1989; 86:7542–46.
14. Wilson A, Petrie HT, Scollay R, Shortman K. Int Immunol 1989; 1:605–12.
15. Hugo P, Waanders GA, Scollay R, Shortman K, Boyd R. Int Immunol 1990; 2:209–18.
16. Crispe IN, Moore MW, Husmann LA, Smith L, Bevan MJ, Shimonkevitz RP. Nature 1987; 329:336–39.
17. Scollay R, Wilson A, D'Amico A, Kelly K, Egerton M, Pearse M, Wu L, Shortman K. Immunol Rev 1988; 104:81.
18. von Boehmer H. Ann Rev Immunol 1988; 6:309–26.
19. Egerton M, Scollay R. Int Immunol 1990; 2:157–63.
20. Budd RC, Miescher GC, Howe RC, Lees RK, Mac Donald HR. J Exp Med 1987; 166: 577–82.
21. Howe RC, Pedrazzini T, Mac Donald HR, Eur J Immunol 1989; 19:25–30.
22. Papiernik M, Pontoux C. Int Immunol 1990; 2:407–412.
23. Bluestone JA, Pardoll D, Sharrow SO, Fowkles BJ. Nature 1987; 326:82–84.
24. Havran WL, Poenie M, Kimura J, Tsien R, Weiss A, Allison JP. Nature 1987; 330:170–73.

29

Thymocyte Differentiation in the Rat Is Disturbed by the Thymus Atrophy–Inducing Compound Dibutyltin Dichloride

Raymond H. H. Pieters, Marianne Bol, Bert W. Lam, Willem Seinen, and André H. Penninks
Research Institute of Toxicology, University of Utrecht, Utrecht, The Netherlands

INTRODUCTION

In the mid-1970s some of the dialkylated organotin compounds like di-n-butyltin dichloride (DBTC), which are used as stabilizer in PVC plastics, were found to be immunotoxic (1). When DBTC was fed to rats for several weeks a depletion of lymphocytes was observed in the thymic cortex and in T-cell areas of peripheral lymphoid organs. In various immune function tests depression of T-cell–dependent immunity was demonstrated (2).

Cortical thymocyte depletion appeared to be the most sensitive criterion of DBTC toxicity. The kinetics of the DBTC-induced thymus atrophy was studied in more detail on several days following a single oral dose (3). Whereas thymus weight reduction was optimal 4–5 days after dosing, thymocyte proliferation and thymoblast count were maximally reduced at days 1 and 2. These results indicated that the thymus atrophy resulted from an antiproliferative effect of DBTC. Subsequent immunohistology studies revealed that DBTC may disturb thymocyte differentiation at an immature stage (4). This hypothesis is further supported by the results of this study, in which CD4/8 double-color flow cytometric analysis was performed on thymocytes isolated various days after a single oral dose of DBTC. In addition, the appearance of blastoid thymocytes was determined in thymus sections with the use of the antitransferrine monoclonal antibody (MAb) OX-26 (5).

MATERIALS AND METHODS

Di-n-butyltin Dichloride

Di-n-butyltin dichloride was kindly provided by Dr. H. A. Meinema, Institute for Applied Chemistry, TNO, Zeist, The Netherlands, and was more than 99% pure.

Animals and Treatment

Male Wistar-derived rats, 4–5 weeks of age, were obtained from the Central Institute for Breeding of Laboratory Animals, TNO, Zeist, The Netherlands, and exposed to an oral dose of 0 or 15 mg DBTC/kg body weight dissolved in corn oil. At each subsequent day, thymus glands of four control and four treated rats were collected. One-half of each thymus gland was snap frozen in liquid nitrogen and the other half was used to prepare thymocyte suspensions.

Monoclonal Antibodies

The OX-8 (anti-CD8) (6) and OX-26 (antitransferrine receptor) (5) cell lines were obtained from the European Collection of Animal Cell Cultures (ECACC, PHLS, Salisbury, U.K.). OX-8 was biotinylated by Mr. R. van Herwijnen, EVL, Amsterdam, The Netherlands. FITC-conjugated ER-2 (7) was kindly provided by Dr. J. Rozing, TNO, Rijswijk, The Netherlands.

Flow Cytometry

For flow cytometric analyses, thymocyte suspensions, prepared by gently pressing the cells through a nylon sieve (3), were washed three times in Dulbecco's phosphate-buffered saline (PBS) supplemented with 2 mM D-glucose (pH 7.4) and suspended in PBS containing 10% FCS and 0.01% NaN_3 at a concentration of 4×10^7 cells/ml. Of this suspension, 25 μl was incubated with a mixture of biotinylated OX-8 and FITC-conjugated ER2 followed by an incubation with Streptavidin-PE (SBA. Inc., U.S.A.). Staining of MAb OX-26$^+$ cells was performed by incubating cells with the MAb OX-26 (IgG_{2a}) and thereafter with a FITC-conjugated GaM IgG_{2a} antibody (SBA. Inc., U.S.A.). Cells were washed and resuspended in physiologic saline containing 5% BSA and 2.7 mM Na_2EDTA (pH 7.4) and analyzed in a flow cytometer (FACScan, Becton Dickinson).

Cell-Size Analysis

The total number of thymocytes and the number of large thymocytes (>8.2 μm diameter) were counted with a Coulter counter using different threshold values as was described before (3).

Immunohistology

Cryosections were sequentially incubated with MAb OX-26, RaM Ig conjugated to HRP (Dakopatts, Copenhagen, Denmark) and 3-amino-9-ethyl carbazole with H_2O_2 as peroxidase substrate.

RESULTS

As was found in previous studies, a single oral dose of 15 mg DBTC/kg body weight caused a reduction in thymus weight in young rats, owing to a decreased number of thymocytes that was maximal at days 4 and 5 after dosing. Although the total number of thymocytes was not affected up to day 2, the frequency of large thymocytes was already maximally reduced (Fig. 1, dark bars). At days 4 and 5, the frequency of thymoblasts from the exposed animals was increased to 300% compared to the frequency of large thymocytes in the daily controls. The pattern by which the number of thymoblasts changed through the

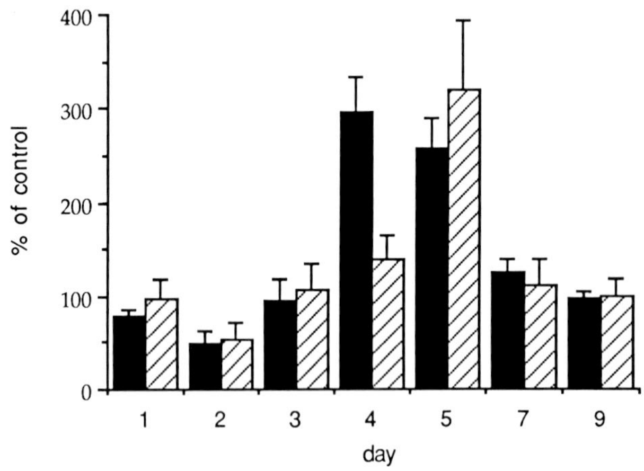

Figure 1 Frequencies of thymoblasts (dark bars) and OX-26^+ cells (hatched bars) in thymocyte suspensions isolated on several days after a single oral dose of DBTC are expressed as percentages of respective frequencies in daily control rats. Values are the mean ± SD of four suspensions.

experimental period was almost completely paralleled by the flow-cytometrically determined number of OX-26-positive thymocytes when the respective frequencies were compared (Fig. 1, hatched bars). In absolute numbers, both the thymoblasts and the OX-26–positive cells were diminished at day 2 and had returned to control level again at day 5. The MAb OX-26, considered to detect active proliferating cells, was used to localize the target thymoblasts of DBTC immunohistologically. Figure 2a shows that in a control thymus section the OX-26–positive cells are scattered throughout the cortex and medulla with a subcapsular rim of weakly positive cells. Two days after DBTC treatment a diminished number of OX-26–positive cells was visible (Fig. 2b) in the subcapsular region and inner cortex. At day 5, the number of OX-26–positive cells was greatly enhanced throughout the cortex (Fig. 2c). In thymocyte suspensions isolated on day 5 after dosing, flow cytometric analysis using the MAbs OX-8 (anti-CD8) and ER2 (anti-CD4) showed an absolute decrease in the $CD4^+8^+$ thymocytes of about 80% (Fig. 3a). Owing to the dramatic decrease in the number of $CD4^+8^+$ thymocytes, the percentages of the $CD4^-8^-$, $CD4^-8^+$, and $CD4^+8^-$ populations were relatively increased (Fig. 3b). In absolute numbers these populations were not changed on any day (Fig. 3a).

DISCUSSION

The decrease in the number of total thymocytes induced by DBTC at days 4 and 5 is preceded by a maximal absolute and relative depletion of OX-26–positive cells and thymoblasts at day 2, as shown in Figure 1. This result is in agreement with the previously observed maximal reduction in deoxyribonucleic acid synthesis of total thymocyte suspensions at days 1 and 2 after DBTC dosage (3). The absolute number of thymoblasts reached control level again at days 4 and 5. The relative increase of thymoblasts is considered to result from the strong decrease in the number of small thymocytes (3). These observations are further confirmed by immunohistological examinations using the MAb OX-26 as a representative marker for proliferating cells. A maximal decrease in the number of

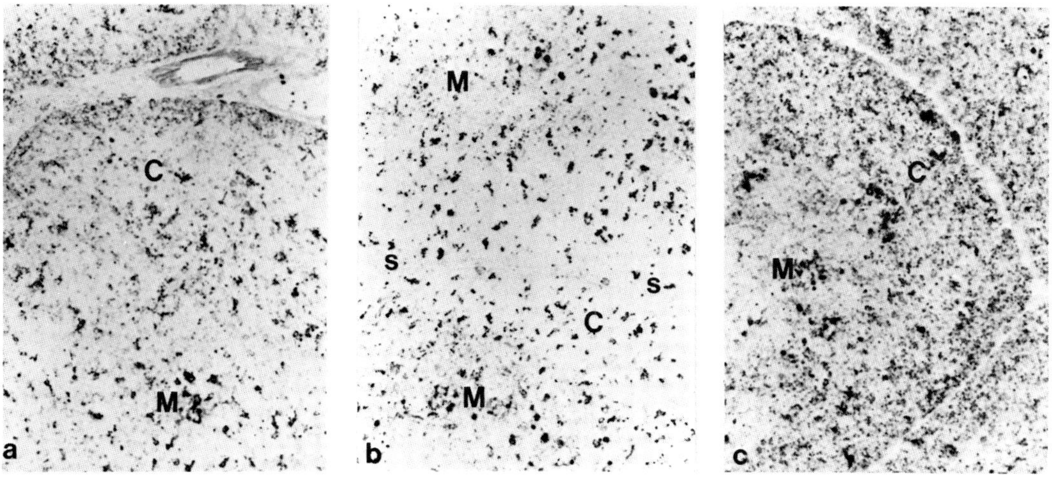

Figure 2 Thymus sections stained with MAb OX-26. (a) Control at day 1, (b) day 2 after dosing, (c) day 5 after dosing. Weak positive cells are thymocytes; strong positive cells are probably myeloid cells (5). C, cortex; M, medulla; s, capsule. Immunoperoxidase staining (33x).

OX-26–positive cells was observed on day 2 and was most obvious in the subcapsular region and the inner cortex. The relative increase of OX-26–positive cells in the cortex at day 5 is also considered to be due to the decreased number of small cortical thymocytes. This was supported by the flow cytometric analysis showing a relative but not an absolute increase of OX-26–positive cells.

To determine the impact of the antiproliferative effect of DBTC on thymocyte differentiation CD4/CD8 double-stained thymocyte suspensions were analyzed by flow cytometry (Fig. 3). Five days after DBTC exposure, $CD4^+8^+$ thymocytes were dramatically increased in relative as well as in absolute numbers. The $CD4^-8^-$, $CD4^-8^+$, and $CD4^+8^-$ thymocytes were relatively enhanced in number but were left unchanged in absolute number. The finding that the single positive cells are not changed in number is well in line with morphological observations showing no effect in the medulla (4). Since the immature $CD4^-8^+3^-$ cells constitute a substantial part of the $CD4^-8^+$ cells (8), it may be concluded that these immature cells are not affected as well.

The previous conclusion that the cortical OX-44–positive cells (4) found to be increased on thymus sections were $CD4^-8^-$ thymocytes is supported by the relative increase of $CD4^-8^-$ thymocytes found in the flow cytometric analysis. The absolute number of $CD4^-8^+$ cells is not changed on any day, indicating that the diminishment of thymoblasts is not within this population. Thymocyte proliferation is detected in the $CD4^-8^-$, the immature $CD4^-8^+$, and in $CD4^+8^+$ thymocyte population (8). However, taken together the above results the majority of the diminished thymoblasts are probably $CD4^+8^+$. The time period between the maximal reduction of thymoblasts (days 1 and 2) and of $CD4^+8^+$ cells (days 4 and 5) is about 3 days. Assuming that the turnover of time of $CD4^+8^+$ thymocytes is equal in rat and in mouse (3–4 days [9]) together with the probability that the decreased thymoblasts are $CD4^+8^+$, the putative target cell of DBTC can be placed prior to or within the early $CD4^+8^+$ thymoblast stage.

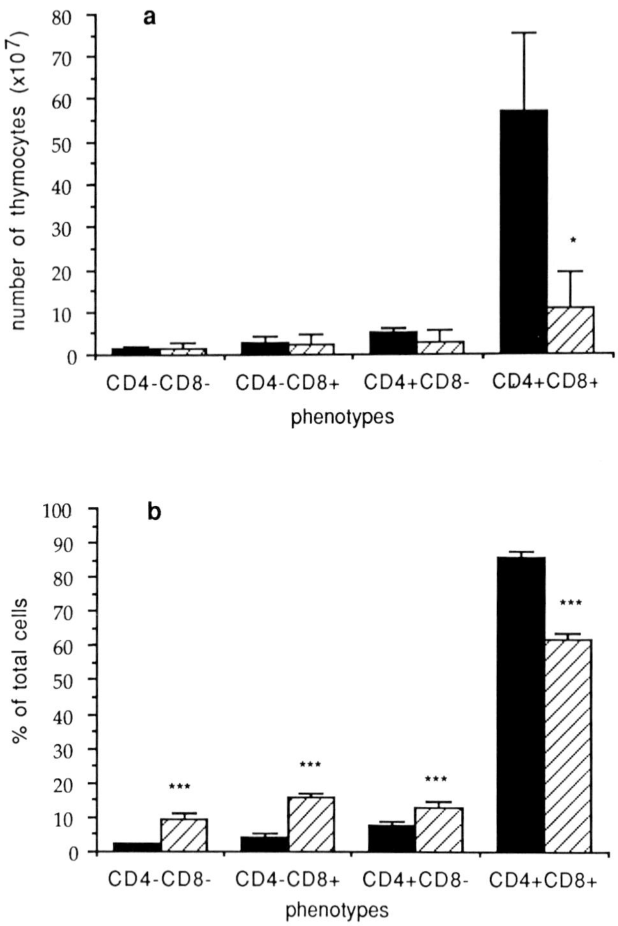

Figure 3 CD4/CD8 characterized phenotypes determined by flow cytometry in thymocyte suspensions isolated 5 days after exposure to a single oral dose of DBTC. (a) Total cell number (cells $\times 10^7$ per organ). (b) Percentage of total cell count. Control, dark bars; DBTC, hatched bars. Each bar represents mean ± SD of four suspensions. *$p < 0.05$, ***$p < 0.001$ in Student's t-test.

These and previous results support our hypothesis that the decrease in the number of small thymocytes was primarily caused by a diminished supply of small thymocytes due to an antiproliferative activity of DBTC on early thymocytes. Together with the high turnover of small cortical thymocytes this will result in the severe thymocyte depletion and thymus weight reduction.

Although the mechanism by which DBTC induces the depletion of thymoblasts is still not clear, a possible explanation can be found in the fact that DBTC has an affinity for sulphydryl groups, in particular dithiol groups (10). SH-dependent processes in the thymus sensitive to DBTC interference may be: receptor/ligand interactions, production or release of growth factors, and signal transduction (11,12). Studies are in progress to investigate possible interactions of DBTC with these processes.

REFERENCES

1. Seinen W, Vos JG, Van Spanje I, Snoek M, Brands R, Hooykaas H. Toxicity of organotin compounds. II. Comparative in vivo and in vitro studies with various organotin and organolead compounds in different animal species with special emphasis on lymphocyte cytotoxicity. Toxicol Appl Pharmacol 1977; 42:197–212.
2. Seinen W, Vos JG, Van Krieken R, Penninks A, Brands R, Hooykaas H. Toxicity of organotin compounds. III. Suppression of thymus-dependent immunity in rats by di-n-butyltindichloride and di-n-octyltindichloride. Toxicol Appl Pharmacol 1977; 42:213–24.
3. Snoeij NJ, Penninks AH, Seinen W. Dibutyltin and tributyltin compounds induce thymus atrophy in rats due to a selective action on thymoblasts. Int J Immunopharmacol 1988; 10:891–9.
4. Pieters RHH, Kampinga J, Bol-Schoenmakers M, Lam AW, Penninks AH, Seinen W. Organotin-induced thymus atrophy concerns the $OX\text{-}44^{+}$ immature thymocytes. Relation to the interaction between early thymocytes and thymic epithelial cells? Thymus 1989; 14:79–88.
5. Jefferies WA, Brandon MR, Williams AF, Hunt SV. Analysis of lymphopoietic stem cells with a monoclonal antibody to the rat transferrin receptor. Immunology 1985; 54:333–41.
6. Brideau RJ, Carter PB, McMaster WR, Mason DW, Williams AF. Two subsets of rat T lymphocytes defined with monoclonal antibodies. Eur J Immunol 1980; 10:609–15.
7. Joling P, Tielen F, Vaessen LMB, Hesse CJ, Rozing J. Intrathymic differentiation in the rat. Adv Exp Med Biol 1985; 186:235–44.
8. Paterson DJ, Green JR, Jefferies WA, Puklavec M, Williams AF. The MRC OX-44 antigen marks a functionally relevant subset among rat thymocytes. J Exp Med 1987; 165:1–13.
9. Scollay R, Wilson A, D'Amico A, Kelly K, Egerton M, Pearse M, Wu L, Shortman K. Developmental status and reconstitution potential of subpopulations of murine thymocytes. Immunol Rev 1988; 104:81–120.
10. Penninks AH, Seinen W. The lymphocyte as target of toxicity: a biochemical approach to dialkyltin induced immunosuppression. In: Haddeb JW, Chedid L, Dukor P, Spreafico F, Willoughby D (eds). *Advances in Immunopharmacology*, Vol 2, Pergamon Press, New York, 1983, pp. 41–62.
11. Loor F, Martin-Pélissard C, Ångman L. Capping Revisited. II. Low sensitivity to sulfydryl reagents. Cell Immunol 1981; 57:73–84.
12. Freed BM, Lempert N, Lawrence DA. The inhibitory effect of N-ethylmaleimide, colchicine and cytochalasins on human T-cell functions. Int J Immunopharmacol 1989; 11:459–65.

30
Evidence for More Than One Type of Nerve Net in the Rat Thymus Gland

Marion D. Kendall,[1] Ali Al-Shawaf,[1] Judy Aberdeen,[2] Peter James,[3] and Tim Cowen[4]

[1]Thymus Research Laboratory and Cell Biology Unit, UMDS, London, England; [2]University College, London, England; [3]Institute of Animal Physiology and Genetics, Agricultural and Food Research Council, Babraham, Cambridge, England; and [4]Royal Free Hospital, London, England

INTRODUCTION

The evidence for a noradrenergic (NA) innervation to the thymus has been presented in Felten and Felten (1), where they also commented on a possible peptidergic innervation. Previous work (2) demonstrating a cholinergic innervation has been challenged (3).

This study was initiated to reinvestigate the presence of acetylcholine esterase fibers previously reported by us (4), to document their distribution in relation to the NA innervation, and to document the presence and distribution of nerves reactive to antibodies raised against a general nerve marker (PGP 9.5), vasointestinal peptide (VIP), neuropeptide Y (NP-Y) and calcitonin gene–related peptide (CGRP) (Fig. 1). The pattern of innervation was examined after chemical sympathectomy using 6-OHDA and guanethidine, and during the recovery period.

MATERIALS AND METHODS

Normal uninjected, vehicle injected and 6-OHDA injected (80 mg/kg) 200-g adult male CSE Wistar rats were used. Full details of the methods are in press (5). Briefly, thymuses for immunocytochemistry were fixed in Zamboni's fluid (24 hr) before being frozen and cut. Primary antibody (Ab) was then applied at optimum dilution and room temperature for 24 hr. After washing with phosphate-buffered saline (PBS), FITC-conjugated secondary Ab was applied for 90 min. Slides were mounted and viewed under fluorescent light, and by confocal laser microscopy. For acetylcholinesterase (AChE) activity, Karnovsky and Root's method was modified and used with comprehensive inhibitory controls (see details in Ref. 5) to block either, both, or none of the specific and nonspecific cholinesterase (ChE). Sympathetic noradrenergic innervation was visualized using De La Torre's method.

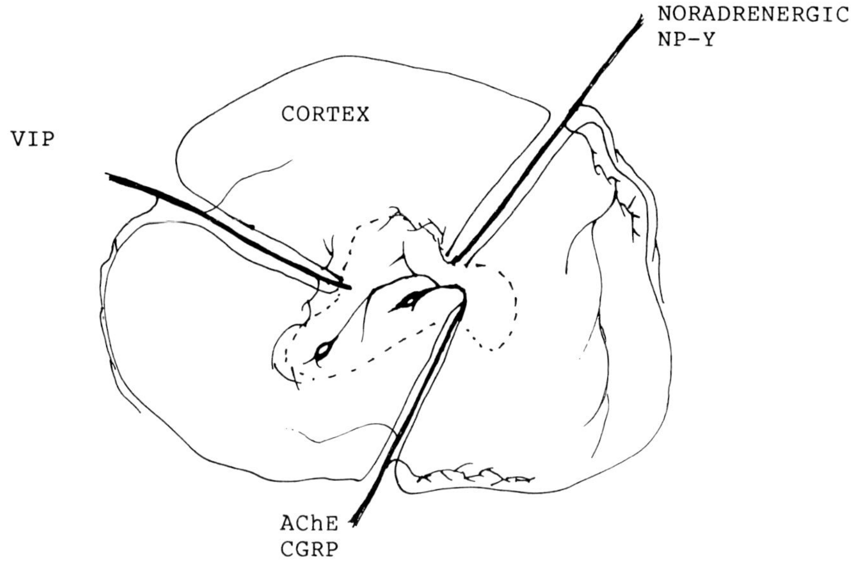

Figure 1 Diagram showing the location of three different types of nerves in the thymus. In reality, the nerves do not run separately as shown here, and the neuropeptides could colocalize or be in cholinergic nerves; e.g., VIP in AChe-positive nerves. All major blood vessels are richly innervated by all three types of nerves.

Random mitotic and pyknotic cell counts were performed on sections from thymuses preinjected with 5-bromodeoxyuridine (BUDR) 4 hr before sacrifice and then processed for paraffin sections.

RESULTS

The AChE activity was found to be specific and located as described previously (4). Its distribution differed from that of NA nerve fibers in being more sparse in the subcapsular cortex and by extending into the medulla where fibers and cells were both found to be positive.

The NA innervation entered the thymus gland with nerves running close to and surrounding major blood vessels in connective tissue septa. From these, fine nerves branched out to form a plexus in the cortex under the capsule, with fibers being seen within the capsule. Other, fewer nerves entered the cortex directly, unaccompanied by blood vessels, and ramified throughout the region, often passing close to autofluorescent macrophages. There was also a plexus at the corticomedullary junction but no NA nerves were observed in the medulla or around any small cortical blood vessels.

In general, the distribution of PGP 9.5 and all neuropeptides examined were similar to that of NA nerves, being found around major blood vessels, in subcapsular and corticomedullary plexuses, and as solitary fibers in the cortex. PGP 9.5 positivity was not as extensive as NA fibers. VIP-positive fibers were usually finer, with fewer in the subcapsular cortex than those of other peptides. CGRP fibers, like AChE-positive fibers, were also found in the medulla. A few medullary cells were CGRP positive.

Four days after chemical sympathectomy, there were no NA fibers in the glands, some were present after 8 days, and by 11 days the gland was fully reinnervated. A second injection of 6-hydroxydopamine (6-OHDA) at this time again abolished any NA reactivity.

Chemical sympathectomy almost entirely abolished PGP 9.5 and NP-Y positivity. Both returned over the following days in a similar manner to that seen in NA fibers. However, VIP and CGRP positivity was not affected at any stage in the experiments, nor was AChE reactivity.

At day 4 after chemical sympathectomy with 6-OHDA, the total weights of thymus glands, and cortical thymocyte numbers were reduced. This was significant by day 8 ($p < 0.001$). Apoptosis was increased in the cortex to reach maximal levels by day 8. Interestingly, cells labeled with BUDR increased in number to day 8 and then dropped again to near previous levels by day 11. Changes in the medulla were not so pronounced, and lagged behind those of the cortex.

DISCUSSION

Thymocytes bear beta-adrenergic receptors (6) which when stimulated with catecholamines cause a reduction in their proliferation and an enhancement of differentiation antigen expression (7). Experiments with sympathectomized animals showed an increase in thymocyte proliferation (8), which as we have observed here is unlike the responses of peripheral lymphocytes to catecholamines where there is a drop in proliferative response (1). However, the presence of other neuropeptides, some of which remained after sympathectomy, (notably VIP) presages a more complex picture.

This study shows that the thymus has an NA innervation (which might also contain NP-Y) that is independent of VIP nerves and of an AChE system. In some nerves, AChe and VIP could be colocalized. There must be at least two and possibly three nerve nets in the gland.

Functionally, abolition of the NA system altered thymocyte numbers and proliferation. These effects may be independent of the VIP innervation, as although mature T cells bear receptors for VIP, there are very few on thymocytes (9). In other systems, VIP has been shown to increase vascular dilatation. The distribution of VIP-positive fibers in the thymus indicates that these interactions should be considered in the thymus too.

REFERENCES

1. Felten DL, Felten SY. Innervation of the thymus. Thymus Update 1989, 2:73–88.
2. Bulloch K, Moore RY. Innervation of the thymus gland by brain stem and spinal cord in mouse and rat. Am J Anat 1981, 162:157–166.
3. Nance DM, Hopkins DA, Bieger D. Re-investigation of the innervation of the thymus gland in mice and rats. Brain Behav Immunol 1987, 1:134–147.
4. Kendall MD, Al-Shawaf A, Zaidi SAA. The cholinergic and adrenergic innervation of the rat thymus. AEMB 1988, 237:255–261.
5. Al-Shawaf A, Cowen T, Kendall MD. Identification of neural profiles containing vasoactive intestinal polypeptide, acetylcholinesterase, and catecholamine in the rat thymus. J Anat (in press).
6. Singh U, Millson, Smith PA, Owen JJT. Identification of beta-adrenergic receptors during thymocyte ontogeny in mice. Eur J Immunol 1979, 6:59–62.

7. Singh U. Effect of sympathectomy on the maturation of fetal thymocytes grown within the anterior eye chambers in mice. AEMB 1985, 186:349–356.
8. Singh U. Lymphopoiesis in the nude fetal mouse thymus following sympathectomy. Eur J Immunol 1985, 93:222–228.
9. Ottaway CA, Greenberg GR. Interaction of vasoactive intestinal peptide with mouse lymphocytes: specific binding and the modulation of mitogen responses. J Immunol 1984, 132: 417–423.

31
Early Processes of Thymocyte Differentiation

A. Sharp, R. Eren, T. Kukulansky, and A. Globerson
The Weizmann Institute of Science, Rehovot, Israel

INTRODUCTION

The decline in T-cell functions in aging has been attributed mainly to thymic involution. However, age-related changes may also occur at the initial prethymic steps of development in the bone marrow, and these could be manifested in seeding of the thymus and in ultimate differentiation. We have investigated the potential of bone marrow cells to give rise to thymocytes in aging in an in vitro thymus-chimera model. It consisted of fetal thymus explants (FT) which were depleted of self-thymocytes, repopulated with bone marrow (BM) cells, and subsequently grown in organ culture. During the culture period, the colonizing cells differentiated, expressed thymocyte surface markers, and manifested certain T-cell functional characteristics (1,2).

By using congenic strains of mice which differed in their expression of the Thy 1 marker, it was possible to simultaneously seed cells from different sources and observe the results of the competitive reconstitution of the FT explants. Thus, when mixtures of cells originating from young and old mice were applied to FT explants, cells originating from the BM of young mice were found to have an advantage in FT colonization and constituted over 80% of the resulting thymocyte population (2). Similarly, when mixtures of cells originating from syngeneic and allogeneic mice which differed in their Thy 1 expression were seeded onto the thymus explants, a major histocompatibility complex (MHC)–linked syngeneic preference was observed (3).

Using the FT colonization model, we determined in the present study the stages at which the age-related advantage of the young cells and the syngeneic preference occurred. For this purpose we applied a number of strategies which enabled separate analyses of the competing cells at their distinct developmental stages.

MATERIALS AND METHODS

Reconstitution of Lymphocyte-Depleted Thymus Lobes

The method of thymus lobe reconstitution was employed as previously described (1–3). Briefly: thymus lobes were obtained from 14-day-old embryos of C57BL/6J or C57BL/Ka mice and depleted of their own thymocytes by incubation in medium containing 1.35 mM 2-deoxyguanosine (4). These explants were reconstituted by being placed individually in Terasaki plates containing $3–6\times10^4$ cells/well. Plates were inverted to form hanging drops, and 3 days later the explants were washed and transferred to organ culture on Nucleopore filters which rested on gelatin sponges. Competitive repopulation experiments were carried out by mixing cells (1:1) expressing the Thy 1.1 marker with cells expressing Thy 1.2 and incubating them with the thymus lobes. The cells were subsequently cultured as above. Cell phenotype analysis was performed after 12 days of incubation by teasing the thymus explants and preparing single cell suspensions for analysis by flow cytometry.

Colonization of FT Stroma by Sequential Seeding

Thymus explants were incubated with BM cells in hanging drops for 24 hr. The explants were then removed, washed in organ culture medium, incubated with the cells of choice in hanging drops for an additional 48 hr, and then transferred to organ culture.

Colonization of FT Stroma by BM-Derived Thymocytes

Thymic explants were colonized by BM cells as described above. After 12 days of incubation, cell suspensions were prepared, washed, and counted. A sample was taken for flow cytometric analysis and the rest of the suspension was incubated with freshly prepared, deoxyguanosine-treated fetal thymuses for 3 days in hanging drops, and transferred to organ culture for an additional 12 days.

Analysis of the Data

Analysis of the data was based on Student's "t" test, paired or independent, as applicable.

RESULTS AND DISCUSSION

Simultaneous Reconstitution of FT with Syngeneic and Allogeneic Cells from Mice of Different Age Groups

In order to determine whether any age-related changes in the MHC-linked recognition of BM cells arise during interaction with the thymic stroma, we colonized FT explants with BM cells of young and old donors with different MHC haplotypes. The chimeric thymuses which we constructed contained syngeneic and allogeneic cells, and we proceeded to determine the levels of T cells originating from each of the donors.

As shown in Table 1, when young and old BM cells were seeded onto an allogeneic thymic stroma (BALB/c seeded onto C57BL/6 or C57BL/Ka FT), at a 1:1 mixture with young BM cells syngeneic with the FT, the Thy 1-positive cells which developed were mainly of the syngeneic BM type. This suggested that homing markers may be associated with MHC determinants. No significant differences were detected when the

Table 1 Colonization of FT Stroma[a] by Mixtures of Syngeneic and Allogeneic Young and Old BM Cells

	Donor cells		% positive cells[b]	
Group	Thy 1.1	Thy 1.2	Thy 1.1	Thy 1.2
A	Syngeneic Young1[c]	Syngeneic Young2[d]	43 ± 3	41 ± 0
B	Syngeneic Young	Syngeneic Old[e]	68 ± 1	24 ± 2
C	Syngeneic Young	Allogeneic Young[f]	69 ± 3	11 ± 1
D	Syngeneic Young	Allogeneic Old[g]	63 ± 5	20 ± 5
E	Syngeneic Old[h]	Allogeneic Old	47 ± 2	43 ± 4

[a]Recipient FT explants were of C57BL/6J or C57BL/Ka origin.
[b]Calculated as follows: [(% Thy 1^+–background)/(100–background)]×100.
[c]C57BL/Ka, 3 months, Thy 1.1.
[d]C57BL/6J, 3months, Thy 1.2.
[e]C57BL/6J, 24 months, Thy 1.2.
[f]BALB/c, 3 months, Thy 1.2.
[g]BALB/c, 24 months, Thy 1.2.
[h]C57BL/Ka, 24 months, Thy 1.1.

competitive capabilities of young and old allogeneic cells vs young syngeneic cells were compared. However, when old syngeneic cells competed with old allogeneic ones (C57BL/Ka vs BALB/c) there was no advantage to either age group. This indicated that the expression of MHC-linked syngeneic preference is reduced with aging.

Two-Step Reconstitution of FT with Cells from Different Sources

To find out whether the reconstituting cells competed at the seeding stage in the thymic stroma, we manipulated the procedure of seeding, when thymocyte progenitors are brought in close contact with the FT stroma in hanging drops. We employed a two-step colonization protocol in which we seeded cells of one group for 24 hr, then rinsed the explants and reincubated them with cells of the competing group. The results of this sequential seeding, presented in Table 2, show that the cells which were incubated with the thymic stroma for the initial 24 hr colonized it to a higher extent, compared with their performance when seeded simultaneously. This occurred regardless of the fact that the second competing group was incubated with the thymic explants for a longer period. These experiments suggested that the initial interactions of the colonizing cells with the thymic stroma are important in determining subsequent development within the fetal thymus.

Reconstitution of FT with Cells from In Vitro Constructed BM-Thymus Chimeras

We analyzed the interactions of the developing thymocytes with the thymic stroma using the recolonization strategy. This consisted in reseeding BM-derived thymocytes which had developed in the FT explants for 12 days into freshly prepared fetal thymuses, in competing groups. We found (Table 3) that when syngeneic young and old cells competed, the age-related differences between them were reduced, although they remained significant.

Table 2 Colonization of FT Stroma by Sequentional Incubation with BM Cells[a]

Group	Source of reconstituting cells		% positive cells[b]	
	0–24 hr	24–72 hr	Thy 1.1	Thy 1.2
A	$Young_1$[c] + $Young_2$[d]	$Young_1$ + $Young_2$	43 ± 3	41 ± 0
B	$Young_1$	$Young_2$	58 ± 1	29 ± 4
C	$Young_2$	$Young_1$	24 ± 1	51 ± 2
D	$Young_1$ + Old[e]	$Young_1$ + Old	53 ± 5	24 ± 1
E	$Young_1$	Old	58 ± 7	13 ± 3
F	Old	$Young_1$	36 ± 4	42 ± 5
G	Syn Young[c] + Allo Young[f]	Syn Young + Allo Young	67 ± 7	14 ± 5
H	Syn Young	Allo Young	76 ± 8	17 ± 9
I	Allo Young	Syn Young	23 ± 9	52 ± 9

[a]Results represent mean ± SE of four experiments.
[b]Calculated as in Table 1.
[c]C57BL/Ka, 3 months, Thy 1.1 (syngeneic to the FT).
[d]C57BL/6J, 3months, Thy 1.2.
[e]C57BL/6J, 24 months, Thy 1.2 (syngeneic to the FT).
[f]BALB/c, 3 months, Thy 1.2.

Table 3 Recolonization of FT Stroma by Thymocytes Derived from Young or Old BM Cells[a]

	Donor cells	% positive cells[b]	
		Thy 1.1	Thy 1.2
First colonization			
A	Syn Young[c]	89 ± 2	0 ± 0
B	Syn Old[d]	88 ± 1	0 ± 0
C	Allo Young[e]	0 ± 0	88 ± 2
D	Allo Old[f]	0 ± 0	87 ± 3
Second colonization[g]			
E	A + B	52 ± 1	38 ± 2
F	A + C	30 ± 8	60 ± 7
G	A + D	51 ± 5	37 ± 7

[a]Recipient FT explants were of C57BL/6J or C57BL/Ka origin.
[b]Calculated as in Table 1.
[c]C57BL/Ka, 3 months, Thy 1.1.
[d]C57BL/6J, 24 months, Thy 1.2.
[e]BALB/c, 3 months, Thy 1.2.
[f]BALB/C, 24 months, Thy 1.2.
[g]BM-derived thymocytes from either young or old mice were obtained after colonizing FT stroma for 12 days and were subsequently used for recolonizations.

Table 4 Kinetics of Competitive Development of Young and Old Cells in Thymus Organ Cultures

	Number of developing cells		
Days in culture	Young[a]	Old[b]	p value
1	1400 ± 360	1520 ± 500	0.73(NS)
3	3470 ± 1660	2420 ± 450	0.30(NS)
5	11110 ± 330	6210 ± 2870	0.08(NS)
7	31100 ± 9300	6600 ± 3630	0.01
10	64480 ± 730	13190 ± 6600	0.01
12	64780 ± 4540	10030 ± 450	0.02

[a]C57BL/Ka (Thy 1.1) or C57BL/6J (Thy 1.2), 3 months old.
[b]C57BL/Ka (Thy 1.1) or C57BL/6J (Thy 1.2), 24 months old.

We also found that following recolonization the allogeneic cells became tolerant to the MHC determinants of the fetal thymus. However, this phenomenon was reduced when old allogeneic cells were employed.

Kinetic Analysis of Thymocyte Development in Mixed BM-Thymus Chimeras

We investigated the causes for the age-related reduction in thymocyte differentiation by analyzing the kinetics of competition of syngeneic young and old cells from the first day in organ culture onwards. We found that the advantage of the young cells was significant from day 7 of culture and on (Table 4). Accordingly, reduced sequential divisions of cells from the old mice may be one of the mechanisms responsible for the age-related change in thymocyte development.

CONCLUSIONS

Our studies of early steps of thymocyte differentiation have shown an age-related decline in the developmental capacity of thymocyte progenitors. This was manifested when either syngeneic young and old, or syngeneic and allogeneic old mouse bone marrow cells were allowed to compete. We investigated a number of distinct developmental phases of the thymocyte progenitors in the FT and found that the initial interactions of cells seeding the thymus stroma were crucial in determining subsequent colonization events. A further analysis of the influence of the thymic stroma on the developing thymocytes showed that allogeneic cells developed a status of tolerance to the recipient's MHC, a phenomenon which declined with age. When we followed the kinetics of Thy 1-positive cell development in organ cultures we found that the old cells manifested a reduced capacity for sequential divisions.

The strategies that we used enabled us to make a separate analysis of distinct phases in the development of thymocyte progenitors, to investigate their interactions with the thymic stroma and to point out several types of age-related changes in their differentiation capacity.

REFERENCES

1. Eren, R., Zharhary, D., Abel, L. and Globerson, A. (1987). Cell Immunol. 108, 76.
2. Eren, R., Zharhary, D., Abel, L. and Globerson, A. (1988). Cell. Immunol. 112, 449.
3. Eren, R., Abel, L. and Globerson, A. (1989). Eur. J. Immunol. 19, 2087.
4. Jenkinson, E.J., Franchi, L., Kingston, R. and Owen, J.J.T. (1982). Eur. J. Immunol. 12, 583.

32

Major Thymocyte Subpopulations of the Thymus in Pregnant Mice Using Flow Cytometry

Ann G. Clarke,[1] **and Nigel G. A. Miller**[2]
[1]*University of Nottingham, Nottingham, England;*
[2]*Agricultural and Food Research Council Institute of Animal Physiology and Genetics Research, Cambridge, England*

INTRODUCTION

During pregnancy there is an involution of the thymus with a loss of cells, apparently precipitated by sex steroids. After pregnancy the thymus returns to its original size. We have shown that the involution is not only affected by hormones, it can be prevented by immunity to paternal antigens (Clarke, 1979) and by an earlier pregnancy (Clarke, 1984). With two-color immunofluorescent analysis in the flow cytometer, four distinct thymic populations are found (Ceredig et al., 1983). About 10% of thymocytes are single positives LY2+L3T4– (cytotoxic/suppressor, CD8+) and about 10% are LY2–L3T4+ (helper precursors, CD8+). These are middle-sized mature cells and are similar to peripheral T cells. The "double positive" nonmature LY2+L3T4+ cells are the commonest (80%). They consist of about 20% large dividing cells and about 80% small nondividing cells. Most small cells, destined to die, are thought to have little function. The fourth subpopulation is made up of 4% LT2–L3T4– double negatives, most large and dividing, and they consist of further minor subsets (Scollay and Shortman, 1985). They are the precursors of all other thymocytes.

This study describes the change in the four sets of thymocytes during pregnancy and their sizes.

MATERIAL AND METHODS

Conventionally raised C57BL/10ScSn and CBA/Ca mice from OLAC Ltd. (Bicester, England) and specific pathogen–free (SPF) BALB/c and C57BL/10ScSn were used. Age-matched mature mice were mated to give syngeneic and allogeneic pregnancies and were killed on day 4 or day 17 of pregnancy; virgin female mice were used as controls. Thymuses, cleared of fat and adhering lymph nodes, were made into suspensions of single

cells. Animals from both types and times of pregnancy and a virgin control were assayed together.

Rat immunoglobulin anti-mouse IgG_{2b} monoclonal antibodies LY2 (YTS 169.4) and L3T4 (YTS 191.2) antibodies were used. For single-color analysis monoclonal antibodies (MAbs) were used with FITC–conjugated rabbit–anti-rat IgG (DAKO, Ltd. High Wycombe, England) as a second stage. For two-color analysis, FITC-conjugated LY2 MAb was used, with rabbit–anti-rat IgG secondary antibody, followed by biotin-conjugated L3T4 MAb with phycoerythrin-strepavidin. Immunofluorescent staining was performed by the method of Cobbold et al. (1984). An IgG_{2b}-irrelevant MAb MAC58 was used as a negative control. Fluorescence was assessed using a FACS 440 (Becton-Dickinson, Abingdon, England) and expressed on an arbitrary logarithmic scale of 2 decades. FITC was examined using a 540-nm short pass filter, and phycoerythrin with a 560-nm long pass filter. Fluorochromes were excited with a 448-nm 400-milliwatt argon laser. Data was analyzed on a Consort 30 system and the results were expressed as a ratio of the percentage of positive cells in the experimental animal compared with that found in the virgin control from the same assay. As the data were not normally distributed, they were expressed as $\log_{10}$ E/C, where E is the experimental value and C is the control value. Forward light scatter (FSC) was expressed on an arbitrary linear scale of 0–225 scatter units (s.u.). Dead cells (FSC <70 s.u.) and the non-lymphoid cells (FSC >220 s.u.) were gated out, and excluded. Data were analyzed in two ways. First, the proportions of the four different subsets (LY2+ L3T4–, LY2– L3T4+, LY2– L3T4– and LY2+ L3T4+) were determined for the small-, medium-, and large-sized cells by setting gates on individual sizes and looking at the phenotypes in each size group. Second, the relative percentages of large, medium, and small cells in the four functionally different populations were measured by setting individual gates on the lineage-specific cell groups; single positives, double positives, and double negatives, and then looking at their size.

RESULTS

All repeat assays gave essentially similar results. There were no major differences between conventionally maintained and SPF mice or between syngeneic and allogeneic pregnancies. The results from a typical assay consisting of 2 day four pregnant, 2 day 17 pregnant, and one virgin control C57BL are given in Figures 1 and 2.

The Phenotype of Total, Small, Medium, and Large Cells

Total Cells

In virgin animals 70–77% of thymocytes were double positives, 4–5% were double negatives, 4–8% were LY2 positive only, and 10–18% were L3T4 positive only. During early pregnancy the proportions of LY2+ L3T4– cells were less than those in the controls, but the proportions of LY2– L3T4+ cells were not changed. In late pregnancy, both showed a value like the control (Fig. 1a). Double positives decreased in late pregnancy though double negatives increased throughout (Fig. 1b).

Small Cells

Seventy-two to eight-three percent of small cells in virgins were double positives, 2–4% were double negatives, 3–7% LY2+L3T4–, and 10–18% were LY2–L3T4+. In pregnancy, small LY2+L3T4– cells are reduced early and return to control levels later. LY2–L3T4+ cells are slightly reduced throughout pregnancy (Fig. 1c). The numbers of double negatives

among the small cells are elevated throughout pregnancy, whereas double positives are lost in late pregnancy (Fig. 1d).

Medium Cells

In the medium-size cells of the controls 55–70% were double positives, 14–15% double negatives, 11–14% LY2+L3T4–, and 14–20% LY2–L3T4+. In early pregnancy the medium cells of both single positives are reduced in numbers. In late pregnancy, LY2+L3T4– are unchanged, whereas LY2–L3T4+ cells are further reduced (Fig. 1e). Double negatives increase early in pregnancy but return to normal later. Numbers of double positives are elevated at the end of pregnancy (Fig. 1f).

Large Cells

Of the large cells in the controls, 64–79% were double positives, 7–10% were double negatives, 10–18% were LY2+L3T4–, and 4–8% were LY2–L3T4+. In early pregnancy, LY2+L3T4– cells are lost early but LY2–L3T4+ show a large gain (Fig. 1g). Both cell groups return to normal in late pregnancy. Double negative levels are increased during the whole of pregnancy and double positives are reduced (Fig. 1h).

These results suggest that in early pregnancy there is a loss of cells carrying the cytotoxic/suppressor marker, and a gain of those of the helper/inducer and precursor groups. In late pregnancy, the cytotoxic/suppressor population returns to normal but there is a loss of middle-sized helper/inducer cells.

Cell Sizes in the Four Phenotypically Different Subsets

In the total thymocyte population of virgin mice, small cells (FSC 58–105 s.u.) make up 85–90% of the total, medium-sized cells (FSC 106-146 s.u.) 9–10%, and large cells (FSC 147–220 s.u.) 2–3%. Figure 2 shows the changes that occur in the distribution of cell size among the four lineage-specific populations during pregnancy.

Total Cells

Small cells are lost early in pregnancy, whereas medium and large are gained. Late in pregnancy, these differences persist but to a lesser extent (Fig. 2a).

The Double Negatives

In the controls, 50–60% of double negative are small, 33–44% are medium, and 6–8% are large. In early pregnancy (Fig. 2b), there are fewer small cells but more medium and large ones. In late pregnancy, these differences persist but to a smaller extent.

The Double Positives

In the controls 95% of double positives are small, 4–5% are medium, and 1% are large. In pregnancy (Fig. 2c), small cells are lost but large cells are gained.

Among "bright" double positives the size distribution is different. In virgin animals, small cells vary from 23 to 52%, medium from 33 to 44%, and large cells from 15 to 37%. In pregnancy, medium-sized cells are lost instead of gained, and the increase in large cells is smaller (Fig. 2f).

The Single Positives

In virgin animals, within the LY2+L3T4– cells, 68–74% were small and 26–32% were medium plus large (medium cells were not measured separately). In early pregnancy, the small cells declined, whereas medium plus large increased. Levels returned to normal

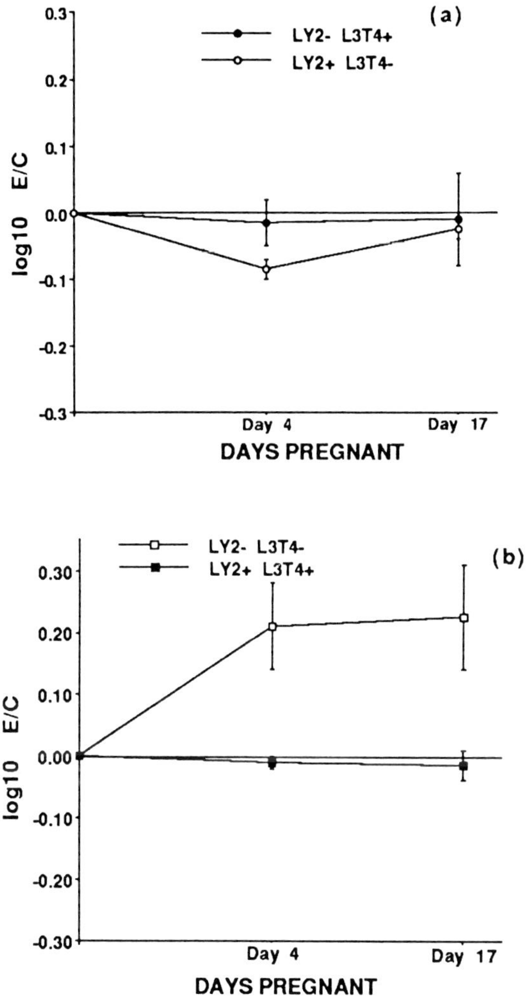

Figure 1 The cell size of the four lineage-specific subsets among the (a) and (b) total thymocyte population; (c) and (d) small cells; (e) and (f) medium cells; and (g) and (h) large cells.

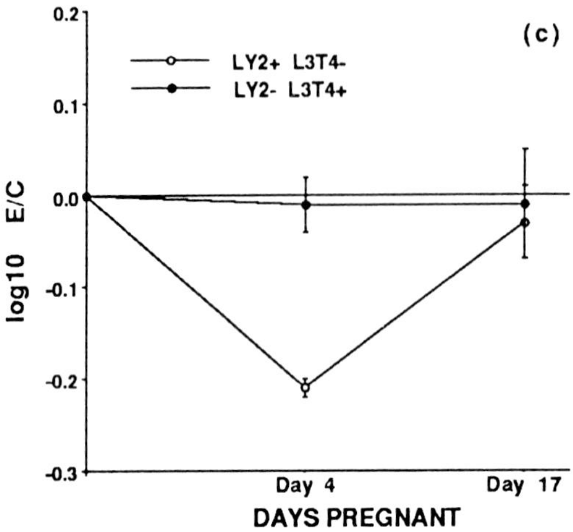

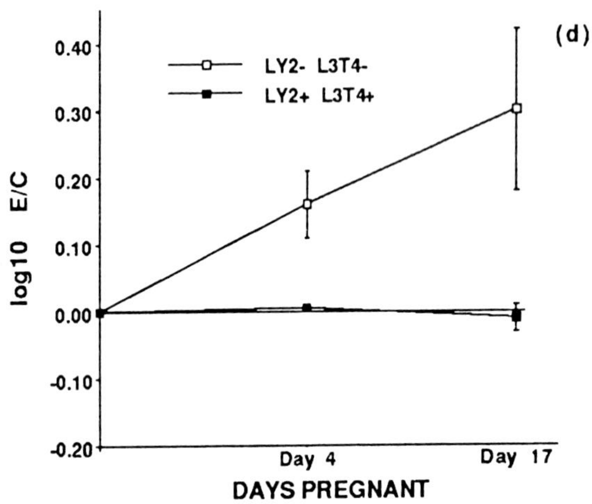

Figure 1 (Continued)

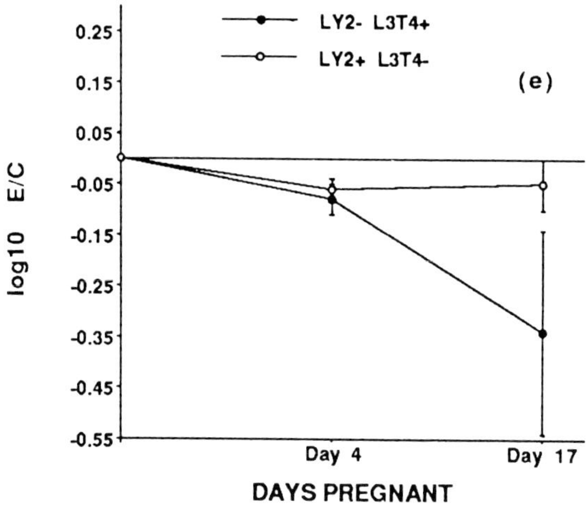

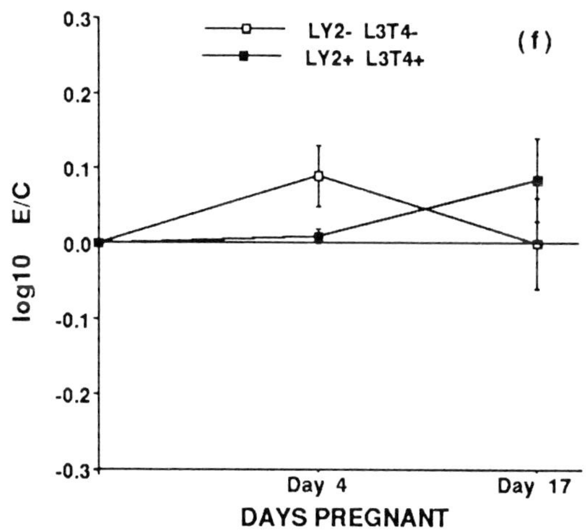

Figure 1 (Continued)

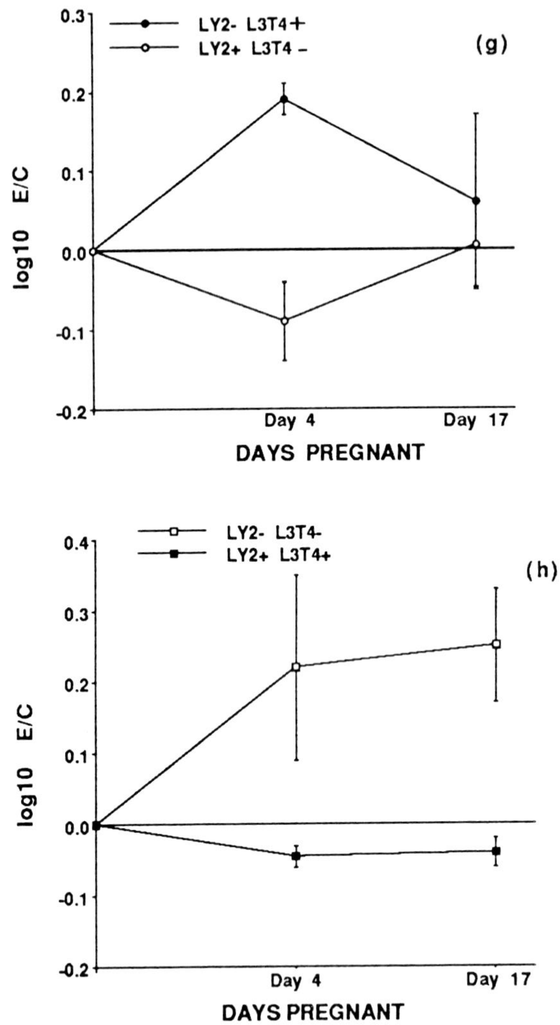

Figure 1 (Continued)

values later (Fig. 2e). In virgins, LY2– L3T4+ are made up of 86–90% small cells and 3–14% medium plus large. In pregnancy, the pattern is similar to that of LY2+L3T4– except the loss of small cells is not much evident (Fig. 2d).

DISCUSSION

It has been thought that the only thymocyte population affected by pregnancy was the small double positive cells. These results, to be reported in full elsewhere, show that there are changes in virtually all major thymocyte populations. In general, numbers of single positive cells increase in early pregnancy. However, among large cells the percentage of LY2+L3T4– declines at the same time. The latter observation reflects an overall proportional increase in the numbers of large LY2–L3T4– during early pregnancy. Thus, there are

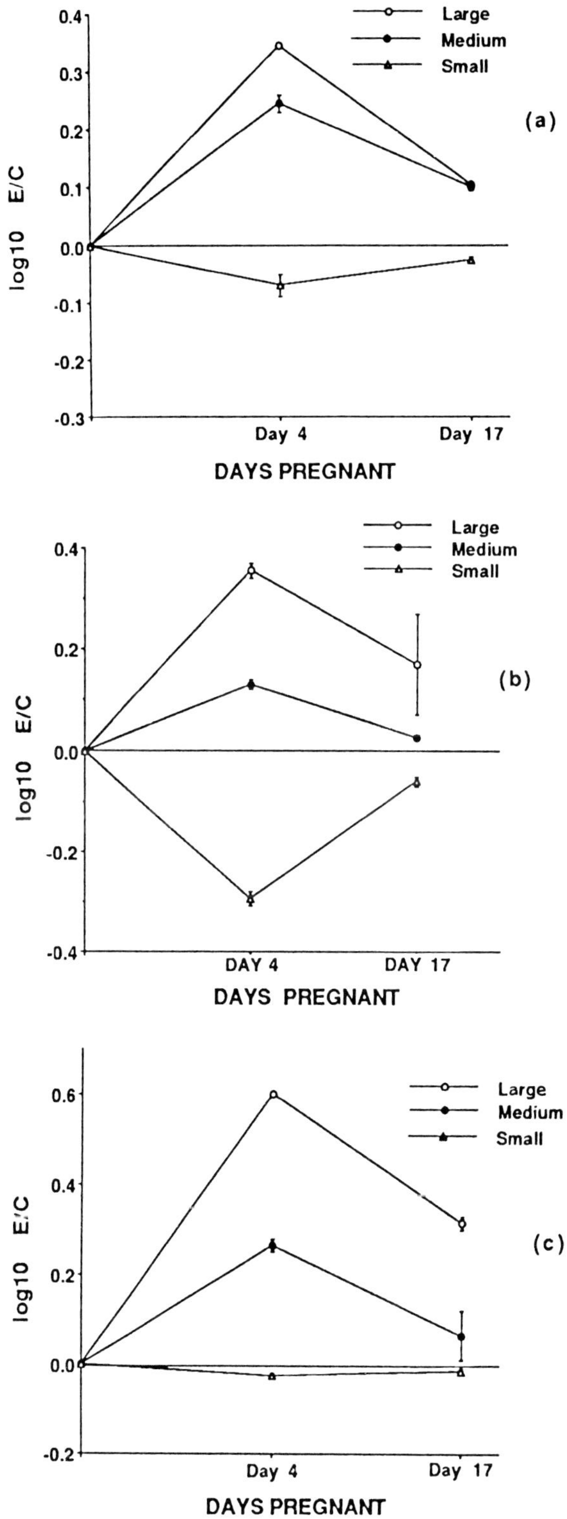

Figure 2 The percentage of fluorescence in the different cell sizes: (a) total thymocyte population; (b) LY2–L3T4–; (c) "major" LY2+L3T4+; (d) LY2–L3T4+; (e) LY2+L3T4–; (f) "bright" LY2+L3T4+.

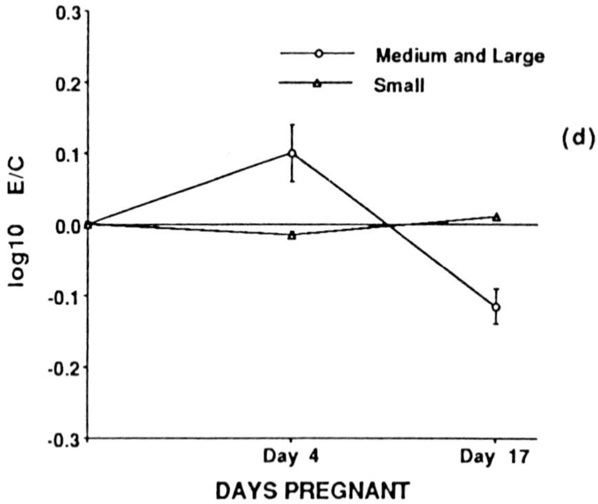

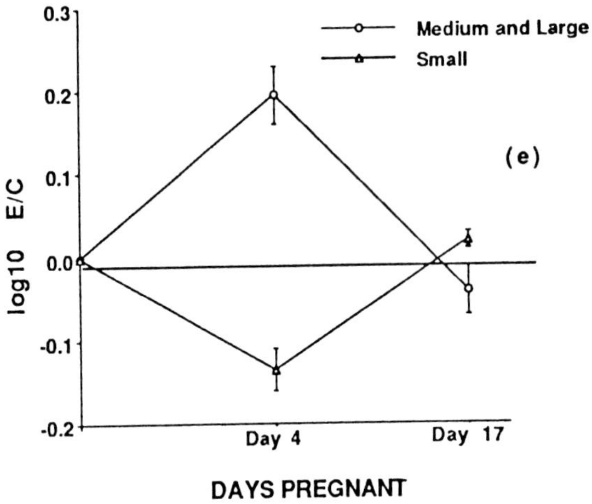

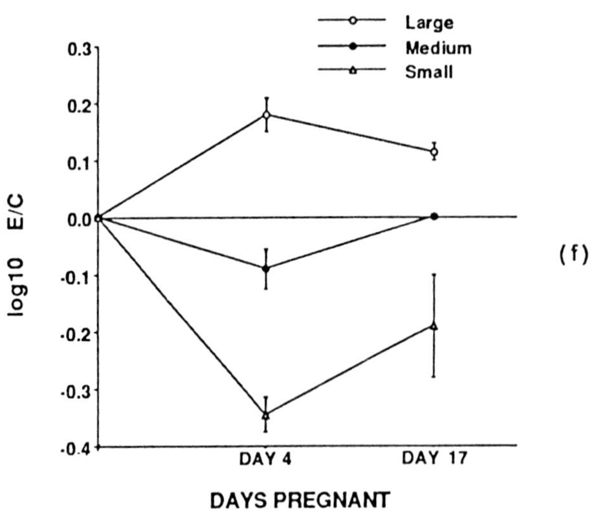

Figure 2 (Continued)

two changes, a shift in the frequencies of size classes among the LY2+L3T4– cells and an overall increase in LY2-negative cells (mainly of large size). The increase in large single positive L3T4 cells in early pregnancy may suggest an increased production of helper/inducer cells at this time. The loss in later pregnancy of medium-sized cells of this group may reflect their loss to the periphery. The corresponding reduction in large single LY2-positive cells in early pregnancy may reflect a decreased production of these cells. The contribution to the changes in mature cells made by immigrating cells is unknown. As the function of the bright double positives is unknown, the changes found in pregnancy are as yet obscure. In general, the retention of the rapidly dividing mature cells and precursor cells suggest that despite losing 75% of its cells the thymus remains fully functional in pregnancy. Indeed, in early pregnancy, the active cells of the thymus are present in greater numbers than normal. These results are in agreement with our observations from histological and cellular studies (Clarke, 1989; Clarke and Kendall, 1989) and FACS analysis (Clarke, 1989a) that activity rather than inactivity is a feature of the thymus in pregnancy. The events that occur soon after mating rather than those that occur later in pregnancy are likely to be significant in the maternal recognition of pregnancy.

ACKNOWLEDGMENTS

The work was supported by a grant from the Nuffield Foundation (AGC). Thanks are due to Professor H. Waldmann for the YTS MAbs and to Dr. G. Butcher for the irrelevant MAb MAC58.

REFERENCES

1. Ceredig R, Dialynas DP, Fitch FW, MacDonald HR. Precursors of T-cell growth factor producing cells in the thymus: Ontogeny, frequency and quantitative recovery in a subpopulation of phenotypically mature thymocytes defined by monoclonal antibody GK-1.5. J Exp Med 1983; 158:1654–71.
2. Clarke AG. Pregnancy induced involution of the thymus can be prevented by immunizing with paternal skin grafts: A strain-dependent effect. Clin Exp Immunol 1979; 35:421–24.
3. Clarke AG. Immunological studies on pregnancy in the mouse. In: Crighton DB (ed). *Immunological Aspects of Reproduction in Mammals*. London, Butterworths, 1984, pp. 153–82.
4. Clarke AG. Structural and cellular changes in the mouse thymus during pregnancy. Ad Exp Med Biol 1989; 237:363–8.
5. Clarke AG, Kendall MD. Histological changes in the thymus during mouse pregnancy. Thymus 1989; 14:65–78.
6. Clarke AG. The thymus in mouse pregnancy. J Dev Comp Immunol 1989a; 13:359.
7. Cobbold SP, Jayasuriya A, Nash A, Prospero TD, Waldmann H. Therapy with monoclonal antibodies by elimination of T-cell subsets in vivo. Nature 1984; 312:548–551.
8. Scollay R, Shortman K. Thymocyte subpopulations: an experimental review including flow cytometric cross-correlations between the major murine thymocyte markers. Thymus 1983; 5:245–295.
9. Scollay R, Shortman K. Identification of early stages of T lymphocyte development in the thymus cortex and medulla. J Immunol 1985; 134:3632–42.

33
T-Cell Subsets in the Human Spleen

Ulrike Brede,[1] Klara Tenner-Racz,[2] R. Kuse,[2] G. Janossy,[3] and P. Racz[1]
[1]*Bernhard-Nocht-Institut für Tropenmedizin, Hamburg, Federal Republic of Germany;*
[2]*AK St. Georg, Hamburg, Federal Republic of Germany;*
[3]*Royal Free Hospital, London, England*

INTRODUCTION

The spleen plays a predominant role in initiating primary immune responses to blood-borne pathogens. Recent observations have described the tissue organization of the human spleen (1–3). In addition to the classic morphological methods, immunohistochemistry has been utilized to characterize the distribution of T, B, and accessory cells in order to give further insight into the functional morphology of this organ. A series of monoclonal antibodies (MAbs) have been developed that are directed against the different components of the leukocyte common antigen (LCA, CD45), a complex of high molecular weight polypeptides expressed on all leukocytes (4). Those monoclonal antibodies further subdivide T Lymphocytes of either lineage into largely nonoverlapping subpopulations. UCHL1 recognizes the 180-kD molecule (CD45RO), whereas 2H4 is directed toward the 220-kD molecule (CD45RA) (6). Functional studies have shown that the expression of different CD45 polypeptides very likely reflects sequential stages of maturation: Resting, unstimulated T cells expressing the 220-kD molecule lose this antigen upon stimulation and acquire expression of the CD45RO molecule.

Thus, very likely the CD45RA positivity corresponds with the "virgin" cells, whereas the expression of CD45RO is a feature of primed cells (5). The difficulty of this kind of investigations in terms of immunohistology is that single labeling does not detect the localization of the different T-lymphocyte subsets. In order to clearly identify each subset double, immunoenzymatic labeling is required. The tissue distribution of lymphocytes expressing the different CD45 polypeptides has indeed been performed only on lymph nodes and thymus (7). The aim of our work was to examine the distribution of these T-cell subsets in the human spleen, and to thus add new data to the understanding of the normal histology of the human spleen. In previous studies, differing terminology has been used by different authors for the splenic architecture, and in this chapter the designation of van Krieken and te Velde has been applied (1).

Table 1 Clinical Data of the Patients

Case	Age	Diagnosis	Spleen wt (g)
1	60	ITP	180
2	41	ITP	110
3	27	ITP	220
4	55	HL	170
5	55	HL	190
6	67	HL	150
7	38	HL	400
8	60	HL	160
9	52	HL	300
10	48	NHL	240
11	78	NHL	180

MATERIALS AND METHODS

Our material (Table 1) consists of three groups:

1. Spleens removed for ITP (three cases)
2. Spleens removed during staging laparotomy for Hodgkin's lymphoma (HL, six cases)
3. Spleens removed during staging laparotomy for non-Hodgkin's lymphoma (NHL, two cases)

For further details see Table 1.

On all spleens routine histology was performed including Giemsa, hematoxylin-eosin, and Gomori stains. Careful examination of the paraffin histology showed no pathological involvement in groups 2 and 3. The material was snap-frozen in liquid nitrogen and stored at −70°C. Serial sections of 6 μ microns were obtained, fixed in acetone for 10 min, and air-dried at room temperature for 2 hr prior to staining.

Single immunoenzymatic labeling was performed using the streptoavidin-biotin method (strept-AB), applying the following antibodies: anti-DRC, anti-IgD, anti-IgM, anti-Leu-8, anti–Leu-7. For the double labeling the strept-AB and an alkaline phosphatase–antialkaline–phosphatase method (APAAP) were combined. Reciprocal combinations of antibodies with the following specificities were used: CD8, CD4, CD45RO, CD45RA, CD22, CD5.

RESULTS AND DISCUSSION

The percentage of white (WP) to red pulp (RP) of the total splenic volume is subject to change under physiological and pathological conditions (8,9). In our material, the estimated WP/RP ratio ranged from 0.1 to 0.3

The white pulp can be divided in two major subcompartments that differ not only in their cellular composition, but also functionally. The malpighian bodies are B-dependent areas and the periarteriolar lymphocyte sheath (PALS) is a T-dependent area. According to van Krieken et al., in humans the structures comparable to the PALS of the rodent spleen are irregular areas occupied by small polymorphic lymphocytes (1). In all spleens we found well-organized PALS. They consisted of several layers of tightly packed lymphocytes

surrounding an arteriole in a cylindrical arrangement and a meshwork of concentrical reticular fibers.

In all spleens, we found several primary follicles per section, and in all but one spleen, at least one secondary follicle. Especially in group 1 (ITP), the number and size of germinal centers (GCs) was striking. The GC is surrounded by the mantle zone. The mantle zone cells display prominent morphological and immunohistological features (3). The mantle zone is bordered by the marginal zone. Splenic marginal zone cells do also show a characteristic marker pattern (3). The GC and, to a smaller extent, mantle zone and marginal zone contain few scattered T cells, most of which belong to the CD4 subset. Since, in contrast to observations made in lymph nodes, the number of Leu-7^+ was very limited we did not perform any double staining with Leu-7^+. In the GCs, a predilection of the localization of T cells to the sparsely populated area like in the lymph node follicles was not observed.

Double immunoenzymatic labeling reveals that the great majority of these T cells are primed cells ($CD45RO^+$). About two-thirds of the cells forming the PALS belong to the CD4 subset. Only few CD8 cells can be found in the PALS. Double labeling for CD45RA and CD45RO revealed that cells with the $CD45RO^+,RA^-$ phenotype were dominant in the PALS region, demonstrating that these T cells are likely to be primed cells. In most cases, only about one-third or even less of the PALS cells belonged to the $CD45RA^+,RO^-$ "virgin" population. In one case, however, the $CD45RA^+,RO^-$ cells were more numerous than the CD45RO virgin cells. This finding tentatively suggests that the splenic T cells may change dynamically depending on the actual immune status.

The cellular composition of the red pulp differed considerably from that seen in the WP: the estimated CD4/CD8 ratio within the RP was about 1:3. Among these T cells only few cells displayed the virgin immunophenotype ($CD45RA^+$); an estimated 80% of cells showed the "primed" feature ($CD45RA^+$). In the RP, both virgin and primed cells were observed in small clusters rather than evenly distributed. Additionally, CD8 staining has also been seen on splenic endothelial lining cells, as described previously (10), but these nonlymphoid cells were $CD45R^-$.

The great number of primed cells in the spleen underlines the importance of the human spleen in the immune system. Further studies on the localization and distribution of the different T-cell subsets under several pathological conditions are in progress.

ACKNOWLEDGMENTS

This collaborative work was supported by the BMFT (Bundesministerium für Forschung und Technologie), and by the Körber Stiftung and by the EC concerted action Pathology and Immunology of HIV Related Diseases.

REFERENCES

1. van Krieken JHJM, te Velde. Normal Histology of the Human Spleen. Am J Surg Pathol 1988; 12:777–785.
2. Tanaka H, Takasaki S, Sakata A, Muroya T, Suzuki T, Ishikawa E. Lymphocyte subsets in the white pulp of human spleen in normal and diseased cases. Acta Pathol Jpn 1984; 34(2):251–270.
3. van Krieken JHJM, von Schilling C, Kluin M, Lennert K. Splenic Marginal Zone Lymphocytes and Related Cells in the Lymph Node. Hum Pathol 1989; 20:320–325.
4. Beverley PCL, Merkenschlager M, Wallace D. Identification of Human Naive and Memory T Cells. In: F. Melchers (ed). *Progress in Immunology VII*, Berlin, Springer, 1989, p. 432–438.

5. Akbar AN, Terry L, Timms A, Beverley PCL, Janossy G. Loss of CD45R and gain of UCHL1 reactivity is a feature of primed T cells. J Immunol 1988; 140:2171–2178.
6. Wallace DL, Beverley PCL. Phenotypic changes associated with activation of CD45RA$^+$ and CD45RO T cells. Immunology 1990; 69:460–467.
7. Janossy G, Bofill M, Rowe D, Muir J, Beverley PCL. The tissue distribution of T lymphocytes expressing different CD45 polypeptides. Immunology 1989; 66:517–521.
8. van Krieken JHJM, te Velde J, Hermans J, Welvaart K. The splenic red pulp; a histomorphometrical study in splenectomy specimens embedded in methylmethacrylate. Histopathology 1985; 9:401–416.
9. van Krieken JHJM, te Velde J, Hermans J, Cornelisse CJ, Welvaart C, Ferrari M. The amount of white pulp in the spleen; a morphometrical study done in methacrylate-embedded splenectomy specimens. Histopathology 1983; 7:767–782.
10. Buckley PJ, Dickson S. Monoclonal antibodies to T-helper/inducer and T-suppressor/cytotoxic lymphocyte subsets recognize antigens on splenic sinusoidal lining cells. AJCP 1984; 12:167–172.

LYMPHOCYTE ACTIVATION AND REGULATION OF THE IMMUNE RESPONSE

34
Immunoregulation by Cytokines

Joost J. Oppenheim[1] **and G. Jeanette Thorbecke**[2]
[1]*Lab. Molec. Immunoregulation, BRMP, NCI-FCRF, National Institutes of Health, Ft. Detrick, Frederick, Maryland;*
[2]*New York University Medical Center, New York, New York*

The session on "Lymphocyte Activation and Regulation of the Immune Response" dealt with a large variety of the immunoregulatory agents, ranging from cytokines to adhesion molecules. Indeed, the effects of the cytokine network and the role of adhesion molecules in the interaction and localization of lymphoid cells need to be addressed by in vivo studies. The exact localization of cytokine-producing cells in the tissues under various conditions seems an appropriate beginning of such work, nicely complementing the studies of in vivo effects of injected cytokines.

Of interest were studies of the production of cytokines such as interleukin-1 (IL-1), IL-2, IL-3, IFN-γ, and IL-6 in various cell types present in the normal and myasthenia gravis thymus. Surprisingly, both soluble CD23 and IL-3 were produced by thymic epithelial cells (under IL-4 control), and promoted thymocyte differentiation (Dalloul). While IL-2–producing cells were found in the follicular and perifollicular areas in the thymus of myasthenia gravis patients, IFN-γ–producing cells were rare there (Emilie). This contrast with the relatively high representation of both IL-2 and IFN-γ producing cells in LN and virtually absent interleukin production in normal thymus (Emilie, Eertwegh).

Upregulation of cytokine production was shown in vivo even after T-independent type II antigen administration (IFN-γ; Eertwegh). It was not clear whether the T cells were directly or indirectly affected by the antigen, since the investigators had not established that the preparation of TNP-Ficoll they used immunized in a truly T-independent fashion. Le Gros showed an increase in IL-4–producing cells when anti-CD3 stimulation was performed in the presence of IL-2 in vitro or after injection of anti-immunoglobulin D (IgD) in vivo. Such IL-4–producing cells were rare in spleen cells taken directly from uninjected mice.

Functional effects of cytokines highlighted included: (a) the cytotoxic effect of IFN-γ and tumor necrosing factor α on intestinal epithelial cells in vitro, postulated to explain graft-vs-host–induced damage to intestines and apparently mediated by activation of NK cells (Garside); (b) the impressive recruitment of mononuclear cells after injection of IL-2 into lepromatous skin, causing rapid clearance of the locally accumulated lepra bacilli (Kaplan); and (c) the protective effect against lethal doses of γ-irradiation of IL-1, which is counteracted by transforming growth factor β (Oppenheim).

Functions of adhesion molecules discussed included: (a) the protective effects of ligands for CD40 and of soluble CD23 with IL-1 on germinal center B cells in vitro, preventing them from undergoing apoptosis (Liu); (b) the characterization of IgD receptors on T cells and of their lectinlike specificity for N-linked glycans of IgD. Upregulation by IgD of these receptors augments T-B cell interaction, leading to enhancement of primary and secondary responses as well as germinal center formation (Thorbecke).

Overall, this session illustrated the merits of evaluating the in vivo production, distribution and effects of cytokines and adhesion molecules. Although such studies are inevitably difficult to interpret, in vivo rather than in vitro studies are more likely to reveal the relevant pathophysiological roles of these molecules.

35

In Vivo Detection, Kinetics, and Characterization of Interferon-γ–Producing Cells During a Thymus-Dependent Immune Response

An Immunohistochemical Study

Alfons J. M. van den Eertwegh, Marianne J. Fasbender, Wim J. A. Boersma, and Eric Claassen
TNO Medical Biology Laboratory, Rijswijk, The Netherlands

INTRODUCTION

Interferon-γ (IFN-γ) is a cytokine of central importance in the regulation of the immune system that also displays nonimmune effects (1). The knowledge concerning the mechanisms of production and action of IFN-γ is mainly based on in vitro experiments. This is somewhat surprising considering the fact that in vitro manipulations like cell separation and culture may introduce artefacts and essentially change the microenvironment of the cells. Immunohistochemical techniques, on the contrary, enable the study of the cells in their unchanged original microenvironment, which is of great importance, since regulation of immune responses by cytokines is most likely a local and strongly compartmentalized process.

There are several reports which describe the detection of cytokine-producing cells at the single cell level (2), in human tissues (3–5), and in tissues of mice (6,7) with cytokine-specific antibodies. In the present study, we investigate the potentials of immunohistochemical techniques in the in vivo analysis of a cytokine-mediated immune response. Therefore, we conducted an experiment analogous to the in vitro experiments performed by Wada et al. (8) and in particular with reference to the in vivo activity and cellular source of IFN-γ.

MATERIALS AND METHODS

Animals

Male BALB/c mice were bred at T.N.O., Rijswijk, The Netherlands, and were used at the age of 20–26 weeks.

Bacteria and Mitogen

Live lyophilized BCG (bacille Calmette-Guérin), a kind gift of Dr. I. Claassen (RIVM, Bilthoven, The Netherlands), were killed by exposure to 60°C for 90 min and were suspended in phosphate-buffered saline (PBS). Concanavalin A (Con A) was purchased from Pharmacia, Fine Chemicals Inc., Uppsala, Sweden.

Treatment of Mice

Three groups of mice were injected i.p. with heat-killed BCG (3.3×10^7) in 400 μl PBS, and stimulated 3 weeks later with 200 μg Con A i.v. Subsequently, mice were bled and sacrificed 0, 1.5, 3.0, 4.5, 6.0 hr after Con A stimulation. Three mice were injected i.p. with 400 μl PBS. Subsequently, these mice were stimulated with 200 μg Con A i.v. Control mice were treated with PBS. Mice were bled and sacrificed after 3 hr.

Reagents

DB-1, a mouse antirat monoclonal antibody (MAb) with a high specificity for mouse IFN-γ, was a kind gift of Dr. P. H. van der Meide (9). DB-1 was conjugated to alkaline phosphatase (AP) according to the procedure described by Claassen et al. (10). The rat MAb Lyt-2^+ (CD8) (clone 53.6.7.2) (11), L3T4 (CD4) (clone GK-1.5) (12), and MOMA2 (panmacrophage marker) (13), kindly provided by Dr. G. Kraal (Amsterdam, The Netherlands), were used as cell markers. Rabbit antiasialo GM_1 serum (natural killer [NK] cell) (14) was obtained from WAKO Chemicals GmBh, West Germany. As control antibodies, the mouse MAb directed to human immunoglobulin (Ig) G_1 (clone 3-1.1) (15) and IgG3 (clone 330-2.2) (16) conjugated to alkaline phosphatase (AP) were used. Second-step conjugates were rabbit antirat conjugated to horseradish peroxidase (HRP) (Dakopatts, Copenhagen, Denmark) and goat antirabbit-HRP (Miles-Yeda, Ltd., Rehovot, Israel).

Immunocytochemistry

Spleens were removed and snap-frozen in liquid nitrogen. Cryostat sections (8 μm) were fixed for 10 min in fresh acetone, containing 0.02% H_2O_2. Slides were rinsed with PBS and incubated overnight at 4°C with Db-1-AP. For the double-staining experiments, Db-1-AP was simultaneously incubated with one of the above-described reagents. Slides were again washed with PBS and incubated for 30 min at room temperature with second-step conjugates. Sections were washed three times with PBS and histochemical revelation of AP was performed prior to the histochemical revelation of HRP, as described previously (10). Slides were counterstained with hematoxylin for 15 sec, and mounted in glycerol/gelatin.

IFN-γ ELISA

Serum samples were assayed for IFN-γ according to the procedure described by Cherwinski et al. (17).

RESULTS AND DISCUSSION

We investigated cryostat sections of spleens of three groups of BALB/c mice after priming with heat-killed BCG and stimulation with Con A. After incubation with DB-1-AP and histochemical revelation the IFN-γ–producing cells characterized by a blue cytoplasm, were detected (Fig. 1a). No staining was seen in control slides from any specimen treated by omission or substitution of primary antibody. Preincubation of DB-1-AP with IFN-γ completely abolished the cytoplasmic staining. The IFN-γ–producing cells were found in small clusters of two to five and were located in the T-cell–dependent areas like the periarteriolar lymphocyte sheaths and the coaxial sheaths of lymphoid tissue surrounding the terminal arteriolar branches (Fig. 1b). Analysis of the kinetics of the IFN-γ–producing cells showed that the maximum number of IFN-γ–producing cells was detected in spleens of BCG-primed mice that were not stimulated with Con A (Fig. 2). The IFN-γ–producing cells in the Con A–stimulated and BCG-primed mice had an enlarged cytoplasm, staining more intensively than in the unstimulated BCG-primed mice, suggesting an increased IFN-γ production. In unprimed mice there were hardly any IFN-γ-PC detectable at 0 and 3 hr after Con A stimulation. The kinetics of the IFN-γ serum levels and of the IFN-γ–producing cells developed according a similar pattern after the first 4.5 hr of Con A stimulation (Fig. 3). However, the IFN-γ serum levels of mice 6 hr after Con A stimulation showed a striking increase, whereas the number of IFN-γ–producing cells remained at the same level.

Possibly the BCG sensitizes a part of the spleen cells to produce and secrete IFN-γ in low concentrations. Con A may stimulate these cells to assemble and secrete IFN-γ in larger quantities, causing an increase of the IFN-γ serum levels after 6 hr. Double staining of the spleen sections for IFN-γ and surface antigens revealed that ± 60% of the IFN-γ–producing cells were expressing the CD4 antigen (see Fig. 1c) and ± 30% the CD8 antigen. NK cells and macrophages producing IFN-γ were not demonstrated. These results are in agreement with the experiments of Wada et al. (8), who found in BCG-primed and Con A–stimulated mice, after in vivo T-cell depletion with MAb, that T cells were the principal cells directly or indirectly responsible for the IFN-γ production, without important participation of macrophages and NK cells. In our experiments we demonstrated directly in vivo that T cells were the main IFN-γ producers in the immune response to heat-killed BCG.

In conclusion, this study demonstrates the potentials of the immunohistochemical approach in the in vivo analysis of a cytokine-mediated immune response. We demonstrated its value for the investigation of the in vivo activity of IFN-γ in a thymus-dependent immune response. Moreover, this technique enables the study of the in vivo localization and cellular origin of IFN-γ. Provided that specific antisera are available, this method is also suitable to detect and characterize other cytokine-producing cells in vivo, thereby opening the way for validation of in vitro findings. Furthermore, this technique will facilitate, in combination with other techniques, the analysis of the local events and interactions of B-, T-, and antigen-presenting-cells during an in vivo immune response.

ACKNOWLEDGMENT

The technical assistance of Mr. A. Van Oudenaren is gratefully acknowledged.

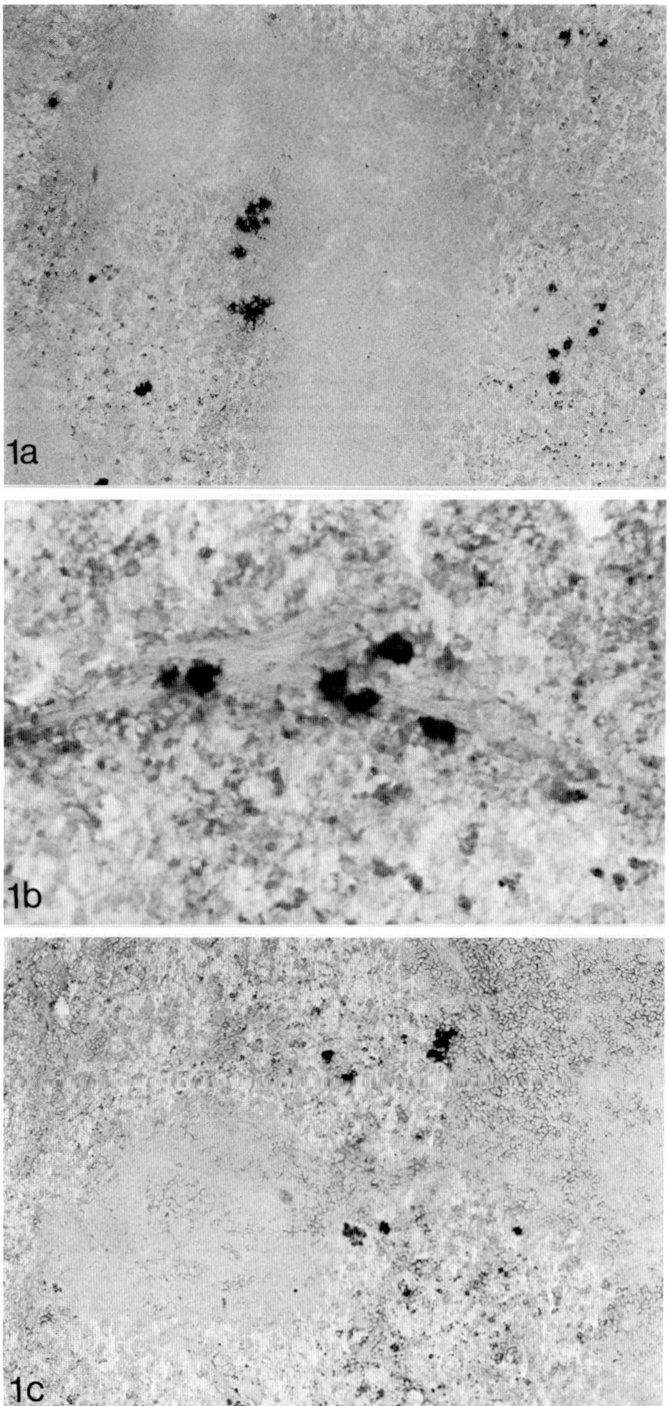

Figure 1 (a) IFN-γ–producing cells in a cryostat section of a spleen of a BCG-primed and Con A–stimulated mouse. Section was incubated with DB-1-AP (MAb specific for IFN-γ) and after AP cytochemistry the IFN-γ–producing cells with a blue cytoplasm were detected. Sections were counterstained with hematoxylin. For double-staining experiments, the sections were simultaneously incubated with DB-1-AP and rat MAb directed to different cell markers, followed by rabbit antirat-

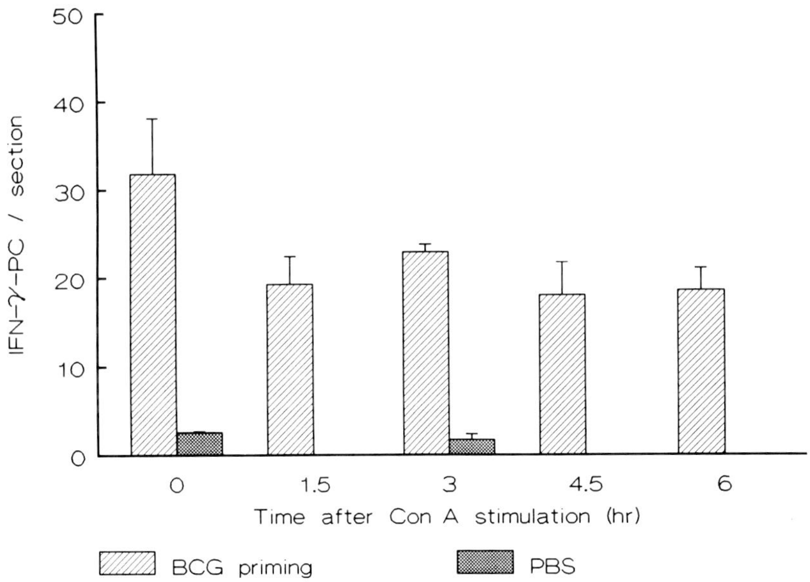

Figure 2 Kinetics of the IFN-γ–producing cells in spleens of mice after BCG priming and Con A stimulation. BALB/c mice were primed i.p. with heat-killed BCG (3.3×10^7) and stimulated i.v. with 200 μg Con A 3 weeks later. Subsequently, mice were sacrificed at the indicated intervals. Control mice were injected i.p. with 400 μl PBS. The INF-γ–producing cells in cryostat sections of spleens were stained and counted. Data presented are expressed as the mean ± SD of three different mice from each group.

HRP. (b) After AP and HRP cytochemistry, the IFN-γ–producing cells and macrophages (MOMA2) were detected. Note the IFN-γ–producing cells in the coaxial sheath of lymphoid tissue surrounding the terminal arterioles in the spleen. (c) After AP and HRP cytochemistry, the IFN-γ–producing cells (cytoplasmic staining) and CD4 (membrane staining) were detected.

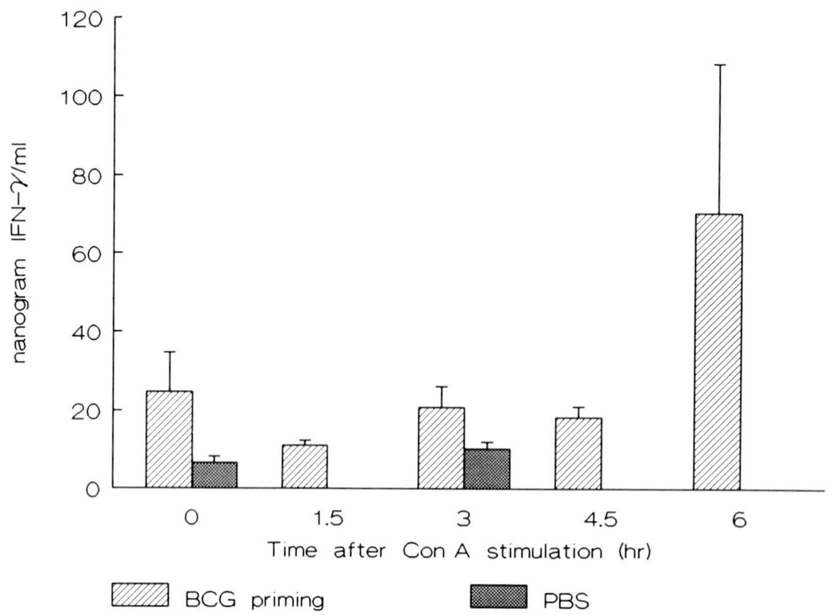

Figure 3 Kinetics of the IFN-γ serum levels of mice after BCG priming and Con A stimulation. BALB/c mice were primed i.p. with heat-killed BCG (3.3×10^7) and stimulated i.v. with 200 μg Con A 3 weeks later. Control mice were injected i.p. with 400 μl PBS. Subsequently, mice were bled at the indicated intervals. Sera were assayed for IFN-γ by a two-site sandwich ELISA. Data presented are expressed as the mean ± SD of three different mice from each group.

REFERENCES

1. Schellekens H. Animal models in interferon research: Some current trends. Experientia 1989; 45:558–62.
2. Laskay T, Andersson U, Andersson J, Kiessling R, Deley M. An immunofluorescent method for identifying individual IFN-γ producing lymphocytes. J Immunol Methods 1986; 95:1–7.
3. McCall JL, Kankatsu Y, Funamoto S, Parry BR. In vivo immunohistochemical identification of tumor necrosis factor/cachectin in human lymphoid tissue. Am J Pathol 1989; 135(3):421–25.
4. Ruco LPR, Stoppacciaro A, Pomponi D, Boraschi D, Santoni A, Tagliabue A, Uccinni S, Baroni CD. Immunoreactivity for IL-1 beta and TNF Alpha in human lymphoid and non lymphoid tissues. Am J Pathol 1989; 135(5):889–97.
5. Husby G and Williams RC. Immunohistochemical studies of interleukin-2 and γ-interferon in rheumatoid arthritis. Arthritis Rheum 1985; 28:174–81.
6. Cleveland MG, Annable CR, Klimpel GR. In vivo and in vitro production of IFN-β and IFN-γ during graft-versus-host disease. J Immunol 1988; 141:3349–56.
7. Gessner A, Drjupin R, Löhler J, Lother H, Lehmann-Grube F. IFN-γ production in tissues of mice during acute infection with lymphocytic choriomeningitis virus. J Immunol 1990; 144:3160–65.
8. Wada M, Okamura H, Nagata K, Shimoyama T, Kawade Y. Cellular mechanisms in in vivo production of gamma interferon induced by lipopolysaccharide in mice infected with mycobacterium bovis BCG. J Interf Res 1985; 5:431–43.
9. Van der Meide PH, Borman AH, Beljaars HG, Dubbeld MA, Botman CAD, Schellekens H. Isolation and characterization of monoclonal antibodies directed to rat interferon-gamma. Lymphokine Res 1989; 8:439–49.
10. Claassen E, Adler LT, Adler FL. Double immunocytochemical staining for the in situ study of allotype distribution during an anti-TNP immune response in chimeric rabbits. J Histochem Cytochem 1986; 34:989–94.
11. Ledbetter JA, and Herzenberg LA. Xenogeneic monoclonal antibodies to mouse lymphoid differentiation antigens. Immunol Rev 1979; 47:63–90.
12. Dialynas DP, Quan Zs, Wall KA, Pierres A, Quitans J, Loken MR, Pierres M, Fitch FW. Characterization of the murine T cell surface molecule designated L3T4, identified by monoclonal antibody GK1.5: similarity of L3T4 to the Leu-3/T4 molecule. J Immunol 1983; 131:2445–51.
13. Kraal G, Rep M and Janse M. Macrophages in T and B cell compartments and other tissue macrophages recognized by monoclonal antibody MOMA 2. An Immunohistochemical study. Scand J Immunol 1987; 26:653–61.
14. Habu S, Fukui H, Shimamura K, Masataka K, Yoshitaka N, Ko O, Tamaoki N. In vivo effects of anti-asialo GM1 I. Reduction of NK Activity and enhancement of transplanted Tumor Growth in Nude Mice. J Immunol 1981; 127:34–38.
15. Boersma WJA, Van Leeuwen JEM, Deen C, Radl J, Claassen E. A monoclonal anti-human IgG1 subclass antibody produced with secondary in vitro immunization. Prot Biol Fluids 1989; 36:157–61.
16. Boersma WJA, Haaijman JJ, Radl J, Claassen E. Antibodies to short synthetic peptide related to the hinge segment of human IgG3 recognizes thermally induced or fixative induced conformational changes in the human IgG3 molecule. Immunology 1989; 68:427–30.
17. Cherwinski HM, Schumacher JH, Brown KD, Mosmann TR. 1987. Two types of mouse helper T cell clone. III Further differences in lymphokine synthesis between Th1 and Th2 clones revealed by RNA hybridization, functionally monospecific bioassays, and monoclonal antibodies. J Exp Med 1987; 166:1229–42.

36
Splenic T-Lymphocyte Subsets in Chicken Embryos Undergoing Graft-vs-Host Reaction

Barbara Fedecka-Bruner, Pierre Vaigot, Marcelle Gendreau, and Guido Kroemer
Institut d'Embryologie du CNRS et du Collège de France, Nogent-sur-Marne, Paris, France

INTRODUCTION

When allogeneic immunologically competent T cells are transferred into an immunocompromised host incapable of rapidly eliminating the grafted T cell by an immunological counterattack (host-vs-graft reaction) a graft-vs-host reaction (GVHR) develops. Although GVHR appears to result from a rather artificial experimental manipulation, it is a clinically relevant phenomenon; chronic or acute GVHR may be one of the complications when bone marrow that is not fully histocompatible is grafted to immunosuppressed patients. In addition, the study of GVHR has greatly contributed to our understanding of major and minor histocompatibility loci, and has allowed the establishment of animal models for systemic autoimmune diseases. In the avian system, GVHR is usually induced either by placing immunocompetent allogeneic T cells onto the chorioallantoic membrane or by injecting them intravenously (1–3). Whereas the former procedure induces mainly a local reaction in form of the so-called "pock," the latter manipulation entails a systemic response whose most spectacular manifestation is splenomegaly. For many years, the mechanism of the GVHR-induced splenomegaly observed in chicken (*Gallus domesticus*) embryos has been a matter of debate (4). Serial transfer experiments suggested that donor T cells stimulated by host alloantigens would proliferate or, alternatively, give rise to a microenvironment which favors the growth of host splenocytes and accelerates the maturation of the host immune system. The recent availability of allospecific serological reagents as well as monoclonal antibodies specific for the chicken equivalents of T cell markers like CD3 (ref. 5), CD4,CD8 (ref. 6), CD25 (ref. 7), and the T-cell receptor αβ (TCR 2, ref. 8) or γδ (TCR 1, ref. 9) has prompted us to investigate the phenotype of donor and recipient splenocytes in the course of the development of splenomegaly.

DISSOCIATION OF SPLENOMEGALY AND T-CELL EXPANSION IN SERIAL TRANSFER EXPERIMENTS

As demonstrated in Table 1, splenomegaly of chicken embryos undergoing GVHR is accompanied by an increased percentage of splenocytes expressing a pan–T-cell differentiation antigen. In serial transfer experiments (10), however, this phenomenon may be dissociated from the increase in splenic weight. Whereas, one allogeneic recipient in a two-step transfer experiment is sufficient to induce splenomegaly, only the maintenance of an allogeneic environment allows significant T-cell recruitment and/or expansion. Although the origin (host or donor?) of the T cells encountered in the spleen remains unknown, this experiment indicates that both nonspecific (non–T lymphocytic) and presumably specific antigen-driven T-cell proliferation are involved in the development of splenomegaly. Since more than two-thirds of the cells contributing to splenomegaly do not express T-cell markers (CD3, CD4, CD8, TCR 1 or 2, antigen recognized by TIIA4; ref. 11) or B cell–specific antigens (Ig, 319-D3), the nonspecific component appears to prevail in quantitative terms.

BOTH HOST AND DONOR CELLS CONTRIBUTE TO SPLENOMEGALY

Using alloantisera specific for class I antigens of either the highly inbred B^4 or B^{12} major histocompatibility (MHC) haplotypes (11a), we found that high 10–20% of splenocytes were of the donor phenotype when 1×10^6 peripheral blood lymphocytes (PBL) of B^4 origin were injected into 13-day-old B^{12} embryos. At day 20, i.e., 1 day before hatching, the spleen contained a total of $27 \pm 5 \times 10^6$ lymphoid cells, indicating that the injected donor cells had proliferated by a factor of about 5. Given that probably only a fraction of the injected PBL population is capable of homing into the recipient's spleen, the expansion of donor cells may be even more important. Nonetheless, the majority of cells present in the

Table 1 T-Cell Proliferation in Serial Transfer Experiments

Experimental manipulation[a]	Splenic/total body mass × 10^5	% T cells in spleen[b]
untreated control B^{14} E or B^{19} E	42	1.4
B^{14} PBL–B^{14} E	80	4.3
B^{14} PBL–B^{19}E	299[c]	17.2[c]
B^{14} PBL– B^{14} E–B^{14}E	70	3.4
B^{14} PBL–B^{19} E–B^{14} E	143[c]	5.4
B^{14} PBL–B^{14}E–B^{19} E	129[c]	4.5
B^{14} PBL–B^{19} E–B^{19} E	147[c]	14.0[c]

[a]13-day-old chicken embryos (E) of either the B^{14} or B^{19} MHC haplotypes were injected i.v. with 1×10^6 peripheral blood lymphocytes (PBL). At day 20 of embryonic development, spleens were removed, dissociated into single cells suspensions, and transferred (1×10^6 cells i.v.) into 13-day-old B^{14} or B^{19} embryos, followed by autopsy on day 20. Untreated controls and one-step transfer experiments are also shown. Each experimental series was repeated for five to 11 times.
[b]Percentages of T cells were evaluated by indirect immunofluorescence staining with the monoclonal antibody TIIA4, a pan–T-cell marker (11).
[c]Significantly different from respective syngeneic control experiment.

hyperplastic spleen (about 10 times control weight) is of host origin. By consequence, in situ proliferation of recipient cells in the enlarging spleen and/or recruitment of such cells from other lymphoid organs quantitatively outnumber the contribution of donor cells. This finding is in accordance with experiments involving local GVHR in which host cells predominated over cells expressing the donor MHC haplotype in pocks (12,13).

INCREASE OF CD4 DONOR AND CD8 RECIPIENT CELLS

Splenomegaly produced in the above-mentioned donor (B^4)–recipient (B^{12}) combination was characterized by an increase of CD8-positive cells (from about 2×10^4 to 5×10^6) as well by the presence of CD4-positive cells and B cells (approximately 2×10^6 each), which are practically absent in control spleens. Double-staining experiments revealed that CD4-positive cells were predominantly of the donor and CD8-positive cells of the recipient MHC haplotype (Table 2). More detailed analysis suggests that most of the CD4-positive cells expressed surface TCR 2 molecules, whereas the bulk of CD8-positive lymphocytes were negative for either TCR 1 or TCR 2. These CD8-positive cells probably belong to the $CD4^-CD8^{dull+}$ TCR 1^- TCR 2^- TCR 3^- surface $CD3^-$cytoplasmic CD3-positive lineage (so called TCR 0 cells) developing in the unmanipulated embryonic spleen independently of the thymus (14). This phenotype may represent the avian equivalent of the mammalian natural killer (NK) cell (15).

INTERLEUKIN-2 RECEPTOR (IL-2R) EXPRESSION ACCOMPANIES T- AND NK-CELL EXPANSION

The monoclonal antibody INNCh16 recognizes the inducible light chain (Mr = 50 kD) of the chicken IL-2 receptor (CD25) (7,16). Under normal conditions, CD25 is faintly expressed only on a small (<5%) subpopulation of embryonic spleen cells. In contrast, up

Table 2 Lymphocyte Subpopulations on 18- to 20-Day-Old GVHR Splenocytes[a]

	% of spleen cells (x ± SEM) from	
Surface antigen	untreated animals	animals undergoing GVHR
CD4[b]	0 (n = 6)	5.8 ± 0.8 (n = 10)
CD8[c]	0.5 ± 0.5 (n = 6)	9.8 ± 0.7 (n = 15)
TCR 1	0 (n = 6)	1.3 ± 0.4 (n = 19)
TCR 2	0 (n = 6)	4.7 ± 1.0 (n = 12)
CD25 (IL-2R light chain)	ND	13.4 ± 1.2 (n = 15)

[a]GVHR was induced by injecting 1×10^6 adult B^4 donor PBLs into 13-day-old B12 embryos. Spleens from treated or control embryos were removed at day 18–20 and subjected to cytofluorometric analysis of T-lymphocyte subpopulations.
[b]$CD4^+$ cells from GVHR spleens predominantly expressed the donor MHC haplotype and are $CB8^-$. Two-thirds of $CD4^+$ cells are $CD25^+$.
[c]$CD8^+$ cells from GVHR spleens predominantly express the host MHC haplotype and $TCR1^-TCR2^-CD25^+$.

to 25% of all cells strongly express CD25 in spleens of chicks undergoing GVHR. In our hands, most of the CD25-positive subpopulation bears class I antigen of the recipient phenotype. Practically all CD8 and the majority (65%) of CD4-positive cells express CD25 on day 18; i.e., 5 days after injection of allogeneic adult PBL. These findings strongly suggest IL-2–mediated proliferation and/or differentiation to be implicated in the events leading to manifest splenomegaly.

CONCLUSIONS

The data discussed above may be integrated into the following hypothetical scenario of GVHR-induced splenomegaly. After injection, a significant portion of donor lymphocytes home into the embryonic spleen where they are activated and start proliferating in response to allogeneic antigens, mainly MHC determinants. Most of these donor lymphocytes are of the CD4-positive ("helper") T-cell phenotype, express the high-affinity IL-2R, produce their own IL-2, and thus proliferate in an autocrine fashion via the IL-2/IL-2R pathway. Simultaneously, $CD8^{+}$TCR 0 (NK?) cells of the recipient become activated either by the antigenic make-up of the donor cell population or the presence of T-helper–derived lymphokines, including IL-2. These $CD8^{+}$TCR 0 cells express the IL-2R and proliferate in response to IL-2 in an auto- or paracrine fashion. In accordance with the hypothesized pivotal role of IL-2 in the pathogenesis of splenomegaly, local as well as systemic GVHR of the mouse (17) and local GVHR of the chicken (12) have been successfully suppressed by monoclonal antibodies directed against the IL-2R. The unphysiological presence of activated CD4 donor cells and/or activation of recipient lymphocytes in the spleen undergoing GVHR gives rise to nonspecific proliferation of stromal and hematolymphopoietic cells. Although it is tempting to imply additional cytokines (e.g., T-helper cell–derived interferon-γ, IL-3, or multi-CSF, GM-CSF, IL-4, etc.) in this process, future studies will be needed to clarify the exact nature of such factors. It is quite conceivable that growth factors are also produced by host cells in an autonomous fashion, explaining why such cells may transfer splenomegaly to syngeneic recipients (see Table 1).

During the course of events traced above, the proliferation of donor lymphocytes is outnumbered by the expansion and/or recruitment of host cells either of lymphoid (CD8-positive, TCR 0), prelymphoid or nonlymphoid type. Whether the GVHR spleen truly represents a more "mature" phenotype as compared to normal control spleens remains a matter of debate.

ACKNOWLEDGMENTS

The authors are grateful to Drs. Cooper, Hála, and Bouret for the gift of valuable serological reagents, and to Mrs. A. Lehmann for expert technical assistance. This work was supported in part by fellowships of the Austrian Research Council and by the Spanish Ministry of Education and Science.

REFERENCES

1. Simonsen M. The impact in the developing embryo and newborn animal of adult homologous cells. Acta Pathol. Microbiol. Scand. 1957, 40:480–491.
2. Desveaux-Chabrol J, Dieterlen-Lièvre F. A comparative study of the GVH-R in the chicken embryo: effects of various allogeneic cells and various administration routes. Dev. Comp. Immunol., 1987, 11:179–190.

3. Desveaux-Chabrol J, Gendreau M, Dieterlen-Lièvre F. Ontogeny of the GVH-R inducing capacity in conventional and germ-free chickens. Dev. Comp. Immunol., 1989, 13:65–71.
4. McBride RA, Coppleson LW, Nisbet NW, Simonsen M, Skowron-Cendrzak A, Wigzell HLR. Accelerated immunological maturation in the chick. Immunology 1966; 10:63–79.
5. Chen CH, Ager LL, Gartland GL, and Cooper MD. Identification of a T3/T cell receptor complex in chickens. J. Exp. Med. 1986, 164:375–380.
6. Chan MM, Chen CH, Ager LL, and Cooper MD. Identification of the avian homologues of mammalian CD4 and CD8 antigens. J. Immunol. 1988, 140:2133–2138.
7. Hàla K, Schauenstein K, Neu N, Kroemer G, Wolf H, Boeck G, Wick G. A monoclonal antibody reacting with a membrane determinant expressed on activated chicken T lymphocytes. Eur. J. Immunol. 1986, 16:1331–1336.
8. Chen CH, Cihak J, Lösch U, Cooper MD. Differential expression of two T cell receptors, TcR1 and TcR2, on chicken lymphocytes. Eur. J. Immunol. 1988, 18:539–543.
9. Sowder JT, Chen CH, Ager LL, Chan MM, and Cooper MD. A large subpopulation of avian T cells express a homologue of the mammalian Tγ/δ receptor. J. Exp. Med. 1988; 167:315–322.
10. Fedecka-Bruner B, Desveaux-Chabrol J, and Dieterlen-Lièvre F. T cells in the spleen of chicken embryos undergoing a graft-versus-host reaction. Progr. Clin. Biol. Res. 1989; 307:19–29.
11. Yassine F, Fedecka-Bruner B, Dieterlen-Lièvre F. Ontogeny of the chick embryo spleen—a cytological study. Cell Diff. Dev. 1989; 27:29–45.
11a. Kroemer G, Bernot A, Béhar G, Chaussé A-M, Gastinel L-N, Guillemot F, Park I, Thoraval P, Zoorob R, Auffray C. Molecular genetics of the chicken MHC: current status and evolutionary aspects. Immunol. Rev. 1990; No. 113:119–145.
12. Penninger J, Klima J, Kroemer G, Dietrich H, Hàla K, Wick G. Intra thymic nurse cell lymphocytes can induce graft-versus-host reactions with high efficiency. Dev. Comp. Immunol. 1989; 13: 313–327.
13. Penninger J, Hála K, Wick G. Intra-thymic nurse cell lymphocytes can induce a specific graft-versus-host reaction. J. Exp. Med. 1990 (in press).
14. Bucy RP, Coltey M, Chen CH, Char D, LeDouarin NM, Cooper MD. Cytoplasmic $CD3^+$ surface $CD8^+$ lymphocytes develop as a thymus-independent lineage in chick-quail chimeras. Eur. J. Immunol. 1989; 19:1449–1455.
15. Bucy RP, Chen CH, Cooper MD. Development of cytoplasmic CD3+/T cell receptor-negative cells in the peripheral lymphoid tissue of chickens. Eur. J. Immunol. 1990, 20:1345–1350.
16. Schauenstein K, Kroemer G, Hàla K, Boeck G, Wick G. Chicken-activated-T-lymphocyte-antigen (CATLA) recognized by monoclonal antibody INN-CH 16 represents the IL-2 receptor. Dev. Comp. Immunol. 1988; 12:823–831.
17. Volk H-D, Brocke S, Osawa H, Diamantstein T. Suppression of the local graft-vs.-host reaction in rats by treatment with a monoclonal antibody specific for the interleukin 2 receptor. Eur. J. Immunol. 1986; 16:1309–1312.

37
T-Cell Proliferation Induced by Murine Monoclonal Anti-idiotypic Antibody

Ljiljana Dimitrijević,[1] Snežana Živančević-Simonović,[2] Marko Radulovic,[1] Tatjana Odrljin,[1] Dragan Jovanovic,[1] and Katarina Isakovic[1]
[1]*Immunology Research Center, Belgrade, Yugoslavia;*
[2]*Zastava-Yugomedica, Kragujevac, Yugoslavia*

INTRODUCTION

B-cell responses to most antigens require T cells. After antigen stimulation, several types of T-helper (Th) cells (5) may be induced: some recognizing antigen in the context of the major histocompatibility complex (MHC) product (Th1 and Th2 or anti-idiotypic T-helper [anti-idTh]), and the others recognizing idiotypic determinants of soluble antibodies expressed on induced B cells (ThId). The antigen-specific Th cells (ThAg) should induce differentiation of B cells and a subsequent increase in idiotype-specific Th cells (ThId or anti-IdTh). In the present study, we investigated the induction of ThId in the case of BALB/c mice immunized with immunoglobulin M (IgM)λ DJ idiotype with phosphorylcholine (PC) paratopic specificity (2).

MATERIALS AND METHODS

Mice

Six- to eight-week-old male and female BALB/c mice were obtained from a breeding colony at the Military Medical Academy, Belgrade, Yugoslavia.

ANTIGEN AND IMMUNIZATION

Mice were immunized with IgMλ DJ immunogen in the hindfoot pads and base of the tail. The immunogen derived from a serum of a patient with Waldenstsröm's macroglobulinemia was used as a 98% purified preparation. The first, second, and third injections (50 μg each) were applied weekly in complete and incomplete Freund's adjuvant and phosphate-buffered saline (PBS), respectively.

Monoclonal Anti-Id

A monoclonal antibody (MAb), designated as Y7, was used in these studies. Y7 is an IgG_1, kappa immunoglobulin of BALB/c origin. The Y7 MAb was obtained from the fusion between the nonsecreting myeloma cell line X63-Ag8.653 and spleen cells from mice immunized with IgMλ DJ (4), and was used as affinity purified over the IgMλ DJ immunoaffinity column. The epitope specificity of Y7 MAb was localized in the unreduced Fab fragment of IgMλ DJ and was characterized as anti-Id based on its ability to produce 100% inhibition of IgMλ DJ–PC binding.

In Vitro Cell Proliferation Assay

T lymphocytes from periaortic, popliteal, and inguinal lymph nodes were isolated on nylon wool column (6) 7 days after the last injection. An overnight incubation at 37°C in 5% CO_2 atmosphere, in RPMI 1640 medium with 10% FCS, was performed to remove the adherent cells. The nonadherent cells were used for proliferation assay in the same medium. T lymphocytes (4×10^5/well) were stimulated for 96 hr by increasing concentrations of different stimuli: soluble IgMλ DJ immunogen, Y7, and murine monoclonal antibody Ei, or irrelevant specificity but with the same IgG_1 isotype as Y7 MAb. The cell proliferation assay was performed in the presence or absence of mitomycin C–treated spleen cells as a source of APC. Besides, T lymphocytes were stimulated with a different number of mitomycin C–treated Y7 hybridoma cells. Proliferative response in each experiment was measured in triplicate cultures 24 hr after 1 μCi [^{3}H]thymidine per well was added.

RESULTS AND DISCUSSION

It was shown that T lymphocytes do proliferate in the presence of IgMλ DJ immunogen. By increasing the concentration of soluble antigen in culture, the higher proliferation response was obtained (Fig. 1). Moreover, a dose-dependent proliferative response of T lymphocytes was shown in the presence of murine monoclonal anti-idiotypic antibody Y7 (Fig. 1). As these proliferations were obtained without the APC being present in the system, the principal question was: What type of T cells proliferate? It is generally accepted that T lymphocytes recognize the immunogen in the context of self-MHC determinants. In the case of ThId, there appears to be no MHC restriction for either immunogen (1) or idiotype (7,8).

However, these T cells are dependent on the presence of anti-IdTh cells. On the other hand, Dun and Bottomly (3) showed one subset of ThId lymphocytes requiring self-Ia recognition. Dose-dependent proliferation of T lymphocytes, obtained after stimulation with soluble IgM or Y7 MAb without addition of antigen-presenting cells, suggests that no MHC presentation and restriction exists in our experimental model. Therefore, T-lymphocyte proliferation could be induced by direct complementary interaction between the T-cell receptor and immunogen or Y7 MAb. The role of antigen-presenting cells could not be completely excluded even in our model, as far as removal of adherent cells was performed by overnight adherence.

The involvement of different ThId cells in the regulation pathways of PC paratopes could explain the obtained proliferation in the presence of soluble IgMλ DJ immunogen. By adding the mitomycin C–treated spleen cells, as the source of antigen-presenting cells, proliferative response of the T lymphocytes was not significantly different (Table 1). Slightly lower proliferation values were obtained with the use of IgMλ DJ for proliferating stimulus. The proliferation was also obtained in the presence of mitomycin C–treated Y7

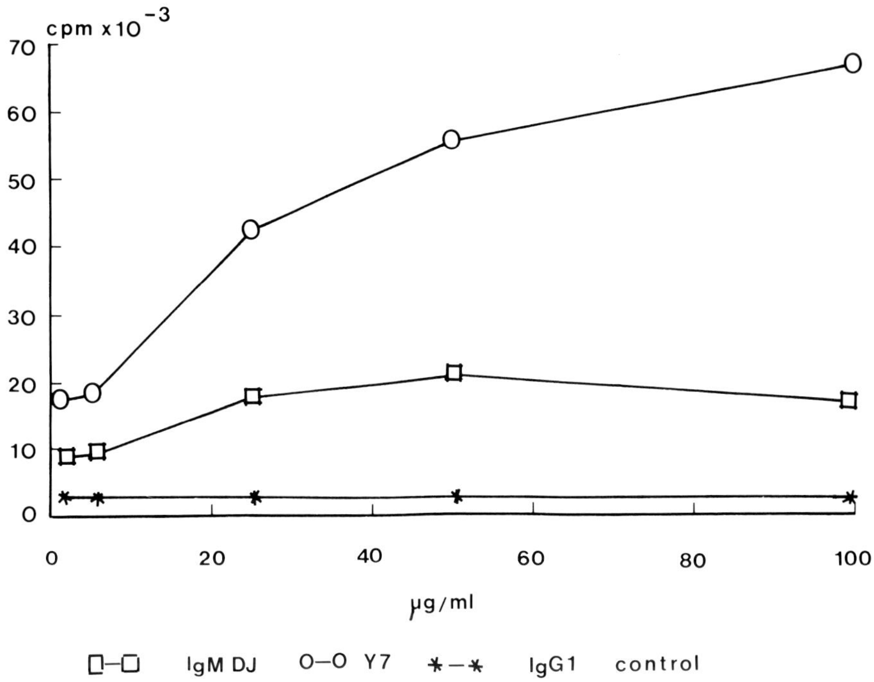

Figure 1 Proliferation of T lymphocytes, isolated from lymph nodes of IgM λ DJ–immunized animals, in the presence of different stimuli: IgM λ DJ (□—□), Y7 (O—O) monoclonal antibody and Ei (x—x), IgG_1 κ, monoclonal antibody of irrelevant specificity. Proliferation was assessed 96 hr later by [^{3}H]TdR incorporation. Results are expressed as mean cpm ±SD of triplicate cultures.

Table 1 In Vitro Proliferation of Murine T Cells in the Presence of APC (5×10^5 Cells/Well)

Stimulus[a]	μg/ml	cpm[b]
Y7 anti-Id	10	36260
	50	47000
	100	77142
IgM λ DJ	10	28330
	50	38229
	100	29329
Medium		277

[a]Proliferative value of lymphocytes without stimuli was 25824 cpm.
[b]Values expressed are cpm of [^{3}H]TdR incorporation of means of triplicate wells.

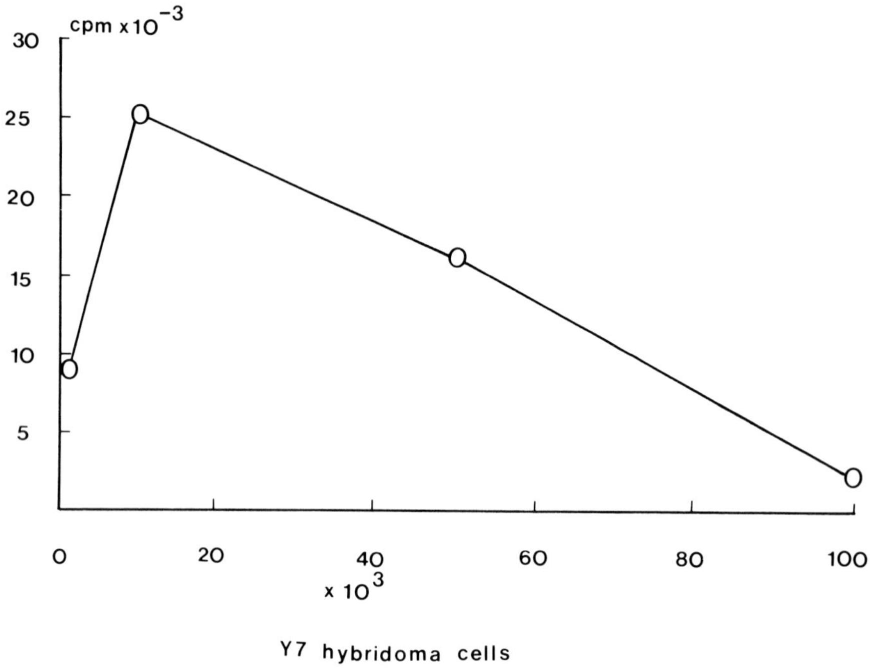

Figure 2 Proliferation of T lymphocytes, isolated from lymph nodes of IgM λ DJ–immunized animals, cocultured with a different number of mitomycin C–treated Y7 hybridoma cells. Proliferation was assessed 96 hr later by [^{3}H]TdR incorporation. Results are expressed as mean cpm ±SD of triplicate cultures.

hybridoma cells (Fig. 2). One may suggest that the simultaneous presence of MHC restricted (anti-IdTh) and unrestricted (ThId) T cells in our system may explain the obtained proliferation irrespectively of the presence of APC. The induction of Y7 ThId cells could imply the existence of a network regulation in the murine immune response against human IgMλ DJ idiotype with PC paratope, and also open the question about the possible suppressive mechanism of "natural" PC anti-IdTh during the IgMλ DJ immunization.

REFERENCES

1. Bootomly K, Maurer PH. Antigen-specific helper T cells required for dominant production of an idiotype (ThId) are not under immune response (Ir) gene control. J. Exp. Med. 1980; 152:1571–82.
2. Dimitrijević Lj, Ratković M, Kovačina K, Jankov R, Isaković K. Anti-idiotypic characteristics of murine monoclonal antibody. Perio. Biol. 1990; 92:120–1.
3. Dun BE, Bootomly K. T15-specific helper T cells: Analysis of Idiotype specificity by competitive analysis. Eur. J. Immunol. 1985; 15:728–32.
4. Ivanović V, Popović Lj, Kovačina K, Dimitrijević Lj, Ilić D, Pirožkov A, Baltić V. Detection of cross-reacting idiotypes in sera of lymphoma patients by inverse monoclonal radioimmunoassay. Acta. Haematol. 1990; 84:64-67.

5. Janeway CA Jr, Rojo R, Portoles P, Dumm E, Bootomly K. Idiotypic interactions between B- and T-lymphocyte receptors. In: Osterhaus A, Uytdehaag F. (eds.). *Idiotype Networks in Biology and Medicine*. Elsevier Science, Amsterdam, 1990, pp. 125–3.
6. Kappler JW, Marrak PC. The role of H -2 linked genes in helper T cells function. In vitro expression in B cells of immune response gene controlling helper T-cell activity. J. Exp. Med. 1977; 146:1748–64.
7. Eichmann K, Falk I, Rajewsky K. Recognition of idiotypes in lymphocyte interactions. II Antigen-independent cooperation between T and B lymphocytes that possess similar and complementary idiotypes. Eur. J. Immunol. 1978; 8:853–7.
8. Woodland R, Cantor H. Idiotype-specific T helper cells are required to induce idiotype-positive B memory cells to secrete antibody. Eur. J. Immunol. 1978; 8:600–6.

38
Influence of Maturation on T-Cell Reactivity

Lex Nagelkerken, Anita Hertogh-Huijbregts, and Ruud Dobber
Institute for Experimental Gerontology, TNO, Rijswijk, The Netherlands

INTRODUCTION

Aging is accompanied by a decrease in the functional capacity of the immune system. With regard to the T cells, this appears from low proliferative responses as well as from a decreased level of interleukin-2 (IL-2) production (1). It has been suggested that the age-related decline in immune reactivity is related to signal transduction defects, which are responsible for a decrease in the ability of T cells to increase cytoplasmic calcium after triggering of the T-cell receptor (2). However, we have recently demonstrated in aging mice that the above-mentioned phenomena may also be related to maturation of the immune system: The age-related decrease in IL-2 production is accompanied by an increased production of IL-4 and interferon-γ (IFN-γ) (2a). Since the production of these cytokines is suggested to be a function of different subsets within the CD4-positive T-cell compartment (3), we investigated whether our observations are in line with phenotypic changes within the CD4-positive T-cell population. Therefore, we studied the expression of CD45R by antibody 16A, which discriminates between IL-2– and IL-4–secreting T-cell clones (4), and Pgp-1 (CD44), the expression of which is associated with IFN-γ production (5). Our data suggest that within the CD4-positive T-cell compartments at least three subsets exist; the relative contribution of each of these subsets to the total CD4-positive T-cell population changes during aging.

MATERIALS AND METHODS

Mice

Young (2 and 3 months of age) male CBA/BrARij and C57BL/KaLwRij mice were derived from the SPF colonies of the TNO Institutes (Rijswijk, The Netherlands). Aged mice under investigation were 14 or 30 months old; these mice were originally derived from the SPF stock and—from an age of 3 months—housed under clean conventional conditions behind a physical barrier. All mice received sterilized pelleted food.

Isolation of Cells

For phenotypic analysis, spleen cells as well as peripheral blood lymphocytes were studied after lysis of the erythrocytes by ammonium chloride treatment. CD4-positive T cells were isolated as described previously (1), by enrichment of T cells over nylon wool and depletion of Lyt-2^+ T cells, employing indirect "panning" techniques.

Phenotypic Analysis

To determine the relative contribution of $CD45R^{high}$ cells or CD44-positive cells to the CD4-positive T cells, spleen cells or peripheral blood lymphocytes (PBLs) were incubated with anti-CD45R (16A) or anti–Pgp-1 (1M7.8.1), respectively, after which the binding of antibody was tested with FITC-labeled mouse–antirat immunoglobulin (Ig). After blocking the free binding sites with rat serum, the cells were incubated with biotin-labeled anti-L3T4 (GK1.5) or with biotin-labeled anti-Lyt-2 (53-6.7), both in combination with avidin-phycoerythrin. Analysis was performed with the use of a FACScan.

Calcium Mobilization

Calcium mobilization experiments were performed with INDO-1–labeled CD4-positive T cells as described elsewhere (6) using a FACS-analyzer, equipped with a mercury arc lamp. Cells were stimulated with anti-CD3 antibody 2C11 at a concentration of 100 μg/ml or with 1 μM ionomycin, and data were collected over a period of 10 min. Data were analyzed with the use of INCA-1 software. Cells in which the ratio INDO-bound/INDO-free was at least 2 SD above this ratio in resting cells were scored as responding cells.

RESULTS AND DISCUSSION

It is well established that proliferative T-cell responses decline during aging. As far as the CD4-positive T cells are concerned, this may be due to a lower production of IL-2. One of the major intracellular signals for expression of the IL-2 gene is the increase in cytoplasmic calcium. We therefore studied in CD4-positive T cells from 3-month-old and from 30-month-old C57BL/Ka mice, rather than in total T cells, the ability to mobilize calcium after stimulation with anti-CD3 or with ionomycin.

As can be seen in Figure 1, CD4-positive T cells from young and old mice display a different response after anti-CD3 stimulation. About 70% of the young cells responded by a calcium flux; the responding fraction in cells from old mice was twofold lower. Stimulation with the calcium-ionophore ionomycin was more effective, resulting in a calcium flux in 95% of the young cells and in 55% of the old cells. In addition, the maximal cytoplasmic calcium concentration induced in the young responding cells by anti-CD3 reached levels of 3.7 μM as compared to 1.6 μM in the responding cells from old mice.

No differences were found when splenic B cells from young or old mice were stimulated with anti-Ig antibodies or with ionomycin (data not shown). Therefore, CD4-positive T cells from old mice may display an intrinsic defect that is related to the lower IL-2 production. However, the lower level of calcium mobilization may also be related to a change in the composition of the CD4-positive T cells, as we demonstrated previously on the basis of cytokine production. In these studies, we observed an age-related shift from

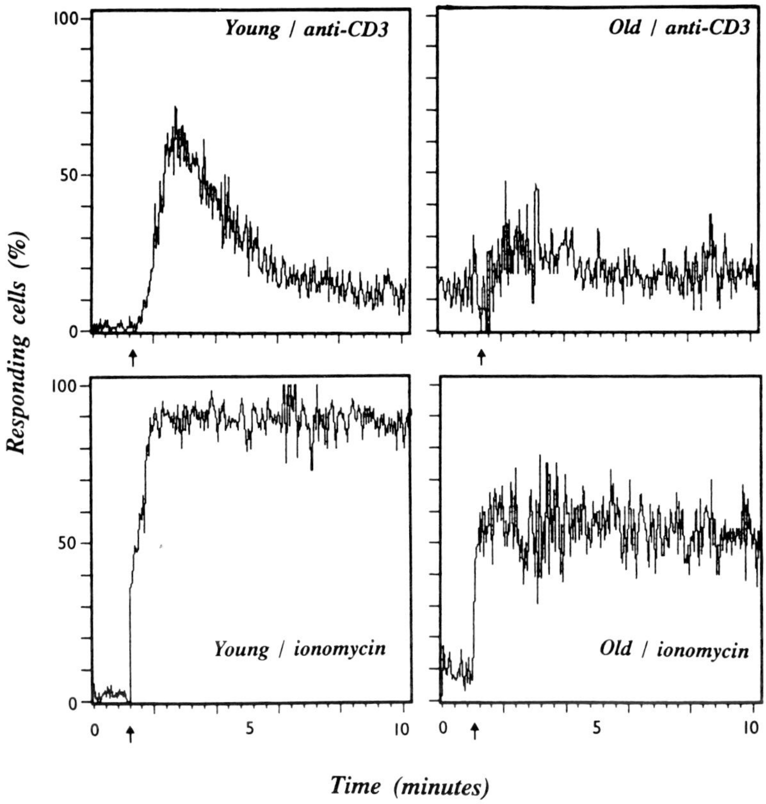

Figure 1 The fraction of CD4$^+$ T cells that responds to activation by calcium mobilization is decreased in old mice. CD4$^+$ T cells from 3-month-old (left) or 30-month-old (right) C57BL mice were stimulated with anti-CD3 (top) or ionomycin (bottom). Arrows indicate the addition of the stimuli.

IL-2 to IL-4 production which correlated well with the loss of CD45R expression as measured with antibody 16A. Since CD4-positive T-cell clones that produce IL-2 (and not IL-4) express 16A in high density, whereas clones producing IL-4 (and not IL-2) express 16A in low density (4), our findings indicate that the percentage of IL-2–producing CD4-positive T cells decreases in favor of IL-4–secreting CD4-positive T cells. Our data did not fit with the distinction of CD4-positive T cells into T-helper cells Th1 and Th2, because IFN-γ production increased during aging and this did not correlate with the decreased IL-2 production (2a). Since IFN-γ production is associated with Pgp-1–expressing cells (5), which are suggested to increase during aging (7), we further studied to what extent our results from functional studies could be explained by the expression of 16A and Pgp-1.

As shown in Figure 2, staining of CD4-positive T cells for Pgp-1 reveals a negative, a weakly positive, and a strongly positive subset. On the basis of these representative data, it can already be concluded that during aging the expression of Pgp-1 increases. In Table 1, the distribution of Pgp-1, as well as of 16A, over the CD4-positive T cells from CBA/Rij mice of different ages is given in more detail. It can be concluded that major changes occur

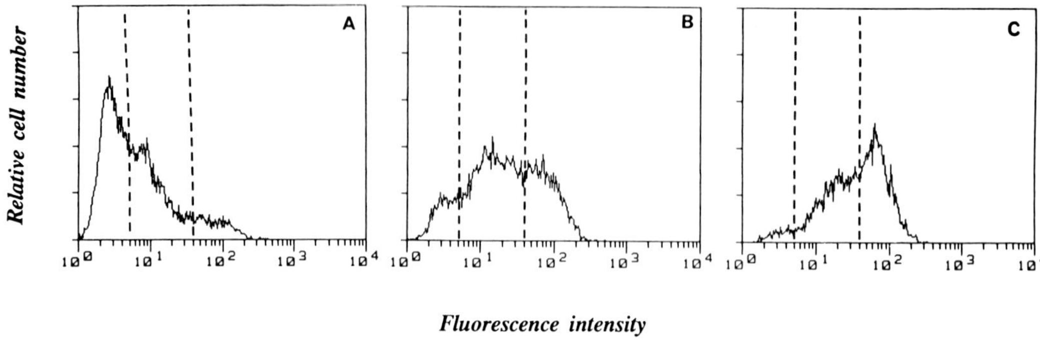

Figure 2 Pgp-1 expression on CD4$^+$ T cells increases during aging. Histograms represent Pgp-1 intensity on CD4$^+$ T cells from a 2-month-old (A), a 14-month-old (B), and a 30-month-old (C) CBA/Rij mouse.

during the first 14 months of life with a decrease in 16A^{high} expression from 20 to 14%, and a reduction of Pgp-1–negative cells from 16.5 to 3%. From 14 to 30 months of age, a further decline in 16A expression is noted, whereas only slight changes occur in Pgp-1 expression. Our results did not allow the conclusion that 16A and Pgp-1 detect fully complementary subsets. Within the CD4-positive T-cell population, which are either 16A^{high} or 16A^{low}, it was possible to discriminate three populations on the basis of Pgp-1 expression. This is obvious for 14-month-old mice with about 14% 16A^{high} CD4-positive T cells, whereas only 3% of the cells were Pgp-1 negative. In 2-month-old mice, about 8% 16A^{low} CD4-positive T cells were found, whereas only 2% of the cells expressed Pgp-1 in high density. Similar observations were made for CD4-positive T cells from peripheral blood. In contrast to CD4-positive T cells, the majority of CD8-positive T cells expresses 16A in high density, in which no changes occurs during aging. In 2-month-old mice, about 5% of the CD8-positive T cells was Pgp-1 positive as compared to 60% of the CD8-positive T cells from 30-month-old mice.

It is likely that at least three subsets can be discriminated within the CD4-positive T-cell compartment: (1) 16A^{high} Pgp-1$^-$, (2) 16A^{high} Pgp-1^{low}, and (3) 16A^{low}Pgp-1^{high}. Most likely, the first subset represents virginal CD4-positive T cells that exclusively produce IL-2, whereas subset 2 may represent cells capable of the production of a variety

Table 1 Age-Related Phenotypic Changes in CD4$^+$ T Cells from CBA/Rij Mice

		Fraction of CD4$^+$ T cells			
Age (months)	CD4$^+$ (%)	16A^{high}	Pgp-1$^-$	Pgp-1^{low}	Pgp-1^{high}
2	28.3 ± 1.7[a]	20.0 ± 2.1	16.5 ± 1.6	9.3 ± 0.9	2.3 ± 0.4
14	24.3 ± 1.6	14.1 ± 1.6	3.1 ± 0.4	12.1 ± 2.7	9.2 ± 1.1
30	20.8 ± 3.7	5.8 ± 2.0	0.8 ± 0.3	8.4 ± 2.5	11.8 ± 1.9

[a]Mean ± SD, n=5; results are expressed as a percentage of total spleen cells.

of cytokines as a consequence of previous activation (not necessarily antigen specific) in vivo; subset 3 may represent memory cells capable of the production of IL-4. The relative contribution of each of these subsets to the CD4- positive T-cell compartment depends on the age of the animals, probably due to the antigens they have encountered. Indeed, preliminary experiments showed that in aged germ-free mice, the percentage of CD4-positive T cells is lower than in conventional mice, and this could in part be attributed to a lower percentage of cells with a mature phenotype. Definite proof of the relation between age-related changes, such as calcium mobilization, cytokine production and proliferation, and the composition of the CD4-positive T-cell compartment will be obtained by studying sorted cell populations derived from mice of different ages.

REFERENCES

1. Hertogh-Huijbregts A, Vissinga C, Rozing J, Nagelkerken L. Impairment of CD3-dependent and CD3-independent activation pathways in $CD4^+$ and in $CD8^+$ T cells from old CBA/Rij mice. Mech Ageing Dev 1990; 53:141–55.
2. Proust JJ, Filburn CR, Harrison SA, Buchholz MA, Nordin AA. Age-related defect in signal transduction during lectin activation of murine T lymphocytes. J Immunol 1987; 139:1472–78.
2a. Nagelkerken L, Hertogh-Huijbregts A, Dobber R, Dräger A. Age-related changes in lymphokine production related to a decreased number of $CD45RB^{hi}CD4^+$ T cells. Eur J Immunol 1991 (in press).
3. Street NE, Schumacher JH, Fong TAT, Bass H, Fiorentino DF, Leverah JA and Mosmann TR. Heterogeneity of mouse T helper cells. Evidence from bulk cultures and limiting dilution cloning for precursors of Th1 and Th2 cells. J Immunol 1990; 144:1629–39.
4. Bottomly K, Luqman M, Greenbaum L, Carding S, West J, Pasqualini T, Murphy DB. A monoclonal antibody to murine CD45R distinguishes CD4 T cell populations that produce different cytokines. Eur J Immunol 1989; 19:617–23.
5. Budd RC, Cerottini J-C, MacDonald HR. Selectively increased production of interferon-γ by subsets of $Lyt2^+$ and $L3T4^+$ T cells identified by expression of Pgp-1. J Immunol 1987; 138:3583–96.
6. Rabinovitch PS, June CH, Grossmann A, Ledbetter JA. Heterogeneity among T cells in intracellular free calcium responses after mitogen stimulation with PHA or anti-CD3. Simultaneous use of INDO-1 and immunofluorescence with flow cytometry. J Immunol 1986; 137:952–61.
7. Lerner A, Yamada T, Miller RA. $Pgp\text{-}1^{hi}$ T lymphocytes accumulate with age in mice and respond poorly to concanavalin A. Eur J Immunol 1989; 19:977–82.

39
A *Mycoplasma* Product Induces Cytolytic T Cells in Thymocyte Cultures by Stimulating Accessory Cells to Release Interleukin-6

Peter F. Mühlradt and Hilmar Quentmeier
Gesellschaft für Biotechnologische Forschung, Braunschweig, Federal Republic of Germany

INTRODUCTION

In search of "factors" that might induce the differentiation of cytolytic T lymphocytes (CTLs) from resting T cells, we discovered an activity in the culture medium of *Mycoplasma fermentans*–infected cell lines which allows mitogen-stimulated thymocytes to differentiate to CTLs. This substance was shown to be derived from the mycoplasmas, not the cell lines, and was accordingly named MDHM (mycoplasma-derived high molecular weight material). It acts indirectly by inducing interleukin-1 (IL-1) and interleukin-6 (IL-6) from adherent accessory cells such as macrophages (1). The mode of action will be described, and possible implications for the etiology of arthritis discussed.

METHODS

Production of MDHM

MDHM was prepared from culture media of *M. fermentans*–infected HL60 or, more recently, from host cell–free *M. fermentans* cultures in GBF-1 medium. This medium consists of RPMI 1640 supplemented with FCS and sonicates from P815 mastocytoma cells. Culture media were freed of debris and mycoplasmas by high-speed centrifugation, and MDHM was precipitated with the bulk of protein by 80% saturated ammonium sulfate. The redissolved precipitate was dialyzed and filter sterilized. In some cases, MDHM was fractionated on G100 Sephadex and eluted near the exclusion volume.

Thymocyte Cultures and Induction of CTLs

Thymocytes from CBA/J or C57BL/6 mice were cultured at 2–3 × 10^6/ml with 4 μg/ml concanavalin A (Con A). MDHM or cytokines were added at the beginning of the culture period. In some cases, thymocytes were depleted of adherent accessory cells by passage over columns of G10 Sephadex or nylon wool. Where shown, such depleted thymocytes were reconstituted with either 4% mitomycin C–poisoned syngeneic splenocytes or the indicated numbers of resident peritoneal macrophages. Cells were harvested after 3 days, and antigen-unspecific cytolytic activity was determined in the presence of PHA at different effector/target ratios during a 4-hr incubation period, using ^{51}Cr-labeled P815 mastocytoma cells as target cells.

Stimulation of Macrophages to Release Mediators

Peritoneal exudate cells were adjusted to 5×10^5/ml in RPMI 1640, 1% FCS, 2.5×10^{-5} M mercaptoethanol, and seeded in 0.6-ml portions into 24-well tissue culture plates. Nonadherent cells were removed after overnight culture, and the remaining macrophages cultured in 0.6 ml medium in the presence of MDHM or other stimulants. Cell-free culture supernatants, or in the case of IL-1, culture supernatants after repeated freezing and thawing of the cells, were tested for monokines. Interleukin-1 was assayed with an IL-1–dependent helper T cell line D.10G4.1 (2), IL-6 with the IL-6–dependent hybridoma 7TD1 (3).

RESULTS

Effects of MDHM on Thymocytes

MDHM caused a dose-dependent increase in CTL formation in Con A–stimulated thymocyte cultures (Fig. 1). The following experiments were designed to clarify its mode of action. MDHM did not act on adherent cell-depleted thymocytes. Reactivity, however, could be restored by adding small numbers of mytomycin C–poisoned spleen cells. This MDHM-mediated response was abolished by addition of a neutralizing αIL-4 monoclonal antibody (MAb) (4) (Fig. 2). To clarify whether MDHM acted directly on helper T cells, thus causing IL-4 release, or more indirectly on macrophages, inducing monokine release, peritoneal macrophages were added in increasing numbers to adherent cell-depleted thymocytes which were then stimulated with Con A and MDHM (Fig. 3). The response to MDHM could be restored by small numbers of macrophages, larger numbers increasing the control levels, presumably because of spontaneous cytokine release. These data pointed to monokines as limiting mediators for CTL development in this system. Figure 4 illustrates that IL-6 is involved in MDHM action, and that the inhibitory effect of an αIL-6 MAb can be overcome by IL-4. In accordance with data from Renauld et al. (5), IL-6 could indeed induce CTLs in adherent cell-depleted thymocyte cultures (1).

Effects of MDHM on Peritoneal Macrophages

The MDHM-mediated release of monokines could be directly demonstrated in macrophage cultures. Interleukin-1 activity (including cell-bound IL-1), and IL-6 (secreted) were maximal 6 hr after stimulation with MDHM, reaching levels of 1024 U/ml and 1280 U/ml, respectively, with control values in unstimulated cultures of 160 U/ml and 16 U/ml, respectively. It should be emphasized that these effects were not due to endotoxin, as MDHM also acts on macrophages from LPS-nonresponder mice (1).

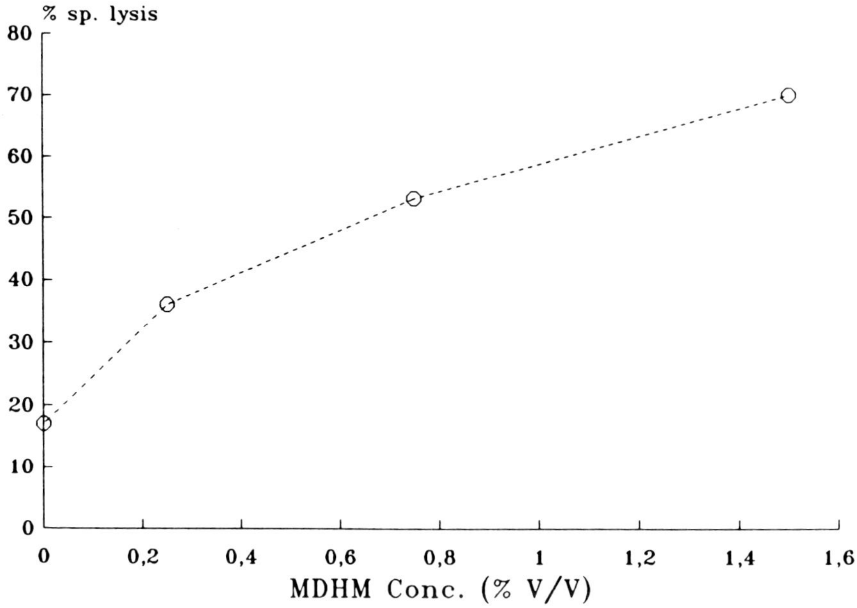

Figure 1 CTL formation in Con A–stimulated thymocyte cultures at different concentrations of MDHM. CTLs were determined after a 3-day culture period at an effector/target ratio of 10:1 in the presence of PHA, using P815 mastocytoma as target cells.

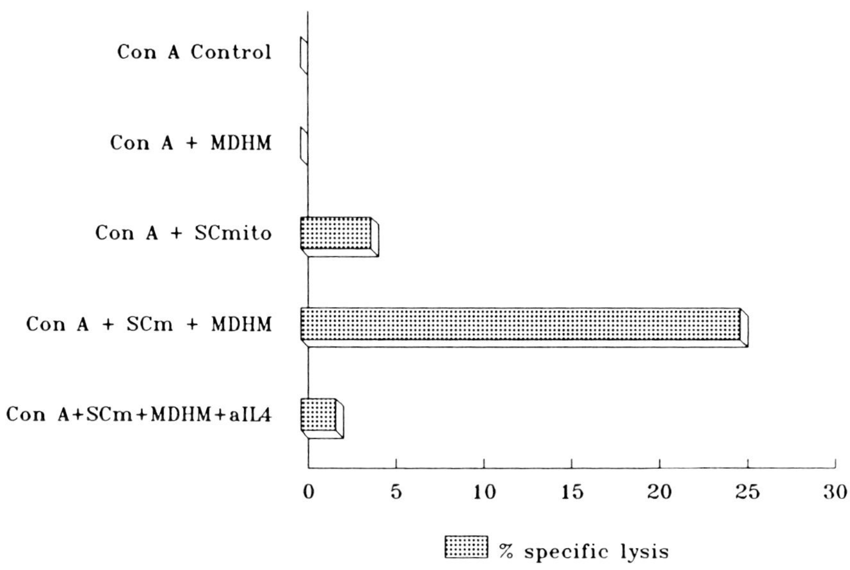

Figure 2 Reconstitution of MDHM response of accessory cell-depleted thymocytes by mitomycin C–treated splenocytes; effect of neutralizing αIL-4 MAb. Thymocytes were depleted of adherent accessory cells by passage over G10 Sephadex. Where indicated, they were reconstituted with 4% mitomycin C–treated syngeneic spleen cells. CTLs were determined as in Figure 1.

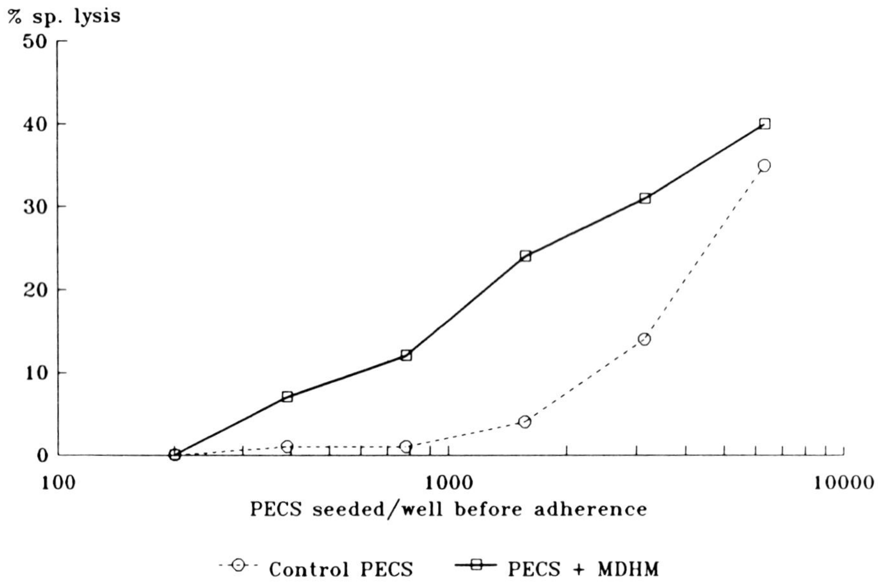

Figure 3 Reconstitution of MDHM response of accessory cell-depleted thymocytes by peritoneal macrophages. Resident peritoneal macrophages comprised in the indicated numbers of peritoneal cells (~40%) were allowed to adhere to microtiter wells, and nonadherent cells were removed. Thymocytes, after passage over nylon wool, were added and stimulated with Con A. Where indicated, MDHM was added. CTLs were determined after 3 days. PECS = peritoneal exudate cells.

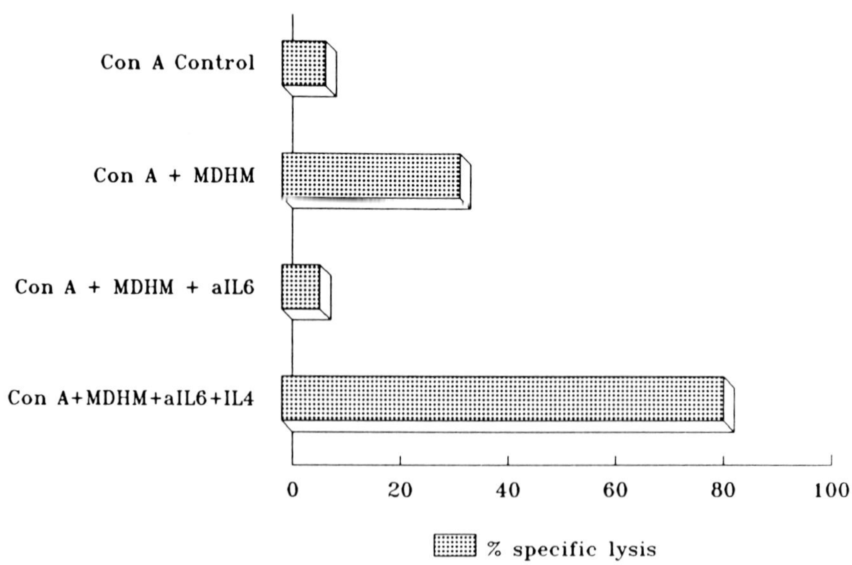

Figure 4 Involvement of IL-4 and IL-6 in the MDHM-mediated formation of CTLs from Con A–stimulated thymocytes. All additives were present from the beginning of the 3-day culture period. CTLs were determined as in Figure 1.

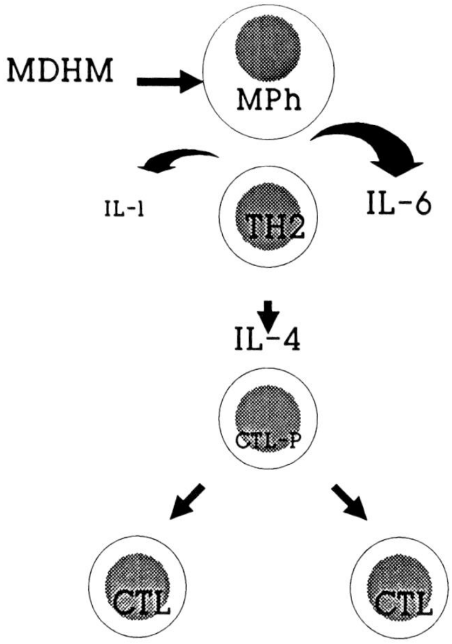

Figure 5 Sequence of events leading to the development of CTLs in Con A–stimulated thymocyte cultures in response to MDHM.

SUMMARY AND CONCLUSIONS

The action of MDHM and the sequence of events leading to CTLs is summarized in Figure 5. Our findings may be a relevant contribution to the ongoing discussion about possible pathogenic mechanisms responsible for reactive and chronic arthritides. Whereas there is no uncertainty about the pathogenic role of some mycoplasma species in animal systems, the situation is less clear for mycoplasma species that can infect man. Early reports implicated *M. fermentans* as a possible cause of rheumatoid arthritis in humans (6), but data have been conflicting and a safe correlation of, e.g., arthritic conditions, with isolation of mycoplasma from synovial fluid has not yet been established. Since a product of *M. fermentans*, MDHM, causes in vitro release of pleiotropic inflammatory mediators capable of inducing fever and causing polyclonal activation of T and B cells, a role of *M. fermentans* in reactive arthritis would be plausible. Biologically active IL-6 and IL-1 have indeed been shown to present in synovial fluid of rheumatoid joints (7,8).

REFERENCES

1. Quentmeier H, Schmitt E, Kirchhoff H, Grote W, Mühlradt PF. Mycoplasma fermentans-derived high molecular weight material induces interleukin-6 release in cultures of murine macrophages and human monocytes. Infect Immun 1990; 58:1273–1280.
2. Günther C, Röllinghoff M, Beuscher HU. Proteolysis of the native murine IL 1β precursor is required to generate IL 1β bioactivity. Immunobiol 1989; 178:436–448.

3. van Snick J, Cayphas S, Vink A, Uyttenhove C, Coulie PG, Ruber MR, Simpson RJ. Purification and NH2-terminal amino acid sequence of a T-cell-derived lymphokine with growth factor activity for B-cell hybridomas. Proc Natl Acad Sci USA 1986; 83:9679–9683.
4. Ohara J, Paul WE. Production of a monoclonal antibody to and molecular characterization of B-cell stimulatory factor-1. Nature (Lond) 1985; 315:333–336.
5. Renauld J-C, Vink A, van Snick J. Accessory signals in murine cytolytic T cell responses. Dual requirement for IL-1 and IL-6. J Immunol 1989; 143:1894–1898.
6. Williams MH, Brostoff J, Roitt IM. Possible role of mycoplasma fermentans in pathogenesis of rheumatoid arthritis. Lancet 1970; 2:277–280.
7. Houssiau FA, Devogelaer J-P, van Damme J, de Deuxchaisnes CN, van Snick J. Interleukin-6 in synovial fluid and serum of patients with rheumatoid arthritis and other inflammatory arthritides. Arthritis Rheum 1988; 31:784–788.
8. Hopkins SJ, Humphreys M, Jayson MIV. Cytokines in synovial fluid. I. The presence of biologically active and immunoreactive IL-1. Clin Exp Immunol 1988; 72:422–427.

40
Influence of Prenatal Administration of Dexamethasone on the Developing Immune System

Emmelien P. van Rees, Marja B. van der Ende, and Taede Sminia
Vrije Universiteit, Amsterdam, The Netherlands

INTRODUCTION

Glucocorticosteroids are known to affect macrophages and T and B cells. The expression of major histocompatibility complex (MHC) class II gene products is decreased on macrophages (1) and on B cells (2), the production of interleukin-1 (IL-1) is diminished, and in accordance antigen presentation is inhibited (1). The number of cortical thymocytes is reduced (3) by affecting multiple steps in thymocyte differentiation pathways (4). The proliferation of immature B cells is suppressed (5,6). In adult rats, these effects are reversible and demonstrable during 2 days following corticosteroid treatment (3).

Most studies on the effects of steroids on the immune system have dealt with adult animals, whereas in hospital, children receive corticosteroid treatment for several indications. Pregnant women are given corticosteroids if delivery of a very premature infant is at hand to improve the production of surfactant factor in the fetal lung. Bronchopulmonary dysplasia, a form of chronic lung disease, threatens preterm infants in particular and is treated with dexamethasone, a corticosteroid with predominantly glucocorticoid activity (7). The neonatal treatment of rats with glucocorticoids has been shown to induce endocrine and behavioral abnormalities in adulthood (8,9). As 17β-estradiol, also a steroid hormone, when administered perinatally affects T-cell functions in adulthood (10), corticosteroids given to neonatal rats may cause irreversible effects on the immune system as well. Therefore, the aim of the present study is to obtain information on the long-term effects of perinatally administered dexamethasone (DEX) on lymphoid and nonlymphoid cells.

MATERIALS AND METHODS

Pregnant Wistar rats, bodily weight 250 g, were obtained from Harlan (Zeist, The Netherlands). Dexamethasone, 500 μg (4 mg/ml, dilution 1:10), was administered intraperitoneally on days 17 and 19 of gestation. Litters were not treated with DEX after birth. At several points of time after birth pups were sacrificed (on the day of birth, days 3, 5, 7, 10, 14, and 21 after birth) by intraperitoneal administration of pentobarbital. Thymus and lymph nodes were collected. Half of the organs were used for a two-step immunoperoxidase technique on cryostat sections (11), applying various monoclonal antibodies (MAbs). Cell suspensions for fluorescence-activated cell sorter (FACS) analysis on a Becton Dickinson FACStar PLUS were made of the remaining organs.

Ox6 was used to detect Ia antigen; Ox8 and W3/25 were used against T-suppressor and T-helper cells, respectively; Ox19 was used as a pan–T-cell marker. All aforementioned MAbs were obtained from Serotec. To characterize macrophage subpopulations ED1, 2, and 3 were applied (12), raised in our laboratory but also commercially available. For FACS analysis fluoresceinated rabbit-antimouse (DAKO) was used to detect Ox8 and W3/25; to label biotinylated Ox19 streptavidine-PE (Southern Biotech. Ass.) was used.

RESULTS

The number of pups in litters of DEX-treated mothers and control mothers did not differ. After prenatal DEX treatment, pups had normal weights and sizes, and showed the same development in bodily weight as control pups.

Immunohistochemistry

Thymus

Regarding macrophage subpopulations, applying the ED MAbs, no differences could be found in the developmental pattern after DEX treatment. The development of thymic macrophage subpopulations has been described in detail in a previous report (13). In short, ED1 "recognized" many cells in the medulla and cortex on the day of birth. During development, especially the number of medullary ED1-positive cells increased. ED2 and ED3 label differentiation antigens (14). ED2-positive macrophages were present in the medulla on day 0. During development, ED2-positive cells tended to concentrate in the corticomedullary area. In adult thymus, ED2 labeled a continuous rim of macrophages along the border between the medulla and cortex, and many macrophages were scattered over the cortex.

On the day of birth, the expression of Ia antigen on the epithelial reticulum of the thymus was decreased after prenatal DEX treatment. Only a few Ia-positive dendritic cells were demonstrable in the medulla, labeled very weakly. Dendritic cells were present in normal numbers, as they were recognized by MAb ED1, but only few of them were weakly stained by Ox6.

The thymic cortex contained only a few Ox19-positive cells, Ox8-positive, or W3/25-positive cells on day 0. The medulla appeared to contain the same ditributional pattern of T cells as in controls.

On day 10 after birth the epithelial reticulum and the dendritic cells in the medulla of the thymus showed normal Ia expression in prenatally DEX treated rats. The number of Ox19-positive cells in the cortex had increased, but it still was less than in controls. On day 14 the staining pattern with Ox19 in the cortex had become normal. Also, the distribution of Ox8-positive cells had regained its normal pattern. Yet, W3/25 still recognized less cells, and the cells that were labeled by W3/25 only reacted weakly. On day 21 no differences were demonstrable anymore between DEX-treated and control thymus.

Lymph Nodes

During the first week after birth, lymph nodes derived from DEX-treated rats were developed less than controls. A corticomedullary differentiation was not visible until the end of the first week. Lymphoid cells were spread over the lymph node during the first week, with only very few lymphoid cells expressing Ia as compared to controls. Only few Ia-positive dendritic cells were displayed in the neonatal lymph nodes. During development, the expression of Ia antigen on lymphoid and nonlymphoid cells increased. On day 10 no difference could be made between DEX-treated rats and control rats regarding Ia expression. The development of primary and secundary follicles in the lymph nodes appeared to be normal.

The development and distributional patterns of macrophage subsets were completely normal, that is, as described before in untreated lymph nodes (15).

As for T cells, on the day of birth almost no cells were labeled in DEX-treated lymph nodes by either Ox19, Ox8, or W3/25. Gradually the numbers of these cells increased during further development. After 2 weeks, the distributional pattern of OX8-positive cells appeared to be normal, but the staining patterns of Ox19 and W3/25 were less dense and less intense as compared to age-matched control rats. On sections of lymph nodes on day 21 after birth, no difference was demonstrable anymore between prenatally DEX-treated rats and controls.

FACS-Analysis

Thymus

FACS-analysis of thymic cell suspensions revealed a decrease in Ox19-positive cells until day 14 after birth and a reduction in W3/25-positive cells until day 21 after birth. The number of Ox8-positive cells already had become normal on day 7 (Table 1).

Lymph Nodes

The numbers of Ox19-positive cells and of W3/25-positive cells still were reduced on day 21 after birth, after prenatal DEX treatment (Fig. 1). Ox8 recognized the normal number of cells on days 14 and 21.

DISCUSSION

In the present study, the effects of prenatal administration of DEX were demonstrable in the thymus on day 14, but not on day 21, whereas in lymph nodes a decrease still was found in

Table 1 Long-Term Effect of Treatment with Dexamethasone on Day 17 and 19 of Fetal Life on T Lymphocytes

	Thymus				Lymph node			
Postnatal day	3	7	14	21	3	7	14	21
Ox19	<	<	=	=	<	<	<	<
W3/25	<	<	<	=	<	<	=	<
Ox8	<	=	=	ND	ND	ND	=	=

Abbreviations: <, Decreased; =, No difference with controls; ND, Not done.

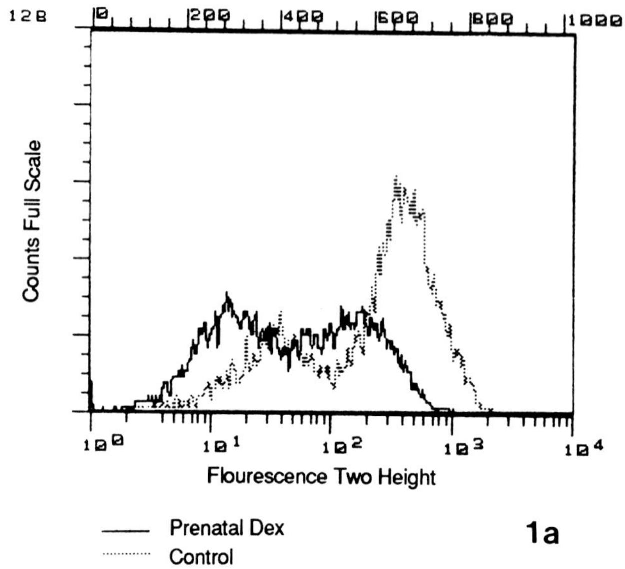

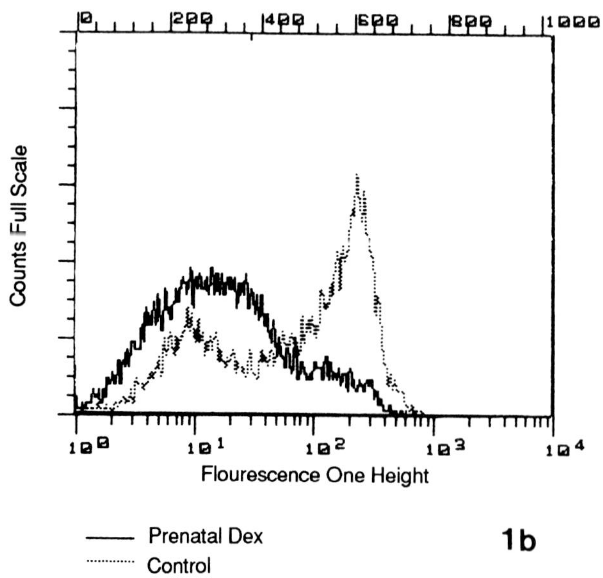

Figure 1 (a) FACs analysis of Ox19-positive cells in lymph nodes from 21-day-old rats. A reduction in Ox19-positive cells is still demonstrable in lymph nodes of rats that received prenatal DEX treatment as compared to control rats. (b) FACS analysis of W3/25-positive cells in 21-day-old lymph nodes. At this stage, a reduction of T-helper cells is shown in the lymph nodes.

Ox19-positive cells and in W3/25-positive cells, but not in Ox8-positive cells on day 21. This points to a long-lasting effect on peripheral T cells with T-helper phenotype. Diabetes-prone BB rats display a profound T-cell lymphopenia, especially of cytotoxic-suppressor T cells, independent of the development of diabetes (16). Macrophages in the cortex of the thymus are thought to play a role in the maturating of thymocytes (17). As in BB rats, the number of thymic macrophages labeled by ED2 is severely reduced (13), and this could induce the T-cell lymphopenia in BB rats. Yet, after DEX treatment in normal Wistar rats, no abnormalities could be observed in the phenotype of thymic macrophages as recognized by the ED MAbs. In the present study, no indications have been found for a role of thymic macrophages inducing T-cell lymphopenia following DEX treatment.

Lymph nodes treated with corticosteroids before injection of labeled lymphocytes, obtained from untreated mice, did not contain any labeled cells (18). The spleen and bone marrow contained normal numbers of labeled lymphocytes. Corticosteroid-treated lymphocytes transferred to untreated animals showed a normal distributional pattern over lymphoid organs (18). These data suggest a redistribution of lymphocytes after corticosteroid treatment, owing to an effect on the vascular adressins on endothelial cells. In adult animals, these effects were temporarily. In the present study, 3 weeks after prenatal DEX treatment W3/25-positive T cells were reduced in lymph nodes but Ox8-positive cells were not. This might indicate a prolonged effect of DEX on the homing of T-helper cells into lymph nodes.

REFERENCES

1. Snyder DS, Unanue ER. Corticosteroids inhibit murine macrophage Ia expression and interleukin 1 production. J Immunol 1982; 129:1803–1805.
2. Dennis GJ, Mond JJ. Corticosteroid-induced suppression of murine B cell immune response antigens. J Immunol 1986; 136:1600–1604.
3. Baxter JD, Harris AW. Mechanism of glucocorticoid action: general features, with reference to steroid-mediated immunosuppression. Transplant Proc 1975; 7:55–65.
4. Screpanti I, Morrone S, Meco D, Santoni A, Gulino A, Paolini R, Crisanti A, Mathieson B, Frati L. Steroid sensitivity of thymocyte subpopulations during intrathymic differentiation. Effects of 17β-estradiol and dexamethasone on subsets expressing T cell antigen receptor or IL-2 receptor. J Immunol 1989; 142:3378–3383.
5. McMillan VM, Dennis GJ, Glimcher LH, Finkelman FD, Mond JJ. Corticosteroid induction of $Ig^{+}Ia^{-}$ B cells in vitro is mediated via interaction with the glucocorticoid cytoplasmic receptor. J Immunol 1988; 140:2549–2555.
6. Cupps TR, Gerrard TL, Falkoff JM, Whalen G, Fauci AS. Effects of in vitro corticosteroids on B cell activation, proliferation and differentiation. J Clin Invest 1985; 75:754–761.
7. Cummings JJ, D'Eugenio DB, Gross SJ. A controlled trial of dexamethasone in preterm infants at high risk for bronchopulmonary dysplasia. N Engl J Med 1989; 320:1505–1510.
8. Turner BB, Newman Taylor A. Persistent alteration of pituitary-adrenal function in the rat by prepuberal corticosterone treatment. Endocrinology 1976; 98:1–9.
9. Angelucci L, Patacchioli FR, Scaccianoce S, Di Sciullo A, Cardillo A, Maccari S. A model for later-life effects of perinatal drug exposure: maternal hormone mediation. Neurobehav Toxicol Teratol 1985; 7:511–517.
10. Novotny EA, Raveche ES, Sharrow S, Ottinger M, Steinberg AD. Analysis of thymocyte subpopulations following treatment with sex hormones. Clin Immunol Immunopathol 1983; 28:205–217.
11. Dijkstra CD, Döpp EA. Ontogenetic development of T and B lymphocytes and non-lymphoid cells in the white pulp of the rat spleen. Cell Tissue Res 1983; 229:351–363.

12. Dijkstra CD, Döpp EA, Joling P , Kraal G. The heterogeneity of mononuclear phagocytes in lymphoid organs: distinct macrophage subpopulations in rat recognized by monoclonal antibodies ED1, ED2 and ED3. Immunology 1985; 54:589–599.
13. Van Rees EP, Voorbij HAM, Dijkstra CD. Neonatal development of lymphoid organs and specific immune responses in situ in diabetes-prone BB rats. Immunology 1988; 65:465–472.
14. Beelen RHJ, Eestermans IL, Döpp EA, Dijkstra CD. Monoclonal antibodies ED1, ED2 and ED3 against rat macrophages: expression of recognized antigens in different stages of differentiation. Transplant Proc 1987; 19:3166–3170.
15. Van Rees EP, Döpp EA, Dijkstra CD, Sminia T. The postnatal development of cell populations in the rat popliteal lymph node. An immunohistochemical study. Cell Tissue Res 1985; 242: 391–398.
16. Woda BA, Like AA, Padden C, McFadden ML. Deficiency of phenotypic cytotoxic-suppressor T lymphocytes in the BB/W rat. J Immunol 1986; 136:856–859.
17. Sminia T, Van Asselt AA, Van der Ende MB, Dijkstra CD. Rat thymus macrophages: an immunohistochemical study on fetal, neonatal and adult thymus. Thymus 1986; 8:141–150.
18. Chung H-T, Samlowski WE, Daynes RA. Modification of the murine immune-system by glucocorticosteroids. Alterations of the tissue localization properties of circulating lymphocytes. Cell Immunol 1986; 101:571–578.

41
Avian Homologue of Mammalian CD2 Antigen

Olli Vainio,[1,2] Brigitte Riwar,[2] Marion H. Brown,[3] and Olli Lassila[1,2]
[1]*Turku University, Turku, Finland;* [2]*Basel Institute for Immunology, Basel, Switzerland;* [3]*The Imperial Cancer Research Fund Laboratories, London, England*

INTRODUCTION

CD2 is a nonpolymorphic surface antigen on human T cells that is involved in cell adhesion and signal transduction (1–3). The natural ligand for CD2 is a broadly distributed molecule, lymphocyte function-associated antigen-3 (LFA-3) (1). Recently, CD2-homologous molecules on mouse, rat, and sheep T cells have been characterized (4–6), and the genes coding for human, mouse, and rat CD2 have been cloned (1–3). A substantial nucleotide and amino acid sequence homology of different CD2 molecules, especially in their cytoplasmic portion, has been demonstrated.

In the present study, we report the characterization of an avian homologue of the mammalian CD2.

MATERIALS AND METHODS

Animals and Antibodies

Chickens and chicken embryos from the inbred CB (*B12* major histocompatibility complex [MHC] haplotype) and partly inbred H.B15 (*B15*).H.B19 (*B19*) and H.B.21 (*B21*) strains from the Basel Institute for Immunology chicken farm, Gipf-Oberfrick, were used.

The following monoclonal antibodies were used: CT3 (immunoglobulin G_1 [IgG_1] isotype), against chicken CD3 molecules (7); TCR 1 (IgG_1), against T-cell receptor $\gamma\delta$ (8) (both a kind gift of Prof. M. D. Cooper, Birmingham, Alabama); TCR 2 (IgG_1) against T-cell receptor $\alpha\beta$ (9) (a kind gift of Dr. Cihak and Prof. Lösch, München, FRG); 2-6 (IgG_1), against a chicken homologue of CD4 (10); 9-8 (IgG_{2b}), against a chicken homologue of CD8 (Vainio et al., manuscript in preparation); M1 (IgG_{2b}), against chicken immunoglobulin mu heavy chain (Southern Biotechnology Ass., Birmingham, Alabama); and 47.5 (IgG_1), against lambda light chain (a kind gift of Dr. G. Koch, Lelystad, The

Netherlands). Production and characterization of a rabbit antiserum, called CD2-300, against a synthetic peptide comprising 18 amino acid residues which are conserved among the cytoplasmic domains of the human, rat, and mouse CD2 antigens has been described earlier (11).

Immunoprecipitation, Gel Electrophoresis, and Cell Proliferation Assay

Cell surface iodination and immunoprecipitation was performed according to Kaufman et al. (12). In cell proliferation assay, 5×10^5 14-day-old embryonic thymocytes and 5×10^5 adult peripheral blood T cells from the H.B21 strain were cultured in 0.2 ml of Isocove's modified Dulbecco's medium adjusted to the correct osmolality for chicken cell cultures (13) and supplemented with 1% normal chicken serum in a flat-bottom 96-well microtiter plate (Costar 3596, Cambridge, Massachusetts) with 10 μg/ml of MAb 2-4 and 25 ng/ml phorbol myristate acetate (PMA) (Sigma) for 48 hr at +40°C in 5% CO_2 humidified atmosphere. Cultures were pulsed for the last 6 hr with 1 μCi [^{3}H]thymidine. [^{3}H]thymidine incorporation was measured using standard scintillation techniques.

RESULTS

Tissue Distribution and Ontogeny of Chicken CD2

The MAb against chicken T-cell surface antigens were raised by immunizing mice with 15-day-old embryonic thymocytes. Initial screening of hybridomas by indirect immunofluorescence revealed two MAbs that reacted with most thymocytes but were negative on bursa cells. The MAbs, designated 2-4 and 2-102, are of IgG_{2a} and IgG_{2b} isotype, respectively. Flow cytometric analysis indicated that these MAbs recognize the same epitope. The antibodies reacted with ~98% of thymocytes and ~60% of the spleen cells and peripheral blood leukocytes but usually less than 1% of bursa cells were positive. Immunohistochemical studies demonstrated that CD2 expression starts intrathymically on day 11.5 of embryonation on mononuclear lymphocytelike cells. Before that time point, no MAb 2-4–positive cells were found in the thymic lobes or anywhere else in the embryo. Two-color immunofluorescence staining using biotinylated MAb 2-4 was applied to detect CD2 expression on CD3, TCR αβ, TCR γδ, CD4- and CD8-bearing cells from the thymus, spleen, and peripheral blood of a 2-month-old CB bird. In the thymus, the expression of CD3, TCR αβ, and TCR γδ was accompanied by the coexpression of the CD2 antigen. However, γδ T cells in spleen and peripheral blood were CD2 negative.

Biochemical Analysis of Chicken CD2

Monoclonal antibodies 2-4 and 2-102 immunoprecipitated from surface-labeled thymocytes material that migrated as a single broad band with M_r 40,000. Rabbit antiserum (CD2-300) against a synthetic peptide corresponding to the conserved portion of cytoplasmic human CD2 immunoprecipitated material from surface-labeled chicken thymocytes whose mobility was coincidental with that of the MAb 2-4–precipitated material. In sequential immunoprecipitation experiments, MAb 2-4 failed to precipitate any material from cell lysates that had been depleted of rabbit antiserum CD2-300–reactive material. From these data we conclude that the antigen detected on chicken T cells by MAb 2-4 is the avian homologue of mammalian CD2.

Chicken CD2 is a single glycosylated polypeptide chain, since reduction of detergent-solubilized material did not change its migration pattern in SDS-PAGE and endo-F digestion of the precipitate increased the migration to M_r of 25,000.

T-Cell Activation

To determine whether activation of deoxyribonucleic acid (DNA) synthesis and triggering of cell division can be induced via CD2 in chicken T cells, we carried out cell proliferation assays. Either one of the anti-CD2 MAbs alone or their combination did not stimulate chicken T cells. However, both MAb 2-4 and 2-102 in the presence of phorbol ester induced a vigorous DNA synthesis by thymocytes and peripheral T cells.

CONCLUSIONS

We describe two mouse monoclonal antibodies recognizing a chicken homologue of mammalian CD2 antigen. These antibodies immunoprecipitate a broad band of M_r 40,000 from lysates of chicken thymocytes and peripheral T cells. Removal of N-linked carbohydrates reveals the core protein size of M_r 25,000. Preclearing experiments using a rabbit antihuman CD2 antiserum (CD2-300) established the conservation of avian and mammalian CD2. This indicates that despite the size difference between mammalian and chicken CD2 antigen, the epitope recognized by CD2-300 antiserum is evolutionary conserved (Table 1). Immunofluorescence analysis showed that anti-CD2 MAb reacts with all thymocytes. In peripheral blood and spleen TCR αβ–bearing cells are all CD2-positive, whereas most γδ T cells lack CD2. Chicken CD2 antigen is also part of the T-cell activation pathway, since anti-CD2 MAb together with PMA triggers both thymic and peripheral T cells into DNA synthesis and cell proliferation.

Table 1 Characteristics of CD2 Antigen in Different Species

Species	Cell distribution	M_r	CD2-300 reactivity	Nucleotide sequence
Human	T cells, natural killer (NK) cells	50-58 K	+	Available
Mouse	T cells, B cells	55-65 K	+	Available
Rat	T cells, subpopulation of macrophages	50-55 K	+	Available
Sheep	T cells, subpopulation of macrophages (most γδ T cells negative)	50-55 K	+	Not determined
Chicken	T cells (peripheral γδ T cells negative)	40 K	+	Not determined

ACKNOWLEDGMENTS

We thank Drs. M. D. Cooper, J. Cihak, U. Lösch, and G. Koch for monoclonal antibodies; Drs. J. Salomonsen and J. Kaufman for helpful suggestions; and E. Nordlund for secretarial assistance. The Turku University Foundation has provided financial support. The Basel Institute for Immunology was founded and is fully supported by F. Hoffmann–La Roche & Co., Ltd., Basel, Switzerland.

REFERENCES

1. Springer TA, Dustin ML, Kishimoto TK, Marlin ST. The lymphocyte function-associated LFA-1, CD2, and LFA-3 molecules: Cell adhesion receptors of the immune system. Ann Rev Immunol 1987; 5:223–52.
2. Moingeon P, Chang H-S, Sayre PH, Clayton LK, Alcover A, Gardner P, Reinherz EL. The structural biology of CD2. Immunol Rev 1989; 111:111–44.
3. Bierer RE, Sleckman BP, Ratnofsky SE, Burakoff SJ. The biological roles of CD2, CD4, and CD8 in T cell activation. Ann Rev Immunol 1989; 7:579–99.
4. Sewell WA, Brown MH, Owen MJ, Fink PJ, Kozak CA, Crumpton MJ. The murine homologue of the T lymphocyte CD2 antigen: molecular cloning, chromosomal assignment and cell surface expression. Eur J Immunol 1987; 17:1015–20.
5. Jefferies WA, Green JR, Williams AF. Authentic T helper CD4 (W3/25) antigen on rat peritoneal macrophages. J Exp Med 1985; 162:117–27.
6. Mackay CR, Hein WR, Brown MH, Matzinger P. Unusual expression of CD2 in sheep: implications for T cell interactions. Eur J Immunol 1988; 18:1681–8.
7. Chen C-LH, Ager LL, Gartland GL, Cooper MD. Identification of a T3/T cell receptor complex in chickens. J Exp Med 1986; 164:374–80.
8. Sowder JT, Chen C-LH, Ager LL, Chan MM, Cooper MD. A large subpopulation of avian T cells express a homologue of the mammalian Tγδ receptor. J Exp Med 1988; 167:315–22.
9. Cihak J, Ziegler-Heitbrock HWL, Trainer H, Schranner I, Merkenschlager M, Lösch U. Characterization and functional properties of a novel monoclonal antibody which identifies a T cell receptor in chickens. Eur J Immunol 1988; 18:533–7.
10. Vainio O, Riwar B, Lassila O. Characterization of chicken CD4-expressing cells. In: Bhogal BS, Koch G (eds). *Recent Advances in Avian Immunology Research*. New York, Liss, 1989, pp. 45–56.
11. Brown MH, Sewell WA, Mason DY, Rothbard JB, Crumpton MJ. Species conservation of the T cell lymphocyte CD2 cell surface antigen. Eur J Immunol 1988; 18:1223–7.
12. Kaufman JF, Flajnik MF, DuPasquier L, Riegert P. Xenopus MHC class II molecules. I. Identification and structural characterization. J Immunol 1985; 134:3248–57.
13. Lassila O, Alanen A, Lefkovits I, Cooper MD, Pink JRL. Immunoglobulin diversification in embryonic chicken bursae and in individual bursal follicles. Eur J Immunol 1988; 18:943–9.

42

Chromatin Disaggregation in Lymphocytes Following Monoclonal Antibody and Immunogold Treatment

Brigid M. Balfour,[1] Nicholas English,[1] John Farrant,[1] A. David B. Webster,[1] John Clark,[1] and Wieslawa Rudnicka[2]
[1]*Clinical Research Centre, Harrow, England;* [2]*Microbiology Institute, Lodz, Poland*

INTRODUCTION

In the course of experiments to examine the induction phase of the immune response in patients with common variable immunodeficiency (CVI) (8), we observed the formation of cell aggregates in cultures containing blood lymphocytes and accessory cells (4) which had been treated with pokeweed mitogen (PWM). To establish the phenotypes of the lymphocytes taking part in these interactions, unfixed cultures were treated with monoclonal antibodies (MAbs) to cell surface markers, followed by immunogold and the cells then examined in the electron microscope (1). This led to the finding of chromatin disaggregation in a proportion of the lymphocytes in CVI cultures (Fig. 1) and to a lesser extent in control cultures.

ANALYSIS OF PROCEDURE RESPONSIBLE FOR NUCLEAR CHANGE

In untreated PWM-stimulated cultures of normal and CVI cells the lymphocytes always showed normal morphology, both in aggregates and in the free cell fraction. Antibodies against surface markers also had no effect by themselves, but gold conjugated antimouse globulin controls showed modest chromatin disaggregation. Both procedures were required to obtain maximum disaggregation.

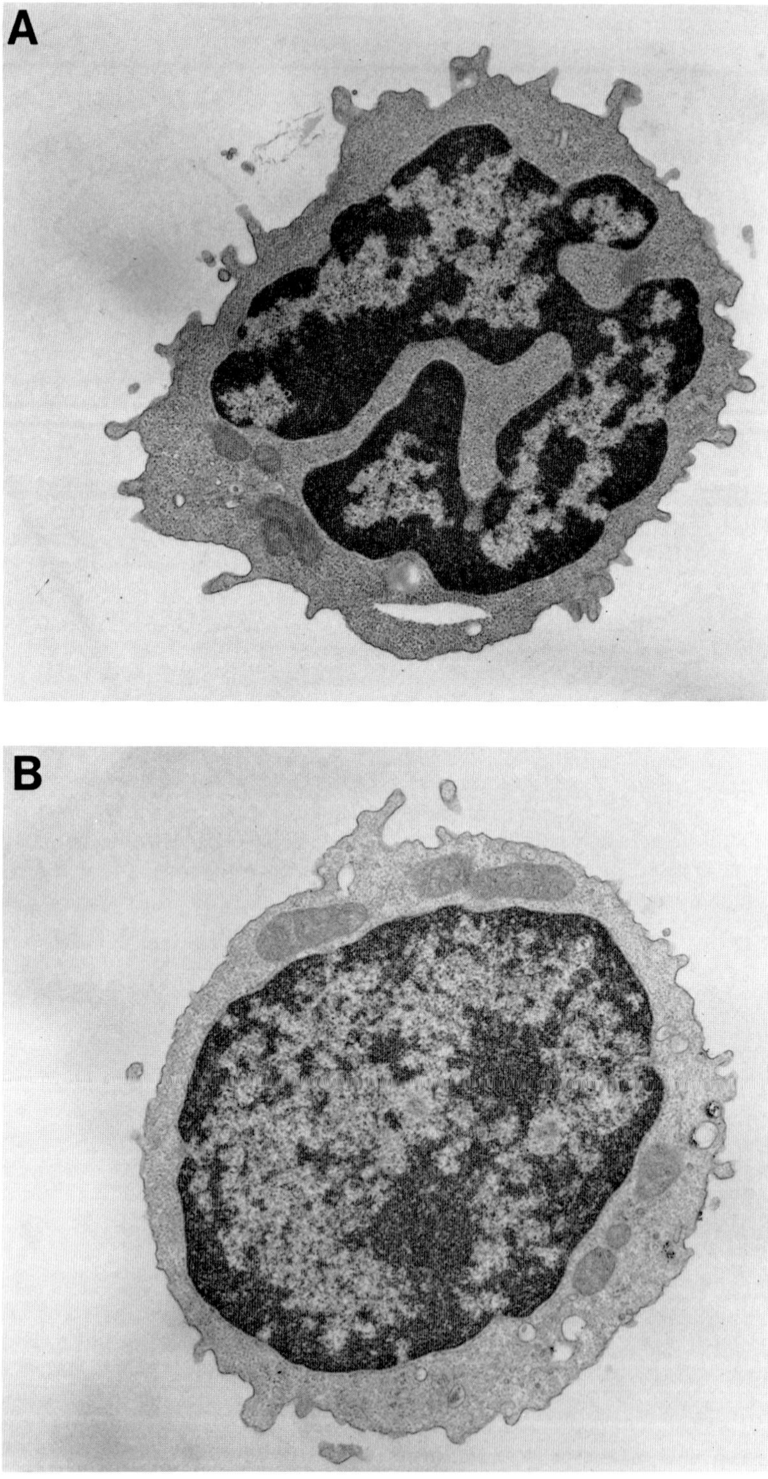

Figure 1 Electron microscopic appearance of lymphocytes following treatment with MAbs and immunogold. Stages in chromatin disaggregation. (A) Normal lymphocyte with somewhat cerebriform nucleus, showing well-defined heterochromatin, the cytoplasm contains organelles, and there are surface microvilli. (B) Stage 1. Slight nuclear change, light and dark areas less well defined, cytoplasm and microvilli normal. This appearance seen in normal and CVI cultures.

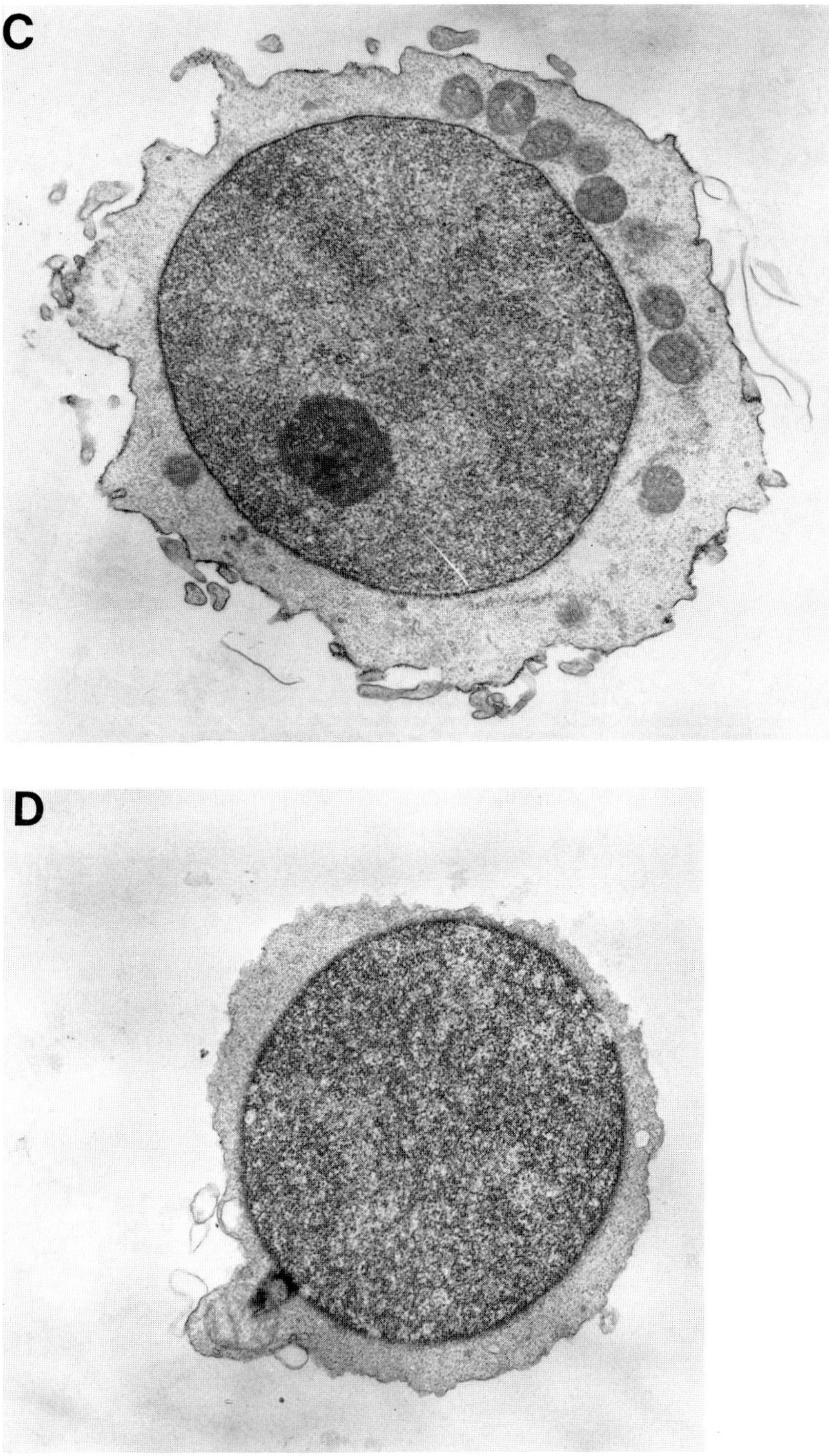

Figure 1 (Continued) (C) Stage II. Heterochromatin ill-defined, enlarged nucleolus, but organelles and microvilli still present. This appearance seen in normal and CVI cultures. (D) Stage III. Chromatin homogeneous, nucleus completely spherical, cytoplasm shrunken with loss of organelles, no microvilli present. This appearance hardly ever seen in normal cultures and most prominent in CVI cultures treated with anti–HLA-DR and immunogold. (Magnification: ×17,250)

EFFECT OF MONOCLONAL ANTIBODY SPECIFICITY ON NUCLEAR CHANGE

Anti–HLA-DR and Immunogold Treatment

In the case of anti-DR, the intensity of labeling as determined by the number of gold particles was correlated with the degree of chromatin disaggregation (Fig. 2a). Since expression of this antigen was increased on CVI, as compared to normal lymphocytes (Fig. 2d), the intensity of labeling was probably responsible for most of the nuclear change.

OKT4 and Immunogold Treatment

Chromatin disaggregation was maximal in CVI cells treated with OKT4 (Fig. 3), although the expression of CD4 antigen was not increased on CVI cells, as compared to normal lymphocytes, and there was no correlation between the intensity of labeling and the degree of nuclear change (Fig. 2b). T4 cells are known to be hypersensitive to gold (3), and this may account for the severity of the nuclear lesions.

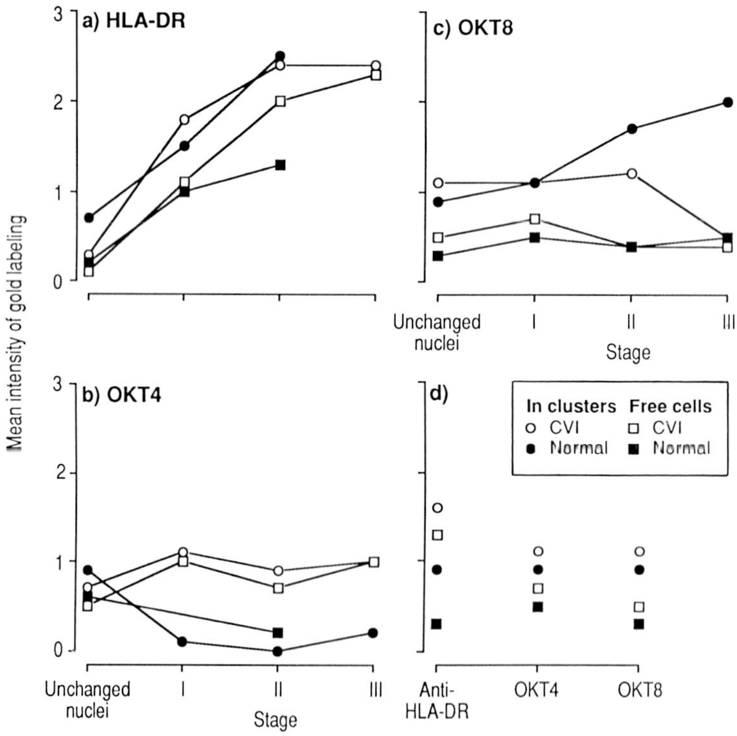

Figure 2 Correlation between intensity of gold labeling and nuclear change, using different MAbs. Labeling assessed by counting gold particles on surface of lymphocytes in EM sections of cell cultures prepared from five normal subjects and five CVI patients. Counts below 20 are not inclued, counts between 20 and 60 = 1 unit, counts between 61 and 101 = 2 units, counts above 101 = 3 units, higher values cannot be accurately determined. Each curve represents the mean value for at least 150 lymphocytes in clusters, or 300 free cells. The degree of chromatin disaggregation of the same cells is indicated on the horizontal axis.

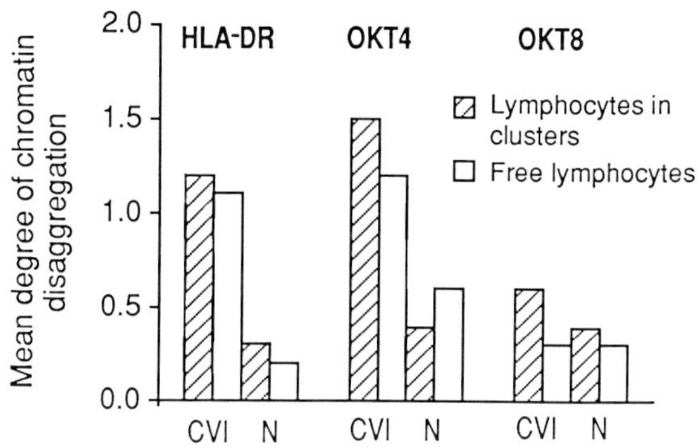

Figure 3 Histogram showing degree of chromatin disaggregation expressed in arbitrary units. Stage I = 1 unit, Stage II = 2 units, Stage II = 3 units. The data is the same as that used to prepare Figure 3.

OKT8 and Immunogold Treatment

This procedure caused minimal chromatin disaggregation and there was no difference between CVI and control cells (see Fig. 3). The intensity of the labeling was correlated with nuclear change in normal lymphocytes, but in CVI cultures, lymphocytes showing the most pronounced nuclear changes had the lowest gold particles counts (see Fig. 2c). Small amounts of CD8 antigen have been found in normal serum (2), and the serum concentration was much higher in the majority of CVI patients (9). It is likely that this antigen is also shed during immunotreatment of CVI cells in vitro, which could explain the lack of correlation between labeling and nuclear change. The fact that T8 cells are not sensitive to gold, or may even be stimulated by it (3), could be due to the lability of many of their surface molecules.

SIMILARITY BETWEEN EFFECTS OF GOLD AND PLATINUM ON NUCLEAR MORPHOLOGY

The nuclear changes seen in these cultures closely resembled those described in tumor cells of rats bearing Yoshida sarcomas after the animals had been treated with cisplatin (6) (Fig. 4A,B). It seems likely that these metals produce similar alterations in chromatin distribution, and that in our cultures traces of gold had dissolved and penetrated the nuclei of the unfixed cells (7). The role of the monoclonal antibodies was probably indirect.

ABSENCE OF CHROMATIN DISAGGREGATION IN ACCESSORY CELLS

Accessory cells never displayed nuclear changes, even when heavily labeled by anti–HLA-DR and immunogold (Fig. 5A,B,C). These cells are also sensitive to gold (5), but the lesions are due to phagocytosis of gold and the formation of aurosomes. Accessory cells are end cells, and it is likely that the chromatin disaggregation produced by gold or platinum occurs only in proliferating cells.

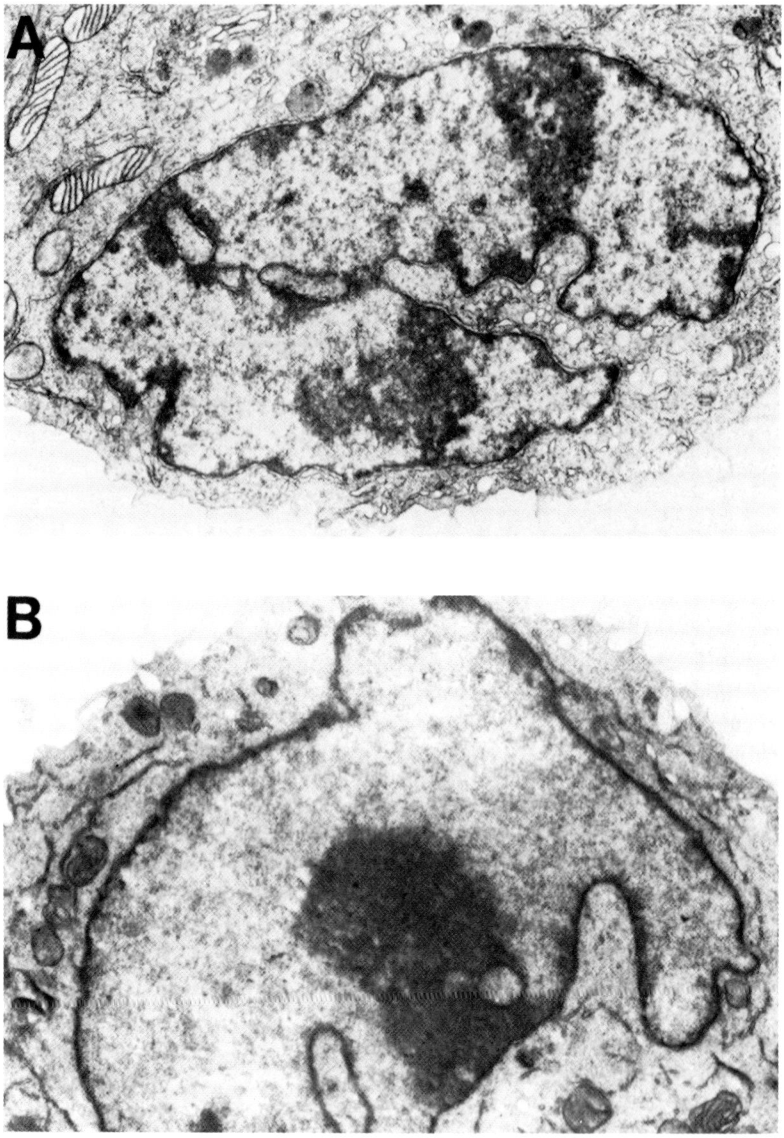

Figure 4 EM appearance of Yoshida sarcoma cells in the rat. (A) Sarcoma cell in untreated animal. (B) Animal treated with cisplatin. Sarcoma cell showing chromatin disaggregation and nucleolar enlargement. (Magnification: ×12,000) (From Ref. 6, used with permission.)

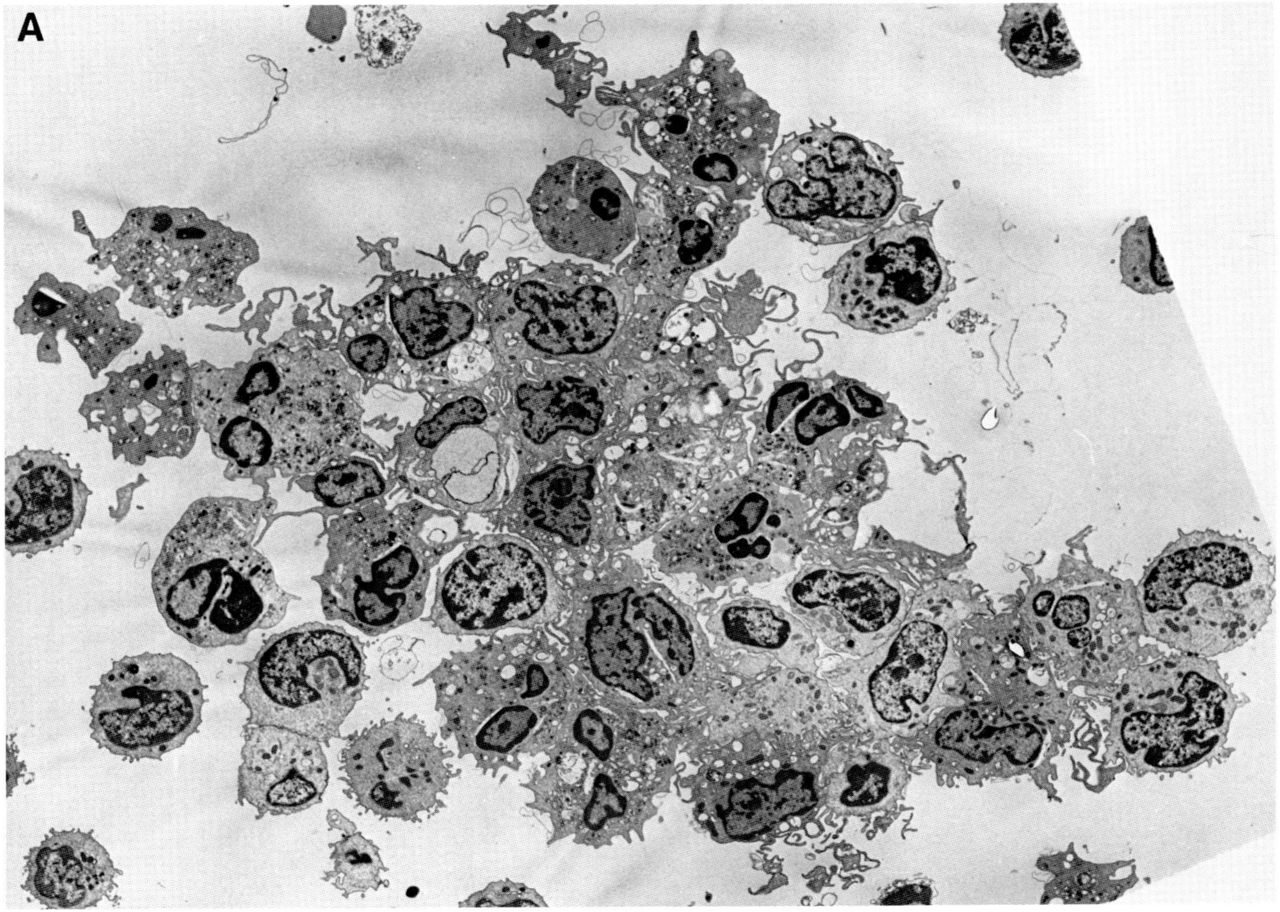

Figure 5 EM appearance of clusters of lymphocytes and PWM-pulsed accessory cells. Cultures treated with anti–HLA-DR and immunogold. (A) Normal culture. The aggregate is large and closely knit; none of the lymphocytes or accessory cells show nuclear change. Neutrophil leucocytes are also present. (B and C) Two clusters in similar preparation made from a CVI patient. The clusters are smaller and cell contacts less close. In B 3/4 lymphocytes display Stage I nuclear change (arrows). In C 2/4 lymphocytes show nuclear change, one being Stage I I (arrow). No nuclear changes seen in accessory cells. (Magnification: ×3,600)

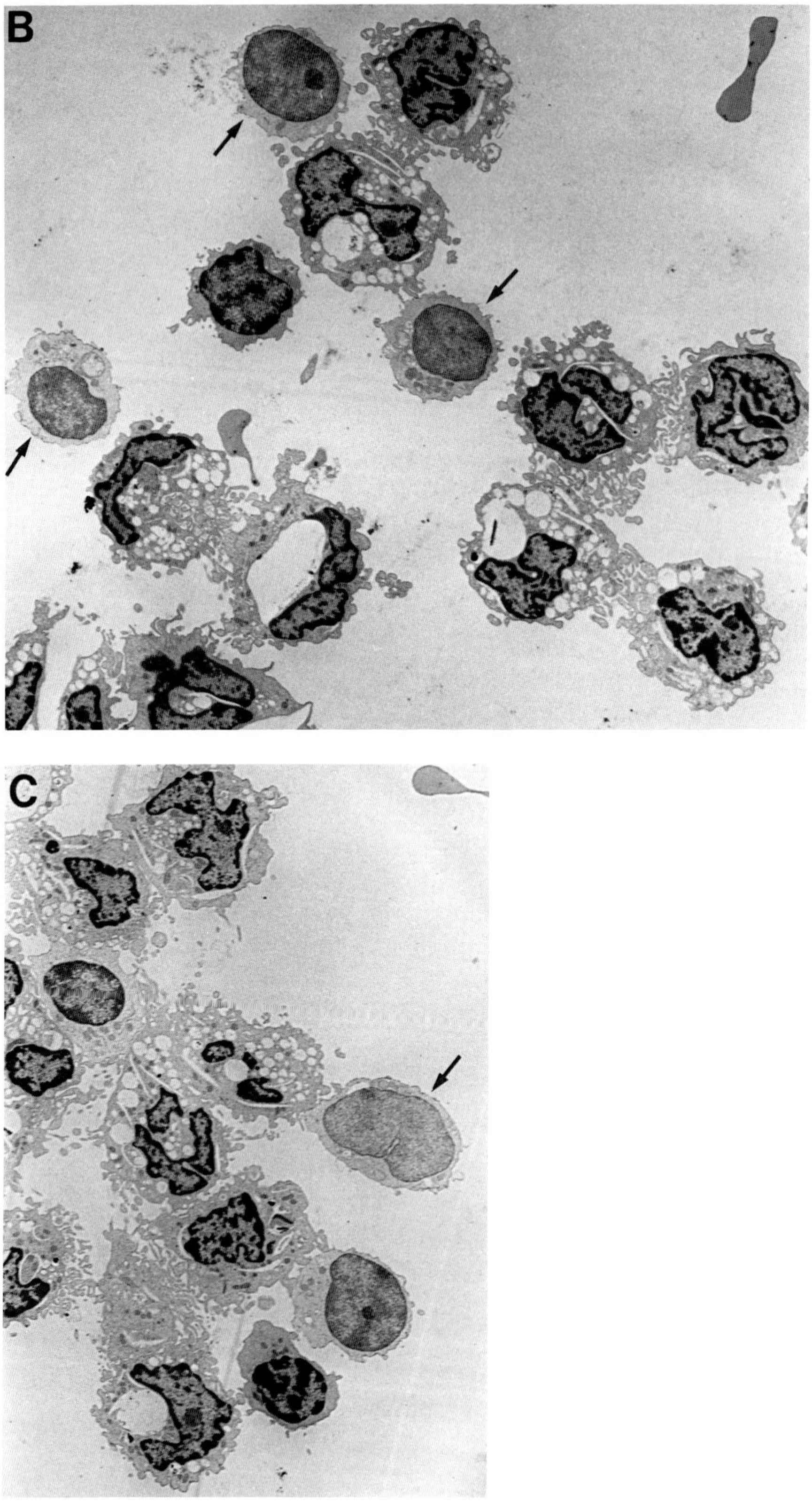

Figure 5 (Continued)

2. Accessory cells pulsed with PWM and incubated for 9 hr with autologous lymphocytes. Cluster formation observed from 3 hr onwards.
3. Cultures treated with OKT4, OKT8, or anti–HLA-DR MAbs and immunogold at 4°C before fixation. Controls treated with MAbs or immunogold alone.
4. Transmission electron microscopic examination (EM) examination of cells. Chromatin disaggregation of lymphocytes seen and classified into three stages (see Fig. 1).

REFERENCES

1. Balfour BM, Goscicka T, MacKenzie JL, Gautam A, Tate M, Clark J. Combined time-lapse cinematography and immuno-electron microscopy. Anat Rec 1990; 12:509–514.
2. Fujimoto J, Levy S, Levi R. Spontaneous release of the Leu 2 (T 8) molecule from human T cells. J Exp Med 1983; 158:752–766.
3. Griswold DE, Lee JC, Poste G, Hanna N. Modulation of macrophage-lymphocyte interactions by the anti-arthritic gold compound, Auranofin. J Rheumatol 1985; 12:490–497.
4. Knight SC, Farrant J, Bryant A, Edwards AJ, Burman S, Lever A, Clark J, Webster ADB. Non-adherent low density cells from human peripheral blood contain dendritic cells and monocytes, both with veiled morphology. Immunology 1986; 57:595–603.
5. Lipsky PE, Ziff M. Inhibition of antigen- and mitogen-induced proliferation by gold compounds. J Clin Invest 1977; 59:455–466.
6. Shepherd T, Kusnierczyk H, Jones M, Harrap KR. Criteria for the selection of second generation Platinum compounds. Br J Cancer 1980; 42:668–676.
7. Snyder R, Mirabelli CK, Crooke ST. Cellular association, intracellular distribution, and efflux of Auranofin via sequential ligand exchange reactions. Biochem Pharmacol 1986; 35:923–932.
8. Spickett GP, Webster ADB, Farrant J. Cellular abnormalities in Common Variable Immunodeficiency. Immunodef Rev (in press).
9 North ME, Farrant J, Webster ADB. Unpublished observations.

43
Localizations and Potential Roles of Leukocyte Proteases

B. Bauvois,[1] J. Gavrilovic,[2] and J. Wietzerbin[1]
[1]*Institut Curie, Paris, France;* [2]*University College, London, England*

INTRODUCTION

In the hematopoietic system, proteolytic enzymes are found intracellularly as well as membrane bound on the surface of cells and secreted in soluble form. They include endopeptidases, which cleave bonds away from the ends of polypeptide chains, and exopeptidases, which cleave bonds within one or two residues from the NH2 ends. Although localizations of these proteases are now well described, their physiological roles remain poorly understood. We report here current knowledge on well-characterized secreted and cell surface enzymes which may be potentially involved in many cell dynamics occurring during ontogeny, tissue invasion, and related and unrelated immunological responses. We present our studies on murine thymocytes and their cell surface–associated proteases.

CHARACTERIZATION OF SECRETED AND CELL SURFACE PROTEASES OF HEMATOPOIETIC CELLS

Secreted Proteases

As summarized in Table 1, a wide spectrum of proteases is secreted from hematopoietic cells. The complex formed following the interaction of α1-protease inhibitor with serine elastase is a chemoattractant for polymorphonuclear (PMN) cells (2). This enzyme is not synthesized by mature cells, but its messenger ribonucleic acid (mRNA) transcripts are found in their precursors (3). When induced to differentiate along the granulocytic lineage, the myelomonocytic cell line HL60 expresses higher levels of elastase mRNA. In contrast, when these cells are differentiated toward the monocytic lineage, no transcripts for elastase are observed. The metalloelastase from macrophages inactivates α1-protease inhibitor (although this is a serine and not a metalloprotease inhibitor), and the cleaved inhibitor

Table 1 Secreted Proteases

Name(s)	Cells	Size (kD)	Degrades	Ref. Nos.
Serine elastase	Granulocytes HL60, U937 cell lines Monocytes	25–28	Elastin, fibronectin Proteoglycans Collagens I, II, III, IV Bacterial cell walls	1
Metalloelastase	Macrophages	25	Elastin Proteoglycans Fibrin Immunoglobulins	4
Collagenase (metalloprotease)	Granulocytes U937 cell line	75	Collagens I, II, III	6 7
Gelatinase (metalloprotease)	Granulocytes Macrophages	92–97	Collagens IV, V Gelatins	8
Plasminogen activator	Macrophages HL60 cells Granulocytes	45	Plasminogen	10
Cathepsin G	Granulocytes Monocytes U937 cell line	28	C components Fibronectin Fibrinogen Immunoglobulins	12
Cathepsin L	Macrophages	?	Elastin	14
Trypsinlike serine proteinase, TSP-1	Activated T cells Malignant T cells	60	Casein Sulfated proteoglycans	15

subsequently becomes chemotactic for PMN cells (5). Gelatinase from granulocytes is closely related to macrophage gelatinase, and is probably involved in the penetration of basement membranes by cells. Upon PMA stimulation, the monoblastic cell line U937 synthesizes both a metallocollagenase and the tissue inhibitor of metalloproteases TIMP (7). This system enzyme/inhibitor is also expressed in macrophages, granulocytes, and HL60 cells which contain both plasminogen activator and plasminogen activator inhibitor (9). Plasmin generated from the action of plasminogen activator on plasminogen enhances macrophage-mediated elastin degradation (10) and activates procollagenase (11). Both cathepsin G and serine elastase are known to prime macrophage superoxide production as well as to stimulate B-cell proliferation (13). The acidic enzyme cathepsin L of macrophages could play a role in the area of close contact between the cell surface and elastin, where such low pH may be generated (14). Activated T cells and malignant T cells possess a serine protease TSP-1, whose regulated release is thought to be important in cell-mediated cytolysis and in activation of B cells. Moreover, from its capacity to release high molecular weight products from sulfated proteoglycans, it has been suggested that TSP-1 may control T-cell migration in vivo (15). Finally, serine proteases secreted from monocytes are able to cleave the platelet-derived connective tissue–activating peptide to generate neutrophil-activating peptide 2, which is chemotactic and induces exocytosis of PMN cells (16).

Cell Surface Proteases

Several endopeptidases and exopeptidases have been characterized (Table 2). Cytolysis of target cells by PMA-activated neutrophils may be attributed in part to the action of the Ca^{2+}-independent neutral serine protease on target cells (18). CD10 antigen (also called CALLA, or common acute lymphoid leukemia antigen) is identical to the human membrane neutral endopeptidase NEP, EC 3.4.24.11 (enkephalinase). Trypsinlike protease and neutral endopeptidase degrade the vasoactive intestinal peptide VIP8, shown to inhibit the proliferative responses of murine lymphocytes to mitogens (20). An arginine-specific serine enzyme on B murine spleen cells is synthesized to a higher level after mitogenic stimulation (21). Dipeptidyl aminopeptidase IV (DPPIV) is identical to CD26. Although not tested for enzyme activity, activated normal B cells and macrophages are CD26 positive. In contrast, DPPIV activity is found on cells belonging to the human myelomonocytic lineage (HL-60, U937, THP-1) as well as on peripheral blood monocytes, which are all CD26 negative (Bauvois, unpublished results). These results suggest that DPPIV/CD26 is expressed all along the differentiation pathway in monocyte/macrophage and B- and T-cell lineages. Specific inhibition of DPPIV suppresses in vitro immunoglobulin (Ig) synthesis, interleukin-2 (IL-2), and interferon-γ (IFN-γ) production by activated mononuclear cells as well as the proliferative response of mitogen-activated T cells to IL-2 (22). CD26 is shown to transduce an activating signal in murine T lymphocytes (24). Leu-aminopeptidase–like activity of human T lymphocytes and murine thymocytes is enhanced upon mitogenic stimulation (23,25). Naquet et al. have shown that Ala-aminopeptidase (THAM) present on thymocytes is involved, like CD26, in antigen- dependent T-cell activation (27).

EXPRESSION OF PEPTIDASE ACTIVITIES BY MURINE THYMOCYTES

Cell migration and thymus invasion by immature cells which migrate from the bone marrow to the thymus involve specific soluble factors, cell-cell and cell-extracellular matrix interactions. The participation of specific cell surface and/or secreted proteases has to be considered. Using sensitive spectrophotometric measurements of the cleavage of synthetic p-nitroaniline peptides, we have recently demonstrated (25) that murine thymocytes express on their surface at least three well-characterized exopeptidases: (a) Leu- and Ala-aminopeptidases are both inhibited by inhibitors for thiol and trypsinlike proteases. Exclusive inhibitions of Leu- and Ala-hydrolase activities, respectively, by pepstatin (specific for carboxyl proteases) and antibodies anti-THAM (specific for aminopeptidase with an Ala-X specificity) strength the view that the peptidase activity detected with Ala-pNA is partly different from Leu-peptidase activity. (b) Dipeptidyl peptidase IV, which cleaves the prolyl bond in the synthetic dipeptide nitroanilide Gly-Pro-pNA is specifically inhibited by a serine inhibitor, PMSF. Less than 10% of its activity is released in the extracellular medium. Whether exopeptidases such as DPPIV can also express endoproteolytic activity is not clearly established. Our results using gelatin-containing SDS gels (Fig. 1) indicate that released DPPIV exhibits endoproteolytic activity toward gelatin

Table 2 Cell Surface Proteases

Name(s)	Cells	Size (kD)	Degrades	Ref. Nos.
Endopeptidases				
neutral serine proteases (elastaselike)	Monocytes	46–65	Serum amyloid protein A	17
Ca^{2+}-independent neutral serine protease	Granulocytes	300	Globin	18
CD10/NEP	Granulocytes Lymphoid leukemia cells Immature lymphoid cells	94–100	Enkephalins Neuropeptides Substance P f-Met-Leu-Phe IL-1	19
trypsinelike serine serine proteinase, TSP-1	T effector cells	60	Casein Sulfated proteoglycans	15
trypsinlike protease	T, B cells	?	VIP 8	20
neutral endopeptidase	T, B cells	?	VIP 8	20
arginine protease	B cells	23	?	21
Exopeptidases				
DPPIV/CD26	Activated T cells (T4) B cells lines Subalveolar macrophages Thymocytes	100	Collagen I ? Fibronectin ?	22 23
Leu-aminopeptidase	Thymocytes, T cells	?	?	23,25
Ala-aminopeptidase/CD13	Macrophages Granulocytes B lymphoid leukemic cells	150	?	26
Ala-aminopeptidase/THAM	Thymocytes	115	?	23,27

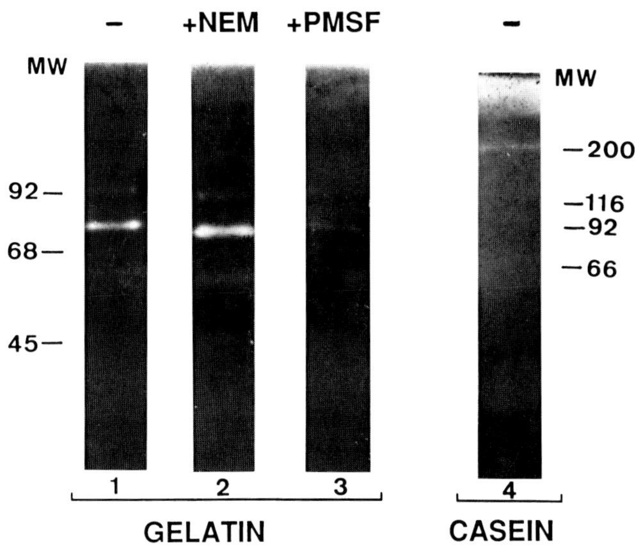

Figure 1 Polyacrylamide substrate gel electrophoresis of the conditioned medium of murine thymocytes. The conditioned medium from 2-hr incubation of murine thymocytes in protease buffer was tested for gelatin-degrading activity or casein-degrading activity in the absence (lanes 1 and 4) and the presence of 1 mM NEM (lane 2), 1 mM PMSF (lane 3). The zymograms were made using 0.5 mg/ml gelatin or 0.5 mg/ml casein incorporated into nonreducing 10% SDS-polyacrylamide gels. After electrophoresis, the gel was shaken in 2.5% Triton X-100 for 1 hr at room temperature before being incubated in protease buffer for overnight at 37°C. The gel was Coomassie-blue stained. The enzyme activities were detected as unstained bands. Gelatin is degraded by a DPPIV-like activity associated with a m.w. of 82 kD. In contrast, casein which does not contain repeated sequences Gly-Pro-X such as in gelatin and collagens is not degraded by DPPIV.

and is associated to a molecular weight of 82 kD. Levels of three cell surface activities are increased by three- to sevenfold in the $CD4^-CD8^-$ thymocyte subset present in the adult thymus (4-week-old mouse), as well as on fetal thymocytes which are > 90% $CD4^-CD8^-$ (from days 14 to 16, during ontogeny). In the presence of concanavalin A, proliferative responses of all thymocyte subsets are also correlated with significant increase (up to fivefold) of peptidase activities.

Considering the potential roles of these proteases detected on the surface of thymocytes, it is possible that they are involved in a vast number of reactions occurring in the thymus. Since CD26/DPPIV and THAM/Ala-peptidase have recently been shown to transduce in vitro activating signals, they probably participate in cell activation in vivo. They may also play a critical role in proliferation and differentiation by processing active/inactive mediators such as growth factors, interleukins, hormones, and their precursors. Secreted or cell surface enzymes may be also involved in the degradation of protein antigens for presentation to T cells and T-cell selection in the thymus. Outside of the hematopoietic system, membrane-bound DPPIV is suggested to participate in cell invasion by binding to fibronectin or collagen, and/or degrading these extracellular components. Further studies on thymocyte surface proteases are needed to substantiate their role in thymopoiesis.

IMPLICATIONS AND CONCLUSIONS

It becomes of fundamental importance to determine whether such specific proteases play critical roles in the hematopoietic development. Together with the present findings, it appears that proteases may have at least three clear functions: (a) signal transduction, (b) degradation, and (c) specific binding and recognition of extracellular matrix components. With regard to degradation, in addition to their importance in producing active/inactive effectors from cytokines, growth factors, hormones, and extracellular matrix components, the proteases may be also involved in the proteolysis of specific cell surface membrane components. Recently, a thiol protease activity has been shown to be associated with the cleavage of FcεR/CD23 on B cells (28). Although they are separated, these three functions probably interfere. One protease may perform all three functions. Through these functions, proteases may potentially be capable of inducing most of biological processes, such as cellular proliferation and differentiation, chemotaxis, cell adherence and invasion, antigen presentation, and cell-mediated cytotoxicity.

Beyond understanding the proteases themselves, their regulatory mechanisms are important. They may involve direct control of the enzyme itself by inhibitors or by activators. Another form of protease control may occur at the level of the expression of the genes (example of the neutrophil elastase gene expressed transiently during cell differentiation (3)). Messenger RNA transcripts may be induced via signal transductions through specific cell surface receptors. Among these receptors, one can include receptors for growth factors, cytokines, and extracellular matrix components such as fibronectin as well as tumor promoters and oncogene products.

Through the literature, it appears that proteolytic enzymes are widely distributed among various cell systems (immune, nervous, endocrine, etc.). It is therefore likely that enzymes which at first were restricted to a given cell type will be found in other cells. Understanding of the roles of leukocyte proteases require comparative protease studies in a variety of normal and malignant cell types outside of the hematopoietic system.

REFERENCES

1. Beith JG. Elastases: Catalytic and biological properties. In: *Regulation of Matrix Accumulation*. Mecham RP, ed. Academic Press, New York, 1986, pp. 217–320.
2. Banda MJ, Rice AG, Griffin GL, Senior RM. The inhibitory complex of human alpha-1 proteinase inhibitor and human leukocyte elastase is a neutrophil chemoattractant. J Exp Med 1988; 167:1608–15.
3. Takahashi H, Nukiwa T, Basset P, Crystal RG. Myelomonocytic cell lineage expression of the neutrophil elastase gene. J Biol Chem 1988; 263:2543–47.
4. Banda MJ, Clark EJ, Werb Z. Selective proteolysis of immunoglobulins by mouse macrophage elastase. J Exp Med 1983; 157:1184–96.
5. Banda MJ, Rice AG, Gaffin GL, Senior RM. α1-proteinase inhibitor is a neutrophil chemoattractant after proteolytic inactivation by macrophage elastase. J Biol Chem 1988; 263:4481–84.
6. Murphy G, Reynolds G, Bretz U, Baglioni M. Collagenase is a component of the specific granules of human neutrophil leukocytes. Biochem 1977; 102:195–97.
7. Welgus HG, Connolly NL, Senior RM. 12-o-tetradecanoyl-phorbol-18-acetate-differentiated U937 cells express a macrophage-like profile of neutral proteinases: High levels of secreted collagenase and collagenase inhibitor accompany low levels of intracellular elastase and cathepsin G. J Clin Invest 1986; 77:1675–81.
8. Mainardi CL, Hasty KA, Hibbs MS. Collagenolytic metalloproteinases of the human neutrophil. In: *The Control of Tissue Damage*. Galuert A, ed. Elsevier Science, Amsterdam, 1988, pp. 139–47.

9. Arndt AD, Gahill J, Rankin K, Houwen B, Hart DA. Differentiation-linked expression of the plasminogen activator inhibitor type 2 gene in the human HL60 promyelocytic cell line. Exp Cell Res 1989; 185:473–81.
10. Chapman HA, Stone OL. Cooperation between plasmin and elastase in elastin degradation by intact murine macrophages. Biochem J 1984; 222:721–28.
11. Gravrilovic J, Murphy G. The role of plasminogen in cell-mediated collagen degradation. Cell Biol Int Rep 1989; 13:367–75.
12. Vartio T, Seppa H, Vaheri A. Susceptibility of soluble and matrix fibronectins to degradation by tissue proteins, mast cell chymase and cathepsin G. J Biol Chem 1981; 256:471–77.
13. Kusner DJ, King CH. Protease-modulation of neutrophil superoxide response. J Immunol 1989; 143:1696–1702.
14. Mason RW. The role of cysteine proteinase in elastin degradation. In: The control of tissue damage. Glauert A, ed. Elsevier Science, Amsterdam, 1988, p. 259–67.
15. Kramer MD, Simon MM. Are proteinases functional molecules of T lymphocytes? Immunol Today 1987; 8:140–42.
16. Walz A, Baglioni M. Generation of the neutrophil activating peptide NAP-2 from platelet basic protein or connective tissue-activating peptide III through monocyte proteases. J Exp Med 1990; 171:449–54.
17. Lavie G, Zucker-Franklin D, Franklin EC. Elastase-type proteases on the surface of human blood monocytes. J Immunol 1980; 125:175–80.
18. Pontremoli S, Melloni E, Michetti M, Sacco O, Sparatore B, Salamino F, Damiani G, Horecker BL. Cytolytic effects of neutrophils: role for a membrane-bound neutral proteinase. Proc Natl Acad Sci USA 1986; 83:1685–89.
19. Letarte M, Vera S, Tran R, Addis JBL, Onizuka RJ, Quackenbush EJ, Jongeneel CV, McInnes RR. Common acute lymphocytic leukemia antigen is identical to neutral endopeptidase. J Exp Med 1988; 168:1247–53.
20. Goetzl LEJ, Kodama KT, Turck CW, Schigolev SA, Sreedharan SP. Unique pattern of cleavage of vasoactive intestinal peptide by human lymphocytes. Immunology 1989; 66:554–58.
21. Ku GSB, Quigley JP, Sultzer BM. The inhibition of the mitogenic stimulation of B lymphocytes by a serine protease inhibitor. J Immunol 1983; 131:2494–99.
22. Schön E, Demuth HU, Eichmann E, Horst HJ, Körner IJ, Kopp J, Mattern T, Neubert K, Noll F, Ulmer AJ, Barth A, Ansorge S. Dipeptidyl peptidase IV in human T lymphocytes. Scand J Immunol 1989; 29:127–32.
23. Bauvois B. Murine thymocytes possess specific cell surface-associated exoaminopeptidase activities. Eur J Immunol 1990; 20:459–68.
24. Hegen M, Niedobitek G, Klein CE, Fleisher B. The T cell triggering molecule TP103 (CD26) is associated with dipeptidyl aminopeptidase IV activity. J Immunol 1990; 144:2908–14.
25. Amoscato AA, Alexander JW, Babcock GF. Surface aminopeptidase activity on human lymphocytes. J Immunol 1989; 142:1245–52.
26. Look AT, Ashmun RA, Shapiro LH, Peiper SC. Human myeloid plasma membrane glycoprotein CD13 is identical to aminopeptidase N. J Clin Invest 1989; 83:1299–1307.
27. Naquet P, Vivier I, Gorvel JP, Brekelmans P, Barad M, Bernard AM, Pierres M. Activation of mouse T lymphocytes by a monoclonal antibody to a developmentally-regulated surface aminopeptidase (THAM). Immunol Rev 1989; 11:177–93.
28. Letellier M, Sarfati M, Delespesse G. Mechanisms of formation of IgE-binding factors (soluble CD23). Mol Immunol 1989; 26:1105–12.

44
B-Cell Proliferation–Suppressing Factors

Dragan Jovanović,[1] Božidar Banićević,[2] Ljiljana Dimitrijević,[1]
Marko Radulović,[1] Ninoslav Nedeljković,[2] and Katarina Isaković[1]
[1]*Immunology Research Center, Belgrade, Yugoslavia;*
[2]*Institute for Blood Transfusion, Belgrade, Yugoslavia*

INTRODUCTION

Activation and proliferation of normal human B lymphocytes are under the control of regulatory T cells which provide both helper and suppressor signals to B cells (1). In the experiment described here, a suppressor activity of normal and leukemic T lymphocytes on the proliferation of normal B cells was investigated. In an in vitro assay, it was demonstrated that normal but not leukemic T cells generated a factor which suppressed B-cell proliferation. Also, it was shown that suppressor activity of T lymphocytes appeared after their helper function.

MATERIALS AND METHODS

Lymphocyte Donors

Lymphocytes were obtained from the peripheral blood (PB) of healthy subjects between 18 and 45 years of age, and from patients with chronic lymphocytic leukemia (CLL), who were not in therapy. Lymphocytes were isolated by centrifugation of heparinized blood on Ficoll-Isopaque gradient, washed three times, and resuspended in RPMI 1640 supplemented with 15% of fetal calf serum (FCS) (Flow Laboratories).

Purified T and B Lymphocytes

Purified T and B lymphocytes were prepared by the method described elsewhere (2). Double rosetting of peripheral blood lymphocytes (PBLs) with SRBC was used to separate T and B lymphocytes. Equal volumes of PBSs (5×10^6/ml) and SRBC suspension (10^8/ml) were mixed, incubated at 37°C for 15 min, centrifugated on 200 × G for 7 min, and incubated thereafter over night at 4°C. Rosettes were sedimented by centrifugation on Ficoll-Isopaque gradient at 600 × G for 40 min. T cells were recovered from the rosettes by addition of Tris-ammonium chloride (0.87%), pH 7.2. Lymphocytes from the interphase were harvested, and B lymphocytes, free of myelomonocytic cells, were obtained by removing adherent and phagocytic cells by adherence in plastic culture dishes at 37°C for 2 hr and by magnetic removal of carbonyl iron–digested cells, respectively.

Supernatants of PHA-TPA–Stimulated T Lymphocytes

Purified T lymphocytes (10^5 cells/well) derived from normal donors and patients with CLL were cultured in RPMI 1640 containing 15% of FCS and stimulated with PHA (1 μg/ml) and TPA (1 ng/ml), (Sigma Chemical Co.) at the initiation of culture. After incubation at 37°C supernatants were harvested either after 48, 72, or 96 hr. After centrifugation (3000 rpm for 10 min), supernatants were passed through a 0.45-μm filter, after that concentrated 10 times using Amicon YM-10 filters. Supernatants were dialyzed against PBS with 0.01% of polyethylene glycol (m.w. 6000), and then sterilized by filtration (0.22-μm filter) and stored at –20°C until use (3).

Assay System of B-Cell Proliferation

Staphylococcus aureus Cowan I strain (SAC)–stimulated cultured of purified normal B cells were used for assessment of activity of supernatants of PHA-TPA–stimulated cultures of normal and CLL T lymphocytes. B cells were cultured in microtiter plastic plates at density 2×10^5 cells/200 μl medium/well, in the presence of 0.04% v/v of SAC. Supernatants of PHA-TPA–stimulated T-cell cultures were added in the concentration of 20% at the initiation of culture. SAC was prepared in our laboratory as formanilized *Staphylococcus aureus* Cowan I strain (4). Proliferation of B cells was measured by incorporation of [^{3}H]thymidine on days 1, 3, 5, and 7. Cultures were pulsed with 0.5 μCi of [^{3}H]thymidine during last 18 hr, and results were recorded as counts per min (cpm) of stimulated cells minus cpm of the background (nonstimulated cells).

RESULTS AND DISCUSSION

This study deals with the suppressive effect of supernatant obtained from 72-hr-old culture of PHA-TPA–stimulated PB T lymphocytes on the proliferation of normal circulating human B cells. To study suppressive activity of regulatory T cells, an assay system for B-cell proliferation developed by Muragushi and Fauci (5) was applied. SAC was used as an activator for cells for several reasons. First, SAC is a competence signal which induces resting B cells to leave the G_0 phase and enter into the cell cycle (6,7). Second, proliferative response of B lymphocytes to SAC is T-cell independent (8,9), and therefore this model is suitable to study involvement of T cell–derived factor(s) in the activation and/or proliferation of B cells. Finally, SAC is interacting with membrane immunoglobulins (10), and therefore the pathway of intracellular transduction of activating signal is like that which occurs after binding of antigen to the immunoglobulin receptors.

It was necessary in a preliminary experiment to determine the optimal number of B cells and concentration of SAC (5). Using various doses of SAC and different numbers of B cells, it was shown that 2×10^5 cells/well and 0.04% v/v of SAC gave the highest level of cell proliferation.

Results concerning activities of supernatants of PHA-TPA–stimulated cultures of normal T lymphocytes taken after 48, 72, and 96 hr after activation on the proliferation of normal B lymphocytes, are summarized in Figure 1. It is evident that supernatant of 48-hr-old culture exerted costimulatory activity on SAC-stimulated B cells, increasing thus incorporation of [^{3}H]thymidine. When supernatant of 72-hr-old cultures was added to the SAC-activated B cells, deoxyribonucleic acid (DNA) synthesis was completely inhibited. On the other hand, a 96-hr-old supernatant did not influence proliferation of B cells induced by SAC.

Suppressive effect of 72-hr-old supernatant was B-cell restricted, since this supernatant did not exert any effect on the proliferation of PHA-stimulated PBLs (Fig. 2).

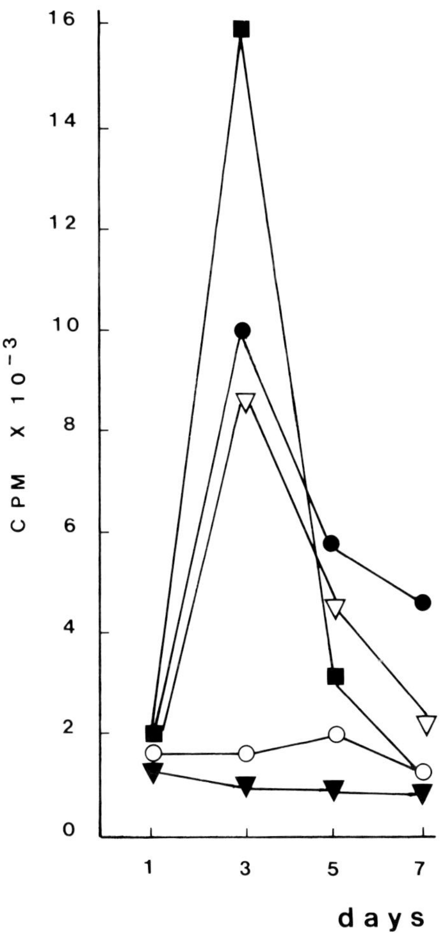

Figure 1 Activity of the supernatants obtained from the cultures of PHA-TPA–stimulated normal human To lymphocytes on the proliferation of normal circulating human B cells. Incorporation of [^{3}H]thymidine by nonstimulated B cells (○—○), B cells stimulated with SPA (●—●), SPA and supernatant taken after 48 hr (■—■), 72 hr (▼—▼), and 96 hr (▽—▽). Results represent the mean of three experiments and each experiment was done in triplicate.

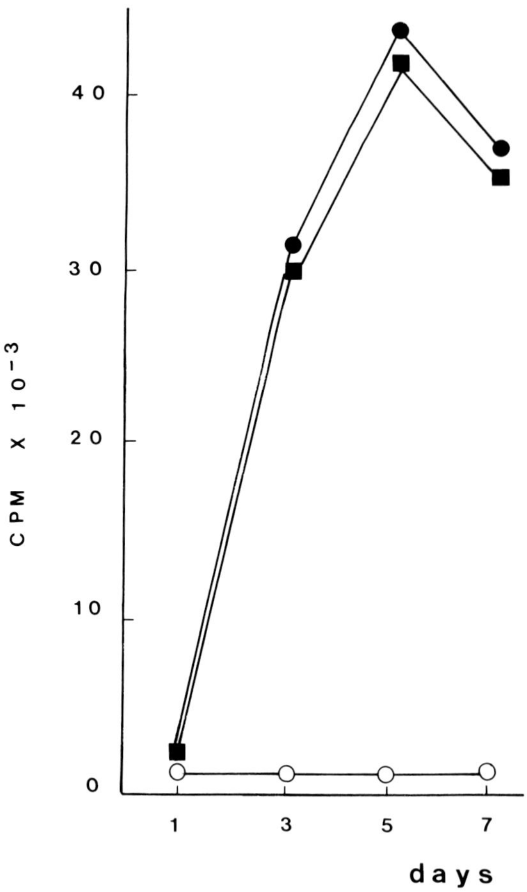

Figure 2 Activity of 72-hr-old supernatant of PHA-TPA–stimulated culture of normal T cells on the proliferation of PBLs activated with PHA. Incorporation of [^{3}H]thymidine by nonstimulated PBLs (○—○), PBLs stimulated with PHA (●—●), and PBLs stimulated with PHA and supernatant (■—■). Results represent the mean of two experiments, and each experiment was done in triplicate.

From these results it is clear that T cells composed of different subsettes of cells, modulate the activation and/or proliferation of B lymphocytes by providing both helper and suppressor activities (1,10). It seems that these two activities of T cells occurring sequentially, thus helper activity proceeds the appearance of suppression. One may assume that the kinetics of the appearance of stimulatory and suppressive functions of regulatory T lymphocytes in the course of B-cell proliferation demonstrated here in an in vitro system may have a physiological significance as well. In this study, no attempt was made to define the cell types generating helper and suppressor activities as well as growth factors contained in 48-hr-old supernatant. It could be proposed that the supernatant which exerted stimulatory activity (48-hr-old) on SAC-stimulated B lymphocytes, contained at least interleukin-2 (IL-2) and IL-4). It is known that both lymphokines drive B cells from the G_1 to S phase of the cell cycle (6), either acting alone or synergistically (11).

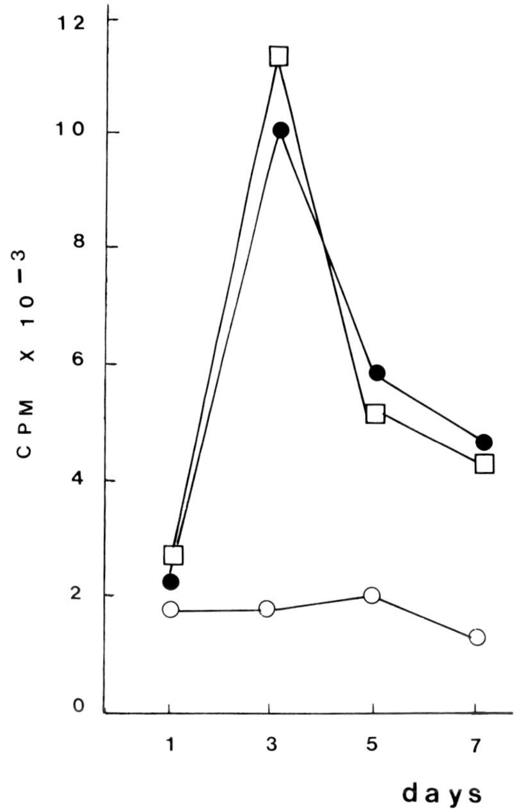

Figure 3 Proliferation of normal human B lymphocytes activated with SPA in the presence of 72-hr-old supernatant of culture of T cells from CLL patients stimulated with PHA-TPA. Nonstimulated B lymphocytes (○—○), SPA-stimulated B lymphocytes (●—●), SPA-stimulated B lymphocytes in the presence of supernatant (□—□). Results represent the mean of triplicates of two experiments.

Results illustrated in Figure 3 showed that circulating T cells derived from patients with CLL did not elaborate suppressor activity after in vitro stimulation with PHA-TPA. Also, 72-hr-old supernatant of stimulated T lymphocytes from these patients did not influence SAC-induced B-cell proliferation. Therefore, these results clearly indicate that in CLL patients there is a defect not only in the population of helper T cells, but also in the suppressor T lymphocytes (10,12). The inability of regulatory T cells to generate a suppressor factor(s) which regulates B-cell proliferation may be one of the mechanisms which are involved in disregulated expansion of a malignant clone of B lymphocytes in CLL (13,14).

REFERENCES

1. Katz DH. *Lymphocyte Differentiation, Recognition and Regulation*. Academic Press, New York, 1977.
2. Ishiazaka A, Sakiyama Y, Talanashi Y, Matsumoto S, The activation of T cells with staphylococcus aureus Cowal I (SAC). Immunol Lett 1985; 10:13–7.

3. Muragushi A, Hishimoto H, Kawanuka N, Hori A, Kishimoto T. B-cell derived BCGF functions as autokrine growth factor(s) in normal and transformed B lymphocytes. J Immunol 1986; 137:179–86.
4. Forsgen A, Svedjelung A, Wigzell H. Lymphocyte stimulation by protein A of Staphylococcus aureus. Eur J Immunol 1976; 6:207–13.
5. Muragushi A, Fauci AS. Proliferative responses of normal human B lymphocytes. Development of an assay system for human B cell growth factor (BCGF). J Immunol 1982; 129:1104–8.
6. Butler J, Muragushi A, Lane H, Fauci AS. Development of a human T-T cell hybridoma secreting B cell growth factor. J Exp Med 1983; 157:60–8.
7. Clark EA, Shu GL, Lüscher B, Draves KE, Banchereau J, Ledbetter J, Valentine MA. Activation of human B cells. Comparison of the signal transduced by IL-4 to four different competence signals. J Immunol 1989; 143:3873–89.
8. Falcoff RJM, Zhu LP, Fauci AS. Separate signals for human B cell proliferation and differentiation in response to Staphylococcus aureus: Evidence for two-signal model of B cell activation. J Immunol 1982; 129:97–102.
9. Romagnini S, Guidili M, Biagiotti R, Almerigna F, Maggi E, Del Prete G, Ricci M. Surface immunoglobulins are involved in the interaction of protein A with human B cells in the triggering of B cell proliferation induced by protein A–containing Staphylococcus aureus. J Immunol 1981; 127:1307–13.
10. Chiorazzi N, Fu SM, Montazeri G, Kunkel HG, Rai K, Gee T. T cell helper defect in patients with chronic lymphocyteic leukemia. J Immunol 1979; 122:1087–90.
11. Miller SL, Hooton JWL, Gillis S, Paetkau V. IL-4 potentiates the IL-2-dependent proliferation of mouse cytotoxic T cells. J Immunol 1990; 144:1331–7.
12. Fu SM, Chiorazzi N, Kunkel HG, Halper JD, Hirris SR. Induction of in vitro differentiation and immunoglobulin synthesis of human leukemic B lymphocytes. J Exp Med 1978; 138:1570–6.
13. Bloem AC, Carien OM, van Hooff EJE, Bast G, Ballieux RE. Mitogenic stimulation of malignant B cells. Clin Exp Immunol 1984; 55:636–42.
14. Rambotti P, Davis S. Lactic dehydrogenase in normal and leukemic lymphocyte subpopulation: evidence for the presence of abnormal T cells and B cells in chronic lymphocytic leukemia. Blood 1981; 57:324–7.

45

Synthetic Peptides

A Unique Model to Analyze the Induction and Regulation of Determinant Specific Immune Responses

W. J. A. Boersma, C. Deen, J. D. Laman, A. Rebel, and E. Claassen
TNO Medical Biological Laboratory, Rijswijk, The Netherlands

INTRODUCTION

Immune complex formation may influence immune responses in a number of ways. Facilitation of antigen presentation is expected in the case of Fc-mediated uptake or binding of complexes by antigen-presenting cells (1). Upregulation of immune responses has been suggested for complexes circulating in the presence of free antigen. In contrast, downregulation is expected when all antigens are complexed (2). Antibodies, like other antigen-binding receptors (major histocompatibility complex [MHC]) also may influence the immune response by protection of specific determinants of the antigen or parts thereof to the activity of proteolytic enzyme which are active in the processing of antigens (3). Modulation of determinant specific processing and presentation is of special importance in the design of vaccines and in the use of peptides to elicit specific antibody responses. Generating antibodies to human immunoglobulin G_2 (huIgG$_2$) using the synthetic peptide approach, we came across SP29, which is a peptide that upon immunization leads to the elicitation of two types of antibodies: one recognizing huIgG$_2$, SP29, and SP10 (which represents the carboxy-terminal part of SP29), and the other type recognizing SP29, only most probably the N-terminal part of the peptide (SP29) (4). Monoclonal antibodies of these two categories of antibodies were used for in vivo investigation of the role of these determinant-specific antibodies in the regulation of humoral responses. SP29 in itself is immunogenic without carrier proteins, and therefore includes a T-cell determinant (4). In this chapter we show that antibodies to the N-terminal part of the SP29 (monoclonal antibody [MAb] 4.1) when complexed with the peptide inhibit SP29 primed T-cell proliferation as well as interleukin-2 (IL-2) production. In addition, MAb 4.1 complexed with SP29 inhibits antibody formation in vivo. Since SP10 does not stimulate T-cell proliferation of SP29 primed T cells, it is concluded that the T-cell determinant will be located on the N-terminal part of the peptide. Masking of the T-cell determinant of SP29 by its specific MAb leads to downregulation of anti-SP29 responses.

MATERIALS AND METHODS

Mice and Immunization

For experiments in which T-cell proliferation and IL-2 were determined, female BALB/c mise, 12–14 weeks old, were immunized with the antigen in a water in oil emulsion (4), of which 50 μl was injected subcutaneously on the upper side of the hind feet of the mice. The spleen and popliteal lymph nodes were used for preparation of the cell suspensions. For systemic antibody production as reflected in serum antibody concentrations, the animals were immunized with antigen in water in oil emulsions intraperitoneally.

Peptides

Sequences were selected and produced as described elsewhere (4,5). SP29 is a sequence from the hinge of HuIgG2 EU-214-235 (6) SP29: DKTVERKCCV*ECPPCPAPPVA* (4). The decapeptide SP10: TCPPCPAPPVA represents the carboxy terminal part of SP29: EU 223-235.

MAbs

Monoclonal antibody 1.2 recognizes the carboxy-terminal part of SP29, SP10, and human IgG_2. It also recognizes the amino-terminal part of SP29, and does not react with $huIgG_2$ or SP10. Antigen-antibody complexes were prepared by mixing them together at the indicated molar ratio (20:1 of 2:1). Complexes were not purified. The immunizations were based on the synthetic peptide content of each preparation.

ELISA

ELISA analysis of serum samples was essentially as performed elsewhere (4,7,8). Alkaline phosphatase conjugates of rabbit antimouse IgG were used throughout.

Cell suspensions of spleens and lymph nodes were cultured at 2.10^6 cells/ml upon addition of the appropriate stimulus (peptide, peptide immune complexes) for 4 days. Cells were stimulated with 10 μl of a solution of antigen for 4 days in RPMI 1640 supplemented with glutamine (200 mM), Na-pyruvate (100 mM), 2-mercaptoethanol (5.10^{-5} M), penicillin (2500 E/ml) and streptomycin (25 mg/ml). [^{3}H]Thymidine (25 μl, 0.5 μCi/well) was added during the last 4 hr. Then cells were harvested on glass fiber filters, dried, and counted by liquid scintillation counting. Proliferation was determined by the incorporation of [^{3}H]thymidine in in vivo primed cells (2.10^6/ml, 200 μl/well) that were restimulated in vitro. Results are expressed as a stimulation index (SI): dpm stimulated cells/dpm non-stimulated cells. The relative concentration of IL-2 in culture supernates was determined by the proliferation of IL-2–dependent CTLL-2 cells essentially as described elsewhere (9). Briefly, CTLL-2 cells were cultured in RPMI 1640 supplemented as described above. To this, IL-2 (±30 IU/ml) was added that consisted essentially of a supernatant of concanavalin A–stimulated rat spleen cells. Before determination of the IL-2 content of a sample, the CTLL-2 cells were starved 24 hr from IL-2 and diluted in microtiter plates (100 μl) at 2500 cells/well. Dilutions of the sample IL-2 were added (100 μl) and incubated for 18–24 hr. The relative proliferation was determined using [^{3}H]TdR incorporation during the last 4 hr of culture. The source of IL-2 was a culture supernatant of in vivo primed spleen or lymph node cells (7 days) after 2 days of stimulation in vitro under conditions as described for the proliferation assay.

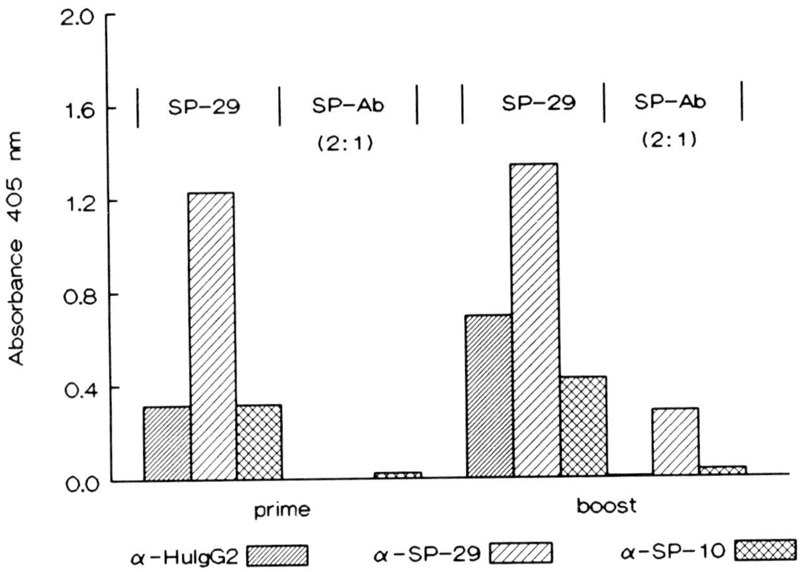

(a)

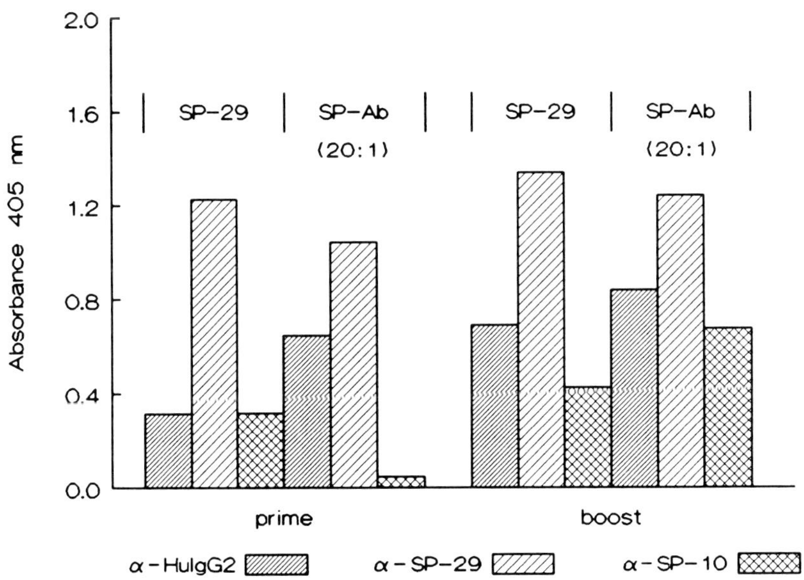

(b)

Figure 1 After i.p. immunization with 50 μg of SP29 (day 21) and subsequent boosting a serum antibody response to SP29, IgG2, and SP10 is observed. Immunization with SP29 (50 μg) complexed with MAb 4.1 (2:1) after priming (day 21) as well as after a booster immunization did not lead to significant levels of specific serum antibodies after priming and only low levels of anti-29 antibodies after a booster immunization (a). Similar immunizations with complexes of SP29 (50 μg) and MAb 4.1 (20:1) did not inhibit determinant-specific responses (b).

RESULTS AND DISCUSSION

Mice immunized i.p. with 50 μg of SP29 from day 14 after immunization show the development of anti-SP29 antibodies which, at least in part, recognize SP10 and huIgG2 to significant levels as determined by ELISA. Figure 1a shows the specific serum antibody levels at 21 days after immunization. As described earlier (4), dependent on the doses of peptide (SP29) used for immunization, the proportion of anti-SP10 and anti-huIgG2 antibodies is lower than observed for anti-SP29 antibodies. Seven days after boosting at 4 weeks after the first immunization this only changes to a limited extent (Fig. 1a). When 2:1 complexes of SP-29 and MAb 4.1 are immunized, antibodies that recognize SP29 only, but do not recognize SP10 or huIgG2, characteristics of MAb 4.1, are detected in serum directly after introduction of the complexes. The levels of these antibodies decrease as expected with typical mouse IgG_1 half-life kinetics. As determined by the anti-SP29 serum antibody level, background levels are reached at about day 14 after introduction of the peptide-antibody complexes (Fig. 2). This means that from this time, the presence of serum MAb 4.1 does not mask specific antipeptide responses. Nevertheless, no anti-SP29 responses are observed after immunization of SP29–MAb 4.1 complexes (2:1) after priming (day 21) and after boost (day 7) with the same antigen (see Fig. 1a). When SP29 and MAb 4.1 are complexed in excess of peptide (20:1), the serum antibody responses are as expected for SP29 immunization, and almost no inhibitive effects are observed after priming nor after boosting with the same antigen preparation (see Fig. 1b). These results might be explained by either protection and masking of the peptide or alternatively by facilitated degradation that prevents stimulation.

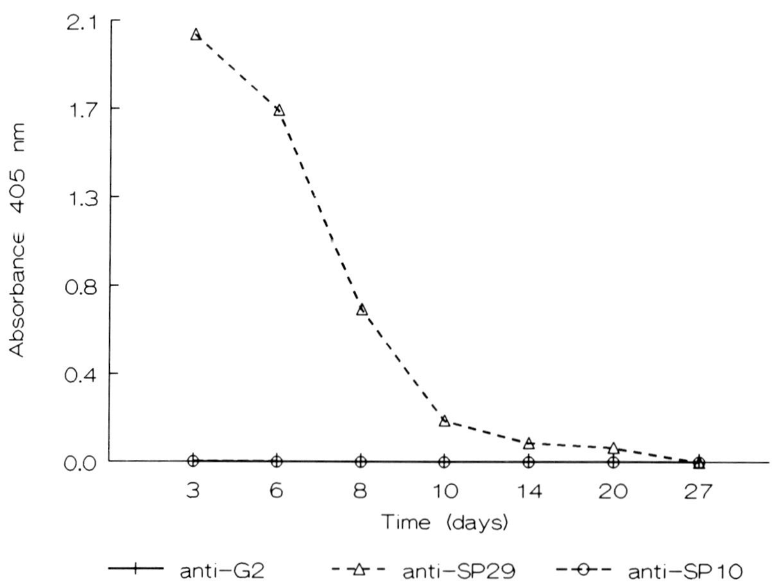

Figure 2 When 2:1 copmlexes of SP29 and MAb 4.1 based on 50 μg of SP29 peptide are used for immunization the antibody recognizing SP29, but not SP10 or IgG2, can be detected in serum until about 14 days after immunization. An antibody response to the peptide is not observed (see also Fig. 1).

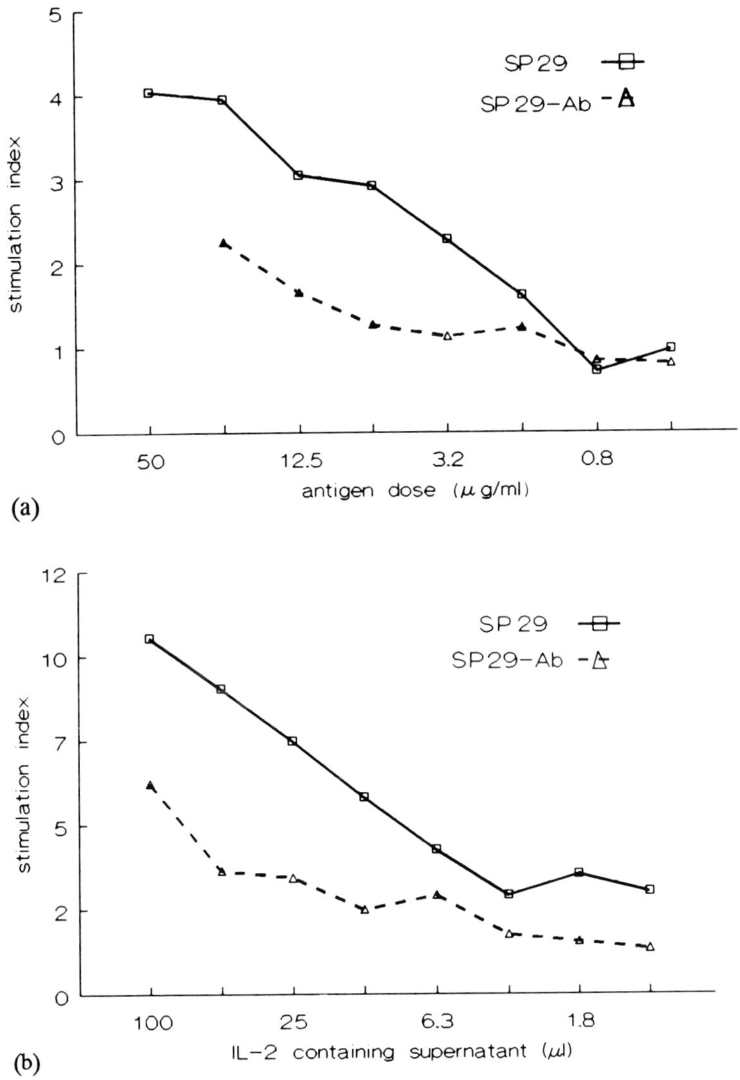

Figure 3 Lymph node cells of mice immunized with SP29 in vivo upon restimulation in vitro proliferate. When the in vitro restimulation is performed with SP29–MAb 4.1 complexes (2:1) proliferation is specifically inhibited (a). Similarly when the SP29-specific IL-2 production is determined atter in vitro restimulation the IL-2 production induced by SP29 is inhibited when instead of the free peptide SP29–MAb 4.1 complexes (2:1) are applied (b).

The lymph node cells of mice immunized with 50 μg SP29 upon immunization in vivo in the hind footpad show a specific proliferation in vitro with a stimulation index of about 4 at 25–50 μg/ml of peptide. When the immune cells of the same lymph node are stimulated in vitro with complexes of 50 μg of peptide with MAb 4.1 (2 mol of antibody: mol of SP29) an inhibition of the proliferative response is observed (Fig. 3a). The antigen-specific production of IL-2 was determined by testing supernatant in vitro restimulated (SP29) lymph node cells. Stimulation with SP29 produces an IL-2 level in the cultures that leads to a stimulation index of about 10 for proliferating CTLL-2. When a 2:1 complex 50 μg SP29 with MAb 4.1 is used for in vitro restimulation a significant inhibition is also observed (Fig. 3b). When spleen cells are isolated from animals locally immunized in the footpad with SP29, the stimulation index for proliferation is lower than observed for the lymph node cells (SI 2.5-3). In this case, only a slight tendency to an inhibition of the anti-SP29 response is observed when the same amount of SP29 is presented to the system in the form of a 2:1 SP29–MAb 4.1 complex. In addition, we found that SP10, the carboxy-terminus of SP29, does not stimulate proliferation of in vivo SP29 primed cells (Fig. 4). From this it is concluded that SP10 does not represent the T-cell determinant of SP29. Therefore, MAb 4.1 probably binds to the T-cell determinant of SP29. The relatively low T-cell response of spleen cells may be the result of the routing of immunization. The injection of the antigens in the footpad leads to optimum stimulation of lymph nodes. The MAb 4.1 antibody in itself (without peptide) does not inhibit or stimulate the proliferation or IL-2 production by cells which are restimulated in vitro (not shown).

In this study instead of a rather complex structure, a peptide representing the most simple model for analysis of response regulation, two B-cell determinants and one T-cell determinant, is used. Our experiments clearly show that antibodies that most probably bind to the T-cell determinant, and thereby may affect the efficiency of the presentation of a two-determinant peptide antigen to T cells with as a result of inhibition of T-cell proliferation and specific IL-2 production. At the same time in vivo, the production of antibodies recognizing this antigen is inhibited.

These results might be explained by alternative processing or inhibition of binding of the T-cell determinant of SP29 to the appropriate receptors (T-cell receptors [TCR], MHC).

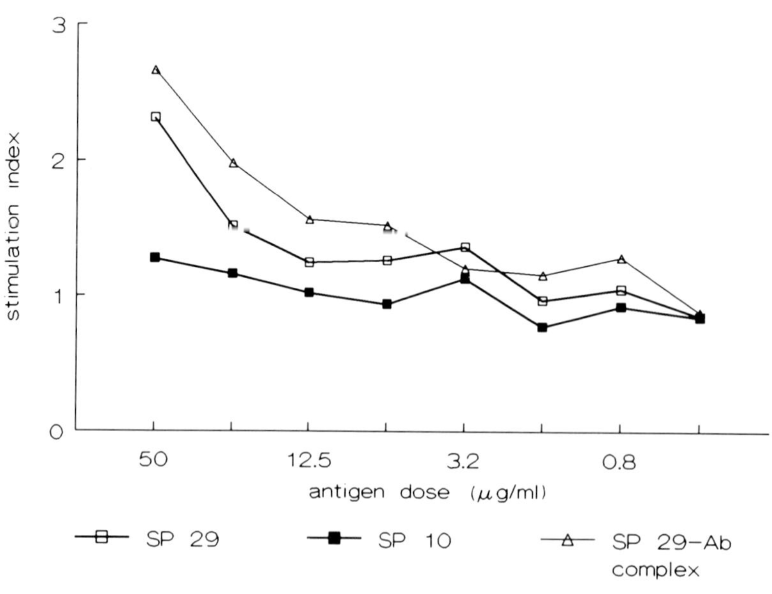

Figure 4 Spleen cells of SP29-immunized mice restimulated in vitro with SP29 proliferate, whereas, the same cells restimulated with complexes of SP29–MAb 4.1 show a limited inhibition. Restimulation with SP10, the C-terminal part of SP29 that is not recognized by MAb 4.1, does not stimulate T-cell proliferation.

Our results are in agreement with processing experiments by Watts et al. (3), who observed that when epitopes other than those involved in receptor (T cells, membrane Ig, MHC) binding are occupied with Fab fragments the processing is altered such that new fragments arise from processing of the antigen. In the case of SP29, the binding of MAb 4.1 may result in processing such that nonimmunogenic fragments are obtained.

REFERENCES

1. Manca F., Fenoglio D, Kunkl A., Cambiaggi C., Sasso M. and Celada F. Differential activation of T cell clones stimulated by macrophages exposed to antigen complexed with monoclonal antibodies. A possible influence of paratope specificity on the mode of antigen processing. J. Immunol. 1988; 130:2893–2898.
2. Manca F., Kunkl A., Fenoglio D., Fowler A., Sercarz E. and Celada F. Constraints in T-B cell cooperation related to epitope topology on E. coli β-galactosidase. I. The fine-specificity of T cells dictates the fine specificity of antibodies directed to conformation dependent determinants. Eur. J. Immunol. 1985; 15:345–350.
3. Watts C., West M.A., Reid P.A., and Davidson H.W. Processing of immunoglobulin-associated antigen in B lymphocytes. In: *Immunological Recognition*, Cold Spring Harbor Symposia on Quantitative Biology, 1989; LIV:345–352.
4. Boersma W.J.A., Deen C., Gerritse K., Zegers N.D., Jaaijman J.J. and Claassen E. Anti-peptide antibodies as subclass specific reagents: epitope mapping of human IgG2. Prot. Biol. Fluids 1989; 36:161–166.
5. Van Denderen J., Hermans A., Meeuwsen T., Troelstra C., Zegers N.D., Boersma W.J.A., Grosveld G. and Van Ewijk W. Antibody recognition of the tumor-specific bcr-abl joining region in chronic myeloid leukemia. J. Exp. Med. 1989; 169:878–98.
6. Kabat, E.A., Wu T.T., Bilofsky H., Reid-Miller M. and Perry H. *Sequences of Immunological Interest.* U.S. Department of Health and Human Services, Washington, D.C., 1984, 1987.
7. Haaijman J.J., Coolen J., Deen C., Kroese C.J.M., Zijlstra J.J. and Radl J. Monoclonal antibodies directed against human immunoglobulins: preparation and evaluation procedures. In: *Reviews on Immunoassay Technology 1.* (S.B. Pal, ed.) Macmillan, London, 1988, pp. 59–93.
8. Boersma, W.J.A., Deen C., Haaijman J.J., Radl J. and Claassen E. Antibodies to a short synthetic peptide related to the hinge segment of human IgG3 recognizes thermally induced or fixative induced conformational changes in the human IgG3 molecule. Immunology 1989; 68:427–430.
9. Vissinga C.S., Dirven C., Steinmeier F., Benner R. and Boersma W.J.A. The deterioration of cellular immunity during aging: the relationship between age dependent IL-2 production ability and the frequency of Thy-1^+,Lyt^- cells in C57bl/ka and CBA/rij mice. Cell. Immunol. 1987; 108:323–334.

46

Protein Kinase C Activation Differentially Regulates Immunoglobulin Isotype Production in Lipopolysaccharide-Stimulated Mouse B Cells

Yue Sheng Li, Edouard Kouassi, and Jean Pierre Revillard
Laboratoire d'Immunologie, Hôpital E. Herriot, Lyon, France

INTRODUCTION

In B lymphocytes, crosslinking of surface immunoglobulins (sIg) initiates hydrolysis of phosphoinositides, leading to the formation of two second messengers: diacylglycerol, which activates protein kinase C (PKC), and inositol triphosphate, which induce mobilization of calcium (Ca^{2+}) from the intracellular stores (1,2). Protein kinase C and Ca^{2+} play an important role in signal transduction in B lymphocyte activation. Activation of PKC and mobilization of Ca^{2+} either by anti-Ig antibodies (3,4) or by a combination of PKC-activating phorbol esters and Ca^{2+} ionophores (5,6) stimulate B-cell proliferation, but do not promote differentiation into Ig-secreting cells (5,7). Furthermore, it was demonstrated that addition of anti-Ig antibodies to lipopolysaccharide (LPS)–stimulated B-cell cultures decreased the number of IgM- and IgG-producing cells (plaque-forming cells) (8,9). However, the effect of PKC activation in the regulation of IgA production as well as the effect of Ca^{2+} mobilization on isotype regulation are still unknown. In this study, we have investigated the differential effects of Ca^{2+} mobilization by a Ca^{2+} ionophore and PKC activation by phorbol esters on the terminal differentiation of LPS-stimulated B cells, and we demonstrate a selective enhancement of IgA production by PKC activation in contrast with a downregulation of IgM, IgG, and IgA production by Ca^{2+} mobilization.

MATERIALS AND METHODS

Mice

Male BALB/c mice, 3 months old, used in this study, were bred in our laboratory.

B-Cell Purification

Resting B cells were prepared as previously described (6). Briefly, spleen cell suspensions were incubated in Petri dishes in medium containing 20% fetal calf serum (FCS, Boehringer, Mannhein, West Germany) for 90 min to remove adherent macrophages. The macrophage-depleted cell population was then depleted of T cells by a mixture of anti–T-cell antibodies (HO13.4, GK1.5, and AD4) and rabbit complement (Low Tox, Cedarlane, Hornby, Canada). Small B cells were separated on a discontinuous Percoll gradient (Pharmacia, Uppsala, Sweden). Cells at band of 65–75% interface were then isolated and used as resting B cells, which contain 80–90% of sIg-positive cells, 2–3% of T cells, and 0.5–1.0% of macrophages as determined by flow cytometric immunofluorescence and May-Grunwald-Giemsa staining.

Preparation of sIgA-Negative Cell Population

To deplete sIgA-positive B cells, purified small B cells were incubated for 2 hr at 4°C in Petri dishes that had been precoated with goat antimouse IgA antibody (Zymed, San Francisco, California) diluted to 5 μg/ml in veronal buffer. Nonadherent cells were collected and used as sIgA-negative B cells; these contained <0.5% sIgA-positive contaminating cells as determined by immunofluorescence staining using a FITC labeled goat antimouse IgA antibody (Southern Biotechnology, Birmingham, Alabama).

Analysis of Ig Production

Resting B cells at 1×10^6 cells/ml were cultured in RPMI 1640 medium containing 5×10^5 M 2ME and 10% FCS in 24-well plates with LPS (Difco, Detroit, California) for 6 days. Phorbol myristate acetate (PMA) or 4α-phorbol 12,13-didecanoate (4α-PDD) (Sigma, St. Louis, Missouri) or ionomycine (Ion) (Calbiochem-Behring Corp. La Jolla, CA) were added at the beginning of culture and the amount of IgM, IgG, and IgA secreted into culture supernatants was measured quantitatively by an ELISA method (10).

RESULTS AND DISCUSSION

It has been reported that anti-Ig antibodies which induce B-cell proliferation by activating PKC and mobilizing Ca^{2+} (1,2) inhibited LPS-stimulated maturation of B lymphocytes into IgM- and IgG-producing cells (7,8). To investigate separately the effects of PKC activation and Ca^{2+} on B-cell isotype differentiation, we measured the production of the three classes of Ig (IgM, IgG, and IgA) by LPS-stimulated spleen B cells in response to PMA, a PKC-activating phorbol, and to the Ca^{2+} ionophore, Ion. As shown in Figure 1 PMA and Ion strongly inhibited IgM and IgG production, in a dose-dependent fashion. Secretion of IgA was also decreased by Ion at concentrations from 0.5 to 1.0 μg/ml (Fig. 1), but unexpectedly, it was dose-dependently enhanced by PMA (Fig. 1). At 10 ng/ml, PMA caused a twofold increase in IgA secretion.

It is well known that PMA is a strong activator of PKC (11). In order to demonstrate that the enhancement of IgA secretion by PMA was mediated by PKC activation but not by other possible activity of phorbol esters, the effect of other phorbol esters was studied, using phorbol 12,13-dibutyrate which activates PKC and 4α-PDD, which is inactive with respect to PKC activation. Only the phorbol 12,13-dibutyrate (data not shown), but not 4α-PDD (Fig. 1), reproduced the effect of PMA, suggesting a selective upregulation of IgA by activation of PKC.

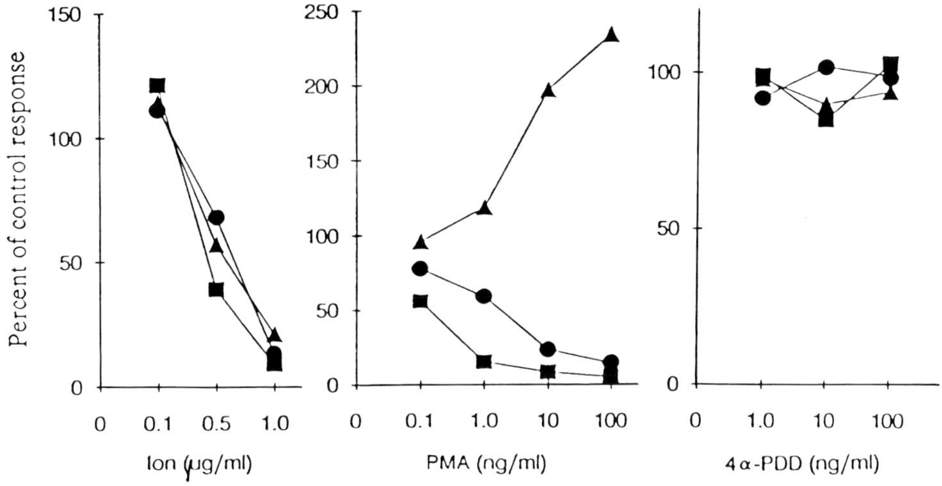

Figure 1 Effects of PMA and Ion on Ig productioan by LPS-stimulated B cells. T-cell– and macrophage-depleted B cells (10^6 cells/ml) were stimulated with LPS (50 µg/ml) for 6 days. Either Ion or PMA or 4α-PDD at the indicated concentrations was added at the beginning of culture. IgM (■), IgG (●), and IgA (▲), secreted into culture supernatants were measured by ELISA. The control cultures received LPS alone and produced 18.96 µg/ml, 4.04 µg/ml, and 2.05 µg/ml of IgM, IgG, and IgA, respectively. Data from one of four similar experiments are expressed as percent of control response.

During the course of B-cell development, two subsequent stages of differentiation have been defined (12). Antigen-dependent differentiation, taking place in fetal liver and then in bone marrow, involves the Ig gene rearrangement and the appearance of B lymphocytes defined by the presence of sIgM and sIgD which function as antigen receptors. Then, these mature B cells migrate to peripheral lymphoid organs, such as the spleen and lymph nodes, where, in contact with antigens and the accessory cells, the second (antigen-dependent) stage of differentiation occurs. sIgM-positive B cells either proliferate and then differentiate into IgM-secreting plasma cells or switch to express other sIg cells with deletion of 5′ C_H sequences (13). Anti-Ig antibodies as well as PKC-activating phorbol esters were demonstrated to inhibit Ig production by downregulating the rate of transcription of the Cµ gene (14,15). The enhancement of IgA by PMA may result either from an increase in switching frequency of sIgA-negative B cells to sIgA-positive B cells, or from a clonal expansion of precommitted sIgA-positive B cells and their progression to terminal differentiation. To distinguish between these two possibilities, the effect of PMA on Ig production by the sIgA-negative population, obtained by depleting sIgA-positive cells from spleen B cell population, was assessed. Comparable levels of IgM secreted by total spleen B cells and by sIgA-negative B cells stimulated by LPS (50 µg/ml) indicated the good viability of sIgA-negative B cells. In contrast to unfractionated spleen B cells, the sIgA-negative cell population did not show any enhancement of IgA production in response to PMA (Fig. 2), which suggested that PKC activation upregulated IgA secretion by stimulating directly the growth and/or terminal differentiation of cells that were already programmed to produce IgA. Whether PKC activation affects selectively the expansion or the terminal differentiation of sIgA-positive B cells is currently being investigated.

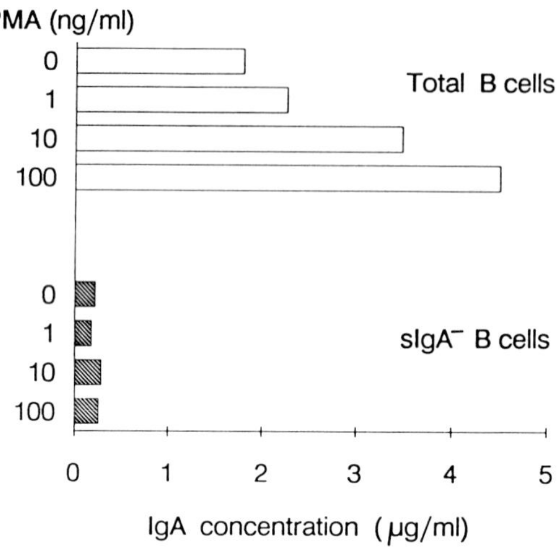

Figure 2 PMA fails to enhance IgA production by LPS-stimulated IgA^- B cells. Total spleen B cells or $sIgA^+$-depleted B cells, which contained <0.5% of $sIgA^+$ B cells (see Materials and Methods section) were cultured with LPS (50 μg/ml) in the presence or absence of PMA at indicated concentrations for 6 days. IgA secretion was determined by ELISA.

Some cytokines, such as interleukin-5 (IL-5) and IL-6, have been shown to enhance preferentially promotion of sIgA-positive B cell differentiation into IgA-secreting cells (16–19). However, we cannot attribute the enhancement of IgA by PKC activation to IL-5 or IL-6 because the residual T cells and macrophages, which represent the major source of IL-5 and IL-6, respectively (20,21), was minimized (2–3% of T cells and 0.5–1.0% of macrophages in the B-cell suspension) by the process of cell preparation. In addition, IL-5 and IL-6 do not inhibit, but rather slightly increase, the production of IgG and IgM (16–19), which is in contrast with the effect of PKC activation. Transforming growth factor β was also reported to enhance IgA secretion, by acting on the sIgA-negative B cell population and enhancing the Ig class switch process (22–24), by a mechanism quite different from that of PKC activation.

PKC and intracellular Ca^{2+} are two essential signals of transduction, which can regulate B-cell activation, proliferation, and differentiation. We provide here evidence that PKC activation and elevation of Ca^{2+} which are concomittantly triggered by aggregation of B-cell antigen receptors have in fact opposite effects on the terminal differentiation of sIgA-positive B cells into IgA-producing cells. Further studies on the differential triggering of B cell in Peyer's patches may provide new clues as regards the yet unknown mechanisms accounting for the predominant production of IgA antibodies in the mucosal-associated lymphoid tissues.

REFERENCES

1. Cambier JC, Justment LB, Newell MK, Chen ZZ, Harris LK, Sandoval MV, Klemsz MJ, Ranson JT. Transmembrane signals and intracellular "second messengers" in the regulation of quiescent B-lymphocyte activation. Immunol. Rev. 1987;95:37–57.

2. Klaus GGB, Bijsterbosch MK, O'Garra A, Harnett MM, Rigley K. Receptor signalling and crosstalk in B lymphocytes. Immunol. Rev. 1987; 99:19–38.
3. Coggeshall KM, Cambier JC. B cell activation VIII. Membrane immunoglobulins transduce signals via activation of phosphatidylinositol hydrolysis. J. Immunol. 1984;133:3382–3386.
4. Ransom JT, Harris LK, Cambier JC. Anti-Ig induces release of inositol 1,4,5-triphosphate, which mediates mobilization of intracellular Ca^{++} stores in B lymphocytes. J. Immunol. 1986;137: 708–714.
5. Klaus GGB, O'Garra A, Bijsterbosch MK, Holman M. Activation and proliferation signals in mouse B cells VIII. Induction of DNA synthesis in B cells by a combination of calcium ionophore and phorbol myristate acetate. Eur. J. Immunol. 1986;16:92–97.
6. Li YS, Kouassi E, Revillard JP. Cyclic AMP can enhance mouse B cell activation by regulating progression into the late G_1/S phase. Eur. J. Immunol. 1989;19:1721–1725.
7. Finkelman FD, Mond JJ, Metcalf ES. Anti-immunoglobulin antibody induction of B lymphocyte activation and differentiation in vivo and in vitro. In: Cambier JC. ed. *B-Lymphocyte Differentiation.* CRC Press, Boca Raton, Florida, 1986, pp. 41–59.
8. Kearney JF, Klein J, Bockman DE, Cooper MD, Lawton AR. B cell differentiation induced by lipopolysaccharide. V. Suppression of plasma cell maturation by anti-μ: mode of action and characteristics of suppressed cells. J. Immunol. 1978;120:158–166.
9. Leanderson T, Forni L. Effects of μ-specific antibodies on B cell growth and maturation. Eur. J. Immunol. 1984;14:1016–1021.
10. Li YS, Kouassi E, Revillard JP. Differential regulation of mouse B cell activation by β-adrenoceptor stimulation depending on type of mitogens. Immunology, 1990;69:367–372.
11. Castagna M, Takai Y, Kaibuchi K, Sano K, Kikkawa U, Nishisuka Y. Direct activation of calcium-activated, phospholipid-dependent protein kinase by tumor-promoting phorbol ester. J. Biol. Chem. 1982;257:7841–7851.
12. Alt FW, Blackwell TK, Yancopoulos GD. Development of the primary antibody repertoire. Science, 1987;238:1079–1087.
13. Davis MM, Kim SK, Hood LE. DNA sequences mediating class switching in α-immunoglobulins. Science, 1980;209:1360–1365.
14. Högbom E, Martensson IL, Leanderson T. Regulation of immunoglobulin transcription rates and mRNA processing in proliferating normal B lymphocytes by activators of protein kinase C. Proc. Natl. Acad. Sci. U.S.A. 1987;84:9135–9139.
15. Hôgbom E, Martensson IL, Funa K, Leanderson T. Effects of phorbol esters on B cell gene expression. Scand. J. Immunol. 1988;28:481–486.
16. Harriman GR, Kunimoto DY, Elliott JF, Paetkau V, Strober W. The role of IL-5 in IgA B cell differentiation. J. Immunol. 1988;140:3033–3039.
17. Schoenbeck S, Mckenzie DT, Kagnoff MF. Interleukin 5 is a differentiation factor for IgA B cells. Eur. J. Immunol. 1989;19:965–969.
18. Beagley KW, Eldridge JH, Lee F, Kiyono H, Everson MP, Koopman WJ, Hirano T, Kishimoto T, McGhee JR. Interleukins and IgA synthesis. Human and murine interleukin 6 induce high rate IgA secretion in IgA-committed B cells. J. Exp. Med. 1989;169:2133–2148.
19. Kunimoto DY, Nordan RP, Strober W. IL-6 is a potent cofactor of IL-1 in IgM synthesis and of IL-5 in IgA synthesis. J. Immunol. 1989;143:2230–2235.
20. Mosmann TR, Cherwinski H, Bond MW, Geidlin MA, Coffman RL. Two types of murine helper T cell clones. I. Definition according to profiles of lymphokine activities and secreted proteins. J. Immunol. 1986;136:2348–2357.
21. Kishimoto T, Hirano T. Molecular regulation of B lymphocyte response. Annu. Rev. Immunol. 1988;6:485–512.
22. Coffman RL, Lebman DA, Shrader B. Transforming growth factor β specifically enhances IgA production by lipopolysaccharide-stimulated murine B lymphocytes. J. Exp. Med. 1989;170:1039–1044.

23. Sonoda E, Matrumoto R, Hitoshi Y, Ishii T, Sugimoto M, Araki S, Tominaga A, Yamaguchi N, Takatsu K. Transforming growth factor β induces IgA production and acts additively with interleukin 5 for IgA production. J. Exp. Med. 1989;170:1415–1420.
24. Lebman DA, Lee FD, Coffman R. Mechanism for transforming growth factor β and IL-2 enhancement of IgA expression in lipopolysaccharide-stimulated B cell cultures. J. Immunol. 1990;144:952–959.

47
Involvement of Interleukin-5 in Response to Thymus-Independent Antigens

Gayle Delmonte Wetzel
Basel Institute for Immunology, Basel, Switzerland

INTRODUCTION

Interleukin-5 (IL-5) enhances plaque-forming cell (PFC) responses by whole and Ly-1-positive large peritoneal B cells stimulated by polyclonal activators (1) and by TNP-LPS (2). Indeed, many responses to IL-5, even from large splenic B cells, can be dominated by Ly-1-positive B cells (1). While this finding is interesting, its interpretation is rather puzzling.

Several alternatives are possible. Ly-1-positive B cells, and their Ly-1-negative "sister population" (3–5), may be special B cells. The IL-5 responsiveness might then be an attribute unique to this rather loosely defined population. Perhaps more attractively, the IL-5 responses of this population may simply result from previous antigenic exposure. This suggests that the form of antigenic stimulation is important and any B cell might become IL-5 responsive, given the appropriate stimulus.

Since IL-5–responsive peritoneal B cells may have encountered bacterial antigens, we stimulated normal, resting splenic B cells with such antigens and analogues to investigate these alternatives.

RESULTS

IL-5 Enhances PFC Responses to TNP-LPS

The influence of several interleukins on the PFC response of resting, B cells to TNP-LPS was assessed. Table 1 shows a typical experiment. This TI-1 antigen (ag) induced a moderate PFC response which was unaffected by IL-3 or IL-4 but was increased more than fivefold by IL-5. Since IL-5 can regulate TNP-LPS responses, the term thymus regulated (TR) (6) is more appropriate than thymus independent for this Ag.

Table 1 Interleukin-5 Enhancement of the Anti-TNP PFC Response Induced by the TR1 Ag TNP-LPS

	Addition to culture			
Stimulus	none	IL-3	IL-4	IL-5
None	28 ± 11	30 ± 13	21 ± 8	42 ± 17
TNP-LPS	400 ± 180	488 ± 160	256 ± 84	2464 ± 650

10^5 Percoll-separated, splenic B cells were cultured 4 days with 0.2 μg/ml TNP-LPS and 6 U/ml interleukins. Direct PFC/10^6 input B cell averages of triplicate cultures are given with standard deviations.

IL-5 Enhances Normal, Resting B-Cell Proliferation Induced by a TR 2 Antigen Analogue

Small, resting B cells do not respond to TNP-Ficoll alone (6), and some form of macrophage help is required (7). Since we wished to avoid the use of accessory cells, we used anti-δ-dextran (anti-IgD coupled to dextran), a TR 2 analog developed by others (8). Table 2 shows that proliferative responses to this analogue were unaffected by IL-2, IL-3, IL-4, or IL-6, but were increased by IL-5, at all TR 2 analogue concentrations. To a smaller extent, IL-1 also enhanced proliferation, whereas interferon-γ (IFN-γ) was inhibitory. Hence, IL-5 can regulate normal B-cell proliferation to TR 2 antigens or analogues. Interleukin-1 and IFN-γ also appear to be active regulators in this system.

Quantitation of Normal, Resting B Cells Induced to IL-5 Responsiveness by TR 1 and TR 2 Antigen Analogues

To quantitate IL-5 responsiveness induced in fresh resting splenic B cells, the filler cell-free clonal proliferation system (1) was chosen. To avoid possible complications involved in the selection of antigen-specific cells, a polyclonal approach was sought. Initial attempts using

Table 2 Effect of Various Interleukins on the Anti-δ-Dextran–Induced Proliferation of Small, Resting B Cells

	ng/ml anti-δ-dextran				
Addition	0.0	0.01	0.1	1.0	10.0
Medium	2.8	2.9	20.6	135.6	146.7
IL-1	*3.8*	*4.9*	*27.7*	*140.7*	*176.3*
IL-2	3.2	2.7	14.3	95.3	139.3
IL-3	1.9	2.5	12.8	102.6	151.2
IL-4	3.0	4.6	23.5	94.2	129.7
IL-5	*6.0*	*9.1*	*34.3*	*161.4*	*187.4*
IL-6	2.0	2.7	15.9	71.2	145.2
IFN-γ	2.3	4.0	15.7	58.2	121.7

10^5 Percoll-separated splenic B cells were cultured 2 days and pulsed with [^{3}H]TdR during the terminal 6 hr. Data are cpm × 10^{-3}. 100 U/ml IL-1, IL-6, and IFN-γ were used and 10 U/ml for other ILs.

Table 3 Frequencies of Normal, Resting B Cells Induced to IL-5 Responsiveness by TR 1 and TR 2 Analogues

Expt	Interleukin	Medium	Anti-IgM+DXS	Anti-IgM+LPS
1	None	<1	12.4 ± 3.8	ND
	IL-4	<1	21.1 ± 5.2[a]	ND
	IL-5	<1	20.2 ± 5.1[a]	ND
2	None	<1	ND[b]	20.1 ± 5.4
	IL-2	<1	ND	11.6 ± 4.0
	IL-4	<1	ND	60.2 ± 11.5[a]
	IL-5	<1	ND	37.5 ± 8.2[a]
	IL-6	<1	ND	21.9 ± 5.7

Percoll-separated small, resting splenic B cells were cultured in Terasaki plates at four different cell inputs (from 1 to about 8 cells/well, with no filler cells) with 60 wells/input dose for each determination. After 4 days, wells were examined for cell growth and Poisson analysis was used to calculate the frequency of input B cells stimulated to proliferate. These frequencies are presented as percentages of the input B cells (i.e., a frequency of 0.1 = 10%) and are given with the associated 95% confidence intervals.

[a]Those frequencies which are statistically different from the appropriate controls at less than the 5% level. LPS was used at 50 μg/ml, the b-7-6 monoclonal anti-IgM at 10 μg/ml, and DXS at 20 μg/ml. Interleukins were used at 10 U/ml except for IL-6, which was used at 1000 U/ml.

[b]ND, not determined.

anti-δ-dextran were unfruitful, hence two alternative systems were employed: anti-IgM plus dextran sulfate (DXS) to model TR 2 Ags and anti-IgM plus LPS to model TR 1 Ags. Table 3 contains two typical experiments. In both systems, a significant fraction of B cells proliferated and these fractions were significantly increased by IL-4 and IL-5. Hence, IL-5 as well as IL-4 appear to regulate B-cell proliferation initiated by TR Ags and their analogues.

CONCLUSIONS

These data provide convincing support for a role for IL-5 in regulating normal, resting B cell responses to TR 1 and TR 2 Ags and their analogues. Since most splenic Ly-1-positive B cells are larger than most resting splenic B cells (3,4), most B cells responding in the systems described here are Ly1 negative. The fractions of at least 10% IL-5–responsive B cells in the TR 2 analogue–driven system, and at least 20% in the TR 1 analogue–driven system are far larger than could be accounted for by residual contaminating LY-1-positive B cells. Hence, normal, resting splenic B cells not belonging to the sister population of Ly-1-positive B cells respond to IL-5 and this responsiveness can be induced by TR 1 and TR 2 Ags and their analogues.

ACKNOWLEDGMENT

The Basel Institute for Immunology was founded by and is supported by F. Hoffmann–La Roche & Co., Ltd., Basel, Switzerland.

REFERENCES

1. Wetzel G. D. Interleukin 5 regulation of peritoneal Ly-1 B lymphocyte proliferation, differentiation and autoantibody secretion. Eur. J. Immunol. 1989;19:1701–7.
2. Wetzel G. D. Interleukin 5 regulation of peritoneal B-cell proliferation and antibody secretion. Scand. J. Immunol. 1990;31:91–101.
3. Herzenberg L. A., Stall A. M., Lalor P. L., Sidman C., Moore W. A., Parks D. R., Herzenberg, L. A. The Ly-1 B cell lineage. Immunol. Rev. 1986;93:81–102.
4. Hardy R. R., Hayakawa K. Development and physiology of Ly-1 B and its human homolog Leu-1 B. Immunol. Rev. 1986;93:53–79.
5. Marcos M. A., Huetz F., Pereira P., Andreu J. L., Martinez-A. C., Coutinho A. Further evidence for coelomic-associated B lymphocytes. Eur. J. Immunol. 1989;19:2031–5.
6. Mond J. J., Brunswick M. A. Role for IFN-γ and NK cells in immune responses to T cell-regulated antigens types 1 and 2. Immunol. Rev. 1987;99:105–18.
7. Chused T. M., Kassan S. S., Mosier D. E. Macrophage requirement for the in vitro response to TNP-Ficoll: a thymic independent antigen. J. Immunol. 1976;116:1579–81.
8. Brunswick M., Finkelman F. D., Highet P. F., Inman J. K., Dintzis H. M., Mond J. J. Picogram quantities of anti-Ig antibodies coupled to dextran induce B cell proliferation. J. Immunol. 1988;140:3364–72.

48
Differentiation and Activation Antigens Associated with Hairy Cell Leukemia

Katalin Pálóczi,[1] Judit Demeter,[1] Éva Pócsik, R. Mihalik,[1] Marianna Magyar,[1] J. Földi,[1] Judit Szelényi,[1] D Lehoczky,[2] M. Benczúr,[1] and G. Gy. Petrányi[1]

[1]*National Institute of Haematology and Blood Transfusion, Budapest, Hungary;*
[2]*Semmelweis University Medical School, Budapest, Hungary*

INTRODUCTION

Defining the expression of various antigens on the surface of neoplastic cells has facilitated the clarification of the cellular origin and differentiation pathways of these cells. In relation to hairy cell leukemia (HCL), however, there has been controversy about the cellular origin of this malignancy (1–3). Most recent evidences are suggesting that in general HCL is an entity of B-cell neoplasms (1,4,5). The leukemic HCL cells appear to be derived from activated B cells or preplasma cells (2,6,7).

In this study, we investigated the expression of differentiation antigens on peripheral blood mononuclear (PBM) cells of 24 HCL patients. Special interest was trended concerning the presence of activation antigens in five leukemic cases.

MATERIALS AND METHODS

Patients

Twenty-four HCL patients, 12 males and 12 females, were studied: age 22–79 years (mean: 54.3). The male-female ratio was 1:1. The diagnosis of HCL was based on the usual cytological, cytochemical, and histopathological, criteria of disease; in the 17 splenectomized cases it was also confirmed by spleen histology. The patients were untreated for at least 3 weeks at the time of study. Peripheral blood from healthy donors (n = 20) served as control samples.

Methods

Binding of the various monoclonal antibodies (MAbs) was assessed with indirect immunofluorescence using FITC-conjugated rabbit antimouse immunoglobulin (Ig), and DAKO as a second antibody. T-cell–associated antibodies (Abs) were CD3(T3), CD2(T11), CD4(T4), and CD8(T8) (Ortho Diagn. System). The B-cell–associated reagents were CD19(B4), CD20(B1), and CD21(B2) (Coulter Corp.). Class II antigens (Ags) were detected with HLA-DR from Becton-Dickinson. Anti-IgM Ab (Heintel) was used as directly conjugated with FITC. RAB-1 MAb was used to detect the hairy cells (Z. Eshhar, Israel) (8). The MAbs from the panel of the IVth International Workshop on human Diff. Antigens (9) were used to detect the activation Ags on PBM cells. Analysis of all samples were done using the FACStar cytometer (Becton-Dickinson). Deoxyribonucleic acid (DNA) rearrangement was determined in 12 cases using the JH and TCR β probes (10). (All DNA probes originated from T. H. Rabbits, Cambridge, England).

RESULTS

The PBM cells from 24 patients with HCL appeared to be of B lineage as shown by cell surface marker determination (CD19, CD20, HLA-DR, sIgM), and as confirmed by gene rearrangement study in 10 out of 12 investigated cases. There was a highly significance between the morphological hairy cells and the RAB-1-positive cells ($p < 0{,}001$). Dual fluorochrome staining of the T cells ($CD3^+/HLA\text{-}DR^+$) demonstrated the proportion of activated T cells to be low as compared to the proportion of other activation antigens.

The activation antigen expression of five leukemic-phase HCL patients was studied using 18 MAbs to activation antigens (belonging to seven different clusters) (Tables 1 and 2). The percentage of hairy cells in these five cases varied between 51 and 97%, whereas the percentage of RAB-1-positive PBM cells was 55–96.2%. The PBM cells carried the interleukin-2 (IL-2) receptor in a significantly increased proportion as shown by three out of four Abs of the CD25 category. The CD40 antibody that reacts with activated B cells showed positivity with the majority of leukemic-phase HCL cells. Two out of four MAbs belonging to the CD69 group were found also to react with cells of these patients. The MAbs belonging to the CD30, CD39, CD70, and CD71 clusters were found not to be increased on the PBM cells.

DISCUSSION

The PBM cells from 24 HCL patients could be characterized by RAB-1, CD19, HLA-DR, and surface IgM positivity and CD21 negativity. This phenotype is similar to the antigen profile of in vitro activated cells. The MAb to hairy cells, RAB-1, was originally described as B-lineage restricted (8). Significant correlation was found between the morphologically hairy cells and RAB-1-positive cells as well as between the RAB-1-positive cells and the B-cell markers (CD19, CD20, HLA-DR, and sIgM). There was no correlation between the presence of CD21 antigen and RAB-1 positivity, showing that the expression of CD21 antigen is not characteristic of HCL.

Using a panel of MAbs directed against activation Ags a significant percentage of the PBM cells of HCL showed positivity with different Abs of the CD25, CD40, and CD69 clusters. Dual fluorochrome staining of the T cells ($CD3^+/HLA\text{-}DR^+$) demonstrated the proportion of activated T cells to be low, suggesting indirectly that the majority of activated cells are B cells (see Table 1). The CD40 molecule has similarities with a number of growth factor receptors. It is a putative receptor for a soluble or a cellular ligand supporting the proliferation of B cells (9). The CD69 antigen is involved in early T- and B-cell activation (9). Two Abs from four monoclonal antibodies belonging to the CD69 cluster were found to react with the activated B-cell population of HCL.

Table 1 Activation Antigens on PBM Cells in HCL I

Patients	Hairy cells (%)	RAB-1 (%)	CD3/DR$^+$ (%)	CD25 (%)				CD30 (%)				CD40 (%)
				25	31	53	Tac	79	102	104	105	35
1.	58.0	56.9	1.53	9.0	4.8	57.8	7.3	1.1	1.1	0.6	2.9	22.7
2.	97.0	96.2	2.50	15.3	22.5	79.2	17.4	2.3	2.9	2.9	14.4	40.6
3.	76.0	83.0	12.27	1.9	1.0	86.0	1.2	0.8	1.4	0.9	3.5	80.2
4.	81.0	55.0	3.7	12.8	17.8	29.7	14.1	20.9	27.8	18.0	19.2	18.1
5.	51.0	68.2	12.75	7.3	4.0	36.2	11.9	7.8	33.5	14.0	17.4	5.7
$\bar{a} \pm SE$	72.6	71.86	6.42	9.3	10.2	57.8	10.4	6.6	13.3	7.3	11.5	33.4
n = 5	±8.2	±12.75	±2.49	±2.3	±4.2	±11.2	±2.8	±3.8	±7.1	±3.6	±3.5	±12.9
Controls												
$\bar{a} \pm SE$	0.0	3.1	5.1	3.1	2.0	15.1	0.8	1.9	4.0	1.1	5.0	2.2
n = 10		±1.1	±2.0	±1.4	±0.6	±5.8	±0.4	±1.2	±2.0	±0.3	±3.1	±0.6
$p <$		0.001	NS	0.05	0.1	0.001	0.01	NS	NS	NS	NS	0.05

NS = not significant.

Table 2 Activation Antigens on PBM Cells in HCL II

	CD69 (%)				CD70 (%)			CD39 (%)	CD71 (%)
Patients	10	40	90	91	92	93	109	47	T9
1.	18.6	0.5	68.0	0.5	0.6	0.5	0.2	0.6	3.0
2.	62.0	2.4	82.1	3.4	2.3	3.4	1.7	10.1	1.8
3.	64.1	1.2	89.8	1.7	1.5	1.1	1.1	8.4	1.5
4.	29.5	14.5	28.7	15.3	14.0	12.2	25.9	15.1	22.6
5.	36.3	16.3	37.5	16.8	14.1	14.7	34.8	15.5	24.1
$\bar{a} \pm$ SE n = 5	42.1 ±9.0	6.9 ±3.3	61.4 ±11.9	7.5 ±3.5	6.5 ±3.1	6.4 ±2.9	12.7 ±7.3	9.9 ±2.7	10.0 ±5.2
$\bar{a} \pm$ SE n = 10	3.7 ±2.7	5.5 ±1.8	4.6 ±1.4	5.2 ±1.8	1.8 ±0.7	1.3 ±0.5	1.8 ±0.7	2.0 ±0.9	3.6 ±0.7
p <	0.001	NS	0.001	NS	NS	NS	NS	0.1	0.1

NS = not significant.

The RAB-1 MAb (although not HCL specific) is a valuable tool in the diagnosis of HCL; on the other hand, it might be regarded as an activation marker based on its positivity on in vitro activated T lymphocytes (8) and in T-HCL (11). The lack of expression of CD70 and CD71 antigens suggests a low tumor proliferative feature with a benign prognostic value in HCL.

REFERENCES

1. Korsmeyer SJ, Greene WC, Waldman TA. Cellular origin of hairy cell leukemia: Malignant B cells that express receptors for T cell growth factor. Semin Oncol 1984; 11:394–400.
2. Anderson KC, Boyd AW, Fischer DC, Leslie D, Schlossman SF, Nadler LM. Hairy cell leukemia: A tumor of pre-plasma cells. Blood 1985; 65:620–629.
3. Al-Katib A, Berman E, Black P, Koziner B. Hairy cell leukemia: A model for studying the B cell family of disease. Semin Oncol 1986; 13:48–54.
4. Foroni L, Catovsky D, Luzzatto L. Immunoglobulin gene rearrangements in hairy cell leukemia and other chronic B cell lymphoproliferative disorders. Leukemia 1987; 4:389–392.
5. Migone N, Giubellino MC, Casorati G, Tassanari A, Lauria F, Foa R. Configuration of the immunoglobulin and T cell receptor gene regions in hairy cell leukemia and B-chronic lymphocytic leukemia. Leukemia 1987; 1:393–394.
6. Posnett DN, Wang CY, Chiorazzi N, Crow MK, Kunkel HG. An antigen characteristic of hairy cell leukemia cells is expressed on certain activated B cells. J Immunol 1984; 133:1635–1640.
7. Posnett DN, Duggan A, McGrath H. Hairy cell leukemia-associated antigen (HC2) is an activation antigen of several hemopoietic cell lineages, inducible on monocytes by IFN-τ. J Immunol 1990; 144:929–933.
8. Berrebi A, Ashar Z, Linder A, Guedj L, Avaraham H. RAB-1: a new monoclonal antibody to leukemic hairy cells. Leuk Res 1986; 10:1071–1078.

9. Stein H, Schwarting R. Activation antigens, Leucocyte typing IV. White cell differentiation antigens. Ed by Knapp W, Dörken B, Gilks WR, Rieber EP, Schmidt RE, Stein H, von dem Borne AEGKr. Oxford University Press, Oxford, 1989; pp. 388–513.
10. Foroni L, Földi J, Matutes E, Catovsky D, O'Connor NI, Baer R, Forster A. α, β and τ T-cell receptor genes rearrangements correlate with hematological phenotype in T cell leukaemias. Br J Haematol 1987; 67:307–318.
11. Demeter J, Pálóczi K, Földi J, Hokland M, Hokland P , Benczúr M, Lehoczky D. Immunological and molecular biological identification of a true case of T-hairy cell leukemia. Eur J Haematol 1989; 43:339–345.

49

Resistant Target Cells Deliver an Inactivating Signal to Natural Killer Cells via LFA-1 (CD11a)

The Impaired NK Activity Is Associated with Defective Tyrosine Phosphorylation of a 190-kD Substrate

Marja Heiskala
University of Helsinki, Helsinki, Finland

INTRODUCTION

We have previously shown that large granular lymphocytes (LGLs) are inactivated by contact with natural killer (NK)–resistant target cells (1). The capacity of the inactivated LGLs to secrete soluble cytotoxic factors (NKCFs) upon stimulation with concanavalin A (Con A) is impaired (2). CD11a-c/CD18, CD54, and an arginine-glycine–aspartic acid sequence (RGD) (3) binding domain, probably CD29, are involved in the binding of LGLs to such inactivating target cells (4). Anti-CD11a antibodies inhibit NK activity by the same mechanism as intact target cells (3,4), suggesting that the target cell–induced inhibitory signal is mediated via CD11a. Recently, signal transduction receptors with tyrosine kinase activity (5,6) and the src gene family products (7), especially $p56^{lck}$ (8) in lymphoid cells, have gained interest as potential regulators of cell growth and differentiation, and signal transductors during cell activation, respectively. The present experiments were designed to show the relationship of tyrosine phosphorylation and the activation/inhibition of NK cells.

MATERIALS AND METHODS

Effector and Target Cells

Large granular lymphocytes were purified as described in detail elsewhere (1,2). The K562 cell line was used as NK-sensitive target cells, and primary cultures of human adult fibroblasts as NK-resistant, inhibitory target cells.

Phosphotyrosine Analysis

Inactivated and control LGLs were labeled with ^{32}Pi, and the phosphotyrosyl compounds from postnuclear cell lysates were separated by P-Tyr (Ab-1) agarose (solid phase–coupled antiphosphotyrosine immunoglobulin G_1 [IgG_1] from mouse, Oncogene Science, Manhasset, New York). Samples were analyzed by 8% SDS-PAGE.

RESULTS

Inhibition of NK Activity by Intact Target Cells and Anti-CD11a Antibodies

As shown before (4), and 18-hr incubation with blocking anti-CD11a antibodies induce a significant inhibition of NK activity. The mechanism of the inhibition is similar to that induced by intact NK-resistant target cells (Fig. 1).

Protein Tyrosine Phosphorylation in Inactivated and Control LGLs

We have previously shown that in addition to diminished (by 59–70%) NK activity, NKCF secretion upon stimulation with Con A is impaired in LGLs inactivated by target cell contact (2). In order to detect concomitant differences in the tyrosine phosphorylation status of the LGL proteins, the postnuclear lysis supernatant was analyzed. As shown in Figure 2, a 190,000-D protein was phosphorylated in tyrosine upon Con A stimulation in control LGLs, but not in LGLs inactivated by contact with fibroblasts. The tyrosine phosphorylation of the 190,000-D protein was also impaired in LGLs inactivated by anti-CD11a antibodies (Fig. 3). In addition, this mini geel preparation revealed another, M_r 150,000- to 160,000-D phosphotyrosyl protein with a weaker labeling intensity in inactivated LGLs. In most of the experiments a third, 90,000- to 100,000-D phosphotyrosyl protein was also distinguished, no matter whether the LGLs were inactivated or not.

	Inhibition of cytotoxicity of uncultured large granular lymphocytes against NK sensitive target cells	Inhibition of antibody dependent cell-mediated cytotoxicity	Inhibition of binding of large granular lymphocytes to NK sensitive target cells	Inhibition of polarization of actin containing filaments in conjugate forming large granular lymphocytes	Inhibition of cytotoxicity of IL-2 treated large granular lymphocytes
Target cells	+	-	-	-	±
anti-CD11a-mAb	+	-	-	-	±

Figure 1 LGLs were preincubated for 18 hr on monolayers of fibroblasts (target cells) or with monoclonal anti-CD11a antibodies (anti-CD11a-MAb, H12, a gift from M. Patarroyo, Karolinska Institut, Stockholm, Sweden; 20 μg/ml). The cytotoxicity (LU 50%) against K562 (NK) and Ab-coated P815 (ADCC), binding capacity, and actin filament polarization of the pretreated LGLs were compared to that of untreated LGLs. (>50% inhibition of cx = +, 10–50% inh. = +/–, <10% inh. = –.) In part of the experiments, LGLs were cultured in the presence of IL-2 (300 U/ml) for 24 hr before the inhibition experiments.

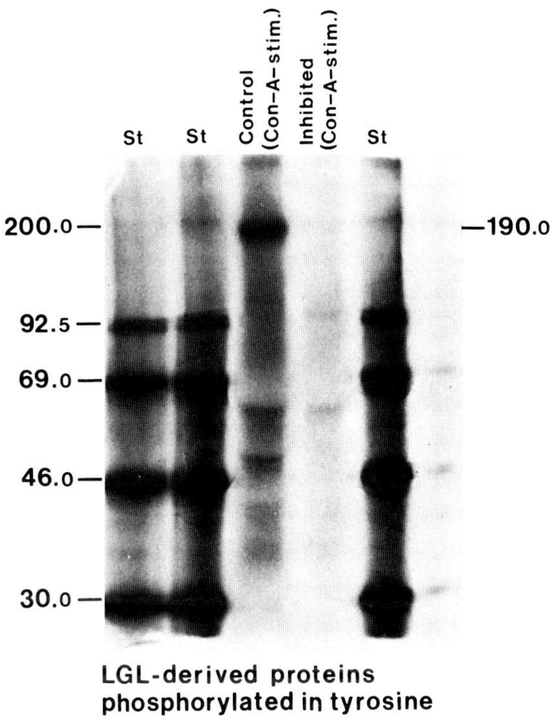

Figure 2 LGLs were incubated in empty plastic wells (=control) or cocultured with monolayers of human skin fibroblasts for 18 hr (=inhibited, cytotoxicity reduced by 88.8%), labeled with ^{32}P in the presence of Con A (3 μg/ml) for 2 hr, and lysed. The postnuclear supernatant was adsorbed with anti-P-tyr-agarose, and the eluate was analyzed by 8% SDS-PAGE. Autoradiograph is shown.

When LGLs were labeled with ^{32}P in the presence of Con A and Na_3VO_4 (30 μM), the 190,000-D phosphotyrosyl protein was constantly detectable, even after a long (3 hr) labeling/stimulation.

DISCUSSION

Intact NK-resistant target cells deliver an inhibitory signal to NK cells (1), and this signal is reproduced by a ligand (= specific antibody) binding to CD11a surface structure (4). Since tyrosine phosphorylation preceeds (9) and is required (10) for phospholipase C activation during T-cell receptor stimulation, it was hypothesized that the same activation pathway is also employed during NK-cell activation, and may show variation in response to inhibitory signals. Indeed, a large 190,000-D protein was found to phosphorylate in tyrosine upon Con A stimulation in control LGLs, but not in LGLs inactivated by target-cell contact. The compound has not been identified, but the molecular size and the evidence that the LCA-associated phosphotyrosine phosphatase (PTPase) is involved in the activation of the 56^{lck} tyrosine kinase (11) suggest that it may be one of the LCA isoforms. In addition, two smaller phosphotyrosyl proteins (150,000 D and 100,000 D) were detected in the LGL lysates, the role and identity of which remain to be defined.

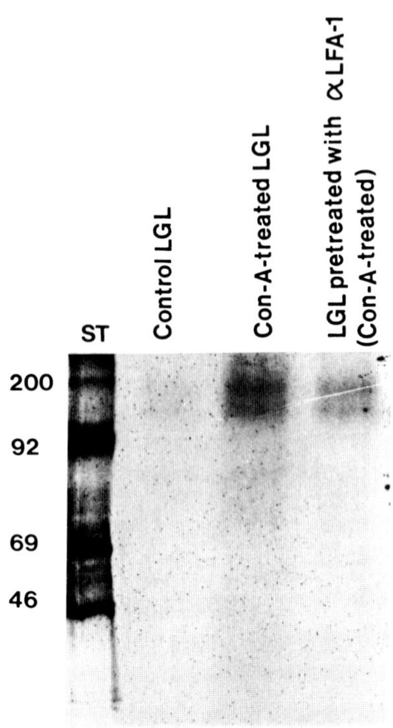

Figure 3 LGLs were incubated in medium only (=control) or in the presence of blocking anti-CD11a antibodies (20 μg/ml, cytotoxicity reduced by 50.3%) for 18 hr before labeling with ^{32}P (1 hr). Part of the control LGLs were labeled in medium only to demonstrate the increased phosphorylation in the presence of Con A (Con A treated). The postnuclear supernatant was analyzed as in Figure 2. The lanes were loaded equally, as shown by Ag staining of the geel (data not shown).

CONCLUSION

As a conclusion, the present work indicates that the NK activity of partially purified LGLs is reduced by contact with resistant target cells, and that the inhibitory signal is mediated via CD11a. Concomitantly with decreased NK activity, the proteins in the postnuclear supernatants of the lysed inactivated LGLs show defective tyrosine phosphorylation upon Con A stimulation. The current experiments support the idea that the tyrosine phosphorylation pathway is involved in the activation of NK cells.

ACKNOWLEDGMENTS

This work was financially supported by the Medical Council of Finnish Academy, Orion Pharmaceuticals Ltd., the National Cancer Institute of Finland, the Life and Pension Insurance Companies of Finland, and the Sigrid Juselius Foundation.

REFERENCES

1. Heiskala, M., Ylikorkala, O. and Timonen, T. Inhibition of human natural killer activity by monolayers of primary cell cultures. Nat Immun Cell Growth Regul 1987, 6:7–11.
2. Heiskala, M., Carpen, O., Saksela, E. and Timonen, T. Mechanism of contact-mediated inhibition of natural killer activity. J Immunol 1987, 139:1414–8.
3. Pierschbacer, M.D. and Ruoslahti, E. Cell attachment activity of fibronectin can be duplicated by small synthetic fragments of the molecule. Nature (Lond.) 1984, 309:30–3.
4. Heiskala, M., Patarroyo, M. and Timonen, T. Participation of Cd11a-c/CD18 and RGD binding adhesion molecules in the binding of LGL to NK-cell inactivating fibroblasts. Evidence for the role of CD11a in the inactivation. Scand J Immunol 1990 (in press).
5. Cohen, S., Ushiro, H., Stoscheck, C. and Chinkers, M. A native 170 000 epidermal growth factor receptor-kinase complex from shed plasma membrane vesicles. J Biol Chem 1982, 257:1523–31.
6. Hanks, S.K., Quinn, A.M. and Hunter, T. The protein kinase family: conserved features and deduced phylogeny of the catalytic domains. Science 1988, 241:42–52.
7. Bolen, J.B. and Veillette, A. A function for the lck protooncogene. TIBS 1989, 14:404–7.
8. Mustelin, T., Coggeshall, K.M., Isakov, N. and Altman, A. T cell antigen receptor-mediated activation of phospholipase C requires tyrosine phosphorylation. Science 1990, 247:1584–7.
9. June, C.H., Fletcher, M.C., Ledbetter, J.A. and Samelson, L.E. Increases in tyrosine phosphorylation are detectable before phospholipase C activation after T cell receptor stimulation. J Immunol 1990, 144:1591–99.
10. Mustelin, T., Coggeshall, K.M., Isakov, N. and Altman, A. T cell antigen receptor-mediated activation of phospholipase C requires tyrosine phosphorylation. Science 1990, 247:1584–7.
11. Mustelin, T. and Altman, A. Dephosphorylation and activation of the T cell tyrosine kinase $pp56^{lck}$ by the leukocyte common antigen (CD45). Oncogene 1990, in press.

50
Cytokine Modulation by FCE 24578, A New Immunoactive Compound

Anna Maria Isetta, Maria Chiara Fornasiero, Mario Ferrari, and Domenico Trizio
Farmitalia Carlo Erba R & D, Nerviano, Italy

INTRODUCTION

Activated macrophages (MOs) are critically involved in both inflammatory and immune responses. Macrophages are activated by a variety of agents, including natural and synthetic immunomodulators. Activation is accompanied by increased cytocidal activity and by the synthesis, expression, and secretion of enzymes, membrane proteins such as class II histocompatibility molecules (Ia), and soluble factors such as cytokines (1).

During a screening program for synthetic immunomodulators, a new class of compounds that are able to activate MOs has been identified. Among these compounds, FCE 24578 (Fig. 1) is under development, on account of its powerful capacity to increase the antitumor MO cytotoxicity, to reduce mortality in mice given P388 leukemia, and to protect neutropenic and normal mice from bacterial infections. Studies were therefore planned to investigate whether FCE 24578 is able to modulate the production of interleukin-1 (IL-1), tumor necrosis factor (TNF), and IL-6, which are some of the most important products of activated MOs (2).

MATERIALS AND METHODS

Animals

Six- to eight-week old, female C57Bl/6 and C3H/HeN mice (Charles River, Calco, Italy) were used.

Compound

FCE 24578, synthetized in our laboratories, was suspended in 0.5% pyrogen-free methocel and administered i.p. or i.m.

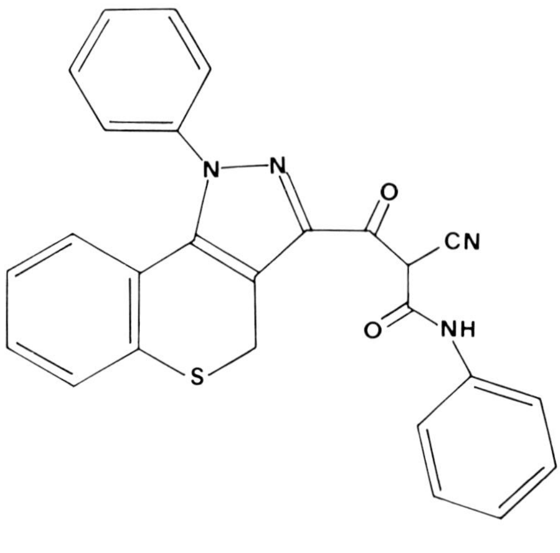

Figure 1 FCE 24578 (2-cyano-3(1,4-dihydro-1-phenil(1)-benzothiopyran(4,3-c)pyrazol-3-yl)-3-oxo-N-(phenylpropanamide).

IL-1, IL-6, and TNF Production and Detection

Adherent cells from PEC were cultured in serum-free medium (IL-1) or in 10% FCS (TNF), in the presence or absence of lipopolysaccharide (LPS) (20 μg/ml) for 2, 6, or 24 hr. Interleukin-1 production was also investigated in the presence of actinomycin D (1 hr contact; 10 μg/ml), a deoxyribonucleic acid (DNA) transcription inhibitor. Soluble and cell-associated IL-1 were measured by lymphocyte-activating factor (LAF) test (3). Culture supernatants and serum TNF levels were evaluated by the L929 cytotoxicity test (4). Serum IL-6 levels were detected by the $7TD_1$ proliferation test (5).

IL-1 and TNF Messenger Ribonucleic Acid (mRNA) Expression

Spleens and livers from FCE 24578– and LPS-treated mice were collected 6 hr posttreatment and immediately frozen in liquid nitrogen. Ribonucleic acid (RNA) was extracted with guanidine thiocyanate (6) and chromatographed on oligo-(dT)-cellulose. The RNA was then electrophoresed in 1.5% agarose, transferred to a Gene Screen membrane, and finally hybridized with murine-radiolabeled IL-1 β or TNF probe. Membranes were then exposed to an x-ray film.

RESULTS

FCE 24578 administered once, 4 days before cell collection, stimulated dose dependently the IL-1 production in 24 hr macrophage supernatant. The LPS was able to modulate this phenomenon positively (Table 1) or negatively (data no shown) depending on the basal cell activation. The IL-1 production by control MOs was similar to that of treated MOs only after LPS exposure (Table 1). The IL-1 activity, both in supernatants and cell extracts, progressively increased from 2 to 24 hr culture time; the IL-1 levels from treated cultures always being significantly higher than that of controls (Table 2). The addition of actinomycin D abolished the IL-1 activity in supernatants, causing also a significant reduction of

Table 1 IL-1 Activity in 24-h Supernatant of Peritoneal MOs from Mice Treated with FCE 24578

FCE 24578 (mg/kg/i.p.)	[^{3}H]thymidine uptake (cpm ± S.E.)					
	– LPS			+ LPS		
	Supernatant dilutions					
	1:8	1:32	1:128	1:8	1:32	1:128
—	1900±185	750±90	560±100	14500±983	9900±451	2500±330
10	13800±1100	3700±200	1000±210	27500±2210	14000±2210	3400±552
2	9200±851	1900±305	1100±198	19500±1920	20300±2100	5200±800

cell-associated IL-1 (Table 3). Negative results were obtained when TNF was measured in MO supernatants and sera from FCE 24578–treated mice, while according to literature data (7), high levels of TNF were observed at 1 and 2 hr post-LPS administration (data not shown). A moderate but significant increase of serum IL-6, dose related with FCE 24578 treatment, was appreciated at 2 and 6 hr posttreatment. The LPS-injected animals produced high levels of IL-6 2 hr posttreatment (Table 4). At 6 hr post–FCE 24578 treatment, a significant amount of IL-1 mRNA was detected in liver (Fig. 2) and spleen (data not shown) of treated mice, whereas TNF signal was negative. Both IL-1 and TNF mRNA proved to be strongly increased in LPS-treated mice (Fig. 2).

DISCUSSION

The results of this study show that FCE 24578 can modulate IL-1 and IL-6 without significantly interfering with TNF production.

The IL-1 production in FCE 24578-activated MOs was a dynamic process, the extracellular and cell-associated IL-1 levels being strongly correlated and both increasing with the culture time. This finding suggests that FCE 24578 can induce IL-1 neosynthesis, not merely stimulate its release from MOs. This hypothesis is also supported by the

Table 2 Time Course of IL-1 Production by FCE 24578–Treated MOs

FCE24578 (mg/kg/i.p.)	Time (hr)	[^{3}H]thymidine uptake (cpm ± S.E.)					
		Supernatant IL-1 dilutions			Cell-associated IL-1 dilutions		
		1:8	1:32	1:128	1:8	1:32	1:128
—	2	1373±131	466±70	343±28	5589±560	1030±88	536±49
	6	2100±181	792±62	464±22	6287±525	1735±123	614±55
	24	1900±150	750±61	560±42	7772±600	1930±110	563±42
10	2	1694±140	428±35	370±30	8699±570	2110±189	410±25
	6	8500±725	2200±250	750±46	9185±650	3926±198	792±65
	24	14500±1100	4315±385	1100±100	9068±725	9577±800	6959±523

Table 3 Effect of Actinomycin D on IL-1 Production by FCE 24578–Treated MOs

FCE24578 (mg/kg/i.p.)	Time (hr)	$[^3H]$thymidine uptake (cpm ± S.E.) Supernatant IL-1 dilutions 1:8	1:32	1:128	Cell-associated IL-1 dilutions 1:8	1:32	1:128
—	2	423±33	301±30	323±28	2968±270	817±90	286±29
	6	1367±101	415±47	330±29	3326±360	506±46	330±40
	2	523±51	377±41	347±33	5261±480	1883±155	551±41
10	6	898±91	368±32	344±35	3936±360	2311±207	675±70

evidence that (a) IL-1 was not detected in supernatants of FCE 24578–activated MOs, cultured in the presence of actinomycin D, probably as consequence of inhibition of protein neosynthesis; and (b) high levels of IL-1 mRNA were expressed in spleens and livers of treated mice. FCE 24578 has also been demonstrated to moderately, but significantly, increase the systemic IL-6 levels in mice. Differently from IL-1 and IL-6, the TNF signal was negative after FCE 24578 treatment, both in terms of mRNA in spleen and liver and of cytokine levels in MOs supernatants and sera of animals.

These results would suggest that FCE 24578, unlike LPS, is capable of inducing the expression of IL-1 and probably also of IL-6 genes without concomitant expression of TNF genes, or alternatively, it can induce the expression of IL-1/IL-6 and TNF genes with a different kinetics. The absence of serum TNF level at any time in FCE 24578–treated mice, compared to the high TNF levels after LPS stimulation, is more consistent with the first hypothesis and in line with recent data (8) on the possibility to regulate differently IL-1 and TNF production in phagocytes. FCE 24578 seems therefore able to activate a subset of MO functions that may be of clinical benefit. Among them, we can include IL-1 production, whose mielorestorative and immunorestorative (9) properties are becoming more and more evident, whereas its role in autoimmune pathologies is still a matter of discussion (10).

Table 4 IL-6 Levels in Sera of Mice Treated with FCE 24578

Compound	mg/kg	IL-6 (U/ml) hr posttreatment 2	6	24
—	—	<50	<50	<50
FCE 24578 i.m.	10	50	250	<50
	2	50	50	<50
LPS i.v.	0.1	1×10^5	ND	ND

ND = Not determined.

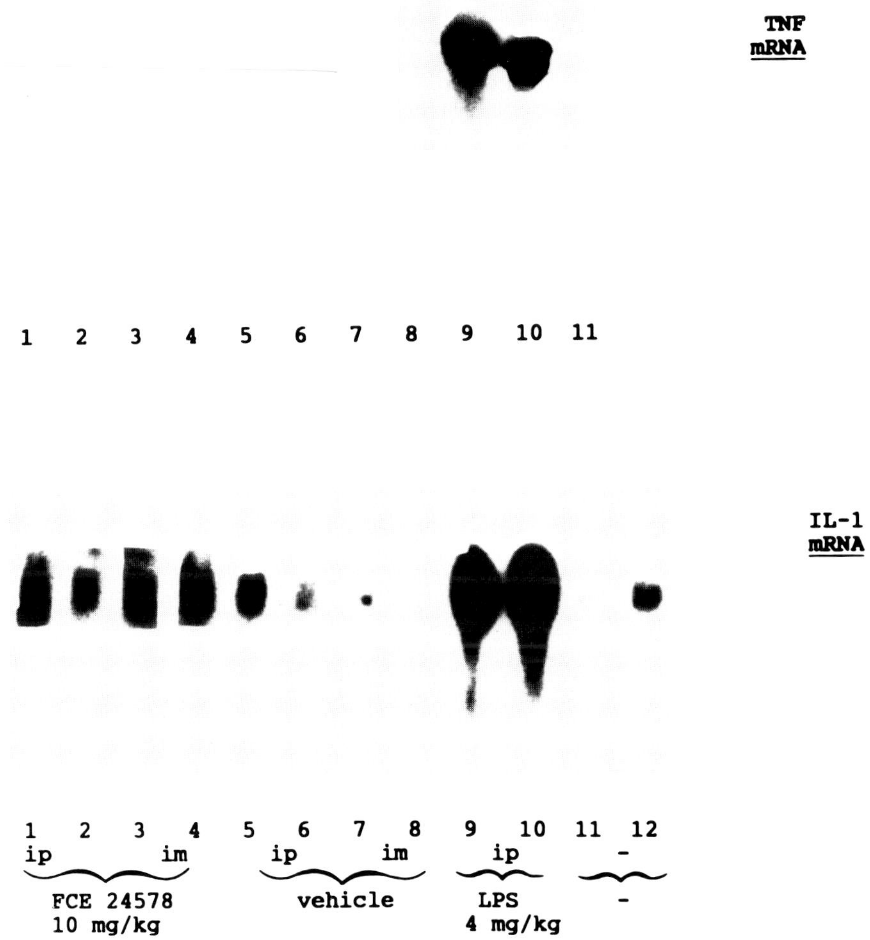

Figure 2 Effect of FCE 24578 on IL-1 and TNF mRNA induction in liver.

REFERENCES

1. Nathan C.F. Secretory products of macrophages. J. Clin. Invest. 1987, 79, 319–26.
2. Dinarello C. IL-1 and its biologically related cytokines. Adv. Immunol. 1989, 44, 153–205.
3. Economou J.S. and Shin S.H. Lymphocyte-activating factor. J. Immunol. 1978, 121, 1446–45.
4. Spofford B., Daynes R.A. and Granger G.A. Cell-mediated immunity in vitro. A high sensitive assay for human lymphotoxin. J. Immunol. 1974, 112, 2111–115.
5. Sironi M., Breviario F., Proserpio P., Biondi P., Vecchi A., Van Damme J., Dejana E. and Mantovani A. IL-1 stimulates IL-6 production in endothelial cells. J. Immunol. 1989, 142, 549–53.
6. Mochizuki D.Y., Einsenman J.R., Conlon P.J., Larsen A.D. and Tushinski R.J. IL-1 regulates hematopoietic activity, a role previously ascribed to hemopoietin-1. P.N.A.S. USA 1987, 84, 5267–271.

7. Beutler B. and Cerami A. Cachectin and TNF as two sides of the same biological coin. Nature 1986, 320, 584–88.
8. Burkett S.K., Weaver W.M., Westall J.A., Larsen A., Kronheim S. and Wilson C.B. Regulation of TNF and IL-1 secretion by human mononuclear phagocytes. J. Immunol. 1988, 140, 3473–481.
9. Morrissey P., Charrier K., Bressler L. and Alpert A. The influence of IL-1 treatment on the reconstitution of the hemopoiesis and immune systems after sublethal radiation. J. Immunol. 1988, 140, 4204–210.
10. Jacobs C., Young D., Tyler S., Callis G., Gillis S. and Conlon P.J. In vivo treatment with IL-1 reduces the severity and duration of antigen-induced arthritis in rats. J. Immunol. 1988, 131, 2967–974.

51
Endogenous Anxiogenic Peptide, ODN-Diazepam Binding Inhibitor, and Benzodiazepine Influence Monokine Production

Véronique Taupin, André Herbelin, Béatrice Descamps-Latscha, and Flora Zavala
Hôpital Necker, Paris, France

INTRODUCTION

Benzodiazepines (BZDs) are widely prescribed molecules endowed with anxiolytic, anticonvulsant, myorelaxant, and sedative properties. These pharmacological activities have been correlated with the affinities for a receptor associated with the γ-aminobutyric acid ($GABA_A$) receptor and the chloride channel in the central nervous system (CNS) (1). On the basis of the displacement of the radiolabeled ligand diazepam from these CNS receptors, an endogenous ligand was purified and termed diazepam-binding inhibitor (DBI). This 11-kD protein displayed anxiogenic properties and was detected not only in CNS, but also in many peripheral organs such as kidney, lung, heart, testis, adrenals, and spleen (2). Interestingly, these peripheral organs were rich in a distinct, GABA-independent, type of BZD receptor (3). Diazepam-binding inhibitor and most BZD molecules were able to bind central type and peripheral-type BZD receptors. Molecules such as Ro 5-4864 and PK 11195, which are mostly deprived of psychoactive properties, were specific for the peripheral-type BZD receptors, whereas by contrast, some anxiolytic BZDs such as clonazepam or anxiogenic ligands (e.g., β-carbolines) showed a strict specificity for the central-type BZD receptor.

The growing body of evidence suggesting the influence of stress and anxiety on immune status (4) prompted us to investigate the possible influence of the different BZD molecules as well as of the endogenous peptide ligands on immune functions. We first demonstrated that phagocytes exhibit a high density of peripheral BZD receptors (PBZDR) (5). Peripheral- and mixed-type BZDs significantly enhanced in vivo the humoral response of mice to sheep red blood cells (5). That phagocyte PBZDR was a functional receptor was further demonstrated in vitro on human monocytes (6) where peripheral and mixed type BZD ligands exerted chemotactic activity at picomolar concentrations. We also demonstrated that in murine macrophagelike P338D1 cells (7) nanomolar concentrations of peripheral- and mixed-type BZD, corresponding to the nanomolar affinity of the ligands for their specific receptors, significantly modulated the respiratory burst activation by arachidonic acid.

We investigated the implication of the peripheral benzodiazepine receptor in human host defense reactions. The production of the bactericidal superoxide anion by normal human polymorphonuclear neutrophils was associated with increased membrane PBZDR expression (8). Moreover, a dramatic alteration of PBZDR expression was encountered on neutrophils of patients with X-linked chronic granulomatous disease, an inherited disorder characterized by the inability of phagocytes to produce superoxide anion, leading to frequent and life-threatening infections (8).

In the present study, we report the influence of BZD ligands on the production of inflammatory monokines. The production of interleukin-1 β (IL-1 β) and tumor necrosis factor α (TNF-α) in vitro by human monocytes stimulated with bacterial endotoxin (lipopolysaccharide [LPS]) was significantly enhanced by peripheral- and mixed- but not central-type BZD molecules. Most interestingly, synthetic peptides corresponding to the pharmacologically active moiety of endogenous DBI were extremely efficient in the modulation of IL-1 and TNF secretion by human monocytes (9).

We also report that in vivo injection of mice with peripheral- and mixed- but not central-type BZDs leads to a significant inhibition in both peritoneal and spleen macrophage production of IL-1, TNF, and interleukin-6 (IL-6) when further stimulated in vitro with LPS (10).

RESULTS AND DISCUSSION

Pharmacological and Endogenous BZD Ligands Stimulate In Vitro Cytokine Production by Human Monocytes

Human monocytes isolated from heparinized peripheral blood were cultured at a density of 5×10^4 cells per well of a 96-well tissue culture dish for 18–20 hr, under stimulation by a suboptimal dose of LPS (1 μg/ml) in the presence or the absence of 10^{-15} to 10^{-5} M BZD ligands. Interleukin-1 and TNF production in supernatants were assessed both by specific ELISA and by biological assays, i.e., lymphocyte-activating factor (LAF) assay for IL-1 and L929 cell lysis for TNF. While no effect was detected in the absence of LPS, a bell-shaped dose-response curve was obtained for the prototypical peripheral ligand Ro 5-4864, which stimulated the LPS-induced production of IL-1 and TNF by 113 and 105%, respectively (mean from six different donors, individual variation was from 50 to 230%) with optimal concentration of 10^{-8} to 10^{-11} M. Approximately 15% of blood donors did not respond to BZD. No correlation could be established between the level of LPS-induced TNF or IL-1 production and the percentage of stimulation by Ro 5-4864 for a given blood donor. Similar results were obtained with ELISA and biological assays.

In order to further confirm that the receptor involved in this in vitro modulation by Ro-5-4864 corresponded to PBZDR, we compared the effect of peripheral-, mixed-, and central-type ligands of the BZD receptor. While the best activity among pharmacological molecules tested corresponded to the peripheral-type ligand Ro 5-4864, no central type ligand, neither the anxiolytic ZK 93423, which is a β-carboline molecule, or clonazepam, nor the anxiogenic β-CCM influenced the monokine production. The mixed-type ligand diazepam (Valium), widely prescribed for its anxiolytic properties, also exhibited immunomodulatory properties, causing a significant, although more moderate, enhancement (+30 to +70%) of LPS-induced TNF and IL-1 production. The mixed-type molecule could thus be considered as a pharmacological probe for possible endogenous messengers between nervous and immune systems. The endogenous anxiogenic peptide, DBI, has been detected and shown to be produced not only in brain, but also in most peripheral organs (2) and Des-(Gly-Ile)-DBI or des-endozepine, extracted from adrenal glands, was able to interact with steroidogenesis via PBZDR (11). We therefore evaluated the influence of synthetic peptide fragments of DBI on monokine production (Fig. 1). A rat sequence of ODN-DBI was tested, which shows close to 80% homology with the human sequence. ODN-DBI, which represents the octadecaneuropeptide active moiety of the anxiogenic DBI, also demonstrated a strong potentiating activity on human monokine production. The pharmacologically active portion of ODN-DBI includes the octapeptidic COOH-terminal sequence of ODN-DBI (octaneuropeptide), which was also active, although not as efficient as the full-length ODN sequence. These results suggest that monocytes represent a privileged site of action of the endogenous anxiogenic ligand of the BZD receptor, where it interacts at pico- to nanomolar concentrations.

In Vivo Treatment of Mice with BZDs Modulates the Capacity of Macrophages to Produce IL-1, TNF, and IL-6

We investigated whether such an influence of BZD ligands on the production of monokines could also be demonstrated in vivo.

CBA/J mice (10- to 12-week-old) were treated with a single intraperitoneal injection of an anxiolytic dose (1 mg/kg) of various BZD ligands. Two days later, peritoneal and spleen cells were collected and washed. After adherence to flat-bottomed wells of 24-well Falcon tissue culture plates (1 ml/well), peritoneal cells (1 × 10^6/ml) and spleen cells (5 × 10^6/ml) were incubated with or without LPS (1 μg/ml). Twenty-four hours later, the supernatant was collected as a source of soluble, secreted cytokines. Cell-associated (intracellular and membrane-associated) cytokines were obtained from the cellular pellets after three freeze-thaw cycles. Murine IL-1 activity was determined by the LAF assay and the

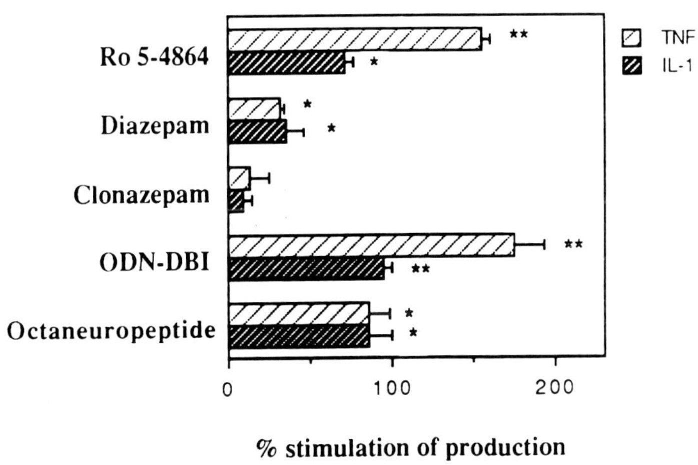

Figure 1 BZD ligands enhance IL-1 β and TNF α production by LPS-induced human monocytes. Human monocytes were incubated for 18 hr with LPS (1 μg/ml) and 10^{-10} M concentration of BZD ligands. TNF α and IL-1 β productions were assessed in culture spuernatants and results are expressed as mean ±SEM of three different experiments. Statistical significance is assed using Student's "t" test (*p <0.05, **p <0.01).

Table 1 Effect of In Vivo BZD Injection on LPS-Induced Production of IL-1, TNF, and IL-6 by Peritoneal and Spleen Macrophages

	Peritoneal macrophages			Spleen macrophages		
	excipient	Ro5-4864	clonazepam	excipient	Ro4864	clonazepam
Secreted IL-1 (U/ml)	10.68±1.76	4.84±0.97** (–55%)	8.37±2.09	3.75±0.75	1.40±0.50* (–63%)	3.80±0.60
Cell-associated	52.61±3.62	47.97±3.76	55.93±9.00	2.96±0.40	1.38±0.20* (–53%)	2.90±0.40
TNF (U/ml)	35±8	7±0.9* (–80%)	27±77	49±4.3	26±2.3*** (–47%)	47±3.7
IL-6 (U/ml)	3167±623	3350±919	3333±471	119±13	54±17*** (–55%)	120±20

Results are expressed as mean ±SEM of three different experiments.
Numbers in parentheses represent percent of inhibition of cytokine production by macrophages of BZD-treated animals as compared to production by cells of animals injected with excipient.
Statistical significance is assessed using Student's "t" test (*p <0.05, **p <0.02, ***p <0.01).

U373 proliferation assay; TNF activity by the lysing activity on L929 cells; and IL-6 activity was measured by the cellular proliferation of B9 cells. As shown in Table 1, the peripheral ligand Ro 5-4864 exerted a systemic effect, detectable both at the site of injection and at a distance, within splenocytes. As compared to excipient-injected animals, animals injected with Ro 5-4864 demonstrated a significant inhibition (–47 to –80%) of the LPS-induced production of all secreted cytokines (IL-1, TNF, and IL-6). However, this effect of Ro 5-4864 was not observed when massive production occurred, as in the case of IL-6 production by peritoneal cells. Similarly, concerning the cell-associated pool of IL-1, a significant inhibition was observed for spleen macrophages but not for peritoneal cells, which produced almost 15-fold the amount of intracellular IL-1 produced by spleen macrophages. In all experiments, the central-type ligand clonazepam remained inactive, demonstrating that this in vivo effect of BZDs was also mediated by the peripheral-type receptor. As already observed in in vitro experiments on human monocytes, the treatment by Ro 5-4864 had no effect in the absence of LPS induction of the monokine production.

CONCLUSIONS

Altogether these results demonstrate that BZD ligands can significantly modulate the production of inflammatory cytokines, both in vivo and in vitro. The activity was restricted to the peripheral- and mixed-type ligands, whereas the different central-type ligands tested displayed no activity, thus demonstrating that phagocyte PBZDR was indeed mediating the observed modulations.

Our results, which may have clinical implications, demonstrate that widely prescribed BZD compounds as well as endogenous anxiogenic ligands interact through the phagocyte PBZDR with molecular networks of immunoregulation.

REFERENCES

1. Schofield PR, Darlison MG, Fujita N, Burt DR, Stephenson FA, Rodriguez H, Rhee LM, Ramachandran J, Reale V, Glencorse JA, Seeburg PH, Barnard EA. Sequence and functional expression of the $GABA_A$ receptor shows a ligand-gated receptor super-family. Nature, 1987; 328, 221–227.
2. Ahlo H, Fremeau Jr RT, Tiedge H, Wilcox J, Bolovin P, Brosius J, Roberts JL, Costa E. Diazepam binding inhibitor gene expression: Location in brain and peripheral tissues of rat. Proc. Natl. Acad. Sci. U.S.A., 1988; 85, 7018–7022.
3. Verma A, Snyder SH. Peripheral type benzodiazepine receptors. Annu. Rev. Pharmacol. Toxicol., 1989; 29, 307–322.
4. Khansari DN, Murgo AJ, Faith RE. Effects of stress on the immune system. Immunol. Today, 1990; 11, 170–175.
5. Zavala F, Haumont J, Lenfant M. Interaction of benzodiazepines with mouse macrophages. Eur. J. Pharmacol., 1984; 106, 561–566.
6. Ruff MR, Pert CB, Weber RJ, Wahl SM, Paul SM. Benzodiazepine receptor-mediated chemotaxis of human monocytes. Science, 1985; 229, 1281–1283.
7. Zavala F, Lenfant M. Peripheral benzodiazepines enhance the respiratory burst of macrophage-like P388D1 cells stimulated by arachidonic acid. Int. J. Immunopharmacol., 1987; 3, 269–274.
8. Zavala F, Veber F, Descamps-Latscha B. Altered expression of neutrophil benzodiazepine receptor in X-linked chronic granulomatous disease. Blood, 1990; 76, 184–188.
9. Taupin V, Herbelin A, Descamps-Latscha B, Zavala F. Endogenous anxiogenic peptide, ODN-diazepam binding inhibitor, and benzodiazepines enhance the production of interleukin-1 and tumor necrosis factor by human monocytes. Lymphokine Res., 1991 (in press).
10. Zavala F, Taupin V, Descamps-Latscha B. In vivo treatment with benzodiazepines inhibits murine phagocyte oxidative metabolism and production of interleukin 1, Tumor Necrosis Factor, and Interleukin-6. J. Pharmacol. Exp. Ther., 1990; 255, 442–450.
11. Besman MJ, Yanagibashi K, Lee TD, Kawamura M, Hall PF, Shively JE. Identification of des-(Gly-Ile)-endozepine as an effector of corticotropin-dependent adrenal steroidogenesis: Stimulation of cholesterol delivery is mediated by the peripheral benzodiazepine receptor. Proc. Natl. Acad. Sci. U.S.A. 1989; 86, 4897–4901.

52
Localization of Interleukin-4 and Interleukin-6 Messenger Ribonucleic Acid in Human Tonsils by ISH

A. Bosseloir,[1] E. Hooghe-Peters,[2] E. Heinen,[1] C. Marcoty,[1] N. Cormann,[1] C. Kinet-DeNoël,[1] and L. J. Simar[1]
[1]*Institute of Histology, University of Liège, Liège, Belgium;*
[2]*Medical School, V.U.B., Brussels, Belgium*

INTRODUCTION

Interleukin-4 (IL-4) and interleukin-6 (IL-6) possess a broad spectrum of biological activities (1,2). Human tonsils are particularly rich in lymphoid follicules, early sites for the humoral immune response (3). Even if the biological activities of IL-4 and IL-6 are well established, the spatial links between these cytokines and the responding cells in a lymphoid organ remain unknown. The aim of this study is to localize IL-4 and IL-6 messenger ribonucleic acid (mRNA) in the different areas of human tonsils by I.S.H.

MATERIALS AND METHODS

Tissue Preparation

Freshly dissected tonsils from four 3- to 10-year-old children with recurrent throat infection were transferred at 4°C in a physiological solution containing 0.4% BSA and frozen at –80°C in OCT compound (Tissue-Tek, Miles Scientific, Naperville, Illinois). Cryosections (6 to 8 μm), prepared at –20°C, were placed on glass slides coated with poly-L-lysine. The sections were then fixed in paraformaldehyde (4%) in phosphate-buffered saline (PBS) containing 20 mM vanadyl ribonucleoside complex (VCR) (Sigma, St. Louis, Missouri) for 10 min at 4°C. After washing, sections were treated with 0.25% Triton X-100 in PBS containing 20 mM VRC for 10 min at room temperature, dehydrated, and stored at 4°C.

In Situ Hybridization

This was performed as described in Bosseloir et al. (4).

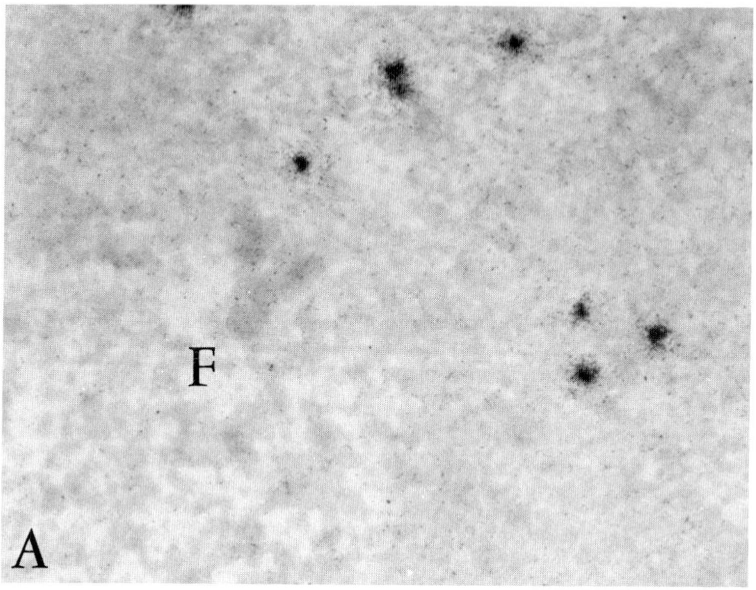

Figure 1 In situ hybridization with ^{35}S-labeled IL-6 cDNA. Exposure time 14 days. Interfollicular zone (A; ×270); conjunctive capsule area (B; ×270); subepithelial zone (C; ×400). F: secondary follicles.

RESULTS

After hybridization with ^{35}S-labeled IL-4 and IL-6 complementary deoxyribonucleic acid (cDNA), small clusters of strongly positive cells were found in three different areas: the interfollicular zone (Fig. 1A and 2A), the conjunctive capsule area (Figs. 1B and 2B), and the supepithelial zone (Fig. 1C). No labeling was found in lymphoid follicles even when large germinal centers were present.

In control sections, pretreatment with ribonuclease before incubation with ^{35}S hIL-6 or hIL-4 cDNA abolished or diminished the autoradiographic signal (data not shown).

CONCLUSIONS

Using ^{35}S-labeled cDNA probes, we could determine the mRNA localization of IL-6 and IL-4 in human tonsils: the interfollicular area, capsular area, and subepithelial zone. Neither IL-6 nor -4 production occurs inside follicles. We suggest that these three sites play a role in the B-cell activation and their differentiation into immunoglobulin (Ig)-secreting cells. B cells, produced in the germinal centers, can only encounter IL-6 and IL-4 during their migration through the perifollicular areas. This hypothesis is compatible with results obtained by Cormann et al. (5) showing that lymphoid cells from tonsils produce less Ig when they are in contact with follicular dentritic cells than with macrophages. Inversely, germinal centers appear as areas isolating B cells from given cytokines.

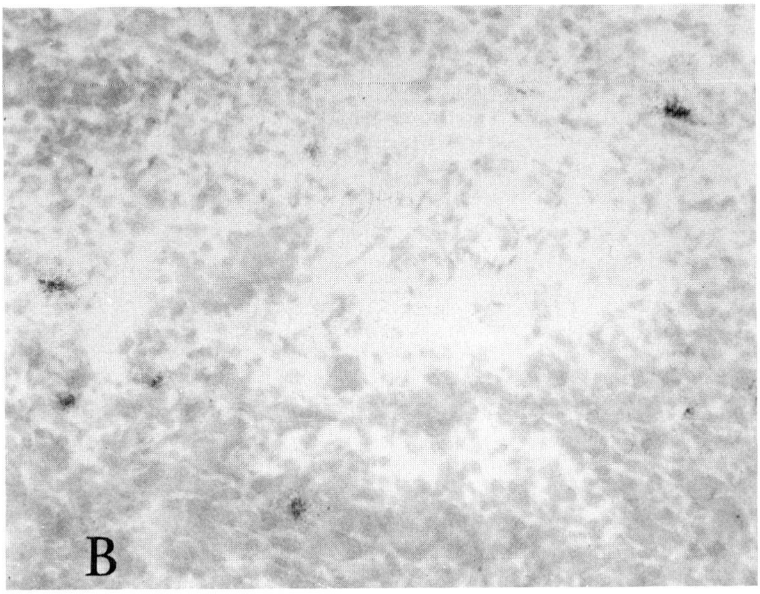

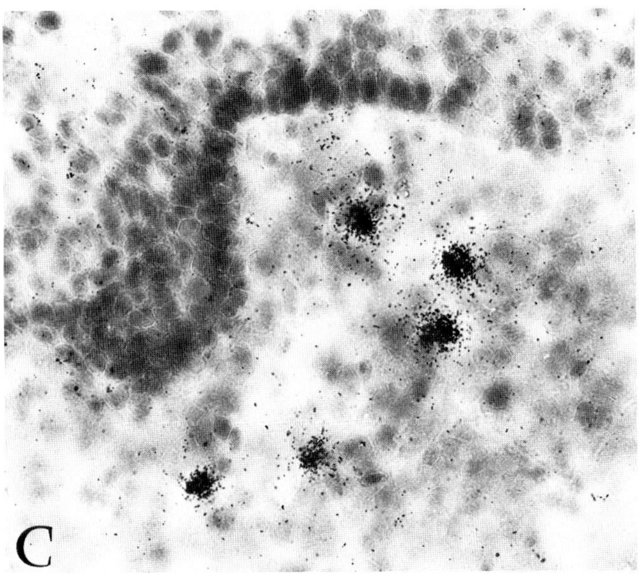

Figure 1 (Continued)

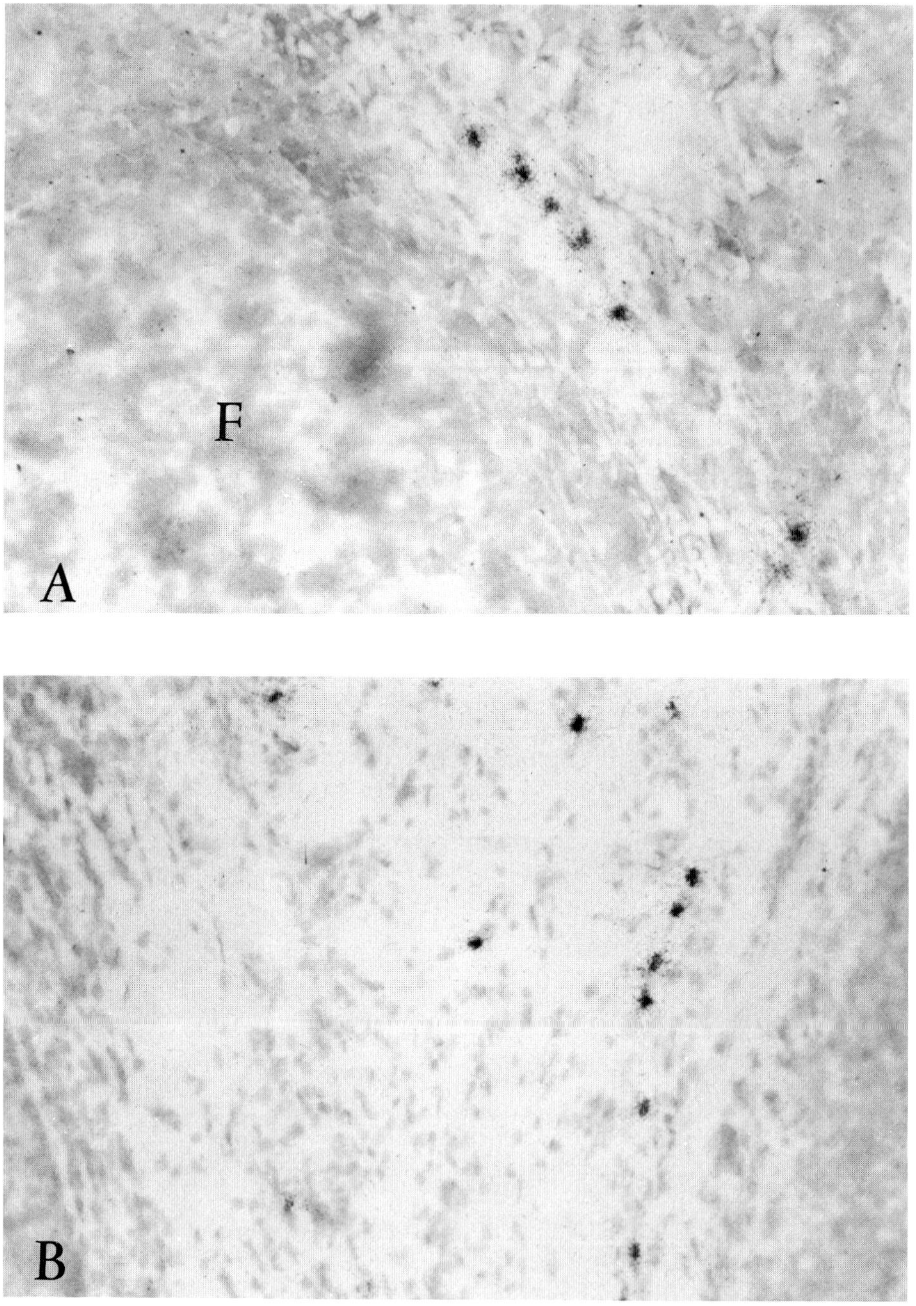

Figure 2 In situ hybridization with ^{35}S-labeled IL-4 cDNA. Exposure time 14 days. Interfollicular zone (A; ×270); conjunctive capsule area (B; ±270). F: secondary follicles.

ACKNOWLEDGMENTS

We would like to express our gratitude to Drs. R. Boniver (Bruyeres), R. Daehl, and D. Malaise (Citadelle) for tonsil supply. We thank P. Verdood, A.M. Greiners, and M. Jackers for expert technical assistance.

This work was supported by the Belgian National Research Foundation (grant 3.0059.85), the Belgian National Lottery (grant 9.0025.84), the Fonds de la Recherche Scientifique Medicale at Liège, and the Institut pour l'encouragement de la Recherche Scientifique dans l'Industrie et l'Agriculture (I.R.S.I.A.).

REFERENCES

1. Hofman F.M., Brock M., Taylor C.R. and Lyons B. IL-4 regulates differentiation and proliferation of human precursor B cells. J. Immunol., 1988, 141:1185.
2. Muraguchi A., Hirano T., Tang B., Matsuda T., Horii Y., Nakajima K. and Kishomoto T. The essential role of B cell stimulatory factor (BSF2/IL-6) for the terminal differentiation of B cells. J. Exp. Med., 1988; 167:332.
3. Thorbecke G., Asofsky R., Hochwald G. and Siskind G. Gamma globulin and antibody formation in vitro. III Induction of secondary response at different intervals after the primary; the role of secondary nodules in the preparation of the secondary response. J. Exp. Med., 1962, 116:295.
4. Bosseloir A., Hooghe-Peters E., Heinen E., Cormann N., Kinet-Denoel C., Vanhaelst L. and Simar L.J. Localization of interleukin 6 mR.N.A. in human tonsils by in-situ hybridization. Eur. J. Immunol., 1989, 19:2379.
5. Cormann N., Lesage F., Heinen E., Schaaf-Lafontaine N., Kinet-Denoel C., and Simar L.J. Isolation of follicular dendritic cells from human tonsils and adenoids. Effect on lymphocyte proliferation and differentiation. Immunol. Lett., 1986/87, 14:29.

53
Production of Epidermal Cytokines During Ontogenesis

Stanislava Stošić-Grujičić, Vesna Stanković, and Miodrag L. Lukić
Institute for Biological Research and Institute of Microbiology and Immunology, School of Medicine, Belgrade, Yugoslavia

INTRODUCTION

Beside barrier function, adult epidermis contains all the components necessary for the immune and inflammatory responses, including a complex network of interacting cytokines. Interleukin-1 (IL-1) and IL-6 appear to be key members of the cytokine network which regulate the growth, development, and function of epidermal, dermal, immunocompetent, and hematopoietic cells. Interleukin-1 is produced constitutively by freshly isolated keratinocytes, including newborn murine keratinocytes (1). Interleukin-6 is known to have similar biological functions to IL-1, and has recently been shown to be secreted by normal human keratinocytes (2,3). Since epidermal cell (EC)–derived products can be differentially expressed during ontogenesis, this led us to investigate the production of IL-1 and IL-6 as well as an inhibitor of these activities in fetal, newborn, and adult rat skin.

CONSTITUTIVE PRODUCTION OF IMMUNOSTIMULATORY CYTOKINES

Single cell suspensions of ECs were prepared from rats of defined ages ranging from day 16 of gestation up to 12 months. The age of fetuses, obtained from timed pregnant rats, was verified by developmental morphology. Cells were obtained either from fetal or newborn back skin, or from ear skin of adult Albino Oxford rats. The optimal conditions for the release of immunostimulatory cytokines were determined by plating 1×10^6 ECs/ml (4). Supernatants were harvested at 24 hr, extensively dialyzed, and tested for their capacity to induce IL-1– and IL-6–dependent cell proliferation.

We have previously shown (4) in the thymocyte costimulation assay that normal freshly removed rat keratinocytes constitutively produced immunostimulatory cytokines. Comparing the levels of their production during ontogenesis, by using the same assay the highest activity was found immediately after birth, and gradually declined in cells obtained with the aging (not shown). During the fetal period, starting from the earliest time when ECs could be obtained (i.e., day 16 of gestation), we have obtained a significant production of IL-1–like activity from the very beginning (data not presented).

In order to discriminate between IL-1 and IL-6 cytokines that are both active in the thymocyte assay (5), in further experiments we used more specific bioassays. To do this, we have used two murine cell lines: the IL-1–dependent subclone D10S (kind gift from C. A. Dinarello, Tufts University, Boston, Massachusetts), and the IL-6–dependent hybridoma subclone B9 (kindly provided by L. Aarden, University of Amsterdam, The Netherlands, through courtesy of M. Colic, Military Medical Academy, Belgrade, Yugoslavia).

IL-1 PRODUCTION MEASURED BY D10S ASSAY DURING ONTOGENESIS

The IL-1 assay was performed by titrating EC supernatants in microcultures of D10S cells, as originally described (6), and was related to a standard preparation of human rIL-1 β. D10S cells have exquisite sensitivity to IL-1, and they do not proliferate to endotoxin, interferon-γ (IFN-γ), tumor necrosis factor (TNF), lymphotoxin (LT), or GM-CSF (6). Obtained results showed (Fig. 1) that during the prenatal period ECs constitutively expressed abundant amounts of IL-1. Interleukin-1 activity reached a peak level on the day of birth. During postnatal life the production of IL-1 steadily declined (Table 1). Thus, our results are in good correlation to the observation that cutaneous IL-1 expression is affected by age (7), and expand this observation to prenatal life.

IL-6 PRODUCTION MEASURED BY B9 ASSAY DURING ONTOGENESIS

Interleukin-6 was assayed by using B9 cells as described by Aarden et al. (8). The specificity of this bioassay is very high, since it has been shown that B9 cells are insensitive to IL-1, IL-2, IL-3, IFN-α, IFN-γ, or TNF-α (8). Epidermal cell–derived samples were compared with a standard preparation of human rIL-6. As shown in Figure 2, fetal ECs are able to produce IL-6. Elevated IL-6 bioactivity can be seen on day 17 of gestation, and is very high until the birth. During postnatal life (Table 2) the production of IL-6 gradually decreased.

Thus, presented results suggest that unstimulated ECs, including fetal cells, release appreciable amounts of IL-1 and IL-6 in the absence of deliberate stimulation. It cannot be excluded that constitutive production is in fact a reflection of in vitro exposure to as yet unidentified stimuli, but it is tempting to speculate that this observation may have in vivo relevance during development.

GLUCOCORTICOID-INDUCED INHIBITORY FACTORS MEASURED DURING ONTOGENESIS

Glucocorticoids (GCs) are known as a potent inhibitors of the production of various cytokines. Beside this effect, we have previously shown that in vivo or in vitro exposure of various accessory cells, among them keratinocytes, to GCs, induced secretion of inhibitory factors which affected lectin-induced IL-1– and IL-6–driven proliferation of T lymphocytes (4,9). Moreover, by combined addition of rIL-1 and rIL-6, it was shown that the

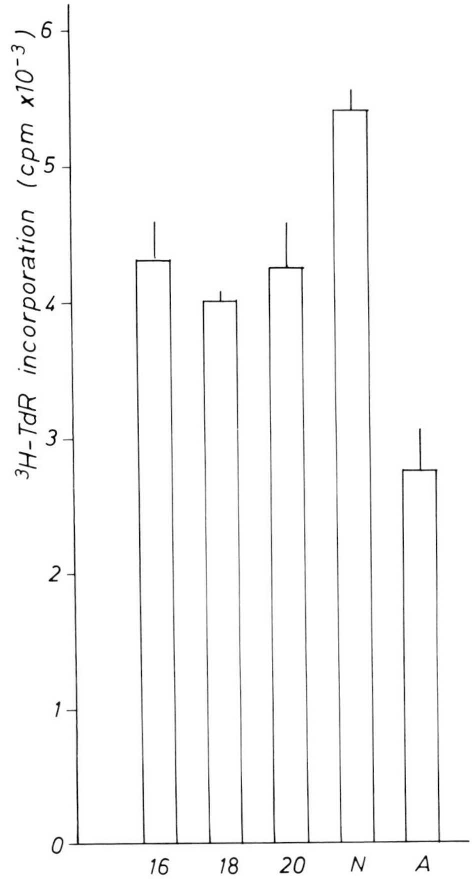

Figure 1 IL-1 production during prenatal period of life. EC culture supernatant (1%, v/v), obtained from fetuses between 16 and 20 days old (as indicated), newborn (N) or adult (A) donor was tested for IL-1 activity in the D10S bioassay (mean ± SE of triplicate cultures).

Table 1 IL-1 Production During Postnatal Period of Life

Reciprocal dilution	EC supernatant: Newborn	EC supernatant: 1 month	EC supernatant: 12 months	Human rIL-1: pg/ml	Human rIL-1: cpm ± SE
	[^{3}H]thymidine incorporation (cpm ± SE)				
20	—	4290 ± 124	3816 ± 126	100	25484 ± 1107
80	10117 ± 623	3921 ± 163	2101 ± 113	25	18242 ± 623
320	3425 ± 225	1251 ± 17	1100 ± 65	6.25	6429 ± 343
1280	1467 ± 66	812 ± 57	694 ± 17	1.5	1810 ± 304

The spontaneous [^{3}H]thymidine uptake of D10S cells was 733 ± 5 cpm.

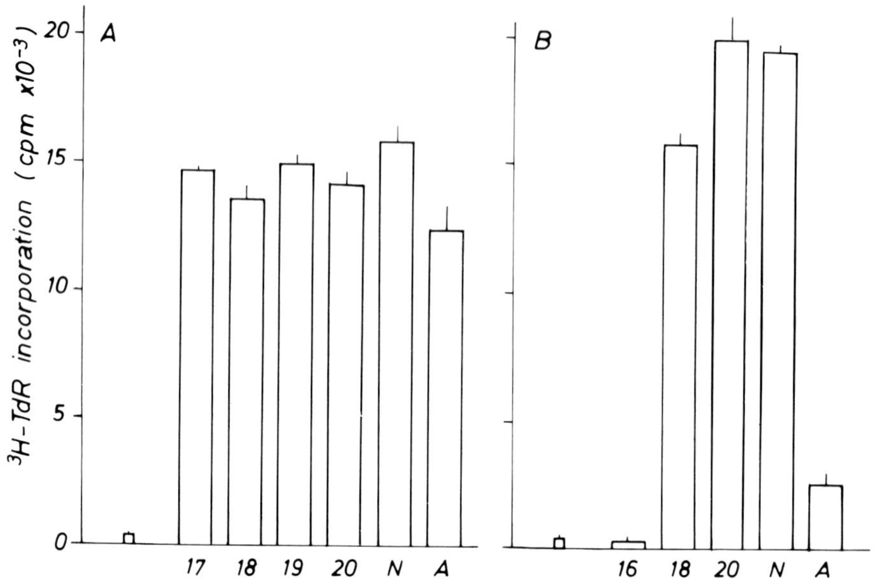

Figure 2 IL-6 production during prenatal period of life. EC culture supernatant (0.3%, v/v), obtained from fetuses between 16 and 20 days old (as indicated), newborn (N) or adult (A) donor was tested for IL-6 activity in the B9 bioassay (mean ± SE of triplicate cultures). A and B: results of two representative experiments.

synergistic interaction of IL-1 and IL-6 in thymocyte proliferation was also inhibited by GC-induced EC-derived products. Glucocorticoid-induced inhibitory factors also affected the direct mitogenic effect of IL-1 on D10S cells, and to a lesser degree on fibroblasts, but did not affect IL-2–dependent proliferation of T-cell blasts (10). Glucocorticoid-induced inhibitor appeared to be a direct receptor antagonist of IL-1.

In the present study, we measured the production of GC-induced inhibitory cytokines in fetal, newborn and adult rat epidermis. In order to detect IL-1–inhibitory activity, thymocytes, or D10S cells were supplemented with human rIL-1 during titration of GC-induced EC products, while for detection of IL-6 inhibitors, human rIL-6 was added to

Table 2 IL-6 Production During Postnatal Period of Life

Reciprocal dilution	EC supernatant: Newborn	EC supernatant: 3 months	EC supernatant: 12 months	Human rIL-6	
	$[^3H]$thymidine incorporation (cpm ± SE)			pg/ml	cpm ± SE
100	33700 ± 1499	28576 ± 417	13909 ± 471	18	40691 ± 708
300	25159 ± 1064	15349 ± 1348	8633 ± 1130	6	25205 ± 720
1000	8771 ± 885	4846 ± 169	3302 ± 10	2	14791 ± 2657

The spontaneous $[^3H]$thymidine uptake of B9 cells was 707 ± 18 cpm.

either thymocytes or B9 cells. Obtained results showed (data not presented) that both IL-1– and IL-6–inhibitory activities are expressed very early, i.e., in epidermis of newborn rats, and decline progressively with age. On the other hand, during the prenatal period GC-induced inhibitors could not be detected until day 20 of gestational age, when tested either on D10S cells or on B9 cells.

CONCLUSION

Thus, our results suggest that immunoregulatory cytokines are differentially and complexly regulated during maturation of epidermis.

REFERENCES

1. Ansel JC, Luger TA, Lowry D, Perry P, Roop DR, Mountz JD. The expression and modulation of IL1α in murine keratinocytes. J Immunol 1988; 140:2274–78.
2. Kupper T, May L, Birchall N, Seghal P. Keratinocytes produce IL6, a cytokine which can provide a 2nd signal in the activation of T cells. J Invest Dermatol 1988; 90:578A.
3. Kirnbauer R, Köck A, Schwarz T., Urbanski A, Krutmann J, Borth W, Damm D, Shipley G, Ansel JC, Luger TA. IFNβ 2, B cell differentiation factor 2, or hybridoma growth factor (IL-6) is expressed and released by human epidermal cells and epidermoid carcinoma cell lines. J Immunol 1989; 142:1922–28.
4. Stošić-Grujičić S, Lalošević Dj, Lukić ML. Modulatory effects of glucocorticoids on immunoregulatory functions of epidermal cells. Int J Immunopharmacol 1987; 9:577–85.
5. Helle M, Boeije L, Aarden LA. IL6 is an intermediate in IL1-induced thymocyte proliferation. J Immunol 1989; 142:4335–38.
6. Orencole SF, Dinarello CA. Characterisation of a subclone (D10S) of the D10.G4.1 helper T-cell line which proliferates to attomolar concentrations of interleukin 1 in the absence of mitogens. Cytokine 1989; 1:14–22.
7. Sauder DN, Ponnappan U, Cinader B. Effects of age on cutaneous interleukin 1 expression. Immunol Lett 1989; 20:111–14.
8. Aarden LA, De Groot ER, Schaap OL, Landsdorp PM. Production of hybridoma growth factor by human monocytes. Eur J Immunol 1987; 17:1411–16.
9. Stošić-Grujičić S, Lukić ML. Immunoregulation in epidermis. II. Immunostimulatory and immunoinhibitory products of keratinocytes. Acta Derm Venereol (Stockh) 1989; 146:16–19.
10. Stošić-Grujičić S, Lukić ML, Simić MM. The mechanisms of action of glucocorticoid-induced interleukin 1 inhibitor. Period Biol 1990; 92:28–29.

54

Subcellular Localization of Cytokines and Their Receptors in Peripheral Lymphoepithelial Organs

B. von Gaudecker,[1] V. Mielke,[1] M. A. Ritter,[2] and W. Sterry[1]
[1]*University of Kiel, Kiel, Federal Republic of Germany;*
[2]*Royal Postgraduate Medical School, London, England*

INTRODUCTION

There is increasing evidence for the central role of cytokines in the functional regulation of various cell types participating in immune responses.

Interleukin 1 (IL-1) is now known to be a product of many cell types, not just macrophages. It has a broad spectrum of biological activities, generally stimulatory, on immune cells (1). Macrophages produce predominantly IL-1β at high levels. Keratinocytes mainly produce IL-1α. Both IL-1α and IL-1β are also secreted by endothelial cells and some B and T cells.

Interleukin 2 (IL-2) and interleukin 4 (IL-4) are produced by T cells, predominantly helper T cells (2). Interleukin-2 promotes growth of activated T cells, B cells as well as cytotoxic T cells, and natural killer (NK) cells. Interleukin-4 was shown to be involved in the early activation of resting B cells, but it also induces both proliferation and maturation of thymocytes, T cells, and B cells.

In the present investigation, we demonstrate immunoreactivity of anti-IL-1β, anti-IL-2, anti-IL-4, and anti-IL-4R monoclonal antibodies (MAbs) in peripheral lymphoepithelial organs.

MATERIALS AND METHODS

The following MAbs were used:

Designation	Reactivity	Source
FIB3	IL-1 β	Prof. H. D. Flad, Borstel, Germany
Bo7	rIL-2	Dr. E. Brand, Borstel, Germany
anti-IL-4	IL-4	Dr. S. Gillis, Seattle, Washington
MR6	IL-4 R	Prof. M. Ritter, London, England

For immuno-electron microscopy small pieces of human tonsils or skin biopsies were fixed for 1 hr in 4% paraformaldehyde, rinsed in buffer, and frozen after cryoprotection with 0.6 M saccharose. Thirty-micrometer cryostat sections were incubated with each of the MAbs. This first antibody was followed by a goat antimouse immunoglobulin G (IgG), coupled with 5-nm gold particles (Janssen, B2430 Olen, Belgium). After postfixation with 2% glutaraldehyde, the sections were silver enhanced, osmicated, and flat embedded in araldite (3,4). These sections have also been evaluated by light microscopy. Controls included omission of first and second antibody, and silver enhancement alone.

RESULTS

In the tonsil, three immunologically important areas were studied; these are the germinal centers (B-cell regions), the parafollicular areas (T-cell dominated), and the crypt epithelium. All investigated MAbs against cytokines revealed an intracytoplasmic localization of the reaction product. Label for IL-1 β was found within the macrophages in all areas. Also interdigitating cells (IDCs) in the parafollicular areas showed intracytoplasmic reaction products, whereas lymphocytes were negative. Some of the reticulated epithelial cells of the crypt epithelium also showed a positive reaction. Anti-interleukin-2 revealed reaction product in the cytoplasm of some lymphocytes; these were medium to large sized, and predominantly found within the T-cell areas. Unexpectedly, some macrophages and IDCs revealed rather strong intracytoplasmic reactivity. Anti-interleukin-4 gave a very weak reaction; few lymphoblasts in the T-cells areas, including some mitotic cells, showed this reactivity.

The MAb MR6, which reacts against IL-4 R, showed clear surface labeling. Particularly macrophages in the follicular centers and the T cell region showed strong reaction, but also follicular dendritic reticulum cells (FDRCs) and IDCs were positive. Only a small fraction of lymphoid cells showed moderate surface reactivity. Such lymphocytes frequently were observed in closed contact to antigen-presenting cells (APCs) both in the T- and B-cell areas; remarkably, the IL-4 R reactivity was strikingly high on those cell surface areas directly opposing the APCs. The crypt epithelium was negative.

Inflamed skin (allergic contact dermatitis) shows dense lymphohistiocytic perivascular infiltrates in the papillary dermis, and some of the mononuclear cells also infiltrated the epidermis. All lymphoid cells exhibited a strongly lobulated nucleus in contrast to the tonsil lymphocytes. Label for IL-1 β was found only in macrophages in the papillary dermis and in indeterminate cells within the epidermis. Endothelial cells, keratinocytes, and lymphocytes were negative. Cells reacting with anti-IL-2 were unevenly distributed. Rarely we found small accumulations of labeled mononuclear cells. However, in most regions, only scattered positive lymphocytes were present, most of them being in close contact with—as in the tonsil—some positively labeled APCs. Cells reacting positively with anti-IL-4 have not been recognized in inflamed skin. The antibody MR6 against the IL-4 R revealed a weak surface label on some macrophages and rarely on medium-sized lymphoid cells in the papillary dermis. In a few instances, a positive macrophage was surrounded by weakly labeled lymphocytes.

DISCUSSION

Our findings show for the first time that ultrastructural localization of cytokines and their receptors is possible using appropriate fixation and staining techniques. Figure 1

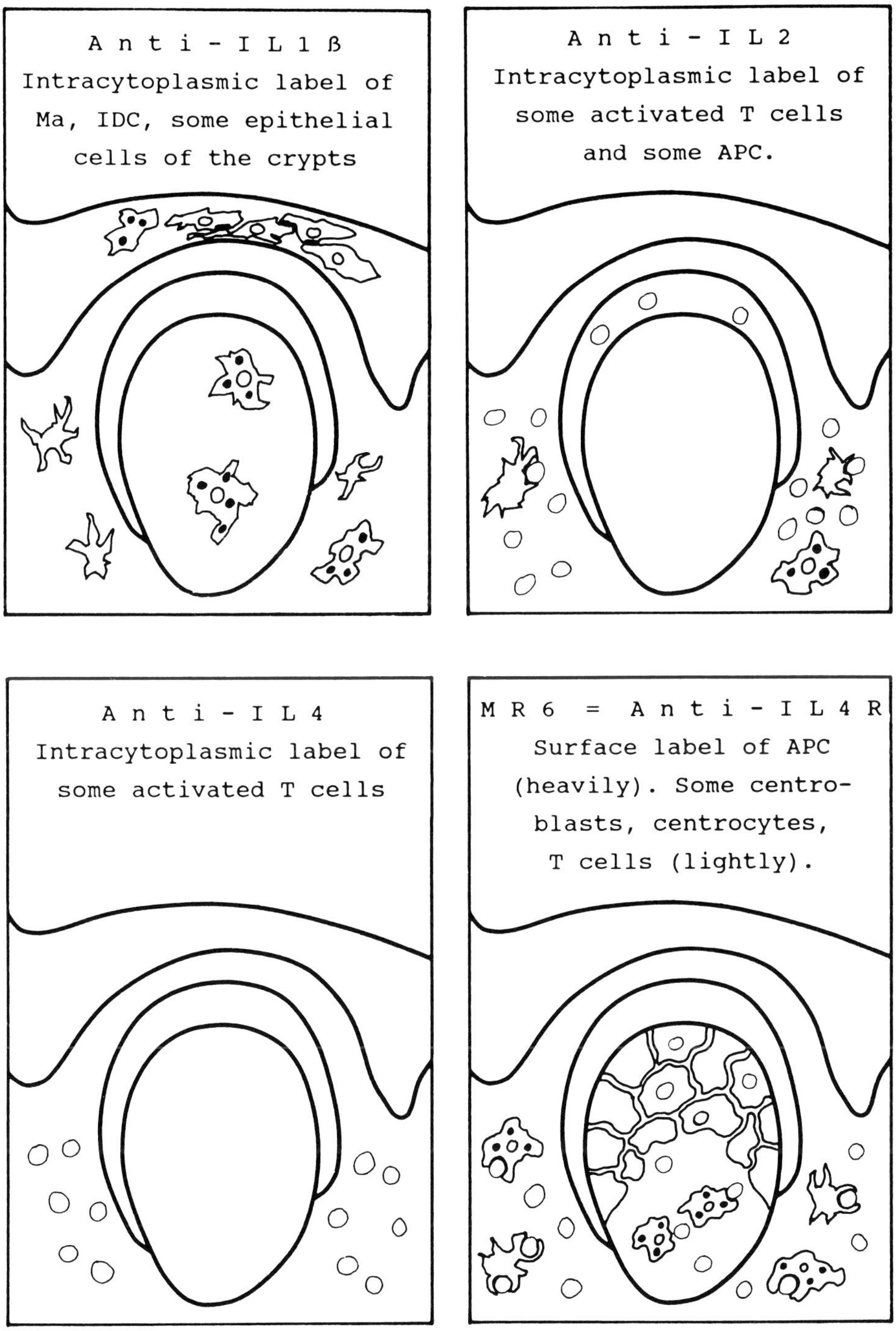

Figure 1 Distribution of positive reacting cells in the tonsillar unit "crypto-lymphon," which consists of one follicle, the parafollicular area at both sides, and the crypt epithelium. The different cell types are specifically labelled by the indicated moAbs. Ma: macrophage; IDC: interdigitating cell; APC: antigen-presenting cell.

summarizes schematically our findings in the "crypto-lymphon," the functional unit of the tonsil (3). The somewhat unexpected finding of both intracytoplasmic and membrane labeling using anti-IL-2 has also been observed in cultured lymphocytes; Steinmann found Jurkat cells to show intracellular IL-2 reactivity, whereas cytotoxic T cells exhibit a membrane reactivity (5). Whether the IL-2 reactivity in macrophages is due to IL-2 presence, or is caused by cross-reacting molecules, remains to be further clarified. The MAb MR6, which reacts with the IL-4 receptor (6), gives a clearcut surface labeling.

Furthermore, an accumulation of cytokine receptors toward neighboring cells has also been observed on thymocytes facing thymic epithelial cells (7). Finally, the fact that a similar staining pattern like in tonsil also has been observed in inflamed skin underlines the importance of ultrastructural cytokine and cytokine receptor demonstration as a powerful tool in the investigation also of pathophysiological conditions in medicine.

ACKNOWLEDGMENTS

This investigation was supported by grants from the Deutsche Forschungsgemeinschaft. The authors appreciate the excellent technical assistance of Mrs. W. Müller, Mrs. K. Schlender, Mrs. H. Siebke, and Mrs. H. Waluk as well as Mrs. J. Schlahn for secretarial assistance.

REFERENCES

1. Durm SK, Oppenheim JJ. Macrophage-derived mediators. In: Paul WE (ed). *Fundamental Immunology*, 2nd ed. New York, Raven Press, 1989, pp. 639–661.
2. Gillis S. T-cell-derived lymphokines. In: Paul WE (ed). *Fundamental Immunology*, 2nd ed. New York, Raven Press, 1989, pp. 621–638.
3. Gaudecker B v. Development and functional anatomy of the human tonsilla palatina. Acta Otolaryngol (Stockh) 1988, Suppl. 454:28–32.
4. Gaudecker B v, Larché M, Schuurman H-J, Ritter MA. Analysis of the fine distribution of thymic epithelial microenvironmental molecules by immuno-electron microscopy. Thymus 1989, 13:187–194.
5. Steinmann GG, Conlou P, Hefeneider S. Serological visualization of IL-2. Science 1983, 220:1188–1190.
6. Larché M, Ritter MA. IL-4, oncogenesis and the thymus. In: Kendall M, Ritter MA, eds. Thymus update, Vol. 2. Harwood Academic Pub. London Paris New York 1989:59–72.
7. Farr AG, Anderson SK, Marrak P, Kappler J. Expression of antigen specific major histocompatibility restricted receptors by cortical and medullary thymocytes in situ. Cell 1985, 43: 543–553.

55
Pathological Effects of Cytokines on the Intestine

Paul Garside, E. Allison Green, and Allan McI. Mowat
Western Infirmary, Glasgow, Scotland

INTRODUCTION

The intestinal lesion which occurs in mice with graft-vs-host reaction (GVHR) provides an experimental model for the immune mediated enteropathy seen in several small intestinal conditions, including, celiac disease, Crohn's disease, and several parasitic infections (1,2). Previous studies have provided indirect evidence that soluble mediators released during a local delayed-type hypersensitivity (DTH) reaction are responsible for the characteristic consequences of this lesion, including villus atrophy, crypt hyperplasia, and increased numbers of intraepithelial lymphocytes (3–6). More recently, we and others have prevented intestinal GVHR by the administration of antibodies against interferon-γ (IFN-γ) (7) and tumor necrosis factor (TNF) (8).

EXPERIMENTAL PROTOCOL

In Vivo

The enteropathic effects of IFN-αβ, IFN-γ, and TNF α in vivo were determined by injecting normal $(CBA \times Balb/c)F_1$ mice with 10^5 U cytokine. Intestinal damage was assessed by measuring jejunal villus and crypt lengths by microdissection and crypt cell production rates (CCPRs) using a metaphase arrest technique (4–6).

The ability of IFN-αβ to enhance natural killer (NK) cell activity was determined using YAC-1 cells in a conventional microcytotoxicity assay as previously described (7).

Natural killer cells were depleted in vivo by treating mice with anti-asialo GM_1 antibody (9).

In Vitro

The rat intestinal crypt cell line (10) (RIE) was used to determine the ability of recombinant IFN-γ and TNF α to be directly cytotoxic or cytostatic to epithelial cells in vitro. Cell numbers were assessed using the MTT colourimetric assay.

RESULTS

Effects of IFN-αβ on NK Cell Activity

Markedly increased NK activity was apparent 24 hr after administration of IFN-αβ (data not shown). This was still present at 48 hr but had subsided by 72 hr postinjection. Maximal effects were seen with a dose of 10^5 U IFN-αβ; therefore this was chosen for the intestinal studies.

Effects of IFN-αβ on Mucosal Architecture

Six hours after injection of 10^5 U IFN-αβ normal (CBA×Balb/c)F_1 mice had some increase in crypt length compared with controls but this did not reach statistical significance; there was no change in villus length. However, by 24 hr, IFN-injected mice had significant increases in crypt length and significant villus shortening (Fig. 1a).

Prevention of IFN-αβ–Induced Enteropathy by anti-asialo GM_1

As IFN-αβ enhanced NK activity, we examined whether these cells were required for its effect on the gut. Depletion of NK cells with anti-asialo GM_1 antibody prevented the villus atrophy and crypt hyperplasia observed in animals given IFN-αβ (Fig. 1b).

Effects of TNF α on Mucosal Architecture

TNF α also caused enteropathy in normal mice, inducing moderate, although not statistically significant villus atrophy and crypt lengthening by 3 hr after injection (Fig. 2a). Significant villus atrophy and crypt hypertrophy were apparent by 6 hr. The increased crypt length was maintained throughout the period examined but the villus atrophy had recovered by 72 hr when villi from TNF α–treated animals were significantly longer than controls (Fig. 2b).

Cytostatic Effects of IFN-γ on Intestinal Epithelial Cells In Vitro

Interferon-γ had no measurable effect in vivo but markedly inhibited the proliferation of RIE cells grown in the presence of serum-containing growth factors (Fig. 3a). Interferon-γ also enhanced the expression of class I (MHC) major histocompatibility complex molecules and induced de novo expression of class II MHC antigens on RIE cells (data not shown).

Toxicity of TNF α for Intestinal Epithelial Cells

In the conventional bioassay rTNF α was equally toxic to actinomycin D treated L929 fibroblasts and RIE intestinal crypt cells (Fig. 3b).

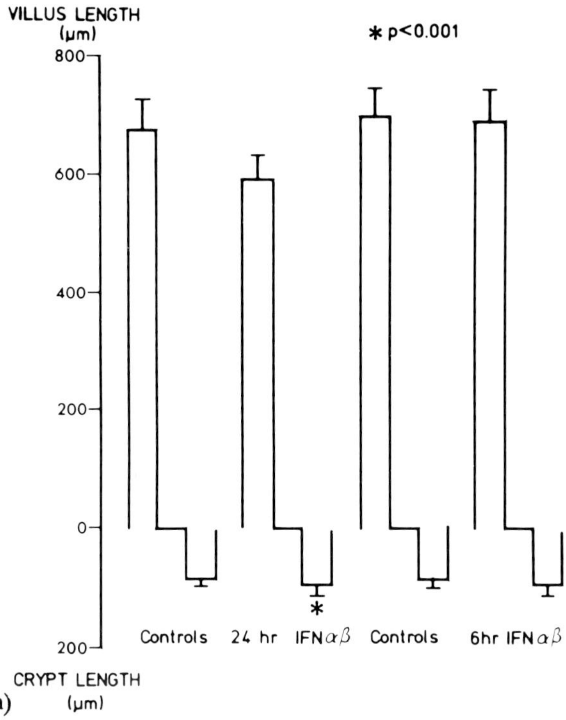

(a)

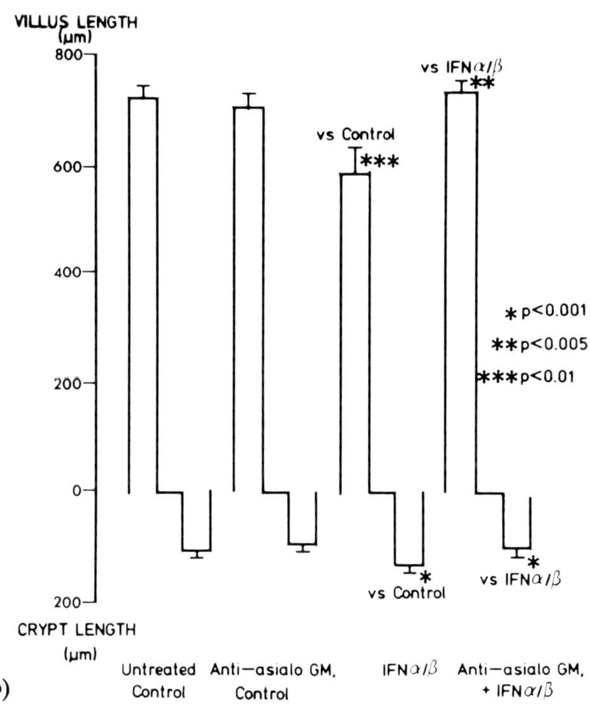

(b)

Figure 1 (a) Induction of enteropathy by IFN-αβ. Villus and crypt lengths in jejunum of mice injected with 10^5 U IFN- αβ 6 or 24 hr previously. (b) Prevention of IFN-αβ–induced enteropathy by antiasialo GM_1. Villus and crypt lengths in jejunum of animals treated with 10^5 U IFN-αβ with or without anti-asialo GM_1 antibody.

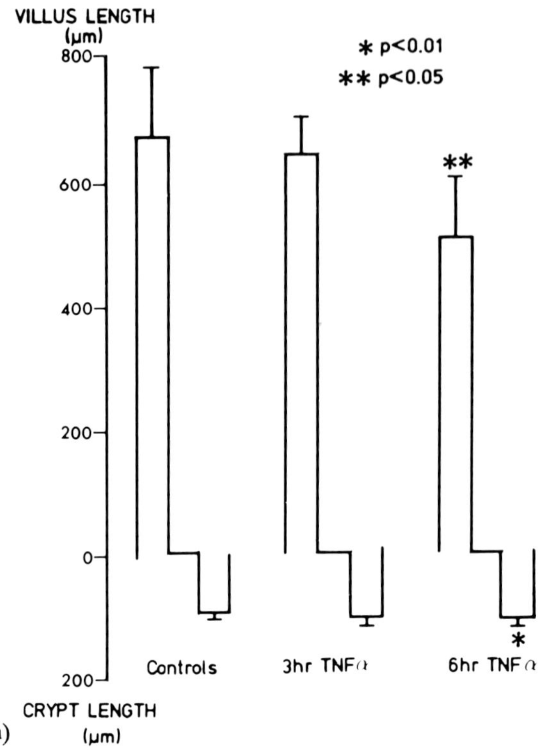

(a)

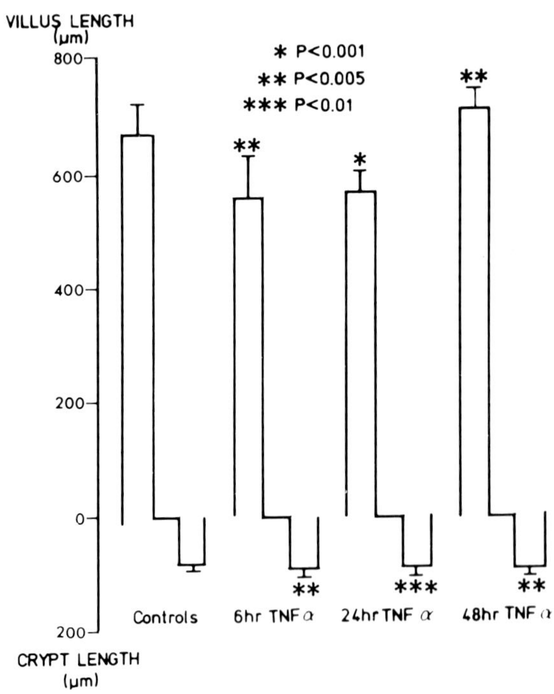

(b)

Figure 2 (a and b) Induction of enteropathy by TNF α. Villus and crypt lengths in jejunum of mice injected with 10^5 U TNF α 3, 6, 24, or 48 hr prior to killing.

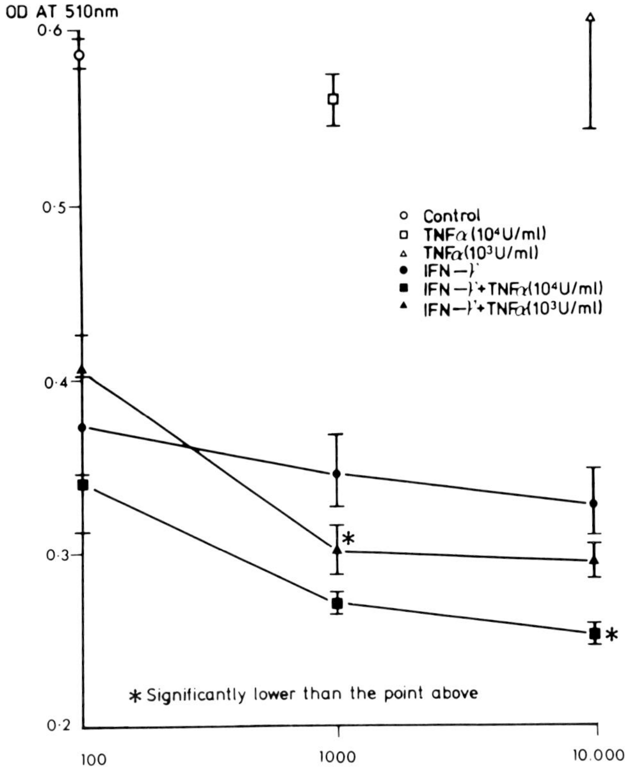

(a)

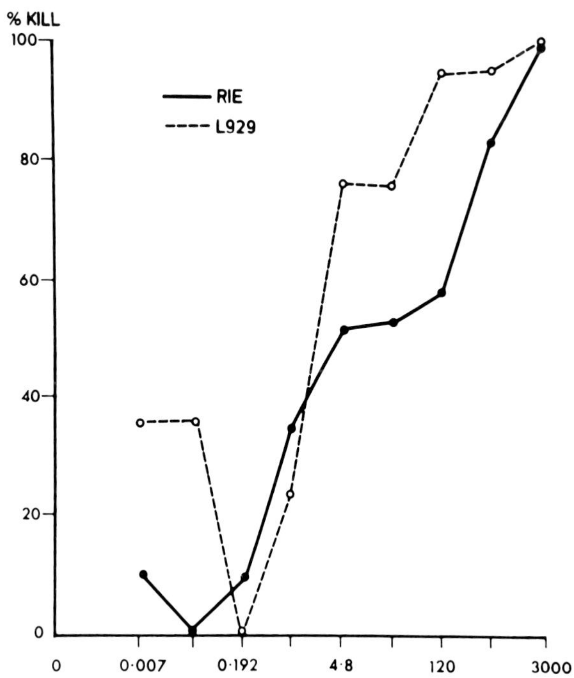

(b)

Figure 3 (a) Cytostatic effects of IFN-γ on RIE cells in vitro. (b) Lysis of actinomycin D–treated L929 fibroblasts or RIE cells by TNF α.

Enhancement of Cytostatic Effects of IFN-γ on Intestinal Epithelial Cells by TNF α

Alone, rTNFα had no effect on the proliferation of RIE cells, but it did enhance the cytostatic effect of IFN-γ on these cells (Fig. 3a).

DISCUSSION

The results provide direct evidence that cytokines are involved in enteropathy.

Production of IFN-γ by lymphoid cells from animals undergoing a GVHR (12) and prevention of the intestinal consequences of GVHR by antibodies against IFN-γ (7) have both been observed. This cytokine may act directly on the gut and/or activate nonspecific immune effector mechanisms such as macrophages and NK cells (13,14), which could damage the intestine by lytic attack on enterocytes or, alternatively, produce further inflammatory mediators. Our study has shown that IFN-γ is cytostatic for epithelial cells in vitro and enhances their expression of MHC antigens. However, IFN-γ had no demonstrable effect in vivo, possibly because it does not reach its site of action when administered in this manner or because its role in immune-mediated enteropathy is to render epithelial cells more sensitive to nonspecific effector mechanisms as a result of enhanced MHC class II expression (15,16).

We also found that IFN-αβ caused significant enteropathy within 24 hr of its administration. Furthermore, this cytokine enhanced NK activity in a dose-dependent manner and the intestinal lesion was prevented by antibodies to NK cells. Increased levels of IFN-αβ (12) have been reported in GVHR, and it is possible that one role of IFN-γ is to stimulate production of IFN-αβ by macrophages with resulting enhanced NK activity which in turn leads to gut damage.

Significant alterations in mucosal architecture were also apparent following injection of TNF α, which was also directly cytotoxic for RIE cells in vitro and enhanced the cytostatic effect of IFN-γ on these cells. Tumor necrosis factor α may act via a variety of mechanisms in GVHR, including direct cytotoxicity, effects on mucosal vascular tissue, or enhanced NK activity.

Overall, this study provides direct support for the hypothesis that inflammatory cytokines are the effector mechanisms responsible for enteropathy associated with local cell-mediated immunity.

ACKNOWLEDGMENTS

E. Allison Green was in receipt of a Wellcome Vacational Scholarship, and the study was supported by The Medical Research Council.

REFERENCES

1. Ferguson, A. & Mowat, A.McI. Immunological mechanisms in the small intestine. In: Wright, R. (ed). *Advances in Gastrointestinal Pathology*. Philadelphia, Saunders, 1980, pp. 93–103.
2. Mowat, A.McI. The immunopathogenesis of food sensitive enteropathies. In: T.J. Newby and C.R. Stokes (eds.). *Local Immune Responses of the Gut*. Boca Raton, Florida, CRC Press, 1984, pp. 199–225.

3. Hedberg, C.A., Reiser, S. & Reilly, R.W. Intestinal phase of the runting syndrome in mice. II. Observations on nutrient absorption and certain disaccharide abnormalities. Transplantation 1968; 6:104–110.
4. MacDonald, T.T. & Ferguson, A . Hypersensitivity reactions in the small intestine. III. The effects of allograft rejection and of GvHD on epithelial cell kinetics. Cell. Tiss. Kinet. 1977; 10:301–312.
5. Mowat, A.McI. & Ferguson, A. Hypersensitivity reactions in the small intestine. VI. Pathogenesis of the graft-versus-host reaction in the small intestinal mucosa of the mouse. Transplantation 1981; 32:238–243.
6. Mowat, A.McI. & Ferguson, A. Intraepithelial lymphocyte count and crypt hyperplasia measure the mucosal component of the graft-versus-host reaction in mouse small intestine. Gastroenterology 1982; 83:417–423.
7. Mowat, A.McI. Antibodies to IFN-γ prevent immunologically mediated intestinal damage in murine graft-versus-host reaction. Immunology 1990; 68:18–23.
8. Piguet, P.-F., Grau, G.E., Allet, B. & Vassalli, P. Tumor necrosis factor/cachectin is an effector of skin and gut lesions of the acute phase of graft-vs-host disease. J. Exp. Med. 1987; 166:1280–1289.
9. Felstein, M.V. "Immunological Mechanisms of Intestinal Graft-versus-host Reactions." 1988 Ph.D. Thesis, University of Glasgow.
10. Blay, J. & Brown, K.D. Characterization of an Epithelioid cell line derived from rat small Intestine: Demonstration of cytokeratin filaments. Cell Biology International Reports 1984; 8:551–560.
11. Heeg, K., Reimann, J., Kabelitz, D., Hardt, C. & Wagner, H. A rapid colorimetric assay for the determination of IL-2-Producing Helper T Cell Frequencies. J. Immunol. Meth. 1985; 77: 237–246.
12. Cleveland, M.G., Annable, C.R. & Klimpel, G.R. *In vivo* and *in vitro* production of IFN-β and IFN-γ during graft vs host disease. J. Immunol. 1988; 141:3349–3356.
13. Spitalny, G.L. & Havell, E.A. Monoclonal antibody to murine gamma interferon inhibits lymphokine-induced anti-viral and macrophage tumoricidal activities. J. Exp.Med. 1984; 159:1560–1571.
14. Trinchieri, G. & Perussia, B. Immune interferon: a pleiotropic lymphokine with multiple effects. Immunol. Today 1986; 6:131–135.

B CELLS

56
Differentiation Stages and Microenvironmental Organization of B-Cell Genesis in Vivo

Dennis G. Osmond
McGill University, Montreal, Quebec, Canada

A plan of the B-lymphocyte lineage is outlined in Figure 1 to illustrate some problem areas which will be addressed in the present chapter.

Within central lymphoid organs (bone marrow in rodents and humans, Peyer's patch in sheep, bursa of Fabricius in birds), self-renewing *stem cells* give rise to B lineage–committed *pro–B cells* which, after rearrangement of V_H gene segments, express free cytoplasmic μ heavy chains as *pre–B cells* and then, after rearranging V_L gene segments, become *primary (virgin) B lymphocytes,* expressing surface membrane immunoglobulin M (sIgM), to which is added sIgD. The existence of B lymphoid–restricted stem cells has been suggested in mouse bone marrow by the use of retrovirus-marked stem cells, but the nature and degree of precommitment of stem cells entering the avian bursa have remained controversial. Cell population dynamic studies have revealed a succession of cell divisions by pro–B and pre–B cells, allowing estimates of the potential daily output of B-cell clones. It has become clear, however, that there is also a major degree of cell loss. The mechanisms of cell death and deletion, and the stages in the differentiation pathway at which they may operate, require further study to examine the role of cell selection, including the clonal deletion of potentially self-reactive cells, in shaping the actual clonal output of primary B cells. In situ immunolabeling methods have begun to explore the tissue organization of primary B-cell genesis in rodent bone marrow. Early B-lineage cells tend to occupy peripheral subosteal microenvironments, and they make intimate associations with stromal reticular cells and macrophages before entering vascular sinusoids from which, after a temporary storage phase, they are discharged into the blood stream. The clonal and spatial arrangement of B-precursor cells in situ, their regulatory interactions with stromal cells, the role of short-range cytokines, and the nature of adhesion molecules, all remain outstanding problems.

Homing via the blood into the peripheral lymphoid tissues, newly formed virgin B cells usually die after a short life span of only a few days. If, in this time, they are appropriately activated, however, they may instead reenter the cell cycle, leading to the

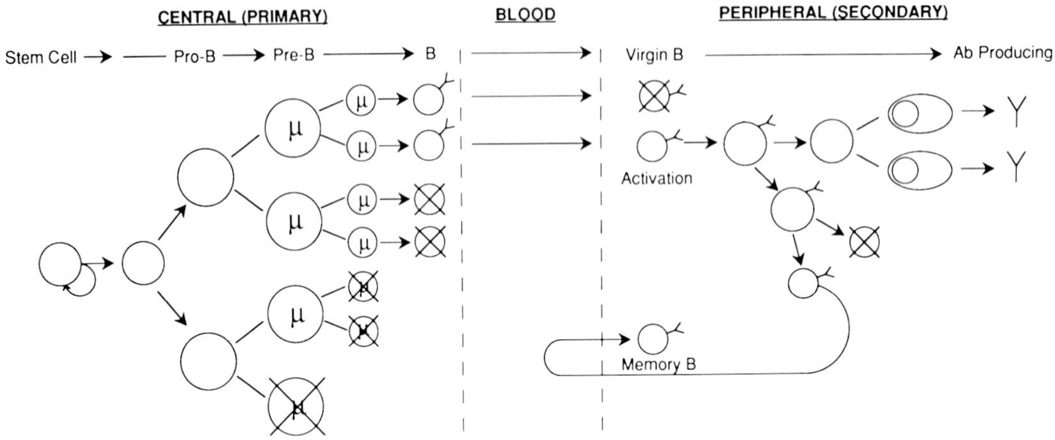

Figure 1 Overview of the B-lymphocyte lineage in vivo.

formation of *antibody-producing cells* and a second wave of B lymphocytes. These *secondary (memory) B lymphocytes* differ from primary B cells in surface Ig isotype, life span, and migratory properties. They now have the capacity to "patrol" the immune system by recirculating between the various peripheral lymphoid tissues and the blood stream. Vital stages in these programmed switches in cell properties occur during a second phase of clonal proliferation and programmed cell death within transient germinal centers. The mutation, regulation, and selection of memory B cells remain incompletely resolved issues. Little is known of the molecular basis for the anatomical localization of lymphocyte subsets in peripheral lymphoid tissues. Although the heterogeneity of B-cell life spans has long been established, methods of multiparameter flow cytometry, combining immunological and cell cycle markers, now make important contributions in correlating B-cell life span and immune function. Other current technologies, including the use of transgenic and mutant mice, immunolabeling by monoclonal antibodies, in situ hybridization, and the availability of recombinant cytokines, are also adding much impetus to studies of the B-cell lineage in vivo.

57
Cell Deletion in B-Cell Genesis and the Role of Bone Marrow Macrophages

Karen Jacobsen and Dennis G. Osmond
McGill University, Montreal, Quebec, Canada

INTRODUCTION

The in vivo production of B lymphocytes in the bone marrow entails a sequence of cell differentiation and proliferation, generating a continuous output of diverse B-cell clones (1). Not all these B-lineage cells are destined to reach the immune system, however. Studies of cell population dynamics have suggested that many cells are lost during B-cell genesis, though this process has not been directly visualized, and the mechanism by which B-lineage cells may be deleted from the bone marrow is not known.

Phenotype and Proliferation of B-Lymphocyte Precursor Cells

The differentiation of B-precursor cells in mouse bone marrow falls into three main stages, based on the expression of the μ heavy chain of IgM; (a) pro–B cells precede the expression of the μ chains, (b) pre–B cells have free μ chains within their cytoplasm, and (c) B cells express μ chains in surface IgM molecules (2–4). Pro–B cells in mouse bone marrow have been subdivided into three stages by the expression of B220 glycoprotein, a B-lineage–associated surface molecule detected by monoclonal antibodies (MAbs), including MAb 14.8, and terminal deoxynucleotidyl transferase (TdT), a nuclear enzyme expressed during μ chain gene rearrangement and apparently involved in inserting nucleotides at the junctions between V-D-J gene segments (3–5). Early pro–B cells express TdT, intermediate pro–B cells express TdT plus B220, and late pro–B cells express B220 alone. Pre–B cells represent the final mitotic step. Large cμ-positive pre–B cells divide to give small cμ-positive pre–B cells, which mature without further division into sμ-positive B cells.

The foregoing cell phenotypes in mouse bone marrow appear to form a continuous differentiation sequence from the stage of heavy chain gene rearrangement to the mature B cell. According to this model, transient expression of TdT precedes and overlaps the onset of B220 expression, which is followed by the synthesis of free μ chains, the rearrangement of light chain genes, and, finally, the synthesis of membrane-form IgM. B220, once expressed, is retained throughout the B-cell lineage. Metaphase arrest techniques have indicated that the B-lineage cells undergo a series of mitoses, at least one mitosis at each pro–B cell stage and large pre–B cell stage, and possibly more than one mitosis (two to three) at the late pro–B cell stage, totaling five to six in all (4).

Cell Loss During B-Cell Genesis

The dynamics of B-cell genesis in mouse bone marrow have been studied by combining mitotic arrest and immunolabeling techniques, determining the rate of production of cells at each of the foregoing phenotypic stages of development (2–4). The resulting values show a progressive expansion in total cell population through the three pro–B cell compartments, which can be reconciled with a flow of cells from one developmental stage to the next. Thereafter, however, marked discrepancies between the predicted and observed number of cells passing through the various differentiation compartments per unit time provide strong circumstantial evidence of a major degree of cell loss. Because the precursor cells themselves are not seen elsewhere in the immune system in normal adult mice, these data imply that the cells are actually lost through local cell death. In the mouse, the calculated cell loss represents approximately 75% of the lineage, mainly evident at the large-to-small pre–B cell stage. In the rat, similar calculations suggest a 60% loss, occurring mainly at the small pre–B to B-cell transition (6,7). These may be minimal estimates, however. The data cannot exclude the possibility that loss may also occur at earlier stages of differentiation. Yet, morphological examination of the bone marrow has shown little evidence of such a massive cell death, and the ways in which B-lineage cells are deleted are unknown.

Two main mechanisms in normal mice may be postulated to lead to B-precursor cell death. First, Ig gene rearrangement is prone to error and is often ineffective. There may be failure of V-D-J joining, nonproductive rearrangement of heavy or light chains, and incompatible heavy and light chains. Second, emerging self-reactive B cells may be deleted if they encounter self-specific antigens locally in high concentration (8). Various perturbations may further enhance the level of cell loss. Differentiating B-lineage cells are unusually sensitive to elevated levels of glucocorticoid steroid hormones and to low doses of ionizing irradiation. In vitro, such stimuli can initiate an actively programmed cell death, termed apoptosis, characterized by endonuclease activation, deoxyribonucleic acid (DNA) fragmentation, and chromatin condensation, followed by lysosomal degradation within phagocytes (9–12). B-cell genesis in the bone marrow occurs within a network of stromal cells, including resident macrophages, many of which actively phagocytose foreign particles and extruded erythroblast nuclei (13–14). Their relationship to B-cell genesis, however, has not been observed.

In previous studies, we have developed methods to examine B-lineage cells in mouse bone marrow at the ultrastructural level in situ, by the radioautographic detection of B-lineage–associated MAbs administered intravenously (15–18). The work has revealed the location and microenvironmental associations of B220-positive cells and sIgM-positive cells in vivo under a variety of experimental conditions.

The present work has been designed to visualize directly the deletion of specifically labeled B220-positive B-lineage cells in the bone marrow of young mice, aiming to examine the possible role of bone marrow macrophages, the various stages of development at which B-lineage cells may be deleted, and the morphological features associated with cell death. In addition to normal mice, we have examined three experimental models of cell deletion which we have previously characterized in terms of cell population dynamics. (a) The scid mutant mouse is unable to produce B lymphocytes, apparently because of a recombinase deficiency leading to an inability to join V, D, and J coding elements and cell death (19), (b) mice treated with anti-IgM antibodies from birth, a process which deletes all newly formed B lymphocytes as they begin to express sIgM in the bone marrow (20), and (c) Eμ-myc transgenic mice which exhibit a preneoplastic expansion of precursor B cells in the bone marrow without a commensurate expansion of the B-cell population (21). These experimental systems permit a comparison between conditions of cell death and deletion at various stages of B-cell genesis.

MATERIALS AND METHODS

Animals

Three- to four-week-old male C3H/H3J mice were purchased from Jackson Laboratories, Bar Harbor, Maine. (C57BL/6XC3H) F_1 hybrid mice were kindly provided by Dr. J. Gordon, Department of Experimental Surgery, McGill University, Montreal, Quebec, Canada, and were injected i.p. with rabbit antimouse IgM (5–10 mg in 0.05–0.10 ml) three times weekly from birth, as detailed previously (20). Control mice received normal rabbit serum. Four-week-old CB.17 scid mice were generously supplied by Dr. R.A. Phillips Ontario Cancer Institute, Toronto, Ontario, Canada, and maintained under sterile conditions. Eμ-myc transgenic mice were used in collaboration with Dr. C. Sidman, Jackson Laboratories, Bar Harbor, Maine.

Antibody and Radioiodination

The rat MAb 14.8 (5), derived from cultures of hybridoma cells, was affinity purified and concentrated to 2 μg/ml. The MAb 14.8 (150 μg) was coupled to 2 mCi Na-^{125}I (specific activity 1.5×10^7 μCi/μg) by a modified chloramine-T method resulting in a final concentration of 50 μg/ml.

In Vivo Labeling with MAb 14.8

Under chloral hydrate anesthesia (1.6% in 0.9% NaCl; 0.75 ml/25 g body weight) mice received a single 100-μl injection of ^{125}I–MAb 14.8 into the jugular vein. Following a 3-min circulation time, whole-body intravascular perfusion was established through the heart to wash out unbound antibody and finally to fix the tissues with a cacodylate-buffered solution of 2.5% glutaraldehyde and 2.0% acrolein (pH 7.4).

Tissue Processing and Radioautography

Perfusion-fixed femurs were decalcified in EDTA (330–340 mOsm, pH 7.4) for 5–7 days and postfixed in reduced osmium tetroxide for 3 h at 4°C. Femurs were then dehydrated in acetone, infiltrated, and embedded in epon 812. Mid-diaphyseal transverse sections were cut and processed for light and electron microscope radioautography, as described (15,16).

Analysis of Light and Electron Microscope Radioautographs

Complete transverse sections of femoral bone marrow were analyzed to quantitate the B220-positive cells as well as the number of macrophages in successive 2160 μm^2 fields as delineated by an ocular grid micrometer. Electron microscope radioautographs were scanned and photographed using a Phillips 301 electron microscope.

RESULTS

Normal Mice

Electron microscopy of bone marrow of normal young C3H/HeJ mice revealed numerous macrophages sending lengthy complex processes between hemopoietic cells throughout the extravascular compartment (Figs. 1 and 2). Sections passing through the cell body and nucleus included copious cytoplasm, electron-dense inclusion bodies, and a variety of lysosomal profiles.

At brief intervals, (2–3 min) after i.v. administration of ^{125}I–MAb 14.8, the B220-positive B-lineage cells showed heavy radioautographic cell surface labeling (see Fig. 1), and accounted for 20% of all nucleated cells. Frequently, labeled B220-positive cells were closely associated with macrophages over considerable portions of their surface membranes, the adjacent membranes sometimes appearing less distinct than usual (see Fig. 1). The macrophage-associated B220-positive cells were heterogeneous in morphology, often,

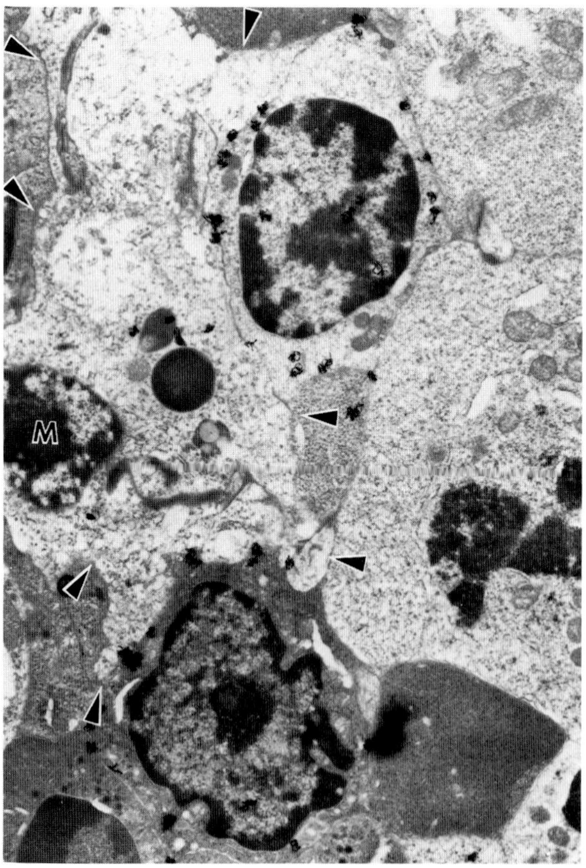

Figure 1 Electron microscope radioautograph of C3H/HeJ mouse bone marrow 3 min after i.v. administration of ^{125}I–MAb 14.8, showing two labeled B220$^+$ cells closely associated with a macrophage (M) (arrow heads). One B220$^+$ cell has increased cytoplasmic and nuclear electron density. (Magnification: ×6120)

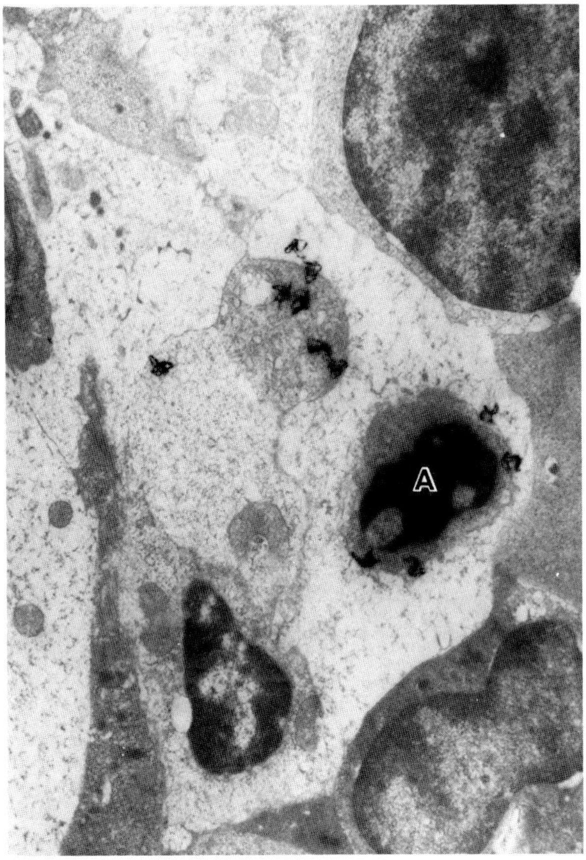

Figure 2 A $B220^+$ lineage cell (A) with an electron dense, apoptotic, nucleus is found within the cytoplasm of a bone marrow macrophage in a C3H/HeJ mouse 20 min after i.v. labeling with ^{125}I MAb 14.8. (Magnification: ×8550)

however, showing a large size and moderate amounts of cytoplasm. They showed an increased electron density of cytoplasm in some cases (see Fig. 1).

When 10–20 min elapsed after i.v. injection of ^{125}I–MAb 14.8, the association of labeled B220-positive cells with macrophages was more readily and frequently seen. Labeled B220-positive cells were often located apparently entirely within macrophages, surrounded completely by macrophage cytoplasm (see Fig. 2), in addition to B220-positive cells associated with the macrophage surface. The nucleus of some of the macrophage-associated B220-positive cells showed condensation of chromatin (see Fig. 2) and the cells, though intact, showed electron-dense cytoplasm. These appearances characterize the process of apoptosis.

Anti-IgM–Treated Mice

The bone marrow of mice treated repeatedly from birth with anti-IgM antibodies, examined by light microscopy, revealed a much reduced incidence of B220-positive cells associated

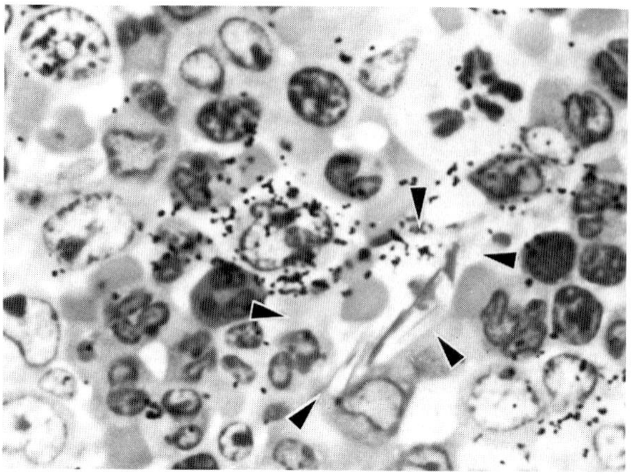

Figure 3 Light microscope radioautograph of bone marrow from an anti-IgM–treated (C57BL/6 × C3H) F_1 mouse, showing a large labeled $B220^+$ cell intimately associated with a macrophage (arrow heads) containing phagocytosed debris and rodlike inclusions. (Magnification: ×1250)

with a strikingly increased prominence of complex macrophages containing large numbers of darkly staining inclusion bodies (Fig. 3).

Scid Mice

B220-positive cells were examined in scid mutant mice at intervals of 10–20 min after i.v. administration of ^{125}I–MAb 14.8. Of the small number of labeled B220-positive cells present, some were in patchy areas near the surrounding bone, some were scattered more centrally, and some were within vascular sinusoids. The scattered B220-positive cells at both time intervals, were often located apparently within macrophages surrounded by macrophage cytoplasm (Fig. 4). These B220-positive cells were sometimes large cells, showing some irregularity of nuclear profile, peripheral chromatin condensation, and a generalized electron density (Fig. 5). These appearances were consistent with those of the early stages of apoptosis. Other cells showed the highly condensed chromatin, shrunken profile, electron density, and endoplasmic vacuoles characteristic of advanced apoptosis. The macrophages exhibited many intracytoplasmic inclusion bodies.

Eμ-myc Transgenic Mice

Electron microscopic examination of bone marrow of Eμ-myc transgenic mice during the prelymphomatous phases of development showed many macrophages, each containing numerous large circular cellular inclusions (Fig. 6). The inclusions exhibited extensive chromatin condensation and generalized electron density. Many macrophages contained linear or sheetlike profiles of crystalloid structures (Fig. 7).

DISCUSSION

The present work has visualized at the ultrastructural level the cellular basis of B-lineage cell deletion in mouse bone marrow. B-cell precursor cells, identified by in vivo immunolabeling of the B220 surface glycoprotein, frequently become closely associated with and internalized by resident macrophages. The various experimental models used reflect the

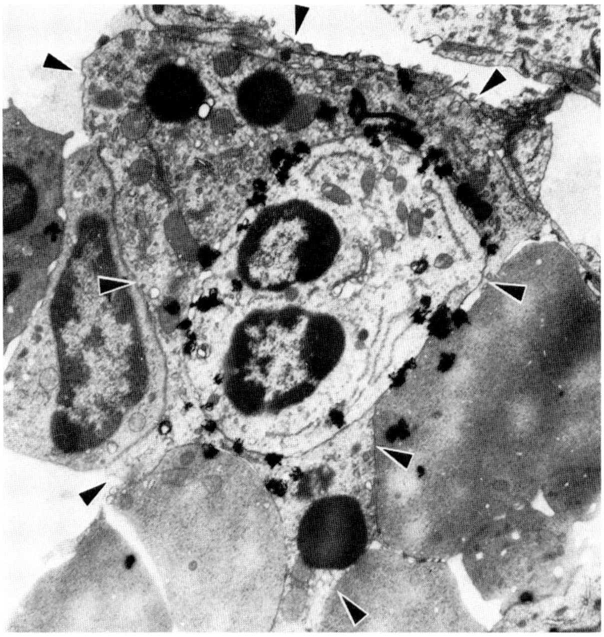

Figure 4 In a scid mouse, an immature B220$^+$ cell containing many mitochondria, evident rough endoplasmic reticulum, and much cytoplasm is virtually surrounded by cytoplasmic processes of a bone marrow macrophage (arrow heads). (Magnification: ×6750)

deletion of cells at various stages of differentiation, yet the role of the macrophage appears to be common to all.

Deletion of B-Lineage Cells by Bone Marrow Macrophages

Bone marrow macrophages have previously been assigned regulatory roles in erythrocytopoiesis and granulocytopoiesis. The present work now indicates that macrophages also play a role in relation to the development of the B-cell lineage, by removing a fraction of the B-precursor cells. The macrophages engaged in this process correspond in distribution with those of acid phosphatase–positive cells and of macrophages with long processes detected by MAb F4/80 binding throughout the extravascular compartment of the bone marrow (14). The cells observed to delete B-lineage cells in the present work show other characteristics of bone marrow macrophages, including prominent lysosomal structures (22) and crystalloid inclusions (23).

The frequency with which B220-positive cell–macrophage associations can be observed in normal mice, and their striking prominence in scid mice, anti-IgM–treated mice, and Eμ-myc mice suggest that macrophage-mediated deletion of B-lineage cells is a major process. This is emphasized by the preliminary evidence revealing the rapidity of B220-positive cell clearance. In the course of 10–20 min, many B220-positive cells which were initially labeled by in situ exposure to radiolabeled MAb 14.8 become ingested by macrophages, a process which is particularly well marked in scid mice in which the entire B-cell lineage aborts. The observations suggest that macrophage activity could readily

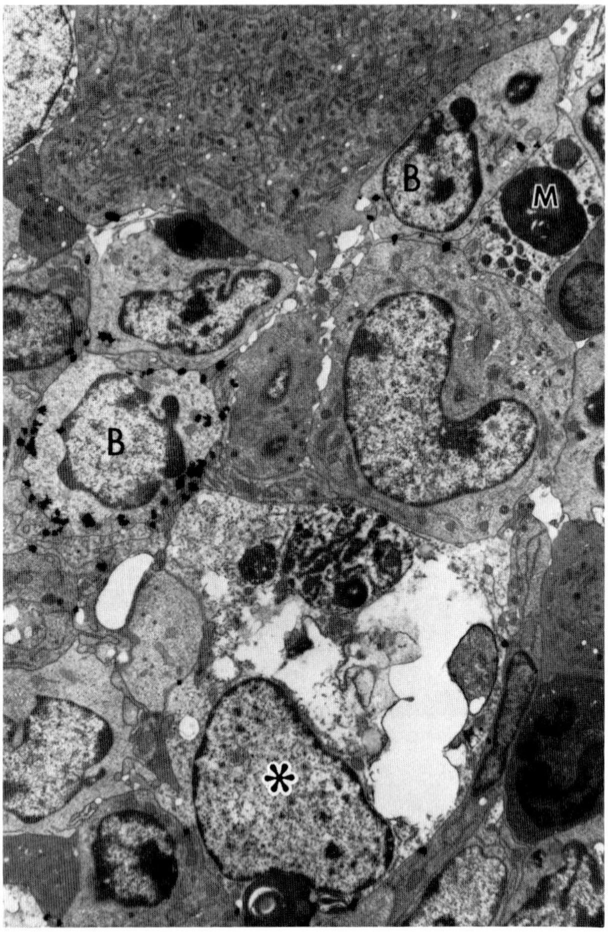

Figure 5 Two $B220^+$ cells (B) adjacent to cytoplasmic processes of two macrophages (M and *), each containing two to three phagosomes, in bone marrow of scid mouse. (Magnification: ×3750)

account for the high rate of B-lineage cell deletion indicated by population dynamic studies in normal mice and in the three experimental perturbations of B-cell loss used in the present work.

Programmed Cell Death of B-Lineage Cells in Bone Marrow

Many of the B220-positive cells associated with or internalized by bone marrow macrophages show morphological features consistent with the programmed form of cell death termed apoptosis (9–12). Further verification of this mode of cell death will require analysis of DNA for evidence of fragmentation.

The apoptotic appearance of macrophage-associated B220-positive cells suggests that they are entering a programmed self-deleting process. The macrophages would not themselves be responsible for killing B-lineage cells but only for rapidly recognizing and

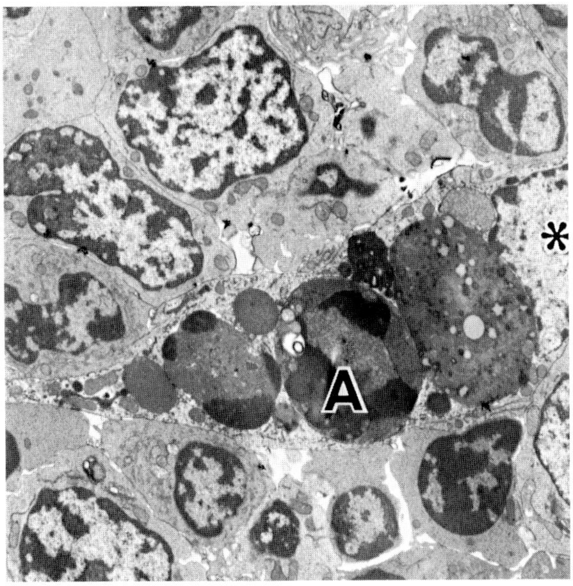

Figure 6 Macrophage (*) containing many ingested apoptotic nuclear profiles (A) in the bone marrow of a Eμ-myc transgenic mouse. (Magnification: ×4200)

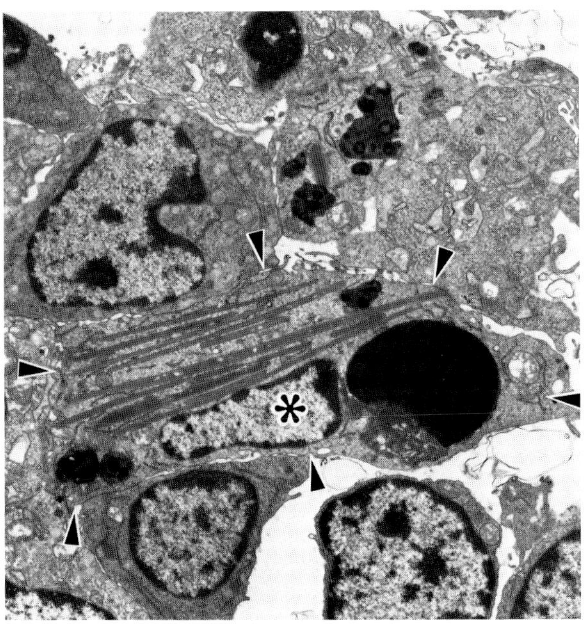

Figure 7 Bone marrow from a Eμ-myc transgenic mouse, showing a macrophage (*) containing phagosomes and crystalloid inclusions. Arrowheads indicate macrophage periphery. (Magnification: ×5400)

disposing of cells which have already been actively triggered into the apoptotic pathway (24).

The stages at which B-lineage cells are deleted and the signals for their deletion may be various. Many B220-positive cells associated with macrophages in the bone marrow of normal mice are relatively large cells rather than terminal small lymphocytes. This accords with kinetic evidence in mice suggesting cell loss at the large-to-small pre–B cell stage (2–4). In scid mice, cells are all deleted at the late pro–B cell stage, when they are apparently rapidly recognized and taken up by local macrophages. In Eμ-myc transgenic mice, the pro–B and pre–B cell compartments are expanded,, but many cells appear to be lost at the pre–B cell stage. This accords with the present findings of multiple apoptotic bodies in prominent macrophages. In anti-IgM–treated mice, however, B-precursor cells of all stages remain but are subsequently deleted at the point at which they would normally begin to express IgM as small postmitotic cells (20). Anti-IgM–treated mice thus provide a model of clonal deletion, which may normally involve the elimination of clones of newly formed B cells which meet high concentrations of appropriate self-antigens in the bone marrow. Transgenic mice have demonstrated that clonal deletion of self-reactive immature B cells can indeed occur in the bone marrow under appropriate circumstances (8).

Cell Selection in Primary B-Cell Genesis

The large-scale loss of cells by programmed cell death and macrophage deletion now appears to be a general phenomenon in primary lymphocytopoiesis. Substantial cell loss by apoptosis has been demonstrated during primary B-cell genesis in Peyer's patches in sheep, and in the bursa of Fabricius in chickens. The process is reminiscent of primary T-cell genesis, in which the great majority of cells die in the thymus. The engagement of the T-cell receptor by antibodies leads to apoptosis, possibly mimicking the mechanism of T-cell self-tolerance by clonal deletion (25).

Lymphocytes undergoing programmed cell death after ionizing irradiation rapidly bind to vitronectin on the surface of macrophages to initiate ingestion (24). The rapid selection and ingestion of B220-positive cells by mouse bone marrow macrophages appear to account for the paradoxical experimental observations of an extensive B-precursor cell loss with no evident accumulation of dying cells. This appears to be part of a general biological mechanism for the deletion of individual cells which become switched into a pathway of programmed cell death in the course of development.

ACKNOWLEDGMENTS

This work was supported by the Medical Research Council of Canada and the National Cancer Institute of Canada.

REFERENCES

1. Osmond DG. Population dynamics of bone marrow B lymphocytes. Immunol Rev 1986; 93: 103–24.
2. Opstelten D, Osmond DG. Pre-B cells in mouse bone marrow: Immunofluorescence stathmokinetic studies of the proliferation of cytoplasmic μ-chain-bearing cells in normal mice. J Immunol 1983; 131:2635–40.
3. Park YH, Osmond DG. Phenotype and proliferation of early B lymphocyte precursor cells in mouse bone marrow. J Exp Med 1987; 165:444–58.

4. Park YH, Osmond DG. Dynamics of early B lymphocyte precursor cells in mouse bone marrow: proliferation of cells containing terminal deoxynucleotidyl transferase. Eur J Immunol 1989; 19:2139–44.
5. Kincade PW. Experimental models for understanding B lymphocyte formation. Adv Immunol 1987; 41:181–267.
6. Deenen GJ, Hunt SV, Opstelten D. A stathmokinetic study of B lymphocytopoiesis in rat bone marrow: Proliferation of cells containing cytoplasmic μ-chains, terminal deoxynucleotidyl transferase and carrying HIS24 antigen. J Immunol 1987; 702–10.
7. Deenen GJ, Balen IV, Opstelten D. In rat B lymphocyte genesis sixty percent is lost from the bone marrow at the transition of nondividing pre-B cell to $sIgM^+$ B lymphocyte, the stage of Ig light chain gene expression. Eur J Immunol 1990; 20:557–64.
8. Nemazee DA, Burki K. Clonal deletion of B lymphocytes in a transgenic mouse bearing anti-MHC class I antibody genes. Nature 1989; 337:562–66.
9. Wyllie AH, Morris RG, Smith AL, Dunlop D. Chromatin cleavage in apoptosis: association with condensed chromatin morphology and dependence on macromolecular synthesis. J Pathol 1984; 142:67–77.
10. Cohen JJ, Duke RC. Glucocorticoid activation of a calcium-dependent endonuclease in thymocyte nuclei leads to cell death. J Immunol 1984; 132:38–42.
11. Sellins KS, Cohen J. Gene induction by γ-irradiation leads to DNA fragmentation in lymphocytes. J Immunol 1987; 139:3199–3206.
12. Clarke PGH. Developmental cell death: morphological diversity and multiple mechanisms. Anat Embryol 1990; 181:195–213.
13. Weiss L, Sakai H. The hematopoietic stroma. Am J Anat 1984; 170:447–63.
14. Hume DA, Robinson AP, MacPherson GG, Gordon S. The mononuclear phagocyte system of the mouse defined by immunohistochemical localization of antigen F4/80. Relationship between macrophages, Langerhans cells, reticular cells, and dendritic cells in lymphoid and hematopoietic organs. J Exp Med 1983; 158:1522–36.
15. Osmond DG, Batten SJ. Genesis of B lymphocytes in the bone marrow: Extravascular and intravascular localization of surface IgM-bearing cells in mouse bone marrow detected by electron-microscope radioautography after in vivo perfusion of ^{125}I- anti-IgM antibody. Am J Anat 1984; 170:349–65.
16. Batten SJ, Osmond DG. The localization of B lymphocytes in mouse bone marrow: Radioautographic studies after in vivo perfusion of radiolabeled anti-IgM antibody. J Immunol Meth 1984; 72:381–99.
17. Osmond DG, Jacobsen K, Park YH, Lamontagne L. In vivo localization of B lymphocyte progenitor cells in mouse bone marrow. In: Fossum S and Rolstad B (eds). *Histophysiology of the Immune System*. New York, Plenum, 1988, pp. 45–51.
18. Jacobsen K, Tepper J, Osmond DG. Early B-lymphocyte precursor cells in mouse bone marrow: Subosteal localization of $B220^+$ cells during postirradiation regeneration. Exp Hematol 1990; 18:304–310.
19. Bosma GC, Custer RP, Bosma MJ. A severe combined immunodeficiency mutation in the mouse. Nature 1983; 301:527–30.
20. Opstelten D, Osmond DG. Regulation of pre-B cell proliferation in bone marrow: Immunofluorescence stathmokinetic studies of cytoplasmic μ chain-bearing cells in anti-IgM-treated mice, hematologically deficient mutant mice and mice given sheep red blood cells. Eur J Immunol 1985; 15:599–605.
21. Langdon WY, Harris AW, Cory S, Adams JM. The c-myc oncogene perturbs B lymphocyte development in Eμ-myc transgenic mice. Cell 1986; 47:11–8.
22. Strausbauch P, Sehgal N. Three-dimensional reconstruction of anomalous beige mouse macrophage lysosomes. J Leuk Biol 1989; 47:11–8.
23. Yamazaki K. Isolated cilia and crystalloid inclusions in murine bone marrow stromal cells. Blood Cells 1988; 13:407–16.

24. Savill J, Dransfield I, Hogg N, Haslett C. Vitronectin receptor-mediated phagocytosis of cells undergoing apoptosis. Nature 1990; 343:170–3.
25. Smith CA, Williams GT, Kingston R, Jenkinson EJ, Owen JJT. Antibodies to CD3/T-cell receptor complex induce death by apoptosis in immature T cells in thymic cultures. Nature 1989; 337:181–4.

58
Differentiation of B Cells in Germinal Centers

Michael Apel and Claudia Berek
Institute for Genetics, University of Cologne, Cologne, Federal Republic of Germany

INTRODUCTION

Germinal centers (GCs) are believed to be the major site of the differentiation of antigen-activated B cells. In this particular microenvironment, they may switch the immunoglobulin (Ig) isotype, hypermutate, and the resulting mutants may be selected to give rise to high affinity memory and plasma cells (1). However, little is known about the changes single B cells undergo in GCs. Germinal center cells (GCCs) make up only a minor part of the B cells found in lymphoid organs; hence a molecular analysis of them is still missing. We have tried to circumvent this problem by immortalization of GCCs by cell fusion. Such cell lines should provide further clues about the differentiation processes happening in GCs.

RESULTS AND DISCUSSION

Kinetics of Germinal Center Development After Immunization

Germinal center cells are characterized by their high binding capacity of peanut agglutinin (PNA^{high} cells). Hence, they can be distinguished from the major low binding population of splenic B cells (PNA^{low} cells) (2). We have used this property to follow the development of GCs during the murine primary immune response against the antigen phenyloxazolone (phox). At different time points after immunization, splenic cells were stained with a monoclonal antibody (MAb) against the B-cell marker B220 (using phycoerythrin) and with FITC-labeled PNA, and thereafter analyzed by two-color fluorescence analysis as recently described (3). Figure 1 shows the kinetics of the GC reaction. The percentage of PNA^{high} B cells increases three- to fourfold up to day 10 of the immune response, and declines within the following 2 weeks to background levels. In frozen sections of spleens, we observed a comparable development in the size of the GCs. The PNA^{high} cells did not express surface immunoglobulin D (IgD), only low levels of other isotypes and high

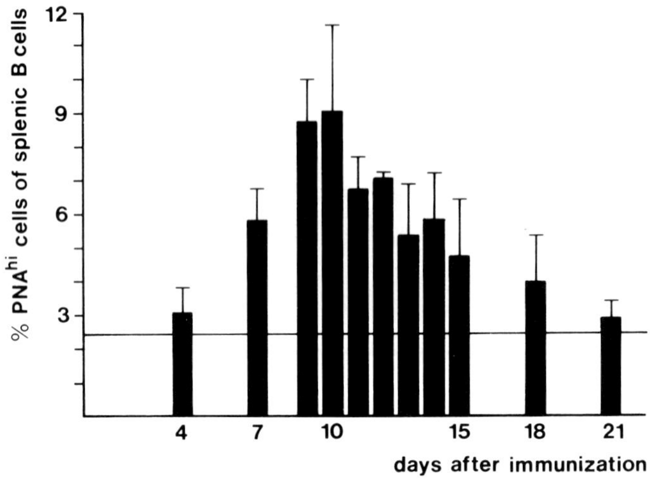

Figure 1 Kinetics of development of PNA^{high} cells. At the indicated days after immunization, the percentages of PNA^{high} B cells were determined by FACS analysis. The horizontal bar designates the background of nonimmunized mice. For each value, at least three experiments were performed.

amounts of major histocompatibility complex (MHC) class II molecules (data not shown). All together, the kinetics and the phenotype are in good agreement with the results of similar studies (4,5).

PNA^{high} Cells Show High Fusion Frequencies, PNA^{low} Cells Do Not

In the second week of the immune response at the height of the GC reaction, PNA^{high} and PNA^{low} splenic B cells were isolated by FACS (fluorescence-activated cell sorter). Reanalysis of the sorted populations revealed that the PNA^{low} cells contained less than 1% PNA^{high} cells, and the PNA^{high} cells 5–15% PNA^{low} cells. From both populations hybridoma lines were produced. Their supernatants were tested by ELISA assays for the production of antigen-specific antibodies and for their isotypes. Although only 2–4×10^5 PNA^{high} cells were isolated from a single mouse, up to 49 hybridoma lines were obtained. In particular, at day 10 PNA^{high} cells fused with a high efficiency (Fig. 2a), a result that could be reproduced in several independent experiments. The control fusions from total splenic cells confirm that the experiments with sorted cells are significant.

GCs Harbor the Antigen-Activated Cells

Whereas the fusion frequency of PNA^{low} B cells is constant, that of PNA^{high} cells increases up to the peak of the germinal center reaction, as demonstrated in Figure 2a. This effect is more dramatically seen if one considers only the antigen-specific lines (Fig. 2b). For instance, at day 10, 10^5 PNA^{high} cells gave rise to 61 times more antigen-specific lines than did the same number of PNA^{low} cells. These high fusion frequencies reflect the rapid rate of division of the antigen-specific cells which leads to the observed increase in GC size.

The conclusion that GCs harbor the antigen-specific B cells was extended by the analysis of the antigenic specificities and isotypes of the antibodies produced. Table 1 gives the numbers and isotypes of antigen-specific hybridomas obtained between 7 and 13 days

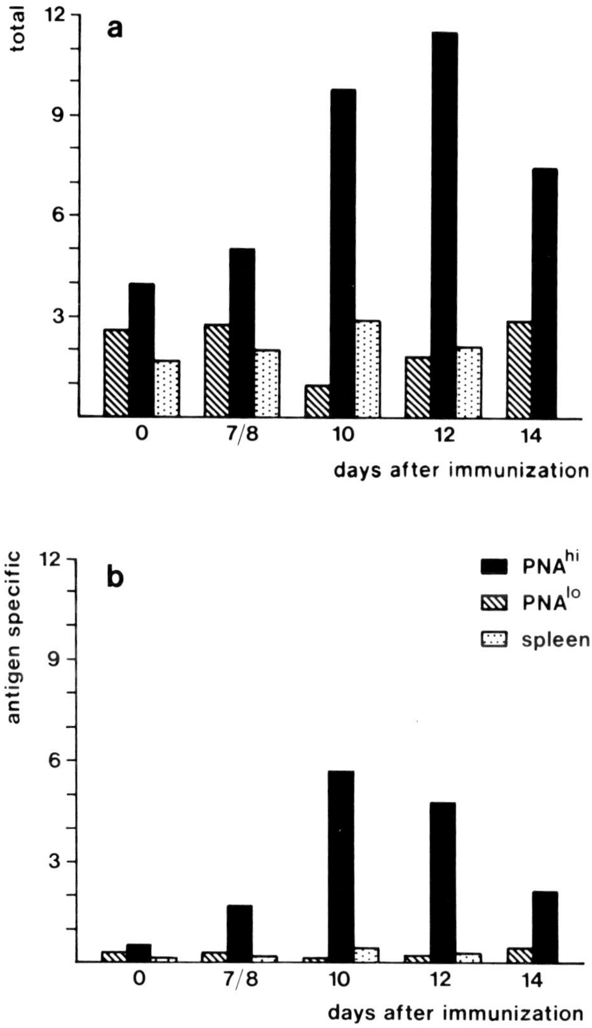

Figure 2 Fusion frequencies. Fusion frequencies were calculated from the total (a) and the antigen specific (b) number of hybridomas per 10^5 fused cells. For each time point values shown are the means of several independent experiments. The numbers of fusion experiments are given Table 1. Data for days 7 and 8 have been pooled.

after immunization from PNA^{high}, PNA^{low} and, total splenic B cells. The total number of hybridomas is given in parentheses; superscripts indicate the number of independent experiments. Although PNA^{high} cells make up only 9% of splenic B cells at day 10, they give rise to 53% of all hybridoma lines and 89% of the antigen-specific ones. With one exception (day 14), all IgG-producing lines were recovered from PNA^{high} cells. The 10–12% IgM-producing lines from PNA^{low} cells may represent the background level of unspecifically activated cells because they are also present in nonimmunized control mice (day 0). At days 10, 12, and 14, all lines from PNA^{low} cells showed cross reactivity with

Table 1 Analysis of Hybridomas Derived From PNA^{high}, PNA^{low}, and Total Splenic Cells

		Day											
	Ig	0		7		8		10		12		14	
	M	20		5		14		8		8		12	
PNA^{low}			(158)^2		(70)^2		(82)^2		(95)^4		(85)^1		(101)^2
	G	—		—		—		—		—		1	
	M	1		2		3		21		17		9	
PNA^{high}			(7)^2				(23)^2		(109)^4		(76)^1		(39)^2
	G	—		3	(9)^2	3		41		14		2	
	M	15				15		18		19			
Spleen			(166)^2				(306)^1		(302)^1		(328)^1		
	G	—				7		24		19			

another antigen (nitrophenyl). In contrast, at day 10, only 25% of the IgM PNA^{high}–derived hybridomas and none of the IgG-producing lines were cross reacting. Only at early stages (before day 10) there may exist a small population of antigen-specific PNA^{low} cells. Such cells, presumably activated outside the follicles, may indeed be the precursors of GCCs.

Antigen-Activated GCCs Switch the Ig Isotype Early During the Primary Response

Already at days 7 and 8, a major part of the PNA^{high}-derived hybridomas expresses IgG. The percentage of IgG-producing lines increases with the number of PNA^{high} cells until day 10, and declines thereafter. The fact that antigen-activated IgG-bearing cells are at this time point exclusively in the GCs supports the hypothesis that the class switch takes place in this microenvironment (2). Thus, even early during B-cell differentiation, a fraction of the cells proliferating in the GCs may switch the Ig isotype. We cannot exclude the possibility that some cells may switch the Ig class before entering the GCs. However, because the fraction of IgG expressing antigen-specific lines increases up to day 10 among PNA^{high}-derived lines, it is likely that the class switch happens during the proliferation in the GCs.

When the GC reaction declines at around days 12–14, we obtained less IgG-producing hybridomas. Two factors may contribute to this. First, many of the cells may have reached a differentiation stage at which they are incapable of fusion (memory or plasma cells). Second, many of the antigen-activated cells may by this time have left the GCs. This may explain why the only IgG-producing line from PNA^{low} cells was recovered from day 14.

CONCLUSIONS

Our data demonstrate that the antigen-activated B cells reside within the GCs during the second week of the immune response. The high fusion frequencies may be due to the rapid proliferation of GCCs, which leads to an enormous expansion of antigen-specific cells within the GCs. Consequently, the percentage of antigen-specific hybridomas among

PNA^{high}-derived lines increases to 57% at day 10. In contrast, we obtained from PNA^{low} cells only a cross-reactive background, which had a lower fusion efficiency.

It has been shown by others that in lymph nodes GCCs are predominantly IgM positive on day 6 after immunization, and predominantly IgG after secondary immunization (2). Our results show that the class switch in the PNA^{high} population occurs early in the primary response. Approximately half of the hybridomas already expresses IgG at days 7 and 8. Those B cells recruited into the GCs express a typical V-gene combination which gives rise to high affinity antibodies (3). We have previously presented evidence that during the ensuing proliferation phase V genes are diversified by somatic mutation (3). Because we find this antigen-specific expansion taking place within the PNA^{high} subset of B cells, our data strongly support the notion that GCs provide the microenvironment for the maturation of the immune response.

REFERENCES

1. Nieuwenhuis P, Opstelten D. Functional anatomy of germinal centers. Am J Anat 1984; 170: 421–435.
2. Kraal G, Weissman IL, Butcher EC. 1982. Germinal centre B cells: Antigen specificity and changes in heavy chain class expression. Nature 1982; 298:377–379.
3. Apel M, Berek C. Somatic mutations in antibodies expressed by germinal centre B-cells early after primary immunisation. Int Immunol 1990; 2:813–819.
4. Coico RF, Bhogal BS, Thorbecke GJ. Relationship of germinal centers in lymphoid tissue to immunologic memory. J Immunol 1983; 131:2254–2257.
5. Butcher EC, Rouse RV, Coffman RL, Nottenburg CN, Hardy RR, Weissman IL. Surface phenotype of peyer's patch germinal center cells: Implications for the role of germinal centers in B cell differentiation. J Immunol 1982; 129:2698–2707.

59
Prebursal Rearrangement of Immunoglobulin Light Chain Genes in the Chicken

Olli Lassila, Antti Mansikka, and Paavo Toivanen
Turku University, Turku, Finland

INTRODUCTION

Commitment to the B-cell lineage during development is a multistep process starting from multipotent hematopoietic stem cells and involving cells which vary in their differentiation potential and their self-renewing capacity. In adults, it is not yet established whether it is the multipotent stem cell or some more restricted progenitor that contributes to the massive daily production of B lymphocytes.

The avian bursa of Fabricius is a unique model to study the entry into the B-cell lineage. The prebursal stem cells, which can be earliest detected at day 7 in the hematopoietic foci of intraembryonic mesenchyme (1), colonize the bursal rudiment between days 8 and 14 of incubation in the chicken embryo. They migrate through the bursal mesenchyme to colonize the bursal follicles. Inside each follicle the bursal cells, which are however already surface immunoglobulin (Ig) positive, divide and give rise to diversified B cells (2).

The rearrangement of chicken immunoglobulin genes occurs only during embryonic development (3). The data so far suggests that the progenitor cells which colonize the embryonic follicles are already committed to a particular Ig gene rearrangement and do not continuously rearrange their genes during the embryonic maturation of the bursa (3).

In this study, we wanted to know whether commitment of the stem cells to the B-cell lineage occurs prior to the colonization of bursal rudiment. We analyzed Ig light chain gene rearrangement during early embryogenesis using a sensitive polymerase chain reaction (PCR). We show that already prebursal stem cells have started to rearrange their light chain genes before bursal colonization, suggesting that Ig-gene rearrangement and B-cell commitment occurs prebursally and independently of bursal influence. Thus, the embryonic bursa of Fabricius acts as a "secondary" lymphoid organ, positively selecting functional B cells for further Ig diversification by somatic gene conversion occurring at the bursal stem cell stage in the bursal follicles (3).

MATERIALS AND METHODS

Cells were prepared from the intraembryonic mesenchyme as described (1) and enriched for mononuclear cells by Ficoll Isopaque gradient. Deoxyribonucleic acid (DNA) was isolated from these cells and subjected to polymerase chain reaction (4). In order to obtain high sensitivity, the amplification was done using four primers in three successive rounds of amplification as described (5). The amplified DNA was also subjected to DNA sequencing using M13 vector and sequence system as described (5).

RESULTS

Rearrangement of Immunoglobulin Light Chain Genes in Embryonic B-Cell Precursors

The aim of the present study was to find out whether the prebursal stem cells which colonize the embryonic bursa would be multipotent or precommitted to the B-cell lineage prior to bursal colonization. This question was addressed by studying the initiation of the V-J joining in the chicken light chain gene locus, a process which is strictly B-cell specific, and in the case of chicken, involves only one V_λ. For detection of cells with rearranged Ig configuration, PCR is a suitable technique that is able to detect a single rearrangement event among 10^5 cells.

Since the hematopoietic foci located in the intraembryonic mesenchyme is the earliest place where B-cell precursors can be detected by adoptive cell transfer studies (1), genomic DNA was isolated from the mononuclear cells of intraembryonic mesenchyme at days 3, 5, 7, and 9 of incubation. During the normal B-cell differentiation, the certain type of V-J recombination occurs, resulting in deletion of a 1.7-kb V-J intervening DNA segment in the chicken light chain locus. Primers for PCR were selected upstream of the $V_{\lambda1}$ gene and downstream of the V-J joint area. The unrearranged germ line light chain locus results in a 2.1-kb fragment which is amplified poorly. In contrast, in the rearranged configuration the primers define a 400-bp DNA fragment. A clear PCR product of a expected molecular size was consistently obtained from cells at days 7 and 9 of incubation, whereas repeated attempts using day 3 or 5 mesenchymal cells were negative (Table 1).

Ig Light Chain Gene Diversification in Prebursal Precursors

In order to find out light chain V-region diversification in the prebursal precursors the specific PCR products obtained were sequenced. The light chain sequences derived from days 7 and 9 of intraembryonic B-cell precursors as well as early bursal cells (up to day 13) were of germ line V_λ type (see Table 1). Concerning the V-J joints, about one-third of the

Table 1 Immunoglobulin Light Chain Gene Rearrangement and V-Region Diversification

	Intraembryonic mesenchyme (d)				Embryonic bursa (d)			
Rearrangement	3	5	7	9	11	13	15	17
V_L–J_L	—	—	+	+	+	+	+	+
Fraction inframe	—	—	1/3	1/3	1/3	1/3	2/3	3/3
$V_{\lambda1}$	—	—	GL	GL	GL	GL	D	D

Abbreviations: GL = germ line, D = diversified.

sequences obtained from prebursal cells were inframe and two-thirds out-of-frame, indicating that the V-J joining is an inaccurate process as shown previously (6). In the bursa, however, a clear increase in the fraction of inframe V-J joints occurs during the late embryonic period so that all the joints are inframe around day 17 of incubation.

DISCUSSION

The present work demonstrates that the prebursal precursor B cells located in the intraembryonic mesenchyme have already started to rearrange their Ig light chain genes at day 7 of incubation. Whether they express the Ig genes is not yet known. However, these precursor cells seem to become committed very early already before bursal colonization, which starts at day 8 of embryonic development. The extrabursal commitment of B cells has been suggested before on the basis of cell transfer studies and the presence of B-cell alloantigen on precursor cells (2,7,8). However, all these studies using precursor cells from days 10 to 15 of incubation have a crucial problem whether they have represented cells which have passed already through the bursa. In the present study, the simultaneous emergence of B-cell precursors capable of bursal homing and the occurrence of light chain gene rearrangement (and most likely also heavy chain gene rearrangements) in day 7 intraembryonic tissue strongly suggest that the commitment of avian B cells is a bursa-independent event. It should be, however, noted that we have not yet directly proven that all the precursor cells show V-J rearrangement, nor do the present results exclude the possibility that some B-cell precursors rearrange their Ig genes during the migration in the bursal mesenchyme. However, our data on extrabursal commitment is in agreement with the observations of some functional B cell clones in chickens surgically bursectomized at days 2–3 of incubation (9). Also, B-cell precursors seem to be equally present in these bursectomized embryos (10).

One interesting point deduced from these studies is that, most likely, the precursor B cells express a germ line type of functional Ig molecule on the cell surface before Ig diversification by somatic gene conversion starts in the bursal follicles. This model resembles the one suggested by Jerne in 1971 (11); i.e., the germ line V region would encode anti-self reactivity. In the case of the bursa of Fabricius, the one and only germ line specificity would be needed for homing and positive selection of B cells into the follicles. Thereafter the somatic gene conversion of Ig receptors would result in mutants acquiring new antigen-binding specificities and being capable of escaping the bursa and generating the peripheral antigen-reactive B-cell compartment. In conclusion, our results indicate that the early embryonic commitment of avian B-cell precursors occurs most likely extrabursally. This picture seems to differ radically from that suggested in mammals where B-cell precursors are produced throughout the lifetime in the adult bone marrow by fresh Ig gene recombination events. However, this species difference seems to become understandable on the basis of the molecular organization of Ig genes. In avians, the Ig gene rearrangement does not create diversity, as is the case in mammals. Instead, the somatic gene conversion in bursal follicles is needed to create a sufficient B-cell repertoire.

REFERENCES

1. Lassila O, Eskola J, Toivanen P. Prebursal stem cells in the intraembryonic mesenchyme of the chick embryo at 7 days of incubation. J Immunol 1979; 1223:2091–94.
2. Pink JRL, Lassila O. B cell commitment and diversification in the bursa of Fabricius. Curr Topics Microbiol Immunol 1987; 135:54–64.

3. Weill JC, Reynaud CA, Lassila O, Pink JRL. Rearrangement of chicken immunoblobulin genes is not an ongoing process in the embryonic bursa of Fabricius. Proc Natl Acad Sci USA 1986; 83:3336–40.
4. Saiki RK, Gelfand DH, Stoffel S, Scharf SJ, Higuchi R, Horn GT, Mullis KB, Erlich HA. Primer-directed enzymatic amplification of DNA with thermostable DNA polymerase. Science 1988; 239:487–91.
5. Mansikka A, Sandberg M, Lassila O, Toivanen P. Rearrangement of immunoglobulin light chain genes in the chicken occurs prior to the colonization of the embryonic bursa of Fabricius. Proc Natl Acad Sci USA 1990; 87:9416–20.
6. McCormack W, Tjoelker L, Carlson L, Petryniak B, Barth C, Humphries E, Thompson C. Chicken IgL gene rearrangement involves deletion of a circular episome and addition of single nonrandom nucleotides to both coding segments. Cell 1989; 56:785–91.
7. Ratcliffe MJ, Lassila O, Pink JRL, Vainio O. Avian B cell precursors: surface immunglobulin expression is early, possibly bursa-independent event. Eur J Immunol 1986; 129–33.
8. Houssaint E, Lassila O, Vainio O. Bu-1 antigen expression as a marker for B cell precursors in chicken embryos. Eur J Immunol 1989; 19:239–43.
9. Mansikka A, Jalkanen S, Sandberg M, Granfors K, Lassila O, Toivanen P. Bursectomy of chicken embryos at 60 hours of incubation leads to an oligoclonal B cell compartment and restricted immunoglobulin diversity. J Immunol 1990; 145:3601–9.
10. Lassila O, Alanen A, Vainio O, Houssaint E, Pink JRL, Weber WT. B cell precursors in chick embryos surgically bursectomized at 72 h of incubation. Eur J Immunol 1988; 18:1867–70.
11. Jerne NK. The somatic generation of immune recognition. Eur J Immunol 1971; 1:1–9.

60
Are Germinal Centers Insulating Microenvironments?

E. Heinen, R. Tsunoda, C. Marcoty, A. Bosseloir, N. Cormann, C. Kinet-DeNoël, and L. J. Simar
Institute of Histology, University of Liège, Belgium; University of Tsukuba, Japan

INTRODUCTION

Among the lymph organs, the thymus appears to be a closed environment: The epithelial barrier of the thymic parenchyma prohibits the access of B cells. Even other cells, such as mature T cells and morphonuclear leukocytes, are not admitted into the cortical zone, which seems to be restricted to bone marrow–derived pre–T cells, dendritic cells, and macrophages.

Considering the peripheral lymph organs, which are open to blood and lymph, thus to various cells and products, we put the question if they also contain protected environments. Here we analyze the fate of the germinal centers (GCs).

Penetration of Nonantigenic Material

Previous experiments based on subcutaneous injections of colloidal carbon showed that draining lymph nodes are, within minutes, charged with this material. It is located in sinuses, lining endothelial cells and macrophages. At the optical level, generally no carbon was found in the lymph follicles nor in their GCs (Sainte-Marie and Peng, 1982).

We conducted similar tests at the ultrastructural level using colloidal gold particles, and were able to draw the same conclusions (Heinen et al., 1983). This indicates that follicles are not as accessible to substances as are the other zones of the lymph organs.

Penetration of Antigens

Nossal and his group showed that antigens are only retained in GCs in animals previously immunized. The antigens remain fixed on follicular dendritic cells in the form of immune complexes for long periods of time (Tew et al., 1979).

Antigens alone apparently do not penetrate the GCs; they must be complexed to specific antibodies. Previously we showed, in accordance with results of Brown et al.

(1981), that lymphoid cells, mainly B cells, transfer immune complexes to GCs (Heinen et al., 1986). Indeed, immune complex–laden B cells attach onto follicular dendritic cells and hand the immune complexes over to these last.

Penetration of Cells

The cell composition of the GCs appears to be controlled. The B cells ($CD5^-$, IgD^-) are at different maturation stages following antigenic stimulation (centroblasts, centrocytes). According to Kroese et al. (1985), only a few clones of B cells are allowed to proliferate per GC. Macrophages, mainly tingible body macrophages phagocyting lymphoid cells, are found in the dark zone, whereas follicular dendritic cells (FDCs), extending long and complex cell projections between the lymphoid cells, are mainly found in the light zone. T cells represent about 5% of the total cells; most of them being CD4-positive (Tsunoda and Kojima, 1987).

Other cells are not admitted: CD8-positive T cells are rare and polymorphonuclear leukocytes, mast cells, dendritic cells, interdigitating cells are absent.

Thus, GCs do not harbor cells at random. Namely, memory B cells are preferentially recruited in comparison to virgin bone marrow cells (Gray et al., 1988). This selection of cells may be due to the restriction of immigration or the nonretention of circulating cells.

Histology of the GCs

The FDCs are the most apparent cells besides the lymphoid cells. They extend long and slender cytoplasmic processes interwoven in a complex network. Desmosomal junctions and macula adherens interconnect these cells. The FDCs surround blood vessels (capillaries with pericytes) and appear in contact with fibrocytes (Radoux et al., 1985).

Intercellular fluid apparently moves in a centrifugal way, from the capillaries in the center toward the periphery. But lymph follicles are frequently located in lymph-drained zones; for example, in the cortex of the lymph nodes or the chorion of the mucosa. The lymph flow may then counteract the exudate arising from the capillaries.

However, the compactness of the FDC network appears to reduce the intercellular fluid displacements. Cells can migrate therein; the selectivity of the cell access to the GCs can be explained by the surface features of FDCs (receptors, charges, glycosyl residues, etc.) (Louis et al., 1990).

Bioactive Substances in GCs

Little information is available concerning the bioactive substances governing the GCs. Using isolated GC cells, we measured in vitro secretion of agents. Briefly, we found TNF α and some interleukin-1 (IL-1) β, no IL-2, IL-4, interferon-γ (IFN-γ) (Tsunoda et al., 1989), no histamine (unpublished), but prostaglandin E_2 (PGE_2) (Heinen et al., 1986). By in situ hybridization we demonstrated that no IL-6 nor IL-4 were produced in the GCs (Bosseloir et al., 1989). Interleukin-5 appears to be secreted and active inside the GCs (Lasky and Thorbecke, 1989).

Experimental and Pathological Alterations of the GCs

Cognate or natural injuries of the GCs can deliver information about their physiology.

Irradiation destroys the lymphoid cell population, leaving FDCs, macrophages, and vascular structures (Kinet-Denoël et al., 1982). Kroese et al. (1987) showed that repopulation then occurs by means of lymphoid cells "importing" immune complexes.

Lipopolysaccharides (LPS) treatment perturbs the general appearance of the follicles: They enlarge and contain abnormally high numbers of plasma cells. This may result from the altered importation or retention of immune complexes (Heinen et al., 1986) and from excessive production of cytokines.

In the acquired immune deficiency syndrome (AIDS), the GCs are enlarged and, in later stages, they are fragmented and impaired, probably as a consequence of an altered T-cell population (increased $CD8^+$ T cells) or of the degeneration of FDCs (Armstrong, 1984).

Another example of perturbed physiology occurs in Castleman's disease, in which IL-6 overproduction forces B cells toward the final differentiation in antibody-secreting cells.

CONCLUSIONS

When considering all aspects of normal or pathological follicles, it appears that GCs are peculiar microenvironments admitting some cell types, whereas barring others, and that they are zones with a defined bioactive molecular composition.

The absence of cells or substances allows given B cells to accomplish peculiar metabolic transformations; for example, in memory cells. The accidental presence of cells or substances modifies these maturation pathways and changes the rate of antibody production and their affinity or isotype.

REFERENCES

Armstrong JA. Horne R. Follicular dendritic cells and virus like particles in AIDS-related lymphodenophaty. Lancet, 1984; 18:370–373.

Bosseloir A. Hooghe-Peters EL. Heinen E. Cormann N. Kinet-Denoël C. Vanhaelst L. Simar LJ. Localization of interleukin 6 (IL6) mRNA in human tonsils by in situ hybridization. Eur. J. Immunol. 1989; 19, 2379–2381.

Brown JC. De Jesus DG. Holbarow EJ. Harris G. Lymphocyte-mediated transport of aggregated human α-globulin into the germinal centre areas of normal mouse spleen. Nature, 1981; 228, 367.

Gray D. Recruitment of virgin B cells into an immune response is restricted to activation outside lymph follicles. Immunology 1988; 65, 73–79.

Heinen E. Braun M. Coulie PG. Van Snick J. Moeremans M. Cormann N. Kinet-Denoël C. Simar LJ. Transfer of immune complexes from lymphocytes to follicular dendritic cells. Eur. J. Immunol. 1986; 16, 167–172.

Heinen E. Cormann N. Braun M. Kinet-Denoël C. Vanderschelden J. Simar LJ. Isolation of follicular dendritic cells from human tonsils and adenoids VI. Analysis of prostaglandin secretion. Ann. Inst. Pasteur Immunol. 1987; 137, 369–382.

Heinen E. Cormann N. Kinet-Denoël C. Simar LJ. Lipopolysaccharide suppresses immune complex retention by follicular dendritic cells without cytological alterations. Immunol. Lett. 1986; 13, 323–327.

Heinen E. Radoux D. Kinet-Denoël C. Simar LJ. Colloidal gold, a useful marker for antigen localization on follicular dendritic cells. J. Immunol. Meth. 1983; 59, 361–368.

Kinet-Denoël C. Heinen E. Radoux D. Simar LJ. Follicular dendritic cells in lymph nodes after X-irradiation. Int. J. Radiat. Biol., 1982; 42, 121–130.

Kroese FGM. Wublene AS. Seijen H. Nieuwenhuis P. Germinal centers develop oligoclonally. Eur. J. Immunol. 1987; 17, 1069–1072.
Lasky JL. Thorbecke GJ. Growth requirements of SJL lymphomas in vitro: effect of BCGF II. Adv. Exp. Med. Biol., 1989; 237, 145–151.
Louis E. Philippet B. Cardos B. Heinen E. Cormann N. Kinet-Denoël C. Braun M. Simar LJ. Intercellular contacts between germinal center cells. Mechanisms of adhesion between lymphoid cells and follicular dendritic cells. Acta ORL, 1990; 43, 297–320.
Radoux D. Heinen E. Kinet-Denoël C. Simar L.J. Antigen/antibody retention by follicular dendritic cells. Adv. Exp. Med. Biol., 1985; 186, 185–191.
Sainte-Marie G., Peng FS. Belisle C. Overall architecture and pattern of lymph flow in the rat lymph node. Am. J. Anat., 1982; 164, 275–309.
Tsunoda R. Cormann N. Heinen E. Onzaki K. Coulie P. Akiyama Y. Yoshizaki K. Kinet-Denoël C. Simar L.J. Kojima M. Cytokines produced in lymph follicles. Immunol. Lett. 1989; 22, 119–134.
Tsunoda R. Kojima M. A light microscopical study of isolated follicular dendritic cell-clusters in human tonsils. Acta Pathol. Jpn. 1987; 37, 575–585.
Tew JG. Mandel TE. Prolonged antigen half-life in the lymphoid follicles of specifically immunized mice. Immunology 1979; 37, 69–76.

61

How Immune Complex on Follicular Dendritic Cells Is Processed in the Germinal Center in the Secondary Response

Kazuo Terashima, Michio Dobashi, Takehiko Aoki, Kohji Saito, and Yutaka Imai
Yamagata University School of Medicine, Yamagata, Japan

INTRODUCTION

Follicular dendritic cells (FDCs) are well known as antigen-retaining cells in germinal centers (GCs), possibly engaging in an immune memory function (1). Recently, Tew and his group introduced the ICCOSOME (immune complex–coated small body) theory (4,5). The ICCOSOMEs are fragments of the cytoplasmic extensions of FDCs and directly deliver immune complex (IC) to GC cells (GCCs). However, it is difficult to find ICCOSOMEs in conventional animals because there are many GCs in varying stages. Fortunately, the present authors could verify the theory in the active secondary response with specific pathogen free (SPF) or semi–germ-free mice immunized against horseradish peroxidase (HRP) (3,7–9). The GC counted only one in one section of the regional lymph node. The popliteal lymph node of the control mice showed neither GCs nor lymphoblasts even after a 70-day observation period. This permitted us to gain more basic and accurate information concerning GCs. The present study disclosed that all immune complex in GCs was not processed merely by the ICCOSOME alternative pathway. The purpose of the present chapter is to describe all types of the immune complex processing, including the alternate pathway, and to understand the secondary response in GCs. In addition, conventional fed mice and rats were comparatively studied.

MATERIAL AND METHODS

Detailed material and methods were described previously on SPF mice (2). The mice were immunized in hind foot pads with HRP (100 μg Sigma, type IV), emulsified in Freund complete adjuvant, and 60 days later boostered with HRP (20 μg) in saline. Conventional mice and rats were similarly immunized. To detect antigen (Ag), microslicer sections of popliteal lymph nodes fixed in paraform glutaraldehyde were incubated with diaminobenzidine (DAB) + H_2O_2 after dipping in 0.1% phenylhydradine. To detect both specific antibody (spAb) and Ag, sections were similarly processed after an incubation with HRP solution. The section were embedded horizontally in Epon-Araldite after osmification and dehydration.

RESULTS AND DISCUSSION (Fig. 1)

FDC and Sequential Changes of Labyrinthlike Structure (7–9)

The cytoplasmic extensions of FDCs compose complicated interwoven structures designated as labyrinthlike structures (LBSs) in the light zone. Before booster injection, LBSs had a somewhat lamellar pattern that more or less contained spAb extensively between the cytoplasmic projections, whereas antigen was disconnectedly disclosed in some intercytoplasmic sites. Immediately after booster injections, LBs were distorted (D-LBSs) by an massive influx of Ag-spAb complex and interstitial edema. The cytoplasmic extensions became atrophic and some FDCs became degenerated. Six hours later, many FDCs had euchromatic nucleolated nuclei and short-running filiform LBSs (F-LBS). At about the twenty-fourth hour, LBS became highly organized or metamorphosed into spherical glomerated LBSs (G-LBSs) as large as small lymphocytes (Fig. 2). This structure has been already described by our present group (3,7–9). At about 24–48 h, G-LBSs became unlaced

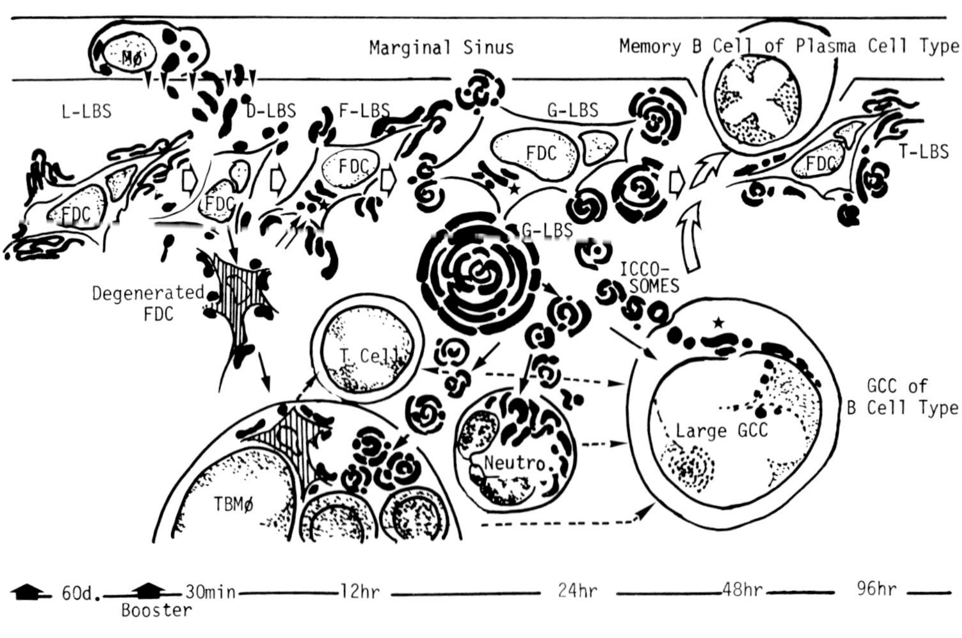

Figure 1 Diagram of the secondary response in the GC (see the text). The relationship of the two tied with a disconnected line remained to be solved.

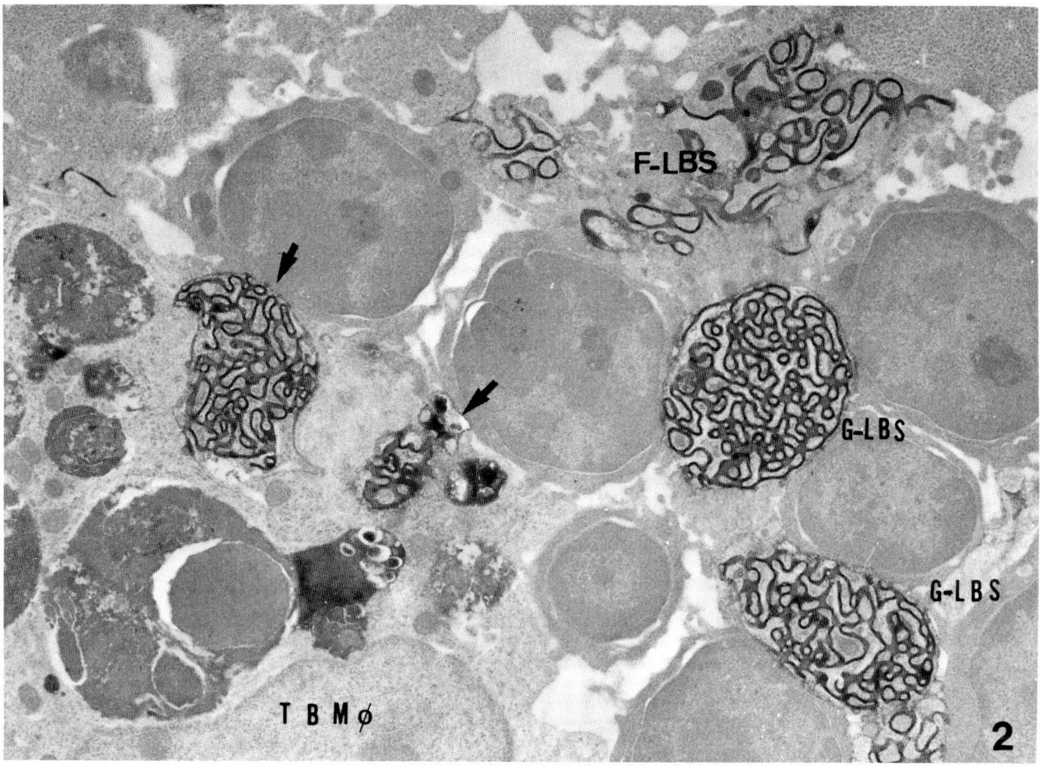

Figure 2 The light zone of a GC 1 day after booster injection showed scattering of G-LBSs and focally F-LBSs. TBMs took fragments of G-LBSs (arrow).

or loosened, giving whorl-like fragments. Finally, this fragments became smaller to form ICCOSOMEs (4,5). The IC of which becomes internalized by GCCs, as described later. Two days afterward, the remaining LBSs gradually reformed or recovered into lamellar structures via transitional forms (T-LBSs) with a mixture of G-LBSs and L-LBSs. The intercellular spaces between the round lymphoid cells and G-LBSs were reoccupied by the extended L-LBSs.

Follicular dendritic cells bore one to multiple euchromatic nuclei. The nuclear matrix was light and homogeneous in electron density when compared with that of lymphoid cells, including T cells. Nucleoli were often observed. As noted above, the cytoplasmic extensions of FDCs were distorted or dissociated immediately after booster injection, and later seemed to become regenerated, whereas some FDCs were phagocytized by tingible body macrophages (TBMs). The nuclei increased in number according to the development of dendrites or LBSs. A giant FDC with four faceted nuclei was seen in conventional-fed mice 2 days after booster injection. Taking release of ICCOSOMEs or fragmentation of G-LBSs into consideration, FDCs seem to be duly analogous to megakaryoblasts in the release of platelets. The multinucleicity has already been confirmed in human lymphoid tissue (8).

Intake of Immune Complex (IC) by GCCs

The smaller, round tips of fragmented G-LBSs have been designated as ICCOSOMEs. IC is decoated from ICCOSOMEs and were internalized in GCCs via pinocytotic vesicles. They were first transported into Golgi sacs and lamellae. This process was first identified by Tew's group (4) as an alternative pathway to process antigen, different from the macrophage system. In some instances, the IC or Ag could reach the perinuclear space and the nucleus, especially near perichromatin area (9).

Finally, LBSs, ICCOSOMEs, and IC in GCCs in conventional-fed mice and rats were compared with SPF mice. In conventional animals, sequential changes of LBSs were difficult to follow. Typical ICCOSOMEs and G-LBSs were difficult to identify though enlarged. LBSs, irregular-expanding outlined, were recognized as large as small lymphocytes. In rats, LBSs were poorly developed. Localization of IC or Ag in the Golgi apparates was identified in GCCs of both conventional mice and rats (Fig. 3).

Intake of IC or Ag by Other Constituents than GCCs

1. A few degenerated FDCs, bearing IC on their cytoplasmic surface, were observed to be phagocytized by TBMs following booster injection. In this stage, TBMs scattered not only in the dark zone, but also in the light zone.
2. At about 24 hr after booster injection, TBMs phagocytized fragments of G-LBSs en bloc (Fig. 2).
3. Neutrophils also phagocytized fragmented G-LBSs. The fragments were more unlaced and undulating than those phagocytized by TBMs. Unlike TBMs, neutrophils do not phagocytize lymphoid cells.
4. Furthermore, some FDCs themselves, when their cytoplasm is conspicuous at around the twelfth hour, ingested IC or Ag in the vesicular system near the contranuclear area (Golgi apparatus). The FDCs have been known to pinocytize a small amount of Ag. The present study of secondary immunization has also disclosed that IC or Ag is engulfed by FDCs in a form of pinocytosis. Such a phenomenon could be observed before the appearance of G-LBSs. The IC or Ag is furthermore transported into the Golgi apparatus in FDCs in a similar manner to that seen in GCCs. The amount ingested by an FDC seems to compare to that by a GCC (Fig. 4).

SPECIFIC ANTIBODY spAb-PRODUCING CELLS AND Ag-INGESTING GCCs

In some instances, large GCCs bearing spAb in their perinuclear space disclosed an intake of immune complex in intracytoplasmic vesicles closely neighboring extracellular fragmented G-LBSs or ICCOSOMEs. This means that immune complex–ingesting GCCs were of the B-cell type but not of the T-cell type. Our previous report noted that spAb-producing GCCs remained as large GCCs without developed rough endoplasmic recitula (rER) throughout the primary response, while they maturate into plasmocytoid cells with an abundance of spAbs around the third day in the secondary response. The latter was also evidenced in the present work. Tew and his colleagues considered the antigen presentation of FDCs to T cells to secrete IL-2 to promote GCCs binarily to be memory B cells and spAb-producing plasma cells within GCs. However, as far as was morphologically detected in the present study, plasmocytoid cells could be observed in the upper end of the light zone and in the marginal sinus (Fig. 5). This means a portion of the memory cells could be spAb-producing plasmocytoid cells themselves, maturated from spAb-producing large

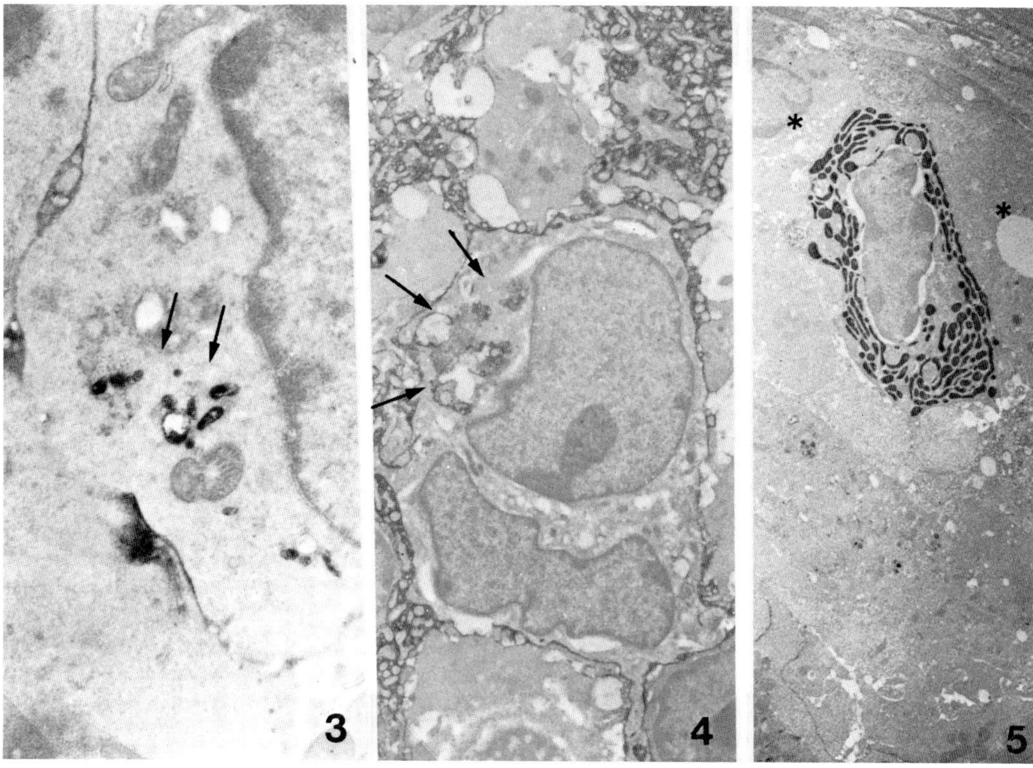

Figure 3 Immune complex was observed in the Golgi apparatus (arrow) in GCCs 2 days after booster injection in conventional-fed mice.

Figure 4 FDCs also contained Ag or IC in the Golgi apparatus (arrow) in some instances.

Figure 5 The marginal sinus (*) showed scattering of plasma cells 3 days after booster injection. They could reach other lymphoid tissues via the blood stream.

GCCs during the booster immunization. They could reach lymphoid tissue through the whole body via lymph and the blood stream.

On the other hand, reflecting upon the IC internalization of B cells, it requires further analysis as to whether another type of plasma cell series outside of or independent of GCs, such as we previously reported (1,2), have the ability to ingest IC or not. When we reached the hypothesis that the GCCs of the B-cell type with IC by themselves maturated into memory B cells in a form of plasma cells, it remained open to question how TBMs and neutrophils intaking more IC or Ag than GCCs participated in their proliferation or maturation.

Recently, B cells have become known to be more potentially endowed with an antigen-presentation ability than are macrophages (11). Direct internalization of IC into GCCs of the B-cell type might further attribute to the potent presentation. On the other hand, the immune complex removed from the surface of the ICCOSOMEs or FDCs was reported to have a special adjuvant effect in addition to an immunogeneity of the uncoated

IC (10). The synergism of the two might engage in proliferation and maturation of GCCs as memory B cells in the secondary response.

CONCLUSIONS

Sequential ultrastructural analysis of GCs of SPF mice lymph nodes secondarily immunized against HRP disclosed time-coursed changes of IC-coated dendrites of FDCs and verified the ICCOSOME theory according to Szakal, Kosco, Tew (4). Immune complex decoated from ICCOSOME was internalized into specific Ab-producing GCCs, some of which mature into plasma cells in the marginal sinus, possibly as a memory B-cell series. Beside GCCs, fragments of the dendrites of FDCs were also phagocytize by TBMs and neutrophils. Some FDCs themselves were phagocytized by TBMs, whereas some FDCs also internalized IC.

REFERENCES

1. Terashima K. Imai Y. Kasajima T. Tsunoda R. Takahashi K. An ultra-structural study on antibody production of the lymph nodes of rats with special reference to the role of germinal centers. Acta Path Jpn 1977: 27: 1–27.
2. Dobashi M. Terashima K. Imai Y. Electron microscopic study of differentiation of antibody-producing cells in mouse lymph nodes after immunization with horse radish peroxidase. J Histochem Cytochem 1982: 30:67–74.
3. Imai Y, Terashima K. Matsuda M. Dobashi M. Maeda K. Kasajima T. Reticulum cells and dendritic reticulum cell. Origin and Function. Rec Adv RES Res 1983:21:51–81.
4. Szakal AK. Kosco MH. Tew JG. A novel in vivo follicular dendritic cell-dependent iccosome-mediated mechanism for delivery of antigen to antigen-processing cells. J Immunol. 1988:140;341–353.
5. Kosco MH. Szakal Ak. Tew JG. In vivo obtained antigen presented by germinal center B cells to T cells in vitro. J Immunol. 1988:140;354–360.
6. Terashima K. Ukai K. Takima K. Yuda F. Imai Y. in Histophysiology of the immune system. Ed. by Fossum S. Rolstad B. Morphological diversity of DRC-1 positive cells: Human follicular dendritic and their relatives. NY. Plenum Publ. Adv Exp Med Biol 1988:168;157–163.
7. Terashima K. Dobashi M. Imai Y. Antigen processing and labyrinth-like structures in germinal centers of mice lymph nodes in the secondary response. In Abstract of 7th International congress of immunology (Berlin). 1989: 57–28.
8. Terashima K. Dobashi M. Imai Y. What happens in the germinal center in the secondary response? In Morphological and functional aspects of accessory cells in retroviral infections. Workshop, Hamburg, November 23/24 1989.
9. Terashima K. Dobashi M. Yuda F. Saito K. Aoki T. Imai Y. Role of the immune complex trapped on follicular dendritic cells (FDC) in the germinal center (GC) in the secondary response. In International symposium on dendritic cells in lymphoid tissue. Yamagata, 7-9 June 1990 Ed. by Imai Y et al. Amsterdam. Elsevier 1990: in press.
10. Burton GF. Maeda K. Szakal A. Tew JG. Immunogenicity of follicular dendritic cell (FDC) associated antigen. In International symposium on dendritic cells in lymphoid tissue. Yamagata 7-9 June 1990. Ed. by Imai Y et al. Amsterdam. Elsevier. 1990: in press.
11. Ashwell JD. Commentary: Are B lymphocytes the principal antigen-presenting cells in vivo? J Immunol. 1988:140:3697–3700.

62
Regulation of Germinal Center Activity

Hendrik G. Seijen, Judoca C.A.M. Bun, Auktje S. Wubbena, Siep Posthuma, and Anita J. Groothuis
University of Groningen, Groningen, The Netherlands

INTRODUCTION

Germinal centers (GCs) are clusters of proliferating B lymphoblasts that appear in peripheral lymphoid organs upon antigenic contact. They provide the organism with B-memory cells, which upon renewed contact with the antigen react more effectively and give better protection than the antibody-forming cells in the primary antibody response. Germinal centers are T-cell–dependent structures (1). Most of the T cells in GCs, as detected by immunohistological methods, are CD4-positive (T-helper) cells. In rats, nearly all these CD4-positive cells also bear a determinant detected by the monoclonal (MAb) ER3, a MAb that reacts in lymph node cell suspensions with only 35% of the CD4-positive cells (and with all CD8-positive cells) (2,3). Very few of the T cells in GCs are CD8-positive T-suppressor and T-cytotoxic cells; i.e., react with the MAb Ox8. We investigated the role of both the $ER3^+$-ve cells and the $Ox8^+$-ve cells in GC formation.

MATERIALS AND METHODS

Experimental procedures were essentially as described previously (4).

RESULTS

$ER3^+$-ve Cells Are Regulatory in GC Formation

The role of $ER3^+$-ve cells in GC formation was investigated in a system, in which thoracic duct lymphocytes (TDLs) are transferred to lethally irradiated rats together with antigen. Specifically, pooled TDLs were depleted for $ER3^+$-ve cells by panning and given to lethally irradiated recipient rats together with sheep red blood cells (SRBCs). Control rats received undepleted TDLs. Spleens were removed 6 days later and their GCs activities

Table 1 ER3$^+$-ve Cells Regulate GC Formation

	Experimental group[a]	Control group
Number of rats	3	3
ER3$^+$-ve cells (%)	1.6	14.4
V (mm^3)[b]	0.53 ± 0.09 ($p < .05$)	1.16 ± 0.20
N[b]	289 ± 15 ($p < .05$)	472 ± 66

[a]TDLs were depleted for ER3$^+$-ve cells by panning, and 3.4×10^7 were given to each of three lethally irradiated rats together with SRBCs. Control rats received 4×10^7 TDLs. .V and N of GCs in the spleens were measured 6 days later.
[b]Mean ± SEM.

were morphometrically assessed. As shown in Table 1, the percentage of ER3$^+$-ve cells remaining in the TDLs after depletion was about one-tenth of the percentage in the original TDLs. Both the volume (V) and the number (N) of the GCs of the animals injected with TDLs, depleted for ER3$^+$-ve cells, reduced to about half those of the control group. Thus, GC activity clearly depends upon ER3$^+$-ve cells, although not in a simple, quantitative way.

Ox8$^+$-ve Cells Suppress Secondary, but Not Primary GC Formation

Thoracic duct lymphocytes were collected from unprimed and 1 month earlier primed rats and depleted for Ox8$^+$-ve cells by panning. Groups of lethally irradiated rats were reconstituted with primed TDLs, unprimed TDLs, Ox8-depleted primed TDLs, or Ox8-depleted unprimed TDL, and challenged with SRBCs. The V and N of the GCs in the spleens were measured 6 days later. Table 2 shows the results with primed TDLs, and Table 3 with unprimed TDLs. As was found earlier (unpublished data), primed TDLs reacted much less vigorously in forming GCs than unprimed TDLs. A marked difference in the effect of depletion for Ox8$^+$-ve cells was observed. The depleted, primed TDLs, although still containing about 40% of the Ox8$^+$-ve cells originally present, reacted almost four times better than without depletion, whereas the depleted, unprimed TDLs, with only about 10% remaining Ox8$^+$-ve cells, reacted equally as well as without depletion. Thus, Ox8$^+$-ve cells,

Table 2 Ox8$^+$-ve Cells in TDLs Suppress Secondary GC Formation

	Experimental group[a]	Control group
Number of rats	3	3
Ox8$^+$-ve cells (%)	4.1	10.1
V (mm^3)[b]	0.60 ± 0.12 ($p < .025$)	0.16 ± 0.03
N[b]	320 ± 55 ($p < .025$)	118 ± 16

[a]TDLs of rats primed with SRBC 1 month earlier were depleted for Ox8$^+$-ve cells by panning, and 5.1×10^7 were given to each of three lethally irradiated rats together with SRBCs. Control rats received 6×10^7 primed TDLs. V and N of GCs in the spleens were measured 6 days later.
[b]Mean ± SEM.

Table 3 $Ox8^+$-ve Cells in TDLs Do Not Suppress Primary GC Formation

	Experimental group[a]	Control group
Number of rats	3	3
$Ox8^+$-ve cells (%)	1.2	12.5
V $(mm^3)^b$	1.88 ± 0.32 (p >.1)	2.48 ± 0.43
N^b	538 ± 79 (p >.1)	612 ± 64

[a]TDLs of unprimed rats were depleted for $Ox8^+$-ve cells by panning, and 5.1×10^7 were given to each of three lethally irradiated rats together with SRBCs. Control rats received 6×10^7 unprimed TDLs. V and N of GCs in the spleens were measured 6 days later.
[b]Mean ± SEM.

as present in TDLs of primed rats, do suppress GC formation, in contrast to the $Ox8^+$-ve cells in TDLs of unprimed rats.

Upon intravenous administration of the MAb Ox8 to rats virtually all $Ox8^+$-ve cells disappeared within 1 day from the blood and the spleen and, moreover, did not reappear within the following 7 days (results not shown). The MAb Ox8 thus effectively eliminates the $Ox8^+$-ve cells, allowing the study of their role in forming GCs in in vivo experiments.

At the age of 2 months, 10 rats were injected intravenously with SRBCs. After 4 months, they were divided into two groups of each five rats. One group received only a second dose of SRBCs, the other group also, 1 day earlier, an injection of the MAb Ox8. Spleens were taken 6 days later to estimate morphometrically the GC activity. A two to three times higher response (Table 4) was seen in the rats depleted for $Ox8^+$-ve cells.

Another group of nine rats were injected with SRBCs at the age of 4 months, and five of them, 1 day earlier, also with the MAb Ox8. Spleens were taken 6 days later to estimate morphometrically the GC activity. No effect of the elimination of the $Ox8^+$-ve cells in these unprimed rats was observed (Table 5). Thus, also in vivo, $Ox8^+$-ve cells suppress secondary but not primary GC formation. As in the reconstitution experiments with TDLs, the GC activity of the secondary response in these in vivo experiments is much less than that of the primary response.

Table 4 $Ox8^+$-ve Cells Suppress the In Vivo Secondary GC Formation

	Experimental group[a]	Control group
Number of rats	5	5
V $(mm^3)^b$	1.65 ± 0.22 (p <.01)	0.72 ± 0.18
N^b	742 ± 60 (p <.01)	472 ± 71

[a]Rats were injected with SRBCs at the age of 2 and 6 months; 1 day before the second SRBC injection, the experimental group also were injected with the MAb Ox8. V and N of GCs in the spleens were measured 6 days later.
[b]Mean ± SEM.

Table 5 $Ox8^+$-ve Cells Do Not Suppress the In Vivo Primary Germinal Center Formation

	Experimental group[a]	Control group
Number of rats	5	4
V (mm^3)[b]	1.74 ± 0.28 (p > .1)	2.13 ± 0.57
N[b]	544 ± 91 (p >.1)	618 ± 88

[a]Rats were injected with SRBCs when 4 months old; the experimental group 1 day earlier also with the MAb Ox8. V and N of GCs in the spleens were measured 6 days later.
[b]Mean ± SEM.

CONCLUSIONS

Our experiments clearly demonstrated that $ER3^+$-ve T-helper cells have a stimulatory role in GC formation. However, no simple relationship was observed between their number and the resulting GC activity. Therefore, we cannot exclude that, beside these cells, also $ER3^-$-ve T-helper cells may be active in GC formation.

Both in reconstitution experiments with TDLs and in in vivo experiments, we found that $Ox8^+$-ve T-suppressor cells suppress the secondary GC reaction. Such an effect was not found with respect to the primary response GC formation. One has to suppose that these T-suppressor cells originate during the primary response and, in particular, in its later phases.

REFERENCES

1. Kroese FGM, Timens W, Nieuwenhuis P. Germinal center reaction and B-lymphocytes, morphology and function. Curr. Topics Pathol. 1990; 84(1):119–64.
2. Kroese FGM, Wubbena AS, Joling P, Nieuwenhuis P. T lymphocytes in rat lymphoid follicles are a subset of T helper cells. Adv. Exp. Med. Biol. 1985; 186:443–9.
3. Vonderheide RH, Hunt SV. T lymphocytes in rat germinal centres belong to an $ER3^+$ subpopulation of $CD4^+$ cells. Immunology 1990; 69:542–7.
4. Seijen HG, Bun JCAM, Wubbena AS, Löhlefink KG. The germinal center precursor cell is surface μ and δ positive. Adv. Exp. Med. Biol. 1988; 237:233–7.

63
Analysis by Confocal Microscopy of the Molecules Expressed by Cells in Follicular Compartments

Gerald D. Johnson, Deborah L. Hardie, and Ian C.M. MacLennan
The Medical School, University of Birmingham, Birmingham, England

INTRODUCTION

In typical, zonally structured germinal centers (GCs), three B-lymphoid cell populations are readily identifiable—centroblasts comprising the lower or dark zone, centrocytes in the upper, light zone, and small lymphocytes which constitute the follicular mantle. Many antibodies are now available which react with cells in GCs, and in the 4th International Workshop of Human Leucocyte Differentiation Antigens (1), we identified additional clusters which show topographically restricted reactivity within GCs. The advent of confocal laser scanning microscopy has provided a precise analysis—particularly in relation to the recognition of coincident/noncoincident reactivity of pairs of antibodies and quantitation of relative intensity. Phenotypic analysis of cells in situ has thus identified new compartments within GCs, and these may be related to their specific roles in the immune response.

MATERIALS AND METHODS

Antibodies

One hundred and forty-one monoclonal antibodies (MAbs) were initially tested through our participation in the studies on the B-lymphocyte panel of the 4th International Workshop (1). The designated clusters of the antibodies which form the basis of this report, their names, and corresponding antigens can be obtained from the Workshop report. BCL2 was a kind gift from Dr. D. Y. Mason, Oxford, England.

Tissues

All antibodies were tested on cryostat sections (5 μ) of tonsil. The tissue was freshly obtained at operation and snap-frozen. Sections were fixed in acetone for 5 min at 20°C.

Staining Procedures

Full details of the immunofluorescence methods have been previously described (2). The following points should be noted: (a) Fluorescent nuclear counterstaining with propidium iodide or bisbenzimide as appropriate facilitated the orientation of GCs. (b) Pairs of antibodies were tested (1) by dual labeling based on mouse immunoglobulin (Ig)–isotype-specific fluorochrome conjugates with MAbs of different isotypes, or (2) by the reversed sequential procedure with MAbs of the same isotype (3). (c) Texas Red linked via streptavidin to biotinylated antibody gives an improved signal—compared with rhodamine—in the 2-channel mode of the confocal microscope operating on the 514-nm argon laser line. (d) All preparations were mounted in glycerol containing diazabicyclooctaine to retard fading during microscopy (4).

Laser Scanning Confocal Microscopy

The Bio-Rad MRC 500 system was employed in order to study the coincident reactivity of pairs of antibodies by merging the separate images obtained by dual fluorescence staining; an additional feature of the system which made a major contribution to this study is the ability to perform visual quantitative analysis of relative intensity on pairs of images by color-banding.

RESULTS

The redistribution of staining obtained with the antibodies is summarized in Table 1, and the GC compartments identified by the reactivity patterns are illustrated in Figure 1.

Established Compartments

The pan–B-specific CD19 antibodies provide a definitive marker confirming the B lineage of subpopulations identified by other antibodies. Mantle, but not GC B cells were stained by CD39; a subset of the mantle cells was stained by CD45R and the CD23 MAbs (except LA1 and LA2). Most GC B cells were stained by CD38 (also present on plasma cells and activated T cells) and anti-Gb3 antibodies (CD77), which showed strongest reactivity with centroblasts.

New Compartments

Four clusters stained cells localized in distinct areas not previously identified within GCs: A subset of B cells at the base of the light zone was identified by CD54 and the new cluster of CDw78 antibodies; a further subset situated at the base of the dark zone and adjacent to the follicular mantle was identified by CDw75 and CD77 antibodies, which also stained cells in the B-blast area of the light zone.

Follicular Dendritic Cells

This study confirmed our previous finding that CD23 antibodies show the strongest reactivity with a subset of the follicular dendritic cell (FDC) network detectable with the FDC-specific MAbs R4/23 (5) and 2BF11,BU-10 (6), which is located in the apical light zone; further heterogeneity within the FDC population was demonstrated by CD73 (anti–ecto-5-nucleotidase) antibodies, which preferentially stained FDCs in the basal light zone with processes extending into the dark zone.

Table 1 Predominant Phenotype in GC Compartments

	Lymphoid cells						FDCs				
	FM	OLZ	ALZ	BLZ	DZ	BDZ	OLZ	ALZ	BLZ	DZ	BSZ
CD19	++	++	++	++	++	++	+	+	+	+	+
CD21	++	+	+	+	+	+	++	++	++	++	+/–
IgG	++	–	–	–	–	–					
Ig	++	+	+	+	+	+	++	++	++	++	+/–
CD39	++										
a FDC BU10							++	++	++	++	+/–
CD23	restr/–						–	++	+	+/–	+/–
CD73	W						–	+/–	+++	+/–	+/–
CD54	W		+	++				+	++		
CDw78	+			++	+	+					
CD38	–	+	+	+	+	+					
CD77	–	+(+)	+	+	++	++					
CDw75	+	++	+	+	+	++					
BCL2 Cyto	++										
BCL2 Nuclear		+	+	+	+	+					
Cell Cycle	NO	YES	NO	NO	YES	YES					
% FDC Area							26	53	69	34	3

Abbreviations: FM: follicular mantle; OLZ: outer light zone; ALZ: apical light zone; BLZ: basal light zone; DZ: dark zone; BDZ: basal dark zone.

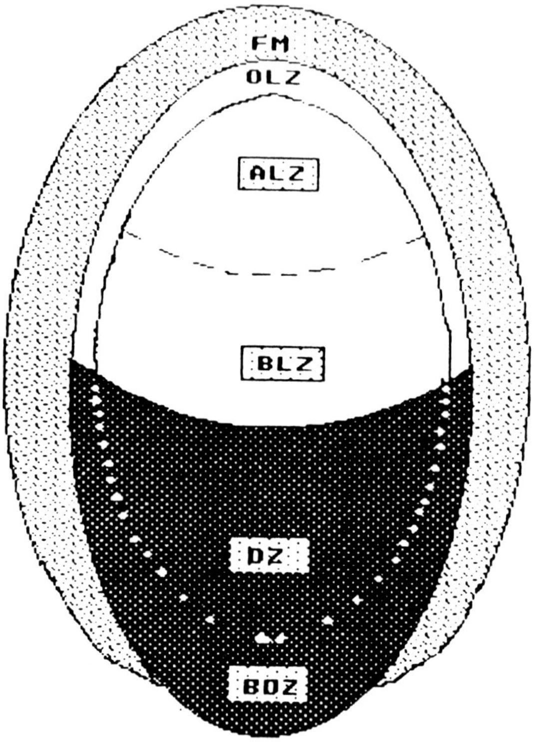

Figure 1 Diagrammatic representation of GC compartments based on the distribution of staining obtained with the antibodies as described in the text. FM = follicular mantle, OLZ = outer light zone, ALZ = apical light zone, BLZ = basal light zone, DZ = dark zone, BDZ = basal dark zone.

DISCUSSION

It is evident from this study that activation and differentiation of B cells in response to antigen involves a greater complexity in the organization of secondary follicles than the original concept of a structure having only three compartments (9). In particular, the discrete population of B cells identified in the outer light zone and the phenotypic heterogeneity of the FDC population may relate to crucial events in the maturation of the immune process. The localization and proliferation of B cells in areas where FDCs are present suggests that FDCs provide an attractive microenvironment to B cells whose activity is driven by the antigen component of immune complexes bound to the surface of FDCs. Elucidation of the molecular events which determine this process will be aided by the detailed in situ analysis provided by laser scanning confocal microscopy.

REFERENCES

1. Knapp W (ed.). *Leucocyte Typing IV*, Oxford University Press, 1989.
2. Johnson GD and Holborow EJ. In: *Handbook of Experimental Immunology*, 4th ed. DM Weir (ed). Oxford, England, Blackwell, 1986.

3. Johnson GD and Walker L. Reversed sequential double immunostaining. J Immunol Methods, 1986, 95:149–152.
4. Johnson GD, Davidson RS, McNamee KC, Russell G, Goodwin D and Holborow EJ. Fading of immunofluorescence during microscopy: A study of the phenomenon and its remedy. J Immunol Methods, 1982, 55:231–242.
5. Naiem M, Gerdes J, Abdulaziz Z, Stein H and Mason DY. Production of a monoclonal antibody reactive with human dendritic reticulum cells and its use in the immunohistological analysis of lymphoid tissue. J Clin Pathol, 1983, 36:167–175.
6. Johnson GD, Hardie DL, Ling NR and MacLennan ICM. Human follicular dendritic cells: A study with monoclonal antibodies. Clin Exp Immunol, 1986, 64:205–213.

64

Expression of Mouse Mammary Tumor Virus Antigen(s) on Pre–B Cells of Balb/c Mice

Mayra Lopez-Cepero, Yang Wang, Richard Riley, and Diana M. Lopez
University of Miami School of Medicine, Miami, Florida

INTRODUCTION

Mouse mammary tumor virus (MMTV) is a type-B retrovirus capable of inducing mammary carcinomas in mice. It is transmitted as a milkborne virus or by germ-line cells in a proviral form (1). Restriction endonuclease mapping and molecular hybridization studies have revealed the presence of MMTV genomes integrated in the deoxyribonucleic acid (DNA) of germinal and somatic normal cells of all inbred mouse strains (2–5). In Balb/c mice, a strain which has a low incidence of mammary tumors and lacks the exogenous milk-transmitted MMTV, there are two genome-size proviruses designated as *Mtv*-8 and *Mtv*-9 and a subgenomic provirus designated as *Mtv*-6 (6–12).

Replication of MMTV and the abundant expression of the gene products are primarily restricted to mammary tissue in animals with a high incidence of mammary tumors such as C3H mice (13). However, studies by Charyulu et al. (14) have shown that the expression of MMTV-related antigen(s) is detectable in 15–20% of spleen cells from Balb/c mice and preferentially in the B lymphocytes. Tax and collaborators (15) reported the expression of an antigen cross reactive with the MMTV-encoded *env* protein, gp52, on a small population (4–6%) of B cells in normal mice. Further studies by Lopez and collaborators (16) showed that a specific subset of highly enriched surface immunoglobulin–positive (sIg^+) spleen cells display MMTV-related antigen(s) on their surfaces. Single and double immunofluorescence experiments using anti-MMTV and anti-sIg antibodies demonstrated the preferential expression of MMTV-related antigens on the surface of 20% of the total splenic B cells from Balb/c mice. Recent unpublished studies in our laboratories by Wang et al. show by Western blot analyses that enriched splenic B-cell populations from Balb/c mice contain a 68-kD membrane protein that cross reacts with polyclonal anti-MMTV antibody. Additionally, *Mtv* ribonucleic acid (RNA) expression can be detected in splenic B cells from these animals (17). No MMTV-related antigen(s) or *Mtv* RNA expression, however, is detected in splenic T cells or in the thymus. Although, Abelson transformed immature B cells and pre–B-cell lines also expresses *Mtv* RNA, most myelomas and B-cell hybridomas express undetectable or very low levels of *Mtv* transcripts (20). Studies by Sharma et al. (18) and King et al. (19) have established a correlation between retroviral gene expression and B-cell differentiation, and indicate that MMTV *env* expression occurs

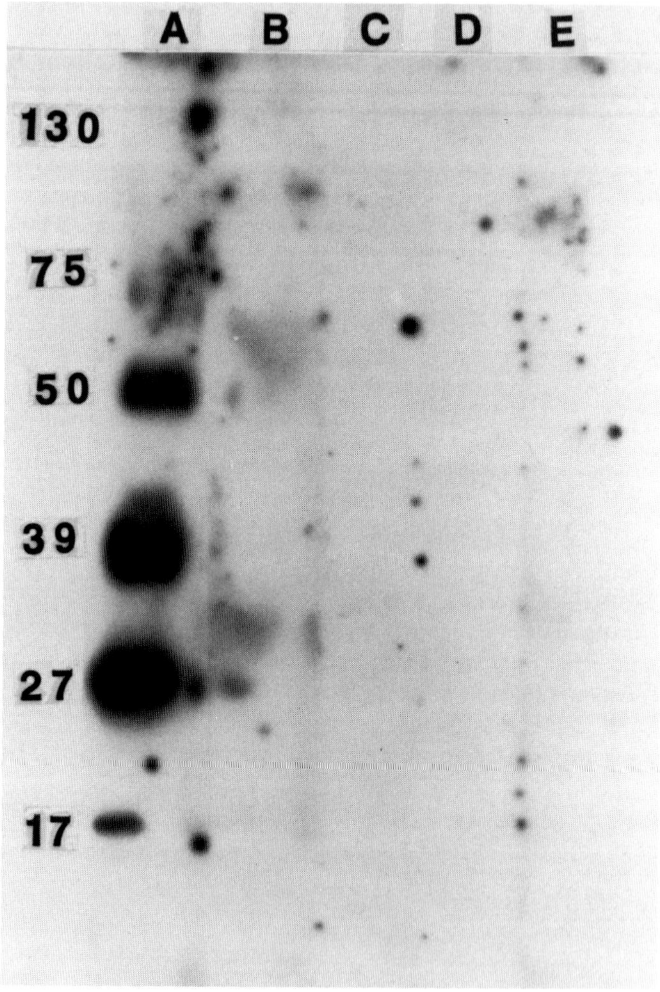

Figure 1 Western blot analyses of MMTV-specific proteins on bone marrow pre–B cells from Balb/c mice. MMTV-specific proteins were detected by Western blot using rabbit antiserum directed against highly purified disrupted MMTV (lanes A, B, and E) and preimmune serum (lanes C and D). Whole-cell proteins of Balb/c bone marrow cell subsets ($B220^{+}sIg^{-}$ and $B220^{-}sIg^{-}$) were extracted in equal volumes of lysis buffer (0.01 M Tris HCl pH 7.4, 1% NP-40, 0.15 M NaCl, 0.001M EDTA) and 4% SDS. The proteins and purified MMTV were electrophoresed on 12.5% poplyacrylamide-SDS gels, transferred to nitrocellulose, and probed sequentially with serum (immune or preimmune) and ^{125}I goat antirabbit IgG. Lane A contains disrupted MMTV, lanes B and C contain $B220^{+}sIg^{-}$ bone marrow cells, lanes D and E contain $B220^{-}sIg^{-}$ bone marrow cells. Molecular weights in kilodaltons are shown at the left.

after Ig gene transcripts are increased but prior to maximal differentiation of the B cell. Further studies by King and coworkers (20) demonstrate that MMTV transcripts are upregulated during cytokine-mediated, as well as lipopolysaccharide (LPS)–mediated, differentiation in CH12 cells, a B-cell lymphoma of B10.A origin.

RESULTS

Since the possible correlation between *Mtv* gene expression and B-cell differentiation has been established (17–20), an enriched pre–B-cell population from the bone marrow of Balb/c mice was examined for the expression of MMTV-related antigens. The bone marrow cell population was separated into B220-positive sIg-negative and B220-negative sIg-negative fractions. Western blot analyses of whole-cell lysates from these populations, probed with polyclonal anti-MMTV, revealed a 68-kD protein in the B220^{+} sIg^{-} subset (Fig. 1), indicating that this subset possess a molecule related to a structural protein of MMTV. Since Northern blot analysis revealed the expression of *Mtv* transcripts in

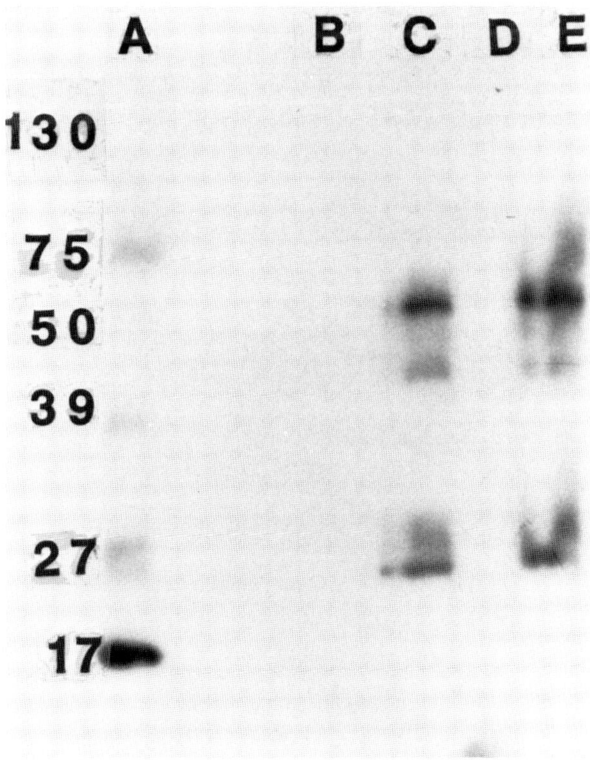

Figure 2 Western blot analysis of MMTV-specific proteins on Abelson-transformed cell lines. MMTV-specific proteins were detected as detailed in Figure 1. Lane A contains disrupted MMTV, lanes B and C contain 2M3 cells (Abelson-transformed Pre–B cells of Balb/c origin), lanes D and E contain A20 cells (Abelson-transformed B cells of Balb/c origin). Rabbit antiserum directed against highly purified MMTV was used in lanes A, C, and E. Rabbit preimmune serum was used in lanes B and D. Molecular weights in kilodaltons are shown at the left.

Abelson-transformed cell lines (10), a pre–B-cell line (2M3) and a B-cell line (A20) were examined for the expression of MMTV-related antigens. Western blot analysis showed that the 2M3 and A20 cell lines contain three MMTV-related proteins, including the 68-kD protein expressed on pre–B and B lymphocytes from Balb/c mice (Fig. 2).

CONCLUSIONS

Our studies in conjunction with the studies performed in other laboratories (18–20) indicate that at least two kinds of murine cells committed to the B-cell lineage express MMTV-related antigens during differentiation: (a) an immature ($B220^+$ sIg^-) B cell from the bone marrow, and (b) a fully mature, immunoglobulin-expressing B lymphocyte. The expression of a 68-kD protein on the surface of pre–B and B lymphocytes appears to be due to a MMTV *env*-related protein or its precursor, which is known to have a corresponding high molecular weight. Furthermore, Abelson-transformed pre–B (2M3) and mature B (A20) cell lines of Balb/c mice origin also express these MMTV-related proteins. Thus, MMTV appears to be a differentiation marker of a subset of cells of B cell lineage.

ACKNOWLEDGMENTS

We thank Lynn Herbert and Mantley Dorsey, Jr., for their excellent technical assistance. Special thanks to Lynn Herbert for the helpful review of this manuscript.

REFERENCES

1. Devaux B. The mouse mammary tumor virus (MMTV). In: Crepin M. (ed). *Research in Retrovirus and Oncogenes*. Vol 1. England, John Libbey, 1988, pp. 141–67.
2. Varmus HE, Bishop JM, Nowinski RC, Sarkar NH. Mammary tumor virus specific nucleotide in mouse DNA. Nature New Biol 1972; 238:189–90.
3. Michalides R, Scholm J. Relationship in nucleic acid sequences between mouse mammary tumor virus variants. Proc Natl Acad Sci USA 1975; 72:4635–39.
4. Morris VL, Medeiros R, Ringold GH, Bishop MJ, Varmus HE. Comparison of mouse mammary tumor specific DNA from inbred, wild and Asian mice and in tumors of normal organs from inbred mice. J Mol Biol 1977; 114–73.
5. Cohen JC, Majors JE, Varmus HE. Endogenous mammary tumor virus DNA varies among wild mice and segregates during inbreeding. Nature 1979; 278:418–23.
6. Cohen JC, Majors JE, Varmus HE. Organization of mouse mammary tumor virus specific DNA endogenous to BALB/c mice. J Virol 1979; 32:483–96.
7. Traina VL, Taylor BA, Cohen JC. Genetic mapping of endogenous mouse mammary tumor viruses: Locus characterization, segregation and chromosomal distribution. J Virol 1981; 40: 735–44.
8. Groner B, Buietti E, Diggelman H, Hynes NE. Characterization of endogenous and exogenous mouse mammary tumor virus proviral DNA with the site specific molecular clones. J Virol 1980; 36:734–45.
9. Peters G, Placzek S, Brookes S, Kozak C, Smith R, Dickson C. Characterization, chromosome assignment and segregation analysis of endogenous proviral units of mouse mammary tumor virus. J Virol 1986; 59:535–44.
10. Pauley R, Parks WW, Popko B. Expression and demethylation of germinally transmitted BALB/c mouse mammary tumor virus DNA in Abelson MuLv B lymphoid cell lines. Virus Res 1984; 1:381–400.

11. Callahan R, Callahan D, Kozak C. Two genetically transmitted BALB/c mouse mammary tumor virus genomes located on chromosomes 12 and 16. J Virol 1984; 49:1005–8.
12. Groner B, Hynes N. Number and location of mouse mammary tumor virus proviral DNA in mouse DNA of normal tissue and of mammary tumors. J Virol 1980; 33:1013–25.
13. Salmons B, Gunzburg WH. Current perspectives in the biology of mouse mammary tumor virus. Virus Res 1987; 8:81–102.
14. Charyulu V, Sigel MM, Durden DL, Lopez DM. Mouse mammary tumor virus (MMTV) antigen(s) are present in B lymphocytes of BALB/c mice. Int J Cancer 1979; 24:813–18.
15. Tax A, Ewert D, Manson LA. An antigen cross reactive with gp52 of mouse mammary tumor virus is expressed on a B cell population of mice. J Immunol 1983; 130:2368–71.
16. Lopez DM, Charyulu V, Paul RJ. B cell subsets in spleens of BALB/c mice: Identification and isolation of MMTV expressing and MMTV responding subpopulations. J Immunol 1985; 134:603–607.
17. Lopez DM, Paul RD, Pauley RJ. Phenotypic expression of endogenous retroviral antigens in B lymphocytes. In: Kaplan JG, Green DR, Bleackley RC, (eds). *Cellular Basis of Immune Modulation.* Vol 9. New York, Liss, 1989, pp. 491–94.
18. Sharma S, King LB, Corley RB. Molecular events during B lymphocyte differentiation. J Immunol 1988; 141:2510–18.
19. King LB, Corley RB. Characterization of a presecretory phase in B cell differentiation. Proc Natl Acad Sci 1989; 86:2814–18.
20. King LB, Lund FE, White DA, Sharma S, Corley RB. Molecular events in B lymphocyte differentiation: Inducible expression of the endogenous mouse mammary tumor proviral gene, *Mtv*-9. J Immunol 1990; 144:3218–27.

65
New Monoclonal Antibodies Identifying Mantle Zone and Marginal Zone B Cells

Juliette Smith-Ravin,[1] Jo Spencer,[2] P.C.L. Beverley,[1] and P.G. Isaacson[2]
[1]*Imperial Cancer Research Fund, Human Tumor Immunology Group, Courtauld Institute, London, England;* [2]*University College and Middlesex School of Medicine, London, England*

INTRODUCTION

B cells are organized in three major populations easily identifiable in tissue sections. The cells of the mantle zone are surface immunoglobulin M–positive (sIgM$^+$) and surface immunoglobulin D–positive (sIgD$^+$) and express mature B-cell markers (CD19, CD20). They belong to a recirculating pool of unprimed B cells which move between peripheral blood (PB) and the mantle zone and primary follicles of lymphoid tissues (1). The second B-cell compartment is the follicle center in which proliferation and somatic mutations occur, leading to the production of high-affinity antibodies (2,3). The third population of B cells is in the splenic marginal zones which contain a mixture of cells at intermediate stages between small lymphocytes and plasmablasts as well as macrophages (4). These B cells express sIgM but not sIgD. Recent studies in rat suggested that the marginal zone contains memory B cells (5,6). We examined the tissue distribution and function of the antigens identified by UCL-3D3 and UCL-4D12. Our preliminary results suggest that these two monoclonal antibodies (MAbs) may be useful in the study of the function and lineage relationship between the different B-cell populations in the mantle zone, marginal zone, and follicle center.

MATERIALS AND METHODS

Production of MAbs

Balb/c mice were immunized (5.10^6 cells/immunization) with cells teased from either a follicular lymphoma (UCL-3D3) or a low-grade lymphoma of mucosal-associated lymphoid tissue (MALT) (UCL-4D12) 17 and 3 days prior to fusion. Fusions were done as described by Waldman (7). Supernatants were screened on frozen sections of normal spleen using indirect immunoperoxidase (8).

Cell Preparation

Mononuclear cells were isolated from peripheral blood (normal, chronic lymphocytic leukemia [CLL], prolymphocytic leukemia [PLL]), tonsils, or spleen by centrifugation on Ficoll Hypaque. T cells were removed by E-rosetting. Tonsil B cells were cultured in RPMI with 10% fetal calf serum and stained at 0, 24, 48, 72 h in culture. Several B- and T-cell lines were tested for 3D3 and 4D12 antigen expression (9).

Immunocytochemistry and Immunofluorescence Staining

Reactivity of the two MAbs was tested on frozen sections of normal tissue (spleen, tonsil, Peyer's patches) and on a panel of lymphomas using the indirect immunoperoxidase method. Single immunofluorescence staining was carried out using MAb supernatant and rabbit antimouse immunoglobulins (Igs) FITC conjugated.

ELISA

ELISA assay was done in flat microtiter plates (Dynatech Immunolon). The plates were coated with rabbit antimouse Igs. Antihuman IgM (HB57 and UCHB1) and UCHT1 were used as positive and negative controls, respectively.

RESULTS AND DISCUSSION

UCL-3D3 recognized specifically mantle zone cells and follicular dendritic cells in normal spleen, tonsil, and lymph node. In contrast, splenic marginal zone B cells were strongly UCL-4D12–positive (Fig. 1). UCL-4D12 recognized a subset of follicle center cells which were concentrated in the light zone of the follicle center. Double immunofluorescence showed that UCL-4D12–positive and UCL-3D3–positive populations were mutually exclusive in splenic white pulp (9). They appear to identify two functionally distinct populations, the mantle zone B cells, which recirculate through blood and lymphoid organs and initiate primary antibody responses, and the marginal zone population of sessile cells. UCL-4D12 or UCL-3D3 did not stain plasma cells or B cells in the dark zone of the follicle center where the centroblasts are concentrated. UCL-3D3 identifies 20–40% of tonsil B cells and 50–60% of spleen B cells. UCL-4D12 stains less than 10% of tonsil B cells and 15–30% of spleen B cells. In normal peripheral blood lymphocytes (PBLs), more than 80% of B cells are UCL-3D3–positive cells and less than 2% UCL-4D12–positive cells (9). None of the cell lines tested by FACS analysis showed reactivity with UCL-3D3 and UCL-4D12. In addition, 3D3 and 4D12 antigens are lost rapidly from the surface of cultured tonsil B cells (Fig. 2). This property has been described with other antigens (10). UCL-3D3 and UCL-4D12 stain CLL and PLL ZB cells. This result is somehow striking as in the case of CLL cells; higher expression of 3D3 and 4D12 antigens seem to correlate with a high expression of CD5 antigen (Table 1). We do not know yet the significance of this correlation.

ELISA assay (Fig. 3) and blocking experiments on spleen sections show that UCL-3D3 and UCL-4D12 do not recognize IgM, D, A, G. The characterization of these two MAbs show that they differ from previously described clusters of differentiation (11). They appear to identify new B-cell antigens and to discriminate between different subpopulations of B cells in the splenic marginal and mantle zones. UCL-4D12 is of particular interest, as it is one of the few B-cell MAbs that recognize specifically human splenic marginal zone. It has been suggested that the marginal zone may contain memory B cells

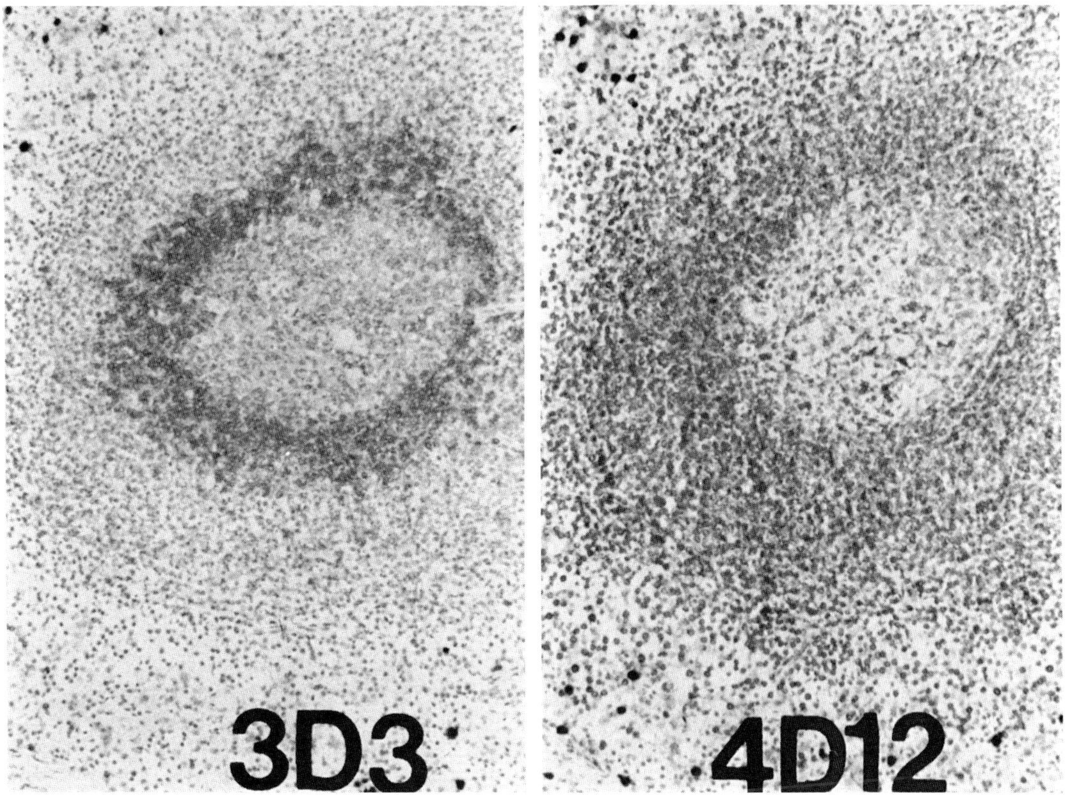

(a) (b)

Figure 1 Spleen sections stained with UCL-3D3 (a) and UCL-4D12 (b) using the indirect immunoperoxidase technique.

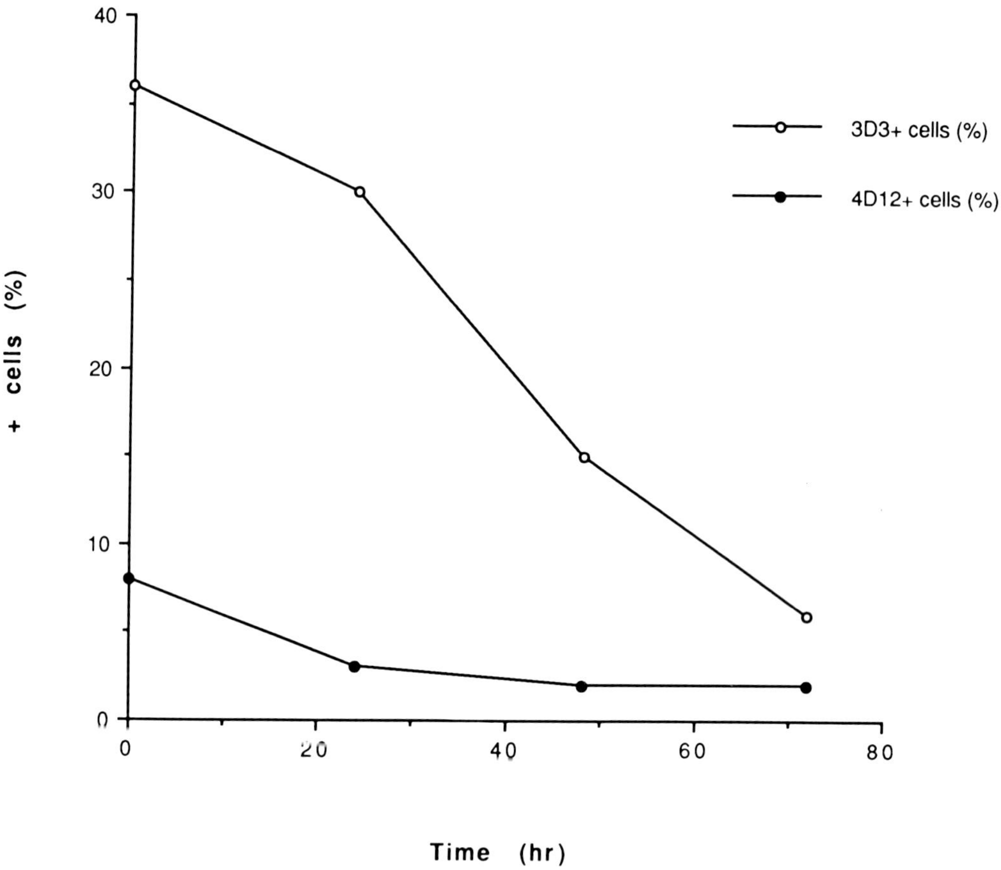

Figure 2 Time course of 3D3 (○) and 4D12 (●) antigen expression on tonsil B cells in culture. Cells were cultured and stained as described in the Materials and Methods section.

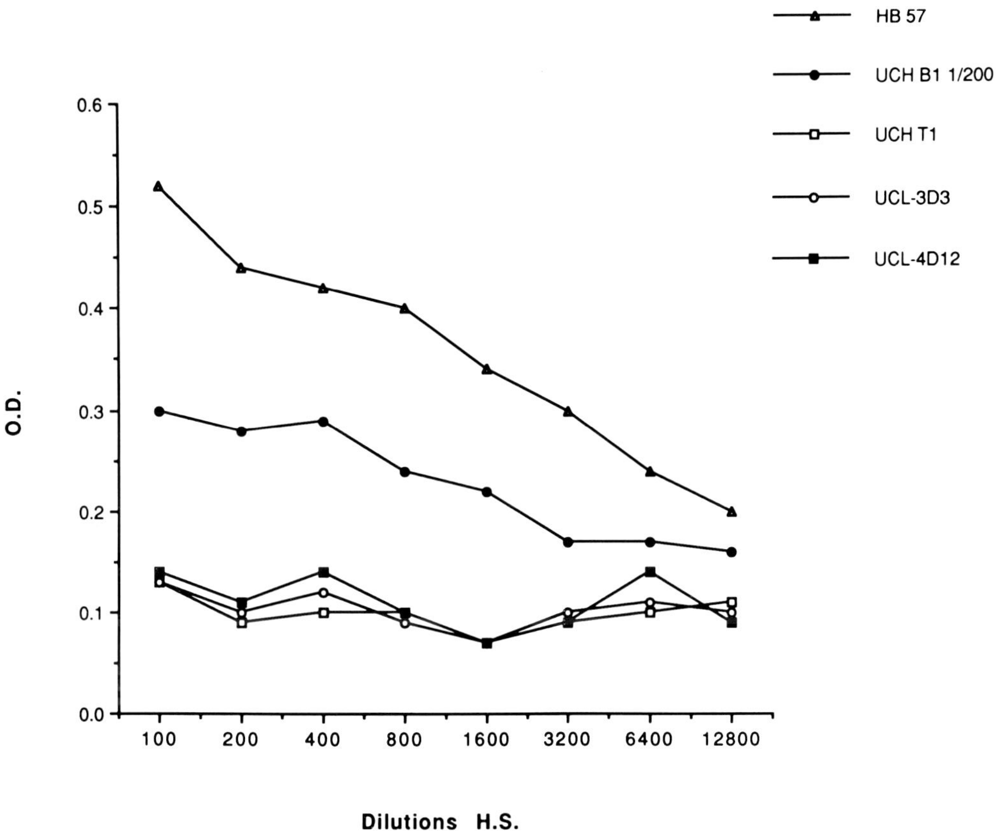

Figure 3 ELISA assay of UCL-3D3, UCL-4D12, and control MAbs. The assay was carried out with different dilutions of human serum (H.S.) and red at 492 nm.

Table 1 Expression of 3D3 and 4D12 Antigens on CLL and PLL Mononuclear Cells: Comparison with CD5 and CD20

	Pan-B (%)	UCL-3D3 (%)	UC-4D12 (%)	CD5 MAb (%)
BR-CLL	68	11	13	10
RC-CLL	87	67	27	77
GC-CLL	60	10	5	10
HL-PLL	90	47	36	90
SC-PLL	80	50	22	85

(5); thus we are currently investigating the functional properties of separated 3D3–positive and 4D12–positive cells of tonsil and spleen. Study is also underway to identify and determine the function of the double-negative population.

REFERENCES

1. Gray D, MacLennan ICM, Bazin H, Khan M. Migrant $\mu^+\delta^+$ and static $\mu^+\delta^-$ B lymphocyte subsets. Eur. J. Immunol. 1982; 12:564–9.
2. Gray D, Kumararatne DS, Lorton J, Khan M, MacLennan ICM. Relation of intrasplenic migration of marginal zone B cells to antigen localization on the follicular dendritic cells. Immunology 1984; 52:659–69.
3. MacLennan ICM, Gray D. Antigen-driven selection of virgin and memory B cells. Immunol. Rev. 1986; 91:61–85.
4. Humphrey JH. Tolerogenic or immunogenic activity of hapten-conjugated polysaccharides correlated with cellular localization. Eur. J. Immunol 1981; 11:212–20.
5. MacLennan ICM, Gray D, Kumararatne DS, Bazin H. The lymphocytes of splenic marginal zones: a distinct B-cell lineage. Immunol. Today 1982; 3:305–7.
6. Zhang J, Liu YJ, MacLennan ICM, Gray D, Lane PJL. B cell memory to thymus-independent antigens type 1 and type 2: The role of lipopolysaccharide in B memory induction. Eur. J. Immunol. 1988; 18:1417–24.
7. Waldmann MCH. Production of monoclonal antibodies. In: *Monoclonal Antibodies*. PCL Beverley (ed). Churchill Livingstone, London, 1986, p 1.
8. Isaacson PG, Wright DH. Immunocytochemistry of lymphoreticular tumours. In: *Immunocytochemistry. Practical Applications in Pathology and Biology*. JM Polak and S Van Noorden (ed). Wright, Bristol, 1983, p .249.
9. Smith-Ravin J, Spencer J, Beverley PCL, Isaacson PG. Characterisation of two monoclonal antibodies (UCL-3D3 and UCL-4D12) that discriminate between mantle and marginal zones B cells. Clin. Exp. Immunol. 1990; 82:181–7.
10. Armitage RJ, Rowe DJ, Beverley PCL. A new antigen identified by the monoclonal antibody UCHB1 delivers a costimulatory signal to a subset of human B cells. Eur. J. Immunol. 1988; 18:67–76.
11. Knapp W, Dorken B, Gilks WR, Rieber EP, Schmidt RE, Stein H, von den Borne WEG (eds). *White Cell Differentiation Antigens. Leucocyte Typing IV*, Oxford University Press, 1989.

66
Rat B-Cell Subsets Identified by Flow Cytometry and Their Anatomical Counterparts

Frans G.M. Kroese,[1,2] Mirjam H. Hermans,[1] Nynke K. de Boer,[1] Eugene C. Butcher,[2] and Leonore A. Herzenberg[2]
[1]*University of Groningen, Groningen, The Netherlands;*
[2]*Stanford University, Stanford, California*

INTRODUCTION

B cells are a heterogeneous population of cells, both with respect to their phenotype, their function, and their anatomical localization. Such a heterogeneity is illustrated in vivo by the presence of two distinct B-cell compartments in spleen: The lymphocyte follicles (primary follicles and, after antigenic stimulation, secondary follicles that are composed of a germinal center and a lymphocyte corona) and the marginal zones (MZs). The MZs are structures that are unique to the spleen; they are not found in other lymphoid organs. In tissue sections, MZ B cells are mainly immunoglobulin M–positive/immunoglobulin D–negative (IgM^+IgD^-) cells in contrast with other (corona) B cells that are mainly IgM^+IgD^+ (Fig. 1) (1). The MZ B cells appear to be involved in the immune response to type-2 T-cell independent antigens and could to be a distinct lineage of B cells (2).

A similar heterogeneity of B cells has been demonstrated in spleen cell suspensions by multiparameter flow cytometry (FACS) stained for IgM and IgD (3). In the mouse, FACS analysis shows that most splenic B cells express relatively low levels of surface IgM (sIgM) and high levels of sIgD. This subset of B cells is called population I. A much smaller population of cells expresses relatively high levels of sIgM and low levels of sIgD. This subset is called population III. In the mouse, population III cells comprise B cells that belong to the Ly-1 B-cell lineage, a self-replenishing, bone marrow–independent population of cells (4). Ly-1 B-lineage cells differ from "conventional" B cells in anatomical localization, function, and phenotype (4).

Apparently both experimental approaches, i.e., flow cytometry and immunohistology, reveal the presence of two IgM/IgD–defined B-cell subpopulations. The relationship between the anatomically defined and FACS-defined B cells is, however, not fully established and is the subject of the present chapter.

IN TISSUE SECTIONS MONOCLONAL ANTIBODIES HIS22 AND HIS24 PREDOMINANTLY REACT WITH FOLLICULAR B CELLS

We previously developed a panel of monoclonal antibodies (MAbs) (HIS14, HIS22, and HIS24) directed to rat B cells (5). These antibodies recognize different epitopes of the B-cell form of the leukocyte common antigen (B220 antigen; CD45R). Figure 1 shows the immunoperoxidase staining pattern of rat spleen sections with HIS22 and HIS24. Both MAbs strongly stain B cells that are located in lymphoid follicles and only (very) weakly MZ B cells. Germinal center B cells are intensely stained by HIS24 but not by HIS 22 (5). Thus, small follicular B cells (i.e., B cells located in primary follicles and in lymphocyte coronas of secondary follicles) are IgM–positive/IgD–positive HIS22-positive and HIS24-positive. This also appears to be the predominant phenotype of B cells located in the splenic red pulp. On the other hand, MZ B cells are $IgM^{+}IgD^{dull}HIS22^{dull}HIS24^{dull}$.

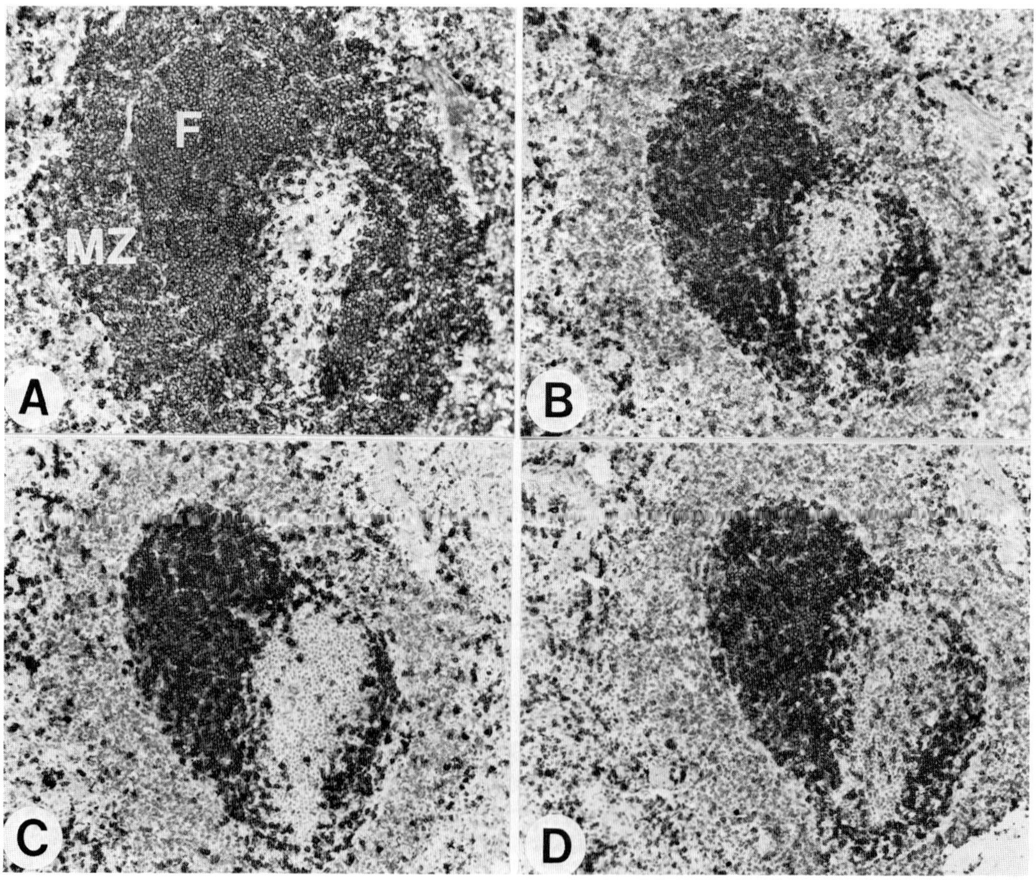

Figure 1 Immunoperoxidase-staining patterns of frozen sections from rat spleen. Serial sections were incubated with (A) monoclonal mouse anti-rat IgM, (B) monoclonal mouse anti-rat IgD, (C) HIS22 or (D) HIS24, followed by polyclonal rabbit anti mouse Ig conjugated to peroxidase. Peroxidase was revealed using diaminobenzidine. F = primary lymphocyte follicle; MZ = marginal zone.

FACS ANALYSIS DEMONSTRATES TWO DISTINCT IgM/IgD–DEFINED B-CELL SUBPOPULATIONS IN RAT SPLEEN

As described in detail elsewhere (6) and is shown in Figure 2, FACS analysis of rat spleen cell suspensions stained for sIgM (MAb HIS40) and sIgD (MAb MARD 3) reveals the presence of two distinct B-cell subsets similar to the mouse; a major population of IgM^{dull}-IgD^{bright} cells (population I) and a smaller population of $IgM^{bright}IgD^{dull}$ cells (population III) (6). In these (not deliberately stimulated) Fisher rats, population III cells account for about 25% of the B cells. A similar proportion of $sIgM^{+}sIgD^{-}$ cells were found in rat spleen cell suspensions using a double-rosette assay (7). In contrast, in the spleen of Balb/c mice the proportion of population III cells is much lower; only 10% of the total B-cell population (3).

Population III cells predominate in adult rat bone marrow (BM) and in neonatal rat spleen (about 70% of the B cells). By contrast, other lymphoid tissues (lymph nodes and Peyer's patches) contain only very few population III cells (<5% of the sIgM/sIgD–defined B cells).

HIS22 AND HIS24 FURTHER DEFINE B-CELL SUBSETS IN RAT SPLEEN BY THREE-COLOR FLOW CYTOMETRY

As described above, MAbs are available (HIS22 and HIS24) that differentially react with morphologically distinguished splenic B-cell compartments in the rat. These antibodies are therefore very useful to further define rat B cells in order to correlate cell

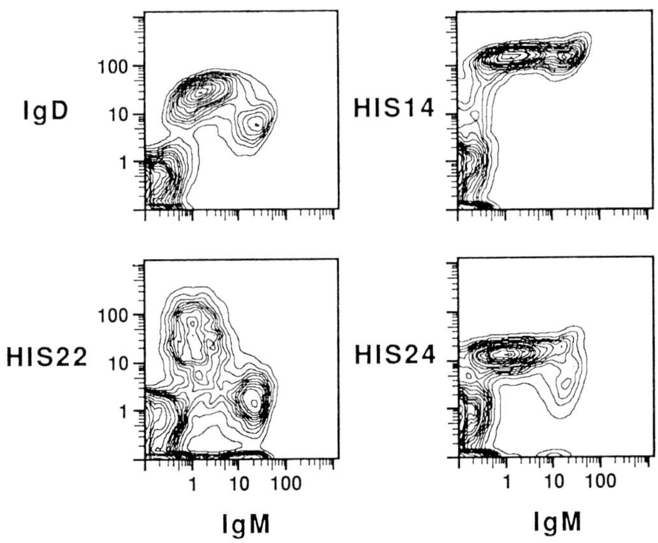

Figure 2 Three-color FACS analysis of rat spleen cells simultaneously stained with monoclonal anti-rat IgM conjugated to FITC, mouse anti-rat IgD conjugated to biotin, and HIS antibody conjugated to allophycocyanin. Biotinylated antibodies were revealed by avidin conjugated to Texas red as a second-step reagent. FACS plots are presented as 5% probably plots of at least 20,000 viable cells.

suspension data with morphological findings. Three-color FACS analysis was performed on spleen-cell suspensions simultaneously labeled with sIgM (conjugated to FITC), sIgD (conjugated to biotin and followed by avidin–Texas Red), and HIS22 or HIS24 (conjugated to allophycocyanin) according to methods described by Hardy et al. (3). FACS analysis shows (6) that HIS22 predominantly reacts with population I cells (see Fig. 2). About two-thirds of these $IgM^{dull}IgD^{bright}$ cells and only about 10% of population III cells express high levels of HIS22 determinant. HIS24 reacts with the vast majority (>95%) of population I cells and subdivides population III into two subpopulations: about one-third for the $IgM^{bright}IgD^{dull}$ cells express high levels of HIS24 determinant, and the remaining two-thirds of these cells only low levels (Fig. 2). These $HIS24^{dull}$ population III cells are relatively large cells, as demonstrated by relatively higher forward scatter profiles (6). In contrast, the majority of $IgM^{bright}IgD^{dull}$ cells (population III) in BM and neonatal spleen are bright for HIS24 (and react only weakly with HIS22).

THE ANATOMICAL LOCALIZATION OF FACS-DEFINED B-CELL SUBPOPULATIONS

FACS analysis shows that in adult rat spleen most B cells are population I cells (IgM^{dull} IgD^{bright}) expressing high levels of both HIS22 and HIS24. These cells also constitute the vast majority of lymph node B cells. In situ, cells with this phenotype are located in lymphoid follicles; i.e., primary follicles and the lymphocyte corona of secondary follicles (see Fig. 1). Most splenic population III cells ($IgM^{bright}IgD^{dull}$) express low levels of both HIS22 and HIS24 and are slightly larger (by forward scatter) than other B cells. These cells are absent in other lymphoid organs. In sections of the spleen, cells with this phenotype are MZ B cells. The $HIS24^{bright}$ (and $HIS22^{dull}$) population III cells are likely to represent B cells that are newly formed. This is based upon the following observations: (a) in rat BM, the vast majority of the IgM/IgD–defined B cells have this phenotype, and (b) these cells are the predominant type of B cells found in neonatal rat spleen.

We do not know the exact anatomical localization of these $HIS24^{bright}$ population III cells (nor of the $HIS22^{dull}$ population I cells). Their phenotype differs from that of the majority of follicular B cells (including IgD-negative germinal centers) and MZ B cells. Some clues about the anatomical localization of $HIS24^{bright}$ population III cells may come from a recently developed MAb, HIS50, recognizing a rat B cell–restricted antigen (M.H. Hermans et al., manuscript in preparation). Three-color FACS analysis of spleen-cell suspensions shows that only population III cells express the HIS50 antigen on their membrane; population I cells express little (if any) HIS50 on their cell membrane. Within population III, both the $HIS24^{dull}$ MZ B cells and the $HIS24^{bright}$ B cells (newly formed B cells) express HIS50. Staining of spleen sections with HIS50 shows that in addition to expected staining of MZ cells (i.e., the $HIS24^{dull}$ population III cells) scattered small follicular B cells (among dull staining B cells), and some cells in the red pulp express high levels of HIS50. Possibly, the scattered HIS50-positive cells observed in the follicles (and/or in the splenic red pulp) represent the $HIS24^{bright}$ population III cells (newly formed B cells).

A MODEL OF B-CELL DIFFERENTIATION IN THE RAT

In Figure 3, we propose a model of B-cell development in rats not deliberately stimulated with antigens. MacLennan and coworkers postulate that follicular B cells and MZ B cells

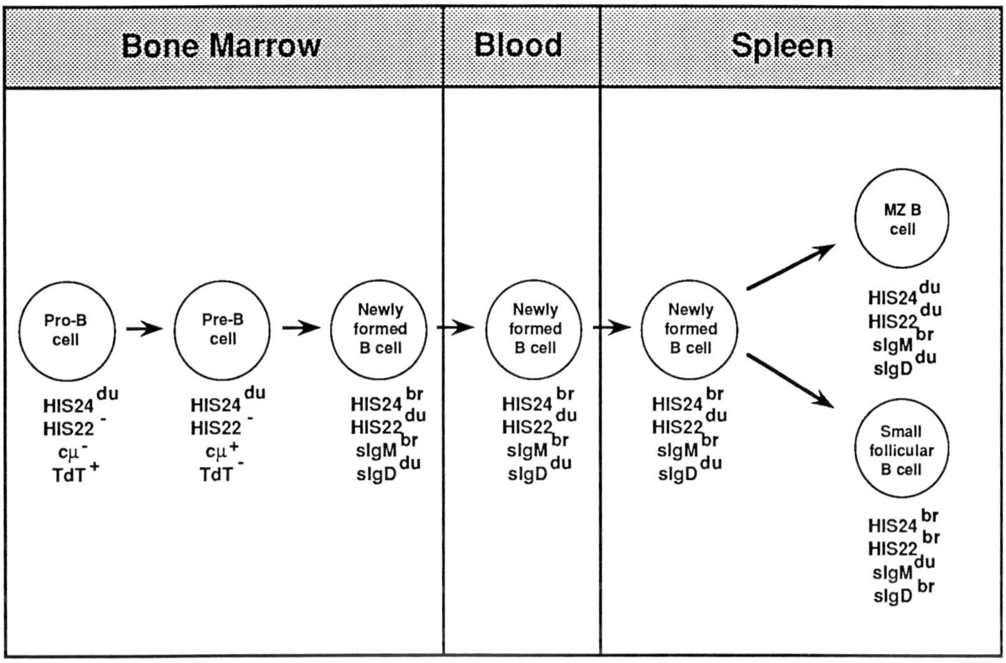

Figure 3 Hypothetical model of B-cell differentiation pathways in the rat. For explanation see text.

represent two distinct lineages of B cells (2). For example, treatment of rats from birth with anti-IgD antibodies leads to the development of spleen with an intact MZ but without lymphoid follicles (1), and the regeneration of B cell follicles precedes that of MZ after x-irradiation with BM shielding (8). These last experiments also demonstrate that precursor cells for both follicular B cells and for MZ B cells are located in the BM. We could not find a major phenotypical heterogeneity of BM B cells (by FACS) that would indicate that there are different precursors for both follicular B cells and MZ B in the BM. In the model shown in Figure 3, we therefore propose that follicular B cells and MZ B cells are derived from a common precursor cell: the newly formed B cell (i.e., $HIS24^{bright}$ population III cell) from which they differentiate independently in the spleen. These newly formed B cells are both found in the BM and in the spleen, which implies that these cells migrate from the BM through the blood into the spleen. Indeed, FACS analysis shows that high numbers of $HIS24^{bright}$ population III cell are found in rat peripheral blood, whereas they are absent in the thoracic duct lymph (N.K. de Boer, manuscript in preparation).

ACKNOWLEDGMENTS

The authors would like to thank Auk Wubbena, Wim Ammerlaan, and Peter van der Sijde for technical help. F.G.M.K. was recipient of a NATO Science Fellowship from the Netherlands Organization for Scientific Research. This work was supported by grants HD-01287 (L.A.H.) and AI-19957 and DK 387076 (E.C.B.).

REFERENCES

1. Bazin H, Gray D, Platteau B. and MacLennan I.C.M. Distinct δ+ and δ-B lymphocyte lineages in the rat. Ann. N.Y. Acad. Sci. 1982; 399:157–173.
2. MacLennan I.C.M. and Gray D. (1986) Antigen-driven selection of virgin and memory B cells. Immunol. Rev. 1986; 91:61–85.
3. Hardy R.R., Hayakawa K., Parks D.R., Herzenberg L.A. and Herzenberg L.A. Murine B cell differentiation lineages. J. Exp. Med. 1984; 159:1169–1188.
4. Herzenberg L.A., Stall A.M., Lalor P.A., Sidman C., Moore W.A., Parks D.R. and Herzenberg L.A. The Ly-1 B cell lineage. Immunol. Rev. 1986; 93:81–102.
5. Kroese F.G.M., Wubbena A.S., Opstelten D., Deenen G.J., Schwander E.H., De Leij L., Vos H., Poppema S., Volberda J. and Nieuwenhuis P. B lymphocyte differentiation in the rat: production and characterization of monoclonal antibodies to B lineage-associated antigens. Eur. J. Immunol. 1987; 17:921–928.
6. Kroese F.G.M., Butcher E.C., Lalor P.A., Stall A.M. and Herzenberg L.A. The rat B cell system: the anatomical localization of flow cytometry-defined B cell subpopulations. Eur. J. Immunol. 1990; 20:1527–1534.
7. Gray D., MacLennan I.C.M., Bazin H. and Khan M. Migrant $\mu^+\delta^+$ and static $\mu^+\delta^-$ B lymphocyte subsets. Eur. J. Immunol. 1982; 12:564–569.
8. Gray D., MacLennan I.C.M. and Lane P.J.L. Virgin B Cell recruitment and the lifespan of memory clones during antibody responses to 2,4-dinitrophenyl-hemocyanin. Eur. J. Immunol. 1986; 16:641–648.

67

Preference for Immunoglobulin A Expression by Germinal Center B Cells in Peyer's Patches Is Likely Due to the Intrinsic Influence of Their Microenvironment

Peter D. Weinstein and John J. Cebra
University of Pennsylvania, Philadelphia, Pennsylvania

INTRODUCTION

Peyer's patches (PPs) are nonencapsulated lymphoid tissue located along the intestinal tract (1). Their chronic stimulation by enteric food and bacterial antigens is believed to lead to the continuous presence of germinal centers (GCs) in PP follicles of conventionally reared mice and also the large number of surface immunoglobulin A–positive ($sIgA^+$) cells within the PP GCs (2–4). In contrast, lymph node (LN) follicles remain quiescent and only display a transient GC reaction following stimulation by an external antigen, which leads to IgG_1 as the primary non-IgM isotype expressed (5–7). The plant lectin, peanut agglutinin (PNA), has been shown to bind to GC B cells, with a high degree of selectivity and avidity (2–6).

Our previous studies using in situ hybridization with C_H-specific riboprobes for IgM, IgG_1, IgG_3, IgE, and IgA have shown that the B-cell population in PPs of conventionally reared mice expressed messenger ribonucleic acid (mRNA) for either IgM or IgA but rarely any other isotype. We were interested in determining whether this apparent preference toward IgA was due to an inherent property of the PP GC microenvironment, or because of the chronic antigenic stimulation PP GC B cells experience; thus driving isotype switching to the 3′ most heavy chain gene. In addition, we were interested in seeing whether the continual presence of GCs in PPs of conventionally reared mice PPs was due to chronic stimulation with the same array of antigens.

RESULTS

A Single Oral Challenge of Reovirus T1 Yields Both a Transient GC Reaction and the Expression of sIgA by PP Cells

Germ-free (GF) mice given 3×10^7 plaque-forming unit (PFU) of reovirus type 1 orally were sampled over a 3-week period to determine whether GCs developed in their PPs, as indicated by the appearance of B cells that bound high levels of PNA (PNA^{high}) and were positive for surface kappa chain ($s\kappa^{+}$). Early after exposure to this enteric virus, no PNA^{high} PP cells were detected by fluorescence-activated cell sorting (FACS), but by day 6 post-immunization (PI), approximately 10% of the total PP cellular population were PNA^{high} and had the surface phenotype $PNA^{high}s\kappa^{high}$. Only 4% of the cells expressed the more typical GC phenotype seen in conventionally reared animals, $PNA^{high}s\kappa^{low}$ (2). By day 11, the $PNA^{high}s\kappa^{high}$ population had increased to about 15% of the total PP population, whereas the $PNA^{high}s\kappa^{low}$ subset rose to around 7%. Soon after, on days 15 and 19, the $PNA^{high}s\kappa^{high}$ population appeared to peak at 16% of the total PP cells, whereas the $PNA^{high}s\kappa^{low}$ subset decreased to around 3–4% of the total PP cellular population. By day 35, the GC reaction had almost completely subsided. The non-GC subset, with surface phenotype $PNA^{low}s\kappa^{high}$, comprised approximately 65% of the total PP cells at day 3, decreased to 55% by day 19, and rose again to the original level by day 35.

Histological examination of PP tissue sections from the primed GF mice over the time course revealed the establishment of GCs in follicles by day 6, at a time coinciding with the first observance of a population of PNA^{high} cells. Also, at day 6, we detected some PNA-binding cells under the dome region of the PPs. Such cells are not detected at this location in PPs of conventionally reared animals. By day 11, all the PNA^{high} cells were located within the GCs of follicles and remained there until about day 19. The establishment of GCs by day 6, and their persistence through day 19 together with FACS analyses, showed that the $PNA^{high}s\kappa^{low}$ population need not be the sole one contributing to the establishment or the maintenance of GCs in follicles.

We examined the heavy chain isotype expression by FACS over the 3-week time course, using labeled antibodies specific for the heavy chains of IgM, IgG_1, and IgA. Early after oral infection, at day 3, the majority (55%) of PP cells were sIgM-positive, and displayed the surface phenotype $PNA^{low}sIgM^{+}$. $PNA^{low}sIgA^{+}$ cells were detected at day 3, comprised about 5% of the total PP cellular population, and remained at this level through day 19. Starting at day 6, $PNA^{high}sIgM^{+}$ cells began to appear, and comprised about 13% of the total PP cells, but this population steadily decreased over time to about 6% of the total PP cells at day 19. This decline was in contrast to the fluctuation of the $PNA^{high}sIgA^{+}$ subset, which at day 6 made up less than 1% of the total PP cellular population, but increased during the time course to around 12% of the total PP cells at day 19. Few if any $sIgG_1$-positive cells were found at any time point.

Immunohistochemical staining of tissue sections of the primed PPs revealed that early in the immune response, at day 3, the B-cell follicles contained sIgM-positive cells, with a few scattered sIgA-positive cells. At day 6, there were sIgM-positive cells in the developing GCs of the follicles and in the mantle zone surrounding the GCs. Few of these cells were found under the dome of the PPs. Many sIgA-positive cells were located under the dome region of the PPs at day 6, but also they could be detected within the GCs. Around day 11 most of the sIgA-positive cells were located within the GCs of follicles, along with a large proportion of sIgM-positive cells. At days 15 and 19, the number of sIgM-positive cells located within the GCs of follicles steadily decreased, but the majority of sIgA-positive cells remained within the GCs.

A Second Oral Challenge with Reovirus Is Unable to Elicit a New GC Response

Since we were able to drive a rapid, transient GC reaction in PPs following a single oral antigenic stimulation of GF mice with reovirus, we were interested in determining whether we could drive a second GC response using the same antigen, again administered orally. We inoculated primed GF mice 5 weeks following the initial stimulation with a dose of virus equivalent to the initial one or a one hundred times higher dose. We analyzed for GC development over a 3-week time course and found that we were unable to stimulate an appreciable second GC reaction with either dose of virus. A small fraction of the cells in PPs that expressed the surface phenotype, $PNA^{high}s\kappa^{high}$ could be detected during this time examined, but this cellular population never amounted to more than a few percent of the total PP cells. Likewise, we were unable to detect any cells that were $PNA^{high}sIgA^{+}$. We believe that the GC response either did not occur, or was extremely muted in comparison to the initial response seen following a primary stimulation of GF mice.

Reovirus Elicits a GC Reaction and Production of IgG_1 in Lymph Nodes Following a Parenteral Immunization

We examined draining lymph nodes following a local challenge with reovirus injected into the footpads to determine whether GC development occurred and which heavy chain isotypes were expressed. We were able to drive a transient GC response as seen by FACS analysis for PNA binding and by histology, and found that within the LN the predominant non-IgM isotype expressed was $sIgG_1$, not sIgA. These observations were further supported by analysis of lymphoid fragment cultures. We were able to detect an appreciable quantity of reovirus specific IgA antibody (Ab) from PP fragment cultures, whereas LN fragment cultures yielded mostly IgM and IgG_1 Ab.

SUMMARY

We have studied the time course of development of a GC response in PPs of orally primed GF mice. We found that the response was transient with the waxing and waning of a GC follicle over a 3-week period of time as shown by both FACS analysis, and histochemical analysis of tissue sections. The time course of the GC reaction in the LN of conventionally reared mice given reovirus by footpad injections was almost identical. These findings support the contention that the chronic GCs in follicles seen within a PP of conventionally reared mice are due to the continual stimulation of the PP by antigens inside the small intestine. However, restimulation of the primed, formerly GF mice, did not perturb a new GC response in the PP. Thus, it appears that not only is continual antigenic stimulation required, but it has to be accomplished using new arrays of antigens. Of course, 6 months or a year PI, the mucosal protection and antigen exclusion we apparently detected may not be as effective as it appears to be at 5 weeks PI.

Finally, we were able to drive expression of IgA following a single, acute stimulation of GF PPs, unlike LN which yielded predominantly IgG_1 following a similar stimuli, thus showing that it probably is not the continual stimulation of the PPs by natural antigen that supports an IgA response in a PP of conventionally reared mice. Rather, some intrinsic property of the PP GC microenvironment may account for the preference for IgA expression in PPs.

ACKNOWLEDGMENT

This work was supported by USPHS Grant AI-17997.

REFERENCES

1. Nieuwenhuis, P. and Opstetelten, D., The functional anatomy of germinal centers. Am J Anat, 170:421 (1984).
2. Butcher, E. C., Rouse, R. V., Coffman, R. L., Nottenburg, C. N., Hardy, R. R. and Weissman, I. L., Surface phenotype of Peyer's patch germinal center cells: Implications for the role of germinal centers in B-cell differentiation. J Immunol 129:2698 (1982).
3. Rose, R. L. and Malchiodi, F., Binding of peanut lectin to thymic cortex and germinal centres of lymphoid tissue, Immunology, 42:583 (1981).
4. Rose, M. L. Birbeck, M. S. C., Wallis, V. J., Forrester, J. A. and Davies, A. J. S., Peanut lectin binding properties of germinal centres of mouse lymphoid tissue, Nature, 284:364 (1980).
5. Kraal, G., Weissman, I. L. and Butcher, E. C., Germinal centre B cells: Antigen specificity and changes in heavy chain class expression, Nature 298:311 (1982).
6. Kraal, G. Weissman, I. L. and Butcher, E. C., Germinal center cells: antigen specificity, heavy chain class expression and evidence of memory, Adv Exp Med Biol, 186:145 (1985).
7. Reichert, R. A., Gallatin, W. M., Weissman, I. L. and Butcher, E. C., Germinal centre B cells lack homing receptors necessary for normal lymphocyte recirculation. J Exp Med, 157:813 (1983).

68
Development of the Intestinal B-Cell Compartment of the Pig

Andre T.J. Bianchi, Bernie Moonen, Jan W. Scholten, and Philip J. van der Heijden
Central Veterinary Institute, AB, Lelystad, The Netherlands

INTRODUCTION

The development of the B-cell compartment has been studied extensively by quantitating the background ("spontaneously" occurring) immunoglobulin (Ig)–secreting cells (Ig-SCs) in various organs of the mouse (1,2). The development of the murine Ig-SC response has been studied both for systemic lymphoid organs (1) and for mucosal lymphoid organs (3,4). These studies provide insight in factors that are important for the development of the Ig-SC response of various organs. The splenic Ig-SC response is hardly affected by external antigens and is relatively high from the first few weeks after birth. In contrast, the development of the Ig-SC response in mucosal lymphoid organs does not depend on age but depends on external antigenic pressure (4). It appears that IgA is the predominant isotype produced along the murine small intestine from the first moment after birth on which a significant number of intestinal Ig-SC is found (3). This type of study has only been done for laboratory animals like mice. In this chapter, we describe the development of the Ig-SC response of different organs in pigs. The Ig-SC response of systemic lymphoid organs was compared with the Ig-SC response of the small intestine. We also studied the dominant Ig isotype of the different organs at the various ages tested. The results of this study are relevant to our knowledge of developmental immunology and also for comparative immunology.

MATERIALS AND METHODS

Animals

Specific pathogen-free (SPF) pigs (crossbred Great Yorkshire × Dutch Landrace) were selected from the breeding stock of our institute. Three littermates were used per age group of 4, 12, and 40 weeks.

Preparation of Cell Suspensions

Pigs were anaesthetized by intravenous injection of hypnodil-stresnil (Janssen, Beerse, Belgium) and subsequently killed by bleeding. Tissue pieces of spleen, prescapular lymph node (PLN), mesenteric lymph node (MLN), jejunal Peyer's patches (PPs-j), and ileal Peyer's patch (PPs-i) were collected and placed in RPMI-1640 medium containing 5% fetal calf serum (FCS), 20 mM HEPES, and 0.1 mg/ml deoxyribonuclease (DNAse) (Sigma, St. Louis, Missouri), then minced with scissors and squeezed through a stainless steel grid (500 μm) followed by nylon gauze filters (200 μm, followed by 100 and 50 μm) to obtain single cell suspensions. Red bone marrow (BM) from femurs or ribs was squirted using a syringe with medium to BM suspensions. Lamina propria (LP) cell suspensions were prepared from pieces of duodenum, jejunum, and ileum essentially according to the method described for the mouse (5).

Enumeration of Ig-SCs

A reversed spot assay (RSA) was used to quantitate Ig-SCs in cell suspensions of the lymphoid organs. The RSA was performed according to the method described for the mouse (6). Monoclonal antibodies (MAbs) specific for the porcine Ig isotypes (CVI-Swμ28.4 specific for IgM, CVI-Swγ23.7 specific for IgG, and CVI-Swα27.9 specific for IgA (7) were used to coat 96-well microtiter plates (Greiner, Alphen a/d Rijn, The Netherlands). The coated plates were incubated with phosphate-buffered saline (PBS) supplemented with 5% FCS to block remaining nonspecific binding sites. The plates were rinsed with PBS, and 10^3, 10^4, 10^5, and 10^6 cells suspended in 0.1 ml RPMI-1640 medium and supplemented with penicillin and streptomycin, which were added in triplicate to the plate and incubated 3–4 hr at 37°C. The plates were rinsed thoroughly with PBS containing 0.5% Tween. The Ig-SCs were detected as follows: optimal dilutions of polyclonal antibodies against the porcine Ig isotypes were made in PBS-Tween supplemented with 1% BSA and were added in aliquots of 0.1 ml to the wells. R-anti-SwIgM(Fc) (Nordic, Tilburg, The Netherlands) was used on plates coated with the anti-IgM MAb to detect IgM-SCs, R-anti-SwIgG(H+L) (Nordic, Tilburg, The Netherlands) was used on plates coated with the anti-IgG MAb to detect IgG-SCs, and R-anti-HuIgA(Fc) (Nordic, Tilburg, The Netherlands) was used on plates coated with the anti-IgA MAb to detect IgA-SCs. After overnight incubation at 4°C or 3 hr at 37°C, the plates were rinsed and incubated with 0.1 ml of the optimal dilution of G-anti-RIg alkaline fosfatase conjugate (Biomakor, Rehovot, Israel) diluted in BSA-PBS-Tween for 1.5–3.0 hr at 37°C. The spots were visualized according to the procedure described for the antigen-specific spot-forming cell assay (8).

RESULTS

Frequencies of Ig-SCs in Various Lymphoid Organs

Suspensions of spleen, MLN, PLN, BM, PPs-j, PPs-i, duodenum, jejunum, and ileum were prepared from 4-, 12-, and 40-week-old SPF pigs. The frequencies of Ig-SCs in each suspension, as determined by the isotype-specific RSA, are shown in Figures 1 and 2. The results per organ are expressed as the mean of each age group (n=3). The results demonstrate that the frequency of Ig-SCs in spleen (see Fig. 1) was already high from the fourth week of life, increased only slightly up to 40 weeks of age, and IgM was the predominant isotype. The same results were found for the MLN, although the IgG and IgA frequencies of MLN were higher compared to IgG and IgA frequencies of spleen, and they

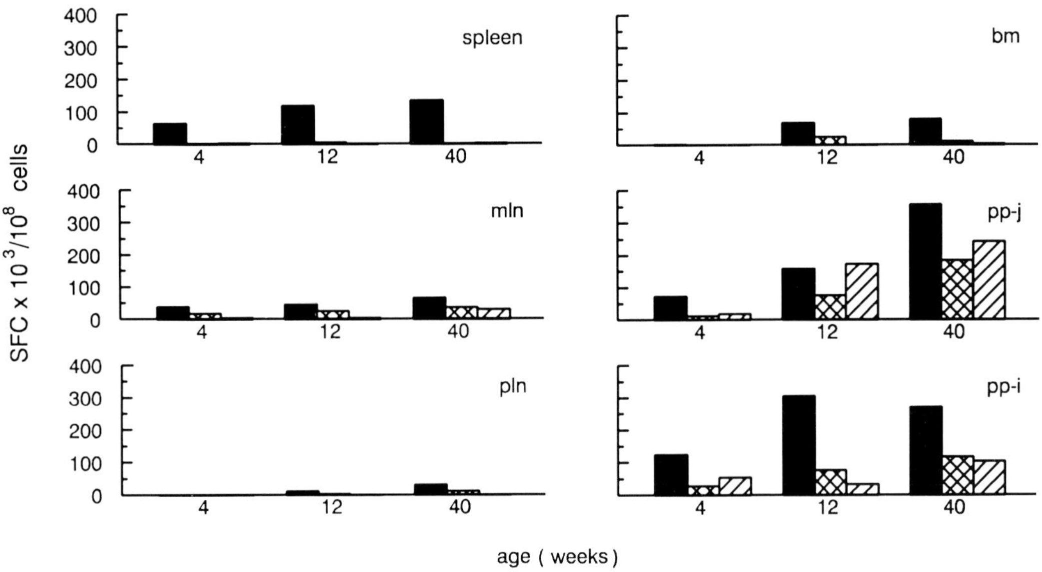

Figure 1 Frequency of Ig-SCs in spleen, MLN, PLN, BM, PPs-j, and PPs-i as a function of age. results are expressed as the mean (n=3). Solid bars represent IgM, cross-hatched bars IgG, and hatched bars IgA.

also increased with age. In PLN and BM cell suspensions, the Ig-SC response started later and significant frequencies of Ig-SCs were only found from 12 weeks of age (see Fig. 1). In PPs cell suspensions, IgM was again the predominant isotype and the frequencies of Ig-SC were higher than in spleen at all ages tested, but in PPs also high frequencies of IgG-SCs and IgA-SCs were found (see Fig. 1). The Ig-SC frequencies of cell suspensions of PPs-j increased clearly from 4 weeks up to 40 weeks of age for all three isotypes, whereas the IgM-SC frequency of PPs-i reached already a maximum of 12 weeks of age and the increase of the IgG-SC and IgA-SC frequencies was less pronounced. The results obtained with the LP cell suspensions are shown separately in Figure 2 because of the much higher Ig-SC frequencies found along the small intestine (SI). The frequency of IgA-SCs increased enormously with age in all three parts of the SI tested. In duodenum and jejunum, the highest (IgA-SC) frequency was reached at 12 weeks, whereas in ileum the highest frequency was reached at 40 weeks of age. The IgM frequency of all parts of the SI was high compared to the other organs tested. Immunoglobulin M was even the predominant isotype in duodenum and ileum at 4 weeks of age, but IgA predominated along the complete SI from 12 weeks of age.

DISCUSSION

The results described in this chapter demonstrate that the development of the Ig-SC frequencies of spleen, PLN, MLN, and BM is compatible with the development of Ig-SC frequencies in mice (3). A difference with mice is the dominant IgM response of these organs in pigs at all ages tested, whereas in mice the IgG-SC and IgA-SC frequencies are relatively higher. This difference can be explained, at least partially, by very clean housing of the SPF pigs. The Ig-SC frequencies of the PPs are higher in pigs than in mice after an

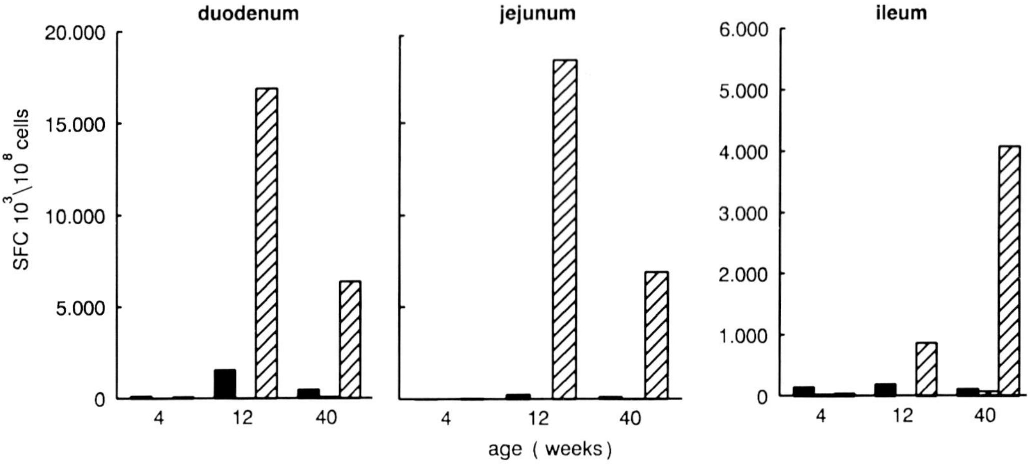

Figure 2 Frequency of Ig-SCs in duodenum, jejunum, and ileum as a function of age. The other details are explained in the legend to Figure 1.

age of 4 weeks. The fast development of PPs-i Ig-SCs fits with the role of PPs-i in the B-cell ontogeny of the pig (9). The most striking differences between murine and porcine Ig-SC responses are found along the SI. The cline of the Ig-SC frequency along the small intestine from cranial to caudal, which is found in mice at all ages (1), disappeared in pigs with age. Further, IgA is also the predominant isotype of the porcine SI, but, in contrast to the murine SI, IgM is relatively important especially at 4 weeks of age.

Our results clearly demonstrate differences between the development of Ig-SCs in pigs and mice, which underlines the importance of comparative immunology.

REFERENCES

1. Benner R, Oudenaren van A, Björkland M, Ivars F. Holmberg D. 'Background' immunoglobulin production: Measurement, biological significance and regulation. Immunol Today 1982; 3: 243–49.
2. Benner R, Haaijman JJ. Ageing of the lymphoid system at the organ level. Dev Comp Immunol 1980; 4:591–603.
3. Heijden van der PJ, Bianchi ATJ, Stok W, Bokhout BA. Background (spontaneous) immunoglobulin production in the murine small intestine as a function of age. Immunology 1988; 65:243–48.
4. Heijden van der PJ, Bianchi ATJ, Heidt PJ, Stok W, Bokhout BA. Background (spontaneous) immunoglobulin production in the murine small intestine before and after weaning. J Reprod Immunol 1989; 15:217–27.
5. Heijden van der PJ, Stok W. Improved procedure for the isolation of functionally active lymphoid cells from the murine intestine. J Immunol Methods 1987; 103:161–67.
6. Czerkinsky CC, Tarowski A, Nilsson LA, Ouchterlony O, Nygren H, Gretzer C. Reversed enzyme-linked immunospot assay (Relispot) for the detection of cells secreting immunoreactive substances. J Immunol Methods 1984; 72:489–96.
7. Zaane van D, Hulst MM. Monoclonal antibodies against porcine immunoglobulin isotypes. Vet Immunol Immunopathol 1987; 16:23–36.

8. Bianchi ATJ, Scholten JW, Jongenelen IMCA, Koch G. The use of monoclonal antibodies in an enzyme immunospot assay to detect isotype-specific antibody-secreting cells in pigs and chickens. Vet Immunol Immunopathol 1990; 24:125–34.
9. Pabst R, Geist M, Rothkötter HJ, Fritz FJ. Postnatal development and lymphocyte production of jejunal and ileal Peyer's patches in normal and gnotobiotic pigs. Immunology 1988; 64:539–44.

69

Dual Pathway for Differentiation of Memory B Cells to Antibody-Forming Cells in the Spleen

Nico van Rooijen
Vrije Universiteit, Amsterdam, The Netherlands

HISTOLOGICAL REACTIONS IN THE SPLEEN AFTER ANTIGEN ADMINISTRATION

Already in the early 1960s, two different histological reactions in the spleen were reported following intravenous administration of antigen (1). The first reaction, comprising the development of numerous blastlike cells from lymphocytes, occurred in the periarteriolar lymphocyte sheath (PALS), and started at about 2 days after antigen injection, whereas the second reaction, in the splenic follicles, was seen from day 5 onward. In the past 3 decades, much evidence has been produced that the early reaction in the PALS corresponds with the production of antibody-forming cells in the spleen (1,2), whereas the second reaction in the follicles corresponds with the generation of memory B cells (3).

Recent studies confirmed that specific antibody-forming cells indeed develop in the PALS irrespective of the type of antigen, the sub(class) of immunoglobulins produced, and the presence or absence of a primed state for the antigen (4). However, antibody-forming cells occasionally developed in the follicles too, their numbers per follicle showing an extremely high degree of variation (5). Such differences in the localization of antibody-forming cells have also been found in lymph nodes after subcutaneous administration of the antigen. Results varied from exclusive follicular localization (6) to exclusive localization in the lymph node medulla (7).

PRODUCTION AND FATE OF MEMORY B CELLS IN THE SPLEEN

Much evidence has been produced that memory B cells are generated in the germinal centers (GCs) of lymphoid follicles (3) under the influence of antigen-antibody complexes that are immobilized on the cell processes of follicular dendritic cells (FDCs). Memory B

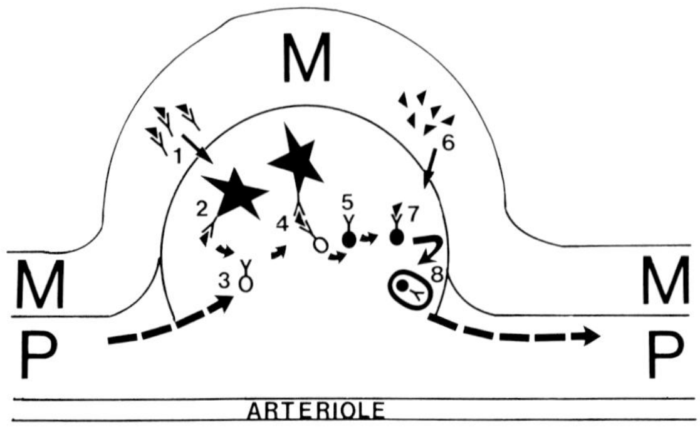

Figure 1 Schematic representation of the events leading to the development of antibody-forming cells in lymphoid follicles of the spleen. (1) Antigen-antibody complexes, formed during the antibody response against the antigen, arrive in the marginal zone, from where they enter into the follicles. (2) Once in the follicles, they are trapped on the surfaces of the cell processes of FDCs. (3) B cells (open circles) with surface Igs that recognize one of the antigenic determinants enter into the follicles from the PALS. (4) They are bound by free antigenic determinants exposed by immune complexes that are immobilized on the FDCs. (5) With the help of follicular T cells (not indicated), these B cells are activated to become memory B cells (closed circles). If no soluble antigen molecules are present at the time that they have completed their differentiation, newly formed memory B cells leave the follicles to enter the marginal zone and the circulation via the PALS. (6) Soluble antigen molecules, if still or again present, enter into the follicles. (7) They are bound by the surface Igs of the newly formed memory B cells. (8) In reaction, these memory B cells are stimulated to become antibody-forming cells (eye).

cells are generally considered to be small resting lymphocytes that are found in the circulating pool and survive for long periods in a quiescent state between each antigen encounter, but recent evidence supports that these are antigen-dependent (8).

After stimulation in the follicle, memory B cells usually colonize the splenic marginal zones (9). It has been shown that in the secondary immune response, just as in the primary response, the development of antibody-forming cells in the spleen is localized in the outer parts of the PALS (4), and a large amount of evidence has been produced that these cells entered into the PALS from the marginal zone (4,9). In conclusion, memory B cells are produced in the follicles, from where they reach the circulation and the marginal zones in the spleen. Upon a new antigen encounter, they leave the marginal zone to enter into the outer PALS and differentiate into antibody-forming cells. The latter cells leave the PALS again via the small sheaths of lymphoid tissue surrounding the terminal arterioles, from where they arrive in the red pulp of the spleen to reach the circulation again.

LABORATORY EXPERIMENTS AND INFECTIOUS DISEASES

After administration of, e.g., a protein antigen, to an animal, an immune response is induced and the antigen molecules are consecutively complexed with the antibodies which are produced by specific-antibody forming cells. The bulk of these immune complexes are ingested and digested by phagocytic cells of the mononuclear phagocyte system, but a very small proportion escapes this destruction and is trapped by FDCs in lymphoid follicles. Here, the complexes are preserved in an undegraded form for long periods of time. As mentioned earlier, these complexes are thought to play a crucial role in the generation of memory B cells. At the time that the first memory B cells have completed their differentiation in the follicles, soluble antigen (or antigen-antibody complexes with free antigenic determinants) is no longer present. These memory B cells may leave the follicles and enter the circulation or colonize the marginal zones in the spleen, and await a new contact with the antigen.

During infectious diseases, however, the antigen can replicate in the body. As a consequence, free antigen is still available in the body at the time that the first memory B cells have completed their differentiation in the follicles. We have recently postulated that in the continuing presence of soluble antigen, these newly generated memory B cells in the follicles may directly continue to differentiate into antibody-forming cells (10). A similar situation can be created if nonreplicating antigens are administered together with an adjuvant with an action based on storage and slow release of antigen. This may well account for the large numbers of antibody-forming cells found in the follicles of lymph nodes in the early studies of Sordat and colleagues (6). These authors administered the antigen horseradish peroxidase (HRP), adsorbed to aluminum phosphate, subcutaneously into the footpads of mice. From the injection site, the antigen is gradually released in the lymph flow toward the draining lymph nodes. Recent studies by Delemarre et al. (Thesis, Vrije Universiteit, Amsterdam, 1990) confirmed that antibody-forming cells may develop in the follicles if soluble antigen and FDC-retained antigen are both present in the follicles.

ANTIBODY-FORMING CELLS IN LYMPHOID FOLLICLES

In conclusion, antibody-forming cells may develop in the follicles from newly formed memory B cells under the following conditions:

1. Antigens are slowly released from an adjuvant serving as an antigen depot.
2. Antigens are repeatedly administered.
3. Antigens can replicate in the body.

However, the simultaneous presence of soluble antigen, or antigen-antibody complexes with free antigenic determinants, and immune complexes immobilized on the FDC surfaces does not automatically induce the follicular production of antibody-forming cells. The antigen should reach the follicles at a time that memory B cells are (still or again) produced in the follicles.

If follicular production of memory B cells has come to an end and all memory cells are in the circulation or the marginal zone, the normal distribution pattern of antibody-forming cells may be expected after antigen injections; that is, in the PALS. On the other hand, during the secondary response, follicular trapping of new immune complexes occurs within some hours. Renewed functional activity in the follicles may well produce new memory B cells at a time when soluble immune complexes with free antigenic determinants are still in the circulation.

REFERENCES

1. Langevoort HL. The histophysiology of the antibody response I. Histogenesis of the plasma cell reaction in rabbit spleen. Lab. Invest. 1962; 12, 106–118.
2. Eikelenboom P, Boorsma DM, Van Rooijen N. The development of IgM- and IgG-containing plasmablasts in the white pulp of the spleen after stimulation with a thymus-independent antigen (LPS) and a thymus-dependent antigen (SRBC). Cell Tissue Res. 1982; 226, 83–95.

3. Klaus GGB, Humphrey JH, Kunkl A, Dongworth DW. The follicular dendritic cell: Its role in antigen presentation in the generation of immunological memory. Immunol. Rev. 1980, 53, 3–28.
4. Van Rooijen N, Claassen E, Eikelenboom P. Is there a single differentiation pathway for all antibody forming cells in the spleen? Immunol. Today 1986; 7, 193–196.
5. Van Rooijen N, Kors N. Specific antibody forming cells in lymphoid follicles of spleen: An aspect of the late immune response. Adv. Exp. Med. Biol. 1988; 237, 221–225.
6. Sordat B, Sordat M, Hess MW, Stoner RD, Cottier H. Specific antibody within lymphoid germinal center cells of mice after primary immunization with horseradish peroxidase: A light and electron microscopic study. J. Exp. Med. 1970; 131, 77–92.
7. Delemarre FGA, Claassen E, Van Rooijen N. Primary 'in situ' immune response in popliteal lymph nodes and spleen of mice after subcutaneous immunization with thymus-dependent or thymus-independent antigens. Anat. Rec. 1989; 223, 152–157.
8. Gray D, Skarvall H. B-cell memory is short-lived in the absence of antigen. Nature 1988; 336, 70–73.
9. Liu Y-J, Oldfield S, MacLennan ICM. Memory B cells in T cell-dependent antibody responses colonize the splenic marginal zones. Eur. J. Immunol. 1988; 18, 355–362.
10. Van Rooijen N. Direct intrafollicular differentiation of memory B cells into plasma cells. Immunol. Today 1990; 11, 154–157.

70

Physiology of Human Thymus-Independent Type 2 Antibody Responses

Lessons from Patients with Selective Failure of Carbohydrate Antibody Responses

D. S. Kumararatne,[1,3] M. Hazlewood,[1] P. Bird,[2] M. Forte,[1]
H. Joyce,[3] S. Misbah,[4] M. Goodall,[1] R. J. Jefferis,[1]
and H. Chapel[4]

[1]*The Medical School, Birmingham, England;* [2]*University of Edinburgh, Edinburgh, Scotland;* [3]*Dudley Road Hospital, Birmingham, England;* [4]*John Radcliffe Hospital, Oxford, England*

INTRODUCTION

High-grade bacterial pathogens like *Streptococcus pneumoniae, Haemophilus influenzae* type b, and *Neisseria meningitidis* possess carbohydrate capsules which inhibit phagocytosis and interfere with binding of the membrane attack complex of complement to the bacterial cell membrane (1). Capsular polysaccharides behave as thymus-independent (type 2) (TI-2) antigens and induce protective antibody responses. B cells responding to TI-2 antigens can be activated independently of T cells but may require T-cell–derived factors for optimum differentiation to antibody-forming cells (2).

Unlike protein antigens, TI-2 antigens are (a) poor immunogens in children, especially those below 2 years of age, (b) they do not induce generation of germinal centers (GCs) and B memory cells, (c) they may be poorly immunogenic in splenectomized individuals (2). Hence, young children (especially those below 5 years of age) are susceptible to invasive disease caused by capsulated bacteria and cannot be effectively protected by bacterial polysaccharide vaccines (3). Circumstantial evidence suggests that TI-2 antibody responses are mainly due to stimulation of a subset of B cells found mainly in the spleen and the acquisition of responsiveness to these antigens coincides with the appearance of an immunoglobulin (Ig) M high, IgD–low, CD21 (CR2)–positive B cell population in the splenic marginal zone of infants around 2 years of age (2). However, the physiological basis for the difference between antibody responses to TD (protein) and T1-2 antigens is unclear. We have identified a spectrum of patients with a selective inability to respond to

TI-2 antigens and in this chapter we discuss the relevance of our findings in an attempt to understand the physiology of human anticarbohydrate antibody responses.

MATERIALS AND METHODS

Patient Selection

1. Patients with a history of invasive disease caused by capsulated bacteria (e.g., *S. pneumoniae, H. influenzae*, type b), or recurrent infections especially involving the upper and lower respiratory tract, referred for investigation during the years 1986–1989 to the Department of Immunology at Dudley Road Hospital, Birmingham or John Radcliffe Hospital, Oxford, England, were studied. During this period, 350 patients of this type were evaluated. Patients with primary immunodeficiency syndromes known to cause antibody deficiency (e.g., X-linked hypogammaglobulinemia, common variable antibody deficiency, the Wiskott-Aldrich syndrome, ataxia telangiectasia), or clinical disorders giving rise to secondary antibody deficiency (e.g., myelomatosis) were excluded from the study. Children below 5 years of age are excluded from this report as physiological deficiency of TI-2 responses are seen in this age group.
2. Sixty-one patients with severe inherited deficiency of single complement components were studied. Details of these patients have been documented elsewhere (4).
3. Serum from two patients with leukocyte adhesion defect, characterized by CD11a,b, and c and CD18 deficiency (5) were kindly provided for study by Dr. R.A. Thompson (East Birmingham Hospital, England) and Dr. A.D.B. Webster (Clinical Research Centre, Northwick Park Hospital, Harrow, England).

Immunological Evaluation

A complete blood count and differential count, serum immunoglobulins (IgG, IgA, IgM) (6) and IgG subclass levels (IgG_1, IgG_2, IgG_3, IgG_4) (6) were measured in all patients. Age-specific normal ranges for these values have been calibrated against WHO reference serum 67/97 and established for the United Kingdom population by the United Kingdom supraregional protein reference service (7). Patients with bacteremic illnesses or severe invasive infection (e.g., meningitis, pneumonia) also had serum total hemolytic complement levels, alternate pathway hemolytic activity, and C3 and C4 levels measured. Where relevant, the presence of a spleen was determined by ultrasound examination and splenic function assessed by counting pitted red cells in peripheral venous blood using darkground microscopy.

Antigen-Specific Antibody Levels

Specific antibody levels to a panel of protein (tetanus toxoid) and polysaccharide (pneumococcal capsular polysaccharide [PCP], *Hemophilus* b polyribose phosphate (Hib prp), *N. meningitidis* type A and C capsular polysaccharide, *Escherichia coli* J5 lipopolysaccharide) were measured by a four-layer solid phase ELISA as described in detail elsewhere (8). Briefly, polystyrene microtiter plates coated with antigen were incubated successively with human sera, mouse monoclonal antibody (MAb) to human Ig classes or IgG subclasses and with a final sheep antimouse-Ig peroxidase conjugate. The binding of conjugate was determined by developing color with OPD substrate at 37°C for 15 min and the absorbance was read at 492 nm. Positive and negative control sera were included in every assay. Positive reference serum for the Hib prp antibody assay was obtained from the Office of Biologics U.S. FDA. (This contained 60 μg/ml antibody, as determined by radioimmunoassay.) The positive reference serum for the other assays was obtained from a serum pool prepared from several healthy donors. The negative control serum was obtained from a panhypogammaglobulinaemic patient. The antibody levels for each individual were expressed as the dilution of antibody giving an optical density reading equivalent to one-third maximum value produced by the standard positive reference serum. Patients with antibody levels below the 5th percentile for an age-matched control population (n = 55) were immunized with the appropriate vaccine and serum retested 4 weeks later.

Statistical Analysis

The statistical analysis was done by the Wilcoxon Rank sum test for unpaired samples.

RESULTS

Patients with Selective TI-2 Antibody Deficiency

Nineteen of 350 patients were found to have low anticarbohydrate antibody levels. The clinical and immunological features are summarized in Tables 1 and 2. Figure 1 shows that these patients as a group had normal antiprotein (TD) antibody levels but selective deficiency of IgG pneumococcal antibodies ($p < 0.05$). Fourteen of 19 patients had IgG_2 antibodies to PCP below the 5th percentile for an age-matched healthy control group. The median and 5th and 95th percentiles of IgG_2 antipneumococcal antibody titers for the control group were 1/223, 1/9, and 1/1500, respectively; the three patients with IgG_2 antipneumococcal antibodies overlapping with the normal group had titers of 1/20, 1/16, and 1/10, respectively; i.e., they had values at the lower end of the normal range.

The largest group of patients had normal serum Ig and IgG subclass levels, normal thymus-independent type 1(TI-1) and TD antibody responses, and deficient antibody levels to PCP, Hib prp, and meningococcal (types A and C) capsular polysaccharides (14/19).

Table 1 Clinical and Microbiological Features of Patients with Selective Anti–Carbohydrate Antibody Deficiency

Clinical problem	No. affected	Infecting organisms	No. affected
Pneumonia	8	Pneumococcus	16
Bronchiectasis	4	*H. influenzae* (b and nontypable)	12
LRTI/URTI	3	*N. meningitidis*	2
Bronchial asthma	5	Group B streptococcus	1
Nonreversible airway		*B. cattarhalis*	4
obstruction	2	Gastrointestinal pathogens	
Otitis media	5	*Giardia*	1
Meningitis	9	Cryptosporidiosis	1
Septicemia	8	*Associated features*	
Peritonitis	2	Congenital heart disease	1[a]
Diarrhea	2	and situs inversus	
Epilepsy	1	Congenital asplenia	1[a]

Total number of patients: 350; number with TI-2 antibody deficiency: 19; age range: 5 to 30 years.
[a]Seen in the same patient.

Table 2 Immunological Abnormalities Associated with TI-2 Antibody Deficiency

	No. patients
Selective IgG_2 deficiency and low anticarbohydrate antibodies following immunization with polysaccharide vaccines	1
Normal total Igs, IgG subclasses, and low anticarbohydrate antibodies following immunization with polysaccharide vaccines	14
Normal total Igs, IgG subclasses, and highly selective antibody deficiency	
1. Normal antibodies to PCP and Hib prp with poor antibody response to *N. meningitidis* (A and C) polysaccharide	1
2. Normal antibodies to PCP, Hib prp, and *N. meningitidis* (A and C) polysaccharide with poor antibody response to group B streptococcal polysaccharide	1
Normal total Igs, and IgG subclasses, and deficient anticarbohydrate antibody response to natural exposure and invasive septicaemic disease with capsulated bacteria	2[a]
Selective IgG_2 deficiency with quantitatively normal anticarbohydrate responses and *no history of infection*	2

[a]These two patients developed good antibody responses following immunization with pneumococcal and Hib capsular polysaccharide vaccines.

They did not respond to immunization with the respective purified capsular polysaccharide vaccines. Two of three patients with poor response to Hib prp vaccine developed good sustained antibody responses to Hib prp conjugated to a protein carrier (tetanus toxoid or mutant diphtheria toxoid CRM157). One patient did not respond to a single dose of Hib-diphtheria toxoid (CRM157) conjugate, in spite of having previous high antibody levels to the carrier molecule (i.e., diphtheria toxoid). Two additional patients (two of 19) with selective deficiency of TI-2 antibodies, in spite of invasive disease by capsulated bacteria, responded to immunization with Pneumovax and Hib prp vaccine with good sustained antibody responses, including antipolysaccharide antibodies of the IgG_2 isotype.

We have also identified two individuals aged 17 and 22 years, respectively, who had selective deficiency of IgG_2 levels and quantitatively normal IgG antibody responses to TI-2 antigens. These antibodies were entirely of the IgG_1 isotype. These two individuals had no history of bacterial infections.

Anticarbohydrate Antibody Levels and Inherited Complement Deficiency

Patients with inherited complement deficiencies leading to impaired C3 activation have low IgG_4 levels, and three of four patients with homozygous C3 deficiency had low IgG_2 levels in addition, as previously reported (4). We therefore measured specific antibody levels in these patients and found that the three of four C3-deficient patients with low IgG_2 levels had no antipneumococcal antibodies. All patients had normal TD responses and antibody levels against Hib prp and *N. meningitidis* (types A and C) capsular polysaccharides (Table 3).

Table 3 TI-2 Antibody Responses in Patients with Inherited Single Complement Component Deficiency[a] or LFA Deficiency

	Number of patients with:	
Type of C′	normal anti-PCP antibodies	low anti-PCP antibodies
C1, C2 or C4	19	0
C5, C6, C7, C8 or C9	16	0
Factor P	9	0
Factor I	4	0
C1 inhibitor	9	0

Type of C′ deficiency: C3

				Anti-PCP antibody titer[b] belonging to following Isotype		
Patient	Age	Serum IgG	Serum IgG_2	Total IgG	IgG_1	IgG_2
ARM	child	normal	low	<5	<5	<5
Ren	8	normal	normal	>2560	10	640
A.V.	24	normal	low	44	12	<5
B.V.	21	normal	low	47	19	<5

Type of deficiency: LFA(CD 11a,b,c deficiency)

	Anti-PCP antibody titer[b] belonging to following Isotype				
Patient	Total IgG	IgG1	IgG2	Anti-Hib prp antibodies	Anti-N.M(A&C) antibodies
JR	>2560	<4	520	normal	normal
JT	>2560	<4	>2560	normal	normal

[a]All patients had normal levels of antiabodies to Hib prp and *N. meningitidis* (A and C) (N.M.,A&C) polysaccharide.
[b]See Figure 1 for normal range.

Leukocyte Functional Antigen (LFA) Deficiency

Two patients with LFA (CD11a,b,c and CD18) deficiency had entirely normal TD and TI-2 antibody levels (see Table 3).

DISCUSSION

The existence of the individuals with selective IgG_2 deficiency with normal levels of anticapsular antibodies and no increase in susceptibility to infection as reported above (see Table 2) and elsewhere (9) casts doubt on the widespread belief that IgG_2 antibodies are critically important for effective immunity against capsulated bacterial pathogens. What is important is the ability to produce anticapsular antibodies of the IgG class, irrespective of the precise subclass composition. Antibodies induce elimination of bacteria by complement-mediated lysis or inducing opsonophagocytic clearance. The IgG_2 isotype is less

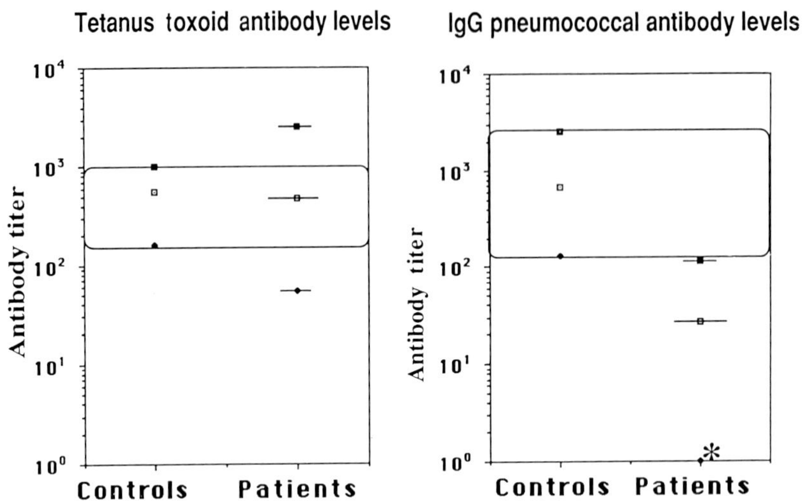

Figure 1 The antibody levels to tetanus toxoid and the TI-2 antigen PCP are shown for a normal healthy control group (n=55) and patients with TI-2 antibody deficiency (n=19). Horizontal bars indicate median values and range for patients. ▣, indicates median value for control group. Horizontal box indicates 5th and 95th percentiles for control group. n *This value was below the limits of detection; i.e., titer <1.

efficient that IgG_1 or IgG_3 (on a molar basis) at activating the classic complement pathway and does not bind to Fc receptors of mononuclear phagocytes (9). Immunoglobulin G_2 binding to Fc receptors of neutrophils is also poor (9). Hence, it is difficult to see from in vitro studies why IgG_2 should be more efficient at inducing protective immunity against capsulated bacteria.

The existence of substantial numbers of patients with normal serum IgG_2 levels but defective TI-2 responses, as demonstrated in this (see Table 2) and other studies (10), rules out the possibility that defective anticarbohydrate antibody responses are due to the inability to synthesize this isotype. Since IgG_2 antibodies are mainly produced in response to carbohydrate antigenic stimulation, low serum IgG_2 levels may be a consequence of TI-2 antibody deficiency.

What are the mechanisms of TI-2 antibody deficiency?

This could be due to (a) a deficiency of antigen-specific B cells (i.e., B cells which are able to generate the appropriate combination of V regions), or (b) a lack of a TI-2 antigen–responsive B-cell subset. The first possibility is very unlikely, as many TI-2 antibody–deficient patients are able to respond to TI-2 epitopes coupled to a protein carrier, as shown in this and other studies (7). Evidence summarized by Maclennan et al. (1990) (2) indicates that a subset of IgM-high, IgD-low, CD21-positive, and CD23-negative B cells, found mainly in the splenic marginal zones, are the only precursors of TI-2 antibody–producing plasma cells. These cells are not present in the marginal zone of infants below 2 years of age, and the tempo of their appearance in this splenic compartment appears to coincide with the acquisition of TI-2 antigen responsiveness.

A further possibility is a failure of accessory signal delivery required for the effective stimulation of TI-2 antigen–specific B cells. This could be due to (a) lack of antigen-processing or -presenting cells. (b) inability to generate C3 breakdown products (e.g., C3d) acting as accessory factors for B-cell stimulation, (c) lack of T-cell–derived accessory factors (11), or (d) lack of B-cell surface receptors for accessory factor(s).

We know very little about in vivo carbohydrate antigen-presenting cells. Humphrey et al. (12) showed that splenic marginal zones (MZs) contain cells with dendritic morphology, which can concentrate and retain neutral polysaccharides like hydroxyethyl starch, dextran, or ficoll. Such cells would be ideally situated to stimulate MZ B cells. However, acidic polysaccharides localize in the splenic red pulp macrophages and are not significantly retained by MZ macrophages. Most PCPs are acidic and would be expected to localize in splenic red pulp rather than in the MZ. It is conceivable that some TI-2 antibody–deficient individuals may lack appropriate accessory cells. It is interesting that TI-2 antigen unresponsiveness of CBA/N mice with an X-linked deficiency of a TI-2–responsive B-cell subset could be corrected by a cloned dendritic cell line (13).

It is likely that polysaccharide antigens with palindromically repeating epitopes are capable of causing sufficient cross linking of B-cell surface Ig receptors to induce B-cell differentiation to antibody-producing cells. Antigen with less repeating units might require accessory signals acting synergistically to induce effective B-cell stimulation.

C3 breakdown products, especially C3d, might act as accessory signals via CD21 surface receptors on B cells (14). This would explain the lack of pneumococcal antibodies in patients with C3 deficiency and the association of the pattern of ontogeny of CR-2-positive ($CD21^+$) B cells and TI-2 antibody responses (2).

Finally, B cells may lack other surface receptors for accessory cell–derived second signals. The CD43 antigen, which is deficient in leukocytes from patients with the Wiskott-Aldrich syndrome, may be such an accessory molecule (5). The results we present also show that cell interactions governed by the LFA family of molecules are not required for effective TI-2 antibody responses.

ACKNOWLEDGMENTS

We are very grateful to our clinical colleagues for providing us with serum samples from their patients for this study and allowing access to clinical case. Funding was provided by the Department of Immunology, the Medical School, Birmingham, England (MH), and the Gulbenkian Foundation, Lisbon, Portugal (MF).

REFERENCES

1. Gold R. Prevention of Bacterial meningitis by immunological means. In: MA Sande, AL Smith, RK Root (eds). Bacterial meningitis. Livingstone, Edinburgh, 1985, pp. 105–122.
2. MacLennan ICM, Liu YJ, Oldfield S, Zhang J, Lane PJL. The evolution of B-cell clones. Curr Topics Microbiol Immunol 1990; 159:37.
3. Granoff DM, Munson RS. Prospects for prevention of Haemophilus influenzae type b disease by immunisation. J Infect Dis 1986; 153:448–461.
4. Bird PAE, Lachmann PJ. Regulation of human IgG subclass production; low serum IgG4 associated with classical pathway C3 activation deficiency. Eur J Immunol 1988; 18:1217–1222.
5. Report of a WHO Sponsored Meeting, Immunodef Rev 1989; 1:173–205.
6. Bird P, Calvert JE, Lowe J, Duggan-Keen M, Forouhi NG, Seppala I, & Ling NR. ELISA measurement of IgG subclass production in culture supernatants using monoclonal antibodies. J Immunol Methods 1987; 104:149.
7. PRU Handbook of Clinical Immunochemistry, 2nd ed. A. Milford-Ward, Sheffield University Press, Sheffield, United Kingdom, 1988, p. 157.

8. Kumararatne DS, Bignall A, Joyce HJ, Hazlewood M. Antibody deficiency disorders. In: *Clinical Immunology: A Practical Approach*. J Gooi, H Chapel (eds). IRL Press, Oxford, England, 1990, pp. 1–22.
9. Jefferis RJ, Kumararatne DS. IgG subclass deficiencies—a review. Clin Exp Immunol 1990; 81:357–367.
10. Knutson AP. Patients with IgG subclass and/or selective antibody deficiency to polysaccharide antigens: Initiation of a controlled clinical trial of intravenous immune globulin. J Allergy Clin Immunol 1989; 84:640–647.
11. Taylor CE, Bright R. T cell modulation of the antibody response to bacterial polysaccharide antigens, Infect Immun 1989; 57:180–185.
12. Humphrey JH, Grennan D. Different macrophage populations distinguished by means of fluorescent polysaccharides. Eur J Immunol 1981; 11:221.
13. Clayberger C, DeKruyff RH, Fay R, Huber B, Cantor H. Evidence for defects in accessory and T cell subsets in mice expressing the xid effect. J Molec Cell Immunol 1985; 2:61–69.
14. Klaus GGB, Humphrey JH. A re-evaluation of the role of C3 in B-cell activation. Immunol Today 1988; 7:165–167.

MUCOSAL IMMUNITY SALT/MALT

71
Mucosal Immunity

Delphine Guy-Grand and Pierre Vassalli
Hôpital Necker-Enfants Malades, Paris, France
University of Geneva, Geneva, Switzerland

Since 1950, when J. Heremans' group (1) isolated an isotype of immunoglobulin from human serum that we call now immunoglobulin A (IgA), and when gut intraepithelial lymphocytes (IELs), which had already been identified, were thought to act in the transport of nutrients through the epithelium, under the name of trephocytes (2), the concept of a mucosal immune system has progressively emerged. Among the first important steps were the demonstration by Gowans and Knight (3) in 1964 of a traffic of lymphocytes toward the gut wall, and their subsequent differentiation; the identification in 1965 by Crabbé (4) of IgA plasma cells localized all along the gut mucosa; and the recognition in 1966 by Enerbäck (5) of mucosal mast cells. In the subsequent years, much has been learned concerning the role of Peyer's patches (PPs) in the generation of IgA plasma cells, and of part of the IELs, as well as on the T-cell nature of this last population. Recently, the observations of Goodman and Le François (6) and of Bonneville, Tonegawa, and coworkers (7) that an unusually high percentage of gut IELs bear T-cell receptors γδ (TCRs γδ) has led a number of immunologists, whose attention had not been particularly focused previously toward mucosal immunity, to take a fresh look at the mucosal system.

In 1990, the mucosal immune system is recognized as being anatomically and functionally part of the immune system in general, but with very particular characteristics of its own. Effector cells of immunity are disseminated all along the gut mucosa: IgA plasma cells in the lamina propria, and T lymphocytes and mast cells or their precursors between the epithelial cells of the villi as well as in the lamina propria. In spite of their common localization, these cells have two different origins.

1. Precursors of IgA plasma cells and of part of the gut T lymphocytes are blasts resulting from antigenic stimulation of the PPs (8–10). For B cells, the PP microenvironment and lymphokines released by T cells induce the IgA class switch leading to the transformation of small B lymphocytes into IgA-bearing blasts (11), a mechanism not existing in athymic mice. These blasts, as well as CD4-positive and CD8-positive T blasts

bearing TCRαβ, migrate from the PPs to the mesenteric lymph nodes, then to the thoracic duct and the blood. From here, displaying gut-homing properties, they seed the whole gut mucosa and, mainly in the case of CD8-positive T cells, become IELs. This special form of traffic leads to the presence in the mucosa of immune effectors specific for antigens they have encountered in the PPs: These cells are especially numerous in adult animals, including humans (12), in whom the gut is chronically infected.

2. In mice, about 50% of the IEL T lymphocytes (13), and also of the gut mast cell precursors (14), do not arise by stimulations in PPs but result from a different circuit. Various labeling experiments have shown that they reach the gut mucosa directly from the bone marrow via the blood. Mast cell precursors proliferate and mature into mucosal mast cells in the gut wall under the influence of lymphokines released by stimulated T cells (i.e., interleukin-3 [IL-3] and interleukin-4 [IL-4]); in athymic mice they never mature. On the other hand, the T IELs belonging to this subpopulation have special features. They are thymic independent, all bear CD8 molecules made only of homodimeric α chains, and they bear either TCR γδ or αβ. In this last case, they bear a repertoire different from that of peripheral positive TCR αβ cells, not displaying the negative selection of T cells found in mice of strains Mls-a and I-E^+. Since these IELs are the only CD3-positive cells detectable in various organs of young nude mice, and because, contrary to mature T cells, they contain a recombinase machinery allowing the rearrangement of their TCR, this thymus-independent population appears to result from an attraction and differentiating activity exerted by the gut epithelium on circulating precursors (13).

As for the functional capacities of the gut mucosal immune cells, some of them are well understood. The IgA molecules released in a polymeric form in the gut lumen, after binding to the secretory piece and crossing through the epithelial cells, prevent the penetration of toxins or microorganisms into the mucosa. Thymus-dependent CD8-positive (bearing heterodimeric α-β chains) and CD4-positive T cells from PPs origin are able to release lymphokines, leading to cascade of events, including, in the case of special antigens, the differentiation of mucosal mast cells favoring parasite expulsion through IgE mechanisms (facilitated by IL-4 local release). What the thymus-independent αα CD8-positive subset recognizes, whether bearing TCR αβ or γδ, is still incompletely understood. Nevertheless, it is important to note that the gut epithelium induces the formation in all IELs, whether thymus-dependent or -independent, of intracytoplasmic granules containing perforin and serine esterases with cytotoxic abilities which are not present in normal unstimulated peripheral lymphocytes. The elimination of altered epithelial cells is probably an essential role of the two populations of IEL T cells. It is also important to realize that the close contact between gut epithelium and mucosal T lymphocytes is a bidirectional relationship. Conditions leading to IEL stimulations induce an acceleration of the epithelium renewal (15), and the epithelium itself induces the terminal differentiation of T lymphocytes (13). Finally, the expression of a new activation molecule (defined in humans by the monoclonal antibody [MAb] HML-1) is triggered on the surface of these cells (12).

Most of the informations concerning the traffic and ontogeny of mucosal T cells refer for the moment to gut T cells, although recent progress has been made concerning the totally different ontogeny of skin positive TCR γδ dendritic epithelial cells (16). The bronchus-associated lymphoid system and the origin of T lymphocytes found in other mucosa are less well understood. A number of essential questions have been raised: What are the surface molecules involved in mucosal homing? Do epithelia, such as the gut, release chemotactic peptides attracting bone marrow precursors, as is the case for thymic epithelium? What are the mechanisms of lymphocyte epithelial interactions and recognition? What role is played by mucosal immunity in human bowel diseases? All these questions are of special interest to immunologists, would it be only when they realize that, considering the very large areas covered by the mucosal immune system, it certainly quantitatively surpasses the totality of the peripheral lymphoid organs.

REFERENCES

1. Heremans JF, Heremans MT, Schultze ME (1959) Isolation and description of a few properties of β_{2A}-globulin of human serum. Clin Chim Acta 4:96.
2. Fergusson A (1977) Intraepithelial lymphocytes of the small intestine. Gut 18:921.
3. Cowans JL, Knight EJ (1964) The route of re-circulation of lymphocytes in the rat. Proc R Soc 159:257.
4. Crabbe P A, Carbonara AO, Heremans JF (1965) The normal human intestinal mucosa as a major source of plasma cells containing γ A-immunoglobulin. Int Acad Pathol 14:235.
5. Enerback L (1966) Mast cells in rat gastrointestinal mucosa. 1. Effects of fixation. Acta Pathol Microbiol Scand 66:289.
6. Goodman T, Le Francois L (1988) Expression of the γ-δ T-cell receptor on intestinal $CD8^+$ intraepithelial lymphocytes. Nature 333:855.
7. Bonneville M, Janeway Jr CA, Ito K, Haser W, Ishida I, Nakanishi N, Tonegawa S (1988) Intestinal intraepithelial lymphocytes are a distinct set of γ T cells. Nature 336:479.
8. Guy-Grand D, Vassalli P (1974) The gut-associated lymphoid system: Nature and properties of the large dividing cells. Eur J Immunol 4:435.
9. Husband AJ, Gowans JL (1978) The origin and antigen-dependent distribution of IgA-containing cells in the intestine. J Exp Med 148:1146.
10. Guy-Grand D, Griscelli C, Vassalli P (1978) The mouse gut T lymphocyte, a novel type of T cell. Nature, Origin and traffic in mice in normal and graft-versus-host conditions. J Exp Med 148:1661.
11. McGhee JR, Mestecky J, Elson CO, Kiyono H (1989) Regulation of IgA synthesis and immune response by T cells and interleukins. J Clin Immunol 9:175.
12. Jarry A, Cerf-Bensussan N, Brousse N, Selz F, Guy-Grand D (1990) Subsets of $CD3^+$ (TcR αβ or γδ) and CD3-lymphocytes isolated from normal human gut epithelium display phenotypical features different from their PBL counterparts. Eur J Immunol 20:1097.
13. Guy-Grand D, Cerf-Bensussan N, Malissen B, Malassis-Seris M, Briottet C, Vassalli P (1991) Two gut intraepithelial $CD8^+$ lymphocyte populations with different T cell receptors: A role for the gut epithelium in T cell differentiationu. J Exp Med 173.
14. Guy-Grand D, Dy M, Luffau G, Vassalli P (1984) Gut mucosal mast cells. Origin, traffic and differentiation. J Exp Med 160:12.
15. Guy-Grand D, Vassalli P (1986) Gut injury in mouse graft-versus-host reaction. Study of its occurrence and mechanisms. J Clin Invest 77:1584.
16. Havran WL, Allison JP (1990) Origin of Thy-1^+ dendritic epidermal cells of adult mice from fetal thymic precursors. Nature 344:68.

72
Effector Limb of T-Cell Immunity in the Gut

Thomas T. MacDonald
St. Bartholomews Hospital, London, England

INTRODUCTION

By virtue of the size and surface area of the gastrointestinal tract, the T cells in the connective tissue of the intestinal lamina propria and the overlying epithelium constitute one of the largest populations in the body. They display considerable heterogeneity in phenotype and T-cell receptor (TCR) usage, which varies according to the microanatomical distribution of the cells within the gut. The presence of most of these cells in the gut mucosa is antigen driven, and thus represents a component of host defenses at mucosal surfaces. In this chapter, the phenotype and function of the T cells in the gut mucosa are outlined.

INTRAEPITHELIAL LYMPHOCYTES

In all species studied so far, intraepithelial lymphocytes (IELs) are mainly $CD3^+$, $CD8^+$ (1) (Fig. 1). Although they are present in the human fetus (2), their numbers increase dramatically after birth. They are mostly $CD45R0^+$ and $VLA\text{-}1^+$ (3,4), and are thus secondary cells. Most detailed immunohistological studies on IELs have been done in man. Four main populations of IELs have been identified (5). Of the CD3-positive cells, 80–90% are CD8-positive, 10–15% are CD4-positive, and 6–10% are $CD4^-$, $CD8^-$. The fourth population is $CD3^-$, $CD7^+$ and constitutes up to 25% of IELs. In rodents, CD8-positive IELs predominate over CD4-positive cells (6); double-negative IELs have not been described; but there is a population of $CD3^-,8^+$ IELs also present in scid mice which may be the murine homologue of the $CD3^-$, $CD7^+$ population in man (7,8).

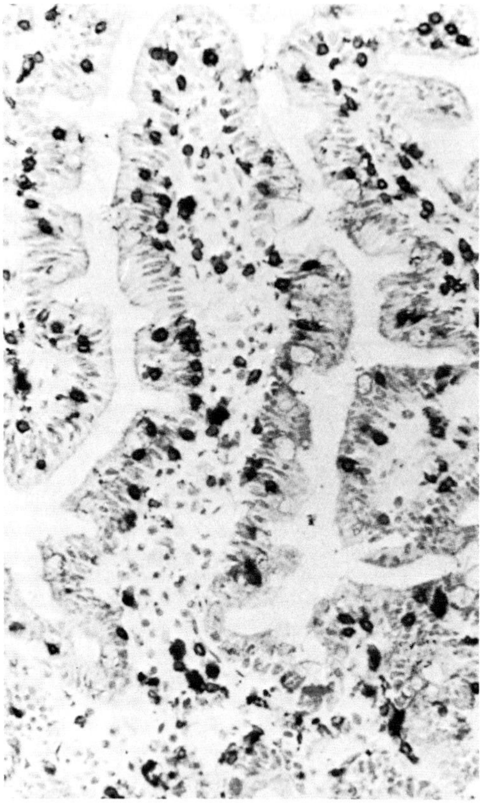

Figure 1 CD3[+] T cells in the lamina propria and epithelium of normal human small intestine (immunoperoxidase, magnification: ×100).

T-CELL RECEPTOR USAGE BY IELs

Biochemical studies indicated that in mouse IELs the major CD3-associated TCR was the γδ heterodimer (9). By FACS analysis and immunohistochemistry it is now clear however that in normal mice about 50–60% of IELs express the TCR-αβ (8–11). These different results may be partly explained by the effects of the gut flora. Germ-free mice have few IELs, but they are mostly TCR-γδ. When these mice are given a bacterial flora the number of IELs increases, but it is mainly the TCR–αβ population which expands (12). Thus, the "bacteriological cleanliness" of the mouse will determine the percentage of TCR–αβ and TCR–γδ IELs. Finally, most of the TCR–γδ IELs in normal mice are Thy1 negative, thymus independent, and only express the α chain of CD8 (10,11).

In humans, the situation is different in that only around 10% of CD3-positive IELs are TCR-γδ (13,14), although there is wide individual variation. In the human fetus, there is an increased percentage of TCR–γδ IELs, all of which are Vδ2 positive (14). In the epithelium in untreated celiac disease, but not other enteropathies, the proportion of TCR–γδ T cells increases to over 30% (13,14) (Fig. 2). The significance of this is unknown. In celiac disease and normal intestine most of the TCR–γδ IELs use $V_{\delta 1}$ (14).

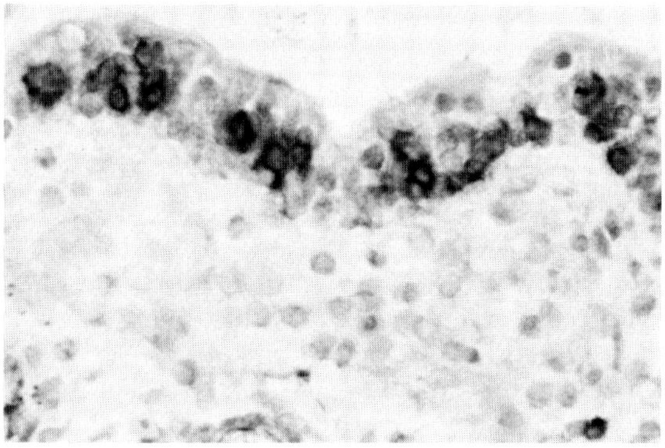

Figure 2 γ/δ T cells in celiac jejunal epithelium (immunoperoxidase with TCRδ1; magnification: ×400).

FUNCTION OF IELs

Functional studies on IELs are almost entirely restricted to rodents. The three papers on the function of IELs in man have shown that they respond poorly to T-cell mitogens, but proliferate well when activated via CD2, and that they do not have natural killer activity (15–17).

In rodents, IELs proliferate weakly to mitogens and alloantigens (18), although antigen-specific T cells which secrete lymphokines (19), and delayed-type hypersensitivity (DTH)–mediating T cells have been described (20). The main function of TCR–αβ CD8-positive IELs would appear to be as cytotoxic effector cells. Using CD3-linked cytotoxicity, TCR–αβ IELs from normal mice are potent effectors at low effector/target cell ratios (9). This activity was originally described to TCR–γδ IELs; however, it is now clear that most of the lytic activity in this assay is due to TCR–αβ IELs (11). TCR–γδ IELs from nude mice are only weakly cytotoxic. The lytic potential of TCR–αβ, CD8-positive IELs has also been confirmed using antigen-specific cytotoxicity. Mice immunized enterally with reovirus develop reovirus-specific, class 1–restricted, CD8-positive TCR–αβ cytotoxic cells in their gut epithelium (21). These cells were probably primed in the Peyer's patches and migrated to the gut epithelium.

The presence of TCR–αβ cytotoxic effector cells in the gut epithelium of normal mice is probably due to Peyer's patch priming with antigens of the gut flora; these cells, however, are not cytotoxic effectors in the epithelium of normal mice because the antigens of the flora are not processed and presented by gut epithelial cells. In contrast, during infection with a pathogen such as rotavirus, which infects epithelial cells, CD8- positive, TCR–αβ IELs will recognize antigen in association with class 1 on epithelial cells and lyse the infected cells.

CD4-POSITIVE LAMINA PROPRIA CELLS

The mucosal T cell which has received least attention is the CD4-positive TCR–αβ cell which is abundant in the lamina propria. Many of these cells are CD45R0 positive (3) and are probably primed cells derived from the Peyer's patches. They are also in close proximity to the abundant accessory cells within the lamina propria. These cells are extremely difficult to isolate from the connective tissue matrix of the lamina propria and there is only limited functional information on them.

Using a novel ex vivo system, lamina propria T cells can be directly activated in situ by the addition of anti-CD3 antibody to explant cultures of human fetal small bowel (22). Using this procedure, the lamina propria CD4-positive T cells rapidly express phenotypic markers of activation such as CD25 and HLA-DR and secrete lymphokines including interleukin-2 (IL-2) and interferon (INF-γ). The most profound consequence of lamina propria T-cell activation, however, is on gut structure. Within 72 hr the villi have disappeared or are reduced in length, the crypts of Lieberkuhn become hypertrophic, and the constituent epithelial cells are hyperplastic (Fig. 3). The mucosa thus resembles that seen in untreated food-sensitive enteropathy or parasitic infection. The mechanisms by which activated T cells cause these morphological changes are not known, although unpublished studies from the author's laboratory make it unlikely that lymphokines have a direct effect

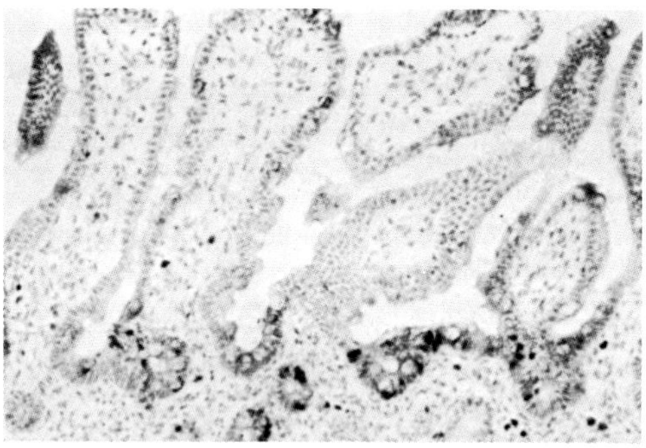

(a)

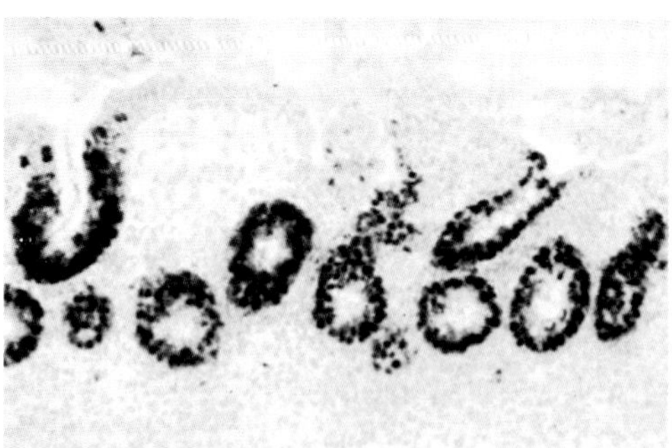

(b)

Figure 3 Ki67 immunoperoxidase staining of fetal small intestine at the onsets of culture (a) and after 3 days in the presence of anti-CD3 (b). Staining in the preculture tissue is restricted to the crypts of Lieberkuhn. In the anti–CD3-treated tissues, the crypts are hypertrophic and there is intense staining of the epithelium, including the surface, with Ki67 (immunoperoxidase; original magnification ×100).

Table 1 The Phenotype and Function of the Main Mucosal T-Cell Populations

Cell type	% of cells	Function
$CD8^+$, TCR $\alpha\beta^+$ IELs	50–70 mouse 90 man	Cytotoxic effectors
$CD8^+\gamma\delta$ TCR IELs	30–50 mouse 10 man	Weakly cytotoxic
$CD3^-$, 7^+ $CD3^-$, 8^+	5–25 man 4 mouse	? ?
$CD4^+$, TCR $\alpha\beta^+$ Lamina propria T cells	90 man 90 mouse	Secrete lymphokines Alter gut structure

on epithelial cell proliferation. It is more likely that these T-cell effects are mediated via the normal mesenchymal/epithelial interactions which regulate epithelial cell proliferation and differentiation. The role that this response plays in host defenses is probably threefold. First, increased epithelial cell division will rapidly replace epithelial cells damaged by infectious agents. Second, those parasites and bacteria which adhere to and live in epithelial cells will be pushed off with the epithelial cells into the hostile environment of the gut lumen. Third, the loss of the villi will make the gut inhospitable to parasites who live between the villi such as some of the parasitic nematodes. The effector functions of mucosal T cells are summarized in the Table 1.

REFERENCES

1. MacDonald TT, Parrott DMV (1990). Mucosal lymphoid tissue. In: *Clinical Aspects of Immunology*, 5th ed. Peter J Lachmann, D Keith Peters, Fred S Rosen, and Mark J Walport (eds). Blackwell, London.
2. Spencer JM, Dillon SB, Isaacson PG, MacDonald TT (1986). T cell subclasses in human fetal ileum. Clin Exp Immunol 65:553–558.
3. Harvey J, Jones DB, Wright DH (1989) Leucocyte common antigen expression on T cells in normal and inflamed human gut. Immunology 68:13–17.
4. Choy M-Y, Richman PI, Horton ME, MacDonald TT (1990). Expression of the VLA family of integrins in human intestine. J Pathol 160:35–40.
5. Spencer J, MacDonald TT, Diss TC, Walker-Smith JA, Ciclitira PJ, and Isaacson PG (1989). Changes in intraepithelial lymphocyte sub-populations in coeliac disease and enteropathy associated T cell lymphoma (malignant histiocytosis of the intestine). Gut 30:339–346.
6. Parrott DMV, Tait C, Mackenzie S, Mowat AM, Davies MDJ, Micklem HS (1983). Analysis of the effector functions of different populations of mucosal lymphocytes. The secretory immune system. Ann NY Acad Sci 307–320.
7. De Geus B, Shulz LD, Van der Enden M, Coolen J, Rozing J. Analysis of intestinal intraepithelial lymphocytes in athymic (nude) and SCID mice. In: *Advances in Mucosal Immunology*. Thomas T MacDonald et al. (eds). Kluwer Academic Press, Lancaster, England, pp. 71–76.
8. De Geus B, Van der Enden M, Coolen C, Nagelkerken L, Van der Heijden P, Rozing J (1990). Phenotype of intraepithelial lymphocytes in euthymic and athymic mice: Implications for differentiation of cells bearing CD3-associated $\gamma\delta$ receptor. Eur J Immunol 20:291–298.

9. Goodman T, Lefrancois L (1988). Expression of the γδ T-cell receptor on intestinal $CD8^+$ intraepithelial lymphocytes. Nature 333:855–858.
10. Viney J, MacDonald TT, Kilshaw PJ (1989). T cell receptor expression in intestinal intraepithelial lymphocyte subpopulations of normal and athymic mice. Immunology 66:583–587.
11. Viney J, Kilshaw PK, MacDonald TT (1990). Cytotoxic α/β^+ and γ/δ^+ T cells in mouse intestinal epithelium. Eur J Immunol 20:1623–1626.
12. Bandeira A, Mota-Santos T, Itohara S, Degermann S, Heusser C, Tonegawa S, Coutinho A (1990). Localisation of γ/δ T cells to the intestinal epithelium is independent of normal microbial colonisation. J Exp Med 172:239–244.
13. Halstensen TS, Scott H, Brandtzaeg P (1989). Intraepithelial T cells of the $TcR\gamma/\delta^+$ $CD8^-$ and $V\delta/J\delta1^+$ phenotypes are increased in coeliac disease. Scand J Gastroenterol 30:665–672.
14. Spencer J, Isaacson PG, Diss TC, MacDonald TT (1989). Expression of disulphide linked and non-disulphide linked forms of the T cell receptor gamma/delta heterodimer in human intestinal intraepithelial lymphocytes. Eur J Immunol 19:1335–1339.
15. Cerf-Bensussan N, Guy-Grand D, and Griscelli C (1985). Intraepithelial lymphocytes of human gut: Isolation, characterization and study of natural killer cell activity. Gut 26:81–88.
16. Ebert EC, Roberts AI, Brolin RE, Raska K (1986). Examination of the low proliferative capacity of human jejunal intraepithelial lymphocytes. Clin Exp Immunol 65:148–157.
17. Ebert EC (1989). Proliferative responses of human intraepithelial lymphocytes to various T-cell stimuli. Gastroenterology 97:1372–1381.
18. Dillon SB, MacDonald TT (1984). Functional properties of lymphocytes isolated from murine small intestinal epithelium. Immunology 52:501–509.
19. Dillon SB, Dalton BJ, MacDonald TT (1986). Lymphokine production by antigen and mitogen activated murine intraepithelial lymphocytes. Cell Immunol 103:326–338.
20. Shields JG, and Parrott DMV (1985). Appearance of delayed-hypersensitivity effector cells in murine gut mucosa. Immunology 54:771–776.
21. London SD, Cebra JJ, Rubin DH (1989). Intraepithelial lymphocytes contain virus-specific MHC-restricted cytotoxic cell precursors after gut mucosal immunization with reovirus serotype 1/Lang. Region Immunol 2:98–105.
22. MacDonald TT, Spencer J (1988). Evidence that activated mucosal T cells play a role in the pathogenesis of enteropathy in human small intestine. J Exp Med 167:1341–1349.

73
Phenotypical Characteristics of Intraepithelial Lymphocytes Isolated from Normal Human Small Intestine

N. Cerf-Bensussan,[1] A. Jarry,[2] N. Brousse,[1] and D. Guy-Grand[1]
[1]*Hôpital Necker–Enfants Malades, Paris, France;*
[2]*Faculté de Médecine X. Bichat, Paris, France*

INTRODUCTION

Intestinal intraepithelial lymphocytes (IELs) represent a special lymphoid population, which displays some morphological and phenotypical features different from those of peripheral blood T lymphocytes (T PBLs) and lamina propria T lymphocytes (1–5). Recent studies have focused on the distribution and function of T cells expressing the γδ type of TCR (TCR γδ). In mice, it was first published that most IELs were CD8-positive TCR γδ positive (6,7). However, in more recent studies, 20–40% of IELs were found to express TCR αβ (8,9). Our own observations indicate that the number of TCR αβ–positive IELs depends on the level of antigenic stimulation in the intestine and can reach 75% in adult mice raised under conventional conditions. We observed that IELs in adult mice raised conventionally consisted of two populations. One is thymus dependent, elicited in Peyer's patches by antigenic stimulations and expresses TCR αβ. The other one is thymus independent and expresses either TCR αβ or γδ. Evidence has been presented that this population acquires the α chain of CD8 (Ly-2) and the TCR under the inductive property of intestinal epithelium (10). Finally, several studies have indicated that most of the murine TCR γδ–positive IELs preferentially use a V_γ gene segment (11,12), a property which may be related with their local differentiation and/or with their capability of interacting with the epithelium (9).

In humans, recent studies have concluded that TCR γδ is expressed on a small number of intestinal IELs (5,13–16). However, controversy persists regarding the exact percentage of TCR γδ–positive IELs. In addition, the variability and nature of γ and δ genes used by human TCR γδ IELs have hardly been studied.

The present study was carried out to calculate accurately the percentage of human IELs bearing the various CD antigens compared with T PBLs when isolated from normal small intestine, or with lamina propria T lymphocytes when studied on frozen tissue sections. Arguments are brought forth concerning the variability of the $V_{\gamma,\delta}$ genes used by human

IELs and concerning the dual origin, thymus dependent or independent, or human IELs. Finally, the expression of IELs of markers associated with the acquisition of immune memory was studied.

MATERIALS AND METHODS

Tissue Specimens

Intestinal samples, duodenum or jejunum, 3–8 cm long, were obtained from 28 adult patients: 18 patients undergoing intestinal surgery for gastric cancers or chronic pancreatitis, samples being taken at least 5 cm away from the lesion, and 10 transplant donors. Samples were found histologically normal. Peripheral blood was obtained from 14 healthy volunteers.

Monoclonal Antibodies (MAbs)

The MAbs used were anti-CD2 (Leu-5), anti-CD3 (Leu-4), anti-CD4 (Leu-3a), anti-CD5 (Leu-1), anti-CD7 (Leu-9), anti-CD8a (Leu-2a) (Becton Dickinson), anti-CD8β (2ST8-5H7) (a kind gift from Dr. E. Reinherz), anti–TCR β (BMA031, Behring, France, or βF1, a gift from Dr. M. Brenner), anti–TCR γδ, TCR δ1 (a gift from Dr. M. Brenner), anti-Ti γA and anti-TiVδ2 (gifts from Dr. T. Hercend), δ TCS1 (T Cell Sciences). The TCR δ1 was shown to reveal all T cells using a TCR δ chain. Anti-TiγA, directed to Vγ9 and anti–Ti $V_{\delta 2}$ directed to $V_{\delta 2}$ encoded proteins recognize almost overlapping subsets of TCR γδ–positive PBLs whereas δ TCS1 directed to proteins encoded by $V_{\delta 1}$–$J_{\delta 1}$ reveals another subset (17). Other MAbs used were antiCD45RO (UCHL-1, Dakopatts), anti-CD45RA (2H4, Coultronics), anti-CD29 (4B4, Coultronics), anti-CD11a (25-3, Immunotech), anti-LFA3 (TS2-9, a gift from Dr. T. Springer). The MAbs were used either unlabeled or when available conjugated to fluorescein or phycoerythrin.

Methods

The methods used for isolation of human PBLs, IELs, CD3-positive, IELs, immuno-cytochemistry on isolated cells, and immunohistochemistry on frozen tissue sections have been previously described (3,5,18,19).

RESULTS AND DISCUSSION

Our studies either of frozen tissue sections or of IELs isolated from normal adult small intestine indicated that human gut IELs are made of three main subsets.

1. The major subset (approximately 75%) (Table 1) expresses TCR αβ and usual markers of the thymus dependent lineage, CD2, CD3, CD7, CD4, or CD8 αβ. In contrast to E-positive PBLs, CD8 (αβ)–positive cells predominated over CD4. Except for the absence of CD5 on some CD8-positive cells, this subset of human IELs appeared, by its phenotype, comparable to the thymus dependent subset of mouse IELs which represents up to 75% of IELs in conventionally raised mice (10).

2. A second subset of variable importance (2–30%) was made of CD3-positive lymphocytes using TCR γδ. Several observations suggested that human TCR γδ lymphocytes preferentially localized in gut epithelium. First, FACS analysis revealed a significantly higher percentage of TCR γδ–positive lymphocytes among IELs than among E-positive PBLs (p=0.04) (Table 2). Second, studies of intestinal frozen tissue sections revealed a

Table 1 TCRαβ$^+$ IEL and E$^+$ PBL Immunofluorescence on Isolated Cells

	CD3	CD7	CD2	BMA031	CD4	CD8	CD5
IEL (n=14 to 28)	87±8	87±10	87±7	73±14	11±8	74±15	61±15
E$^+$ PBL (n=14)	86±9	88±12	ND	79±11	60±14	32±6	86±10

significantly higher percentage of CD3 positive TCR γδ–positive cells (p=0.001) in the epithelium (18 ± 9%) than in the lamina propria (5 ± 3%). Finally, a striking observation was made in a child with severe combined immunodeficiency and circulating nonfunctional T cells, 50% of which were TCR αβ positive and 30% TCR γδ positive (δ TCS1$^+$ $V_{\delta}9^-$ $V_{\delta2}$–). Southern blot analysis of her blood revealed two detectable clones. One TCR αβ positive using Cβ2; one TCR γδ using $V_{\delta1}$–$J_{\delta1}$ and $V_{\gamma1}$ (20). Because of diarrhea, this child had an intestinal biopsy which showed an elevated number of CD3-positive IELs (25/100 EC) in the villous epithelium, 80% of which were TCR δ1$^+$ $V_{\gamma9}$– $V_{\delta}2^-$δTCS1$^+$, 15% βF1 positive, whereas over 90% of CD3-positive lamina propria lymphocytes were βF1 positive and less than 10% TCR δ1 positive. This suggested that the circulating TCR γδ clone using $V_{\delta1}$–$J_{\delta1}$ preferentially localized or expanded in the gut epithelium.

As shown in Table 2, the use of MAbs directed to $V_{\gamma9}$ and $V_{\delta2}$ and $V_{\delta1}$–$J_{\delta1}$ did not allow to detect any statistically significant difference between subsets of TCR γδ–positive cells in peripheral blood and normal adult small intestine. Thus, these data although limited by the lack of MAbs directed to V_{γ}-encoded proteins other than $V_{\gamma9}$, do not favor the hypothesis that a subset of TCR γδ–positive cells is preferentially associated with the normal human gut epithelium. This contrasts with findings in mice where TCR γδ–positive IELs using $V_{\gamma7}$ were found with a high frequency in gut epithelium but not in other sites (11,12).

In mice, it has been observed that TCR γδ–positive IELs (as well as some TCR αβ–positive IELs) are thymus independent. Such cells are characterized by their isolated expression of CD8 α chain (without CD8 β) (10). In humans, double staining experiments with anti–CD8α (Leu-2a) and anti–CD8 β (2ST8-5H7) MAbs revealed that 12 ± 4% of total IELs bore CD8 α but not CD8 β, whereas only 5 ± 3% E-positive PBLs were CD8 $\alpha^+\beta^-$. In blood, double staining experiments suggested that many CD8 $\alpha^+\beta^-$ might be CD16-positive natural killer (NK) cells. Indeed, in two experiments, CD16-positive cells did not express CD8β, whereas 20 and 80%, respectively, were CD8 α positive. In isolated

Table 2 TCRγδ$^+$ IEL, PBL, and LPL

	TCR δ1	Anti-Ti γA	Anti–Ti Vδ2	δ TCS1
IEL[a] (n=28)	13 ± 8	5 ± 7	6 ± 3	5 ± 2
E$^+$ PBL[a] (n=14)	6 ± 4	3 ± 2	3 ± 1	2 ± 1
CD3$^+$ LPL[b] (n=11)	5 ± 3	3 ± 2	3 ± 1	1 ± 1

[a]Data obtained by FACS analysis of isolated lymphocytes.
[b]Data obtained by counting LPLs on frozen tissue sections.

IELs, which contained very few CD16 positive cells (0.5 ± 0.5%), two experiments with induction of capping with 2ST8-5H7 or Leu-2a showed that, respectively, 40 and 45%, of TCR γδ– positive IELs were CD8 α positive, whereas only 8 and 27% were CD8β positive. This suggested that some intestinal TCR γδ–positive IELs are only CD8 positive. In mice, it has been demonstrated that CD8 α (but not CD8 β–positive) can be acquired in vitro independently of the thymic microenvironment by $CD3^+CD4^-CD8^-$ cells (21). The presence of CD8 α but not CD8 β on peripheral blood human CD16–positive NK cells suggests that in humans, CD8 α can also be acquired independently of the thymus. Human TCR γδ– positive IELs might thus acquire CD8 α outside the thymus, and it is possible that in humans as in mice the gut microenvironmental provides factors stimulating expression of CD8 α.

3. Finally, double staining experiments revealed a third minor subset (9.2 ± 6%) of $CD7^+CD3^-$ lymphocytes. Such cells differed from $CD7^+CD3^-$ peripheral blood cells. Indeed, 11.2 ± 9.6%, E-positive PBLs were $CD7^+CD3^-$. However, over 90% were CD16-positive NK cells. By contrast, IELs contained very few CD16-positive cells (see above). Furthermore, isolation of CD3-positive IELs in two experiments confirmed that such cells were $CD7^+CD16^-$. They did not express any T-cell or NK markers except for CD8 present on, respectively, 2 and 30% cells. Such lymphocytes may have a tropism for the epithelium as they were rare not only in the blood, but also in the lamina propria (which contained less than 1% $CD7^+CD3^-$ cells in double staining experiments on frozen tissue sections). This hypothesis is reinforced by an observation in an immunodeficient patient with an early blockage of T-cell differentiation. In this patient, a large number of $CD7^+CD3^-CD2^-CD5^-$ $CD8^-CD16^-CD56^-CD57^-$ cells were observed in the intestinal epithelium but neither in the blood nor in the lamina propria. The nature as well as the function of these cells remain unknown. Cytosmears of $CD7^+CD3^-$ IELs showed that approximately 50% of them contain conspicuous granules, suggesting that they may be non–major histocompatibility (MHC)–restricted cytotoxic cells. However, it should be noted that they differ from PB NK cells by the lack of CD16, CD56, and CD7 antigens, and by the lack of spontaneous cytotoxicity against K562 (18). Their phenotype identical to that of T-cell precursors (22), the recent evidence that mouse gut epithelium can be a site of extrathymic T-cell maturation (10) might also suggest that they represent T-cell precursors capable of differentiation in the human gut epithelium. Studies of immunodeficient patients with a thymic deficiency such as the DiGeorge syndrome may help to solve this issue.

Finally, phenotypical studies provided evidence that human intestinal IELs are in a state of activation different from that of PBLs. Indeed, most IELs stained brightly with anti-CD45RO MAb (83 ± 10%; n = 13), whereas only 6–7% CD3-positive IELs stained with anti-CD45RA MAb. This observation may be related to the fact that a high proportion of intestinal IELs have already encountered an antigen as $CD45RA^-CD45RO$ high peripheral T cells were shown to be memory T cells (23). Studies in mice have indeed shown that a large number of intestinal IELs are the progeny of blasts elicited by antigenic stimulation in Peyer's patches. However, the other antigens strongly expressed by CD45RO high-memory T cells in blood (23) were inconstantly present on CD45RO high IELs. In only six out of 16 intestinal samples tested, a large number of IELs (50–90%) expressed CD29 (VLAβ1). In the 10 remaining cases, CD29 antigen was present only on 2–30% IELs (mean 11%) and preferentially on CD3-negative IELs. CD11a (LFA1) was tested in 10 samples. In eight cases, the percentage of CD11a-positive IELs varied between 2 and 36% (mean 11%). In only two cases, a high percentage of IELs (75%) were found to be CD11a- positive. However, their fluorescence was dim compared to PBLs (data not shown). In contrast, IELs possessed two phenotypical markers absent in resting peripheral

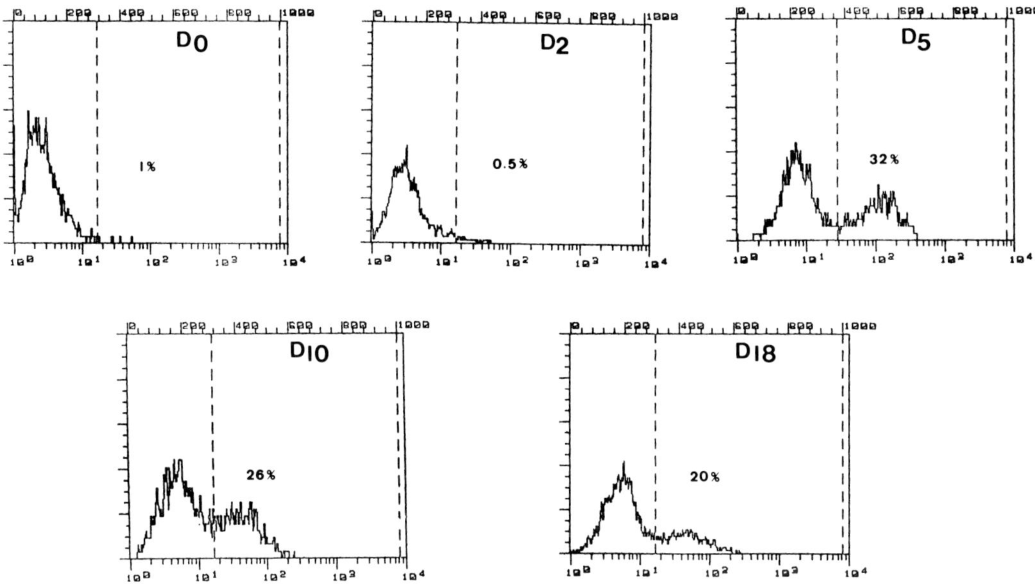

(a)

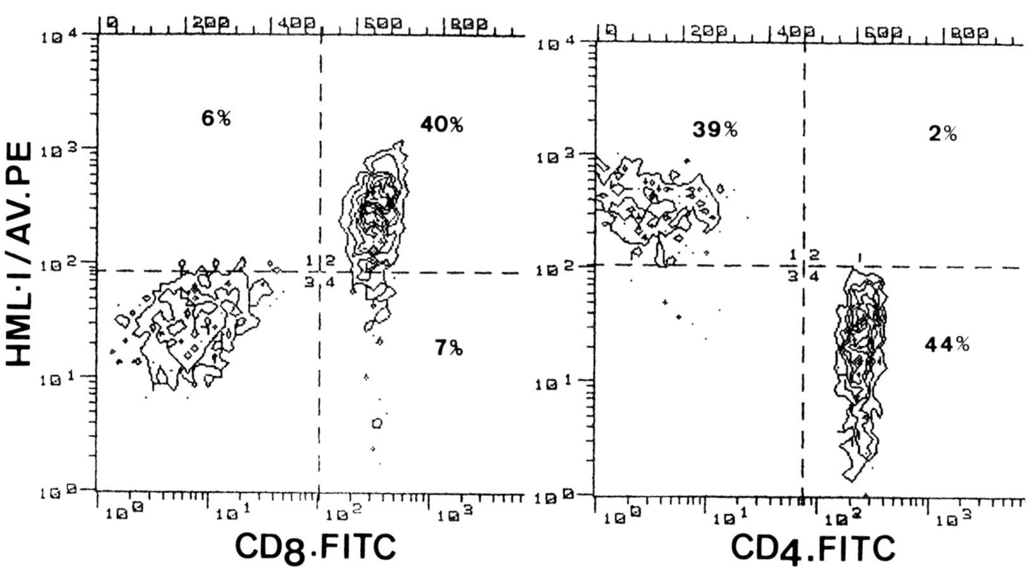

(b)

Figure 1 HML-1 expression by PHA-stimulated PBLs. HML-1 is almost absent from resting PBLs. It appears between days 3 and 5 following PHA stimulation (a); the number of HML-1^+ cells peaks at day 8 (B) and thereafter decreases progressively (A). Double immunofluorescence on day 8 shows that the majority of HML-1^+ cells are $CD8^+$ (b).

T cells. First, approximately 25% contained intracytoplasmic granules similar to those observed in cytotoxic cell lines. Second, over 90% IELs (whatever the subset) were labeled by HML-1 (5). The antigen recognized by this antibody is expressed by lymphocytes in all the normal and tumoral epithelia tested. It is absent on resting peripheral T cells but appears 2 to 3 days following various stimulations (Fig. 1) and (24) on peripheral blood T cells mainly CD8-positive. This antigen is made of two noncovalently bound chains of approximative 110–120 and 150 kD (5). Preliminary data obtained by microsequencing showed that the 110–120-kD band has strong homology with the β chains of integrins. Altogether these data indicate that IELs are a unique population of activated cells. It is possible that the gut microenvironment provides factors inducing this peculiar pattern of activation. A nonexclusive hypothesis is that the state of activation of IELs plays a role in their ability to enter the epithelium or to interact with the enterocytes. The observation that IELs express a unique integrin sustains the latter hypothesis.

REFERENCES

1. Guy-Grand D, Griscelli C, Vassalli P. The mouse gut T lymphocyte, a novel type of T cell. Nature, origin and traffic in mice in normal and graft-versus-host conditions. J Exp Med 148:1866.
2. Janossy G, Tidman N, Selby WS, Thomas JA, Granger S, Kung PC, Goldstein G. 1980. Human T lymphocytes of inducer and suppressor type occupy different microenvironments. Nature 288:81.
3. Cerf-Bensussan N, Schneeberger EE, Bhan AK. 1983. Immunohistologic and immunoelectron microscopic characterization of the mucosal lymphocytes of human small intestine by the use of monoclonal antibodies. J Immunol 130:2615.
4. Ernst PB, Befus AD, Bienenstock J. 1985. Leukocytes in the intestinal epithelium: An unusual immunological compartment. Immunol Today 6:50.
5. Cerf-Bensussan N, Jarry A, Brousse N, Lisowska-Grospierre B, Guy-Grand D, Griscelli C. 1987. A monoclonal antibody (HML-1) defining a novel membrane molecule present on human intestinal lymphocytes. Eur J Immunol 17:1279.
6. Goodman T, Lefrancois L. 1988. Expression of the γδ- T cell receptor on intestinal $CD8^+$ intraepithelial lymphocytes. Nature 336:479.
7. Bonneville M, Janeway CA, Ito K, Haser W, Ishida I, Nakanishi N, Tonegawa S. 1988. Intestinal intraepithelial lymphocytes are a distinct set of γδ T cells. Nature 336:479.
8. Goodman T, Lefrancois L. 1989. Intraepithelial lymphocytes. Anatomical site, nor T cell receptor form, dictates phenotype and function. J Exp Med 170:1569.
9. Bonneville M, Itohara S, Krecko EG, Mombaerts P, Ishida I, Katsuki M, Berns A, Farr AG, Janeway CA, Tonegawa S. 1990. Transgenic mice demonstrate that epithelial homing of γ/δ T cells is determined by cell lineages independent of T cell receptor specificity. J Exp Med 171:1015.
10. Guy-Grand D, Cerf-Bensussan N, Malissen B, Malassis-Seris M, Briottet C, Vassalli P. Two gut intraepithelial $CD8^+$ lymphocyte subpopulations with different T cell receptors: A role for the gut epithelium in T cell differentiation. J Exp Med (in press).
11. Takagaki Y, Decloux A, Bonneville M, Tonegawa S. 1989. Diversity of γδ T-cell receptors on murine intestinal intraepithelial lymphocytes. Nature 339:712.
12. Asarnow DM, Goodman T, Lefrancois L, Allison JP. 1989. Distinct antigen receptor repertoires of two classes of murine-epithelium associated T-cells. Nature 341:60.
13. Bucy RP, Chen CH, Cooper MD. 1989. Localization and CD8 accessory molecule expression of Tγδ cells in humans. J Immunol 142:3045.
14. Groh V, Porcelli S, Fabbi M, Lanier LL, Picker LJ, Anderson T, Warnke RA, Bhan AK, Strominger JL, Brenner MB. 1989. Human lymphocytes bearing T-cell receptor γ/δ are phenotypically diverse and evenly distributed throughout the lymphoid system. J Exp Med 169:1277.

15. Brandzaeg P, Halstensen TS, Scott H, Sollid LM, Valnes K. 1989. Intraepithelial T cells of the TCRγ/δ^+ $CD8^-$ and $V\delta1/J\delta1^+$ phenotypes are increased in coeliac disease. Scand J Immunol 30:665.
16. Spencer J, Isaacson P, Diss TC, McDonald TT. 1989. Expression of disulfide-linked and non-disulfide-linked forms of the T cell receptor γ/δ heterodimer in human intraepithelial lymphocytes. Eur J Immunol 19:1335.
17. Miossec C, Faure F, Ferradini L, Roman-Roman S, Jitsukawa S, Ferrini S, Moretta A, Triebel F, Hercend T. 1990. Further analysis of the T-cell receptor γ/δ^+ peripheral lymphocyte subset. The $V\delta1$ gene segment is expressed with either $C\alpha$ or $C\gamma$ J Exp Med 171:1171.
18. Cerf-Bensussan N, Guy-Grand D, Griscelli C. 1985. Intraepithelial lymphocytes of human gut: Isolation, characterization and study of natural killer activity. Gut 26:81.
19. Jarry A, Cerf-Bensussan N, Brousse N, Selz F, Guy-Grand D. 1990. Subsets of $CD3^+$ (T cell receptor α/β or γ/δ) and $CD3^-$ lymphocytes isolated from normal human gut epithelium display phenotypical features different from their counterparts in peripheral blood. Eur J Immunol 20:1097.
20. De Saint Basile G, LeDeist F, de Villartay JR, Cerf-Bensussan N, Journer O, Brousse N, Griscelli C, Fischer A. Restricted heterogeneity of T lymphocytes in the combined immunodeficiency with hypereosinophilia (Omenn's syndrome). J Clin Invest (in press).
21. McDonald RH, Schreyer M, Howe RC, Bron C. 1990. Selective expression of $CD8\alpha$ (Ly-2) subunit on activated thymic $\gamma\delta$ cells. Eur J Immunol 27:927.
22. Haynes BF, Martin ME, Kay H, Kurtzberg. 1988. Early events in human T-cell ontogeny. Phenotypic characterization and immunohistologic localization of T-cell precursors in early human fetal tissues. J Exp Med 168:1061.
23. Sanders ME, Makgoba MW, Shaw S. 1988. Human naive and memory T-cells: Reinterpretation of helper-inducer and suppressor-inducer subsets. Immunol Today 9:195.
24. Schiefferdecker HL, Ullrich R, Weiss-Breckwoldt AN, Schwarting R, Stein H, Riecken EO, Zeitz M. 1990. The HML-1 antigen of intestinal lymphocytes is an activation antigen. J Immunol 144:2541.

74
Origin and Nature of Heterogeneity Among Murine Intestinal Intraepithelial Lymphocytes

Allan McI. Mowat, Kevin J. Maloy, and Delphine M. V. Parrot
University of Glasgow, Western Infirmary, Glasgow, Scotland

INTRODUCTION

There is considerable controversy over the nature of the large population of intraepithelial lymphocytes (IELs) found in the small intestine. Although the majority are CD3-positive T cells, most are CD8-positive and a large proportion do not possess other pan–T-cell markers including Thy 1 and CD5 (1). Recent studies in mice and chickens have suggested that CD8-positive IELs express the γδ form of the T-cell receptor (TCR) and form a distinct lineage of T cells whose function is to protect mucosal surfaces (2,3). However, much of this evidence has been indirect or dependent on immunoprecipitation analysis, and we and others have found abundant TCR αβ–expressing IELs in rodents (4–6). In addition, normal human IELs appear to be almost exclusively αβ positive T cells (7).

In this study, we have investigated the basis of these discrepancies by using two-color flow cytometry to identify directly subsets of IELs defined by expression of TCR and other T-cell markers. We have also examined whether factors such as age and exposure to local antigen influence the balance of these subsets.

MATERIALS AND METHODS

Animals

Specific-pathogen free (SPF)(CBA×Balb/c) F_1 mice were obtained from Harlan Olac (Bicester, Oxon), aged 3–4 weeks, and maintained under conventional conditions until use.

Phenotypic Analysis of T-Cell Markers by Flow Cytometry

The IELs were obtained by our published method (8), whereas mesenteric lymph node (MLN) cells were used as a source of conventional T cells. 5×10^5-10^6 cells were stained on ice in 50 μl aliquots of phosphate-buffered saline (PBS)/2% newborn calf serum (NCS) for 45–60 min in each step . Between steps, cells were washed in PBS/NCS at 4°C and fixed in 1% paraformaldehyde before analysis on a FACScan i.v. flow cytometer. T cells were detected using FITC-conjugated anti-CD3 (145.2C-11), whereas FITC-anti Lyt-2 (Seralab Ltd.) and PE-anti-L3T4 (Becton Dickinson) were used to detect CD8-positive and CD4-positive T cells, respectively. Hamster antimouse TCR αβ (H57.597) antibody was used to detect αβ-positive T cells in conjunction with PE-goat antimouse immunoglobulin (Ig) (Sigma Ltd.), which cross reacts with hamster Ig. Biotinylated anti–Lyt-3 plus PE-streptavidin (Sigma Ltd.) was used to detect the CD8 χ chain, whereas rat antimouse CD45RB antibody (16A) plus PE or FITC-antimouse Ig was used for analysis of CD45 expression.

Induction of Graft-vs-Host Reactions (GvHRs)

Six-week-old (CBA×Balb/c)F_1 mice were injected intraperitoneally with $6{\times}10^7$ CBA spleen cells.

RESULTS

Phenotypic Heterogeneity of Normal IELs

The results of our analyses of normal IEL and MLN cells are summarized in Table 1. As anticipated, most IEL and MLN cells are CD3-positive T cells. However, whereas the majority of MLN T cells were CD4 positive, most IELs were CD8 positive. In addition, although all CD3-positive MLN cells coexpressed the TCR αβ, a variable but often substantial proportion of CD3-positive IELs were TCR αβ negative.

All CD8-positive MLN cells expressed both the CD8 α (Lyt-2) and CD8 β (Lyt-e) chains and were αβ T cells, but up to 70% of CD8 α–positive IELs did not coexpress the CD8 β molecule (Table 2). In addition, although virtually all the CD8 α^+CD8β^+ IELs expressed the TCR αβ, CD8 α^+CD8 β^- IELs were more heterogeneous, with a large proportion being TCR αβ negative. Thus, three populations of CD8-positive IELs could be discerned on the basis of their expression of TCR and the CD8 heterodimer. All CD4-positive IELs expressed the TCR αβ).

Closer inspection revealed that the exact proportion of these subpopulations depended on the age of the mice used in each experiment (see Table 1). The majority of CD3-positive IELs from mice aged less than 8 weeks did not express the TCR αβ, and these animals had a large proportion (~70%) of CD8-positive IELs, which were TCR αβ negative and were CD8 α^+CD8β^- (see Table 2). In contrast, up to 70% of CD3-positive IELs from mice older than 8 weeks were αβ positive, and there was a much increased proportion of CD8-positive IELs which expressed the TCR αβ. This was attributable to increases in both the CD8 α^+CD8 β^+ and CD8 α^+CD8 β^- populations of αβ-positive T cells.

Influence of Intestinal GvHR on Subsets of IELs

The age-dependent changes in the IEL phenotype seemed likely to reflect the effects of an increased level of local antigen. Therefore, we examined the effects of a more intense local cell-mediated immune response by inducing a GvHR. This resulted in a similar pattern of increased numbers of CD8-positive IELs expressing the TCR αβ and the heterodimeric form of the CD8 molecule (Table 3).

Table 1 Phenotypic Analysis of MLN and IEL Cells from Normal (CBAxBalb/c) F_1 Mice of Different Ages

	% of cells positive from			
Marker	MLN	All IELs	<8-wk IELs	>8-wk IELs
Surface Ig^+	10 (7–15)	9 (6–13)	10 (10,10)	9 (6–13)
$CD3^+$	79 (78–90	79 (75–84)	78 (75,80)	80 (74-85)
$CD3^+$ TCR $\alpha\beta^+$	79 (78–80)	51 (32–70)	34 (32,36)	59 (50–70)
$CD4^+$	55 (52–59)	9 (2–16)	12 (11,13)	7 (2–16)
CD8 α^+	24 (23–25)	72 (62–80)	68 (62,74)	74 (68-80)
CD8 α^+ TCR $\alpha\beta^+$	24 (23–25)	43 (18–59)	22 (18,26)	53 (49–59)
CD8 α^+ CD8 β^+	23 (22–23)	23 (16–30)	17 (16,18)	30 (29–30)
CD8 β^+ TCR $\alpha\beta^+$	23 (22–25)	26 (18–30)	18 (18,18)	30 (29–30)

Values shown are medians and ranges for six (MLN and total IELs), four (8/10-week-old IELs) or two experiments (6- to 8-week-old IELs).

Table 2 Phenotypic Analysis of $CD8^+$ T Cells from MLN and IEL Cells

	% of CD8 α^+ cells coexpressing markers			
Marker	MLN	Total IELs	<8-wk IELs	>8-wk IELs
TCR $\alpha\beta^+$	100	60	32	72
CD8 β^+	96	33	25	41
CD8 β^+ TCR $\alpha\beta^+$	96	33	25	41

Results shown are calculated from the experiments in Table 1 and represent the proportion of all CD8α^+ (Lyt-2^+) cells which coexpress CD8 β and/or the TCR $\alpha\beta$.

Table 3 Phenotype of IELs in (CBAxBalb/c) F_1 Mice with GvHR

	% IELs positive	
Marker	Control	Day 11 GvHR
Surface Ig^+	10	8
$CD4^+$	13	10
$CD3^+$	75	80
$CD3^+$ TCR $\alpha\beta^+$	32	43
% $\alpha\beta^+/CD3^+$	43	54
CD8 α^+	60	70
CD8 α^+ TCR $\alpha\beta^+$	18	27
% $\alpha\beta^+$/CD8 α^+	30	39
CD8 α^+ CD8 b^+	18	28

Results shown are from ILEs pooled from three mice on day 11 of GvHR and from age-matched controls.

Expression of CD45RB by IELs

The rapid antigen-dependent changes in IELs led us to investigate whether IELs would show features consistent with an unusual state of differentiation, using the CD45RB molecule as a marker (9).

Like CD8-positive MLN cells, all CD8-positive IELs were strongly CD45RB positive. However, whereas most peripheral CD4-positive T cells show medium to high expression of CD45RB, the small population of CD4-positive IELs had an unusually high proportion of cells with low expression of CD45RB.

DISCUSSION

Our study has confirmed other indications that CD8-positive IELs are an unusual and heterogeneous population of T cells (1,4,5,7,8,10). The first population we observed were CD8-positive T cells which express the TCR $\alpha\beta$ and both the α and β chains of the CD8 heterodimer. This population is in the minority in young mice, but increases markedly as mice age, presumably reflecting adaptation to an increased level of gut flora from their original SPF status. These cells are identical to CD8-positive T cells in the periphery and their number is further increased during the enteropathy of GvHR. Others have described an analogous population of Thy 1^+CD8^+ cells with cytolytic function which appears after exposure to intestinal flora (11) and we consider our first group of CD8-positive IELs to be conventional cytotoxic T lymphocytes (CTLs).

The second population of CD8-positive IELs we observed were CD8 α^+CD8 β^- TCR $\alpha\beta$–negative T cells. As this was the dominant subset in young mice, our findings support previous suggestions t hat IELs are enriched for $CD8^+\gamma\delta^+$ T cells (2,3). However, this population decreased rapidly in older mice and TCR $\alpha\beta$–negative T cells were in the minority in mature mice. Thus, $\alpha\beta$-positive T cells appear to be recruited into the epithelium in response to antigen, and we propose that $\gamma\delta$-positive IELs have no functional role in this site. In addition, our study may explain discrepancies between previous reports by showing that the relative numbers of αβ-positive and γδ-positive IELs depends on the age and antigen exposure of the mice used.

In contrast to a previous report, we found that not all CD8 β–negative IELs were γδ-T cells (10) as we consistently detected a population of αβ-positive IELs which only expressed the CD8 α chain. They also increased in maturing mice, but their significance is unclear. Conventional CD8-positive T cells express a CD8 αCD8 β heterodimer, but a CD8 α homodimer is sufficient for CTL activity (12). This unique group of IELs may provide a means of investigating the functional roles of the CD8 molecule.

Finally, our analysis of CD45RB expression provided the first evidence that CD4-positive IELs may also differ from their peripheral counterparts. Most CD4-positive IELs expressed low levels of CD45RB, a phenotype which is believed to characterize the T_H2 subset (9). The function of CD4-positive IELs warrants further study.

ACKNOWLEDGMENTS

The authors are grateful to Drs. R. Zamoyska, R. Kubo, and K. Bottomly for the gifts of antibodies.

REFERENCES

1. Mowat, A.McI. Human intraepithelial lymphocytes. In: *Seminars in Immunopathology*. D.P. Jewell (ed.). Springer-Verlag (in press).
2. Lefrancois, L., and Goodman, T. In vivo modulation of cytolytic activity and Thy 1 expression in TcR-$\gamma\delta^+$ intraepithelial lymphocytes. Science 1989; 243:1716–8.
3. Bucy, R. P., Chen, C-L.H., Cihak, J., Losch, U., and Cooper, M.D. Avian T cells expressing γδ receptors localize in the splenic sinusoids and the intestinal epithelium. J. Immunol. 1988; 141:2200–5.
4. Viney, J.L., MacDonald, T.T., and Kilshaw, P.J. T cell receptor expression in intestinal intraepithelial lymphocyte subpopulations of normal and athymic mice. Immunology 1989; 66:583–7.
5. De Geus, B., Van Den Enden, M., Coolen, C., Nagelkerken, L., Van Der Heijden, P., and Rozing, J. Phenotype of intraepithelial lymphocytes in euthymic and athymic mice: Implications for differentiation of cells bearing a CD3-associated γδ T cell receptor. Eur. J. Immunol. 1990; 20:291–8.
6. Mowat, A.McI., Edwards, A.J., and Crispe, N. T cell receptor expression by $CD8^+$ intraepithelial lymphocytes from mouse small intestine. In: *Advances in Mucosal Immunology*. T.T. MacDonald et al. (eds.). Kluwer Academic Press, Lancaster, England, 1990, pp. 83–5.
7. Trejdosiewicz, L.K., Smart, C.J., Oakes, D.J., Howdle, P.D., Malizia, G., Campana, D., and Boylston, A.W. Expression of T-cell receptors TcR1 (γ/δ) and TcR2 (α/β) in the human intestinal mucosa. Immunology 1989; 68:7–12.
8. Davies, M.D.J., and Parrott, D.M.V. Preparation and purification of lymphocytes from the epithelium and lamina propria of murine small intestine. Gut 1981; 22:481–8.
9. Bottomly, K., Luqman, M., Greenbaum, L., Cording, S., West, J., Pasqualini, T., and Murphy, D.B. A monoclonal antibody to murine CD45R distinguishes CD4T cell populations that produce different cytokines. Eur. J. Immunol. 1989; 20:617–25.
10. Guy-Grand, D., Cerf-Bensussan, N., Malissen, B., Malassis-Seris, M., Briottet, C. & Vassalli, P. Two gut intraepithelial $CD8^+$ lymphocyte populations with different T cell receptors: A role for the gut epithelium in T cell differentiation (submitted).
11. Goodman, T., and Lefrancois, L. Intraepithelial lymphocytes. Anatomical site, not T cell receptor form, dictates phenotype and function. J. Exp. Med. 1989; 170:1569–81.
12. Dembic, Z., Haas, W., Zamoyska, R., Parnes, J., Steinmetz, M., and von Boehmer, H. Transfection of the CD8 gene enhances T-cell recognition. Nature 1987; 326:510–1.

75
Analysis of Lymphocytes Infiltrating M Cells in Follicle Epithelium of Rabbit Gut-Associated Lymphoid Tissues

Thomas H. Ermak, Harold J. Steger, and Jacques Pappo
Veterans Administration Medical Center and the University of California, San Francisco, California

INTRODUCTION

M cells in follicle epithelium (FAE) of gut-associated lymphoid tissues (GALT) enclose clusters of mononuclear leukocytes in a supranuclear, cytoplasmic pocket. M cells transport antigens to lymphoid cells in the epithelium and dome (1) and express distinctive surface molecules which are not present on adjacent enterocytes (2). The FAE is a dynamic structure in which epithelial cells are renewed every 3–4 days, and mononuclear leukocytes migrate between FAE cells and localize specifically in M-cell pockets. The FAE cells are replenished from undifferentiated epithelial cells in crypts surrounding the base of each dome and migrate along the basal lamina from the base to the tip of each dome (3,4). Near the crypts, immature M cells are found which lack lymphocyte-containing pockets, whereas fully differentiated M cells further up the dome have large pockets containing groups of more than five lymphocytes (2,4). Circulating lymphocytes enter GALT through high endothelial venules and localize in the FAE (5,6). Although it has been shown that recirculating lymphocytes localize in M-cell pockets, little is known about the phenotype and function of these cells. The development of monoclonal antibodies (MAbs) against rabbit M cells and lymphocytes has enabled investigation of M-cell–lymphocyte associations in follicle epithelium in situ.

LYMPHOCYTE COMPARTMENTALIZATION IN GALT

Lymphocyte compartments in GALT have been identified by MAbs recognizing all lymphocytes (4F3), T cells (L11/135), B cells (6D4), subpopulations of dome lymphocytes (3B6 and 3C10), and class II–positive cells (2C4) (7–9). T cells are concentrated in T-cell–dependent areas (TDA), domes, and FAE, and represent about 40% of lymphocytes in Peyer's patches and 10–20% in appendix by flow cytometry (7). B cells aggregate in follicles and germinal centers and account for the majority of lymphocytes in GALT.

Two subpopulations of lymphocytes have been described in GALT domes. One population is identified by MAb 3B6, which recognizes most dome and FAE lymphocytes and B cells, but not lymphocytes in TDA. The expression of 3B6 antigen overlaps with, but is more restricted than, that of Ia-positive cells in domes. The 3B6 molecule is acquired early in T-cell development, as evidenced by the presence of a subpopulation of 3B6-positive medullary thymocytes, but it is not expressed by T cells in "mature" T-cell compartments of spleen or GALT (7).

A second population of cells is recognized by MAb 3C10, which identifies dome and germinal center macrophages and a subpopulation of dome and FAE lymphocytes. It is unreactive with lymphocytes in TDA or with B cells in coronas and germinal centers.

LYMPHOCYTES IN FOLLICLE EPITHELIUM ARE PRIMARILY Ia-POSITIVE CELLS

In the FAE, the proportion of lymphocytes defined by each MAb was determined in M-cell pockets identified by MAb 5D9 (Fig. 1). Greater than 95% of lymphocytes in the FAE were 4F3 positive and 2C4 positive. T cells represented about 95% of lymphocytes in appendix and 65% in Peyer's patch FAE, with 6D4-positive B cells accounting for the remaining lymphocytes.

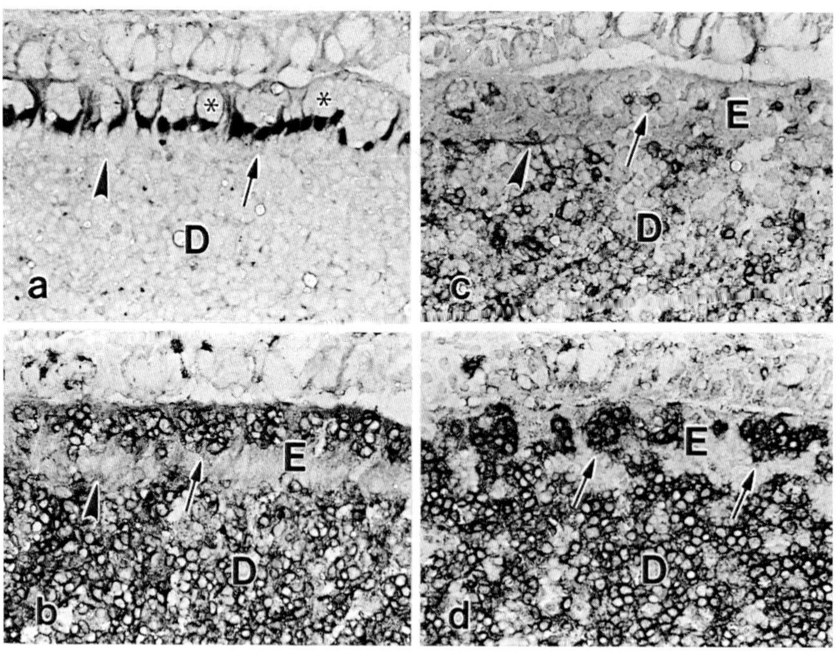

Figure 1 Distribution of appendiceal lymphocytes in M cell pockets (asterisks) of the FAE (E). (a) M cells (arrow) defined by MAb 5D9. (b) 2C4$^+$ cells. (c) 6D4$^+$ B cells. (d) 3B6$^+$ cells. Positive cells in b–d denoted by arrows. Arrowheads point to basal lamina below FAE. Distribution of L11/135$^+$ cells in M-cell pockets similar to 2C4$^+$ cells (b). Lymphocyte counts were made in 350-μm long segments of the FAE where M cells were present in serial sections. An average of 90–110 cells per 500 μm were found. D, Dome (magnification: ×200).

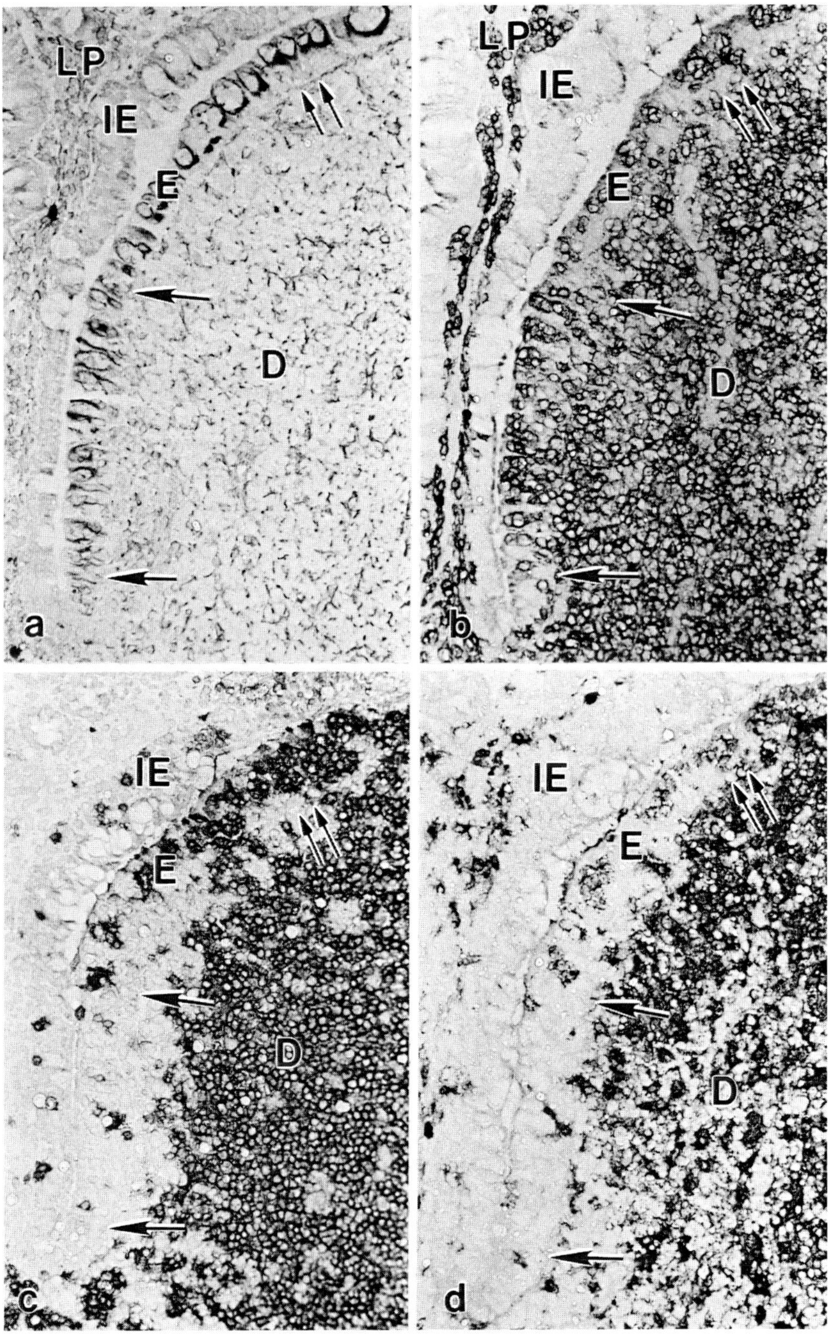

Figure 2 Correlation of lymphocyte subsets populating M-cell pockets on the sides of follicle domes (appendix). (a) $5D9^+$ M cells. Light bands of immature M cells populate the base of dome (area between single arrows). Higher on the dome, mature M cells (double arrows) give a dense reaction product with MAb 5D9 forming a pocket. (b) $L11/135^+$ cells. (c) $3B6^+$ cells. (d) $3C10^+$ cells. Most lymphocytes associated with immature M cells at base of dome are $3B6^-$ (c), $3C10^-$ (d), but $L11/135^+$ (b). Further up the dome, lymphocytes reactive with L11/135, 3B6, and 3C10 are found. Distribution pattern of $2C4^+$ cells in lower and upper FAE similar to $L11/135^+$ cells (b) (magnification: ×160).

Table 1 MAbs 3B6 and 3C10 Define Distinct Populations of Lymphocytes within M-Cell Pockets

	TDA	Lower FAE	Upper FAE
L11/135	+++	+++	+++
2C4	++[a]	+++	+++
3B6	—	—	+++
3C10	—	—	++

[a]Reticular pattern.

3B6-positive cells accounted for about 75% of FAE lymphocytes in appendix and >95% in Peyer's patches (Fig. 1d), whereas 3C10-positive cells accounted for ~30% of lymphocytes in M-cell pockets. Because 95% of FAE lymphocytes in appendix were T cells, these results indicate that M cells harbor phenotypically distinct T-cell subpopulations defined by MAbs 3B6 and 3C10.

In the appendix, the phenotype of lymphocytes correlated with the differentiation stage and position of M cells on the sides of domes (Fig. 2). At the base of the dome, M cells had small pockets or lacked them altogether (Fig. 2a). In this region, lymphocytes were reactive with L11/135 and 2C4 but not 3B6 nor 3C10 (Fig. 2b–d). Higher up on domes, lymphocyte clusters populating pockets of mature M cells were L11/135 positive, 2C4 positive, 3B6 positive, and 3C10 positive.

EXPRESSION OF THE NOVEL ANTIGENS 3B6 AND 3C10 BY GALT LYMPHOCYTES

While most lymphocytes populating M cell pockets of rabbit GALT are a phenotypically discrete population of Ia-positive cells, it is not currently known how expression of the 3B6 and 3C10 antigens relates to the life history of FAE lymphocytes. The finding of 3B6-positive and 3C10-positive T cells in the FAE at areas distant from crypts suggests that acquisition of these molecules correlates with M-cell maturation. Whether 3B6-positive cells recirculate to domes from the thymic medulla and eventually home to M cells, or whether 3B6-negative precursors originate directly in GALT is not clear. However, the absence of 3C10-positive lymphocytes in thymus or spleen suggests that the 3C10-positive T cell subpopulation may be GALT derived. The observation that 3B6 and 3C10 infiltrate specifically mature M cells, which take up and transport luminal antigen across the FAE to pocket and dome lymphocytes, raises the possibility that expression of 3B6 and/or 3C10 molecules may be associated with T-cell activation.

REFERENCES

1. Neutra MR, Phillips TL, Mayer EL, Fishkind DJ. Transport of membrane-bound macromolecules by M cells in follicle-associated epithelium of rabbit Peyer's patch. Cell Tissue Res 1987; 247:537–546.
2. Pappo J. Generation and characterization of monoclonal antibodies recognizing follicle epithelial M cells in rabbit gut-associated lymphoid tissues. Cell Immunol 1989; 120:31–41.

3. Bhalla DK, Owen RL. Cell renewal and migration in lymphoid follicles of Peyer's patches and cecum—an autoradiographic study in mice. Gastroenterology 1982; 82:232–242.
4. Bye WA, Allan CH, Trier JS. Structure, distribution, and origin of M cells in Peyer's patches of mouse ileum. Gastroenterology 1984; 86:789–801.
5. Streeter PR, Lakey Berg E, Rouse BTN, Bargatze RF, Butcher EC. A tissue-specific endothelial cell molecule involved in lymphocyte homing. Nature 1988; 331:41–46.
6. Perey DYE, Milne RW. Rabbit gut-associated lymphoid tissue. Major pathway for thoracic duct lymphocyte circulation. Lab Invest 1975; 33:678–686.
7. Ermak TH, Steger HJ, Pappo J. Phenotypically distinct subpopulations of T cells in domes and M-cell pockets of rabbit gut-associated lymphoid tissues. Immunology 1990; 71:530–537.
8. Jackson S, Chused TM, Wilkinson JM, Leiserson WM, Kindt TJ. Differentiation antigens identify subpopulations of rabbit T and B lymphocytes. Definition by flow cytometry. J Exp Med 1983; 157:34–46.
9. Lobel SA, Knight KL. The role of rabbit Ia molecules in immune functions as determined with the use of anti-Ia monoclonal antibody. Immunology 1984; 51:35–43.

76

Contamination of CBA/RIJ Germ-Free Mice with an Enteropathogenic *Staphylococcus aureus* Strain Results in Changes in the Composition of the Intestinal Intraepithelial Lymphocyte Population

Bernard de Geus,[1] Arno Kleijweg,[1] Margit van den Enden,[1] Peter Heidt,[2] Cor Timmermans,[2] and Jan Rozing[1]

[1]*Institute for Experimental Gerontology TNO, Rijswijk, The Netherlands;*
[2]*Institute for Applied Radiobiology and Immunology TNO, Rijswijk, The Netherlands*

INTRODUCTION

The intestinal intraepithelial lymphocyte (IEL) population consists of lymphocytes with a heterogeneous phenotype. Based on T-cell receptor (TCR) usage, the IEL population can be divided into two populations expressing either the TCR γδ or the TCR αβ. About half of the TCR αβ–positive IELs express also Thy 1 (1). The other half is Thy 1 negative (2). This population is markedly enriched in the TcR αβ–positive intestinal IEL fraction as compared to the TcR αβ–positive population in peripheral lymphoid organs (B. de Geus et al., manuscript submitted). The majority of TcR γδ–positive IELs are Thy 1 negative.

In contrast to the rather abundant knowledge about phenotypical and molecular aspects of the IEL population, hardly anything is known about the functional properties of these cells. In view of the suspected role of IELs in the first line of defense against microorganisms, indications for functional aspects of the IEL population may be found by investigating the response of IELs upon exposure to pathogenic microorganisms. In this chapter, we describe the changes which occur in time within the IEL population when germ-free (GF) CBA/Rij mice are associated with an enteropathogenic *Staphylococcus aureus* strain producing staphylococcal enterotoxin B (SEB).

MATERIALS AND METHODS

Animals

Germ-free CBA/Rij mice, aged 10–16 weeks, were obtained from the breeding facilities at ITRI/TNO Rijswijk, The Netherlands. For experiments, animals were kept in isolators or in laminar flow cabinets. The GF animals which were associated with viable *S. aureus* (*S. aureus* strain 14458 ATCC) were actively contaminated. Pure SEB (Sigma) was given to animals in phosphate-buffered saline (PBS) at 25 ng/ml SEB. As control, formaldehyde-fixed *S. aureus* was given to animals at a quantity of $5 \cdot 10^9$ fixed particles per milliliter water.

Analysis of IELs

Animals were sacrificed for IEL analysis on days 0, 7, 14, 21, and 28 after contamination with viable and fixed *S. aureus* and pure SEB. The IELs were isolated as described previously (1) with some minor modifications with respect to biohazard risks. From each intestine, which was used for IEL isolation, a piece of the duodenum was processed for immunohistology using an anti-CD3 monoclonal antibody (MAb). CD3-positive IELs were counted using a square grid and expressed as the number of IELs per villus area. Isolated IELs were analyzed by two-color flow cytometry using FITC-conjugated or biotinylated MAbs-specific for the TCR αβ, Thy 1, or CD3. The total number of CD3-positive cells was calculated. Subtraction of the number of TCR αβ–positive cells gives the number of TCR γδ–positive cells. Double staining of IELs using MAbs directed to the TCR αβ and Thy 1 allows discrimination between TCR $\alpha\beta^+$Thy 1^+ and TCR $\alpha\beta^+$Thy 1^- IELs.

RESULTS

The changes in time within the intestinal IEL population upon antigenic pressure by pathogenic microorganisms were investigated by contaminating GF animals with viable *S. aureus*, producing SEB, followed by phenotypical analysis of the IEL fraction at various times after the contamination. As controls, two other groups of animals were used, one (a) contaminated with pure SEB, and another group (b) which was treated with killed *S. aureus*. Contamination of GF mice with viable *S. aureus* and pure SEB resulted in rather similar changes within the IEL fraction. The introduction of killed bacteria on the other hand had hardly any effect on the composition of the IEL population during the experimental period studied.

As illustrated in Figure 1, the total number of IELs initially decreased after association of GF animals with viable *S. aureus* by a factor of 3 until day 14. Thereafter, a rise in the number of CD3-positive IELs could be observed. On day 28, the number of CD3-positive IELs had reached again the level before contamination (day 0). The presence of the introduced viable *S. aureus* in the intestine resulted in levels of approximately 100 ng SEB/g feces. Rather similar results were obtained when GF animals were given pure SEB (see Fig. 1). The decrease in the number of CD3-positive IELs in this situation is about a factor of 2 on day 7. As mentioned before, the presence of fixed *S. aureus* did not influence the number of intestinal IELs significantly. The badge of fixed *S. aureus* used in these experiments did not contain any detectable quantities of SEB.

Results of the analysis of TCR αβ–positive and TCR γδ–positive IELs after association of GF mice with viable *S. aureus* are shown in Figure 2. As can be seen in this figure, both subpopulations decreased rapidly in number after the introduction of *S. aureus*. Both

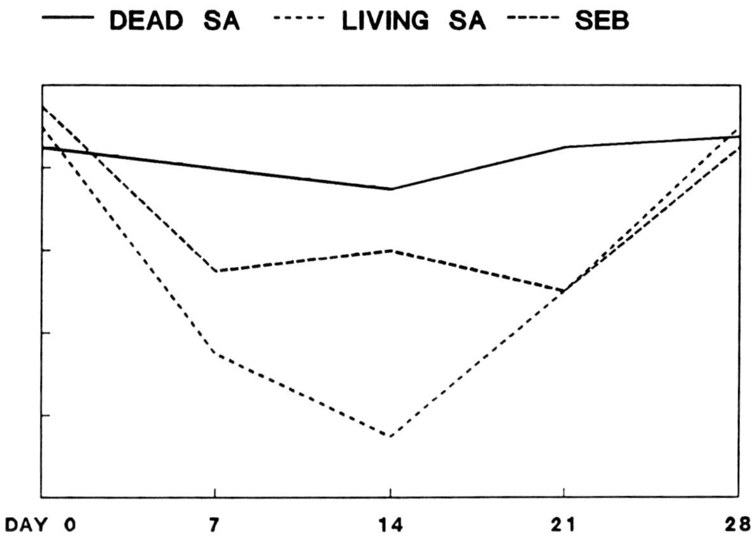

Figure 1 Relative numbers of CD3$^+$ IELs per villus area as determined on time points as indicated after contaminations of GF animals with viable and fixed *S. aureus* (SA) and pure SEB. Numbers of CD3$^+$ IELs were quantified as described in the text.

cell types reached minimal levels at day 14. Thereafter, a differential pattern could be observed for these two subpopulations. The number of TCR γδ–positive cells started to increase, resulting in an overall cellularity at day 28 which was even higher than initially present in these GF mice (day 0). The number of the TCR αβ–positive cells did not restore after day 14, but remained at a rather constant, low level during the rest of the experimental period.

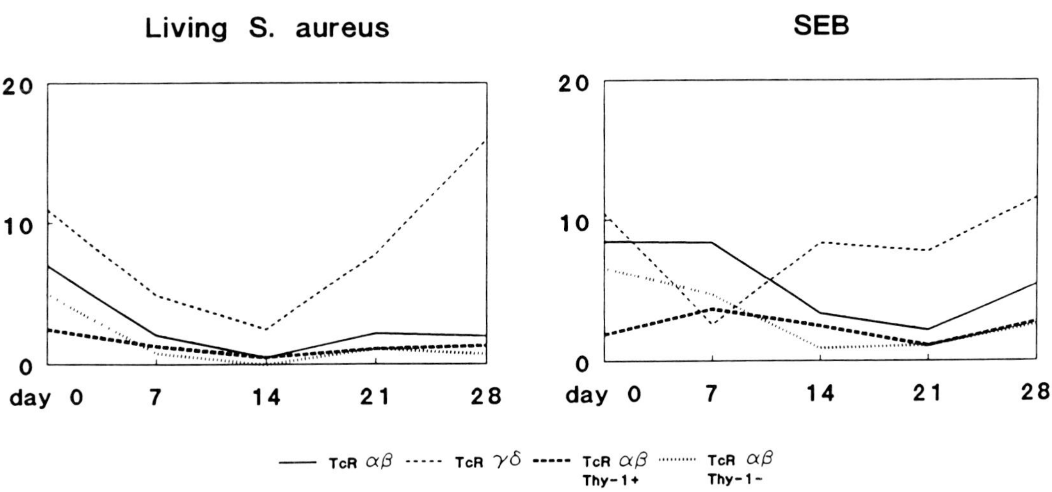

Figure 2 Relative numbers of TCR$^+$ IEL subpopulations after association of GF CBA/Rij mice with viable *S. aureus*. All values are related to the number of CD3$^+$ cells (100%).

Germ-free mice contaminated with SEB displayed again a rather similar response pattern with respect to changes in the two major subsets of IELs when compared with animals which were associated with viable *S. aureus*, though with slightly different kinetics. Minimal levels of TCR γδ–positive cells were already reached at day 7, when the recovery period again started. The decrease in numbers of TCR αβ–positive cells in SEB-treated mice was delayed when compared to mice treated with viable bacteria, but when decreased the numbers of TCR αβ–positive cells also stayed low (see Fig. 2).

Further analysis of the TCR αβ–positive IEL population for Thy 1 expression revealed that after treatment both with viable, SEB-producing *S. aureus* and with SEB directly, the pattern of changes observed for the total TCR αβ–positive IEL population was closely followed by the TCR $\alpha\beta^+$Thy 1^- subset, but not by the TCR $\alpha\beta^+$Thy 1^+ IEL subset. In fact, the number of TCR $\alpha\beta^+$Thy 1^- cells decreased immediately after treatment with SEB in analogy with the situation in *S. aureus*–contaminated mice (see Fig. 2). The observed stabile level until day 7 for the total production of TCR αβ–positive cells proved to be caused by an initial increase of the TCR $\alpha\beta^+$Thy 1^+ IEL population, which compensated for the decrease of the TCR $\alpha\beta^+$Thy 1^- population. In general, the TCR $\alpha\beta^+$Thy-1^+ IEL population remained at a rather constant level throughout the experimental period. No significant changes for neither total CD3-positive cellularity nor subpopulation typing were observed during the experimental period when GE animals were contaminated with fixed *S. aureus* (data not shown).

DISCUSSION

Contamination of GF mice with the pathogenic microorganism *S. aureus* resulted in dramatic changes within the CD3-positive IEL compartment. These changes can probably be attributed to the presence of SEB produced by these bacteria in the intestine, since (a) direct administration of pure SEB had similar effects upon the IEL compartment as the presence of viable *S. aureus*, and (b) killed *S. aureus* introduced no significant changes. The results with inoculation of GF mice with viable *S. aureus* and SEB obtained in the present study are clearly different from the data from other experiments in which GF mice were conventionalized with a conventional (3) or a specific-pathogen free (SPF) flora (B. de Geus et al., manuscript submitted). These protocols resulted in a change in the composition of the IEL population in favor of the TCR αβ–positive IEL population. The present findings indicate, however, that (a) at first both TCR αβ–positive and TCR γδ–positive cells decreased in number, and (b) while TCR αβ–positive cells stayed at a low level, the TCR $\gamma\delta^+$ cell population markedly recovered. It should be noticed, however, that *S. aureus* is a pathogenic microorganism, whereas the other types of flora are not. Furthermore, one has to keep in mind that the presence of viable *S. aureus* and pure SEB in the intestinal lumen also results in villus atrophy with an onset at day 21. Therefore, the increase of TCR γδ–positive IELs at a late stage as described in this report may be related to the pathogenic effect associated with the observed villus atrophy.

It has been reported that SEB induces proliferation of T cells expressing V_β (4). Surprisingly, the presence of SEB in the intestine both after the administration of viable *S. aureus* and of pure SEB did not result in these experiments in an increase of the TCR αβ–positive IEL populations expressing one of the members of the $V_\beta8$ family (results not shown). Several explanations can account for these negative results: (a) T cells of the CBA/Rij strain used in these experiments are nonresponders for SEB; (b) GF animals have a different response to SEB than conventional animals; or (c) TCR $\alpha\beta^+V\beta8^+$ IELs of

CBA/Rij GF mice do proliferate, but cannot be recognized anymore owing to an instant and active migration upon stimulation. These possibilities are currently under investigation.

Taken together, it can be concluded that the response of IELs upon contamination with a viable bacterial flora is still a complicated and poorly understood phenomenon. The strong response of TCR γδ–positive IELs in the case of administration of an enteropathogenic bacterium suggests that these cells may play a role in pathological intestinal situations. Whether these cells are involved in the modulation of the mucosal immune system remains unclear.

REFERENCES

1. De Geus B, Van Den Enden M, Coolen J, Nagelkerken L, Van Der Heijden P, Rozing J. Phenotype of IEL in euthymic and athymic mice; implications for differentiation of cells bearing a CD3 associated γδ TcR. Eur. J. Immunol 1990; 20:291–98.
2. Goodman T, LeFrancois L. Intraepithelial Lymphocytes. J Exp Med 1989; 170:1569–81.
3. LeFrancois L, Goodman T. In vivo modulation of cytolytic activity and Thy-1 expression in TcRγδ IEL. Science 1988; 243:1716–18.
4. White J, Herman A, Pullen A.N, Kubo R. Kappler J.W, Marrack P . The Vβ superantigen SEB: Stimulation of mature T cells and clonal deletion neonatal mice. Cell 1989; 56:27–35.

77

Cytolytic Activity in Murine Intestinal Intraepithelial Lymphocytes Is Largely Attributable to T-Cell Receptor αβ-Positive Cells

Joanne L. Viney and Thomas T. MacDonald
St. Bartholomews Hospital, London, England

INTRODUCTION

Since it was claimed that the majority lymphocytes in the gut epithelium utilize the T-cell receptor (TCR) γδ (1,2), the functional properties of (intestinal intraepithelial lymphocytes) IELs have been attributed to cells expressing this receptor. In redirected cytotoxicity assays with anti-CD3 monoclonal antibody (MAb) IELs were potently cytolytic (3), and it was suggested, therefore, that γδ-positive IELs through this cytolytic activity might have a role in protecting mucosal surfaces from viral and bacterial infection. It is now clear, however, that there are two major populations of IELs in normal mice (4). Approximately half of IELs are thymus derived, are induced by the gut flora, and use the TCR αβ. The remainder are thymus independent, use the TCR γδ and are also present in germ-free mice. The following experiments were designed to determine the relative contribution of αβ-positive and γδ-positive cells in redirected cytotoxicity assays using anti-CD3 and anti–TCR αβ MAb.

MATERIALS AND METHODS

Mice

Ten- to twenty-week-old Balb/c mice were obtained from Olac Laboratories.

Antibodies

Monoclonal antibody anti-CD3 (135-2C11), and anti–TCR αβ (H57.597), and anti–Thy 1.2 (HO.13.3) were used in this study.

IEL Isolation

The gut epithelium was removed in the presence of EDTA and IELs were purified by fetal calf serum (FCS) and Percoll density gradient centrifugation as previously described (4).

Panning

The IELs were treated with anti–Thy 1.2, then panned on a Petri dish precoated with goat antimouse immunoglobulin (Ig). Nonadherent Thy 1–depleted cells were removed by pipetting. Adherent Thy 1–enriched cells were removed by a forced stream of Hank's balanced salt water solution (HBSS).

Cytotoxicity Assay

The IELs were incubated with labeled P815 target cells in a standard 4-hr ^{51}Cr release assay at varying effector to target ratios in the presence or absence of anti-CD3 or anti–TCR αβ MAb. Percent specific lysis was calculated by:

$$\frac{\text{Experimental Cr release} - \text{spontaneous Cr release}}{\text{Maximum Cr release} - \text{spontaneous Cr release}} \times 100\%$$

RESULTS

Cytotoxicity of Unseparated IELs

Unseparated IELs were induced to display cytolytic activity by engaging the TCR with either anti-CD3 or anti–TCR αβ MAb (Fig. 1a). The level of cytotoxic activity was similar with both antibodies. In the absence of antibody there was no cytotoxicity.

Cytotoxicity of Thy 1–Enriched IELs

The IELs were separated by panning with anti–Thy 1 MAb. Adherent Thy 1–enriched cells were 87.9% Thy 1 positive, 86.5% CD3 positive, and 89.3% αβ positive. These cells were induced to display cytolytic activity by engaging the TCR with anti-CD3 and anti–TCR αβ MAb (Fig. 1b). The cytolytic activity was similar with both antibodies, and was comparable to that of unseparated IELs. No cytotoxicity was detected in the absence of antibody.

Cytotoxic Activity of Thy 1–Depleted IELs

After panning, nonadherent Thy 1–depleted cells were 14.6% Thy 1 positive, 69.8% CD3 positive, and 17.1% TCR αβ positive. Lytic activity of Thy 1–depleted cells with anti-CD3 and anti–TCR αβ MAb was greatly diminished compared to unseparated or Thy 1–enriched cell populations (Fig. 1c). In the absence of antibody there was no cytolytic activity.

DISCUSSION

These data demonstrate that most of the cytolytic potential of IELs resides in the αβ-positive cell population (5). Since αβ-positive IELs appear to be induced by the gut flora, it is possible that they may have specificity for gut bacterial antigens. γδ-positive IELs are

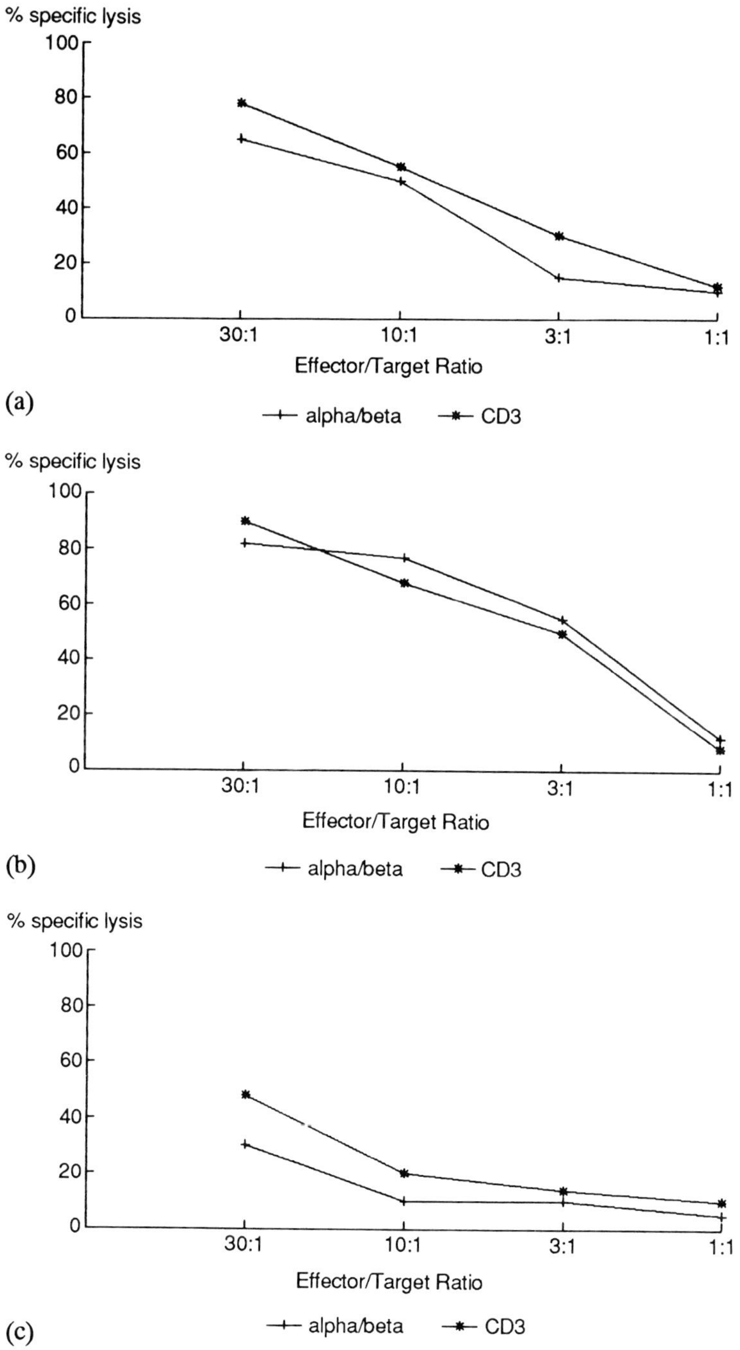

Figure 1 Unseparated (a), Thy 1–enriched (b), and Thy 1–depleted (c) IELs freshly isolated from mice were induced to display cytolytic activity with either anti–TCR αβ or anti–CD3 MAb (representative experiments shown). Comparable levels of cytolytic activity were observed in the presence of both antibodies in unseparated (a) and Thy 1–enriched (b) cell populations. Increased levels of activity can be observed in the Thy 1–enriched cell populations compared to unseparated IELs. In contrast, Thy 1–depleted IELs showed minimal levels of cytolytic activity with anti–CD3 MAb, and no activity with anti–TCR αβ MAb. Similar results were obtained in six other experiments. Together these data would indicate that Thy 1^+, $\alpha\beta^+$ IELs are potent cytolytic effectors, whereas Thy 1^-, $\gamma\delta^+$ IELs are only weakly cytolytic.

thymus independent and their presence does not require bacterial colonization of the gut. Although these cells do have very low levels of cytotoxic activity, the stimulus which induces the cytotoxicity is unknown. It is evident that, at least in the redirected cytotoxicity assay, major functional differences between the two IEL populations can be demonstrated, and that αβ-positive cells are responsible for most of the functional activity detected in IELs. In the absence of defined ligands, it is difficult to assess the role of αβ-positive and γδ-positive IELs in local mucosal immunity.

REFERENCES

1. Goodman T., and Lefrancoi L. (1988) Nature *333*:855.
2. Bonneville M. et al. (1988) Nature *336*:479.
3. Lefrancois L., and Goodman T. (1989) Science *243*:1716.
4. Viney J., MacDonald T., and Kilshaw P. (1989) Immunology *66*:583.
5. Viney J., Kilshaw P., and MacDonald T. (1990) Eur. J. Immunol. (in press).

78

T-Cell Receptor Expression on Intestinal Intraepithelial Lymphocytes During Chronic Graft-vs-Host Disease in the Mouse

Bernard de Geus,[1] Margit van den Enden,[1] Emile de Heer,[2] Jan A. Bruijn,[2] Co Coolen,[1] and Jan Rozing[1]
[1]*Institute for Experimental Gerontology TNO, Rijswijk, The Netherlands;*
[2]*University of Leiden, Leiden, The Netherlands*

INTRODUCTION

Transfer of T cells to semiallogeneic hosts can cause graft-vs-host disease (GVHD). This syndrome is associated with lesions of the kidney, skin, liver, intestinal tract, and lymphoid organs. One of the pathological effects of GVHD on the intestinal tract is chronic active inflammation with villus atrophy and destruction, which is also one of the pathological features of celiac disease in man. In celiac disease, it has been shown that numbers of T-cell receptor (TCR) γδ–positive intraepithelial lymphocytes (IELs) increase in the intestinal epithelium (2). Intestinal IELs in mouse and man can be subdivided upon their TCR usage into two populations of cells. One population expresses the TCR αβ, the other population expresses the TCR γδ [1,2]. To investigate whether chronic GVHD has any influence on the intestinal IEL population in the mouse, chronic GVHD was induced by transfer of DBA/2 lymphocytes into (C57BL10xDBA/2) F_1 hybrids. The results indicate that the destruction of villus epithelial cells in the model studied here is not directly mediated by IELs, since this population remains constant in composition and rapidly decreases in number after the time when GVHD enteropathy becomes apparent.

MATERIALS AND METHODS

Animals

C57BL10 and DBA/2 mice were purchased from Olac (Bicester, England). F_1 (C57BL10XDBA/2) hybrid mice were bred and kept under clean conventional conditions at the animal facility of the University of Leiden, (Leiden, The Netherlands).

Induction of GVHD

The induction of chronic GVHD by transfer of DBA/2 lymphocytes into F_1 (C57BL10XDBA/2) acceptor mice was performed as described in detail previously (3).

Analysis of IELs

Animals were sacrificed for IEL analysis at 0, 5, 6, and 9 weeks after induction of GVHD. Experimental groups were composed of three animals each. The IELs were isolated from the small intestinal epithelium as described previously (1). From each intestine which was used for IEL isolation a piece of the duodenum, ileum, and colon was processed for immunohistology using an anti-CD3 monoclonal antibody (MAb) and standard histology. CD3-positive IELs were counted using a square grid and expressed as number of IELs per villus area. Isolated IELs were analyzed by two-color flow cytometry using FITC-conjugated or biotinylated MAb specific for the TCR αβ, Thy 1, or CD3. The relative number of CD3-positive cells was calculated. Subtraction of the number of TCR αβ–positive cells gives the number of TCR γδ–positive cells. Double staining of IELs using MAbs directed to the TCR αβ and Thy 1 allows to discriminate between TCR $\alpha\beta^{+}$Thy-1^{+} and TCR $\alpha\beta^{+}$Thy-1^{-} IELs.

RESULTS

Pathology of Intestines

Induction of GVHD in (C57BL/10XDBA/2) F_1 hybrid mice resulted in the development of a chronic active disease which was characterized by dispersed infiltration of granulocytes in the lamina propria of the duodenal villi at week 5 after induction of GVHD. At this time point, villus atrophy also developed and small epithelial lymphocyte infiltrates could be observed. At 5 weeks after induction of GVHD, the villus atrophy became more severe and less epithelial lymphocyte infiltrates were visible. Granulocyte infiltration of the villi became more disperse. At 9 weeks after induction of GVHD, the disease developed further, resulting in variable individual differences the degree of villus atrophy and lymphocyte infiltrations. At this time, the animals showed watery diarrhea. Usually most animals died at ±12 weeks after induction of GVHD from immune complex glomerulonephritis [3].

Numbers of IELs During Chronic GVHD

In Figure 1, the mean relative number of CD3-positive IELs at 5 and 6 weeks after induction of GVHD is shown. An increase in the number of CD3-positive IELs could be demonstrated at 5 weeks after induction of GVHD. The increase was small but significant ($p \leq 0.05$, Wilcoxon's signed rank sum test). A sharp decrease in CD3-positive IELs per villus area was observed at 6 weeks after induction of GVHD. The number of CD3-positive IELs at week 6 was ±4 times lower than the number of CD3-positive IELs at week 5. On week 9 after induction of GVHD, the number of CD3-positive IELs varied strongly between individual animals. The observed relative numbers of IELs per villus area at week 9 after induction of GVHD were either equal or higher than the number of CD3-positive IELs at week 5 (data not shown).

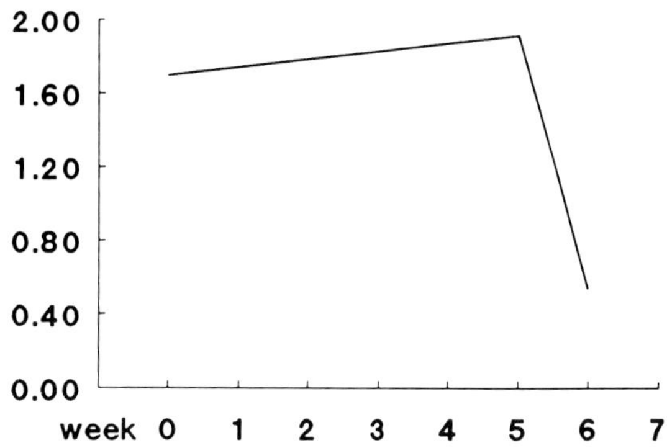

Figure 1 Mean relative numbers of $CD3^+$ IELs after induction of GVHD. Counted numbers per time point (n=3) were compared to those of the next time point using the Wilcoxon's signed rank sum test. Significance levels are at the 5% level.

Composition of the CD3-Positive IEL Population After Induction of GVHD

The TCR usage during chronic GVHD was analyzed by flow cytometry. In Figure 2, the composition of the CD3-positive IEL population is shown.

Figure 2A shows that the ratio of the TCR αβ–positive and the TCR γδ–positive IEL populations did not change during the experimental period. The relative numbers for both populations strongly decreased at week 6 after induction of GVHD. A similar pattern could be observed for the TCR αβ–positive Thy 1-positive population and for the TCR αβ–positive Thy 1^- population (Fig. 2B). At week 9 after induction of GVHD, the composition of the CD3-positive IEL population remained similar when compared to the other time points. No clear changes in the IEL population with respect to CD8 (95% of the CD3-positive cells) or CD4 (5% of the CD3-positive cells) could be observed (data not shown).

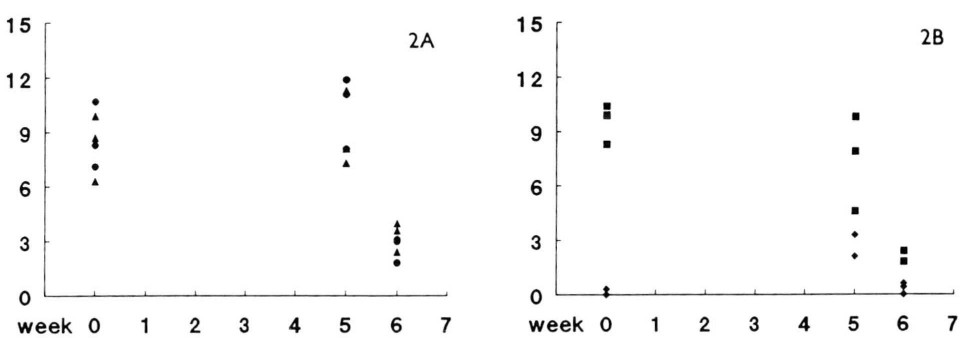

Figure 2 Composition of the $CD3^+$ IEL population at different time points after induction of GVHD. Values are expressed as relative numbers, related to the numbers of $CD3^+$ IELs. (A) Numbers of TCR $\alpha\beta^+$ and TCR $\gamma\delta^+$ IELs are given. (B) Numbers of TCR $\alpha\beta^+$ Thy 1^+ and TCR $\alpha\beta^+$ Thy 1^- IELs. ● = TCR αβ, ▲ = TCR γδ, ■ = TCR $\alpha\beta^+$Thy 1^+ and ♦ = TCR $\alpha\beta^+$Thy 1^- are given.

DISCUSSION

The induction of chronic GVHD as performed by us in (C57BL10XDBA/2) F_1 hybrid mice differs from other GVHD models. In our model, GVHD was induced by multiple injections of a mixture of splenocytes, thymocytes, and lymph node cells from DBA/2 donors into the recipient animals. Using this protocol, it is possible to induce chronic GVHD (3). At week 5 after induction of GVHD, we showed a small increase in numbers of IELs. This observation was consistent with histological data which showed dispersed epithelial lymphoid infiltrates in the villus surface epithelium. At week 6 after induction of GVHD, we observed a sharp decline in numbers of CD3-positive IELs. The decrease in numbers of CD3-positive IELs could not be attributed to loss of IELs through destruction of the villi, since only atrophy of the villi could be detected at week 6 after induction of GVHD. The decrease in numbers of CD3-positive IELs was probably caused by recruitment of IELs leaving their site of localization into the recirculation. The TCR $\alpha\beta^+$Thy 1^- IEL population is probably a true TCR $\alpha\beta$–positive IEL population, since it has a similar response pattern as the TCR $\alpha\beta^+$Thy-1^+ IEL population. The intestinal IEL population changed only in numbers but not in composition. Therefore, we believe that this population was not directly involved in causing the pathological effects of GVHD in the intestine.

The possible role of autoantibodies, which have been shown to play a role in this model (3), remains to be investigated with respect to the intestine. Furthermore, GVHD has been shown to be mediated by donor-received CD4-positive T cells (4). Those cells appeared, however, not to be involved in infiltration of CD3-positive cells at 5 weeks after induction of GVHD, since the percentage of CD4-positive T cells remained equal in the isolated IEL preparations. Apart from the observation that villus atrophy was manifest in this chronic GVHD model, this murine model may be useful for chronic inflammatory enteropathy, but differs from human celiac disease, since TCR $\gamma\delta$–positive IELs appear not to play a pathogenetic role in the model used by us.

REFERENCES

1. De Geus B, Van den Enden M, Coolen J, Nagelkerken L, Van Der Heijden P, Rozing J. Phenotype of IEL in euthymic and athymic mice; Implications for differentiation of cells bearing a CD3 associated γδ TcR. Eur J Immunol 1990; 20:291–98.
2. Savilahti E, Arato A, Verkasalo M. Increased numbers of TcR γδ bearing cells in the epithelium of coeliac patients. In: *Advances in Mucosal Immunology*; Kluwer, The Netherlands, 1990, pp. 61–66.
3. Bruijn JA, Hogendoorn P, Corver W, Van Den Broek L, Hoedemaeker P, Fleuren G. Pathogenesis of experimental lupus nephritis: A role for anti-basement membrane and anti-tubular brush border antibodies in murine GVHD. Clin Exp Immunol 1990; 79:115–22.
4. Thiele D, Eigenbrodt M, Bryde S, Eigenbrodt E, Lipsky P. Intestinal GVHD is initiated by donor T cells distinct from classic cytotoxic T lymphocytes. J Clin Invest 1989; 84:1947–56.

79

Analysis of Functional Potential of Germinal Center B Cells by Lymphoid Fragment Culture, In Situ Hybridization, and T-Dependent, Single Cell Microculture

John J. Cebra, Anna George, Ava C. Logan, Peter A. Schweitzer, and Peter D. Weinstein
University of Pennsylvania, Philadelphia, Pennsylvania

INTRODUCTION

We have been puzzled by the apparent preference for switching to the expression of the immunoglobulin A (IgA) isotype by B cells in Peyer's patches (PPs) compared with B cells in lymph nodes (LNs) after local antigenic (Ag) stimulation (1). Since the earliest expression of non–IgM/IgD isotypes occurs most conspicuously on the surface of germinal center (GC) blasts following Ag stimulation, the GC has been implicated in isotype switching (2). We initially supposed that the chronically present GC in PPs compared with the transient ones in LNs might occasion a difference in their physiological state that could account for the apparent difference in isotype preference exhibited by B cells responding in the two sites to a new, local Ag stimulus (1). To examine this possibility, we sought to initiate GC reactions de novo in both PPs and LNs and to analyze the functional potential of B cells from the two sites to produce antibody (Ab) of various isotypes.

FINDINGS

De Novo Perturbation of PPs and Peripheral Lymph Node GCs by Antigen and the Use of Fragment Cultures to Analyze Ab Isotype Expression

Our approach was to either colonize the intestine of germ-free (GF) mice with *Morganella morganii*, or to inject a heat-killed vaccine of this bacterium into the footpads of conventionally reared mice (3). In either case, we induced a GC reaction in PPs or LNs, respectively, as detected by the appearance of a population of B cells that bound high levels of peanut agglutinin (PNA^{high}). However, the time course of the GC reaction of the two different sites differed markedly: The PNA^{high} cells became obvious in PPs only in the period 12–15 weeks after colonization, whereas the GC reaction waxed and waned over a 3-week period in LNs. To examine the result of these local stimuli, we established PP and LN fragment cultures from tissues taken during the times of the conspicuous GC reactions. Supernatants from the cultures were analyzed for Ab after both 1 day and 6–10 days in vitro. We found that local stimulation with *M. morganii* resulted in a net production of exclusively IgA and IgM Ab in vitro in PP cultures and IgM, IgG_1, and IgG_2 Abs in LN cultures. These findings suggested a site difference in preferences for non-IgM isotype expression, even when the GC reactions at the different sites were initiated de novo. However, because of the marked differences in the time courses of GC development at the different sites we could not exclude intervening but not functionally detectable switching to IgG isotypes in PPs during the prolonged development of GCs there.

Thus, we sought to compare a more acute development of GC reactions in PPs vs LNs, and accomplished this by using oral infection of GF mice with reovirus, type 1 vs footpad inoculation of this virus into conventionally reared mice (see Chapter 67). The GC reaction in both PPs and LNs waxed and waned with the same time course over a 3-week period as judged both histologically or by the appearance of PNA^{high}, surface IgA–positive, or surface IgG_1–positive B cells detected by FACS. Again, fragment cultures of the responding PPs vs LNs showed distinctly different patterns of antireovirus isotypes—PP fragments secreted IgA and IgM Abs, whereas LN fragments made mostly IgM and IgG_1 Abs. These observations made over the same 2-week period of de novo GC development in PPs vs LNs and using the same Ag stimulus delivered at different local sites support an intrinsic difference in microenvironmental sites of the PPs vs LNs.

Use of In Situ Hybridization and Single B-Cell Microcultures to Assess the Functional Potential of GC B Cells

The correlations between histochemical and cytochemical perturbations involving GC cells in PPs or LNs with isotype output of their respective fragment cultures suggest a difference in regulation of isotype switching at the different types of GC sites. However, a direct demonstration of this possibility requires an assay for the functional potential of GC B cells. Essential frequency analyses of specificity and isotype potential of GC cells in vitro has heretofore been unsuccessful—GC cells usually die rapidly in culture—and assessment of their functional potential by adoptive transfer has been confounded by the lack of "homing" receptors on most GC B cells and the impossibility of defining the exact surface phenotype of progenitor cells responsible for any Ig expression in a host (4,5).

Recently, we have developed a haplotype-restricted, antigen-independent, Th 2 cell-dependent assay for the functional potential of single B cells (6). This microculture assay results in clonal outgrowth and Ig production by two of three to three of four single B cells from most lymphatic tissue. About 0.5–2.0 B cells to be tested are plated out in Terasaki wells (10 μl) with $1–3 \times 10^3$ alloreactive Th 2 cells (D10) which respond to $I\text{-}A^b$ determinants. Such microcultures support clonal outgrowth and isotype switching, although mostly only IgM, IgG_1, and IgE are expressed as secreted products. If about 400 dendritic cells (DCs) from spleen or PPs are added to these cultures, IgA is also expressed among other isotypes as a clonal product and IgA memory cells—prevalent in PPs—are also supported to give clones exclusively secreting IgA (7). When we cultured GC cells from PPs (PNA^{high}, $s\kappa^{low}$) under these conditions, we found relatively low frequencies of responding cells, and these gave clones that were not particularly distinctive of the site: secretion of IgM, IgG_1, and only occasionally some IgE and IgA. Since about one-half to two-thirds of PP GC B cells from conventionally reared mice bore surface IgA (sIgA), we supposed these were not responding with Ig secretion in our microcultures. We then sought to probe the possible functional potential of GC B cells from PPs by in situ hybridization for messenger ribonucleic acids (mRNAs) encoding the various isotypes of Ig heavy chains using riboprobes (8). We have identified a novel phenotype characteristic of these GC B cells from the PPs of conventionally reared mice undergoing natural, chronic intestinal stimulation by environmental antigens: The major subset of GC cells that is PNA^{high} $s\kappa^{low}$ contains levels of cytoplasmic mRNA α or mRNA μ that are easily detectable by in situ hybridization and which are intermediate between those of plasma cells and small B lymphocytes. About 38% of this GC subset has easily detectable levels of mRNA α and 51% mRNA μ. Enrichment of sIgA-positive and sIgA-negative PP cells led to a segregation of essentially all the cells with moderate levels of mRNA α in the sIgA-positive fraction (48% positive). We conclude that those cells which are PNA^{high} sIgA-positive account for almost all the cells in unfractionated PP populations (11%) with easily detectable levels of mRNA α and that these are GC blasts. It is likely that IgA memory cells (9) have levels of mRNA α that cannot be detected by our in situ hybridization methods.

We had been unable to reveal a special functional potential to produce IgA by PPs GC cells either by microculture with Th 2 and DC cells or by splenic fragment culture, which involves an initial adoptive transfer of B cells (9). In fact, those cells which gave clones that exclusively secreted IgA (IgA memory cells) were always found among the non-GC cells (PNA^{low} $s\kappa^{high}$) by either assay method. However, we found that our microcultures did allow extensive proliferation of GC B cells, although we could not detect IgA secretion and could not determine whether those cells containing moderate levels of mRNA α were among those that proliferated. Because proliferation and differentiation have often been observed to be seemingly antagonistic processes, we assessed the effect of blocking division on Ig secretion by GC B cells from PPs (10). Untreated GC B cells from PPs, plated at 0.5–2.0 cells/well, show no positive cultures making only IgA in supportive microculture. However, if division of these cells is blocked by either x-irradiation (1600 R) or aphidicolin, a specific inhibitor of deoxyribonucleic acid (DNA) polymerases, a high proportion of the positive cultures (>60%) exclusively express IgA. Both Th 2 and DC cells are required for such expression. Incorporation of [^{3}H]thymidine is blocked by the treatments and positive cultures expressing multiple Ig isotypes become rare. Experiments demonstrating GC B/Th 2 haplotype restriction and assay of secreted IgM by F_1 cells using anti-Ig allotype strongly argue against B cell contaminants of the DC cells being the source of the secreted IgA in these cultures. Finally, purification of sIgA-positive cells from PPs enriches for both the uncommon (13–14%) B cells that give clones secreting exclusively IgA (memory cells) and those that give only IgA when this proliferation is blocked. The former population is seldom detected among the GC B cells, but it is found in the PNA^{low} $s\kappa^{high}$, non-GC subset.

CONCLUSIONS

We hypothesize that microculture of GC B cells from PPs, when their division is blocked, reveals a subset of cells committed to secretion. Our assay for Ig, reverse radioimmunoassay (RIA), is sensitive enough to detect the secreted products of a single plasma cell. The GC cells alone, or without either alloreactive Th 2 or DCs, fail to make detectable product in microculture if their division is blocked. Thus, we presume that our positive cultures result from GC cells maturing to high-level secretion of Ig, the majority (60–70%) making IgA. This approach to assessing functional potential of GC cells should permit frequency analyses for antigen-specific GC cells. It also demonstrates that although many

GC B cells may die in situ by apoptosis, death need not be their immediate fate if their continued division is blocked and they are provided with necessary supportive accessory cells and signals (10). Finally, these observations again emphasize the extraordinary preference for the expression of IgM and IgA isotypes by GC B cells from PPs.

ACKNOWLEDGMENT

This work was supported by USPHS grant AI-17997.

REFERENCES

1. Cebra JJ, Gearhart PJ, Halsey JF, Hurwitz JL, Shahin RD. Role of environmental antigens in the ontogeny of the secretory immune response. J. Reticuloendothel. Soc. 1980; 28:61s–71s.
2. Kraal G, Weissman IL, Butcher EC. Germinal centre B cells: Antigen specificity and changes in heavy chain class expression. Nature 1982; 298:377–379.
3. Logan AC, Chow K-PN, George A, Weinstein PD, Cebra JJ. Peyer's patch fragment cultures to compare local immune responses to *Morganella morganii*. Infect. Immun. 1991; 59(3).
4. Coico RF, Bhogal BS, Thorbecke GJ. Relationship of germinal centers in lymphoid tissue to immunologic memory. VI. Transfer of B cell memory with lymph node cells fractionated according to their receptors for peanut agglutinin. J. Immunol. 1983; 131:2254–2257.
5. Reichert RA, Gallatin WM, Weissman IL, Butcher EC. Germinal center B cells lack homing receptors necessary for normal lymphocyte recirculation. J. Exp. Med. 1983; 157:813–827.
6. Kerlin RL, George A, Kotloff DB, Cebra JJ. Both primary and secondary B cells can be stimulated in clonal microculture to produce diverse immunoglobulin isotypes by haplotype-restricted antigen-dependent and -independent interactions with Th cells. J. Immunol. Methods 1990 (submitted).
7. Schrader CE, Kerlin RL, George A, Cebra JJ. Dendritic cells support production of IgA and other non-IgM isotypes in clonal microculture. Int. Immunol. 1990; 2:563–570.
8. Schweitzer PA, Cebra-Thomas JA, Weinstein PD, Cebra JJ. Distribution of B cells containing mRNAα for IgA heavy chain among subsets of murine Peyer's patch cells determined by *in situ* hybridization. Int. Immunol. 1990 (submitted).
9. Lebman DA, Griffin PM, Cebra JJ. Relationship between expression of IgA by Peyer's patch cells and functional IgA memory cells. J. Exp. Med. 1987; 166:1405–1418.
10. George A, Cebra JJ. Responses of single germinal center B cells in T-dependent microculture. Proc. Natl. Acad. Sci. U.S.A. 1991; 88:11–15.

80

Differentiation of B-Cell Lymphoma with CD38 (Anti–Leu-17)

An Immunohistological Study

Mami Shiota, Yasuyuki Morishita, Keisuke Toyama, and Shigeo Mori
The Institute of Medical Science, University of Tokyo, Japan;
Tokyo Medical College, Tokyo, Japan

INTRODUCTION

The term follicular center cells (FCCs), implying lymphocytes originated from germinal centers (GCs), has been used widely in histopathology. Recent immunological studies have further characterized the phenotype of FCCs. They were reported to bear CD10 (CALLA) and CD21 (CR2). However, available antibodies to these epitopes are not adequate for diagnosis. CD21 is detected on mantle zone (MZ) B cells and follicular dendritic cells (FDCs) as well as FCCs. During a study to find FCC-specific antibodies, we observed that CD38 is rather specific for nontumorous FCCs and plasma cells on immunostaining of human tonsils.

MATERIALS AND METHODS

Five nontumorous tonsils removed from patients suffering from reactive tonsillitis, 43 lymph nodes taken from non-Hodgkin's lymphoma of B-cell malignant lymphoma (B-ML; 13 follicular types and 30 diffuse types), and 10 nodes from T-cell lymphomas (T-MLs) were selected from the file of our frozen tissue library. The unfixed frozen sections of these specimens were studied immunopathologically. Eight anti–B cell antibodies, LN1, CR2, CALLA, NU-N1, NU-N2, Ln100, J5, and anti–Leu-17 (1) were selected in this study. The avidin-biotin peroxidase method (ABC-PO) was employed for immunostaining. The number of Ki67-positive cells, indicating cells in G_1-S phase of the cell cycle (2), was counted and analyzed statistically. In this study, 300 cells in each of three different fields were counted. The t-test was used for comparison of these mean values. Two tonsils were investigated with immunoelectron microscopy.

Table 1 Immunopathological Reactivity of Nontumorous Tonsils

	MZ	PF	DZ	FL
KiM4	–	+	±	–
Ln1	±	+	+	+
CD21	±	+	+	–
CD38[a]	–	–	+	–

Abbreviations: MZ, mantle zone; PF, primary follicle; DZ, dark zone; FL, FDC-depleted area in follicle lysis.
[a]Heavily stained cells were excluded.

RESULTS

Immunoreaction on Nontumorous Tonsils (Table 1)

The LN1 antibody reacted heavily with FCCs and lightly with MZ cells and primary follicles that lack KiM4-positive FDCs. It also reacted with lymphocytes of GCs that were in follicle lysis from which FCCs were mostly lost. CR2 reacts more specifically with FCCs than LN1. Meanwhile, CR2 showed some additional reaction on a small portion of non-FCCs; namely, MZ B cells. With all five anti-CALLA antibodies, the reactions on GC were too faint to use it for further study of FCCs. With anti–Leu-17, two types of immunoreactive cells, heavily stained cells, and lightly stained cells were present in GCs mostly. Such cells were not observed in primary follicles, MZs, nor GCs that were in the FDC-depleted area in follicle lysis (FL). The heavily stained cells were present mostly in perifollicular areas and GCs. T zones were stained very weakly; far weaker than GCs but more than MZ.

Electron microscopically, a heavy immunoreaction was observed in smaller cells with round nuclei and well-developed rough endoplasmic reticulum, corresponding to plasma cells and their immediate precursors. Such cells were found in perifollicular areas and in GCs. Meanwhile, a much weaker immunoreaction was noted on larger lymphocytes with cleaved nuclei that were located in GCs, corresponding to FCCs (Fig. 1). Thus, anti–Leu-17 was shown to differentiate FCCs as well as plasma cells and their immediate precursors from other nontumorous lymphocytes.

Immunoreactions of B-Cell Lymphoma with Anti–Leu-17 and CR2

The reaction of 43 B-MLs with anti–Leu-17 and CR2 are listed in Table 2, together with the results of immunoreaction with KiM4. These B-cell lymphomas are classified here into four groups. The first group, follicular lymphoma with complete tumor follicles, indicates follicular lymphomas on which over 75% of tumor tissue was occupied by tumor follicles. The second group, follicular lymphoma with partial diffuse area, implies the follicular lymphoma with a diffuse area of less than 75%. The third group, diffuse lymphoma with a trace of tumor follicles, indicates diffuse ML with partial tumor follicles in less than 25%, and the fourth group, diffuse lymphoma without tumor follicles.

Follicular Lymphoma with Complete Tumor Follicles

Leu-17–positive cells were observed in tumor follicles exclusively. The intensity of reaction was apparently weaker than that of normal FCCs. Tumor follicles were covered by the

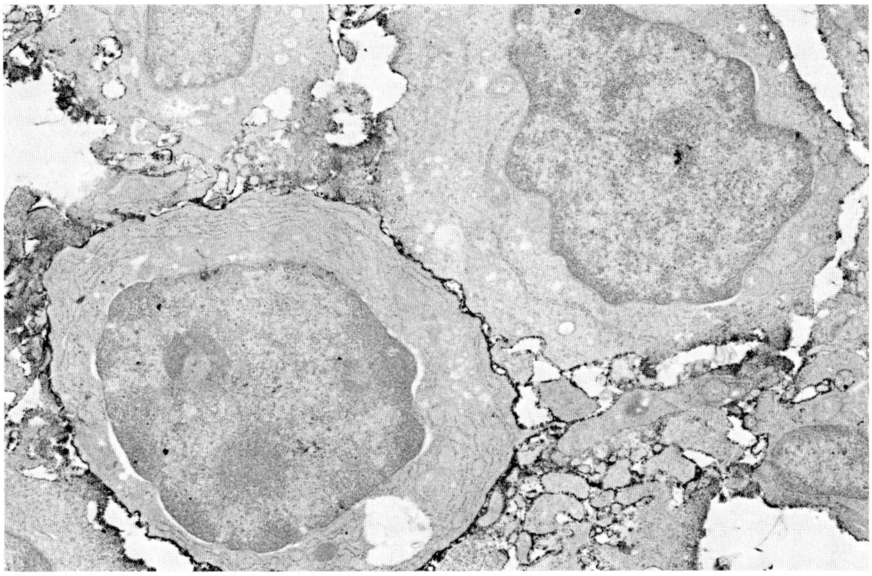

Figure 1 An immunoelectron microscopic examination of nontumorous tonsil. There are heavily stained cells (left) and lightly stained cells (right). The heavily stained cells are thought to be plasma cells or their precursors.

well-developed cytoplasmic projections of FDCs, as were shown by KiM4. However, the number of FDCs in tumor follicles was much less than in normal FCs (Fig. 2).

Follicular Lymphoma with Partial Diffuse Area

Leu-17–positive cells were distributed in tumor tissue much more widely than in the area where FDCs were present. Such Leu-17–positive cell clusters seemed to constitute tumor follicles with FDCs in the center. These tumor follicles were stained with CR2 as well.

Diffuse Lymphoma with Trace of Tumor Follicles

In nine out of 10 cases, tumor cells were stained well with anti–Leu-17 diffusely and distinctly. In six cases that were stained with anti–Leu-17, KiM4-positive FDCs were

Table 2 Immunopathological Reactivity of B-MLs

	F	FD	DF	D
	Positive cases/total cases			
KiM4	4/4	9/9	6/10	0/20
CD21	4/4	9/9	6/10	2/20
CD38	4/4	9/9	9/10	8/20

Abbreviations: F, follicular lymphoma with complete tumor follicles; FD, follicular lymphoma with partial diffuse areas; DF, diffuse lymphoma with trace of tumor follicles; D, diffuse lymphoma without tumor follicles.

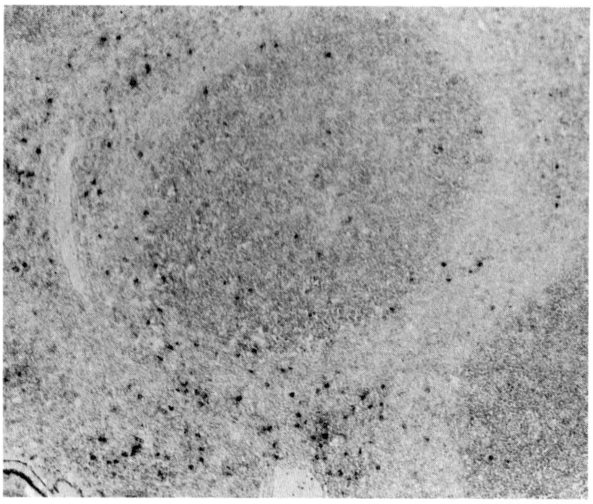

(a)

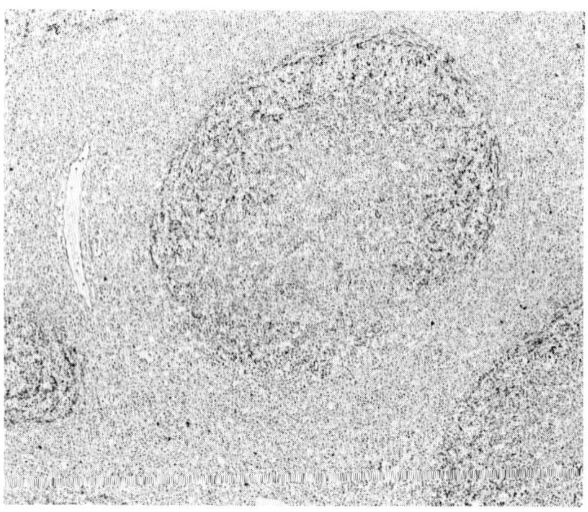

(b)

Figure 2 Serial sections of follicular lymphoma immunostained with KiM4 (b) and anti–Leu-17 (a). The Leu-17–positive cells were observed mostly in tumor follicles.

present rudimentarily to form incomplete follicles. In each of these cases, the cytoplasmic networks of FDCs were heavily degenerated. CR2 reacted with much fewer cases (6/10).

Diffuse Lymphoma Without Tumor Follicles

Out of 20 cases constituting this group, eight MLs were stained with anti–Leu-17 diffusely. On histological typing, two of them were of Burkitt's type (small noncleaved cell type) and others were of the large noncleaved cell type. No phenotypic differences were noted between Leu-17–positive and –negative cases. KiM4-positive cells were not demonstrated in any of these cases.

Ki67 Positivity in B-MLs

The number of Ki67-positive cells on different histological types and phenotypes were studied. Many more Ki67-positive cells, indicating cells in the G_1-M phase of the cell cycle, were noted in diffuse lymphoma than follicular lymphoma ($p<0.001$), and in Leu-17–negative diffuse lymphoma than Leu-17–positive diffuse lymphoma ($p<0.001$). Also, in FDC-negative DLs, many more Ki67-positive cells were found in Leu-17–negative cases than in Leu-17–positive cases. These data clearly indicate that Leu-17–positive MLs have much lower mitotic rates than Leu-17–negative MLs.

Immunoreaction of T-Cell Lymphomas with Anti–Leu-17

In 10 T-cell lymphomas, one case was found to be Leu-17^{++}, two cases Leu-17^{+}, four cases Leu-17 positive and negative and three cases Leu-17 negative. No histopathological or phenotypical differences were noted between Leu-17–positive and Leu-17–negative cases.

DISCUSSION

CD38 (anti–Leu-17) was shown by study with flow cytometry to react at low intensity with most normal human natural killer (NK) cells, most B cells, subsets of Leu-2 CD8-positive and Leu-3 CD4-positive T cells and monocytes, and at high intensity with plasma cells, mitogen-activated T cells, and several B- and T-cell lines (1). Even though this antibody has been commonly used for flow cytometry, there have been published a very limited number of reports on immunopathology (3).

In a trial to find FCC-specific monoclonal antibodies, we noted that CD38 demonstrates FCCs and FCC-derived MLs at a satisfactory level. First, we stained five non-tumorous human tonsils and found that CD38 demonstrated plasma cells as heavily stained cells, FCCs rather weakly but clearly, and T zone T cells very faintly. Meanwhile, CD38 did not show any immunoreaction with MZ B cells and primary follicles. When the antibody was used on MLs, a clear reaction was noted on all of the follicular lymphomas; all of the follicular lymphomas with partial diffuse areas; a large number of diffuse lymphomas, which still keep follicular characteristics like the process of FDC nests, and eight of 20 diffuse B-MLs, which lack follicular characteristics. In follicular lymphomas with partial diffuse areas, Leu-17 was demonstrated on all the tumor tissues, while the FDC nests were lost in a part of such lesions. These areas were the very areas where the transformation into follicular to diffuse pattern occurred. Thus, this finding suggested that the lymphoma cells tended to keep CD38 during the transformation of follicular to diffuse pattern. The present study also showed diffuse B-MLs can be differentiated into two groups, CD38 positive and CD38 negative. It is possible that CD38-positive MLs are originated from FCCs, although we could not present direct evidence for this assumption.

The present data with Ki67 suggested that CD38-positive diffuse B-ML seemed to have a lower mitotic rate than CD38-negative cases. As the Ki67 positivity seems to correlate with the prognosis of the patients, it is probable that such CD38-positive diffuse MLs might favor better prognosis (4–6). However, many more cases will have to be studied for evaluation of its clinicopathological significance.

REFERENCES

1. Tedder TF, Crain MJ, Kubakawa H, Clement LT, Cooper MD. J Immunol 1985; 135:1786–1791.
2. Gerdes J, Lemnke H, Baish H. J Immunol 1984; 133:1710–1715.

3. Ling NR, Mc Lennan ICM, Mayson DY. Oxford, England, New University Press, 1987, pp. 302–335.
4. Schwartz BR, Pinkus G, Bacus S, Toder M, Weinberg DS. Am J Pathol 1989; 1134:327–336.
5. Vago JF, Weisenburger DD, Armitage JO. Hematol Pathol 1987; 1:217–225.
6. Weiss JM, Strickler JG, Medeiros LJ, Gerdes J, Stein H, Warnke RA. Hum Pathol 1987; 18: 1155–1159.

81
Decrease of Immunoglobulin A–Secreting Lamina Propria Cells in Aging Mice

Jan Rozing,[1] Co Coolen,[1] Philip van der Heijden,[2] Wil Stok,[2] Jitske Weegenaar,[1] and Andre Th.J. Bianchi[2]
[1] *Institute for Experimental Gerontology, Netherlands Organization for Applied Scientific Research, Rijswijk, The Netherlands;*
[2] *Central Veterinary Institute, Lelystad, The Netherlands*

INTRODUCTION

Most aging studies deal with the systemic immune system, while only a few aging studies have focused on the mucosal immune system. Contradictory results have been reported with respect to changes in humoral response patterns of gut-associated lymphoid tissues (GALT) during aging, varying from a decrease in the ability to respond, as reported by Schmucker et al. (1), to a persistent normal level of responsiveness, as described by Wade et al. (2) in old animals. Direct quantitative data for the number of antibody-producing cells in the GALT and changes during aging are only available for mesenteric lymph nodes and Peyer's patches (3). These tend to decline with age. However, we showed previously that in young adult mice the vast majority (≥90%) of immunoglobulin-secreting cells (IgSCs) in the body is located in the lamina propria (LP) along the gut (4). Therefore, the study of especially this population of IgSCs during aging is of great interest.

In the present study, the intestinal B-cell compartment was investigated in CBA/Rij mice varying in age between 3 and 30 months. Immunoglobulin-secreting cells were quantitated in the lamina propria and the localization of these cells was examined in immunohistological sections of the gut. The number of LP IgSCs was compared with the number of IgSCs of spleen, bone marrow, and Peyer's patches.

MATERIALS AND METHODS

Mice

CBA/Rij mice were bred and maintained in the mouse colonies of ITRI/TNO in Rijswijk, The Netherlands. Female mice were obtained from a specific-pathogen free (SPF) and barrier-maintained aging colony and were used in groups of six mice at the age of 5, 12, 18, and 30 months.

Quantitative IgSC Assay

Mice were killed by carbon dioxide exposure. Cell suspensions of spleen, Peyer's patches, bone marrow (BM), and lamina propria (LP) lymphocytes were prepared as described previously (5,6). A modified protein A PFC assay (7) was used to quantitate the number of IgSCs in the isolated cell suspensions. Rabbit–anti-mouse IgM and IgA (Nordic Lab., Tilburg, The Netherlands) and rabbit–anti-mouse IgG (ICN, Lisle, USA) were used for isotype determination.

Immunohistology

Small pieces of mesenteric lymph nodes and Swiss rolls of the small and large intestine were fixed in formalin–acetic acid–mercury chloride fixative. Immunohistology on paraplast section was performed as described previously (8), using the following antisera and conjugates: Sheep–anti-mouse IgM (Serotec Ltd., Blackthorn Bicester, England), goat–anti-mouse IgG (Fc)7S and IgA (Fc)7S (Nordic Lab., Tilburg, The Netherlands), and peroxidase-labeled rabbit–anti-sheep Ig and rabbit-goat Ig (Dakopatts, Glostrup, Denmark). Total numbers of Ig-containing cells (IgCCs) were counted in sections of mesenteric lymph nodes and small and large intestines.

RESULTS

Serial sections of mesenteric nodes and small and large intestines of 5-, 12-, 18-, and 30-month-old CBA/Rij mice were made and the frequencies of IgM-, IgG-, and IgA-containing cells were determined. As shown in Figure 1, the majority, i.e., 80%, of intestinal IgCCs was of the IgA class in all the age groups. A different pattern could be observed in the mesenteric lymph nodes. Aging caused in this organ a clear shift from IgM- to IgG-containing cells, with IgA-containing cells at a rather constant level. A similar pattern was observed for the spleen (data not shown). These data confirm earlier findings that IgA is the dominant isotype produced by LP lymphocytes (4). The IgCCs in the small intestine were located almost exclusively in the lamina propria in the villi and around the crypts. In the large intestine, IgCCs were found scattered throughout the lamina propria surrounding the crypts both in the proximity of the intestinal lumen as well as near the muscularis mucosae. We observed no major changes in the localization and in the isotype distribution of the IgCCs in the lamina propria during aging. However, for IgG-containing cells it was observed that these cells in old mice preferentially were located in the lamina propria in the large intestine near the muscularis mucosae (data not shown).

The number of LP IgSCs increased up to 10^7 in CBA/Rij mice until the age of 12 months. Thereafter, the number of LP IgSCs decreased, as illustrated in Figure 2. The distribution of IgSCs along the gut did not change during aging. At all ages, the vast majority of intestinal LP IgSCs were located in the small intestine and produced IgA (data not shown). As is obvious from Figure 2, the kinetics of IgSCs in spleen and BM during aging was different from the small intestine: Numbers of IgSCs in spleen and BM increased also up to 12 months, but remained at the same level thereafter. Moreover, there was almost a 10-fold difference between the total number of IgSCs along the intestine as compared with the other organs. The isotype patterns of IgSCs in spleen and BM during aging were comparable to the pattern as shown for the IgCCs in mesenteric lymph nodes (see Figure 1), though with a more outspoken increase in IgA-secreting cells (data not shown) in old mice.

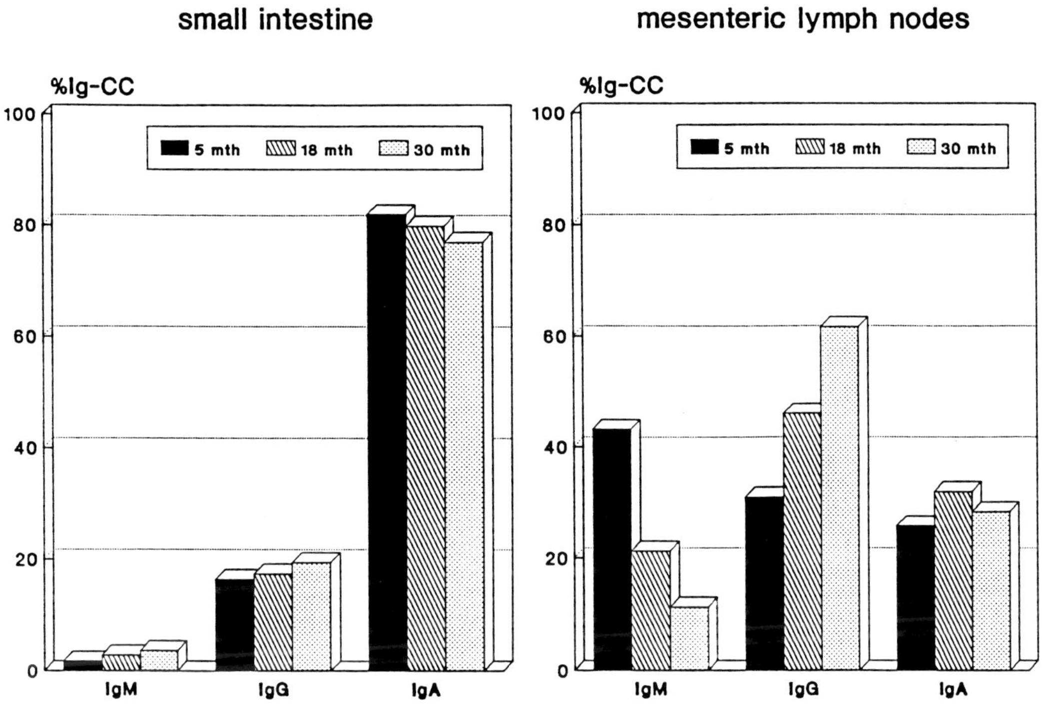

Figure 1 Effect of aging on the frequency of IgM-, IgG-, and IgA-containing cells in small intestine and mesenteric lymph nodes of 5-, 18-, and 30-month-old CBA/Rij mice. Each bar represents the mean percentage of Ig-containing cells (IgCCs) (n=3).

DISCUSSION

It can be concluded that the spontaneous IgSC response in the small intestine differs from other lymphoid organs in total number, isotype distribution, and kinetics during aging. Immunohistological examination of IgM-, IgG-, and IgA-Ig-containing cells in spleen, mesenteric lymph nodes, and intestine of CBA/Rij mice of various ages showed that the localization and isotype distribution of IgCCs was not seriously affected by aging.

In studies on the effect of aging on the enteric antibody response decreased levels of luminal IgA in the intestine have been reported (9). Different mechanisms can account for such a decrease, since the IgA concentration in the intestinal lumen depends on: (a) the number of IgSCs in the LP, (b) the efficiency of the transport mechanisms of dimeric IgA toward the lumen, and (c) the proteolytic degradation of IgA in the lumen. Although our results do not provide direct information about the effect of aging on the luminal IgA concentrations in our mice, it is obvious that the declined numbers of IgSCs in the LP contribute significantly to the diminished enteric humoral responsiveness during aging.

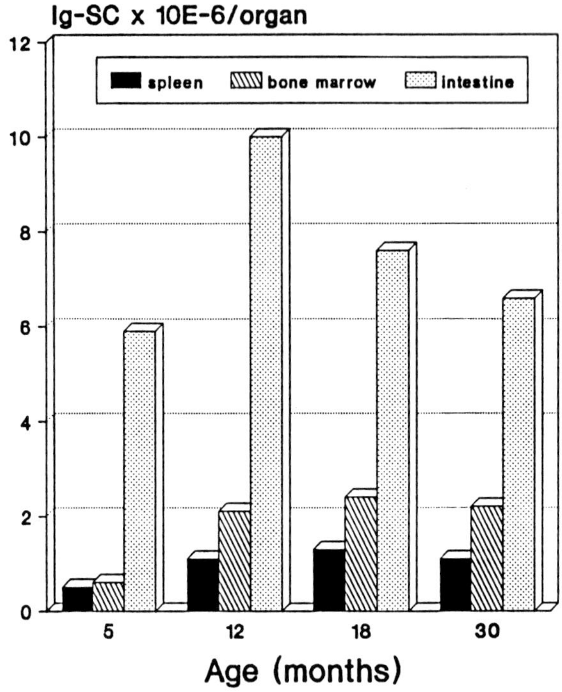

Figure 2 Effect of aging on the total number of Ig-secreting cells (Ig-SCs) in spleen, bone marrow, and small intestine of CBA/Rij mice. Each bar represents the mean number of IgSCs per organ (n=6).

REFERENCES

1. Schmucker DL, Daniels CK, Wang RK, Smith K. Mucosal immune responses to cholera toxin in ageing rats. I Antibody and antibody-containing cell response. Immunology 1988; 64:691.
2. Wade AW, Green-Johnson J, Szewczuk MR. Functional changes in systemic and mucosal lymphocyte repertoires with age: an update review. Aging Immunol Infect Dis 1988; 1:65.
3. Benner R, Van Oudenaren A, Björklund M, Ivars F, Holmberg D. Background immunoglobulin production: measurement, biological significance and regulation. Immunol Today 1982; 3:243.
4. Van der Heijden PJ, Stok W, Bianchi ATJ. Contribution of immunoglobulin secreting cells in the murine small intestine to the total "background" immunoglobulin production. Immunology 1987; 62:551.
5. Van der Heijden PJ, Stok W. Improved procedure for the isolation of functionally active lymphoid cells from the murine intestine. J Immunol Meth 1987; 103:161.
6. De Geus B, Van Den Enden M, Coolen J, Nagelkerken L, Van Der Heijden P, Rozing J. Phenotype of IEL in euthymic and athymic mice; implications for differentiation of cells bearing a CD3 associated gamma delta TcR. Eur J Immunol 1990; 20:291.
7. Van Oudenaren A, Hooijkaas H, Benner R. Improvement of the protein-A plaque assay for immunoglobulin secreting cells by using immunoglobulin depleted guinea pig serum as source of complement. J Immunol Meth 1981; 43:219.

8. Haaijman JJ, Coolen C, Deen C, Krose JM, Zijlstra J, Radl J. Monoclonal antibodies directed against human immunoglobulins: Preparation and evaluation procedures. In: *Reviews on Immunoassay Technology*. Vol. 1. S. B. Bal, ed. Macmillan, London, 1988, p. 59.
9. Lim TS, Messiha N, Watson RR. Immune components of the intestinal mucosae of ageing and protein deficient mice. Immunology 1981; 43:401.

82
Functional and Morphological Aspects of Proximal Colonic Lymphoid Tissue

Greg A. Perry and J. Graham Sharp
University of Nebraska Medical Center, Omaha, Nebraska

INTRODUCTION

Approximately 3 years ago, we became interested in an aggregate of lymphoid tissue found in the proximal colon of mice and rats. During the course of studies examining the synergy between irradiation and carcinogens in the induction of colon cancers, we found that greater than 75% of the adenocarcinomas observed in the right colon were in direct association with a nodule of lymphoid tissue. In addition, we found this nodule in both untreated and carcinogen-treated groups, suggesting that the lymphoid nodule preexisted the local carcinogenic event. This aggregate was consistently located 25% of the distance from the cecum to the rectum in all animals examined. We have spent much of the past 3 years examining and characterizing this proximal colonic lymphoid tissue (PCLT), and present an overview of this work here.

MORPHOLOGICAL CHARACTERISTICS OF PCLT

One of the most striking morphological features of PCLT is that it is consistently located 25 ± 2% of the distance from the cecum to the rectum. Our original observations of this tissue were carried out in rats (1); however, its consistent location allowed us to find it in mice as well. The formation of the lymphoid aggregate in this location does not appear to be random, nor does it appear to be in response to luminal antigenic stimulation. Grafts of this segment of fetal colon under the kidney capsule of syngeneic adult recipients developed lymphoid tissue in the appropriate location, indicating that exogenous luminal antigen is not a stimulus for the formation of this tissue (1).

Grossly, PCLT is a small nodule found in the lateral aspect of the plicae near the center of the antimesenteric side of the colon. On light microscopic examination, the lymphocytes in PCLT were generally unremarkable, being very regular in size and shape (2). Plasma cells and mitotic figures were rarely seen. When examined by transmission electron microscopy (TEM) the lymphocytes are very tightly packed. The lack of plasma cells and mitotic figures seen by light microscopy was confirmed with TEM. Few if any cytoplasmic organelles or granules could be observed, and the nuclei were generally heterochromatic with no mitotic activity. In this respect, these cells resembled the lymphocytes seen in small lymphocytic lymphoma/chronic lymphocytic leukemias associated with the intestinal tract.

The phenotype of the cells within PCLT does not appear to be extremely unique among intestinal lymphoid tissues (3). Approximately 85% of the cells in PCLT are B lymphocytes. The great majority of these cells are B220-positive, immunoglobulin M^{high} (IgM^{high}), IgD-positive, Ia-positive B cells. A minor population of IgM^{low}, IgD-negative cells also exists. Less than 2% of the B cells in PCLT appear to be of the IgA or IgG isotype. In addition, initial experiments demonstrated that approximately 10–15% of the IgM^{high} B cells are of the CD5-positive lineage (3). Approximately 10–15% of the cells in PCLT are T cells, as characterized by being either CD4-positive (~8%) or CD8-positive (~4%). In addition to B cells and T cells, there is also a small number (2%) of "accessory" cells, which we have characterized as either Mac-1-positive or ER-TR4-positive in tissue sections. The majority of these accessory cells appear to localize in the periphery of the nodule, as demonstrated by immunohistochemical analysis.

In addition to the lymphocyte populations within PCLT, at least two types of accessory cells could be identified (2). Most prominent was a population of "tingible body" macrophages. These cells were characterized at the light microscopic level as large cells (15–20 μm) with dark and prominent inclusion bodies within their cytoplasm. In addition, a second population of cells could also be identified, which was characterized by their large size (~18 μm) and a high nucleus to cytoplasm ratio. No cytoplasmic inclusions could be distinguished in this second population at the light microscopic level. On TEM analysis, the second population of cells displayed an amorphous cytoplasm with few mitochondria and no obvious cytoplasmic organelles. In addition, these cells had a euchromatic nucleus. Owing to their lack of distinguishing characteristics, we have termed these cells "clear" cells. In many respects these cells somewhat resemble the dendritic Langerhans cells described in the skin and other lymphoid organs (4,5).

On microscopic examination it is immediately apparent that PCLT is covered by a specialized follicle-associated epithelium (FAE). This epithelial border is different from that lining the crypts or villi of the colon, as there are no crypts or goblet cells in this epithelial layer. In this regard it is identical to that described in the small bowel covering the domes on the luminal aspect of Peyer's patches. Owen and others (6–9) have described the presence of specialized M cells in the epithelium overlying Peyer's patches of the ileum. These M cells appear to play a unique role in the transport of luminal antigen and virus across the epithelial border. Using scanning electron microscopy, we have been able to confirm the presence of M cells in the FAE overlying PCLT (G. A. Perry, manuscript submitted). As an obvious route for luminal antigenic entry, these cells may play an important role in driving B-cell proliferation. In addition, they may be important in the generation of the B-cell repertoire within the gut. Clearly a more detailed examination of the role of M cells in the formation and maintenance of intestinal lymphoid tissues is in order.

FUNCTIONAL CHARACTERISTICS OF PCLT

One of the most surprising initial findings about PCLT was its extreme sensitivity to treatment with hydrocortisone in vivo. In both rats (1) and mice (3) treatment with hydrocortisone resulted in an approximately 75% decrease in tissue weight. Similar decreases in

Table 1 Effects of Recombinant Growth Factors on the LPS Responsiveness of Intestinal Lymphoid Tissues

	Recombinant factor added			
Tissue	None	IL-1 β	IL-4	IL-5
Spleen	+++	Not tested	+++	+++
Jej. PP	++	++	++	++
Ileal PP	+	+	+	+
PCLT	+/–	++	+/–	+/–

tissue weight were seen in thymus (77%); however, no significant decrease in tissue weight was observed when Peyer's patches were tested (8%). Although a crude measure, these results would suggest that PCLT may contain a large number of relatively immature, steroid-sensitive B cells. In this light, it is interesting to note that a similar decrease in tissue weight has been observed in the bursa of Fabricius (71%) after steroid treatment (10,11).

In our initial efforts to characterize the functional repertoire of the B cells within the PCLT, simple lipopolysaccharide (LPS) mitogen-stimulation experiments were performed. Much to our surprise, the lymphocytes within PCLT are generally unresponsive to LPS, even though the majority of the cells are phenotypically B cells. We suspected that the lack of LPS responsiveness might be linked to a lack of cytokine-producing helper or accessory cells, and thus added recombinant lymphokines to the LPS-stimulated cultures. Results of these experiments are presented in Table 1, and demonstrated that neither interleukin-4 (IL-4) nor IL-5 appeared to significantly increase the proliferative response by PCLT. However, treatment of the cultures with recombinant IL-1 β significantly increased the LPS response of PCLT lymphocytes.

It was apparent that the lack of LPS responsiveness by PCLT B cells could be attributed to a lack of accessory cell–produced cytokines, thus we decided to test the hypothesis that spleen adherent cells could increase the LPS responsiveness of PCLT-derived lymphocytes. Single cell suspensions of normal adult spleen and PCLT were allowed to adhere to plastic 96-well microtiter plates. After 1 hr at 37°C nonadherent cells were removed, the adherent cells gently washed, and PCLT nonadherent cells placed into wells containing spleen adherent cells and LPS. In addition, spleen nonadherent cells were placed into wells containing LPS and adherent cells from PCLT. Three days later, the cultures were harvested for [^{3}H]thymidine uptake. Results of these experiments (Table 2) demonstrated that PCLT B cells were capable of responding to LPS in the presence of spleen adherent cells, as PCLT nonadherent cells on spleen adherent cells showed a greater proliferative response than spleen nonadherent cells on spleen adherent cells. In addition, these experiments demonstrated that splenic B cells did not respond well to LPS when placed on PCLT adherent cells. When the number of adherent cells from each tissue was quantitated, it was found that for an equal number of cells plated, spleen cell suspensions contain approximately four times as many adherent cells. Subsequent experiments in which we titered spleen adherent cells into LPS-stimulated PCLT cultures showed a synergistic effect of the spleen adherent cells. Similar results were obtained when adult spleen cells were added to LPS-stimulated cultures of neonatal spleen cells, but not when added to cultures of adult spleen or Peyer's patch cells. These results demonstrate that the lack of LPS responsiveness by B cells from specific tissues may not necessarily indicate an

Table 2 LPS Responsiveness of PCLT and Spleen Nonadherent Cells Plated in the Presence of PCLT or Spleen Adherent Cells

Nonadherent cell donor	Adherent cell donor	Stimulator	Magnitude of response
Spleen	Spleen	LPS	++
PCLT	PCLT	LPS	– or +/–
PCLT	Spleen	LPS	++++
Spleen	PCLT	LPS	+ or +/–

inability of the B cells to respond, but may in fact also be influenced by the accessory cell populations within that tissue.

Further experiments using isolated individual Peyer's patches and aggregated lymphoid nodules along the length of the intestine demonstrated that there is a gradual decrease in LPS responsiveness along the length of the gut (Fig. 1). The response to LPS is highest in the proximal most Peyer's patches of the jejunum, and gradually decreases to reach a nadir in the area of the terminal ileum and proximal colon. This low response in the proximal colon is reversed in distal lymphoid aggregate near the rectum, which is again LPS responsive. It is interesting to note that this pattern of responsiveness is generally the inverse of the *Escherichia coli* content in the bowel, which reaches its maximum in the terminal ileum, cecum, and proximal colon. It is possible that this pattern of reactivity is reflected in changes in the distribution of accessory cell populations along the gut, and this hypothesis is currently being tested. However, it is also possible that this pattern of nonresponsiveness may reflect clonal anergy, tolerance, or specific unresponsiveness on the part of the intestinal B cells to simulation by bacterial cell wall products. This raises a number of interesting hypotheses which can be tested; however, our results would tend to emphasize a central role for adherent accessory cell populations in this unusual pattern of response.

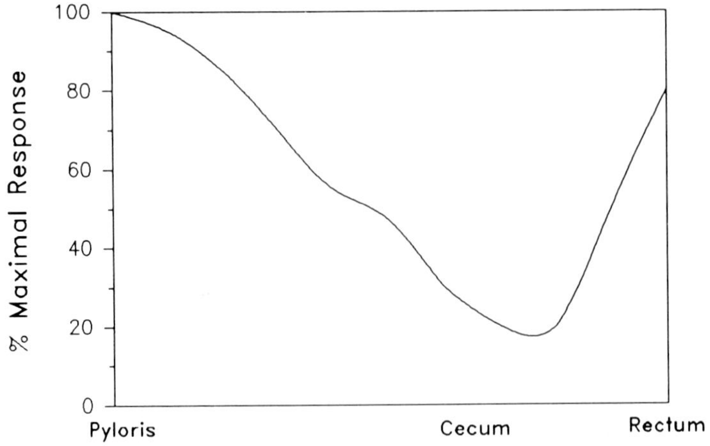

Figure 1 Relative LPS responsiveness along the length of the intestine.

Finally, we would like to speculate on the role of intestinal antigens and pathogens (specifically murine hepatitis virus, MHV) in the maintenance and stimulation of intestinal lymphoid tissues. One of our initial unique observations about PCLT was its consistent lack of germinal centers. Although small in size, we could recover an average of 10^6 lymphocytes/mouse. These mice were housed under extremely good conditions in an MHV-free facility on laminar air flow hoods. During the past year we changed our animal quarters, and began to notice several changes in the issue. In these mice, PCLT consistently contained germinal centers, was larger in size, and yet yielded only an average of 10^5 lymphocytes/mouse. These mice did not display MHV titers on entering the colony, but had high titers to MHV several months later. The murine hepatitis virus is a corona virus which resides in the intestine and can be passaged via oral ingestion of fecal material (12). Clearly PCLT contains M cells in the FAE, which have been shown to passage reovirus across the epithelial border (13), and could presumably pass MHV as well. The B-cell target for MHV is a B220-positive (14.8^+) IgM-positive B cell (14), a population which constitutes the majority of cells within PCLT. Viral infection of this B-cell population results in a lysis of the infected cell and a significant decrease in the number of 14.8^+IgM-positive cells within 48–72 hours after infection (14). In addition, the virus appears to reside and replicate in bone marrow–derived adherent cells (15–17). Our observations, in conjunction with the observations of others, serve to emphasize the dynamic nature of intestinal lymphoid tissues. The intestinal tract is continuously exposed to a seemingly infinite number of antigenic and pathogenic stimuli. The ever changing palate of human consumption serves as a glorious example of the variety of antigens that can be encountered, and the antigenic stimulus more than likely will change with every meal. Changes or intrinsic differences in diet or intestinal bacterial flora and/or viral pathogens may represent a significant problem when various laboratories attempt to definitively define those immune cell populations found in the "normal" intestine. Clearly this could explain already published discrepancies in the frequency of $\alpha\beta$ and $\gamma\delta$ T-cell populations in the gut (18–22), and may similarly influence B-cell populations. It is, therefore, important to consider the dynamic nature of the intestine and its lymphoid component when making conclusions about the mucosal immune system.

REFERENCES

1. Crouse, DA, Perry, GA, Murphy, BO, Sharp, JG. Characteristics of submucosal lymphoid tissue located in the proximal colon of the rat. J. Anat. 1989; 162:53–65.
2. Perry, GA, Eccleston-Joyner, C. Ultrastructural characterization of microenvironmental elements associated with proximal colonic lymphoid tissue (PCLT) in the mouse. Proc. Int'l. Symp. Mucosal Immunology, London (1989).
3. Perry, GA, Sharp, JG. Characterization of proximal colonic lymphoid tissue in the mouse. Anat. Rec. 1988; 220:305–12.
4. Stingl, G., Tamaki, K., Katz, SI. Origin and function of epidermal Langerhans cells. Immunol. Rev. 1980; 53:149–74.
5. Silberberg-Sinakin, I, Gili, I, Baer, RL, and Thorbecke, GJ. Langerhans cells: Role in contact hypersensitivity and relationship to lymphoid dendritic cells and to macrophages. Immunol. Rev. 1980; 53:203–32.
6. Owen, RL. Sequential uptake of horseradish peroxidase by lymphoid follicle epithelium of Peyer's patches in normal unobstructed mouse intestine: An ultrastructural study. Gastroenterology 1977; 72:440–51.
7. O'Leary, AD, Sweeney, EC. Lymphoglandular complexes of the colon: Structure and distribution. Histopathology 1986; 10:267–73.

8. Jacob, E, Baker, SJ, Swaminathan, SP. 'M' cells in the follicle-associated epithelium of the human colon. Histopathology 1987; 11:941–52.
9. Bland, PW, Britton, DC. Morphological study of antigen-sampling structures in the rat large intestine. Infect. Immun. 1984; 32:693–99.
10. Glick, B. The effect of bovine growth hormone, desoxycorticosterone, and cortisone on the weight of the bursa of Fabricius, adrenal glands, heart, and body weight of young chickens. Poultry Sci. 1960; 39:1527–33.
11. Glick, B. Experimental modification of the growth of the bursa of Fabricius. Poultry Sci. 1957; 36:18–23.
12. Thigpen, JE, Lebetkin, EH, Dawes, ML, Amyx, HL, Caviness, GF, Sawer, BA, Blackmore, DE. The use of dirty bedding for detection of murine pathogens in sentinel mice. Lab. Animal Sci. 1989; 39:324–7.
13. Wolf, JL, Rubin, DH, Finberg, R, Kauffman, RS, Sharpe, AH, Trier, JS, Fields, BN. Intestinal M cells: A pathway for entry of reovirus into the host. Science 1981; 212:471–2.
14. Jolicoeur, P, Lamontagne, L. Mouse hepatitis virus 3 pathogenicity expressed by a lytic viral infection in bone marrow 14.8$^+$ μ^+ B lymphocyte subpopulations. J. Immunol. 1989; 143:3722–30.
15. Schindler, L, Klimetzek, V, Kirchner, H. Bone marrow derived macrophages as targets for the replication of mouse hepatitis virus type 3. Immunol. Lett. 1983; 7:107–10.
16. Morahan, PS, Connor, JR, Leary, KR. Viruses and the versatile macrophage. Br. Med. Bull. 1985; 41:15–21.
17. Lamontagne, L, Decarie, D, Dupuy, JM. Host cell resistance to mouse hepatitis virus type 3 is expressed in vitro in macrophages and lymphocytes. Viral Immunol. 1989; 2:37–45.
18. Goodman, T, Lefrancois, L. Expression of the $\gamma\delta$ T-cell receptor on intestinal CD8$^+$ intraepithelial lymphocytes. Nature 1988; 333:855–6.
19. Bonneville, M, Janeway, CA, Ito, K, Haser, W, Ishida, I, Nakanishi, N, Tonegawa, S. Intestinal intraepithelial lymphocytes are a distinct set of $\gamma\delta$ T cells. Nature 1988; 336:479–81.
20. Bonneville, M, Itohara, S, Krecko, E, Mombaerts, P, Ishida, I, Katsuki, M, Berns, A, Farr, AG, Janeway, CA, Tonegawa, S. Transgenic mice demonstrate that epithelial homing of γ/δ T cells is determined by cell lineages independent of T cell receptor specificity. J. Exp. Med. 1990; 171:1015–26.
21. Brandtzeg, P, Halstensen, TS, Scott, H, Sollid, LM, Valnes, K, Bosnes, V. Epithelial homing of γ/δ T cells? Nature 1989; 341:113.
22. Brandtzeg, P, Brosnes, V, Halstensen, TS, Scott, H, Sollid, LM, Valnes, KN. T lymphocytes in human gut epithelium preferentially express the α/β antigen receptor and are often CD45/UCHL1-positive. Scand. J. Immunol. 1989; 30:123–8.

83

The Immune Response of the Rat to Intestinally Administered Thymus-Dependent and Thymus-Independent Antigens

Role of Peyer's Patches in the Regulation of Specific Antibody Production

Marsetyawan Soesatyo, Jeike Biewenga, Nico van Rooijen, and Taede Sminia
Vrije University, Amsterdam, The Netherlands

INTRODUCTION

It has been generally accepted that Peyer's patches (PPs) play an important role in the regulation of the immune response in the gut (1). Besides induction of immunoglobulin A (IgA) specific T-helper cells (2), PPs are responsible for the generation of local suppressor cells leading to systemic tolerance (3). After oral antigen feeding, specific suppressor T cells are generated in PPs (4,5), which migrate to the spleen (6). The exact mechanism of suppression remains uncertain, although many investigators have studied the immunoregulatory functions of PPs using a wide range of methods and antigens.

The present study deals with the role of PPs in the regulation of the systemic antibody response. Peyer's patches were inactivated in situ, and the effects on local and systemic immune responses were studied. For this purpose, the development of specific antibody-forming cells to thymus-dependent trinitrophenyl-KLH [TNP-KLH]), and thymus-independent type 1 and type 2 (TNP-lipopolysaccharide-LPS [TNP-LPS] and TNP-Ficoll, respectively) antigens in situ was determined using immunohistochemistry.

MATERIALS AND METHODS

Animals

Adult Wistar rats, weighing 250–280 g, were obtained from the Harlan Sprague Dawley-CPB (Zeist, The Netherlands). Animals were kept under routine laboratory conditions.

Immunization Procedures

One day before PP inactivation by cauterization (for details see Ref. 7), groups of four to five rats were primed intraperitoneally (i.p.) with 100 μg of either TNP-KLH, TNP-LPS, or TNP-Ficoll. Another group of 4 rats was primed intragastrically (i.g.) with 1 mg of these antigens. Two weeks later, the rats received a booster immunization intraduodenally. Sham-treated controls were immunized in the same manner as treated groups. Five days after antigen challenge, the animals were sacrificed, and in addition to the spleen, parts of the intestinal villi and mesenteric lymph nodes (MLNs) were collected and snap frozen in liquid nitrogen.

Immunohistochemistry for the Detection of Total and Isotype-Specific Anti-TNP Antibody-Forming Cells In Situ

In short, anti-TNP–AFCs were detected by incubation of 8 μm cryostat sections with TNP-alkaline phosphatase (AlPh) followed by staining for phosphatase activity. Isotype specificity was detected in a double staining technique by incubation with TNP-AlPh and anti-isotype–specific antibody (Ab). Staining for phosphatase activity preceded incubation with horseradish peroxidase (HRP)–conjugated anti-Ig and HRP reaction with 3-amino-9-ethylcarbazole (AEC, Sigma Chemical Co.) (7).

RESULTS

Immune Response to TNP-KLH, TNP-LPS, and TNP-Ficoll

TNP-KLH

Anti-TNP–AFCs were found in high numbers in the spleen of PP-inactivated rats, whereas in the control groups only few specific AFCs were detected (Table 1). Anti-TNP–AFCs were mostly found in the outer part of the periarteriolar lymphocyte sheath (PALS); only a few cells could be detected around the terminal arterioles. With respect to the antibody isotypes, anti-TNP–AFCs of the IgM, IgG, and IgA classes were found in the spleen of PP-inactivated group (Table 2).

Table 1 Number of Specific AFCs per Tissue Section of the Spleen After Primary and Secondary Immunization with TNP-KLH, TNP-LPS, and TNP-Ficoll[a]

	Spleen[b]	
Antigens	Controls	PP-inactivated rats
TNP-KLH (TD)	±	++
TNP-LPS (TI-1)	±	±
TNP-Ficoll (TI-2)	±	±

[a]Intraperitoneal priming followed by intraintestinal booster immunization 2 weeks later; four rats per group.
[b]–, No anti-TNP–AFCs; +/–, 1–10; +, 10–50; ++, >50 anti-TNP–AFCs/section.

Table 2 Number of AFCs of Different Isotypes per Tissue Section of the Spleen After Primary and Secondary Immunization with TNP-KLH[a]

	Spleen	
Isotype	Controls (n±SE)	PP-inactivated rats (n±SE)
IgM	0	55 ± 3
IgG	0	39 ± 3
IgA	0	47 ± 4

Abbreviation: SE, standard error of the mean; four rats per group.
[a]Intraperitoneal priming followed by intraintestinal booster immunization 2 weeks later.

In MLNs and in the mucosa of the gut, very few anti-TNP–AFCs were found. For example, only one to two AFCs were found in a tissue section of the lamina propria of the intestine.

TNP-LPS

Antibody-forming cells could only be detected in one rat out of six animals used per group. Anti-TNP–AFCs were mainly found in the spleen of the PP-inactivated and sham-treated controls. No differences were observed in the numbers of AFCs in the spleens of either group of rats. In addition, anti-TNP–AFCs were neither found in MLNs nor in the gut.

TNP-Ficoll

Antibody-forming cells against TNP-Ficoll were not elicited in any rat investigated. Hardly any anti-TNP–AFCs were found either in the spleen, MLN, or mucosa of the gut.

DISCUSSION

This study demonstrates the contribution of PPs to the local and systemic immune response to thymus-dependent and thymus-independent antigen. After inactivation of PPs, an extensive splenic reaction to TNP-KLH occurs, whereas only a weak immune response was found in the spleen of rats with normal PPs. In contrast, PP inactivation has almost no effect on the immune response to thymus-independent antigens TNP-LPS and TNP-Ficoll. These findings indicate that PPs play a major part in the regulation of thymus-dependent systemic immune response. A possible explanation for the observations may be as follows. Peyer's patches might be responsible for immunosuppression to thymus-dependent antigens by generating suppressor cells (4,5). These suppressor cells were removed or affected following PP inactivation by cauterization (7). This leads to an enhanced immune response in the spleen. The immunological suppression was mainly found in the spleen because PP-suppressor cells only function effectively after their migration to this organ (6). This may also be the explanation that specific immunosuppression does not occur against thymus-independent antigens.

Since we do not have any direct evidence, it is difficult to say that suppressor T cells are the only cells responsible for the observed phenomenon. Often cell types like macrophages can also be involved. Splenic non–T suppressor cells (8), which have a glass-adherence property, have been reported in in vitro studies to play a role in immunosuppression. In addition, the suppressive effector function of alveolar macrophages has also been documented (9). Furthermore, we have found recently that peritoneal macrophages of the rat displayed a suppressive activity in the in vitro immune response to TNP-KLH (unpublished observation). We found an elevated immune reaction to intraperitoneally administered TNP-KLH in the draining parathymic lymph node after depletion of peritoneal macrophages with dichloromethylene diphosphonate (C12MDP)–containing liposomes.

In conclusion, PPs and also peritoneal cells are involved in the regulation of the immune response to intestinally administered antigen. The present study emphasizes the important role of PPs in controlling the splenic immune response against thymus-dependent antigen. Most probably this effect was caused by the generation of specific suppressor T cells.

REFERENCES

1. Kawanishi H, Saltzman LE, Strober W. Mechanisms regulating IgA class-specific immunoglobulin production in murine gut-associated lymphoid tissue. I. T cells derived from Peyer's patches that switch sIgM B cells to sIgA B cells in vitro. J Exp Med 1983, 157:433–43.
2. Richman LK, Graeff AS, Yarchoan R, Strober W. Simultaneous induction of antigen-specific IgA helper T cells and IgG suppressor T cells in the murine Peyer's patch after protein feeding. J Immunol 1981, 126:2079–83.
3. Challacombe SJ, Tomasi TB Jr. Systemic tolerance and secretory immunity after oral immunization. J Exp Med 1980, 152:1459–72.
4. Mattingly JA, Waksman BH. Immunologic suppression after oral administration of antigen. I. Specific suppressor cells formed in rat Peyer's patches after oral administration of sheep erythrocytes and their systemic migration. J Immunol 1978, 121:1878–83.
5. MacDonald TT. Immunosuppression caused by antigen feeding. I. Evidence for the activation of a feedback suppressor pathway in the spleen of antigen-fed mice. Eur J Immunol 1982, 12:767–73.
6. Ngan J, Kind LS. Suppressor T cells for IgE and IgG in Peyer's patches of mice made tolerant by the oral administration of ovalbumin. J Immunol 1978, 120:861–5.
7. Soesatyo M, Biewenga J, Jeurissen S, Sminia T. The effects of Peyer's patches inactivation in the rat on the development of antibody-forming cells to intestinal antigen. Immunol Biol 1990, 187:97–107.
8. Kirchner H, Chused TM, Herberman RB, Holden HT, Lavrin DH. Evidence of suppressor cell activity in spleens of mice bearing primary tumors induced by moloney sarcoma virus. J Exp Med 1974, 139:1473–87.
9. Thepen T, Van Rooijen N, Kraal G. Alveolar macrophage elimination in vivo is associated with an increase in pulmonary immune response in mice. J Exp Med 1989, 170:499–509.

84

Mucosal Immune Responses and Systemic Immunological Memory After Oral Administration of Trinitrophenyl-*Lactobacillus* Conjugates in Mice

K. Gerritse, M. Posno, M. J. Fasbender, M. M. Schellekens, W. J. A. Boersma, and E. Claassen
TNO Medical Biological Laboratory, Rijswijk, The Netherlands

INTRODUCTION

The oral route is a very convenient route of vaccination in comparison with the more frequently used parenteral routes, especially in vaccination programs in which large numbers of subjects are involved. In addition, the activation of the mucosal immune system as well as systemic responses can be obtained by oral application of antigens. Although this sometimes results in an adequate local expression of immunoglobulin A (IgA) responses in various mucosal tissues and secretions (1), the oral administration is generally very inefficient, requiring large quantities of immunogen and yielding only modest systemic antibody responses. With regard to numerous pathogens, a local response only is not sufficient and a systemic response obligatory.

Owing to a digestive processing, many antigens loose their immunogenic potential. A suboptimal amount of antigen reaches the mucosal immune system and, therefore, requires an adjuvant to evoke or enhance the immune response. Transformed microorganisms can be used as antigen carriers, but most of these microorganisms (e.g., *Escherichia coli, Streptococcus mutans, Salmonella typhi*; [2]) are generally recognized as pathogens and are not acceptable for general application. In this respect, the use of a GRAS (Generally Recognized as Safe) organism like *Lactobacillus* may be preferred.

The use of *Lactobacillus* as a vector antigen delivery system has several other potential advantages over other microorganisms besides the above-mentioned GRAS status. *Lactobacillus*, in mammals, is able to pass the digestive tract and colonize in the gut. In addition, adjuvant properties of *Lactobacillus* have been described (3). As for many other microorganisms, it is possible to produce transformations of *Lactobacillus* with foreign deoxyribonucleic acid (DNA). Strains of *Lactobacillus* which produce a foreign antigen epitope, which is expressed on the membrane surface or is secreted intra- or extracellularly, can be constructed.

Considering the findings mentioned above, we recently initiated investigations on: (a) development of gene-transfer and gene-expression systems for the introduction and efficient expression of antigens in *Lactobacillus* species which are (natural) inhabitants of the gastrointestinal tract, and (b) immunological evaluation and optimization of the immune responses (mucosal and systemic) that are generated through presentation of *Lactobacillus*-associated antigens by the oral route.

The aim of the work presented here was a comparative study on the effects of *Lactobacillus* administered by the oral or peritoneal route on the generation of the systemic response. To evaluate this a small hapten, trinitrophenyl (TNP), coupled to *Lactobacillus* was used for oral immunization purposes, serum titers were determined, and lymphoid tissues were screened for specific antibody forming cells (AFCs).

Although life antigen carriers are more immunogenic at mucosal surfaces than non-replicating antigen carriers (4), most live antigen carriers have an undesirable potentiation of an immune response to a large number of bystander antigens found in the gastrointestinal tract. For this reason, the *Lactobacillus* microorganisms were heat killed prior to trinitrophenylization. Furthermore, Bloksma et al. (5) revealed that viable *Lactobacillus* microorganisms stimulate exclusively delayed hypersensitivity, whereas heat-killed bacteria had an adjuvant effect on antibody formation.

The potential use of *Lactobacillus* as an antigen carrier system will be discussed.

MATERIALS AND METHODS

Cultivation of *Lactobacillus*

Lactobacillus acidophilus (strain NCK89) was grown on MRS broth (Difco). After aerobic incubation at 37°C overnight, the organisms were harvested by centrifugation at 3640 g for 15 min at room temperature and resuspended in phosphate-buffered saline (PBS) (1×10^{10} CFU·ml^{-1}). Subsequently, the suspension was heated for 30 min at 60°C.

Conjugation

In order to obtain TNP-*Lactobacillus* conjugate, 50 μl of a 2,4,6-trinitrophenyl sulphonic acid (TNBS) solution (20 mg·ml^{-1} PBS) was added to 1 ml *Lactobacillus* suspension (53 mg·ml^{-1} PBS). The suspension was incubated for 1 hr at room temperature in the dark, washed, and resuspended in 1 ml PBS.

The TNP–alkaline phosphatase (TNP-AP) conjugates were obtained essentially according to the method of Claassen and Van Rooijen (6).

Trinitrophenylated ovalbumin was used for the detection of anti-TNP antibodies in a direct enzyme-linked immunosorbent assay (ELISA). The TNBS (100 mg) was added under gentle stirring to 100 mg ovalbumin in 10 ml borate buffer (0.1 M, pH 9). The solution was incubated in the dark for 2 hr at room temperature, and dialyzed against PBS.

Immunization

Lactobacillus-TNP conjugates were orally administered three times on alternating days to groups of female mice (Balb/c, 12–15 weeks old). Each oral administration contained 50 μg *Lactobacillus* suspended in 500 μl 0.2 M $NaHCO_3$ to neutralize hydrochloric acid in the stomach and reduce degradation of the antigen determinants to a minimum (7). Four weeks after the last administration, the mice were boosted orally three times on alternating days. Control groups were both i.p. primed and boosted with 500 μg TNP-*Lactobacillus* conjugates suspended in 250 μl PBS. The mice were sacrificed 3, 5, 7 and 21 days after the last oral administration or i.p. prime injection and 5 days after the last booster administration or booster injection. Blood samples of the mice were collected by heart puncture. The sera were screened for anti-TNP and anti-*Lactobacillus* antibody (Ab) reactivity. The spleen (SP) and mesenteric lymph nodes (MLNs) were removed and stored in liquid nitrogen. Tissue sections of the organs were screened for anti-TNP–specific AFCs and antigen trapping.

Direct ELISA

Polyvinyl chloride (PVC) microtiter plates (Titertek) were coated with TNP-ovalbumin (5 $\mu g \cdot ml^{-1}$ PBS, 50 μl/well). To block nonspecific binding a second coating of gelatine (5 $mg \cdot ml^{-1}$, 50 μl/well) was applied. The plates were incubated for 1 hr at 25°C with dilutions of TNP-induced antisera and preimmunization sera to correct the TNP-induced antisera for background reactivity. Sera dilutions were added to three separate plates. The plates were washed and separately incubated with either alkaline phosphatase–labeled goat-antimouse IgA, IgM, or IgG (H + L) (KPL, Inc., Gaithersburg, MD) 1:2000 in PBS. After washing 50 μl para-nitrophenylphosphate (Boehringer, Mannheim, West Germany) solution (1 $mg \cdot ml^{-1}$) in 10 mM diethanolamine (1 mM $MgCl_2$, pH 9.8) was added to each well. After 30 min, the absorption at 405 nm was determined.

The anti-*Lactobacillus* serum titer was determined on glutaraldehyde-preactivated polystyrene microtiter plates (NUNC). The ELISA was performed as was indicated for the TNP-ovalbumin–coated microtiter plates.

Tissue Preparation and Immunocytochemical Staining

Mice were sacrificed by CO_2 euthanasia, SP and MLNs were removed and snap frozen in liquid nitrogen. Eight micrometer cryostat tissue sections were fixed for 10 min in acetone containing 0.02% (v/v) hydrogen peroxidase.

For determination of the antigen specificity of the AFCs in MLNs or SP, tissue sections were incubated overnight with TNP-AP dilutions in 0.1% bovine sera albumin (BSA) in PBS (w/v). The AP activity was revealed according to the method of Burstone (8) with some modifications (9).

Trapped *Lactobacillus* conjugate was detected in a two-step staining procedure. Slides were incubated overnight at 4°C with purified rabbit anti-*Lactobacillus* Abs (2 $mg \cdot ml^{-1}$) diluted 1/15 to 1/50 in a solution of BSA (1 $mg \cdot ml^{-1}$ PBS). After washing, the slides were incubated for 60 min at RT with goat-antirabbit IgG–horseradish peroxidase (HRP) conjugate diluted 1/100 in a solution of BSA (1 $mg \cdot ml^{-1}$ PBS) and normal mice sera (1% v/v). The HRP activity was revealed as described previously (9).

RESULTS

ELISA Analysis of the Sera Antibody Titers

In both oral- and intraperitoneal-primed animals, a specific anti-TNP antibody response (IgM) was observed with a peak level on day 7 after prime. Only in the intraperitoneal-primed mice, a low IgM anti-*Lactobacillus* response was detected (Fig. 1). No specific

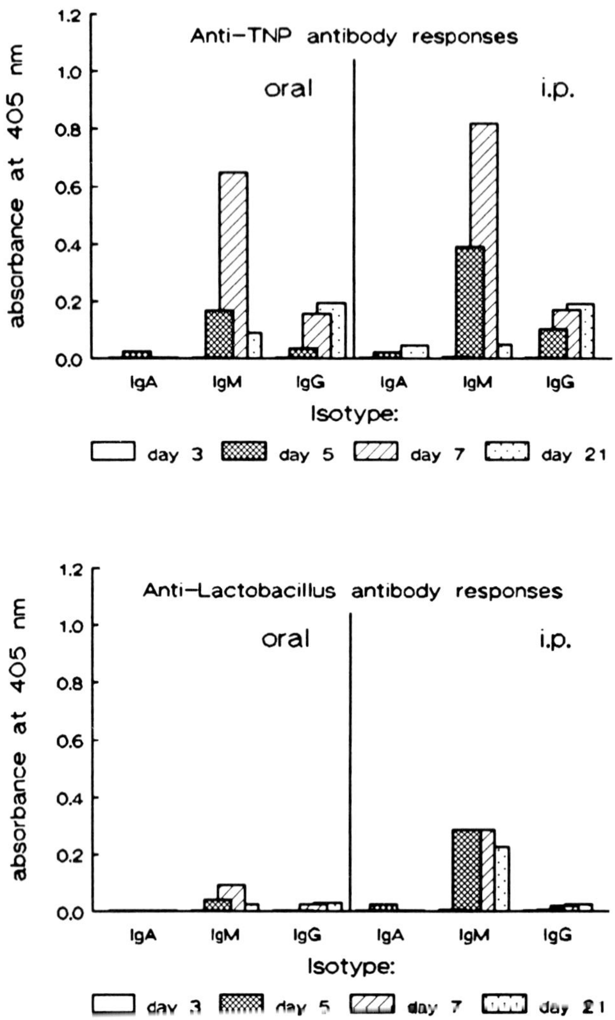

Figure 1 Sera of the mice were screened for specific anti-TNP and anti-*Lactobacillus* Abs in a direct ELISA on a coating of ovalbumin-TNP and *Lactobacillus*, respectively. Alkaline phosphatase–labeled goat-antimouse IgA, IgM, and IgG Abs and para-nitrophenylphosphate as substrate were used for detection. The results of 1:50 dilutions of sera collected on days 3, 5, 7, and 21 after prime are shown.

anti-TNP and anti-*Lactobacillus* serum antibodies of the IgA or IgG isotype could be detected after both oral or i.p. prime. In both groups, the booster administration or injection resulted in a specific anti-TNP as well as a low specific anti-*Lactobacillus* response (Fig. 2). Immunoglobulin G is the prevailing isotype of the anti-TNP and anti-*Lactobacillus* antibodies after boost in both groups. In the oral boosted animals, also a significant anti-TNP IgA response was detected. The anti-TNP IgG response of the orally primed and boosted mice is of similar strength as compared to the specific anti-TNP IgG response of the animals immunized twice i.p.

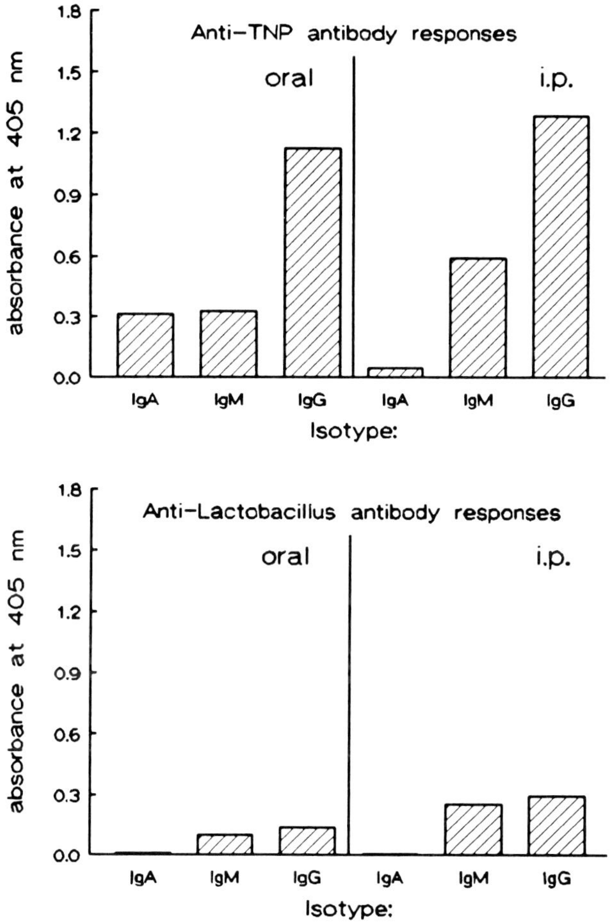

Figure 2 Analysis of serum anti-TNP and anti-*Lactobacillus* antibodies in ELISA. The assay conditions are as indicated for Fig. 1. The results of 1:50 dilutions of sera collected on day 5 after booster injection or last booster administration are shown.

Immunocytochemical Detection of TNP-Specific AFCs

In the spleens of both the oral- and intraperitoneal-immunized mice, specific anti-TNP antibody-forming cells were detected on all sample days (Fig. 3). The number of AFCs in the spleen sections is of the same magnitude in both groups (Table 1). Specific AFCs in the MLNs are only observed in the oral-primed animals (Fig. 3). The greatest number of AFCs were found in the tissue sections of the MLNs removed on day 5 after the last oral administration. Antigen trapping in immune complexes was observed in MLN tissue sections of the oral-immunized animals by staining with TNP-AP (see Fig. 3). The antigen trapping was verified by staining alternating tissue sections with anti-*Lactobacillus* antibodies (results not shown). The immune complexes were detected in the lymphoid follicles; this observation is in accordance with the normal localization of immune complexes as reviewed by Van Rooijen et al. (10).

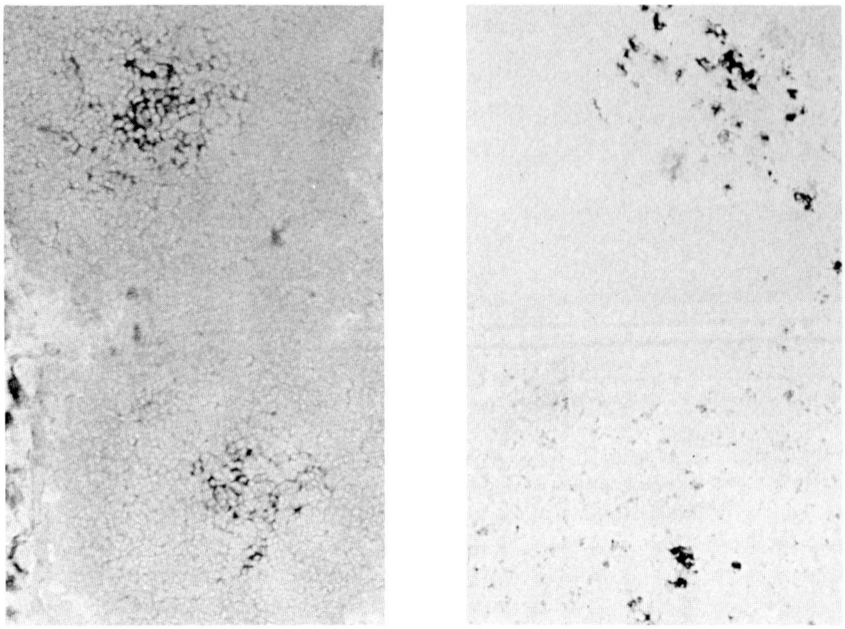

(a) (b)

Figure 3 MLNs and SP of the animals, fed with a suspension of TNP-*Lactobacillus* conjugate, were removed on day 5 after the last oral prime administration. Tissue sections of mesenteric lymph nodes (a) and spleen (b) were stained with TNP-AP conjugate.

DISCUSSION

In a previous study, we demonstrated that orally administered TNP *Lactobacillus* conjugates evoke a specific anti-TNP IgG antibody response in serum after an i.p. booster injection (11). We now demonstrate that oral priming followed by an oral booster administration also results in a specific anti-TNP response, as could be revealed from the serum IgG antibody titers. This response was of the same magnitude as the antibody response in serum of the animals immunized twice i.p. This implies that an anti-TNP response is equally effective elicited by oral administration of TNP-*Lactobacillus* conjugates as by i.p. immunization. In addition, the enumeration of the anti-TNP AFCs in tissue sections of the spleen led to similar results.

To get similar levels of serum antibody responses, it is necessarily to administrate orally three times the *Lactobacillus* conjugate. Oral administration of the TNP-*Lactobacillus* conjugate only once or twice is not sufficient to evoke a specific response (results not shown). This could be explained in two ways. One possibility is that only a small part of the total amount of TNP-*Lactobacillus* reaches the mucosal epithelium and is only partly internalized by either the epithelium cells or the specialized M cells, whereas the greater part passes the digestive tract. Another possibility is that when antigens enter the mucosa, they mainly stimulate IgA precursor lymphocytes owing to the fact that the greatest population of B cells in the GALT are IgA lymphocytes. For this reason, it is not surprising

Table 1 Number of Specific Anti-TNP Antibody–Forming Cells in MLNs and SP Tissue Sections After Oral or i.p. Priming[a,b]

Time (days)	Immunization Tissue	Oral MLN	I.p. MLN	Oral SP	I.p. SP
3		0	0	3.4	1.7
5		1.4	0	7.9	6.2
7		1.2	0	3.1	5.1
21		0.4	0	2.0	2.1

[a]The number of AFCs was calculated per square mm^2 on days 3, 5, 7, and 21 after immunization.
[b] Cells were detected by TNP-AP staining.

that there is a larger amount of antigen needed to stimulate the relatively small population of non-IgA lymphocytes.

Only in the sera of the orally boosted mice was a specific IgA response observed. In previous experiments, no IgA response was observed after oral priming subsequently followed by an i.p. booster injection, suggesting that IgA-producing lymphocytes can only be restimulated via the oral route.

The occurrence of an IgA response could be explained in two ways. The majority of the IgA precursor cells are derived from Peyer's patches (12). After these cells are stimulated for the first time they migrate via the MLNs and thoracic duct into the circulation. Finally, they return to the mucosal tissues with a preference for the organ they were initially stimulated by (13). After restimulation, the greater part of the Abs produced will be excreted as secretory IgA in the intestinal lumen, whereas a small amount will be released as monomeric Iga to the circulation. Alternatively, it is possible that some of the precursor IgA cells do not return to the mucosal lymphoid tissues after the first stimulation but remain in the MLNs. Since trapped TNP-*Lactobacillus* could be detected in the MLNs after oral immunization, restimulation might occur. Determination of the isotype of the specific AFCs in the MLNs which occur during the time course between prime and boost could help to clarify this issue.

In both groups, low IgM and IgG and no specific IgA anti-*Lactobacillus* responses were measured after boost. This observation confirms the low intrinsic antigen properties reported by other investigators (14). The low responses could be due to the use of a heat-killed *Lactobacillus* as carrier. Usually, life antigens induce better immune responses than nonreplicating antigens (15).

When antigens are internalized in the mucosal tissue it is believed that antigen is processed by antigen-presenting cells and are subsequently presented to T lymphocytes or B lymphocytes in the lamina propria or Peyer's patches, respectively. In this study, it has been shown that at least a part of the TNP-*Lactobacillus*, whether or not processed, is transported directly to the MLNs, as could be concluded by the presence of antigen complexes after staining with TNP-AP and anti-*Lactobacillus* in alternating MLN tissue sections.

The low intrinsic antigenic properties of the *Lactobacillus* together with the observation that oral prime and booster administrations led to a comparable specific antibody response obtained after i.p. immunization suggests the possible usage of the *Lactobacillus* as an antigen carrier for oral immunization purposes.

REFERENCES

1. Mestecky, J. The common mucosal immune system and current strategies for induction of immune responses in external secretions. J. Clin. Immunol. 1987; 7:265–279.
2. Leclerc, C., A. Charbit, A. Molla and M. Hofnung. Antibody response to a foreign epitope expressed at the surface of recombinant bacteria: importance of the route of immunization. Vaccine 1989; 7:242–248.
3. Perdigón, G., M. E. Nader de Macias, S. Alvarez, G. Oliver and A. A. Pesce de Ruiz Holgado. Effect of perorally administered lactobacilli on macrophage activation in mice. Infect. Immun. 1986; 53,404.
4. Lycke, N. and J. Holmgren. Strong adjuvant properties of choleratoxin on gut mucosal immune response to orally presented antigens. Immunology, 1986; 59;301.
5. Bloksma, N., E. de Heer, H. van Dijk and J. M. Willers. Adjuvanticity of lactobacilli. I. Differential effects of viable and killed bacteria. Clin. Exp. Immunol. 1979; 37:367–375.
6. Claassen, E. and N. Van Rooijen. TNP-enzyme conjugate for the detection of anti-TNP antibody producing cells in vivo. J. Immunol. Meth. 1984; 75:181.
7. Black, R., M. M. Levine, C. Young, J. Rooney, S. Levine, M. L. Clements, S. O'Donnell, T. Hughes and R. Germainer. Immunogenicity of Ty21a attenuated *Salmonella typhi* given with sodium bicarbonate or in enteric-coated capsules. Dev. Biol. Stand. 1983; 53:9–14.
8. Burstone, M. S. Histochemical comparison of naphthol-phosphates for the demonstration of phosphatases. J. Natl. Cancer Inst. 1958; 20:601.
9. Claassen, E., D. M. Boorsma, N. Kors and N. Van Rooijen. Double enzyme conjugates, producing an immediate colour, for the simultaneous and direct detection of three different intracellular immunoglobulin determinants with only two enzymes. J. Histochem. Cytochem. 1986; 34:423.
10. Van Rooijen, N., E. Claassen, G. Kraal and C. D. Dijkstra. Progress in histochemistry and cytochemistry. Cytological basis of immune functions of the spleen. Progr. Histochem. Cytochem. 1989; 19:3.
11. Gerritse, K., M. Posno, M. M. Schellekens, W. J. A. Boersma and E. Claassen. 1990. Oral administration of TNP-*Lactobacillus* conjugates in mice: A model for evaluation of mucosal and systemic immune responses and memory formation elicited by transformed lactobacilli. Res. Microbiol. 1990; 141:955–962.
12. Craig, S. W. and J. J. Cebra. Peyer's patches: An enriched source of precursors for IgA-producing immunocytes in the rabbit. J. Exp. Med. 1971; 134:188-200.
13. Pierce, N. F., W. C. Cray Jr. Determinants of the localisation, magnitude and duration of a specific mucosal IgA plasma cell response in enterically immunized rats. J. Immunol. 1982; 128:1311–1315.
14. Carlsson, P. & Bratthal D. Secretory and serum antibodies against *Streptococcus lactis, Streptococcus thermophilus* and *Lactobacillus bulgaricus* in relation to ingestion of fermented milk products. Acta Odontol. scand. 1985; 43,3:147–153.
15. Fuhrman J. A. and Cebra J. J. Special features of the priming process for a secretory IgA response. J. Exp. Med. 1981; 153:534.

85
Uptake of Soluble and Particulate Antigen by the Gut

Taede Sminia, Kees Twisk, Ineke van der Ven, and M. Soesatyo
Vrije University, Amsterdam, The Netherlands

INTRODUCTION

Gut-associated lymphoid tissue (GALT), represented by Peyer's patches (PPs), is composed of lymphoid follicles, interfollicular T-cell areas, and a specialized follicle-associated epithelium (FAE) overlying the B-cell follicles (3,9). The FAE contains M cells, which ingest intestinal antigen and transport the antigen to intraepithelial antigen-presenting cells and lymphocytes (6,7). There are strong indications that PPs are mainly involved in the uptake and translocation of particulate antigen, whereas the villus epithelium (enterocytes) is an important site of uptake of soluble antigen (4.8).

This study deals with antigen handling in the gut. Using labeled soluble and particulate antigens we have investigated the passage of antigen through the wall of the gut. The experiments were based on the hypothesis that (a) soluble antigen is primarily taken up by enterocytes and subsequently is transported to the spleen, free or bound to antigen-presenting cells; and (b) particulate antigen is endocytosed by FAE and transported from PPs to mesenteric lymph nodes (MLNs).

MATERIALS AND METHODS

Animals

For the experiments, female Balb/c mice, female Wistar rats, and female New Zealand white rabbits were used.

Soluble and Particulate Antigen

For the experiments, the following "model" antigens were used: latex microspheres (500 nm, 750 nm, and 1 μm; Polysciences Ins., Warrington, Pennsylvania) coupled to fluorescein isothiocyanate (FITC) or tetrarhodamine isothiocyanate (TRITC), and solved FITC (not particle bound).

Injection of Antigen

The animals were fasted overnight. After anesthetization, laparotomy was performed and intestinal segments, with or without PPs, were ligated. Antigen was injected into these intestinal loops. In one experiment, particles were injected into PPs. After different periods of time (between 10 min and 48 hr), the animals were sacrificed. Villi, PPs, spleen, and MLNs were harvested, rinsed extensively with physiological salt, and frozen in liquid nitrogen. Cryostat sections were viewed with a Zeiss fluorescence microscope or after staining with monoclonal antibodies (MAbs) raised to rat and mouse macrophages (2,10,11) with a conventional light microscope.

RESULTS

The experiments show that the villi had taken up the soluble FITC. A clear green band could be recognized when viewing the villi under the fluorescence microscope. In contrast, only some uptake of solved FITC had taken place by the FAE above PPs. Occasionally, slight fluorescence could be observed in the spleen (Table 1). There was almost no influence of the time period between the injection of FITC and collecting the tissues, although there was a tendency toward a brighter fluorescence in the enterocytes after short time periods. The FITC- and TRITC-latex particles were mainly endocytosed by FAE; almost no fluorescent particles were observed inside the villus epithelium or lamina propria. After short time periods (10–30 min), the majority of the particles were localized inside the epithelium. Later on, particles were also found in PPs. Immunohistochemistry showed that it was PP macrophages and dendritic cells that had taken up the fluorescent particles. After 24 hr, the first particles were seen in MLNs. Fluorescence was not found in villi and spleen. Only after longer periods (48 hr), fluorescent particles could be found in the spleen. When the particles were directly injected into PP far more particles were found inside MLNs than after injection into the lumen of the intestine.

It must be stressed that, in general, the uptake of the used artificial particulate and soluble antigens in both FAE and enterocytes is small. Besides the techniques and materials used, the species is important. The best uptake was found in rabbits, whereas in rats the lowest uptake of particulate and soluble markers occurred. We have tried to stimulate the uptake by adding 10% glucose to the antigen solution but this did not lead to a better uptake.

Table 1 Results of FITC and TRITC Experiments

	PPs	Villi	MLNs	Spleen
FITC	–	++	–	+
FITC-latex	+	–	+	–
TRITC-latex	+	–	+	–
FITC-latex injected into PP	++	–	++	–

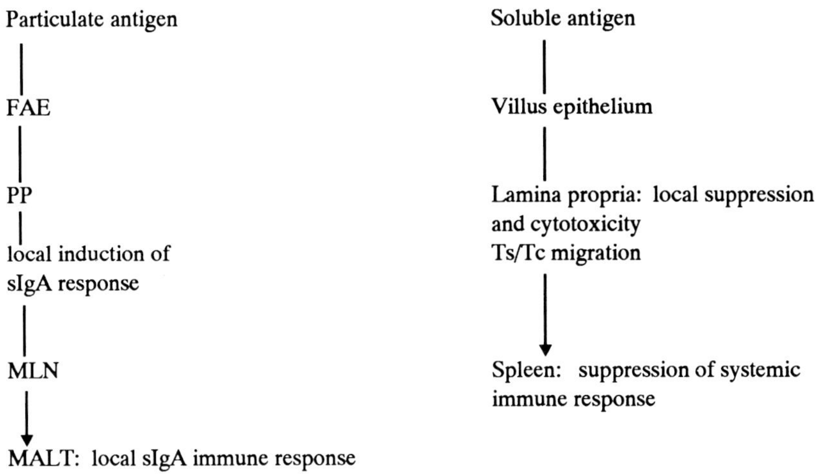

Figure 1 Schematic drawing of effects of antigen uptake by the gut.

DISCUSSION

The present results show that (a) FITC and TRITC bound to latex particles are endocytosed by PPs, and (b) free FITC and TRITC are mainly taken up through the villus epithelium. These two routes may lead to different immune responses, as shown in Figure 1. Particulate antigen taken up by FAE will be transported to MLNs via the lymphatics. The result will be a local secretory immunoglobulin (IgA) immune response and in addition systemic suppression by the local generation of suppressor T cells. Soluble antigen processed by enterocytes (villus epithelium) may stimulate the T-cell suppressor and/or cytotoxic circuit. Within the gut epithelium numerous intraepithelial lymphocytes comprising suppressor and cytotoxic T cells occur. Recent studies on the gut have provided evidence that enterocytes are capable of presenting antigen to T cells of the suppressor phenotype (1,5). Migration of these cells to the spleen leads to systemic suppression. This hypothesis on the relation between the site of antigen uptake and the immune response is currently under investigation using not only inert particles and soluble substances but also "true" antigens.

REFERENCES

1. Bland PW, Warren LG. Antigen presentation by epithelial cells of the rat small intestine. II. Selective induction of suppressor T cells. Immunology 1986; 58:9–14.
2. Dijkstra CD, Döpp EA, Joling P, Kraal G. The heterogeneity of mononuclear phagocytes in lymphoid organs: Distinct macrophage subpopulations in the rat recognized by monoclonal antibodies ED1, ED2 and ED3. Immunology 1985; 54:589–599.
3. Ermak TH, Owen RL. Differential distribution of lymphocytes and accessory cells in mouse Peyer's patches. Anat. Rec. 1986; 136:455–461.
4. Jeurissen SHM, Kraal G, Sminia T. The uptake of particles by Peyer's patches. In: *Recent Advances in Mucosal Immunology*, Part A: Cellular interactions. Mestecky J, McGhee JR, Bienenstock J, Ogra PL, eds. Plenum, New York, 1988, pp. 257–265.

5. Mayer L, Shlien R. Evidence for function of Ia molecules on gut epithelial cells in man. J. Exp. Med. 1987; 166:1471–1483.
6. Neutra MR, Phillips TL, Mayer EL, Fishkind DJ. Transport of membrane bound macromolecules by M cells in follicle associated epithelium of rabbit Peyer's patch. Cell Tissue Res. 1987; 247:537–542.
7. Owen RL, Pierce NF, Apple RT, Cray WC. M cell transport of *Vibrio cholerae* from the intestinal lumen into Peyer's patches, a mechanism for antigen sampling and microbial transepithelial migration. J. Infect. Dis. 1986; 153:1108–1115.
8. Pappo J, Ermak TH. Uptake and translocation of fluorescent latex particles by rabbit Peyer's patch follicle epithelium: A quantitative model for M cell uptake. Clin. Exp. Immunol. 1989; 76: 144–148.
9. Sminia T, Janse EM, Plesch BEC. Ontogeny of Peyer's patches of the rat. Anat. Rec. 1983; 207:309–316.
10. Kraal G, Janse M. Marginal metallophilic cells of the mouse spleen identified by a monoclonal antibody. Immunology 1986; 58:665–669.
11. Kraal G, Rep M, Janse M. Macrophages in T and B cell compartments and other tissue macrophages. Recognized by monoclonal antibody MOMA-2. An immunohistochemical study. Scand. J. Immunol. 1987; 26:653–661.

86
Tissue-Specific Expression of ε and α Messenger Ribonucleic Acid in Allergy-Prone C3H Mice

A. O. Anderson, M. L. M. Pitt, J. D. Cooley, and M. Vahey
USAMRIID, Fort Detrick, Frederick, Maryland

INTRODUCTION

Intraperitoneal inoculation of Rift Valley fever virus (RVFV) in C3H substrains of mice resulted in acute respiratory distress of all C3H/HeJ mice upon repeat exposure on day 14. In contrast, no C3H/HeN mice were affected by reexposure to RVFV. This phenomenon was never observed until C3H/HeJ mice were substituted for other strains because of increased immunoglobulin A (IgA) responses (1,2). We examined immunoglobulin heavy chain gene expression by in situ hybridization in sections and by Northern blot analysis of extracted tissue ribonucleic acid (RNA) from control and RVFV-immunized mice.

MATERIALS AND METHODS

Animals

Adult female C3H/HeJ, C3H/HeN (OuJ), mice were vaccinated intraperitoneally (i.p.), subcutaneously (s.c.), and by intranasal (i.n.) instillation. Mice were killed via CO_2 exposure. Blood IgA and IgE levels were determined by ELISA.

In conducting the research described in this report, the investigator(s) adhered to the Guide for the Care and Use of Laboratory Animals, as promulgated by the Committee on Care and Use of Laboratory Animals of the Institute of Laboratory Animals Resources, National Research Council. The facilities are fully accredited by the American Association for Accreditation of Laboratory Animal Care.

The views of the author(s) do not purport to reflect the positions of the U.S. Department of Defense.

Vaccine

Rift Valley fever virus vaccine (IND 365) was prepared from Entebbe strain virus grown on fetal rhesus lung cells and formalin inactivated (2).

RNA Isolation—Mouse Tissues

Peripheral, mediastinal, and mesenteric lymph nodes (LNs), spleens, intestines, and lungs were removed and immediately frozen in liquid nitrogen (organs from each group were pooled). Ribonucleic acid was isolated from frozen mouse tissue by the method of Chirgwin et al. (4). Concentrations of RNA were adjusted to 10 μg per lane. Samples were heated to 65°C for 2 min and loaded onto 1.5% agarose gels containing 0.66 M formaldehyde, 20 mM MOPS, 5 mM EDTA, 6.6 μg ethidium bromide. Gels were electrophoresed at 18–20 V for 18 hr.

Cyclic Deoxyribonucleic Acid (DNA) Probes

The chimeric plasmid $C^3$30 containing 1300 bp cDNA for the mouse IgE heavy chain was the kind gift of Dr. Fu-Tong Liu (5). The α660 plasmid (6) was the generous gift of Dr. John Cebra and Peter Weinstein. This construct is a Gemini plasmid (Promega, Madison, Wisconsin) containing α660 bp cDNA for mouse IgA.

Northern Blots

Ribonucleic acid gels were blotted overnight onto nitrocellulose. Filters were baked under vacuum at 80°C for 2 hr. Prehybridization was carried out for 20 min at 47°C in 40% formamide, 4X SSC, 1X Denhardt's solution, 7 mM Tris pH 7.4, and 25 μg salmon sperm DNA. Hybridization was carried out in the same buffer at 47°C for 20 hr. Radiolabeled probe was added to a final concentration of 1×10^8 dpm. Posthybridization washes were done for 30 min each in 2.0x, 1.0x, 0.1x SSC; 0.1% SDS; and for 5 min at 68°C.

In Situ Hybridization

Lung tissue sections from each strain/treatment group were exposed to the above probes according to the method of Singer et al. (7) using the Genius kit.

RESULTS AND DISCUSSION

C3H/HeJ mice that died within 30 min of i.p. or i.n. secondary inoculation 14 days after i.p. immunization with RVFV exhibited antimortem and postmortem signs of acute respiratory distress. C3H/HeN mice were completely resistant to this phenomenon. Mouse models of hypersensitivity are exceedingly complex (8), with networks of immunoregulatory cells, cytokines (interleukin-4 [IL-4] vs interferon-γ [IFN-γ]) differences in mediator responsiveness (9), IgE Fc receptor expression, and IgE binding factors. We examined messenger RNA (mRNA) expression for α and ε heavy chains in total RNA extracted from lymph nodes, spleen, lung, and intestines of untreated and i.p. vaccinated mice (Table 1).

Low levels of mRNA were found in all tissues of control C3H/HeJ and higher levels in the C3H/HeN mice. However, we found increased α and ε mRNA levels in lungs and spleen of C3H/HeJ, whereas there was decreased or unchanged α and ε mRNA levels in all organs except the spleens of C3H/HeN mice 14 days after i.p. immunization with RVFV. In situ hybridization of lungs from C3H/HeJ and C3H/HeN mice with the same cDNA

Table 1 Effect of I .P. Vaccination with RVFV on α and ε mRNA Levels

	Intestine		Lung		Med LN		Mes LN		Per LN		Spleen	
Mouse strain	α	ε	α	ε	α	ε	α	ε	α	ε	α	ε
CeH/HeJ	D	D	I	I	=	I	=	I	D	D	I	I
C3H/HeN	D	D	=	D	D	D	D	D	=	D	I	I

Comparison between control and immunized mice by using densitometry of Northern blots. Abbreviations: D, decreased; I, increased; =, is unchanged; Med, mesiastinal, Mes, mesenteric; Per, peripheral; LN, lymph node.

probes revealed peribronchial distribution of cells bearing α and ε mRNA, whereas ε mRNA was distributed throughout the lung interstitium only in C3H/HeJ mice (Table 2).

There were no significant differences among total serum IgE levels (ng/ml) of control or immunized C3H/HeJ (9.8 ± 1.4) and C3H/HeN (5.1 ± 1.2) mice. Both strains showed at least double the control IgE levels after immunization.

The concentration of total IgA in serum increased from 73 μg/ml in control C3H/HeJ mice to 142 μg/ml in the immunized mice. The concentration of IgA in bronchial lavages also increased dramatically in C3H/HeJ mice after immunization, from 71 ng/ml to 90 ng/ml. There was no significant change in the concentration of IgA in bronchial lavage from C3H/HeN mice.

We have shown that substrains of the C3H mouse have potential as a model of vaccine-induced acute hypersensitivity. Although this strain is intermediary between SJL and Balb/c mice with regard to IgE antibody levels (7), there are organ-specific differences in IgA and IgE commitment after i.p. immunization which correlate with differences in expression of mucosal immunity and/or allergy in the mouse strains tested. Furthermore, in situ hybridization suggests that interstitial B cells are responsive for the increased IgE expression in the lungs of C3H/HeJ mice which had been vaccinated i.p. We have recently observed significant transdiaphragmatic traffic of peritoneal LY-1 B cells into the lungs interstitium (Pitt and Kroese, unpublished data), and suggest that they may be the target population for i.p. stimulation.

Table 2 In Situ Hybridization of α and ε mRNA[a] in Lungs from C3H/HeN and C3H/HeJ Mice

	C3H/HeN				C3H/HeJ			
	Untreated		S/P RVFV[b]		Untreated		S/P RVFV[b]	
Tissue pattern	α	ε	α	ε	α	ε	α	ε
Peribronchial	+	–	++	+	++	+	+++	+
Interstitial	–	–	+	–	–	+	+	++

[a]Mouse IgA heavy chain αmRNA was probed with α660 cDNA, and Weinstein. IgE heavy chain εmRNA was probed with $C^2$30 cDNA.
[b]14 days after i.p. RVFV.

REFERENCES

1. Kiyono H, Babb JL, Michalek SM, McGhee JR. Cellular basis for elevated IgA responses in C3H/HeJ mice. J Immunol 1980; 125:732–737.
2. Anderson AO, Snyder LF, Pitt MLM, Wood OL. Mucosal priming alters pathogenesis of Rift Valley fever. Adv Exp Med Biol 1988; 273:727–733.
3. Randall R, Binn LN, Harrison VR. Immunization against Rift Valley fever virus. Studies on the immunogenicity of lyophilized formalin-inactivated vaccine. J Immunol 1964; 93:293–301.
4. Chirgwin JJ, Przbyla AE, MacDonald RJ, Rutter WJ. Isolation of biologically active ribonucleic acid from source enriched in ribonuclease. Biochemistry 1979; 18:5294.
5. Liu FT, Albrandt K, Sutcliffe JG, Katz DH. Cloning and nucleotide sequence of mouse immunoglobulin chain cDNA. Proc Natl Acad Sci USA 1982; 79:7852–7856.
6. Marcu KB, Banerji J, Penncavage NA, Lange R, Arnheim N. "5" flanking region of immunoglobulin heavy chain constant region genes displays length heterogeneity in germlines of inbred mouse strains. Cell 1980; 22:187–196.
7. Singer RH, Lawrence JB, Villnave C. Optimization of in situ hybridization using isotopic and nonisotopic methods. BioTechniques 1986; 4:230–250.
8. Katz DH. IgE antibody responses *in vitro*: from rodents to man. Prog Allergy 1982; 32:105–160.
9. Levitt RC, Mitzner W. Expression of airway hyperreactivity to acetylcholine as a simple autosomal recessive trait in mice. FASEB J 1988; 2:2605–2608.

87
Comparison of Two Methods for Collecting Murine Intestinal Secretions to Detect Antigen-Specific Antibodies

Philip J. van der Heijden, Andre T. J. Bianchi, Maike Dol, and Bernard A. Bokhout
Central Veterinary Institute, Lelystad, The Netherlands

INTRODUCTION

The in vivo expression of the intestinal mucosal immune response can be studied by measuring secretory immunoglobulin A (sIgA) responses in intestinal secretions. Some of the methods used to sample intestinal secretions are to lavage the intestine in vivo by inducing a mild diarrhea in the animal (3), to flush isolated loops of intestine in vivo, or to flush intestinal sections in vitro (5), to scrape intestinal tissue (1), or to homogenize the entire intestine in a blender (2). Most sampling methods, except for the lavage procedures, have not been well standardized. Some investigators have found only antigen-specific IgA antibodies in intestinal secretions (3), whereas others have found antigen-specific IgG antibodies as well (2). These differences may be due to the sampling methods used.

The purpose of the present study was to determine whether the scraping technique contaminates intestinal Ig with Ig from the blood. In an earlier article (6), we described antigen-specific B-cell responses in the small intestine after an immunization regimen that induced both mucosal and systemic immune responses. Using the same immunization regimen as in the earlier study, we compared the gentle lavage technique (3) with the rougher scraping technique for recovering intestinal Ig. The distribution of antigen-specific IgM, IgG, and IgA in serum and intestinal secretions was compared with the distribution of total IgM, IgG, and IgA in these fluids.

MATERIALS AND METHODS

Mice

Female C3H/He mice were purchased from Harlan-Olac Ltd., Bicester, Oxon, England, housed conventionally, and used at the age of 12–20 weeks.

Antigens and Immunization

Mice were injected intraperitoneally (i.p.) with 0.1 ml of a water-in-oil emulsion containing 0.1 mg polymerized ovalbumin (OA; Sigma, St. Louis, MO) (6). Four weeks later, the mice were given booster immunizations either orally with 80 mg monomeric OA in 0.5 ml 0.2 M $NaHCO_3$ or i.p. with 0.1 mg polymerized OA in 0.1 ml saline.

Intestinal Secretions

Intestinal washings were obtained in vivo by lavage according to the method of Elson et al. (3). Intestinal scrapings were obtained in the following manner. Mice were killed with carbon dioxide and the small intestines were removed and flushed with phosphate-buffered saline (PBS). The contents of the intestine were pushed out by squeezing the intestine between a Petri dish and the round tip of a pair of forceps. The squeezing was standardized, so that afterwards 34 ± 9% (w/w) remained in the intestinal tissues and 66 ± 5% (w/w) was scraped out. The scrapings, about 1 ml per small intestine, were dissolved in 2 ml PBS containing 50 mM EDTA and 0.1 mg/ml trypsin inhibitor and mixed vigorously. The solution was clarified by centrifugation (10 min, 650 × g) and 10 µl of 1% NaN_3 was added before storage. Samples collected this way could be stored at –20°C without detectable decrease in titer. The addition of PMSF did not enhance the recovery of Ig or the storage life of the samples.

Antigen- and Isotype-Specific Detection of Ig

Ovalbumin-specific antibodies in intestinal secretions and sera were assayed in an ELISA on microtiter plates coated with polymerized OA as described (6). Total Ig in intestinal secretions and sera were assayed in an ELISA on microtiter plates coated with rabbit anti-mouse IgM, IgG, or IgA (Nordic, Tilburg, The Netherlands). Total Ig levels were expressed as arbitrary units/ml; the amount of Ig that gave an extinction of 0.300 at 450 nm was set on 0.1 units/ml.

RESULTS

Mice were primed i.p. with OA in a water-in-oil emulsion and were given booster immunizations orally 4 weeks later. Intestinal secretions were collected from one-half of the mice by lavage, and from the other half by scraping. Serum samples were collected by heart puncture. Table 1 shows the isotype-specific anti-OA titers and total Ig units/ml. In scrapings the OA-specific IgA titer equaled the IgG titer, whereas in washings only low titers of OA-specific IgA were measured. Serum samples had relatively high titers of OA-specific IgG and low titers of IgA and IgM. To determine whether IgA in intestinal secretions was produced locally or had leaked from blood, we calculated the ratios of total IgM, IgG, and IgA units/ml in sera to those in scrapings and the ratios of those in sera to those in washings (Table 2). The serum/scraping ratios for IgM and IgG (on average 250 and 170, respectively) and the serum/washing ratios for IgM and IgG (on average >2118 and 4703, respectively) were much higher than the serum/scraping and serum/washing ratios calculated for IgA (on average 0.59 for scraping and 2.1 for washing). Next, from Table 1, we calculated the ratios of total IgA units to total IgG units in sera, scrapings, and washings. The IgA/IgG ratio in washings (82:1) was more than four times as high as in scrapings (20:1) and more than 800 times as in serum (0.07:1). Thus, IgA in scrapings and washings was not derived from blood and, therefore, must have been produced locally.

Table 1 Total and OA-Specific Ig Content in Sera, Scrapings, and Washings After Oral Booster Immunization

	Total IgM[1]	Spec. IgM[2]	Total IgG	Spec. IgG	Total IgA	Spec. IgA
Serum						
Day 7	566 (80)	13.1 (6.0)	2830 (400)	8000 (2800)	200 (0)	30.3 (24.2)
Day 8	492 (65)	8.7 (2.4)	4660 (640)	18400 (5500)	318 (50)	40.0 (40.0)
Scrapings						
Day 7	2.3 (0.8)	<2.0 (–)	21.1 (3.7)	52.8 (14.3)	420 (40)	69.6 (19.8)
Day 8	2.0 (0.7)	<2.0 (–)	22.6 (4.1)	56.6 (10.0)	450 (20)	28.3 (12.1)
Washings						
Day 7	<0.20 (–)	<2.0 (–)	0.67 (0.4)	<2.0 (–)	80 (0)	5.0 (1.0)
Day 8	0.35 (0.06)	<2.0 (–)	0.90 (0.6)	<2.0 (–)	40 (10)	4.4 (1.2)

Results are expressed as the mean (n=10 for sera, n=5 for scrapings and washings) with the SEM in brackets. 1) Total IgM, IgG, and IgA are expressed as units/ml; 2) OA-specific IgM, IgG and IgA are expressed as titers.

Theoretically, if IgG in scrapings was derived from blood, the ratio of OA-specific IgG titers to total IgG units/ml should be the same in both fluids. From Table 1, we calculated that the ratio of OA-specific IgG to total IgG for serum (3.0) was almost the same as that for scrapings (2.5). Thus, IgG measured in scrapings probably originated from blood.

To determine whether or not the IgG was derived from the blood, in another series of experiments we immunized mice to induce a systemic but not a mucosal immune response. Mice were primed i.p. with OA in a water-in-oil emulsion and given a booster immunization i.p. 4 weeks later. Results are shown in Table 3. After parenteral booster immunization, the OA-specific IgG titer in serum was more than two times as high as after oral booster immunization. In scrapings, the OA-specific IgG titer after parenteral booster was the same as after oral booster. In contrast, the IgA titer in scrapings after parenteral booster (see Table 3) was five times less than the IgA titer after oral booster immunization (see Table 1). After parenteral booster, the ratios of OA-specific IgG to total IgG for scrapings (8.1) was nearly the same as that for serum (8.0). Ovalbumin-specific antibodies were not detected in washings.

Table 2 Ratios of Total Ig (Units/ml) in Serum to Those in Scrapings and in Washings

	Serum/scraping ratios		Serum/washing ratios	
	Day 7	Day 8	Day 7	Day 8
IgM	250	250	>2,830	1,406
IgG	134	206	4,230	5,177
IgA	0.48	0.71	1.9	2.3

Table 3 Total and OA-Specific Ig Content in Serum, Scrapings, and Washings at Day 7 After Parenteral Booster Immunization

	Total IgM[1]	Spec. IgM[2]	Total IgG	Spec. IgG	Total IgA	Spec. IgA
Serum	700 (105)	4100 (1400)	4900 (750)	39450 (11250)	340 (40)	<10 (–)
Scrapings	4.6 (1.3)	6.1 (0.8)	6.9 (1)	56 (29)	220 (30)	9 (3)
Washings	<0.2 (–)	<2.0 (–)	<0.4 (–)	<2.5 (–)	37 (5)	<2.5 (–)

Results are expressed as in Table 1.

DISCUSSION

We compared two methods for sampling intestinal secretions; namely, lavage and scraping. Scrapings had antigen-specific IgA titers that were 10 times those measured in washings (see Table 1). Antigen-specific IgG titers were measured in scrapings but not in washings.

From the ratios of total IgM, IgG, and IgA Units/ml in serum to those in scrapings and to those in washings (see Table 2) and the ratios of total IgA titers to total IgG titers in the various fluids, it can be concluded that IgA detected in scrapings and washings was mainly produced locally and transported actively to the intestinal lumen.

Antigen-specific IgG in scrapings may be locally produced or may be derived from blood; the latter as a consequence of the method used to collect the intestinal secretions. We calculated the ratios of antigen-specific IgG titers to total IgG titers in serum and in scrapings. It was assumed that proteolytic degradation of IgG would affect antigen-specific IgG titers and the total IgG titers equally and, therefore, would not alter the ratio between these two values. Indeed, the ratios of the antigen-specific IgG titers to the total IgG titers in both serum and scrapings were nearly the same (3.0 and 2.5, respectively). We concluded, therefore, that most of the IgG detected in scrapings originated from blood. To confirm this hypothesis, we determined the antigen-specific antibody titers and total Ig titers after an immunization regimen that induced a systemic response only (6). Again, the ratios of OA-specific IgG to total IgG were equal in serum and scrapings (8.0 and 8.1, respectively).

In conclusion, intestinal secretions collected by the lavage techniques reliably indicate the isotype distribution of luminal antigen-specific Igs. This isotype distribution agrees with the isotype distribution of the Ig-secreting cells isolated from the small intestine (6). However, only luminal IgA can be detected, whereas intestinal IgA tends to reside in the mucus layer (4). Scraping is less laborious and provides the possibility to detect mucus-bound IgA. Therefore, scraping is the more sensitive technique for detecting intestinal IgA. However, most IgG detected in intestinal secretions collected by scraping is due to an artefact.

REFERENCES

1. Aizpurua de HJ, Russell-Jones GJ. Oral vaccination. Identification of classes of proteins that provoke an immune response upon oral feeding. J Exp Med 1988;167:440.
2. Clements JD, Lyon FL, Lowe KL, Farrand AL, El-Morshidy S. Oral immunization of mice with attenuated *Salmonella enteritidis* containing a recombinant plasmid which codes for production of the B subunit of heat-labile *Escherichia coli* enterotoxin. Infect Immun 1986;53:685.

3. Elson CO, Ealding W, Lefkowitz J. A lavage technique allowing repeated measurement of IgA antibody in mouse intestinal secretions. J Immunol Meth 1984;67:101.
4. Magnusson K-E, Stjernström I. Mucosal barrier mechanisms. Interplay between secretory IgA (SIgA), IgG and mucins on the surface properties and association of salmonellae with intestine and granulocytes. Immunology 1982;45:239.
5. Nedrud JG, Liang X, Hague N, Lamm ME. Combined oral/nasal immunization protects mice from Sendai virus infection. J Immunol 1987;139:3484.
6. Van der Heijden PJ, Bianchi ATJ, Bokhout BA, Dol M, Scholten JW, Stok W. Quantitation of antigen-specific antibody-secreting cells in the small intestine and other lymphoid organs of mice after oral booster immunization. Immunology 1989;66:404.

88
Milky Spots Can Be Considered as Omentum-Associated Lymphoid Tissue

R. H. J. Beelen, R. J. B. M. Hendrickx, I. L. Eestermans, and J. F. A. M. Wijffels
The Free University, Amsterdam, The Netherlands

INTRODUCTION

Milky spots in the mouse and rat appear as opaque patches in the transparent omentum, first described by Ranvier (1). Our earlier studies showed that milky spots in the omentum must be regarded as strongly reactive structures originating in part from perivascular effusions in the omentum (2,3). We also concluded that at least part of the free peritoneal macrophages was derived from these milky spots, which was confirmed later by others (4). Mandache et al. (5) mentioned the presence of plasma cells and lymphocytes in the milky spots, and Dux et al. (6) noted a change in the number of B and T lymphocytes after immunization. Moreover, the omentum is used in surgery as a very potent tissue in wound healing, which suggests besides a very good vascularization pattern also a very important immunological function (7). Clearly, milk spots might be involved in this immune process, as has already been suggested by Fischer et al. (8), and it has recently been shown without doubt that the milky spots are present in the human system (9). Therefore, we investigated the immunological characteristics of milky spots in the rat after stimulation with newborn calf serum (NBCS) and found that milky spots not only are very reactive structures, but also have more or less lymphoid characteristics (10).

In this study, we have further investigated the question whether milky spots in the mouse (using a panel of monoclonal antibodies [MAbs]) can be considered as omental lymphoid organs by specific immunization with NCBS and specific primary and secondary immunization with trinitrophenyl-KLH [TNP-KLH] and TNP-Ficoll. The results clearly show that milky spots in the omentum can be considered as omentum-associated lymphoid tissue and, therefore, are renamed as OALT.

MATERIALS AND METHODS

Animals

Male Balb/c mice weighing 20–25 g (and Wistar rats weighing 180–200 g) were used.

Immunization

An acute inflammatory state was induced by intraperitoneal (i.p.) administration of 1 ml NBCS according to Beelen et al. (2). For the primary stimulation, we looked after 2 days and for the secondary stimulation we repeated the i.p. administration of NCBS after 6 days. A specific immunization was given by i.p. administration of 0.5 ml TNP-KLH (1 mg/ml) or TNP-Ficoll (1 mg/ml) according to Claassen et al. (11). For the primary immunization, we looked after 5 days and for the secondary immunization we repeated the i.p. administration after 1 month.

The omentum was dissected free and processed for immunohistochemistry.

Immunochemistry

Peroxidase immunochemistry was done exactly according to Dijkstra et al. (12). Briefly: cryostat sections were fixed in aceton, incubated in diluted ascites fluid, washed, incubated with rabbit antirat (Ig) peroxidase in phosphate-buffered saline (PBS) with 1% bovine serum albumin (BSA) and 1% normal mouse serum for 60 min and stained for peroxidase using diaminobenzidine as trapping agent. Alkaline phosphatase histochemistry was done according to Claassen et al. (11). Briefly: cryostat sections were fixed in aceton, incubated with anti TNP-AP in PBS with 1% BSA (over night) and stained for alkaline phosphatase in ASMX-naftol and Fast-Blue.

RESULTS AND DISCUSSION

Number and Cellular Composition

In the omentum of normal steady-state mice (and rats) milky spots are always present. After i.p. administration of NBCS, the number and size of the milky spots increased strongly, indicating the omentum as a very reactive tissue. The number of cells isolated after collagenase digestion increased enormously. Besides macrophages, lymphocytes were found in relatively large numbers. This observation fits very well with the findings of Dux et al. (6), who also noted the presence of plasma cells and lymphoblasts after i.p. immunization with sheep red blood cells (SRBCs). In the milky spots, plasma cells are even seen in the normal steady state, as shown in Figure 1, indicating their importance as possible lymphoid tissue.

Immunochemistry

With a panel of monoclonal antibodies recognizing mouse macrophage and lymphocyte subsets (13), we found, already after NBCS, clusters of both T and B cells in discrete areas in the milky spots. Moreover, MOMA-1 (Fig. 2) and ERTR-9–positive macrophages were found, as normally seen in the lymphoid organs (spleen, lymph node) but not in the free peritoneal cavity. Finally, NLDC-145, which stains interdigitating cells in situ in lymphoid organs (14), was recognized on dendriticlike cells in situ in the milky spots in T-cell areas. Altogether, these results (milky spot present in steady state, plasmacellular

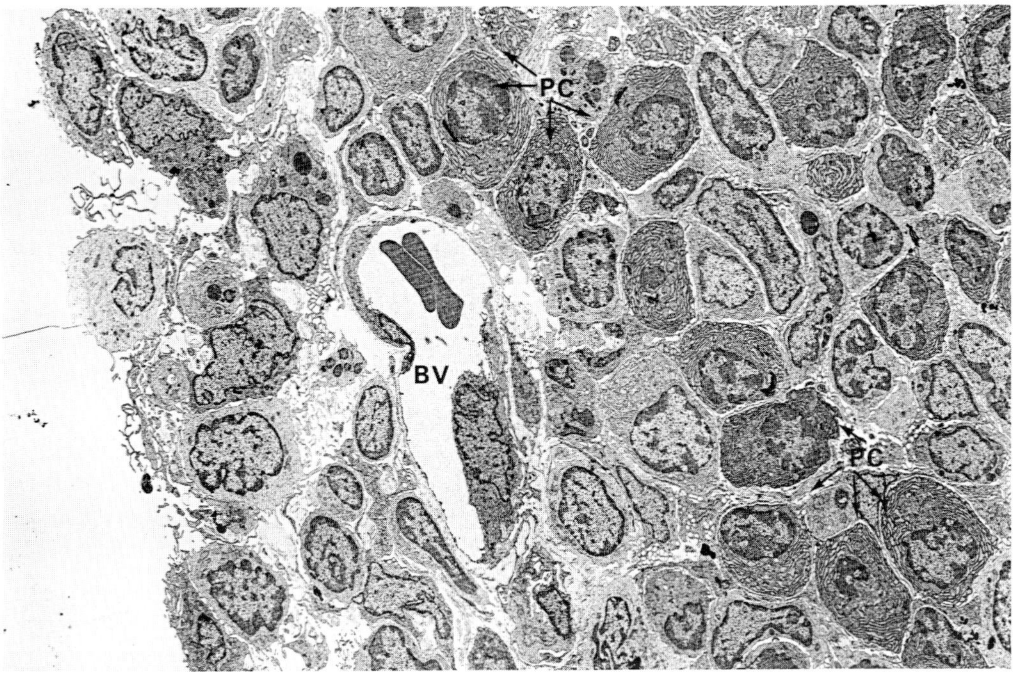

Figure 1 Milky spot obtained from normal steady state, processed for electron microscopy, showing cluster of plasma cells (Pc). BV = blood vessel (magnification: ×3000).

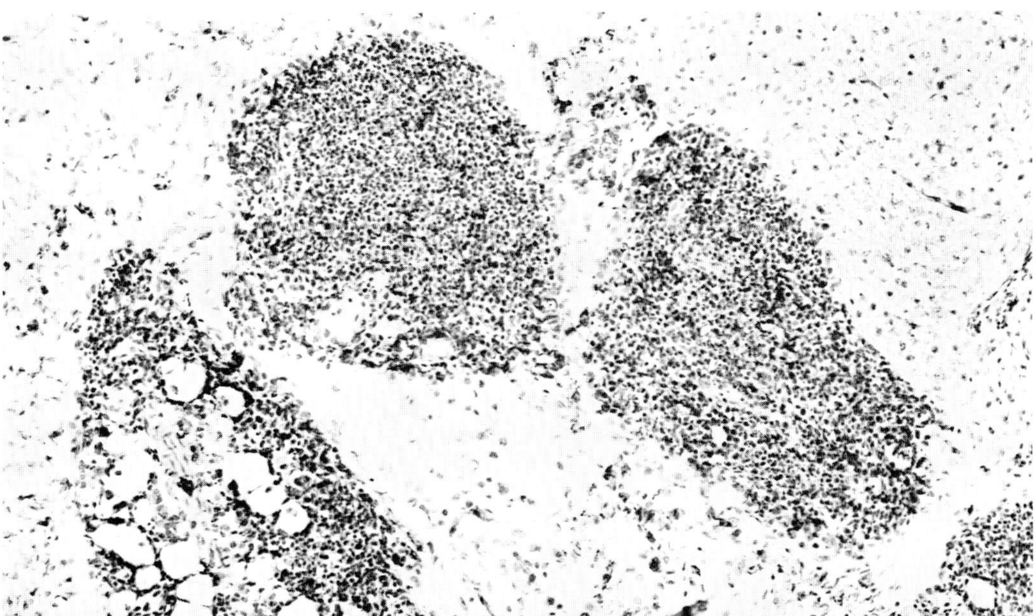

Figure 2 Mouse milky spot after secondary stimulation with NBCS stained with MOMA-1. Note the presence of many positive macrophages (magnification: ×100).

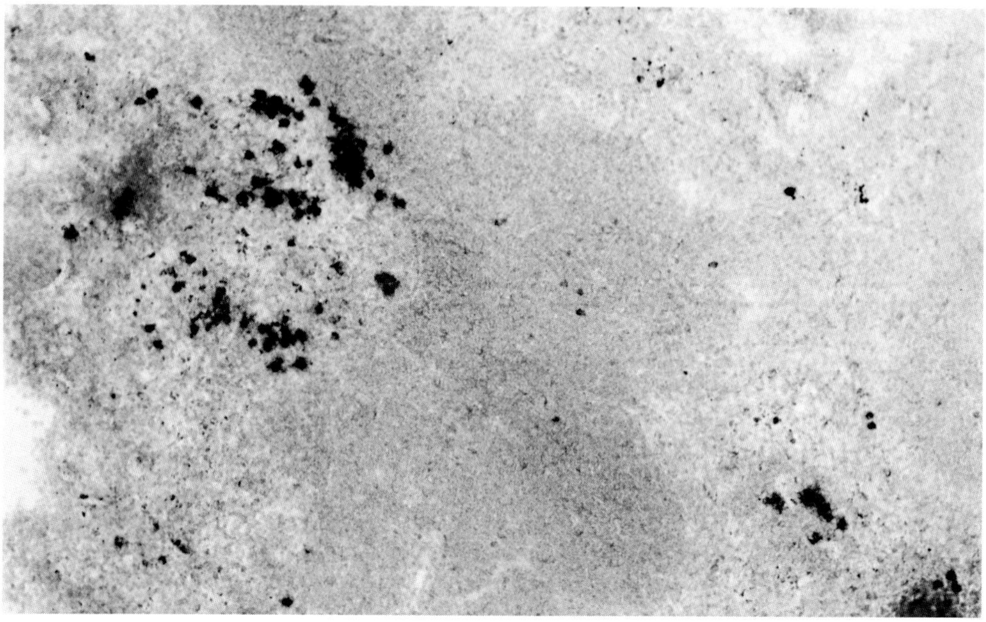

Figure 3 Milky spots (a), spleen (b), and parathymic lymph node (c) after secondary immunization with TNP-Ficoll stained for anti-TNP–forming cells. Note the most prominent effect in the milky spots (magnification: ×100).

reaction, T- and B-cell areas, specific macrophage subsets) strongly support the concept that milky spots are not only reactive inflammatory tissue, but potentially might be considered as omentum-associated lymphoid tissue (OALT) comparable with, for instance, the gut-associated lymphoid tissue (GALT), mucosa-associated lymphoid tissue (MALT), and bronchus-associated lymphoid tissue (BALT).

Specific Immunization

After specific i.p. immunization with TNP-KLH and TNP-Ficoll both in the rat and mouse, we found fairly the same results: Primary immunization results in an increase in the size but not in the number of the milky spots, whereas secondary immunization resulted in a strong increase in both the size and the number of the milky spots.

Anti-TNP–forming B cells could be found in low numbers in the primary response and in relatively high numbers in the secondary response as compared with the spleen and the draining parathymic lymph nodes (Fig. 3; Table 1). These results clearly show a specific immune reaction in the milky spot (most pronounced after TNP-Ficoll) and even more pronounced than in the common peripheral lymphoid organs.

All together, our results stress the importance of the milky spots as "immune factories" (8) or as "omental lymphoid organ" (6), and therefore must be renamed as OALT (omentum-associated lymphoid tissue).

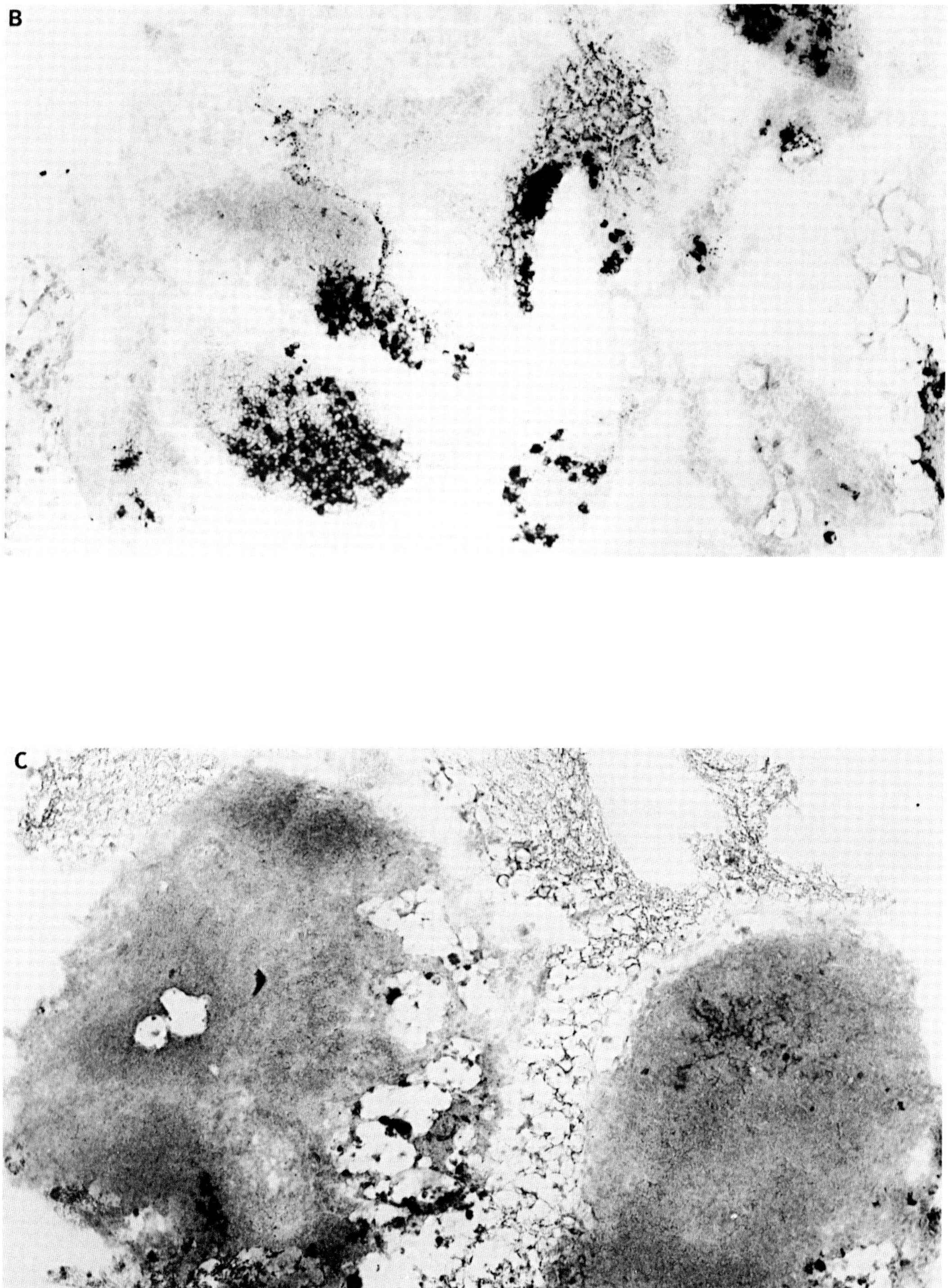

Figure 3 (Continued)

Table 1 Number of Anti-TNP–Producing B Cells in the Spleen, Parathymic Lymph Node, and Milky Spots After Immunization with TNP-KLH and TNP-Ficoll

	Lymph node	Spleen	Milky spots
TNP-KLH			
primary	±	–	±
secondary	±	±	+
TNP-Ficoll			
primary	–	+	±
secondary	±	+	+++
PBS (control)			
primary	–	–	–
secondary	–	–	–

REFERENCES

1. Ranvier 1. Du development et de l'accroisement de vaisseaux sanguins. Arch. Physiol. 1874; 1:429.
2. Beelen RHJ, Fluitsma DM, Hoefsmit ECM. Cellular composition of milky spots and fine structure of milky spot macrophages and reticulum cells. J. Reticuloendothel. Soc. 1980; 28:585.
3. Beelen RHJ, Fluitsma DM, Hoefsmit ECM. Peroxidatic activity of mononuclear phagocytes developing in milky spots. J. Reticuloendothel. Soc. 1980; 28:601.
4. Bakker JM de. Thesis, Leiden, The Netherlands. 1983.
5. Mandache E, Moldoveany E, Savi G. Cellular changes in the omentum after stimulation. Rev. Roum. Morphol. Embryol. Physiol. 1985; 23:137.
6. Dux K, Rouse RV, Kyewski B. Composition of the lymphoid cell population from omental milky spots during the immune response in C57BL/Ka mice. Eur. J. Immunol. 1986; 16:1029.
7. Lieberman-Meffert D and White H (eds.). *The Greater Omentum. Anatomy, Physiology, Pathology, Surgery*. Springer-Verlag, Heidelberg, 1983.
8. Fischer H, Ax W, Malchow H. Die Immunfabrik. Klin. Wochenschr. 1969; 47:19.
9. Shimotsuma M, Kawata M, Hagiwara A, Takahashi T. Milky spots in the human greater omentum. Acta Anat. 1989; 136:211.
10. Beelen RHJ, Eestermans IL, Dopp EA, Dijkstra CD. Immunological characteristics of milky spots in the omentum of rats. Adv. Exp. Med. Biol. 1988; 237:745.
11. Claassen HJHM. Antibodyforming Cells in the Spleen. Thesis. Amsterdam, The Netherlands, 1987.
12. Dijkstra CD, Dopp EA, Joling PP, Kraal G. The heterogeneity of mononuclear phagocytes in lymphoid organs: distinct macrophage subpopulations in the rat recognized by monoclonal antibodies ED 1, ED 2 and ED 3. Immunology 1985; 54:589.
13. Wijffels JFAM, Rover Z de, Rooyen N van, Kraal G, Beelen RHJ. Clonal expansion of bone marrow derived macrophage cell lines, which can be repopulated in vivo. In: *Lymphatic Tissues and In Vivo Immune Responses*, Imhof et al. (eds.), Marcel Dekker, New York, 1991.
14. Breel M, Mebius RE, Kraal G. Dendritic cells of the mouse recognized by two monoclonal antibodies. 1987; 17:1555.

89
The Unique Role of the Lung in the Mucosa-Associated Lymphoid Organs

Reinhard Pabst, Ilse Gehrke, and Sabine Delventhal
Centre of Anatomy, Medical School of Hannover, Hannover, Federal Republic of Germany

INTRODUCTION

In reviews on the cells of the lung, lymphocytes are often only mentioned in passing. Similarly, in lymphocyte migration studies, the lung is only regarded as a filter for removing damaged cells. Moreover, the organized lymphoid tissue of the lung, as best characterized in rabbits, has been taken as typical for all species. For characterization of the role of the lung in the immune system, lymphocytes in the lung have to be attributed to four major compartments, each of which seems to consist of a typical composition of lymphocyte subsets, differing in their migration kinetics (1). These compartments are (a) The bronchoalveolar space, nowadays often sampled in man by bronchoalveolar lavage. (b) Organized follicularlike lymphoid tissue, associated to bronchi with a specialized covering epithelium (BALT). (c) Lymphocytes in the interstitium of the lung. (d) Lymphocytes in the lung vascular bed, consisting of huge numbers and seemly different from lymphocytes of the general blood pool.

BRONCHOALVEOLAR SPACE

Bronchoalveolar lavage can be performed in experimental animals and also routinely in man (2). In healthy nonsmokers, about 10–15% of the nucleated cells are lymphocytes with very few B cells. Very little is known about the origin and rate of influx of lymphocytes from the blood into the alveolar space. Normal adult rats were injected with thoracic duct lymphocytes, labeled with fluorescein isothiocyanate (FITC) in vitro. In a total of 20 rats, the lungs were lavaged immediately after sacrifice at intervals between 15 min and more than 4 days. The frequency (%) of FITC-labeled cells in the peripheral blood was initially several percent and similar levels were found in the lung vascular pool (see below). In the bronchoalveolar lavage, however, the FITC labeling index was always ≤0.01%. This indicated a very low rate of influx of lymphocytes from the blood into the pool in the bronchoalveolar space or a very long delay in the interstitium.

BALT

In a previous study (3), it had been documented that no organized lymphoid tissue was detected in the lung tissue of 34 patients (with no known chronic respiratory tract disease). In rabbits and rats, however, BALT was present in all animals after 2 months of age. In mice and guinea pigs, about 50% of the lungs contained BALT. It was hypothesized that infections of the lung might initiate the development of organized lymphoid tissue associated with bronchi. This concept was substantiated by the following findings: In germ-free pigs of ~2 months of age, BALT had not developed. In conventionally reared pigs of 4 months of age, about 20% of the animals had small amounts of BALT. In contrast, in pigs of similar age studied 3 weeks after an infection with *Haemophilus pleuropneumoniae*, all lung sections contained prominent BALT.

In some respects, BALT has a similar structure to Peyer's patches (PPs) and the similarities in function have often been stressed (e.g., see Ref. 4). BALT in rabbits and rats does not consist of well-defined compartments for T and B lymphocytes, lymphocyte traffic and lymphocyte production (1,5) as is well known for PPs (6). Other aspects, however, are similar. For example, the epithelium covering rabbit BALT does not express the secretory component for immunoglobulin A (IgA) transport, similar to human and rabbit PPs (1). The lack of BALT in normal human lungs and its variability in many species has to be considered when planning experiments for aerosol immunization in animal models. It is important for future experiments to define the factors which regulate the appearance of BALT at its specific sites and under certain conditions.

INTERSTITIAL PULMONARY LYMPHOCYTES

Holt et al. (7,8) digested lung tissue with enzymes and recovered surprisingly high lymphocyte numbers. In rats, there were ~10^8 cells/g lung, which consisted of about 44% lymphocytes (7). In human peripheral lung tissue, 15–48 × 10^6 lymphocytes/g were determined with a different subset composition from that of blood lymphocytes. Contamination by lymphocytes from the vascular pool was found to be negligible. Extrapolation to the total number of lymphocytes in the interstitial space of the lungs would result in ~10 × 10^9 lymphocytes, which is equivalent to the total pool of lymphocytes in the blood (8). Thus, the interstitial lung lymphocyte pool is of considerable size.

INTRAVASCULAR LYMPHOCYTE POOL IN THE LUNG

For a long time the localization of lymphocytes in the lung shortly after i.v. injection had been taken as an artifact of filtering in vitro–damaged cells on their passage through the lung capillaries, as discussed recently (1). The physiological size of this pool was demonstrated in young pigs when during an in vitro perfusion period of up to 4 hr lymphocytes were released continuously, resulting in about 1.5 × 10^9 lymphocytes (9). In adult rats, similar experiments have been performed. Despite the huge volume of up to 400 ml perfusing the small rat lung lymphocytes were still released in the last fraction. The number of nucleated cells released was ~15 ×10^6. The ratio of red cells to mononuclear cells in the perfusate fractions showed that it was not only peripheral blood washed out of the lung vasculature (ratio ~1000). When lymphocyte subsets were determined in early and late samples, there were some differences in the numbers of T and B lymphocytes. In a further series of experiments on rats in vitro, FITC-labeled thoracic duct lymphocytes were injected i.v. and the lungs were perfused at 15 min and 1, 24, and 48 h later. The index of FITC-labeled lymphocytes in the lung vascular bed decreased rapidly from 15 min to 1 hr but later remained relatively constant (15 min: 21.1 ± 1.0%; 1 hr: 4.6 ± 2.8%; 1 day: 3.8 ± 0.7%; 2 days: 2.8 ± 0.7%). Taking all these data together, it can be concluded that the pulmonary pool in the rat lung is of considerable size and shows a rapid exchange with the circulating blood pool. This marginal pool seems to be typical for organs with protease-insensitive homing characteristics as the spleen, lung, liver, and bone marrow and is in contrast to organs with high endothelial venule (HEV)–mediated, protease-sensitive homing characteristics such as the lymph nodes, Peyer's patches, and tonsils, as discussed recently (10).

DISCUSSION

In conclusion, the normal lung contains larger numbers of lymphocytes than previously thought. They can be attributed to four major pools: alveolar space lymphocytes, organized lymphoid tissue, interstitial lymphocytes, and the marginal pool in the vascular bed. The subset composition and the migration kinetics between these pools seem to be different and need further investigation. In understanding the lung immune system, it is important to note that BALT is not a constitutive structure of the lung in all species, e.g., in man. Thus, lymphocytes of the lung differ from those in other mucosa-covered organs in many aspects.

ACKNOWLEDGMENTS

These studies were supported by a grant from the German Federal Ministry of Research (O1KE88141).

REFERENCES

1. Pabst R. Compartmentalization and kinetics of lymphoid cells in the lung. Reg Immunol 1990; 3:62–71.
2. Reynolds HY. Bronchoalveolar lavage. Am Rev Respir Dis 1987; 135:250–63.
3. Pabst R, Gehrke I. Is the bronchus-associated lymphoid tissue (BALT) an integral structure of the lung in the normal mammals including man? Am J Respir Cell Mol Biol 1990; 3:131–35.
4. Bienenstock J, Befus D. Gut- and bronchus-associated lymphoid tissue. Am J Anat 1984; 170:437–45.
5. Sminia T, Brugge-Gamelkoorn GJ van der. Structure and function of bronchus-associated lymphoid tissue (BALT). Crit Rev Immunol 1989; 9:119–50.
6. Pabst R. The anatomical basis for the immune function of the gut. Anat Embryol 1987; 176: 135–44.
7. Holt PG, Degebrodt A, Venaille T, O'Leary C, Krska K, Flexman J, Farrell H, Shellam G. Preparation of interstitial lung cells by enzymatic digestion of tissue slices: preliminary characterization by morphology and performance in functional assays. Immunology 1985; 54:139–47.
8. Holt PG, Robinson BWS, Reid M, Kees UR, Warton A, Dawson VH, Rose A, Schon-Hegrad M. Extraction of immune and inflammatory cells from human lung parenchyma: Evaluation of an enzymatic digestion procedure. Clin Exp Immunol 1986; 66:188–200.

9. Pabst R, Binns RM, Licence ST, Peter M, Evidence of a selective major vascular marginal pool of lymphocytes in the lung. Am Rev Respir Dis 1987; 136:1213–8.
10. Pabst R, Binns RM. Heterogeneity of lymphocytes homing physiology: several mechanisms operate in the control of migration to lymphoid and non-lymphoid organs in vivo. Immunol Rev 1989; 108:83–109.

90

Paired Nasopharyngeal Lymphoid Tissue in the Rat

An Experimental Model for Waldeyer's Ring Lymphoid Tissue

P. Koornstra, A. Duijvestijn, F. De Jong, L. Vlek, E. Marres, and P. Van Breda Vriesman
Medical Faculty, University of Limburg, Maastricht, The Netherlands

INTRODUCTION

The nasopharyngeal lymphoid tissue of man consists of tonsils, nodules, and diffuse lymphoid tissue, and is called Waldeyer's ring (WR). For years the tonsils were clinically considered to be pharyngeal structures provoking infection rather than preventing and combating infection, and as a result, tonsillectomy was, and in fact still is, a common approach in the treatment of enlarged (reactive) tonsils. More recently, however, indications have been found that tonsillectomy is a risk factor for the development of Hodgkin's disease, autoantibodies, and serum immunoglobulin A (IgA) deficiency (1–3), requiring clinicians to reconsider the necessity of this surgical approach. The WR, as a mucosal lymphoid structure, is probably involved in regulatory processes effecting IgA responses and mucosal tolerance induction (4,5). However, as the precise role of the nasopharyngeal mucosa-associated lymphoid tissue in local or systemic immune responses is not yet clear, immunological investigations are needed. Therefore, we decided to develop a rat experimental model for studying the immunological function of nasopharyngeal lymphoid tissue. In this chapter, we describe the characterization of Waldeyer's ring–equivalent (WRE) lymphoid tissue in the rat with respect to anatomical position, cellular composition, and T- vs B-cell binding potentials of WRE high endothelial venules (HEVs).

MATERIALS AND METHODS

Animals

Lewis rats were obtained from the Central Animal Research Facility at the University of Limburg, The Netherlands. Animals had free access to food and water, and were used at the age of 8 weeks.

Tissue Extirpation

Rats were ether anesthetized. Under a surgical microscope, the palatum between the two molar rows was removed, exposing the rod-shaped lymphoid organs in the left and right first nasal choana. The organs were carefully removed and kept in buffered saline on ice until they were processed. Other lymphoid organs such as cervical and mesenteric lymph nodes, spleen, and Peyer's patches were routinely removed.

Tissue Treatment

Tissues were either snap-frozen in isopentane and stored at –70°C, or routinely fixed with formalin and embedded in paraffin.

Immunohistochemistry

Immunohistochemistry was performed on frozen sections using a two-step immunoperoxidase technique as previously described (6). Briefly, 4-μm thick sections were incubated with specific mouse monoclonal antibodies (MAbs). After washing, the sections were incubated with a peroxidase-conjugated second-step antibody directed at mouse Ig (DAKO, Denmark). Staining was visualized using a diaminobenzidin/hydrogen peroxide solution. For cytoplasmic Ig detection (plasma cells), 4-μm thick paraffin sections were used. Sections were deparaffinized and rehydrated before applying immunoperoxidase staining as described. All sections were counterstained with hematoxylin.

Fluorescent Flow Cytometry

Cell suspensions from various lymphoid organs were prepared from extirpated tissues. Lymphocytes were collected from the tissues by teasing precut tissue pieces on a metal gauze under frequent flushing with buffer containing 2% bovine serum. Using a Percoll gradient, dead cells were removed, resulting in cell suspensions with more than 95% cell viability. Cell suspensions were stained in a two-step immunofluorescence technique using specific mouse MAbs in the first step. In the second step, fluorescinated antibodies directed at mouse Ig (Cappel, USA) were used. Stained cell suspensions were fixed in 1% paraformaldehyde and kept in the dark at 4°C until they were analyzed using fluorescent flow cytometry.

Antibodies

All antibodies were used at saturation concentrations. The following MAbs of mouse origin were used:

MAb	Specificity	Source[a]
W3/13	T cells (granulocytes)	A. Williams
W3/25	T-helper cells (some macrophages)	A. Williams
OX-8	T-cytotoxic/suppressor cells	A. Williams
R73	T-cell receptor αβ (TCR)	T. Hünig
MARK	Ig κ light chain	H. Bazin
MARL	Ig λ light chain	H. Bazin
MARA-2	Ig α heavy chain	H. Bazin
MARG1,2a,2b,2c	Ig (subset) γ heavy chain	H. Bazin

MAb	Specificity	Source[a]
ED-1	Monocytes/macrophages	C. Dijkstra
ED-3	Lymphoid tissue macrophages	C. Dijkstra
ED-5	Follicular dendritic cells	C. Dijkstra
OX-6	Nonpolymorphic Ia determinant	A. Williams
RECA-1	Rat endothelial cell antigen	Our laboratory

[a]MAbs were kindly donated by the persons mentioned.

HEV Binding Assay

To define the binding preference of HEV in the rat WRE for T vs B cells, we used the in vitro HEV-binding assay, slightly modified from the original technique described by Stamper and Woodruff (7). Briefly: freshly cut sections of various lymphoid organs were overlayered with 100 μl suspensions of 10^6 mesenteric lymph node cells, with known T/B ratios in the presence of MAb W3/13. Cells were allowed to bind to HEV for 30 min at 7°C under rotation. Subsequently, the sections were carefully washed in buffer and fixed in 0.2% glutaraldehyde for 10 min followed by 1% paraformaldehyde fixation for 30 min. The sections were then incubated with fluorescinated antibody directed to mouse Ig (Cappel, USA), washed, and examined in an epifluorescent microscope. Fluorescinated T cells vs unlabeled B cells bound to HEV were counted in multiple sections, and the T/B binding ratio was calculated for the various organs studied.

RESULTS

Anatomy and Morphology of Nasopharyngeal Lymphoid Tissue in the Rat

To define lymphoid tissue in the oronasopharynx, cross sections were made of the whole head-neck area of decalcified paraffin-embedded material. Lymphoid tissue was exclusively observed in the left and right first nasal choana. The tissue was rod shaped, about 8 mm in length, and located at the bottom of the nasal choana extending caudally into the nasopharyngeal duct (Fig. 1). Because no other lymphoid tissue could be detected in the nasopharynx, these organs were considered the Waldeyer's ring equivalent (WRE) in the rat. Morphologically, the WRE lymphoid tissue was located directly underneath cuboidal to columnar mucosal epithelium. This epithelium contained intraepithelial lymphocytes, and was sometimes invaginated to cryptlike structures such as observed in human tonsils. The lymphoid mass was organized into follicles and interfollicular areas in which HEV were present.

Immunohistochemistry

Immunoperoxidase staining with MAbs detecting the various lymphocyte B- and T-cell subsets showed the presence of organized T- and B-cell compartments in WRE as known from other lymphoid organs such as lymph nodes and Peyer's patches. B-cell areas were larger than T-cell areas and normally had germinal center (GC) activity as demonstrated by the presence of follicular dendritic cells (ED-5 positive) and the negative appearance of GCs in IgD staining (Fig. 2A,B). T-helper and T–cytotoxic/suppressor cells constituted the T-cell areas which were located predominantly at the nonmucosal side of the WRE

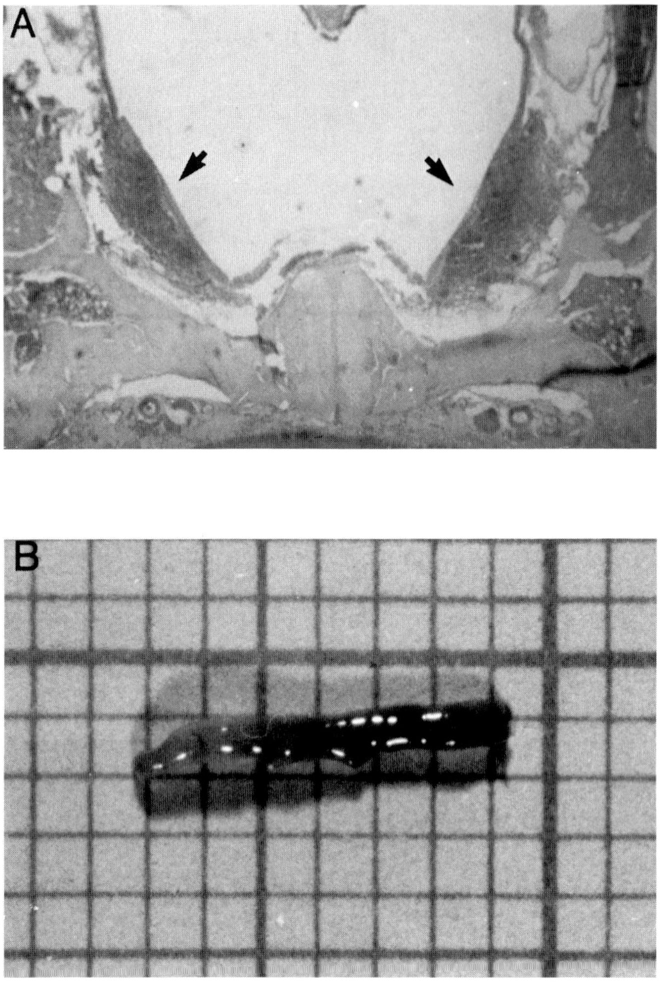

Figure 1 Frontal section through the rat nose/mouth, hematoxylin & eosin stained. Arrows indicate the paired nasopharyngeal lymphoid tissues. (B) An extirpated WRE organ. A small square measures 1 mm^2.

(Fig. 2C,D). T-helper cells, in contrast to T–cyt/sup cells, were also observed in germinal centers.

Staining with ED-1 and ED-3 (see Fig. 1E,F) showed that, in addition to lymphoid tissue macrophages (ED1 and ED3 positive) located at the connective tissue side of the organ, a distinct population of cells of monocyte/macrophage origin (only ED-1 positive) was scattered throughout the lymphoid tissue, especially in the T-cell areas. The HEV and Ia-positive interdigitating cells were present in T-cell areas, as shown by staining with RECA-1 and OX-6, respectively (Fig. 3A,B).

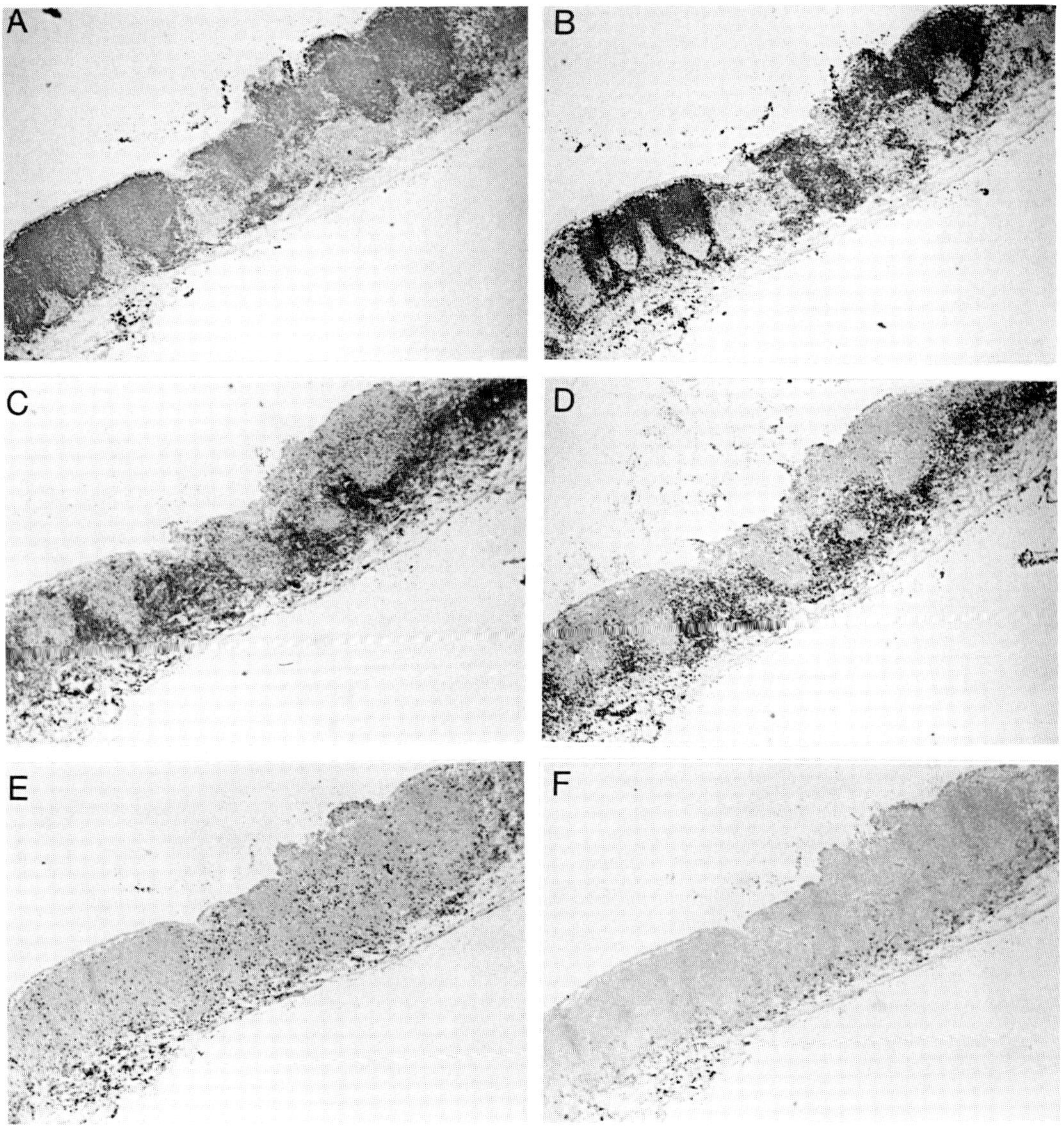

Figure 2 Immunoperoxidase staining on frozen sections of rat WRE tissue. Sections were counterstained with hematoxylin. (A) B-cell staining with MAb MARK. (B) IgD staining with MAb MARD shows germinal centers (IgD negative) in the B-cell areas. (C) T-helper cell staining with MAb W3/25. (D) T–cytotoxic/suppressor cell staining with MAb OX-8. (E) Monocyte/macrophage staining with MAb ED-1. (F) Lymphoid tissue macrophage staining with MAb ED-3.

Staining for plasma cells with either anti-Ig κ chain (MARK) detecting all plasma cells or anti-Ig α chain (MARA) detecting IgA plasma cells, clearly showed: (a) these cells are predominantly located at the connective tissue side and almost never in the covering mucosal epithelium (Fig. 3C); and (b) IgA plasma cells make up a considerable proportion of the total plasma cells present in this area (Fig. 3D).

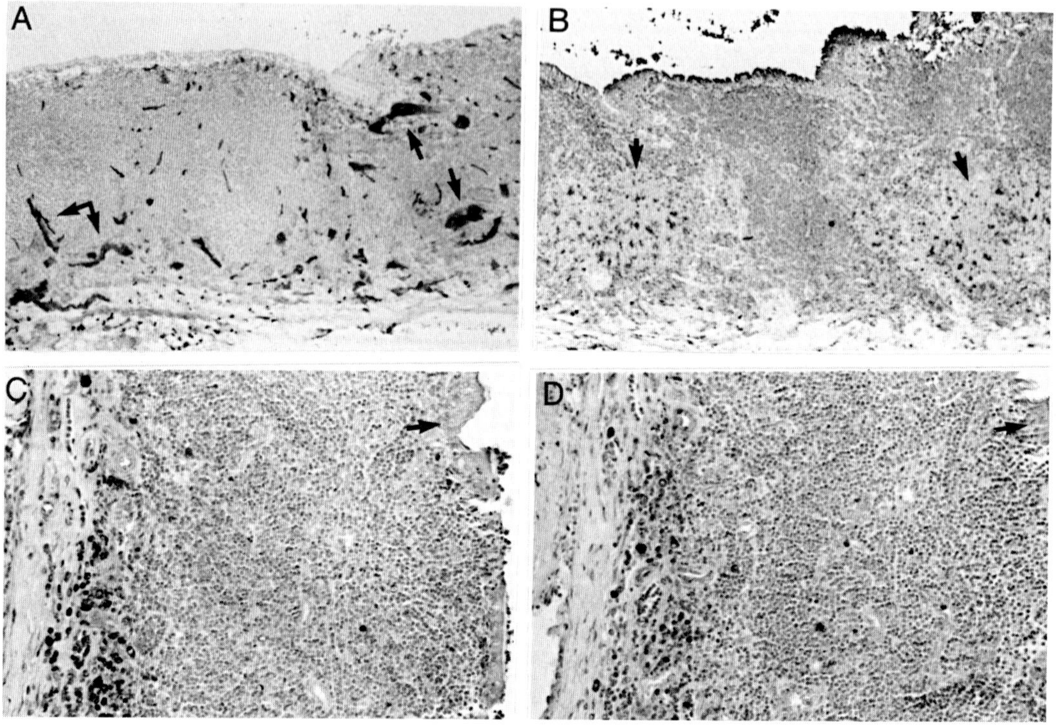

Figure 3 Immunoperoxidase staining on sections of WRE tissue. Sections were counterstained with hematoxylin. (A) Frozen section. Staining of vascular endothelium with MAb RECA-1. Notice the HEV (arrows) in the interfollicular areas. (B) Frozen section. Staining of Ia-positive cells with MAb OX-6 shows strongly positive interdigitating cells in the T-cell areas (arrows). (C) Paraffin section. Staining of plasma cells with MAb MARK. Arrow indicates the mucosal epithelium. (D) Consecutive section stained for IgA plasma cells with MAb MARA-2.

Fluorescent Flow Cytometry

Distribution profiles of lymphocyte subsets in WRE tissue in comparison to other lymphoid organs are shown in Table 1. Because limited numbers of cells could be obtained from single WRE tissues, the data presented for the various lymphoid organs result from cell suspensions pooled from 4–5 animals.

In Vitro Binding of Lymphocytes by HEV in WRE

To define the specificity of HEV in WRE tissue with respect to their potential to mediate T- and B-cell immigration from blood, we measured the adherence of T vs B cells to HEV in frozen WRE sections and compared these data with those obtained from various other lymphoid tissues. The following T/B ratios were obtained:

HEV in WRE: 1.8
HEV in cervical lymph nodes: 3.2
HEV in mesenteric lymph nodes: 1.8
HEV in Peyer's patches: 0.4

Table 1 Distribution Profiles of Lymphocyte Subsets in WRE and Other Lymphoid Tissues

	% of membrane-positive cells						Ratio	
Tissue	T cells	B cells	Th	Tc,s	IgG	IgA	T/B	Th/Tc,s
WRE	36.0	53.7	26.9	5.3	0.1	0.3	0.7	5.1
CLN	73.8	19.5	55.3	14.4	1.1	0.4	3.8	3.8
MLN	76.1	21.1	54.7	12.9	0.1	<0.1	3.6	4.2
PP	11.9	63.9	11.3	1.7	0.7	0.5	0.2	6.6
Spleen	51.2	30.0	38.7	15.5	0.4	1.7	1.7	2.5

Specific MAbs used: R73 (T cells); MARK+MARL (B cells); W3/25 (Th cells = T-helper cells); OX-8 (Tc,s cells = T–cytotoxic/suppressor cells); MARG1+2a+2b+2c (IgG); MARA-2 (IgA).
Abbreviations: WRE, Waldeyer's ring equivalent; CLN, cervical lymph node; MLN, mesenteric lymph node; PP, Peyer's patch.

DISCUSSION AND CONCLUSIONS

Nasopharyngeal lymphoid tissue in the rat appeared to consist of paired rod-shaped lymphoid organs located in the first nasal choana. We consider this lymphoid tissue to be an equivalent of human tonsillar structures, and because no other lymphoid tissue was found in the rat oronasopharynx, these lymphoid organs comprise the Waldeyer's ring equivalent in the rat. The WRE tissue is a well-organized lymphoid structure containing all immunological prerequisites for adequate immune responding in case of antigenic challenge. B cells are obviously preponderant over T cells (T/B ratio of 0.7), as was demonstrated by histological and flow cytometrical analysis. In this respect, WRE tissue most resembled Peyer's patches (PPs). In addition, WRE is closest to PPs with respect to the high ratio of T-helper cells to T–cytotoxic/suppressor cells of both organs. This, in combination with its association with the mucosal epithelium, classifies the WRE among the mucosa-associated lymphoid tissues, and thus suggests an important role of this tissue in characteristic mucosal immunological aspects such as IgA production and induction of mucosal tolerance. However, the HEV-binding data show that, with respect to T- and B-cell immigration from blood, WRE tissue is distinct from PPs, e.g., there is a preferential T-cell adherence to HEV in WRE in contrast to the preferential B cell adherence to HEV in PPs. In this respect, the WRE more resembles bronchus-associated lymphoid tissue and the mesenteric lymph nodes (8). Such HEV specificity has previously been demonstrated for human tonsillar HEV (9). We conclude that: (a) the rat has distinct, anatomically defined nasopharyngeal lymphoid organs, (b) the organs appear as immunocompetent lymphoid structures belonging to the mucosa-associated lymphoid tissues, (c) this nasopharyngeal lymphoid tissue has also properties distinct from other mucosal lymphoid tissues, suggesting a special function in local immune responses, (d) these organs can be considered to be Waldeyer's ring equivalent lymphoid tissue in the rat, and as such, the rat WRE seems a useful experimental model for exploring the immunological significance of Waldeyer's ring in man.

ACKNOWLEDGMENTS

The authors thank H. van Rie for technical assistance in histological work, and N. Genders for secretarial support.

REFERENCES

1. Vianna NJ, Greenwald P, Davies JNP. Tonsillectomy and Hodgkin's disease: The lymphoid tissue barrier. Lancet 1971; 2:431–2.
2. Yoshida Y, Yamauchi S, Miyaki H, Okamoto K, Ozawa A. Tonsillectomy and autoantibodies in patients with habitual tonsillitis. Auris Nasus Larynx (Tokyo) 1980; 7:151–7.
3. D'Amelio R, Palmisano L, Le Moli S, Seminara R, Aiuti F. Serum and salivary IgA levels in normal subjects: Comparison between tonsillectomized and non-tonsillectomized subjects. Int Arch Allergy Immunol 1982; 68:256–9.
4. Mestecky J, Russell MW, Jackson S, Brown TA. The human IgA system: A reassessment. Clin Immunol Immunopathol 1986; 40:105–14.
5. Mattingly JA, Wakson BH. Immunologic suppression after oral administration of antigen. I. Specific suppressor cells formed in rat Peyer's patches after oral administration of sheep erythrocytes and their systemic migration. J Immunol 1978; 121:1878–83.
6. Duijvestijn AM, Kerkhove M, Bargatze RF, Butcher EC. Lymphoid tissue- and inflammation-specific endothelial cell differentiation defined by monoclonal antibodies. J Immunol 1987; 138:713–9.
7. Stamper HB, Woodruff JJ. Lymphocyte homing into lymph nodes: in vitro demonstration of the selective affinity of recirculating lymphocytes for high endothelial venules. J Exp Med 1976; 144:828–33.
8. Van der Brugge-Gamelkoorn GJ, Kraal G. The specificity of the high endothelial venule in bronchus associated lymphoid tissue (BALT). J Immunol 1985; 134:3746–50.
9. Pals ST, Kraal G, Horst E, de Groot A, Scheper RJ, Meijer CJLM. Human lymphocyte-high endothelial venule interaction: organ selective binding of T and B lymphocyte populations to high endothelium. J Immunol 1986; 137:760–3.

91

Ontogeny of Macrophages and Dendritic Cells in the Mucosal Immune System of the Rat

Emmelien P. van Rees, Marja B. van der Ende, and Taede Sminia
Vrije Universiteit, Amsterdam, The Netherlands

INTRODUCTION

Many studies have dealt with the existence of a common mucosal immune system, reviewed by Mestecky (1), including the gastrointestinal, respiratory, and female urogenital tracts. Respiratory and intestinal tissue have in common that both are heavily challenged with antigens immediately after birth. The ability to generate a sufficient systemic or mucosal immune response to pathogenic microorganisms is limited during early postnatal life. As a consequence, neonates of most species are highly susceptible to infections by viruses and bacteria, which can have a systemic or mucosal portal of entry.

Macrophages and dendritic cells (DCs) play a significant role in the immune response as regulator and antigen-presenting cells. As many antigens challenge the mucosal surfaces of newborns, the contribution of mucosal macrophages and DCs in antigen uptake and in the induction and regulation of local and systemic immune responses is of importance.

The aim of the present study was to compare the development of macrophages and DCs in pulmonary tissue and bronchus-associated lymphoid tissue (BALT) (2) to that in intestinal tissue and gut-associated lymphoid tissue (GALT) (3).

A panel of monoclonal antibodies (MAbs) has been described that recognize rat macrophage subpopulations (ED-1, ED-2 and ED-3) (4). Nonlymphoid cells were considered macrophages if they were recognized by one of these MAbs, showed strong acid phosphatase activity, weak or no expression of Ia-antigen, and did not have a dendritic morphology. Dendritic cells were defined by weak acid phosphatase activity, abundant expression of Ia, and a dendritic morphology; i.e., a cell shape in which dendrites and veils of cytoplasm extend in several directions from the cell body. Using the mentioned criteria to distinguish macrophages and DCs, the ontogeny in respiratory and intestinal tissue was compared.

MATERIALS AND METHODS

Pregnant Wistar rats were obtained from Harlan, (Zeist, The Netherlands). After cesarian section whole fetuses from 15, 16, 17, 18 and 20 days after conception were frozen in liquid nitrogen and stored at –70°C. Neonatal rats were sacrificed on the day of birth (day 0), and on several points of time after birth. Lungs and gut were taken out; before being frozen in liquid nitrogen, the lungs were filled by injection in the main bronchus with gelatin in aquadest (4%) to prevent collapse of the lung tissue. A two-step immunoperoxidase method was used (6,7) on cryostat sections, applying various monoclonal antibodies (MAbs). Stainings for Ia expression (MAb Ox6, Serotec) and ED-positive macrophages (all MAbs are commercially available) were carried out on consecutive sections. Acid phosphatase activity was demonstrated (8). Double-staining procedures for immunoperoxidase and acid phosphatase activity were also carried out.

Quantification of cells was carried out on at least 10 microscopic fields of three sections for each specimen. Owing to the filling of neonatal lungs with gelatin dissolved in aquadest, it was possible to make a clear distinction between alveolar cells and cells attached to alveolar walls or in mesenchymal lung tissue.

RESULTS

Macrophages

Intestinal Tissue

These results have been described before in detail (3). In summary: The first macrophages to be recognized by ED-1 appeared in the liver, being the hemopoietic organ in fetal animals, on day 15 of gestation (Table 1). These cells did not express Ia antigen and did not have a dendritic morphology, but showed abundant acid phosphatase activity. In developing mesenteric lymph nodes and in the gut wall, ED-1–positive macrophages were found for the first time on days 17 and 18 of gestation, respectively. On day 21, an accumulation of ED-1–positive cells was visible in the gut wall under slightly dome-shaped epithelium, representing developing Peyer's patches.

Table 1 Ontogeny of Macrophages and Dendritic Cells in the Rat Gut

Days	15F	17F	20F	0	4	14
ED-1 liver	+	++	++	++	++	++
mesench.	–	+	+	+	+	+
gut wall	–	–	+	+	+	+
ED-2 liver	–	±	++	++	++	++
mesench.	–	–	±	++	++	++
gut wall	–	–	–	+	+	+
aIa liver	–	–	–	±	±	±
mesench.	±	+	++	++	++	++
gut wall	–	+	++	++	++	++

Symbols: –, not seen; ±, 1–5 cells per microscopic field (magnification: ×400); +, 5–10 cells per field; ++, 10–20 cells per field.

Until birth, ED-2 recognized few cells in the gut-associated tissue; on the day of birth this subpopulation showed a sudden increase. Peyer's patches also contained ED-2–positive cells from the day of birth. In mesenteric lymph nodes, the first ED-2–positive cells were present on day 2 after birth.

The distribution pattern of the macrophage subpopulation that is recognized by ED-3 appeared to be similar in fetal and adult rats; in gut-associated tissue, it was confined to developing mesenteric lymph nodes (from day 19 of gestation) and Peyer's patches (from day 21 of fetal life).

Respiratory Tissue

Early fetal lung tissue was composed of loose mesenchymal tissue with epithelial tubules in it. From day 17 of gestation, saccular extensions of the tubules were formed, compressing the mesenchymal tissue to septal walls between the luminal spaces. On day 17 of gestation, ED-1 recognized cells that were dispersed in the mesenchymal tissue of the lung (Table 2). These cells displayed the same features as the early ED-1–positive cells in the liver and in mesenchyme surrounding the intestine. Alveolar macrophages, appearing in large numbers directly after birth, always were ED-1 positive. As soon as BALT was recognizable, it contained many scattered ED-1–positive cells; i.e., after the fourth postnatal day.

Only a few ED-2–positive macrophages were found from day 20 of gestation scattered over the mesenchyme, but immediately after birth the number of these cells showed a conspicuous increase. From the day of birth ED-2 recognized many cells, evenly spread over the tissue surrounding the alveolar pouches. Yet, after postnatal day 4, the number decreased, and from day 10 ED-2–positive macrophages were only present in peribronchial or perivascular tissue. ED-2 reactivity could not be detected in BALT.

Respiratory tissue, including BALT, was almost devoid of ED-3 throughout development.

Dendritic Cells

Intestinal Tissue

Ia-positive cells appeared very early in ontogeny, on day 15. The first Ia-positive cells recognized by MAb Ox6 had a dendritic morphology with veils of cytoplasm extending in several directions. They were found in the mesenchymal tissue between the intestinal loops. From day 18, many Ia-positive cells with a dendritic appearance were demonstrable in the

Table 2 Ontogeny of Macrophages and Dendritic Cells in the Rat Lung

Days	15F	17F	20F	0	4	14
ED-1 interst.	–	±	±	+	±	–
alveolar	–	–	–	–	+	++
ED-2 interst.	–	–	+	++	++	±
alveolar	–	–	–	–	–	–
aIa interst.	+(16F)	+	+	+	+	++
alveolar	–	–	–	–	–	–

Symbols: –, not seen; ±, 1–5 cells per microscopic field (magnification: ±400); +, 5–10 cells per field, ++, 10–20 cells per field.

gut wall and in developing mesenteric lymph nodes. From day 21 of gestation, prospective Peyer's patches contained Ia-positive dendritic cells under dome-shaped epithelium.

Respiratory Tissue

Ia-positive cells with a dendritic morphology were found on day 16 of gestation. During ontogeny, the number of cells labeled by MAb Ox6 gradually increased, and they were always found in the mesenchymal tissue of the lung and in perivascular or peribronchial areas. Alveolar macrophages did not reveal any expression of Ia antigen. As soon as BALT was found, it contained cells with a distinct dendritic morphology and an abundant expression of Ia antigen.

DISCUSSION

ED-1 labeled macrophages in respiratory and in intestinal tissue from day 17 of gestation, as in brain and kidney (3). Earlier, on days 15 and 16, ED-1 recognized cells in the liver only, which organ has a hemopoietic function at that time. As ED-1 recognizes macrophages and monocytes (4), it can be concluded from these data that this subpopulation of macrophages is dispersed over the fetal organs on day 17.

Nasal-associated lymphoid tissue (NALT), which was not included in the present study, accounts for the mucosa-associated lymphoid tissue of the upper respiratory tract. This is located near the anterior orifice of the nasopharyngeal duct (12). As on the day of birth already many ED-1–positive cells were found on these locations (13), nasal-associated lymphoid tissue probably exists before birth. As BALT could not be found before day 4 after birth, this implies that the upper respiratory tract plays a more important role in the immunological defense of neonatal rats than the lower respiratory tract.

ED-2 recognizes a differentiation antigen on mature macrophages (5). It was remarkable that in lung tissue from 1 day before birth until day 10 after birth, many macrophages in septal walls were reactive to ED-2, contrary to the situation in older rats. ED-2 also appeared around birth in gut-associated tissue and thymus (9), but on these locations the number of ED-2–positive cells increased during further development and did not decrease as in the lung. Probably this is related to the relative lack of connective tissue in adult lung, apart from small amounts of peribronchial and perivascular connective tissue.

ED-3–positive macrophages are present at distinct sites in lymphoid organs; i.e., in the marginal zone of the spleen and in the marginal sinus and medulla of lymph nodes (4), and to a lesser extent also in Peyer's patches (3). Functional studies have shown that marginal zone macrophages are engaged in the antibody response against thymus-independent type 2 antigens (10,11). Neonatal lymph nodes and Peyer's patches contained ED-3–positive macrophages, as did NALT (13). As ED-3 did not recognize any cell in BALT, this may indicate that BALT does not play a role of importance in the mucosal defense against bacterial thymus-independent antigens.

Ia-positive cells with a dendritic morphology appeared in large numbers early in ontogeny (day 15 of gestation) in the mesenchymal tissue surrounding the gut (3). A comparable early occurrence of Ia-positive cells (day 16) was found in respiratory tissue. The only other organ where Ia is demonstrable at this stage in fetal life is the thymus (14). Lu et al. (15) suggested that the early Ia-positive cells in the thymus might be important in the restriction of autoimmunity via suppression, whereas the later developing Ia-positive dendritic cells may play a role in the development of immunocompetence. Comparable to this possible suppressive function of early thymic Ia-positive cells, the function of similar cells, found on day 15-16 in respiratory and intestinal tissues, also might be a suppressive one. The induction of tolerance to nonpathogenic antigens in the aeroalimentary tract is an important phenomenon in neonatal life.

REFERENCES

1. Mestecky J. The common mucosal immune system and current strategies for induction of immune responses in external secretions. J Clin Immunol 1987; 7:265–276.
2. Van Rees EP, Van der Ende MB, Sminia T. Ontogeny of macrophage subpopulations and Ia-positive dendritic cells in pulmonary tissue of the rat. Cell Tissue Res (in press).
3. Van Rees EP, Dijkstra CD, Van der Ende MB, Janse EM, Sminia T. The ontogenetic development of macrophage subpopulations and Ia-positive non-lymphoid cells in gut-associated lymphoid tissue of the rat. Immunology 1988; 63:79–85.
4. Dijkstra CD, Döpp EA, Joling P, Kraal G. The heterogeneity of mononuclear phagocytes in lymphoid organs: Distinct macrophage subpopulations in rat recognized by monoclonal antibodies ED1, ED2 and ED3. Immunology 1985; 54:589–599.
5. Beelen RHJ, Eestermans IL, Döpp EA, Dijkstra CD. Monoclonal antibodies ED1, ED2, and ED3 against rat macrophages: expression of recognized antigens in different stages of differentiation. Transplant Proceed 1987; 19:3166–3170.
6. Dijkstra CD, Döpp EA. Ontogenetic development of T and B lymphocytes and non-lymphoid cells in the white pulp of the rat spleen. Cell Tissue Res 1983; 229:351–363.
7. Graham RC, Karnovsky MC. The early stages of absorption of injected horseradish peroxidase in the proximal tubules of mouse kidney: ultrastructural cytochemistry by a new technique. J Histochem Cytochem 1966; 14:291–302.
8. Burstone MS. Histochemical comparison of naphthol phosphates for the demonstration of phosphatases. J Natl Cancer Inst 1958; 20:601–616.
9. Van Rees EP, Voorbij HAM, Dijkstra CD. Neonatal development of lymphoid organs and specific immune responses in situ in diabetes-prone BB rats. Immunology 1988; 65:465–472.
10. Van Rooijen N, Van Nieuwmegen R. Elimination of phagocytic cells in the spleen after intravenous injection of liposome-encapsulated dichloromethylene diphosphonate. An enzyme-histochemical study. Cell Tissue Res 1984; 238:355–360.
11. Claassen E, Kors N, Van Rooijen N. Influence of carriers on the development and localization of anti-TNP antibody forming cells in the murine spleen. II. Suppressed antibody response to TNP-Ficoll after elimination of marginal zone cells. Eur J Immunol 1986; 16:492–496.
12. Spit BJ, Hendriksen EGJ, Bruijntjes JP, Kuper CF. Nose-associated lymphoid tissue (NALT) in the rat. Ultramicroscopy 1987; 21:201–210.
13. Hameleers DMH, Van der Ende M, Biewenga J, Sminia T. An immunohistochemical study on the postnatal development of rat nasal-associated lymphoid tissue (NALT). Cell Tissue Res 1989; 259:371–377.
14. Duijvestijn AM, Sminia T, Köhler YG, Janse EM, Hoefsmit ECM. Ontogeny of the rat thymus micro-environment: development of the interdigitating cell and macrophage populations. Dev Comp Immunol 1984; 8:451–460.
15. Lu CY, Beller DI, Unanue ER. During ontogeny, Ia-bearing accessory cells are found early in the thymus but late in the spleen. Proc Natl Acad Sci USA 1980; 77:1597–1601.

IMMUNOLOGICAL TOLERANCE

92
What Do We Know About Immunological Tolerance?

Rolf M. Zinkernagel
University Hospital, Zurich, Switzerland

The question of how immunological tolerance is induced and maintained is an obviously crucial one to understand the immunological discrimination between self and nonself. The word *tolerance* reflects more the idea, *responsiveness* is what we measure, and *unresponsiveness* is the experimental finding indicating that tolerance may be operative (1). These definitions make the difficulties of many experiments on tolerance obvious: the attempt to prove something, i.e., the idea of tolerance, with the absence of something, i.e., the absence of responsiveness. However, negative results have rarely if ever convinced scientists, whereas positive findings do so much more readily. For this reason T-cell receptor (TCR) studies in transgenic mice have been very gratifying (2,3); here unresponsiveness has been positively correlated with unequivocal evidence: A particular TCR is genetically there or expressed in early thymocytes and disappears thereafter upon contact with appropriate antigens in the thymus. Therefore, clonal abortion—elimination—is generally accepted. Most other evidence that attempts to illustrate or prove tolerance are on much less safer experimental grounds.

Immunologists distinguish between central and peripheral tolerance; while central (thymic) tolerance is well documented and accepted, phenotypes and mechanisms of peripheral tolerance remain elusive (4). On one side it is argued that peripheral tolerance of T cells is necessary to inactivate those T cells specific for epitopes that may not be presented in the thymus or the T cells that express possibly generated somatic variants of TCR. On the other extreme side, one might argue that the absence of somatic variants found in T cells so far is a hint at the "genetic stability" or short livedness of effector T cells, rendering a peripheral tolerance mechanism superfluous.

In our view, there are two important experimental issues which appear to blurr the views of tolerance, particularly with respect to central (in the thymus) versus peripheral (thymus-independent) T-cell tolerance. First, we do not know what measurement in vitro does reflect the affinity and avidity situation relevant in vivo. Is a proliferative response measured by [^{3}H]thymidine uptake or interleukin-3 (IL-2) release a reflection of a low-affinity cross-reactive stimulation, which has little to do with the specific response? Unless biologically relevant readouts in vivo can be linked directly to the readout systems in vitro, we will probably not know the answer to this question. Therefore, we may risk the playing immunological games as *art pour l'art* to have results but not to understand the self/nonself discrimination. Immunology has gone through similar states before. Once, chemically defined haptens and antibody responses against them had been thought to truly reflect immunological specificity rules (5), now we have learned that this may not necessarily be so because too many heterogeneous receptors with vastly different affinities can bind to haptens. Maybe proliferation assays in vitro with poorly defined T-cell–containing populations may be similarly nondiscriminatory with respect to affinity-avidity requirements. Nevertheless, there are certain experiments that may be revealing: One key experiment should be to have an antigen expressed in the periphery that can be shown to be recognized by biologically relevant *effector* T cells but that fails to induce tolerance; i.e., relevant effector T cells can be induced in the host despite the presence of the antigenic epitope in the periphery. Such an experimental result should be a strong point against peripheral tolerance-anergy to exist generally as postulated.

Second, antigen unprocessed or processed (alone or associated with secreted major histocompatibility complex products) may reach the thymus on antigen-presenting cells or otherwise without becoming detectable experimentally. For example, if an alloantigen is expressed in one specific tissue without rejection, then tolerance may be operative, but it remains unclear whether the alloantigens have found the way to the thymus or whether unresponsiveness truly reflects what is called peripheral anergy. Therefore, unless peripheral tolerance studies with a negative (i.e., "anergic") readout can be done in thymectomized mice, this issue remains open. Also for this question, positive demonstration of antigen in the periphery *without* T-cell anergy again should be a decisive experiment disproving a general role for peripheral anergy.

The papers presented in this session and the chapters in this section reflect the exciting side of new experiments but they illustrate well the experimental problems and limitations mentioned. Probably we all must still think, work hard, and do simple experiments before we understand immunological tolerance better than in Compiègne.

REFERENCES

1. Cohn, M. 1986. The ground rules determining any solution to the problem of the self/nonself discrimination. In: *The Tolerance Workshop*. P. Matzinger et al. (ed). Editiones <Roche>, Basel, Switzerland, p. 3.
2. von Boehmer, H., and P. Kisielow. 1990. Self-nonself discrimination by T cells. Science 248:1369–1372.
3. Arnold, B., C. Goodnow, H. Hengartner, and G.J. Hämmerling. 1989. The coming of transgenic mice: Tolerance and immune reactivity. Immunol. Today 11:69-72.
4. Schwartz, R. H. 1990. A cell culture model for T lymphocyte clonal anergy. Science 248: 1349–1356.
5. Roitt, I., J. Brostoff, and D. Male. 1985. *Immunology*. Gower, London, p. 1.1.

93

Donor Haplotype Tolerance in Athymic Nude Rats After Implantation of Allogeneic Cultured Thymic Fragments

Cees de Heer,[1] **Roel Broekhuizen,**[2] **Henk-Jan Schuurman,**[1,2] **and Jan Rozing**[3]

[1]*National Institute of Public Health and Environmental Protection, Bilthoven, The Netherlands;* [2]*University Hospital, Utrecht, The Netherlands;* [3]*TNO Institute for Experimental Gerontology, Rijswijk, The Netherlands*

INTRODUCTION

After implantation of cultured thymic fragments (CTFs), congenitally athymic (nude) rats develop an immunocompetent T-cell system (1–3). This immunocompetence includes the in vivo and in vitro reactivity after allogeneic stimulation. For CTF of allogeneic origin, this in vitro alloreactivity is to donor haplotype, but not to host haplotype. In contrast, skin grafts of donor haplotype are not rejected, and the CTF graft (with restored thymic architecture) shows no signs of rejection (2,3). Thus, there is a state of in vitro alloreactivity but in vivo tolerance to the donor haplotype after allo-CTF implantation. This discrepancy was subsequently investigated by implantation of CTFs from two different donor strains. In this experiment, skin transplants of both the donor strains were rejected (3). From these data it was suggested that T cells with alloreactivity to one particular donor haplotype were generated in the CTFs coming from the other donor strain. In addition, this experiment indicated that the observation of in vivo tolerance in the presence of in vitro alloreactivity cannot be explained by peripheral tolerance or suppression, but rather by selection processes of precursor T lymphocytes in the grafted CTFs. The graft shows a chimeric state, with the stationary epithelium being of donor type, and the passenger leukocytes (including medullary interdigitating dendritic cells) being of recipient type. The medulla area in the graft shows RT1 class I expression of both donor and recipient, and RT1 class II of only the recipient. Assuming that negative selection occurs in the medullalike area, cells reactive to donor class II are not negatively selected. Such cells in the periphery can manifest in vitro alloreactions to donor haplotype, but are unable to mediate in vivo rejection of donor skin grafts.

This phenomenon was further explored in the present study, in which CTFs from two different donor strains were implanted not only separately, but also after mixing.

EXPERIMENTAL DESIGN

Twelve rnu/rnu rats (10 weeks old) of the WAG/CPB strain ($RT1^u$) were implanted either with CTFs from heterozygous +/rnu littermates (designated +/rnu-CTF, n=3), CTFs from BN/BiRij ($RT1^n$) origin (BN-CTF, n=3), +/rnu-CTF at one kidney and BN-CTF at the other kidney (double-CTF, n=3), or a mix of +/rnu and BN-CTF (ratio 1:1) at each kidney (mix-CTF, n=3). The preparation of CTFs was done as described earlier (1). Four rnu/rnu animals and 2 +/rnu littermates serves as controls.

Eighteen weeks after implantation immune competence was analyzed by ovalbumin (OA) immunization. All but three animals showed anti-OA antibodies. These three animals (2 +/rnu-CTF and 1 mix-CTF animal) did reject allogeneic skin, and were therefore considered to have developed immunocompetence. The ^{2}log titers at 25 days after immunization in responding animals ranged between 5 and 9, which values were in the same range as those in +/rnu animals. Thirty-two weeks after transplantation, skin transplants of WAG/Rij, BN/BiRij, and PVG/Ola ($RT1^c$) origin were performed on the back. Rejection was scored by regular macroscopic reading of the graft until autopsy 5 weeks later.

All animals were sacrificed at 37 weeks after CTF implantation. The CTFs, mesenteric lymph nodes, and spleen were removed. Immunohistology was performed on 6-μm sections of snap-frozen CTF transplants and mesenteric lymph nodes, to detect T-cell differentiation antigens, RT1 class I ($RT1^u$, U9-F4-B1; $RT1^n$, OX27) and class II ($RT1^u$, HIS19; $RT1^n$, F17-23-02) expression. Mixed lymphocyte cultures (MLCs) were performed using spleen cell suspensions. All techniques were done as described elsewhere (1–3).

RESULTS AND DISCUSSION

All CTF-treated animals responded in in vitro MLC to both BN and third-party (PVG) stimulator cells (Table 1). Differences were observed when the MLC data were expressed in ratio of response after BN over PVG stimulation. Animals that had received a BN-CTF (with or without +/rnu-CTF) showed a lower BN/PVG ratio than animals with only a +/rnu-CTF or +/rnu control animals. Following the negative selection hypothesis (mentioned above), this phenomenon may be related to a less frequency of anti-$RT1^n$ reactive cells compared to anti-$RT1^c$ reactive cells in animals with a BN-CTF. One animal in the mix-CTF group showed a BN/PVG ratio of 1.15 (see Table 1). The CTF of this animal at autopsy did not show (epithelial) cells expressing $RT1^n$ major histocompatibility complex molecules, and should therefore be considered as a +/rnu-CTF rather than a mix-CTF animal. This conclusion fits with the 1.15 BN/PVG ratio. Stimulation indexes (ratio allogeneic/syngeneic stimulation) ranged between 2.9 and 10.2, which is in the same range as +/rnu controls (6.1): rnu/rnu controls were negative in MLC.

All CTF-treated and +/rnu control animals rejected the third-party (PVG) skin graft, which confirms the T-cell immunocompetence generated after CTF implantation. The +/rnu controls and +/rnu-CTF animals showed rejection of the $RT1^u$ graft (see Table 1). This is presumably due to minor differences between the Wag substrains used for CTF preparation (WAG/CPB +/rnu) and for skin grafts (WAG/Rij +/+). None of the animals with BN-CTF generated such reactivity; WAG/Rij skin was not rejected.

The +/rnu-CTF and double-CTF animals showed rejection of BN skin. This observation confirms our previous data using CTF-transplants from two different allogeneic strains

Table 1 In Vivo and In Vitro Alloreactivity of Athymic Nude Rats After Implantation of CTF from Different Origin and Control Rats

Animal	n	Skin graft rejection[a] WAG ($RT1^u$)	BN ($RT1^n$)	PVG ($RT1^c$)	In vitro reactivity: ratio BN/PVG alloreactivity[b]
rnu/rnu animals					
+/rnu-CTF	3	±[d]	+	+	1.08 (0.94–1.30)
BN-CTF	3	–	–	+	0.56 (0.20–0.77)
Double-CTF[c]	3	–	+	+	0.72 (0.45–0.97)
Mix-CTF[c]	3	–	–[e]	+	0.55 (0.18–0.92)[d]
Control animals					
+/rnu	2	+[d]	+	+	0.97 (0.93–1.01)
rnu/rnu	4	–	–	–	–[f]

[a]Rejection was monitored macroscopically. + denotes rejection within 10–12 days after grafting, – denotes acceptance until 5 weeks after grafting.
[b]In vitro alloreactivity was measured in mixed lymphocyte cultures and is given as the ratio of alloreactivity to BN (in cpm) over the alloreactivity to PVG (in cpm). Data as mean values, within brackets ranges. (3×10^5 responders with 2×10^5 stimulators, 5 days culture, final 6-hr incorporation of [^{3}H]thymidine).
[c]Double-CTF animals were implanted with +/rnu-CTF at one kidney and BN-CTF at the other kidney; mix-CTF animals received a mixture of +/rnu and BN-CTF (ratio 1:1) at each kidney.
[d]Rejection probably due to minor differences between the Wag substrains used for CTF preparation (WAG/CPB) and skin donation (WAG/Rij).
[e]Data from two animals: The third one with a value of 1.15 did not show $RT1^n$ expression in CTF at autopsy and therefore was representing a +/rnu-CTF. This animal rejected BN skin.
[f]BN/PVG ratio is not calculated because the MLC responsiveness was negative.

(3). The animal with a mix-CTF, showing at autopsy no expression of $RT1^n$ in the graft, did reject BN skin. This fits with the status of a +/rnu-CTF rather than of a mix-CTF, and accords with the 1.15 BN/PVG ratio in MLCs. The other two mix-CTF animals did not reject BN skin. This observation can be explained by the negative selection hypothesis mentioned above because BN-derived components are present in a similar way in the mix-CTF as in a BN-CTF. The mix-CTF represents a chimeric state of the epithelial component (both $RT1^u$ and $RT1^n$ haplotype): In this condition $RT1^n$-derived cells apparently are effective in mediating negative selection of cells with anti-$RT1^n$ class I reactivity. Obviously our data do not exclude the possibility of only partial negative selection. In this condition, anti-$RT1^n$ alloreactive cells are allowed to pass this chimeric CTF owing to the lower density of $RT1^n$-expressing cells, but are present in the periphery at a too low frequency to mediate $RT1^n$ skin graft rejection. We were unable to perform limiting dilution experiments to investigate this possibility in detail.

In conclusion, the model of allogeneic CTF implantation in athymic animals is useful to study intrathymic selection events for alloreactive T-cells. When combined with our previous studies, both the stationary epithelium and passenger leukocyte population (interdigitating cells) have a function in negative selection of such alloreactive cells. Even in condition of a less density of the stationary phase involved (mix-CTF), this micro-environment is sufficient to induce tolerance, as seen by the acceptance of the respective skin graft.

REFERENCES

1. Schuurman H-J, Vaessen LMB, Vos JG, Hertogh A, Geertzema JGN, Brandt CJWM, Rozing J. Implantation of cultured thymic fragments in congenitally athymic nude rats: Ignorance of thymic epithelial haplotype in generation of alloreactivity. J Immunol 1986; 137:2440–7.
2. Schuurman H-J, Vaessen LMB, Broekhuizen R, Brandt CJWM, Holewijn MC, Vos JG, Rozing J. Implantation of cultured thymic fragments in congenitally athymic (nude) rats. Influx of lymphocytes and dendritic cells. Scand J Immunol 1987; 26:129–39.
3. Schuurman H-J, Rozing J, Broekhuizen R, Tielen F, Van de Bergh P. Implantation of cultured thymic fragments in athymic nude rats: studies on tolerance towards donor haplotype. Thymus 1989; 13:123–8.

94
Tolerance to Embryonic Tissue Grafts in Avian Chimeras

Claude Martin,[1] Hiroko Ohki-Hamazaki,[2] and Catherine Corbel[1]
[1]*Institut d'Embryologie cellulaire et moléculaire du CNRS et du Collège de France, Nogent-sur-Marne, France;* [2]*Chiba University, Chiba, Japan*

INTRODUCTION

It is widely accepted that tolerance to self-antigens is acquired during ontogeny (Owen, 1945). Self–major histocompatibility complex (MHC) tolerance and self-MHC restriction result from interactions of lymphoid precursors with other cells in the thymus (Ready et al., 1984; Jenkinson et al., 1985; von Boehmer and Hafen, 1986; Sprent et al., 1988). Deletion of autoreactive clones by the thymus seems to be the main mechanism by which the animal is rendered tolerant to self-components (Kisielow et al., 1988; Kappler et al., 1987; Kappler et al., 1988; MacDonald et al., 1988). However, the respective roles of the different thymic stroma cells, thymic epithelium of endodermic origin, and hemopoietically derived dendritic cells in this process remain unclear. In addition to the decisive role played by the thymus, the possibility of extrathymic mechanisms for inducing tolerance has repeatedly been proposed (Lafferty et al., 1983; Allison et al., 1988; Lo et al., 1988; Markmann et al., 1988; Morahan et al., 1989; Böhme et al., 1989; Lo et al., 1989). Does there exist a "fail safe" mechanism which prevents potentially autoreactive cells that happen to escape deletion in the thymus to be activated?

Classic as well as recent microsurgical techniques have made the avian embryo accessible to manipulations not only during early embryogenesis, but also throughout the period of organogenesis. Avian chimeras can be constructed by transplantation of defined anlagen in the embryo, thus offering a tool to study the immunological status of an adult host somatically modified before the development of the immune system (Martin, 1990). Moreover, taking advantage of the characteristic structure of the quail nucleus, in quail-chick chimeras the precise participation of the grafted tissue in the host can be defined (Le Douarin, 1969). We report here the fate of early grafted wings in allogeneic and xenogeneic combinations. Tissue tolerance has been obtained in chick-chick and chick-quail but not in quail-chick chimeras. However, the graft of the quail thymic epithelium along with the quail wing bud results in permanent tolerance of both organs.

MATERIAL AND METHODS

Eggs of quails and white Leghorn chicks from commercial sources were used in this study. We also used the congenic lines CC and CB (MHC haplotypes B4 and B12, respectively) and F_1 from a cross between two inbred lines B15 × B21. These eggs were kindly provided by Dr. Hlozanek (Institute of Molecular Genetics, Praha, Czechoslovakia).

The wing rudiment was retrieved from a donor embryo (stages 15–18 according to Zacchei [1961] for the quail, stages 19–25 according to Hamburger and Hamilton [1951] for the chick) and substituted to its counterpart in a stage-matched recipient. The rudiment was maintained by platinum staples according to Hampé (1959).

Thymic chimeras result from isochronic and isotopic transplantation of the rudiment of the thymus from quail at 4.5 day of incubation (E4.5) to E5 chicks after partial thymectomy of the recipient. The surgical procedure has been previously described in detail (Martin, 1983).

RESULTS

Quail-Chick Wing Chimeras

During embryonic and first posthatching days, the grafted wing developed in a healthy condition. But in all the 30 chimeras observed, edema, the first sign of rejection, was recorded before day 15 after hatching (Fig. 1A). Suppuration, necrosis, and finally auto-amputation occurred (Ohki et al., 1987).

Quail-Chick Wing plus Thymus Chimeras

To challenge the ability of the thymic epithelium to induce tolerance we made double chimeras: Chick hosts were engrafted with a wing bud and thymic epithelial rudiments from the same quail donor. Among the 21 chimeras that hatched, six exhibited a full tolerance to the grafted wing for 2 months. In 13 chimeras, signs of rejection appeared later than in quail-chick wing chimeras and were moderate. In one chimera, the wing was rejected acutely 12 days after hatching (Fig. 1B)

Chimerism of the thymus was determined using species-specific monoclonal antibodies (MAbs) against class II antigens of the MHC (Guillemot et al., 1984) and anti-MB1 that recognize quail hemopoietic and endothelial cells (Péault et al., 1983). No dendritic cells, macrophages, or thymocytes of quail origin were found in the thymus of the chimeras, confirming that the colonization of the quail rudiment had not yet begun at the time of transplantation of the quail thymus. Induction of tolerance in the chimeras correlates with the presence of quail epithelial cells in the thymic stroma. The thymic lobes were chimeric in two respects: They contained hemopoietically derived cells from the chick, whereas the epithelium was either from quail or chick origin according to the thymic lobe considered. The presence of the thymic epithelium from the chick host indicates that the thymectomy of the host was not complete. The quail thymus undergoes physiological involution 5 weeks after hatching, making it difficult to identify the quail epithelial component in adult chimeras. Nevertheless, in all tolerating chimeras studied before complete involution of the quail component, at least a third of the thymic lobes contained quail epithelial cells, emphasizing the decisive role of the thymic epithelium in inducing tolerance (Ohki et al., 1988).

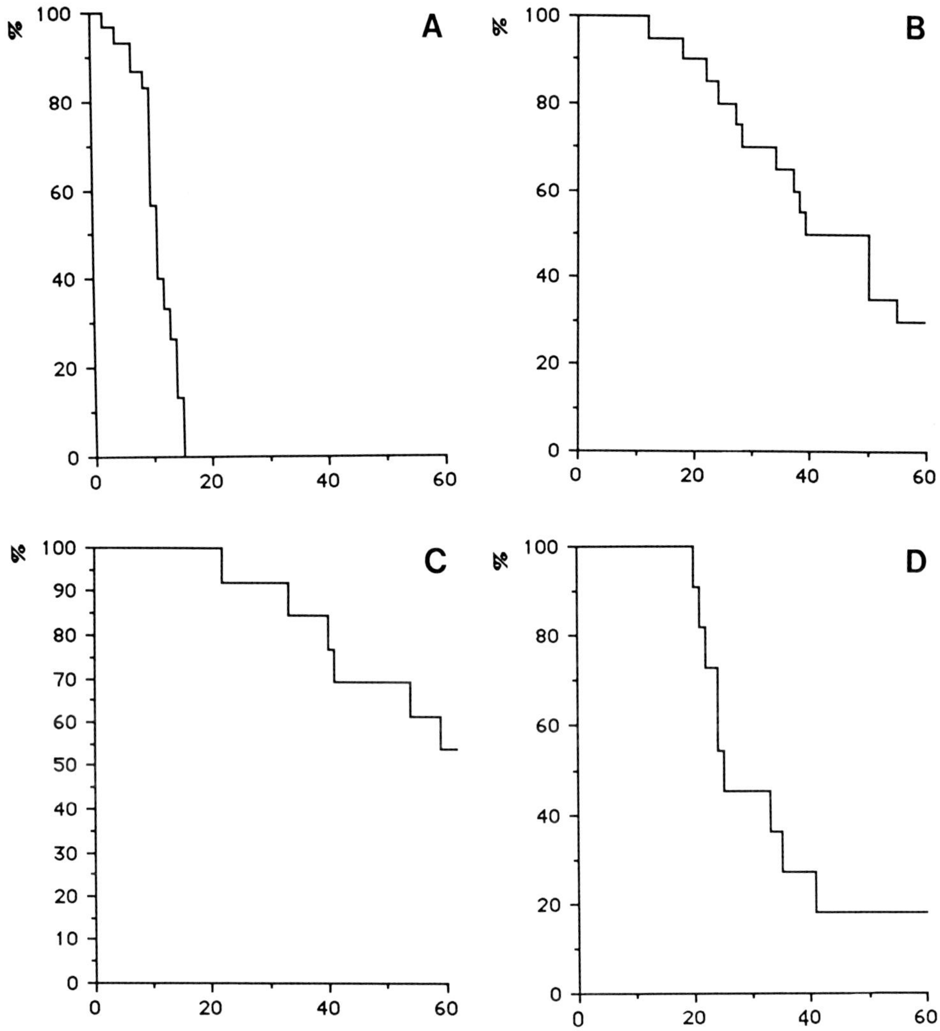

Figure 1 Percentage of chimeras without signs of rejection during 2 months post-hatching. Percentage: vertical axis. Days: horizontal axis. A: Quail-Chick wing chimeras. B: Quail-Chick wing plus thymus chimeras. C: Chick-chick wing chimeras. D: Chick-quail wing chimeras. Two chimeras were not included in this data, one in B and one in D because they died without any signs of rejection at 48 days and 49 days, respectively.

Chick-Chick Wing Chimeras

We wondered if tolerance could be achieved by transplanting embryonic tissues between chick embryos differing at the MHC level. We grafted a wing rudiment from either the CC or CB line on a (B15 × B21) F_1 host. Thirteen allogeneic wing chimeras hatched. All exhibited a prolonged state of tolerance (Fig. 1C). Five chimeras never showed acute signs of rejection. In seven chimeras, a period of strong rejection occurred followed by cicatrization. Only one chimera had an acute rejection crisis starting early (22 days). However

Adult skin graft of the same genotype as the grafted limb and from a third-party (i.e., B4 genotype when the limb graft was from B12 and vice versa) were performed. All chimeras, except the one that severely rejected the wing, tolerated limb-type skin graft in some cases with transient and moderate signs of rejection. In contrast, third-party skin grafts were always acutely rejected, meaning that the tolerance induced was MHC specific. Chimeras were assayed for tolerance in vitro by mixed lymphocyte reaction (MLR). All chimeras had a strong proliferative response when their peripheral blood leukocytes were stimulated by mitomycin C–treated leukocytes of graft limb type (Corbel et al., 1990).

Chick-Quail Wing Chimeras

Preliminary results showed unexpectedly that chick wings grafted on quail recipients has been perfectly tolerated in three chimeras, whereas moderate and chronic alteration of the transplant appeared in three other chimeras (Fig. 1C). Even in six chimeras that exhibited strong signs of rejection, autoamputation never occurred. In five chimeras, adult skin grafts of the same genotype as the embryonic grafted wing were performed. One acutely rejected this adult skin, whereas four accepted it. In contrast, no tolerance was observed in MLR assays: In the two chimeras tested, proliferative responses of the quail peripheral blood leukocytes against mitomycin C–treated cells were similar when stimulator cells were of the graft type or from a third party.

CONCLUSIONS

In the experiments reported here, isotopic and isochronic transplantation of wing buds and thymic rudiments had modified the somatic environment of the future lymphoid cells without introducing foreign hematopoietic stem cells, making the system different from the experiments of Billingham et al. (1953) in mammals, Hasek (1956) and Lehtonen et al. (1987) in birds, showing that the presence of allogeneic hematopoietic cells can induce tolerance in embryos or neonates.

When the wing grafts were performed between closely related embryos, i.e., in allogeneic combinations, partial and, in some chimeras, permanent tissue tolerance was observed. This tolerance was MHC specific and not observed in vitro assays.

Our experiments demonstrate that in quail-chick wing chimeras, despite the early presentation of the foreign antigens, no tolerance is induced. But if a quail thymic epithelium is grafted along with the quail wing bud, a permanent state of tolerance could be induced in this xenogeneic combination.

Unexpectedly, the fate of the chick wing bud grafted on a quail embryo is fundamentally different from that of the opposite combination. As the chick is much bigger than the quail at hatching, the size of the graft could influence the response. Experiments are in progress to test this possibility.

Altogether these experiments show that besides the decisive role played by the thymic epithelium in inducing tolerance, a peripheral mechanism also exists.

REFERENCES

Allison, J., Campbell, I.L., Morahan, G., Mandel, T.E., Harrison, L.C. and Miller, J.F.A.P. (1988). Diabetes in transgenic mice resulting from over-expression of class I histocompatibility molecules in pancreatic beta cells. Nature 333:529.

Billingham, R.E., Brent, L. and Medawar, P.B. (1953). Actively acquired tolerance of foreign cells. Nature 172:603–606.

Böhme, J., Haskins, K., Strecha, P., van Ewijk, W., Le Meur, M., Gerlinger, P., Benoist, C. and Mathis, D. (1989). Transgenic mice with I-A on islets cells are normoglycemic but immunologically intolerant. Science 244:1179.

Corbel, C., Martin, C., Ohki, H., Coltey, M., Hlozanek, I. and Le Douarin, N.M. (1990). Evidence for peripheral mechanisms inducing tissue tolerance during ontogeny. Int. Immunol. 2:33–40.

Guillemot, F.P., Oliver, P.D., Péault, B.M., and Le Douarin, N.M. (1984). Cells expressing Ia-antigens in the avian thymus. J. Exp. Med. 160:1803–1819.

Hamburger, V. and Hamilton, H.L. (1951). A series of normal stages in the development of the chick embryo. J. Morphol. 88:49–92.

Hampé, A. (1959). Contribution à l'étude du développement et de la régulation des déficiences et des excédents dans la patte de l'embryon de Poulet. Arch. Anat. Micros. Morphol. Exp. 48:345–478.

Hasek, M. (1956). Tolerance phenomena in birds. Proc. R. Soc. B. 146:67–77.

Jenkinson, E.J., Jhittay, P., Kingston, R. and Owen, J.J.T. (1985). Studies of the role of the thymic environment in the induction of tolerance to MHC antigens. Transplantation 30:331.

Kappler, J.W., Roehm, N. and Marrack, P. (1987). T cell tolerance by clonal elimination in the thymus. Cell 49:273.

Kappler, J.W., Staerz, U., White, J. and Marrack, P.C. (1988). Self-tolerance eliminates T cells specific for Mls-modified products of the major histocompatibility complex. Nature 332:35.

Kisielow, P., Bluthmann, H., Staerz, U.D., Steinmetz, M. and von Boehmer, H. (1988). Tolerance in T-cell-receptor transgenic mice involves deletion of non mature $CD4^{+}8^{+}$ thymocytes. Nature 333:742.

Lafferty, K.J., Prowse, S.J. and Simeonovic, C.J. (1983). Immunobiology of tissue transplantation: a return to the passenger leukocyte concept. Annu. Rev. Immunol. 1:143.

Le Douarin, N.M. (1969). Particularités du noyau interphasique chez la Caille japonaise (Coturnix coturnix japonica). Utilisation de ses particularités comme "marquage biologique" des recherches sur les interactions tissulaires et les migrations cellulaires au cours de l'ontogenèse. Bull. Biol. Fr. Belg. 103:435–452.

Lehtonen, L., Vainio, O. and Toivanen, P. (1987). Transplantation tolerance to total chicken Major Histocompatibility Complex (B-Complex) antigen disparity is impaired by interleukin 2. Transplant. Proc. 19:508–510.

Lo, D., Burkly, L.C., Widera, G., Cowing, C., Flavell, R.A., Palmiter, R.D. and Brinster, R.L. (1988). Diabetes and tolerance in transgenic mice expressing Class II MHC molecules in pancreatic beta-cells. Cell 53:159.

Lo, D., Burkly, L.C., Flavell, R.A., Palmiter, R.D. and Brinster, R.L. (1989). Tolerance in transgenic mice expressing class II major histocompatibility complex on pancreatic acinar cells. J. Exp. Med. 170:87.

MacDonald, H.R., Schneider, R., Lees, R.K., Howe, R.C., Acha-Orbea, H., Festenstein, H., Zinkernagel, R.M. and Hengartner, H. (1988). T-cell receptor V beta use predicts reactivity and tolerance to Mlsa-encoded antigens. Nature 332:40.

Markmann, J., Lo, D., Naji, A., Palmiter, R.D., Brinster, R.L. and Heber-Katz, E. (1988). Antigen presenting function of class II MHC expressing pancreatic beta cells. Nature 336:476.

Martin, C.S. (1983). Total thymectomy in the early chick embryo. Arch. Anat. Micros. 72:107–115.

Martin, C., LeDouarin, N., Dieterlen-Lievre, F., and Smith, J. (eds.) (1990). Quail-chick chimeras, a tool for developmental immunology. In: *The Avian Model in Developmental Biology: From Organism to Genes*. ed. du CNRS, pp. 207–217.

Morahan, G., Allison, J. and Miller, J.F.A.P. (1989). Tolerance of class I histocompatibility antigens expressed extrathymically. Nature 339:622.

Ohki, H., Martin, C., Corbel, C., Coltey, M., and Le Douarin, N.M. (1987). Tolerance induced by thymic epithelial grafts in birds. Science 237:1032–1035.

Ohki, H., Martin, C., Coltey, M. and Le Douarin, N.M. (1988). Implants of quail thymic epithelium generate permanent tolerance in embryonically constructed quail/chick chimeras. Development 104:619–630.

Owen, R. D. (1945). Immunogenetic consequences of vascular anastomoses between bovine twins. Science 102:400–401.

Péault, B.M., Thiery, J.P. and Le Douarin, N.M. (1983). Surface marker for the hemopoietic and endothelial cell lineages in the quail that is defined by a monoclonal antibody. Proc. Natl. Acad. Sci. U.S.A. 80:2976–2980.

Ready, A.R., Jenkinson, E.J., Kingston, R. and Owen, J.J.T. (1984). Successful transplantation across major histocompatibility barrier of deoxyguanosine-treated embryonic thymus expressing class II antigens. Nature 310:231–233.

Sprent, J., Lo, D., Gao, E.K. and Ron, Y. (1988). T cell selection in the thymus. Immunol. Rev. 101:173–190.

von Boehmer, H. and Hafen, K. (1986). Minor but not major histocompatibility antigens of thymus epithelium tolerize precursors of cytolytic T cells. Nature 320:626–628.

Zacchei, A.M. (1961). Lo sviluppo embrionale della quaglia giapponese (Coturnix coturnix japonica T.e S.). Arch. Ital. Anat. Embryol. 66:36–62.

95

Tolerance and Immunocompetence in Murine Semiallogeneic Complete and Mixed Chimeras

Peter Leenaerts, Halina Sobis, Michael Vandeputte, and Mark Waer
University of Leuven, Leuven, Belgium

INTRODUCTION

After bone marrow (BM) transplantation, chimeric mice are considered to be tolerant and immunocompetent when they respectively do not respond to host (absence of graft-vs-host reaction [GVHR]) or donor (absence of host-vs-graft [HVGR]) major histocompatibility complex (MHC) molecules and, when after adequate reconstitution of the lymphoid organs, normal cellular, and humoral responses to foreign proteins (e.g. viral antigens) or third-party MHC molecules can be induced. In complete allogeneic chimeras (no host lymphohematopoietic cells), immunocompetence may be severely impaired by two phenomena, chronic graft-vs-host disease (GVHD) and MHC restriction problems, which may both be related to each other, and which are both claimed to be responsible for the long-term mortality (so called secondary disease) seen in these animals (1,2). Chronic GVHD is a poorly understood disease which, apart from clinical and histological findings, is accompanied by a profound immunosuppression of cellular and humoral immunity (3). Its severity can be reduced by T-cell depletion (TCD) of the BM inoculum, but this procedure may have a high risk of engraftment failure (4). The MHC restriction problems are due to the fact that donor T lymphocytes mature in an allogeneic thymus, acquire MHC restriction for host MHC molecules, and consequently may have an impaired collaboration between donor T cells and antigen-presenting cells (APCs) or B cells (5,6). To avoid both problems of GVHD and MHC restriction, mixed instead of complete chimerism has been propagated (7,8). In semiallogeneic chimeras such as the combination P into F_1 hybrids, MHC problems do not occur, but these mice may not be protected against chronic GVHD. The aim of the present study was to investigate whether there is any difference in tolerance and immunocompetence in mixed and complete semiallogeneic chimeras.

MATERIALS AND METHODS

Animals

Adult (7- to 10-week-old) inbred male Balb/c(H-2^d), C57Bl/6 (H-2^b), C3H/He (H-2^k), and Balb/cxC57Bl F_1 hybrids (H-$2^{d,b}$) were used throughout the experiments. Mice were kept in conventional housing conditions, but received antibiotics the first 6 weeks after BM transplantation.

Chimeras

Mixed semiallogeneic chimeras (H-$2^{d,b}$, H-2^b)F_1 were obtained by using TLI (34 Gy) followed by 20×10^6 untreated C57Bl BM cells (9) or by using 10.5 Gy WBI and 5×10^6 TCD F_1 cells and 15×10^6 untreated C57Bl cells (7). Complete chimeras (H-2^b)F_1 received 20×10^6 untreated C57Bl cells. Chimerism was scored with flow cytometry using anti-MHC monoclonal antibodies (MAbs) or hyperimmune serum and antimouse immunoglobulin G (IgG) second-step reagent as described (10). The percentage of host-type lymphoid cells (F_1 cells) in mixed chimeras varied between 5 and 60%; no host cells were found in complete chimeras.

Experimental Protocol

Subgroups of chimeric mice and control animals were primed and boostered i.p. on days 75, 82, and 90 with 50×10^6 cells of either parental (Balb/c or C57Bl) or third-party (C3H) origin. Cellular immunity of the spleen cells and alloantibody formation in the serum was examined on day 100. Tolerance was further assessed by animal survival rate, and development of clinical (general appearance and weight evolution) and histological findings (infiltrates in liver, gut, and skin) indicative for GVHD.

Examination of Cellular and Humoral Immunity

Cellular immunity was assessed by the mixed lymphocyte reaction (MLR) using parental and third-party 30-Gy irradiated spleen cells as stimulators and nylon wool–treated spleen cells from each chimeric animal as responders. Humoral immunity was evaluated by determining the alloantibody titer, using a flow cytometry method as described (11). The method detects IgG alloantibodies in the serum of primed and boostered mice by incubating target cells with this serum.

RESULTS

The results are summarized in Table 1. Mixed as well as complete semiallogeneic chimeras showed excellent survival. Two animals died due to the i.v. injection of bone marrow, whereas the other five died during the first 2 weeks. None of the mice developed clinical signs that were indicative for GVHD and all animals seemed perfectly healthy when they were sacrificed. Histology of skin, liver, and gut in BM-transplanted mice did not differ from the histological findings seen in control mice. Priming with lymphoid cells did not alter the MLR reactivity and, therefore, the mean stimulation index ± 1 SD of all mice from a group was represented. All chimeras were tolerant to parental stimulator cells but showed vigorous responses to third party cells. A similar result was found for the humoral response; only the mice that were primed with C3H cells developed alloantibody titers which did not

Table 1 Tolerance and Immunocompetence of Mixed and Complete Chimeras

Group	Survival	MLR (stimulators)[a]			Alloantibody $\log^2$ titer
		Balb/c	C57BI	C3H	
Control F_1	10	1.3 ± 0.3	1.7 ± 0.5	33 ± 11	10.6 ± 1.2 (n=5)
Mixed F_1 (TLI)	16/18	1.2 ± 0.4	1.8 ± 0.4	48 ± 17	10.3 ± 0.8 (n=6)
Mixed F_1 (WBI)	15/18	1.2 ± 0.2	1.4 ± 0.5	39 ± 12	10.8 ± 1.4 (n=6)
Complete F_1	10/12	1.2 ± 0.6	1.6 ± 0.3	38 ± 8	10.2 ± 0.6 (n=4)

[a]The proliferative response is expressed as stimulation index (SI).

significantly differ from each other. Representative examples of mice primed with parental and third-party cells are shown in Figure 1.

Together, the results suggested that both groups of chimeras were tolerant and immunocompetent on cellular and humoral levels. However, when target cells of the nontransplanted parental strain were incubated with serum from third-party primed complete chimeric mice, a clear shift of the class II–bearing cells was seen, demonstrating that

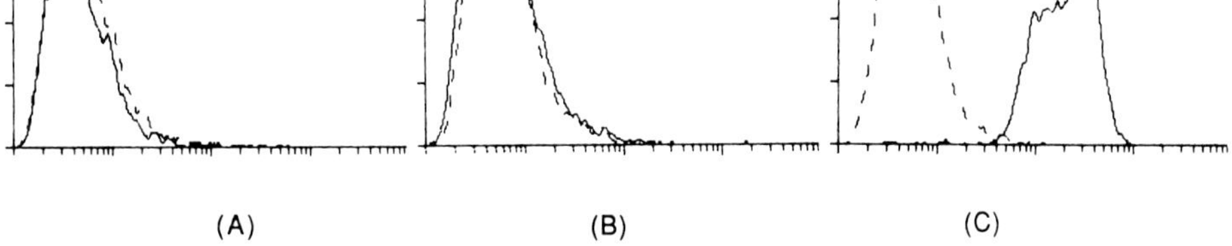

Figure 1 Demonstration by flow cytometry of alloantibody production in primed mice. Target cells incubated with serum from F_1 chimeras primed with Balb/c (A) or C57BI (B) (solid lines) did not differ from those incubated with irrelevant serum (dashed lines). The fluorescense along the horizontal axis was obtained by using a fluorescein-conjugated goat antimouse IgG(Fc) as second-step reagent. Serum from mice primed with C3H lymphoid cells (C) contained IgG alloantibodies that shifted the histogram. The titer was the last serum dilution that caused a significant shift.

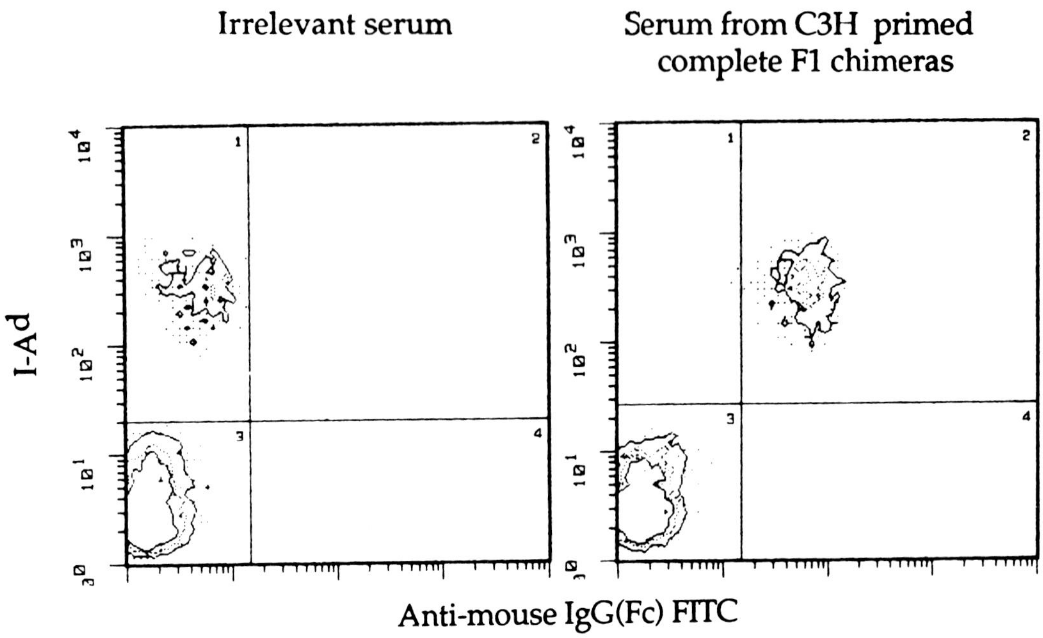

Figure 2 Cross-reactivity of alloantibodies raised against third-party antigens in complete chimeras. Spleen target cells of the nontransplanted parental were incubated with serum from complete chimeras primed with C3H lymphoid cells. Alloantibody binding is represented along the horizontal axis and class II molecule staining along the vertical axis.

cross-reactive antibodies to host were evoked in these mice (Fig. 2). Such cross-reactive antibodies were not found in mixed chimeras and no evidence was present for in vivo absorption in these mice.

DISCUSSION

The results show that mixed and complete semiallogeneic chimeras were tolerant and immunocompetent and on first view reacted indistinguishably from control mice. Apparently, in semiallogeneic BM transplantation T-cell depletion is not required to obtain healthy immunocompetent animals. While administration of large amounts of immunocompetent C57Bl/6 lymphoid cells in F_1 animals is an established model for acute lethal GVHD (12), the small amounts of immunocompetent cells in the bone marrow seem to have no detrimental effects on lethally irradiated F_1 hybrids. Whether this is also true for other donor-recipient combinations needs further assessment. Indirectly, this observation also argues in favor for the hypothesis that MHC restriction problems are the major cause for the lack of immunocompetence in fully allogeneic chimeras, as has been claimed (2,5).

While all chimeras showed perfect T-cell tolerance to parental cells, cross-reactive alloantibodies to class II antigen-expressing cells of the nontransplanted parental were found in the serum of third-party primed complete chimeras. Thus, host reactive B cells were not eliminated in these animals. The nature of the target antigens has yet not been

96
Modulation of T-Cell Response by Self–Major Histocompatibility Complex Peptides

Gilles Benichou,[1] Peter A. Takizawa,[1] Philip T. Ho,[1] Catherine C. Killion,[2] Clifford A. Olson,[1] Minnie McMillan,[2] and Eli E. Sercarz[1]
[1]*University of California at Los Angeles, Los Angeles, California;*
[2]*University of Southern California, Los Angeles, California*

INTRODUCTION

It is now well established that T lymphocytes recognize protein antigens in the form of peptides presented in association with self–major histocompatibility complex (MHC) molecules (1,2). While the immune response to foreign molecules has been extensively studied at both molecular and cellular levels, very little is known about the recognition of self-antigens. It has been proposed by Kourilsky et al. that self-proteins are processed and presented as peptides in the context of class I or class II MHC molecules for interaction with T lymphocytes (3). Experimental evidence for this hypothesis has been recently obtained in several laboratories and presentation of self-peptides is now generally accepted. The self-peptides which are readily processed and can bind efficiently to self-MHC should be continuously presented at the surface of antigen-presenting cells (APCs) and may play a critical role in the immune system. In this chapter, we will address the possible role of self-peptides in different contexts: tolerance induction and acquisition of the T-cell repertoire, modulation of the T-cell response to a foreign antigen, and induction of autoimmune disease.

ROLE OF SELF-PEPTIDES IN T-CELL TOLERANCE INDUCTION

Tolerance Is Not Induced to Certain Self-Peptides

It has been clearly shown that self-molecules such as hemoglobin are regularly processed and presented to induce T-cell responses in the periphery (4). Mechanisms of self-antigen processing and presentation must be crucial in the induction of self-tolerance in the thymus, where self-antigens presented to developing T cells cause deletion of autoreactive T cells. One would therefore predict that examination of a panel of self-peptides expressed in the thymus would reveal a subset of peptides which bind with high affinity to self-MHC but are

Table 1 Immunogenicity and Binding Properties of Self-MHC Peptides

Immunization with		Proliferative response (cpm ± SD)	Class II binding
Class II peptides	A^{k}_{α} 1–18	30,291 ± 3,928	+
	A^{k}_{α} 49–63	1,959 ± 209	–
	A^{k}_{α} 68–81	2,150 ± 344	–
	A^{k}_{β} 1–16	32,396 ± 4,042	+
	A^{k}_{β} 58–71	2,052 ± 263	–
Class I peptides	L^{d}_{1} 61–85	78,620 ± 8,630	+
	D^{d}_{1} 61–85	1,600 ± 660	+
	L^{d}_{1} 148–162	2110 ± 418	–

B10.A mice were immunized in both footpads and at the base of the tail with 50 μg of MHC peptides in CFA. Popliteal and inguineal lymph node cells were used 10 days later in antigen-induced proliferation assays. All the peptides were tested for their capacity to inhibit the in vitro interleukin-2 production of a class II–restricted HEL–peptide–specific T-cell hybridoma. Inhibition under these conditions is attributed to competitive binding to the appropriate MHC restriction element by the extrinsic peptide. The background values (cells without antigens) ranged from 1,122 to 4,670 cpm. The positive control responses to PPD ranged from 88,134 to 157,017 cpm.

not immunogenic owing to the deletion of the corresponding T cells. We confirmed this hypothesis and showed that an MHC class I–derived peptide, D^{d} 61-85, binds to self-MHC class II (A^{k}) with high affinity but is not immunogenic in B10.A mice (H-2^{a}) owing to the elimination/inactivation of the autoreactive T cells. This peptide was capable of triggering T-cell proliferative responses when seen as an allopeptide in B10.BR mice (H-2^{k}) in the context of the same restriction element, confirming that this peptide can bind efficiently to A^{k} molecules. However, we found that several other self-MHC class I and class II peptides, capable of binding to self-MHC, induce T-cell responses. These results indicate that certain self-MHC peptides are not physiologically presented by MHC-expressing cells in sufficient density to induce T-cell tolerance. This could be attributed to incomplete antigen

Table 2 MBP-Induced T-Cell Response Can Be Blocked In Vivo by a Self-MHC Peptide

	Proliferative response to (cpm ± SD)		
Immunization with	Medium	A^{k}_{β} 58–71	MBP
MBP	3,850 ± 3,500	ND	102,548 ± 28,334
MBP / A^{k}_{β} 58–71	3,336 ± 570	27,440 ± 5,842	3,708 ± 1,545

(SJL ± B10.PL) F_1 mice were immunized in both footpads with 100 μg of guinea pig MBP, or with a mixture containing MBP + A^{k}_{β} 58–71 added at a 1/1 molecular ratio. Popliteal lymph node cells were used in antigen-induced proliferation assays. The results are expressed as counts per minute (cpm) ± SD, and they represent six mice tested individually. ND = not determined.

processing or competition with other self-peptides (5). Similar failure to induce tolerance by a self-protein has been described by Stockinger et al. In this case, presentation of the pro-C5 self-peptide in the context of class II MHC was not efficient enough to ensure tolerance (6). This has been also observed for certain self-hemoglobin fragments presented in the context of MHC class I molecules (7). Despite the risk of autoimmune disorders, a system permitting such inefficiency of tolerance induction to self-peptides could have survived so that many self-reactive T cells cross-reactive with exogenous antigens would remain and not be purged from the T cell repertoire.

"Idiopeptides" from Variable Portions of the Self May Shape the T-Cell Repertoire

It is now well accepted that the T-cell repertoire is acquired through a complex positive and negative process of recognition of self-molecules in the context of self-MHC (8,9). How can T cells highly specific for a very large number of different foreign antigen peptides be positively selected in the absence of the foreign antigens themselves? It is possible that peptides derived from variable regions of polymorphic molecules such as the MHC on the one hand and "idiopeptides" from the antibodies or TCR on the other, could represent an important driving force for shaping the T-cell repertoire. The polymorphic portions of MHC peptides themselves would be ideally suited for this role, since there is evidence that they have access to the binding site of complete molecules. In this way, maximal diversification of repertoire in the species would occur. Idiopeptides from the TCR and antibodies described by Kourilsky et al. as "immune-self" also represent an intrinsic source of diversity which would mimic the external world of foreign peptides (3). Each idiopeptide is available only at a much lower concentration than conserved sequences because of clonal or oligoclonal expression. In any case, it seems unlikely that the idiopeptides would be engaged in negative selection.

IN VIVO REGULATION OF T-CELL RESPONSES TO FOREIGN OR AUTOANTIGENS BY SELF-PEPTIDES

Self-peptides which are readily processed and bind to self-MHC with high affinity may represent a source of potent agents capable of competing with other self-components during the induction of self-tolerance or with foreign antigens during an immune response. It has been shown by Adorini et al. that administered self-peptides can compete efficiently in vivo with foreign peptides to block T-cell activation (10). This in vivo competition was found to act at the level of the binding to MHC molecules. Recently, several groups have succeeded in modulating the response to autoantigens involved in autoimmune diseases by using peptides capable of competing for MHC recognition (11–14). Similarly, in our laboratory we have found that one MHC class II peptide, derived from the second polymorphic region of the β chain, can block the in vivo T cell response to myelin basic protein (MBP) very efficiently in (SJLxB10.PL)F_1 mice, and can cause an extensive delay in the onset of experimental autoimmune encephalomyelitis (EAE) disease. Of course, during the normal progression of the immune response, self-peptides play a still unknown role in modulating or regulating the response to foreign determinants by competitively occupying the MHC binding sites.

SELF-PEPTIDE RECOGNITION AND AUTOIMMUNE DISEASES

As we have mentioned earlier, tolerance is not induced to certain self-peptides. Gammon et al. (15) have demonstrated that the induction of adult tolerance to hen eggwhite lyzozyme (HEL) is directed only toward major (dominant) determinants present on this molecule. T cells specific for minor determinants on the same protein escape clonal deletion/inactivation, owing presumably to inefficient processing of these peptides. Accordingly, self-MHC peptides capable of inducing T-cell responses in vivo can be considered minor determinants that did not induce T-cell tolerance. The presence of this self-directed repertoire is not expected to cause autoreactive T-cell activation under normal circumstances because it is directed toward minor determinants that usually remain unexpressed. Nevertheless, when dysregulation of the expression of self-proteins modifies the nature of the level of processing and presentation of determinants on this molecule, or in the case of mimicry between a foreign component and certain self-peptides, T-cell responses to minor self-determinants may occur and induce autoimmune disorders.

CONCLUSIONS

As shown in this chapter, self-peptides play a crucial role in determining the specificity of at least the T-cell branch of the immune system. They are certainly involved in the induction of T-cell tolerance and acquisition of the T-cell repertoire. They may also regulate the response to foreign antigens and become involved under certain conditions in autoimmune disease. In the not distant future, the nature of the self-peptides present in the binding site of self-MHC molecules will become elucidated and thus clarify an important aspect of T-cell immunology. Furthermore, this knowledge should provide a powerful tool for manipulation of the immune response for therapeutic purposes.

ACKNOWLEDGMENTS

Work was supported by NIH grants to E.E.S. and to M.M. Gilles Benichou is a fellow of the Ministère Français des relations extérieures (Lavoisier fellowship).

REFERENCES

1. Townsend, A.R.M., S. Rothbard, F.M. Gotch, G. Bamadur, D. Wraith, and A.J. McMichael. The epitopes of influenza nucleoprotein recognized by cytotoxic T lymphocytes can be defined with short synthetic peptides. Cell 1986; 44:959–968.
2. Babbitt, B.P., P.M. Allen, G. Matsueda, E.P. Haber, and E.R. Unanue. Binding of immunogenic peptides to Ia histocompatibility molecules. Nature 1985; 317:359–361.
3. Kourilsky, P., G. Chaouat, C. Rabourdin-Combe, and J. Claverie. Working principles in the immune system implied by the "peptidic self" model. Proc. Natl. Acad. Sci. U.S.A. 1987; 84:3400–3404.
4. Lorenz, R.G., and P.M. Allen. Direct evidence for functional self protein/Ia complexes in vivo. Proc. Natl. Acad. Sci. U.S.A. 1988; 85:5220–5223.
5. Benichou, G., P.A. Takizawa, P.T. Ho, C.C. Killion, C.A. Olson, M. McMillan, and E. Sercarz. Immunogenicity and tolerogenicity of self-MHC peptides. 1990 (submitted).
6. Stockinger, B., and Rong Hwa Lin. An intracellular self protein synthesized in macrophages is presented but fails to induce tolerance. Int. Immunol. 1989; 1:592–597.
7. Schild, H., O. Rotzschke, H. Kalbacher, and H. Rammensee. Limit of T cell tolerance to self proteins by peptide presentation. Science 1990; 247:1587–1589.

8. Kappler, J.W., N. Roehm, and P. Marrack. T cell tolerance by clonal elimination in the thymus. Cell 1987; 49:273–280.
9. Kisielow, P., H. Bluthmann, U.D. Staerz, M. Steinmetz, and H. Von Boehmer. Tolerance in T cell receptor transgenic mice involves deletion of immature $CD4^+8^+$ thymocytes. Nature 1988; 333:742–746.
10. Adorini, L., S. Muller, F. Cardinaux, P.V. Lehmann, F. Falcioni, and Z.A. Nagy. In vivo competition between self peptides and foreign antigens in T cell activation. Nature 1988; 334:623.
11. Kumar, V., J.L. Urban, S.J. Horvath, and L. Hood. Amino acid variations at a single residue in an autoimmune peptide profoundly affect its properties: T-cell activation, major histocompatibility complex binding, and ability to block experimental allergic encephalomyelitis. Proc. Natl. Acad. Sci. U.S.A. 1990; 87:1337–1341.
12. Singh, V.K., H.K. Kalra, K. Yamaki, T. Abe, L.A. Donoso, and T. Shinohara. Molecular mimicry between a uveitopathogenic site of S-antigen and viral peptides. J. Immunol. 1990; 144: 1282–1287.
13. Gautam, A.M., and P. Glynn. Competition between foreign and self proteins in antigen presentation. Ovalbumin can inhibit activation of myelin basic protein-specific T cells. J. Immunol. 1990; 144:1177–1180.
14. Sakai, K., S.S. Zamvil, D.J. Mitchell, S. Hodgkinson, D.B. Rothbard, and L. Steinman. Presentation of experimental encephalomyelitis with peptides that block interaction of T cells with major histocompatibility complex proteins. Proc. Natl. Acad. Sci. U.S.A. 1989; 86:9470–9474.
15. Gammon, G., and E.E. Sercarz. How some T-cells escape tolerance induction. Nature 1989; 342:183–185.

97
Involution of the Thymus Medulla by Cyclosporin

Henk-Jan Schuurman,[1,2] Henk Van Loveren,[2] J. Gerard Loeber,[3] Aalt Van Dijk,[1] Jan Rozing,[3] and Joseph G. Vos[2]
[1]*University Hospital, Utrecht, The Netherlands;* [2]*National Institute of Public Health and Environmental Protection, Bilthoven, The Netherlands;* [3]*Institute for Experimental Gerontology, Netherlands Organisation for Applied Scientific Research, Rijswijk, The Netherlands*

INTRODUCTION

Under specified experimental conditions, the immunosuppressive agent cyclosporin A (CsA) can induce autoimmune-like symptoms resembling graft-vs-host reactions. This so-called syngeneic graft-vs-host disease emerges in rodents after a short-term CsA administration during the recovery phase after whole-body irradiation and syngeneic bone marrow transplantation (1). Congenitally athymic (nude) recipients develop similar symptoms after implantation of thymus from CsA-treated animals (2). This observation points to a role for the thymus in this process. The thymus after CsA administration manifests an almost incomplete disappearance of the medulla compartment (3). Since this compartment is considered to be the site where negative selection occurs (inhibition of immature T lymphocytes with potential self-reactivity to further development), its disappearance may be associated with the loss of negative-selection potential, yielding autoreactive T-cell clones in the periphery.

We performed a detailed (immuno)histochemical analysis of the thymus in rats immediately after a 2-week course of CsA administration and during the subsequent recovery phase. Special attention was paid to changes in the medulla compartment.

EXPERIMENTAL DESIGN

Eight male PVG ($RT1^c$) rats and eight male WAG/CPB ($RT1^u$) rats, aged 6 weeks, received daily subcutaneous injections of 15 mg CsA/kg body weight (1.5 mg/ml, diluted from the stock reagent Sandimmun [Sandoz, Basel, Switzerland] injection fluid 50 mg CsA/ml) for 14 days. Two PVG and 2 WAG/CPB animals were sacrificed immediately after this period, and after a subsequent 2, 4, and 6 weeks. The whole-blood CsA concentration was determined for three animals at day 3 and day 13 during the treatment period. Samples taken at 0, 1, 2, 4, 6, and 24 hr after CsA injection were analyzed using a specific monoclonal antibody (MAb) in the Sandimmun Kit (Sandoz). Two PVG and two WAG/CPB animals served as control. At autopsy part of thymic tissue was processed for conventional histology (formalin fixation, paraffin embedding), and part was snap-frozen in liquid nitrogen for frozen tissue section immunohistochemistry. This was done using a three-step immunoperoxidase method on acetone-fixed sections. Mouse monoclonal antibodies applied were MRC OX-19 (CD5, detecting all thymocytes and all peripheral T cells); ER-2 (CD4, T-helper–inducer phenotype); MRC OX-8 (CD8, T-suppressor–cytotoxic phenotype); R73 (T-cell receptor αβ [TCR αβ positive]); ER-13 and MRC OX-6 (common determinant of major histocompatibility complex [MHC] class II molecule); ED-2 (macrophages, in thymus strong expression on macrophages in the cortex); ED-7 and ED-8 (macrophages, in the thymus present on a very few cells in the cortex, and in a somewhat higher density in the medulla); HIS-37 (epithelial cells in the thymus cortex, part of medullary epithelium); HIS-38 (epithelial cells in the thymus cortex); and HIS-39 (epithelial cells in the subcapsule and medulla). Antibodies in the second and third step were horseradish peroxidase–conjugated rabbit antimouse immunoglobulins and swine antirabbit immunoglobulins, respectively (Dakopatts, Glostrup, Denmark); the staining was done using 3,3-diaminobenzidine tetrahydrochlorid with H_2O_2 as substrate. Keratin expression by epithelial cells was documented by a two-step immunoperoxidase reaction using a rabbit antikeratin antibody (Dakopatts) and conjugated swine antirabbit immunoglobulin.

RESULTS

Cyclosporin Concentration

Just before CsA injection on day 3, blood concentrations (mean ± SD) were 4.6±0.3 mg/l; at day 13, these values were 6.3±0.6 mg/l. Peak levels were observed at 6 hr after CsA injection on day 3 (7.5±0.8 mg/l) and at 2 hr after CsA injection on day 13 (9.1±1.1 mg/l). These values are in the same range as those reported by others (4).

The Thymus Immediately After CsA Treatment

Conventional histology showed the almost complete absence of the medulla. The whole section was densely filled by small lymphocytes like the cortex in the normal thymus. In frozen sections, these lymphocytes showed the cortical phenotype (CD4 positive, CD8 positive, low CD5 positive, low TCR αβ positive). Also the microenvironment was compatible with that of the normal thymus cortex, consisting of keratin-positive, MHC class II–positive epithelium. ED-2–positive macrophages were observed at scattered location, and some ED-7–positive and ED-8–positive macrophages were present. A diffuse MHC class II–labeling pattern, present in the normal thymus medulla, was not observed, except for some small foci. Serial section analysis showed that these foci contained lymphocytes of medullary phenotype (high expression of CD5 and TCR αβ, some CD8-positive cells and some CD4-positive cells), and comprised in addition HIS-39–positive epithelial cells. Just like the normal thymus medulla, ED-7–positive and ED-8–positive macrophages occurred in a somewhat higher density in these foci. In addition to these foci, there were some small-sized areas lacking the expression of keratin, epithelial antigens, and class II expression. In serial section analysis, these areas were filled by lymphocytes of cortical phenotype. From these observations we conclude that both the stationary (epithelial) and the passenger leukocyte (lymphocytes, interdigitating cells [IDCs]) cell population disappeared from the normal medulla during CsA treatment. Only some small remnants remained, and in addition small "holes" in the microenvironment occurred. These holes are discussed below in more detail.

Thymus (Immuno)histology During Recovery

An apparent normal thymus architecture was observed in rats sacrificed 2, 4, and 6 weeks after the end of CsA administration. Cortex and medulla areas were observed in relative proportions similar to those in the normal thymus. The phenotype expression of lymphocytes, macrophages, and epithelial microenvironment in the cortex was as in the normal thymus. In contrast, the medulla-like areas, defined on the basis of conventional histology, revealed some striking abnormalities. Three different appearances of this microenvironment were noted:

1. A normal medulla microenvironment was observed, with confluent MHC class II expression compatible with that by medullary IDCs, and plump HIS-39 and keratin compatible with that by medullary epithelium. These areas were filled by lymphocytes of normal medulla phenotype, and comprised ED-7–positive and ED-8–positive macrophages at scattered location.

2. "Holes" were observed in the microenvironment in which there was no expression of MHC class II expression and epithelial markers. ED-2–positive macrophages did not occur at these locations. The lymphocytes showed the cortex phenotype, which makes it unlikely that these areas represent perivascular spaces. In conventional histology, lymphocytes in these areas showed the cytology of medium-sized cells. These holes in the microenvironment were prominently present in the thymus obtained 2 weeks after the end of CsA administration, and gradually disappeared later on. They were still present, but in smaller size, in the thymus at 6 weeks after the end of CsA treatment.

3. Areas with an intermediate composition between a "true-medullary" area and holes did occur. These areas lacked epithelial antigens, but showed cells with plump MHC class II expression compatible with IDCs. The density of these cells was less than in the normal thymus medulla. Lymphocyte phenotyping at this location gave the impression of a mixed population of cells with the cortical phenotype (low CD5 positive, low TCR $\alpha\beta$ positive, most cells being CD4-positive and CD8-positive) and medullary phenotype (high CD5-positive, high TCR $\alpha\beta$ positive, the majority being CD4-positive and incidentally CD8-positive). This type of medullary-like area was observed in two out of four specimens at 2 weeks after the end of CsA treatment. It was also present in specimens obtained later on, but here the density of cells expressing MHC class II appeared to be higher, and the lymphocyte population was more shifted toward the medullary phenotype.

DISCUSSION

The recovery of the thymus medullary area after discontinuation of CsA treatment is associated with the reappearance of IDCs, defined on the basis of MHC class II expression. This may represent the influx of cells originating in the bone marrow. The cells occupy areas without an epithelial microenvironment: Apparently the regeneration of the medullary epithelium occurred at a lower speed. The areas comprising IDCs were filled with lymphocytes of mixed cortical and medullary composition. In case of a higher density of IDCs, the proportions of cells with the cortex phenotype seemed to be lower: At the other end of the spectrum, holes completely lacking MHC class II expression contained almost exclusively lymphocytes of cortex phenotype. Thymus medullary lymphocytes most likely originate from the cortex stage in T-cell development. Thus, it is tempting to speculate that after CsA discontinuation at first lymphocytes in the cortical stage are allowed to further development, thereby leaving the cortex microenvironment and filling holes that lack a defined microenvironment. These areas give the impression of a medulla-like area because the lymphocytes do not show the cytology of small cortex thymocytes, but rather that of medium-sized cells. Then, IDCs enter these holes and create the first medullary environment; this process is accompanied by changes in lymphocyte marker expression from cortical into medulla phenotype. This process can occur without the presence of medullary epithelium. Finally, epithelial regeneration occurs and the original medulla architecture is restored.

These changes in the composition of the microenvironment and lymphocytes after a course of CsA treatment may have relevance for the generation of syngeneic graft-vs-host disease. It is generally assumed that negative selection has its tissue location in the thymus medulla, and is primarily mediated by medullary IDCs. The holes in the medulla found in the present study may be the site where T cells (after positive selection in the cortex) emigrate from the thymus, without having been subjected to negative selection owing to the absence of IDCs at this site, and hence have potential autoreactivity. This explanation would imply that the transition from cortex into medullary phenotype before emigration as autoreactive cell does not require the presence of IDCs.

In conclusion, this detailed (immuno)histological analysis of the rat thymus after CsA treatment and subsequent recovery presents data that may in part explain the role of the thymus in CsA-induced syngeneic graft-vs-host disease. These data may further serve as a basis to design studies focusing on the antigen-recognition repertoire of lymphocytes in different compartments of the thymus generated by CsA treatment.

ACKNOWLEDGMENTS

The authors gratefully acknowledge the expert technical assistance of Roel Broekhuizen, Bert Elvers, Cees de Heer, and Joke Robinson in various parts of the experimental work. Antibodies in the MRC OX series were provided by Dr. A.F. Williams, Oxford, UK; those in the ED series by Dr. C. Dijkstra, Amsterdam, The Netherlands; those in the HIS series by Dr. J. Kampinga, Groningen, The Netherlands; and R73 by Dr. T. Hünig, Würzburg, Germany. This study was supported in part by the Foundation for Technical Sciences, Utrecht, The Netherlands.

REFERENCES

1. Glazier A, Tutschka PJ, Farmer ER, Santos GW. Graft-versus-host disease in cyclosporin A-treated rats after syngeneic and autologous bone marrow reconstitution. J Exp Med 1983; 158:1–8.
2. Sakaguchi S, Sakaguchi N. Thymus and autoimmunity. Transplantation of the thymus from cyclosporin A-treated mice causes organ-specific autoimmune disease in athymic nude mice. J Exp Med 1988; 167:1479–85.
3. Beschorner WE, Namnoum JD, Hess AD, Shinn CA, Santos GW. Cyclosporin A and the thymus. Immunopathology. Am J Pathol 1987; 126:487–96.
4. Attridge S, Eccles SA, Alexander P. Serum cyclosporin A levels in rats and mice. In: *Cyclosporin A*. White DJG (ed). Elsevier, Amsterdam, 1982; 173–5.

EXPERIMENTAL MODELS FOR AUTOIMMUNE DISEASES

98
The NOD Mouse as a Model of Local Autoimmunity

Jean-François Bach
INSERM U25, CNRS URA122, Hôpital Necker, Paris, France

The NOD mouse develops insulin-dependent diabetes mellitus (IDDM) at 5–8 months of age, with a marked predominance in females. The disease is characterized by a selective destruction of insulin-secreting β cells with preservation of other cellular constituents of the pancreas (exocrine tissue, α and γ cells). Long before β-cell destruction, the islets of Langerhans are infiltrated by mononucleated cells that essentially include T cells and to a lesser extent monocytes and macrophages. Converging arguments indicate that β-cell destruction is exclusively mediated by T cells and their products. IDDM is prevented by neonatal thymectomy, anti-CD4 monoclonal antibodies (MAbs) and cyclosporine and can be transferred into healthy (nondiabetic) syngeneic recipients by purified T cells even in mice rendered agammaglobulinemic by perinatal treatment with anti-μ antibodies. Importantly, the disease onset is controlled by a class II major histocompatibility complex (MHC) gene, but other non-MHC genes are also involved. Based on this data, one may assume that β cell aggression results from T-cell autosensitization against β-cell islet antigens that are presented to T cells by MHC class II antigens. Such activated CD4-positive T cells may act locally within the islets by producing various pharmacologically active lymphokines, which attract and activate macrophages, or by helping the differentiation of cytotoxic CD8-positive T cells, the reality of which, however, has never been formally demonstrated. In this scheme, several questions remain largely unsolved.

The nature of the target β-cell autoantigen is ill-defined. Several molecules have been characterized as a target of anti-islet autoantibodies, notably a 58-kD and a 64-kD proteins but there is no evidence that the antibodies directed against these antigens are specific to NOD mice and related to IDDM pathogenesis. In fact, one would like to know what are the antigens that are recognized by pathogenic T cells. A number of islet-specific T-cell clones have been generated in several laboratories but the antigen recognized by these clones has not been characterized. One should note, however, the recent work by I. Cohen indicating that the 65-kD hear-shock protein may accelerate IDDM onset in NOD mice, which suggests that this antigen shows cross-reactive epitopes with the β-cell antigen that pathogenic T cells recognize.

The T-cell receptor (TCR) usage of T cells is another important question. TCR αβ–bearing cells play a major role, since the disease is prevented by treatment with an anti–TCR αβ monoclonal antibody. This observation does not exclude a role for TCR γδ–bearing T cells. The putative restriction of V_{α} or V_{β} gene usage is still under scrutiny. Results obtained in our laboratory by C. Carnaud indicate that pathogenic T cells, as assessed in a diabetes transfer model, preferentially use the $V_{\beta 6}$ gene, but other studies using different approaches do not show the same restriction.

Regulatory T cells control the development of the disease. Diabetes onset is accelerated by thymectomy performed at 3 weeks of age or by cyclophosphamide treatment. The existence of suppressor T cells is further suggested by the prevention of diabetes transfer afforded by injecting spleen cells from nondiabetic mice before infusing diabetogenic spleen cells in irradiated recipients. It has been established that these suppressor T cells are CD4-positive, but much remains to be learned about their antigen specificity, T-cell receptor usage, and mechanism of action. It is interesting to note that the disease frequency is much lower in male than in female NOD mice, but males show a similar incidence to females after combined castration and thymectomy (each operation done alone being inefficient). These data suggest a sex hormone control of the T-cell–mediated suppression just mentioned.

Local islet immune phenomena should be investigated with regard to T-cell homing and trafficking. Data obtained from transfer studies indicate that CD4-positive T cells are first present within the islet and are necessary for attracting and probably activating CD8-positive T cells. The intimate mechanisms of T-cell homing to the islets and the stimuli that trigger the entry of T cells in the islet (passage from the periinsulitis that precedes by several weeks to true insulitis) must be determined. The mode of action of effector T cells must also be studied. The responsibility of cytokines is suspected but not proven. A role had been given recently to interleukin-1 (IL-1), but the specificity for β cells of the toxic effect of IL-1 is questionable and one has to explain why IL-1 therapy protects NOD mice from diabetes rather than promotes the disease.

In conclusion, very significant progress has been achieved on the complex T-cell–mediated anti-islet autoimmune response that leads to β-cell destruction in NOD mice. One may hope that the efforts in progress to generate T-cell autoreactive clones directed against the relevant β-cell autoantigen will permit us to reproduce in vitro the islet aggression that takes place within the islets and analyze in depth its cellular and molecular basis.

99

Analysis of the Acetylcholine Receptor Epitope–Bearing Protein p153 in Thymomas Favors "False-positive T-Cell Selection" as a Mechanism of Paraneoplastic Myasthenia Gravis

A. Marx,[1] K. I. Geuder,[1] R. Schoepfer,[2] S. Tzartos,[3] U. Kristoffersson,[4]
B. Schalke,[1] T. Kirchner,[1] and H. K. Müller-Hermelink[1]
[1]University of Würzburg, Federal Republic of Germany; [2]The Salk Institute, San Diego, California; [3]The Helenic Pasteur Institute, Athens, Greece; [4]Institute of Clinical Genetics, University of Lund, Sweden

INTRODUCTION

Myasthenia gravis (MG) is a model autoimmune disease as the late steps of the autoimmune process are well documented: the mechanisms of muscle weakness produced by autoantibodies to the muscle nicotinic acetylcholine receptors (AchRs); the production of autoantibodies by autoaggressive B cells, and their control by AchR-specific autoaggressive T cells (1). In addition, the target of the autoimmune process, the nicotinic AchR, has been completely cloned (2), the epitopes most relevant for autoantibody binding have been defined (3), and epitopes functioning as immunogens for autoaggressive T cells have been identified (4). However, the autoantigen triggering the autoimmune process and the place where primary autosensitization occurs are not known. In addition, an explanation linking the pathogenesis of MG to the thymic alterations associated with MG—thymic hyperplasia, atrophy, or thymoma—has been conclusive only in MG associated with thymic hyperplasia: AchRs on thymic myoid cells have been assumed as the autoantigens that are presented by thymic antigen-presenting cells to AchR-specific T cells, which in turn support autoaggressive B cells (5,6). In contrast, the initial pathogenesis of paraneoplastic MG has been unclear, as tumor autoantigens that share an extended homology with the AchR have not been identified (7–11). Here we give an update of our findings concerning a 153-kD thymoma protein (p153) that exhibits only a limited homology with the AchR (10). From our findings we derive a model how AchR-specific immature T cells may enter the T-cell repertoire.

MATERIALS AND METHODS

The classification of thymomas (12), the immunohistochemical (6), and most biochemical (8,9) procedures were published elsewhere. For affinity chromatography monoclonal antibody (MAb) 155 (3) was coupled to tresyl-activated Sepharose (Pharmacia, Freiburg, West Germany). Protein extracts were incubated with the affinity gel for 15 hr at 4°C and bound proteins eluted by boiling in gel-running buffer. For selective cyclic deoxyribonucleic acid (cDNA) synthesis a kit from Pharmacia was used. An oligonucleotide coding for the AchR alpha 371-378 amino acid sequence was used as primer to start cDNA synthesis from oligo(dT)-purified messenger ribonucleic acid (mRNAs) as templates. The cDNAs were cloned into the EcoR1 site of lambda-gtll phages and multiplied by infection of *Escherichia coli* Y1090.

RESULTS

Recent immunohistochemical investigations of thymomas with anti-AchR MAbs have confirmed previous findings of a positive correlation between the intrathymomatous expression of the AchR epitope alpha 371-378 and the occurrence of MG (Table 1). This correlation becomes even more significant when biochemical techniques are used to identify this epitope in p153 (Fig. 1a). Although this finding has suggested a role of p153 in the pathogenesis of anti-AchR autoimmunity, biochemical analysis of p153 has failed to demonstrated extensive structural homology between p153 and the nicotinic AchRs (Table 2). Molecular biological and electrophysiological experiments were therefore designed to identify thymoma proteins that might share a more extended homology with the AchRs. However, neither mRNAs similar to the AchR alpha subunit mRNA (Fig. 2) nor mRNAs similar to the other AchR subunit RNAs were identified (not shown), nor could ion channels be detected which share homologies with the AchRs (neuronal-type AchRs, gamma-aminobutyric acid [GABA] and glycine receptors) (11).

On the other hand, p153 is not unique to thymomas: In neuroblastomas we found a 153-kD protein as well (9), and its biochemical features (see Table 2) and partial cDNA (Fig. 3) strongly suggest that this protein is identical to p153. Obviously, the expression of p153 in these tumors is not associated with MG.

Table 1 Correlation Between the Expression of the AchR Epitope Alpha 371-378 in Various Thymoma Types and the Occurrence of Myasthenia Gravis (MG) in Thymoma Patients

Tumor type	Tumors with alpha 371-378	Tumors without alpha 371-378
Medullary thymoma	0	1
Mixed thymoma	1	10
Predominantly cortical thymoma	6	5
Cortical thymoma	10	0
Well-differentiated thymic carcinoma	8	2
Tumors with MG	23	4
Tumors without MG	2	12

The AchR epitope was detected immunohistochemically with anti-AchR Mab 155 (3). Thymomas were classified according to Kirchner and Muller-Hermelink (8).

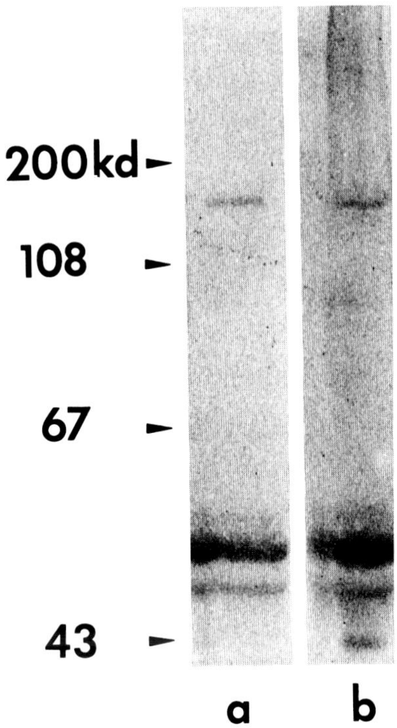

Figure 1 Identification of small quantities of p153 in an MG-associated thymoma that was not stained with MAb 155 immunohistochemically (lane a). p153 as a constituent of normal human thymus (lane b). p153 was enriched by MAb 155–Sepharose affinity chromatography. 7.5% SDS-PAGE was performed under reducing conditions. Western blots were probed with MAb 155. The bands at about 50 kD are due to MAb 155 eluted from the affinity gel. The band at 42 kD in lane b is due to the AchR alpha subunit from thymic myoid cells.

Table 2 Different Biochemical Features of the Nicotinic AchR (12,18); and of p153 from Thymomas and Neuroblastomas (8,9) Suggest a Lack of Structural Homology Between the Two Proteins

	Molecular weight	Isoelectric point	Compound structure	Sugar residues	Alpha-Btx[a] binding	MIR[b]
AchR	42–66	5.0	+	+	+	+
p153	153	5.0	–	–	–	–

[a]Alpha-Bungarotoxin.
[b]Main immunogenic region (3).

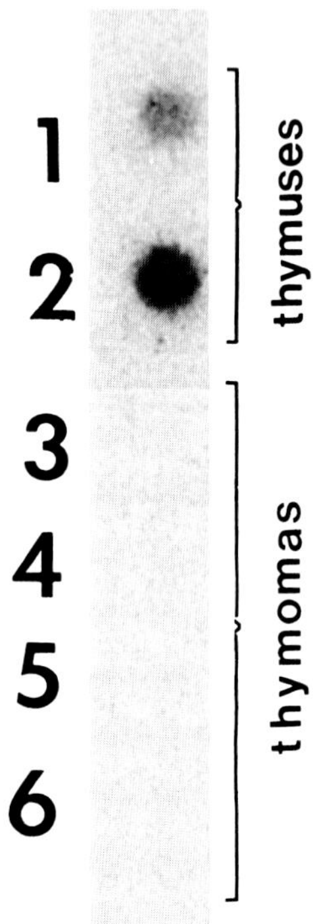

Figure 2 Occurrence of mRNA coding for the AchR alpha subunit in normal thymuses (dots 1 and 2) but not in MG-associated thymomas (dots 3–6). The thymus represented in dot 2 had considerably more myoid cells immunohistochemically than the thymus represented in dot 1. The Northern dot blot with 20 μg RNA per dot was probed with the AchR alpha subunit cDNA (15).

CONCLUSIONS

The correlation between the expression of p153 in thymomas and the occurrence of MG in thymoma patients strongly suggests the pathogenetic relevance of p153 (7). However, the immunogenicity of p153 alone obviously is not a sufficient prerequisite to trigger autoimmunity: otherwise neuroblastomas should be associated with MG, which is not the case. Therefore, we suggest that it is an essential additional prerequisite for triggering autoimmunity that p153 is expressed in a thymoma microenvironment (9). This microenvironment, has at least one unique feature not found in nonthymic tumors: It maintains the homing function for immature CD1-positive T cells (unpublished) that otherwise is only provided by the normal thymic microenvironment. The relevance of this property of MG-associated thymomas is supported by our observation that undifferentiated thymic tumors without maintenance of the homing function are not associated with MG (unpublished). However, there is also a striking difference between the microenvironments of the normal thymus and of MG-associated thymomas: On the one hand we show here (see Fig. 1b) that it is p153 that causes immunoreactivity of a few normal thymic medullary (!)

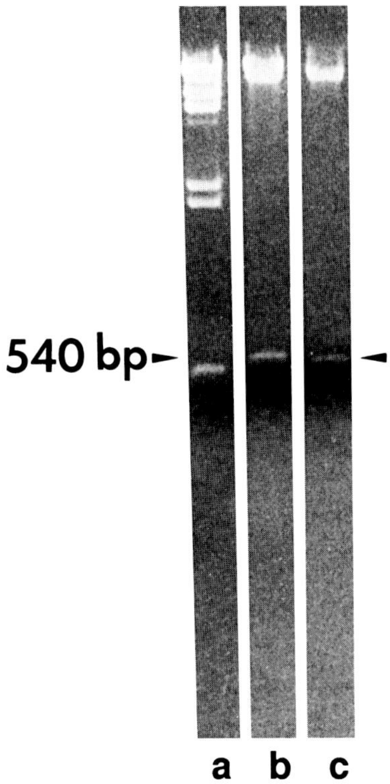

Figure 3 Selective synthesis of a 540-bp cDNA from thymoma (lane b) and neuroblastoma (lane c) mRNA using oligonucleotides as primers that code for the AchR amino acid sequence alpha 371-378. Molecular weight markers in lane a. The identical length of the cDNAs suggests that thymoma and neuroblastoma share an identical protein with the AchR epitope alpha 371-378.

epithelial cells with MAbs to the AchR epitope alpha 371-378 (7). On the other hand, p153 in thymoma is coexpressed with cortical (!) epithelial cell markers (13). From these findings we conclude that both the homing function and a specifically defective selection mechanism may be required to develop autoimmunity: As self-peptides expressed in the context of cortical epithelium contribute to the match of the MHC with a given T-cell receptor (TCR) (14), we suggest that it is only inside thymomas that epitopes of p153 serve as the "self-components" of MHC-self complexes. These pathological complexes could contain an AchR epitope as the self-component, and may therefore have an increased avidity for AchR-specific TCR, causing the very specific "false-positive selection" of autoaggressive AchR-specific T cells (Fig. 4).

ACKNOWLEDGMENTS

This work was supported by DFG grant Ki370/1-1 (A. Marx and T. Kirchner) and the Greek General Secretariat of Research and Technology (S. Tzartos).

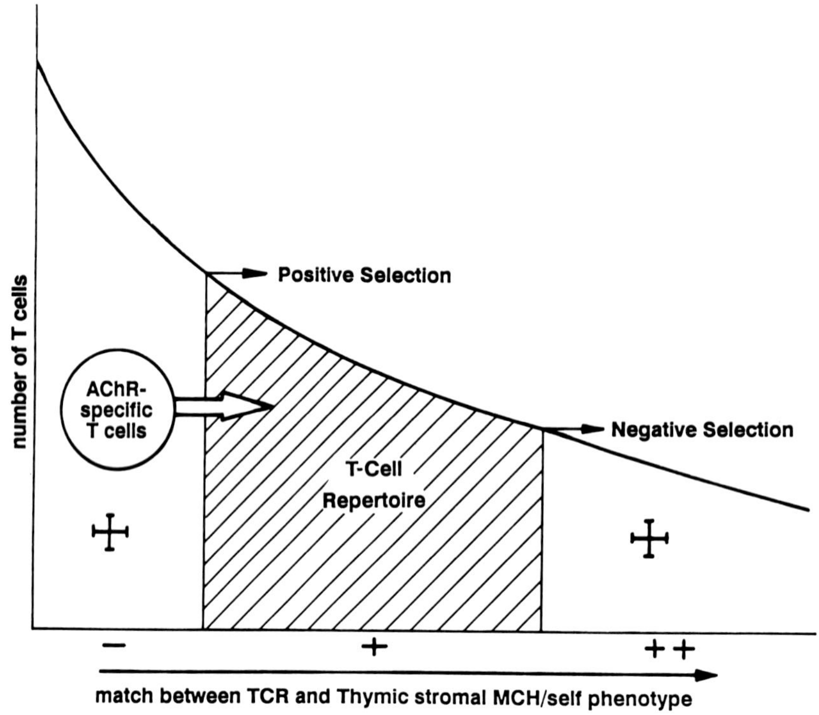

Figure 4 "False-positive selection" as disease mechanism: AchR-epitopes of p153 abnormally expressed on thymoma cortical type epithelial cells could serve as "self-peptides" in abnormal MHC-self complexes, thereby improving the match of otherwise mismatching AchR-specific TCRs with the thymic stroma

REFERENCES

1. Hohlfeld R. Myasthenia gravis and thymoma; paraneoplastic failure of Neuromuscular transmission. Lab Invest 1990;62:241–243.
2. Mishina M, Takai T, Imoto K, Noda M, Takahashi T, Numa S, Methfessel C, Dakmann B. Molecular distinction between fetal and adult forms of muscle acetylcholine receptor. Nature 1886;321:406–411.
3. Tzartos SJ, Kokla A, Walgrave SL, Conti-Tronconi BM. Localization of the main immunogenic region of human muscle acetylcholine receptor to residues 67-76 of the alpha subunit. Proc Natl Acad Sci USA 1988;86:2899–903.
4. Harcourt G, Jermy A. Mapping the autoimmunizing epitopes on acetylcholine receptors. Immunol Today 1987; 8:319–321.
5. Wekerle H, Ketelsen UP, Zurn AD, Fulpius BW. Intrathymic pathogenesis of myasthenia gravis: Transient expression of acetylcholine receptors on thymus derived myogenic cells. Eur J Immunol 1978;8:579–581.
6. Kirchner T, Hoppe F, Schalke B, Müller-Hermelink HK. Microenvironment of thymic myoid cells in myasthenia gravis. Virchows Arch B Cell Pathol 1988; 54:295–302.
7. Kirchner T, Tzartos S, Hoppe F, Schalke B, Wekerle H, Müller-Hermelink HK. Pathogenesis of myasthenia gravis: Acetylcholine receptor-related antigenic determinants in tumor-free thymuses and thymic epithelial tumors: morphological and immunocytochemical characterization. Am J Pathol 1988;130:268–280.

8. Marx A, Kirchner T, Hoppe F, O'Connor R, Schalke B, Tzartos S, Müller-Hermelink. Proteins with epitopes of the acetylcholine receptor in epithelial cell cultures of thymomas in myasthenia gravis. Am J Pathol 1989;134:865–877.
9. Marx A, O'Connor R, Geuder KI, Hoppe F, Schalke B, Tzartos S, Kalies I, Kirchner T, Müller-Hermelink HK. Characterization of a protein with an acetylcholine receptor epitope from myasthenia gravis-associated thymomas. Lab Invest 1990;62:279–286.
10. Geuder KI, Schoepfer R, Kirchner T, Marx A, Müller-Hermelink HK. The gene of the alpha-subunit of the acetylcholine receptor: Molecular organization and transcription in myasthenia gravis-associated thymomas. Thymus 1989;14:179–186.
11. Siara J, Rüdel R, Marx A. Absence of acetylcholine-induced current in epithelial cells from thymus glands and thymomas of myasthenia gravis patients. Neurology 1990 (in press).
12. Kirchner T, Müller-Hermelink HK. New approaches to the diagnosis of thymic epithelial tumors. In: *Progress in Surgical Pathology*. Vol 10. Fenoglio-Preiser CM, Wolff M, and Rilke F (eds). Philadelphia, Field and Wood, 1989, pp. 167-186.
13. Willcox N, Schluep M, Ritter MA, Schuurman HJ, Newsom-Davis J, Christensson B. Myasthenic and non-myasthenic thymoma. An expansion of a minor cortical epithelial cell subset. Am J Pathol 1987;127:447–460.
14. von Boehmer H, Teh HS, Kisielow P. The thymus selects the useful, neglects the useless and destroys the harmful. Immunol Today 1989;10:61–67.
15. Schoepfer R, Luther M, Lindstrom J. The human medulloblastoma cell line TE671 expresses a muscle-like acetylcholine receptor: Cloning of the alpha-subunit cDNA. FEBS Lett 1988;226:235–240.
16. Momoi MY, Lennon VA. Purification and biochemical characterization of nicotinic acetylcholine receptors of human muscle. J Biol Chem 1982;257:12757–12764.
17. Luther MA, Schoepfer R, Whiting P, Casey B, Blatt Y, Montal MS, Montal M, Lindstrom J. A muscle acetylcholinereceptor is expressed in the human cerebellar medulloblastoma cell line TE671. J Neurosci 1989;9:1082–1096.

100
Myasthenia Gravis
Modulation by Hormones

Evelyne Morel,[1] Béatrice Vernet-der Garabedian,[1] Ana Cardona,[1] Tapan Audhya,[2] Hervé Lefèvre,[1] Gideon Goldstein,[2] and Jean-François Bach[1]
[1]*INSERM U25, CNRS URA122, Hôpital Necker, Paris, France;*
[2]*Immunobiology Research Institute, Annandale, New Jersey*

INTRODUCTION

Although it is evident that the symptoms of myasthenia gravis (MG) are caused by an antibody-mediated autoimmune response to the nicotinic acetylcholine receptor (AchR), what initiates and regulates the autoimmune reactivity in MG is still unclear. Several studies used experimental autoimmune myasthenia gravis (EAMG) that can be induced in animals by immunization with purified AchR and which is an interesting model to answer the unresolved questions about the disease.

Among the numerous factors that would be involved in the human or the experimental disease, the role of hormones is poorly known. Recent interest has concerned the putative neuroendocrine-neuroimmune interactions (1).

In order to seek such a role, we attempted to modulate EAMG in high- and low-responder mice using steroid, gonadotropic, and thymic hormones. We found that they can account for the heterogeneity of clinical and biological expression in MG.

MATERIALS AND METHODS

Animals

Four-week-old C57Bl/6 (male and female) and Balb/c (female), high- and low-EAMG responders, were obtained from the IFFACREDO Company. Mice were studied in groups of five or 10.

Antigens

Triton X-100 solubilized AchR were prepared from human, rat, or mouse muscles, from human TE671 cell line, and from *Torpedo* (an electric ray) (2). For the immunizations the preparations were extensively dialyzed against phosphate-buffered saline (PBS) buffer to eliminate triton X-100.

Protocols

Immunizations

Mice were immunized twice at 1-week intervals by subcutaneous injections of 20 μg of Torpedo. AchR emulsified in complete Freund's adjuvant (Gibco Labs.). Rat antigen was used alone in the preliminary protocol. For some experiments human TE671 or mouse antigens were added to the immunizing preparations. Dialyzed buffer was used as control.

Pretreatments

Steroid (β-estradiol, progesterone), gonadotropic (prolactin, PRL; luteinizing hormone–releasing hormone, LHRH) and thymic (thymopoietin, Tpo, thymopentin, TP5) hormones were used for pretreatment.

In the first protocol, low doses (10 ng/mouse) of β-estradiol, progesterone, and prolactin were given subcutaneously twice a month for 6-months to male and female C57Bl/6 mice before immunization by rat AchR. In the second protocol, mice received, twice a week for 4 weeks, hormones or saline in intraperitoneal injections. Final doses were: 20 μg/mouse for PRL and LHRH, 10 μg/mouse for TP5, and 1 μg/mouse for Tpo.

Assays

Mice were bled at various intervals by retro-orbital plexus puncture; sera were isolated and stored at –20°C until use. Mice were killed between 8 and 10 weeks after the beginning of the protocol.

Total IgG concentrations were determined using an ELISA method with anti-mouse immunoglobulin G (IgG) (H+L) peroxidase–conjugated antibody (Biosys). Purified mouse IgG was used to establish standard curves.

Anti-AchR antibody levels were measured on 1–5 μl of mouse serum by a standard double antibody radioimmunoassay using the various antigens bound to 125I–α-bungarotoxin. The antibody titers were determined from the linear region of the dilution curve, and expressed as nM of radioactive toxin binding sites precipitated per liter of serum (3).

Lymphocytes were harvested from mouse spleens and cultured for a week in the presence or not of mitogens. Anti-AchR antibody levels were measured by the radioimmunoprecipitation method on 100 μl of supernatants (4).

Fatigability of mice was estimated by testing their capacity to repeat subsequent grips (20) and to rotate in a roller after a preliminary series of training.

RESULTS

The data obtained according to the first protocol are summarized in Table 1. No changes were observed in anti-AchR antibody titers after pretreating with β-estradiol. On the contrary, progesterone and prolactin enhanced the anti-AchR antibody titers: about two times in males and three times in females for progesterone, about three times in males and five times in females for prolactin.

We used females for subsequent protocols. Figure 1 shows a representative distribution of IgG levels in C57Bl/6 mice. These levels were generally enhanced by pretreatments 6 weeks after immunization. The mean values were for control AchR: 2.84+0.83 mg/ml;

Table 1 Anti-Rat AchR Antibody Titers[a] in C57BL/6 Mice

Hormonal pretreatment	Male	Female
None	4.70 + 0.10	6.00 + 0.52
+ β-estradiol	4.67 + 0.05	6.33 + 0.25
None	5.90 + 0.27	5.80 + 0.30
+ Progesterone	12.27 + 0.05	18.70 + 0.14
None	6.70 + 0.40	5.50 + 0.35
+ Prolactin	18.40 + 0.27	28.38 + 1.57

[a]Expressed as nM.

Tpo+AchR: 4.97+1.95 mg/ml; PRL+AchR: 3.04+1.20 mg/ml; TP5+AchR: 4.18+1.30 mg/ml. This was also observed throughout the protocol in low-responder mice.

Evolution of anti-AchR antibody titers (mean) in C57Bl/6 mice against the immunizing antigen were measured throughout the protocol. Positive titers were observed 1 month after the immunization. The maximum was reached 6 weeks after starting. Responses toward auto- and xenoantigens were enhanced in some cases of pretreated mice, as shown in Fig. 2. This reactivity was variable among the animals without a relationship between the level of the responses toward the immunizing antigen for mice pretreated by Tpo (Fig. 3). Similar results were found in Balb/c mice.

We looked for activation in spleens of some mice at the end of experiments. Data for mice having received gonadotropic hormones are given in Table 2. Weak anti-AchR antibody responses were observed in LPS-stimulated cultures of mice without hormonal pretreatment. In mice having received PRL or LHRH, weak anti-AchR antibody responses were found in non- or concanavalin A (Con A)–stimulated cultures. Furthermore, the responses were enhanced in LPS-stimulated cultures.

The clinical status of mice was checked between 6 and 8 weeks after the first immunization. A typical result is shown in Figure 4. The scores were lower in immunized

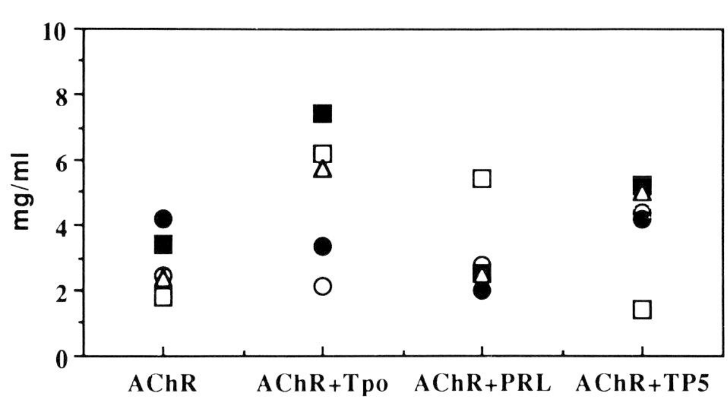

Figure 1 Evolution if IgG concentrations in C57Bl/6 mice pretreated with hormones and immunized with Torpedo AchR.

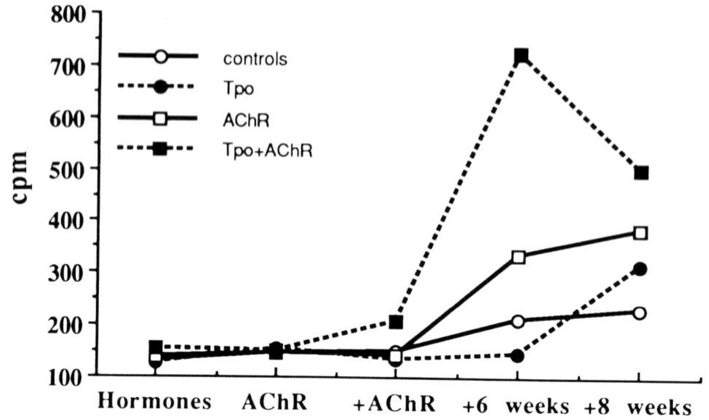

(a)

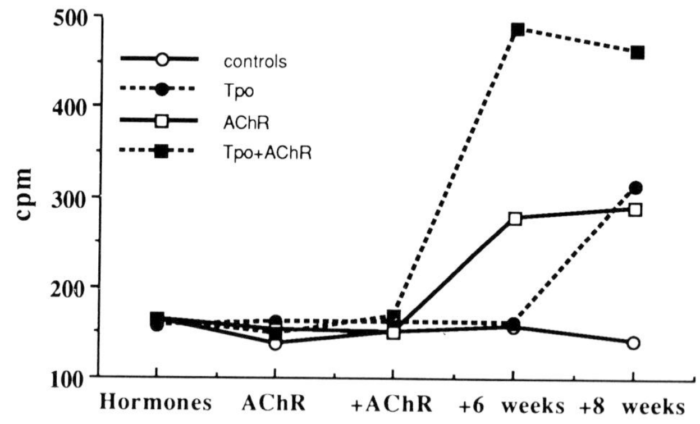

(b)

Figure 2 Evolution of anti-AchR antibody levels in C57Bl/6 mice: (a) against human AchR; (b) against mouse AchR.

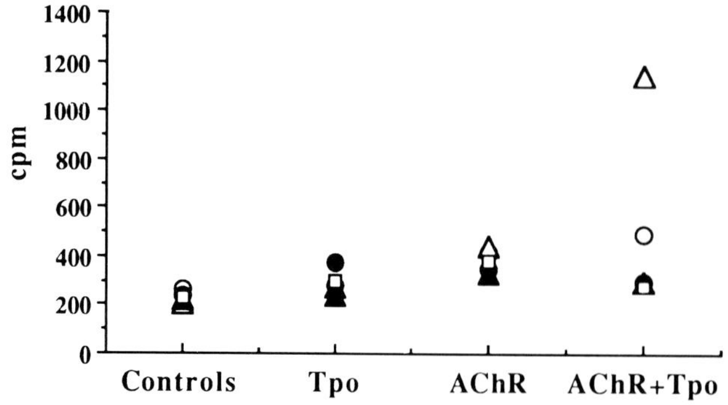

Figure 3 Individual anti-AchR antibody levels in controls and immunized C57Bl/6 mice.

Table 2 Anti-AchR Antibody Level in C57Bl/6 Spleen Culture Supernatants

	Mitogens		
Immunization groups	None	Con A	LPS
Controls	0.31 + 0.30	0.45 + 0.34	1.48 + 1.02
PRL + AchR	0.11 + 1.09	1.10 + 0.98	11.30 + 18.76
LHRH + AchR	2.42 + 2.03	2.52 + 1.76	9.39 + .822

mice than in others. The lowest were observed in the LHRH pretreated mice, but the data were not statistically significant.

CONCLUSIONS

Immunization with mammal or Torpedo AchR can provide EAMG in mice, with a great variability in the biological and the clinical parameters depending on the animals and on other factors.

The capacity to produce specific and nonspecific IgG is higher in females than in males. The nonspecific IgG and the anti-AchR antibody responses can be enhanced by pretreatment with steroid hormones, such as progesterone, gonadotropic hormones, and releasing hormones PRL and LHRH and by thymic hormones such as Tpo and a pentapeptide (TP5).

In some mice it is possible to observe, besides the responses toward the immunizing antigens, cross-reactivity toward auto- and xenoantigens favored by the pretreatment. It is also possible to observe production of anti-AchR antibody by spleens from mice having received some pretreatment.

Polyclonal and specific activation can be found in high (C57Bl/6) and weak (Balb/c) EAMG-responder mice.

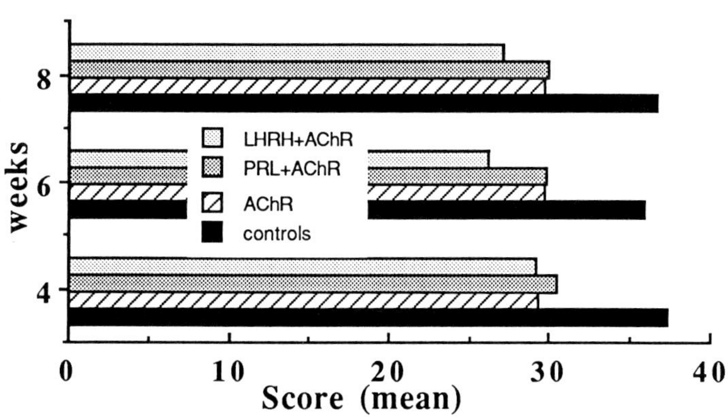

Figure 4 Evolution of fatigability scores in C57Bl/6 mice.

The clinical observation of EAMG is not constantly associated with the anti-AchR antibody titers whether the mice were pretreated or not. In some cases, we have observed more fatigability in mice having received pretreatment. However, as in human MG, great variability was observed among the animals.

All these data need support by further experiments in order to determine how, among all the hormones, hormones of the "neuroendocrinoimmunological axis" could be involved in the etiology of MG. By stimulating the humoral response, it could trigger the production of pathogenic autoantibodies.

ACKNOWLEDGMENTS

This work was supported by grants of the Association Française contre les Myopathies. We greatly thank Mrs. M. Turpin for helpful technical assistance.

REFERENCES

1. Jarvis, D.W. Neuroimmuno-Neuroendocrine Interactions. Prog Neuroendocrinolmmunol 1990;3:65–67.
2. Morel E, Raimond F, and Bach J.F. Increased reactivity with the thymus acetylcholine receptor antigen in myasthenia gravis associated with other disease. J. Neuroimmunol., 1987;14:221–227.
3. Morel E., Raimond F., Goulon-Goeau C., Berrih S., Vernet-der Garabedian B., Harb J. and Bach, J.F. Le dosage des anticorps anti-récepteur de l'acétylcholine dans la myasthénie. Etude de 329 sérums. Nouv. Presse Méd., 1982; 11:1849–1854.
4. Safar D., Berrih-Aknin S., Morel E. In vitro anti-acetylcholine receptor antibody synthesis by myasthenia gravis patient lymphocytes. Correlations with thymic histology and thymic epithelial cell interactions. J. Clin. Immunol. 1987;7:225–234.

101

Decreased Soluble Interleukin-2 Receptor After Thymectomy in Patients with Myasthenia Gravis

Sylvia Cohen-Kaminsky,[1] Yannick Jacques,[2] Christine Aime,[1] and Sonia Berrih-Aknin[1]
[1]*CNRS URA-1159, Hôpital Marie-Lannelongue, Le Plessis-Robinson, France;* [2]*INSERM U-211, Nantes, France*

INTRODUCTION

Myasthenia gravis (MG) is the prototype of acquired organ-specific autoimmune disorders, characterized by alteration of neuromuscular transmission (1). The basic defect is caused by autoantibodies against the acetylcholine receptor (AchR), which circulate at variable levels in the sera of more than 85% of the patients and neutralize their specific target at the neuromuscular junction (1,2). However, anti-AchR antibody (Ab) titers do not strictly correlate with disease severity (1,3). Because of the beneficial effect of thymectomy (4) and the finding of thymic abnormalities (5), a role for the thymus has been proposed in the pathogenesis of MG. Few studies have documented the activation state of T and B cells in MG by both phenotypic and functional criteria. Recently, we have shown that thymic and peripheral blood T cells are activated as reflected by their increased response to recombinant interleukin-2 (rIL-2) without previous stimulation (6,7), and the data suggested a possible aberrant mechanism of the regulation and/or expression of the IL-2 receptor in MG. Thymic B cells are also activated as demonstrated by expression of various activation markers and spontaneous response to 12-kD B-cell growth factor (8). Since soluble IL-2 receptor (sIL-2) serum level represents a very early sign of cellular activation and is thought to serve an immunoregulatory function during cell growth (9), we explored the activation state in MG patients by measurement of serum levels of sIL-2R before and after thymic surgery. We also evaluated the usefulness of sIL-2R as a marker of disease severity in the follow-up of MG patients.

MATERIALS AND METHODS

Patients

Thirty-three patients with myasthenia gravis diagnosed on the basis of clinical features, electromygraphic decrement, and positive effect of anticholinesterase (females, age range: 16–74 years; males, age range: 15–57 years) were followed-up at various periods after thymectomy (3– to 8 points during 2–6 years). On the whole, 138 MG sera were tested for their sIL-2R content. Sera of age- and sex-matched normal subjects (n = 24) from the blood transfusion center (Marie-Lannelongue Hospital, Le Plessis Robinson, France) served as controls.

Quantification of Serum-Soluble IL-2R

A quantitative immunoradiometric assay for human sIL-2R was set up essentially as previously described (9) using two monoclonal antibody (MAb)–directed against two distinct epitopes on the 55-kD chain of the human membrane IL-2R. The results were referred to a calibration standard curve obtained with purified sIL-2R from a high-producer T-cell clone as previously described (9), and expressed as pM IL-2R in serum. The detection limit of this assay was about 5 pM (or 0.2 ng/ml). Levels of sIL-2R in MG sera were considered significantly positive when higher than 2 SD above the mean of healthy controls (>58.53 nM).

RESULTS

Follow-up of Soluble IL-2R Levels After Thymectomy

The analysis of the MG sera samples indicated a gradual decrease in the frequency of significantly high sIL-2R levels with time after thymectomy. Before thymectomy, 42.4% of MG patients presented high levels of sIL-2R, then it decreased gradually to reach 13% 3 years or more after thymectomy (Table 1). Significantly higher sIL-2R levels compared to the control group were found before thymectomy as well as 6 months and 1 year after thymectomy ($p<0.001$, $p<0.001$, and $p<0.01$, respectively, by the Mann-Whitney test), whereas patients tested 2 years or more after thymectomy were not significantly different from controls. Accordingly, these patients had significant lower levels than when tested before thymectomy ($p<0.02$, Wilcoxon matched-pair test). All together the data indicate a significant decline of sIL-2R levels within 2 years after thymectomy.

Relationship of Serum IL-2R to Clinical Parameters

Before thymectomy, all the patients monitored presented generalized symptoms and were classified into clinical subgroups according to disease severity: IIA (mild disease) or IIB (severe disease). MG patients from the IIA subgroup presented lower sIL-2R levels than patients from the IIB subgroup (Fig. 1). The difference between the tow subgroups was statistically significant ($p<0.05$, chi-squared test). Indeed in the IIA subgroup, two of 10 (20%) patients had levels significantly higher than control values ($p<0.02$, Mann-Whitney test), whereas in the IIB subgroup, 14 out 23 (61%) presented such higher sIL-2R titers ($p<0.001$, Mann-Whitney test). After surgery, a significant and progressive decrease of sIL-2 receptor levels was observed in severely affected patients (see Fig. 1). In addition, all the 16 patients who improved from grade IIA or IIB to grade I or to remission within 2

Table 1 Frequencies of MG Sera with Significant Titer of Soluble IL-2 Receptors

	Number of positive[a] MG sera	Frequency (%)	Significativity: vs controls	Significativity: vs patients before thymectomy
Before thymectomy	14/33	42.4	p<0.001	
6 months postthymectomy	11/26	42.3	p<0.001	NS
1 year postthymectomy	8/31	25.8	p<0.01	NS
2 years postthymectomy	7/24	29.2	NS	p<0.02
>3 years postthymectomy	3/24	13.0	NS	p<0.02

[a]Positive sera are defined as samples with soluble IL-2R levels higher than 2 SD above the mean of healthy controls (>58.53 pM).

years after thymectomy had low levels of sIL-2R. For the patient group slightly improved or not after surgery, the frequency of high sIL-2R level (eight of 17 patients, 47%) was similar to the one observed before thymectomy (42%), and conversely all the patients still presenting high serum sIL-2R levels after surgery (eight of 33) showed generalized symptoms. Interestingly, in individual patients the decrease of sIL-2R took place before clinical improvement and was observed whether the patients were treated by corticosteroids or not (data not shown). Together these data indicate that the decrease of frequency of high sIL-2R is related to clinical improvement of the patients and establish a clear association between high sIL-2R levels and disease severity.

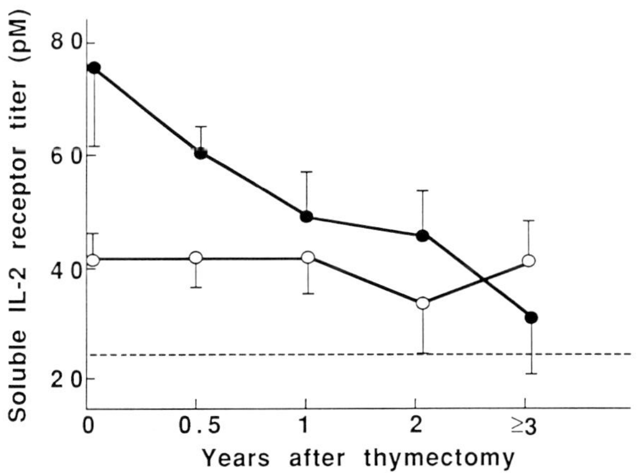

Figure 1 Effect of thymectomy on serum levels of sIL-2R in relation with disease severity. Mean values of sIL-2R levels are represented. Vertical bars represent SEM. Subgroups of patients are defined according to disease severity: (O) patients with mild disease (IIA) before surgery, 10 cases; (●) patients with severe disease (IIB) before surgery, 23 cases. Disease severity was graded according to Osserman's classification as previously described (6–8). The broken line represents the mean value of the healthy controls.

DISCUSSION AND CONCLUSIONS

This chapter reports the presence of sIL-2R in sera of patients with myasthenia gravis. Our conclusions are the following: (a) Soluble IL-2 receptor titer is high in a significant number of patients when tested before thymectomy. (b) A significant and progressive decline of sIL-2R titers is observed after surgery, which is well correlated to clinical improvement in individual patients.

These findings represent an additional evidence of high-activation state in MG patients and are in accordance with the previously observed occurrence of high serum levels of sIL-2R in various autoimmune disorders, including lupus erythematosus (10), multiple sclerosis (11), and rheumatoid arthritis (12). In these diseases, although sIL-2R does not represent a specific marker, it was well correlated to disease severity and closely paralleled clinical improvement.

Because of its capacity to bind IL-2 (9), the physiological role of the sIL-2R might be the homeostatic control of the immune response. Several in vitro studies has suggested a role for sIL-2R in downregulation of the IL-2–dependent responses by decreasing the density of cell-associated IL-2R and/or by competing with cellular IL-2R for IL-2 binding (9), thus preventing the ongoing pattern of the immune response. It remains to be determined whether quantitative or qualitative abnormalities of sIL-2R in diseases associated with chronic cellular activation, including autoimmune diseases, have any pathophysiological implication in the immunological aberrations observed; that is, whether they may in themselves mediate an impairment of the immune system regulation that could contribute to pathogenesis. Nevertheless, the most simple hypothesis is that the elevated titer of sIL-2R may only reflect the immunopathogenic activation in the course of the disease.

The high levels of sIL-2R in the periphery before thymectomy and its decrease after surgery with a concomitant clinical improvement underline the role of the thymus in MG, which is thought to be involved in many aspects of disease pathogenesis (6,8,13). The possibility that the thymus could play a role in the occurrence of sIL-2R in the periphery could be raised. As one hypothesis, the thymus gland could be the source of sIL-2R production. However, this is not supported by the kinetics of sIL-2R decreases after thymectomy (significant decline after 2 years). Alternatively, the thymus could be involved in the exacerbation of the autoimmune process by generating a long-lived activated cell fraction, which might be slowly eliminated after thymectomy. These activated cells could result from primary autosensitization against an AchR-like molecule demonstrated in the thymus by several groups (13).

The evaluation of serum sIL-2R, may represent a good marker of disease severity in the follow-up of individual patients and of the effect of thymectomy. Further sampling during acute exacerbations will determine the usefulness of sIL-2R in monitoring disease progression, in particular to assess it interest for predicting relapse or clinical aggravation, and in following response to therapy.

SUMMARY

Serum samples from 33 patients with myasthenia gravis followed after thymectomy were titrated for their soluble interleukin-2 receptor content. High levels of interleukin-2 receptor were found in 42.4% of the patients before thymectomy. Patients severely affected presented the highest sIL-2R titers. A significant and progressive decline of soluble interleukin-2 receptor levels within 2 years after surgery, which was well associated with clinical improvement of remission was observed. The decline after thymectomy of soluble interleukin-2 receptor titers suggests a possible role of the thymus in the occurrence of soluble interleukin-2 receptor in the periphery.

ACKNOWLEDGMENT

This work was supported by grants from AFM (Association Française contre les Myopathies) and CNAMTS (Caisse Nationale d'assurance Maladie des Travailleurs Salariés).

REFERENCES

1. Engel AG. Acquired autoimmune myasthenia gravis. In: *Myology*. A.G. Engel and B.Q. Banker eds. McGraw-Hill, Yew York, 1986, pp 1925–1954.
2. Fambrough DM, Drachman DB, Satyamuri S. Neuromuscular junction in myasthenia gravis: Decreased acetylcholine receptor. Science 1973; 182:293–295.
3. Berrih S, Morel E, Gaud C, Raimond F, Le Brigand H, Bach JF. Anti-AChR antibodies, thymic histology, and T cell subsets in myasthenia gravis. Neurology 1984; 34:66–71.
4. Genkins G, Kornfeld P, Papatesta AE, Bender AR, Matta RJ. Clinical experience in more than 2000 patients with myasthenia gravis. Ann. N.Y. Acad. Sci. 1987; 505:500–513.
5. Levine G, Rosai J. Thymic hyperplasia and neoplasia: A review of current concepts. Hum. Pathol. 1978; 9:495–515.
6. Cohen-Kaminsky S, Levasseur P, Binet JP, Berrih-Aknin S. Evidence of enhanced recombinant interleukin-2 sensitivity in thymic lymphocytes from patients with myasthenia gravis: Possible role in the autoimmune pathogenesis. J. Neuroimmunol. 1989; 24:75–85.
7. Cohen-Kaminsky S, Gaud C, Morel E, Berrih-Aknin S. High recombinant interleukin-2 sensitivity in peripheral blood lymphocytes from patients with myasthenia gravis: Correlations with clinical parameters. J. Autoimmun. 1989; 2:241–258.
8. Leprince C, Cohen-Kaminsky S, Berrih-Aknin S, Treton D, Galanaud P, Richard Y. 1989. Thymic B cells from myasthenia gravis patients are activated B cells: Phenotypic and functional analysis. J. Immunol. 1990; 145:2115–2122.
9. Jacques Y, Le Mauff B, Boeffard F, Godard A, Soulillou JP. A soluble interleukin 2 receptor produced by a normal alloreactive human T cell clone binds interleukin 2 with low affinity. J. Immunol. 1987; 139:2308–2316.
10. Huang Y, Perrin LH, Miescher PA, Zubler RH. Correlation of T and B cell activities in vitro and serum IL-2 levels in systemic lupus erythematosus. J. Immunol. 1988; 141:2612–2618.
11. Greenberg SF, Marcon L, Hurwitz BJ, Waldmann TA, Nelson DL. Elevated levels of soluble interleukin-2 receptors in multiple sclerosis. N. Engl. J. Med. 1988; 319:1019–1020.
12. Symons JA, Wood NC, Di Giovine FS, Duff GW. Soluble IL-2 receptor in rheumatoid arthritis: Correlation with disease activity, IL-1 and IL-2 inhibition. J. Immunol. 1988; 141:2612–2618.
13. Berrih-Aknin S, Morel E, Raimond F, Safar D, Gaud C, Binet JP, Levasseur P, Bach JF. The role of the thymus in myasthenia gravis. Immunohistological and immunological studies in 115 cases. Ann. N.Y. Acad. Sci. 1987; 505:50–70.

102
Functional Properties of Thymic Nonlymphoid Cells in Myasthenia Gravis

Katarina Isaković, Ljiljana Popesković, Slobodan Apostolski, Nevena Arsenović, and Jelena Gospavić
Immunology Research Center, Faculty of Pharmacy, and University Clinical Center, Belgrade, Yugoslavia

INTRODUCTION

In our earlier studies (1,2) it was demonstrated that in myasthenia gravis (MG) thymuses, epithelial cells present in inner cortex were numerically and functionally affected. Decreased in number, those cells showed a lower synthesis and ability to interact with autologous thymocytes. On the other hand, medullary thymic epithelial (TE) cells in MG exerted an increased synthesis, while interaction with thymocytes was altered. In this experiment, it was shown that cortical epithelial cells in MG thymuses, cultured for 10 days, expressed class II major histocompatibility complex (MHC) components in a significantly lower extent. However, expression of Ia antigens on medullary TE cells was increased. The role of Ia molecules expressed on cortical and medullary TE cells, in induction of tolerance and/or autoimmunity as well as their role in autoimmune processes in MG was discussed.

MATERIALS AND METHODS

Thymuses

Myasthenia gravis thymuses were obtained from female patients between 19 and 30 years of age after thymectomy. Only hyperplastic thymuses derived from patients not receiving immunotherapy were used in this study. Thymuses obtained from individuals (females) who underwent heart surgery, 12 to 15 years old, served as controls.

Thymus Culture

In order to estimate thymic nonlymphoid cells (epithelial cells and macrophages), a confluent monolayer culture was established according to the method of Pyke and Gelfand (3), which was slightly modified (2). Cultures were harvested on day 10, and single cell suspension was prepared as it is described elsewhere (4).

Expression of Ia Antigens on Epithelial Cells and Macrophages

Thymic epithelial cells were identified by following monoclonal antibodies (MAbs): anti-cytokeratin (Immunotech, Marseille, France), reacting with all TE cells; and anti-MR6 and anti-MR19 (gift of Dr. M. Ritter, London), specific for cortical and medullary TE cells, respectively (5). Cells expressing M1 antigen were considered as macrophages, which were detected by MAb OKM1 (Ortho Dyagnostic System). Anti-Ia MAb was used for detection of Ia molecules. Ia-positive TE cells and macrophages were determined by a double-staining technique, combining immunoperoxidase staining with immunofluorescence. Smears of cultured nonlymphoid cells were first stained by MAbs specific for TE cells and macrophages using the immunoperoxidase technique (6). This procedure was followed by immunofluorescent staining with anti-Ia MAb overnight at 4°C. After several washings with phosphate-buffered saline (PBS) pH 7.2, smears were treated with fluorescein isothiocyanate (FITC)–conjugated antimouse immunoglobulin (Ig) for 1 hr washed with (PBS), and mounted for microscopic analysis.

Rosette Test

The rosette test was used to assay interaction of Ia-positive TE cells and macrophages with autologous thymocytes (7). In order to identify the cell type–forming rosettes, smears of rosettes prepared by cytocentrifuge were processed for immunoperoxidase and/or immunofluorescent staining (2) with appropriate MAbs.

RESULTS

The activity of thymic epithelial cells and macrophages in MG was studied in thymus organ culture by assessment of expression of class II MHC antigens on these cells, and by interaction of TE cells and macrophages bearing Ia molecules with autologous thymocytes. Expression of Ia antigens on nonlymphoid cells of MG thymus cultures was significantly higher (21%) than in control cultures (10%). When double staining was applied in order to identify the cell type expressing Ia molecules, the following results were obtained (Fig. 1). In MG thymuses there was a significant decrease in the number of keratin-positive TE cells compared to the control thymuses (Fig. 1A). However, these cells were more efficient in expressing Ia molecules, and more than 30% were Ia-positive, whereas in control thymuses only about 12% of keratin-positive cells expressed Ia (Fig. 1B). It should be examined that in both thymus cultures Ia molecules were less expressed on cortical MR6-positive TE cells than on medullary MR19-positive cells. However, in comparison to the control thymuses, in MG thymuses the number of $MR6^{+}Ia^{+}$ TE cells were numerically reduced. On the other hand, medullary TE cells in MG thymus cultures expressed Ia antigens in a significantly higher extent, thus 60% were Ia-positive (32% in controls).

Regarding the macrophages in MG thymus cultures, a decreased expression of Ia molecules on M1-positive cells was observed.

Results related to the rosette-forming ability of TE cells and macrophages expressing Ia antigens are summarized in Figure 2. Cortical MR6-positive cells in MG thymus cultures were less able to interact with thymocytes in comparison to the controls. Nevertheless, $MR6^{+}Ia^{+}$ cortical epithelial cells formed rosettes in a similar extent in both MG and normal thymus cultures. On the other hand, MR19-positive TE cells either from normal and MG

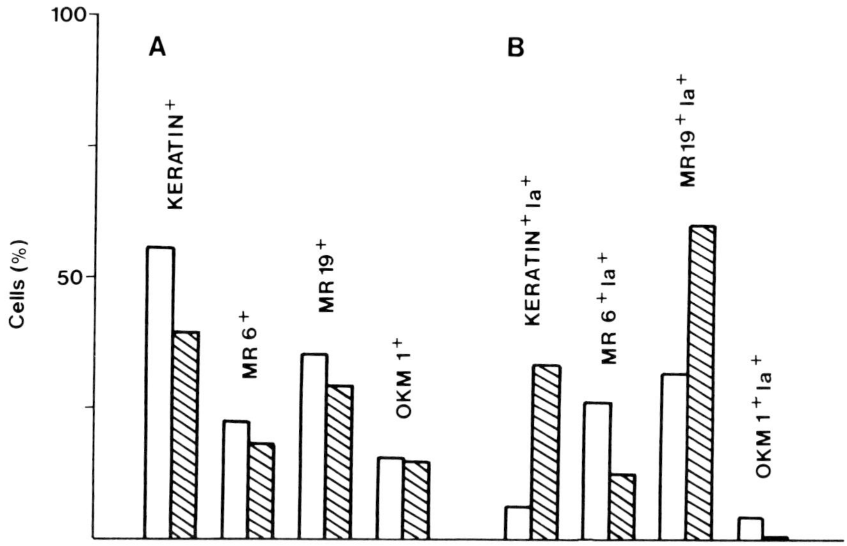

Figure 1 (A) Epithelial cells and macrophages in 10-day-old cultures of normal (▭) and MG (▨) thymuses. Results represent the percentages of appropriate cell type within a population of nonlymphoid cells. (B) Expression of Ia antigens on epithelial cells and macrophages in 10-day-old cultures of normal (▭) and MG (▨) thymuses. The percentages of Ia^+ cells within each cell type was determined by double-staining technique (immunoperoxidase staining combined with immunofluorescence).

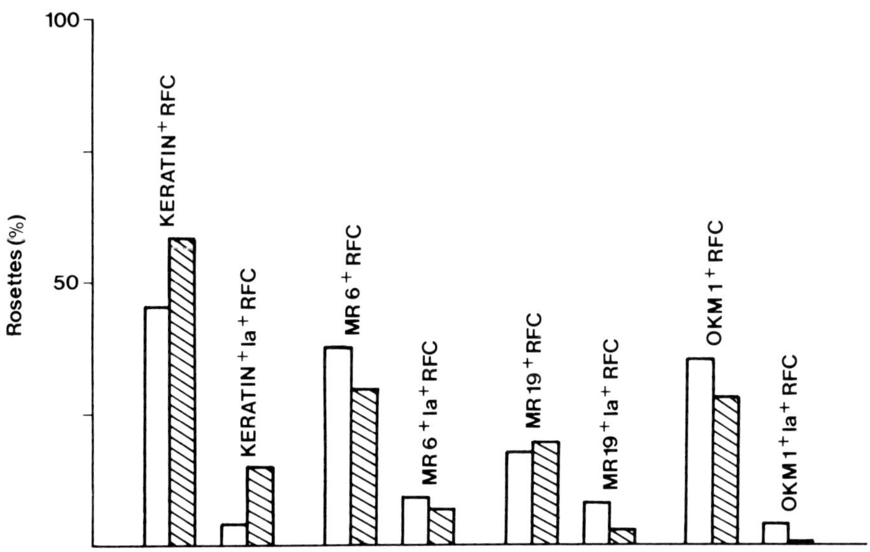

Figure 2 Ability of epithelial cells and macrophages from normal (▭) and MG (▨) thymus cultures to form rosettes with autologous thymocytes. Cell type-forming rosettes were defined either by immunoperoxidase staining or by double-staining technique (immunoperoxidase staining combined with immunofluorescence). Results represent the percentages of cells forming rosettes within each cell type.

thymus cultures exerted similar activity on thymocytes. However, the number of MR19$^+$Ia$^+$ rosettes was lower in MG than in control thymus cultures.

DISCUSSION

The following results obtained in this study have to be emphasized. First, cortical MR6-positive TE cells from MG thymuses expressed Ia antigens in a significantly lower extent compared to the control. The ability of MR6$^+$Ia$^+$ TE cells from MG thymuses to interact with autologous thymocytes was similar to the control. Second, medullary MR19-positive TE cells showed increased expression of class II MHC components. Nevertheless, MR19$^+$Ia$^+$ TE cells were less able to interact with autologous thymocytes. Finally, within the population of macrophages bearing Ia antigens, expression of Ia molecules as well as interaction of those cells (M1$^+$Ia$^+$) with thymocytes was similar in MG and normal cultures.

It was known that T cells during their development within thymic microenvironment gain the ability to recognize self-MHC molecules (8), which are involved in the development of MHC-restriction. Thus, T-helper cells recognize determinants of foreign antigen in the context of class II MHC antigens, whereas cytotoxic T cells recognize foreign epitopes in the context of MHC class I antigens (9). Further, it was demonstrated that TE cells bear both classes of MHC antigens (9). The involvement of class II MHC components, expressed on TE cells, either in the maturational events of T cells or in immunological processes, depend on the subpopulation of Ia-bearing TE cells. Decreased expression of Ia molecules by cortical TE cells in MG thymuses, as shown in this experiment, together with our earlier results showing functional insufficiency of these cells (1,2), support our hypothesis that in MG thymuses early events of T-cell maturation occurring in the inner cortex are altered (1,2). Therefore, a deficient cortical microenvironment induces a generation of untolerized T-helper lymphocytes which initiate autoimmune response. Similar results concerning the role of Ia antigens in the development of functional T cells in vitro were also obtained in a murine system (10).

Increased expression of Ia antigens by medullary TE cells in MG detected in this experiment is in accordance with our earlier findings showing an increased synthesis in these cells (1). An increased expression of Ia antigens on nonlymphoid cells in autoimmune disorders was also observed by other investigators (11,12). Thus, these results suggested that expression of Ia molecules by medullary TE cells to a higher extent in MG may be due to autoimmune processes which are going on in the medulla (13).

REFERENCES

1. Apostolski S, Micic M, Popeskovic Lj, Stojkovic M, Gospavic J, Isakovic K. Thymic microenvironment in myasthenia gravis. J Neuroimmunol 1989; 24:1–8.
2. Apostolski S, Gospavic J, Isakovic K, Micic M, Popeskovic Lj, Stojkovic M. Functional differences between cortical and medullary thymic epithelial cells in patients with myasthenia gravis. Ann NY Acad Sci 1987; 496:707–10.
3. Pyke KW, Gelfand EW. Morphological and functional maturation of human thymic epithelial cells in culture. Nature 1974; 251:421–3.
4. Loor F. Mouse reticulo-epithelial (RE) cells in vitro: isolation, cultivation and preliminary characterization. Immunol 1979; 37:157–77.
5. Ritter MA, Souvage CA, Cotmore CR. The human thymic microenvironment: in vitro identification of thymic nurse cells and other antigenically distinct subpopulations of epithelial cells. Immunology 1981; 44:439–46.

6. Horowitz DA, Allison AC, Ward P, Knight N. Identification of human mononuclear leucocyte population by esterase staining. Clin Exp Immunol 1977; 30:289–98.
7. Volger LW, Tuck DT, Springer TA, Haynes BF, Singer KH. Thymocyte binding to human thymic epithelial cells is inhibited by monoclonal antibodies to CD2 and LFA-3 antigens. J Immunol 1987; 138:358–63.
8. Zinkernagel RM, Callahan GN, Althage A, Cooper S, Klein PA, Klein J. On the thymus in the differentiation of "H-2 self-recognition" by T cells: Evidence for dual recognition? J Exp Med 1978; 147:882–96.
9. Rouse RV, van Ewijk W, Jones PP, Weissman. Expression of MHC antigens by mouse thymic dendritic cells. J Immunol 1979; 122:2508–15.
10. DeLuca D. IA-positive nonlymphoid cells and T cell development in murine fetal thymus organ cultures: monoclonal anti-IA antibodies inhibit the development of T cells. J Immunol 1985; 136:430–9.
11. Micic M, Damjanovic M, Apostolski S, Popeskovic Lj, Gospavic J, Isakovic K. Increased expression of HLA-class II molecules on the thymic epithelial cells in myasthenia gravis. FASEB J 1988; 2:A1175.
12. Tayton L, Lottean V, Turmel P, Arenzana-Seisdedos F, Virelizier JL, Pujol JP, Layou G, Piaher-Tanneau P, Auffray C, Charrou DJ. HLA DR, DQ and DP antigen expression in rheumatoid synovial cells: a biochemical and quantitative study. J Immunol 1987; 138:1730–8.
13. Pizzighela S, Riviera AP, Tridente G. Thymic involvement in myasthenia gravis. Study by immunofluorescent and immunoperoxidase staining. J Neuroimmunol 1984; 6:31–40.

103
A Mouse Model for the Cellular Immunology of Myasthenia Gravis

A. N. Brown and H. N. A. Willcox
Royal Free Hospital, London, England

INTRODUCTION

In most young myasthenia gravis (MG) patients, the thymic medulla shows typical germinal centers (GCs) and T-cell areas (1). In addition, the rare myoid cells there express acetylcholine receptors (AchR); the similar AchR in muscle is the target of these patients' pathogenic autoantibodies. Cultured MG thymus (and bone marrow) cells spontaneously synthesize these antibodies—at rates that correlate very well with the serum anti-AchR titer (2). When conventional (CONV) single-cell suspensions are prepared, many fine clumps are discarded. If they are rescued and dispersed with the neutral protease Dispase (D/C cells), much more activity is recovered, mainly because of a greater yield of thymic plasma cells rather than of GC cells as we initially suggested (1).

To test whether this is a general phenomenon, we have immunized mice with soluble AChR purified from the electric ray *Torpedo*. We gave it in repeated low doses, the better to mimic the recurrent release of AchR from damaged endplates that presumably occurs chronically in MG, and we now report the strikingly close parallels with our findings in MG.

MATERIALS AND METHODS

Immunization

Two- to three-month-old Balb/c, CBA/Ca, C57Bl/6, and F_1 hybrid mice (Olac Ltd., Bicester, England) were injected with 1 μg of purified soluble AchR, either intrasplenically (i.s.) (3), or i.p. + 2.10^9 *Bordetella pertussis* (Wellcome), and were boosted fortnightly with 1 μg i.p.

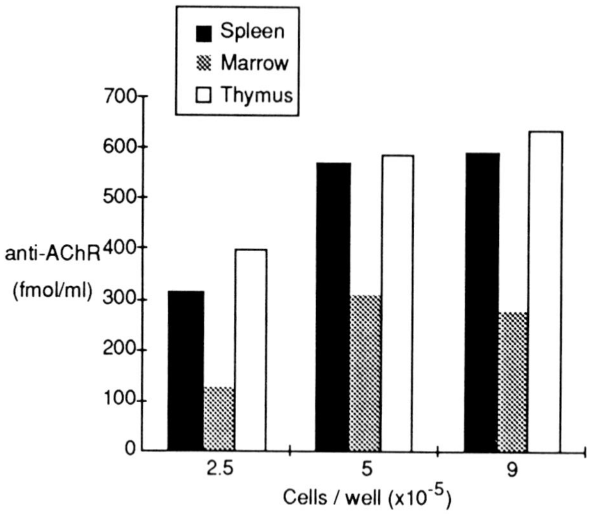

(a)

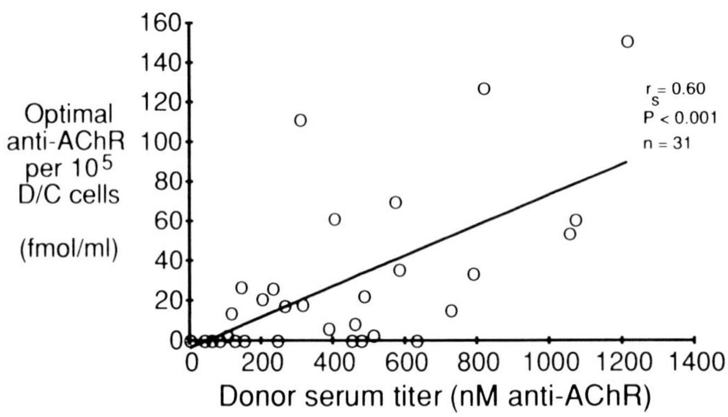

(b)

Figure 1 (a) Spontaneous in vitro anti-AchR production by spleen, bone marrow, and thymus cells from AchR-immunized mice. Balb/c mice primed with AchR plus *B. pertussis* i.p. were used 5 days after their sixth i.p. boost. (b) Correlation of in vitro anti-AchR production by D/C spleen cells with donors' serum anti-AchR titers in 31 experiments.

Cell Suspensions and Cultures

Spleens were gently teased in Hank's medium/5% fetal calf serum (FCS), and pressed through a 0.5-mm^2 mesh. The remaining clumps were thrice pelleted at 40xg for 20 sec to remove single cells, which were pooled, washed again, and designated conventional (CONV) suspension.

The clumps were incubated with 0.5–0.8 mg/ml dispase (grade II) plus 50 U/ml deoxyribonuclease (DNAase) (staphylococcal nuclease, both Boehringer Mannheim) in RPMI 1640/10% FCS at 37°C for 20 min with frequent aspiration with a Pasteur pipette. The resulting D/C suspension was washed twice, and any remaining clumps discarded (4).

Femoral bone marrow, thymus, and peripheral lymph nodes were all dispersed identically; 2.5, 5, and 9×10^5 cells were cultured in triplicate in 200 µl of RPMI/15% FCS in round-bottomed Nunclon microtiter plates (5) ± pokeweed mitogen (PWM, Gibco) at 1/100. We sampled/replaced 150 µl medium on days 8 and 15, and *assayed supernatants for anti-AchR* by radioimmunoassay, and for *total IgG* by ELISA as previously described (5), but using reagents specific for mouse immunoglobulin G (IgG).

RESULTS

In response (in vivo) to only 3 × 1 µg AchR (i.s. and then i.p.) without adjuvant: (a) Serum anti-AchR levels rose to about 150 nMol at week 6 (3), a higher titer than in most MG patients (1), and then fell sharply. On further boosting (3), they reached a plateau of 200–300 nMol, and then declined more gradually (not shown). (b) When $2.0\text{–}5.10^6$ cells from mice similarly immunized four to six times were transferred to irradiated recipients, the brisk antigen-dependent responses (titers 70–1400 nMol) were very similar for D/C and CONV cells (6).

Spontaneous in vitro anti-AchR production was consistently high with unstimulated spleen D/C and bone marrow cells, and was seen with thymus cells in one of three groups of mice tested (Fig. 1a). Lymph node cells produced no detectable antibody, either with or without PWM, in the four groups of mice tested (not shown).

With spleen D/C cells of the four mouse strains immunized by a range of protocols, spontaneous anti-AchR production was detected in 22/31 experiments (7). It apparently depended on at least four immunizations, the latest within the previous 12 days, and correlated strongly with the serum titer above a threshold of about 100 nMol (Fig. 1b). Anti-AchR production was detected within 24 hr, reached a plateau in 3–4 days (Fig. 2), and was sustained for at least 2 weeks (not shown).

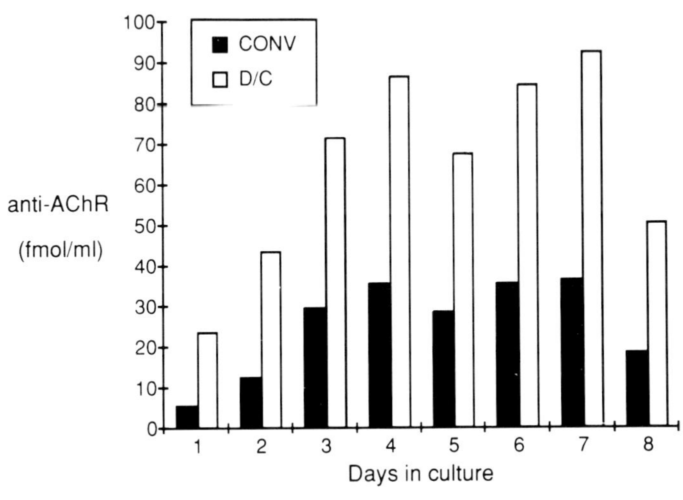

Figure 2 De novo production of anti-AchR on successive days. Balb/c mice primed as for Figure 1a were used 7 days after their sixth i.p. boost.

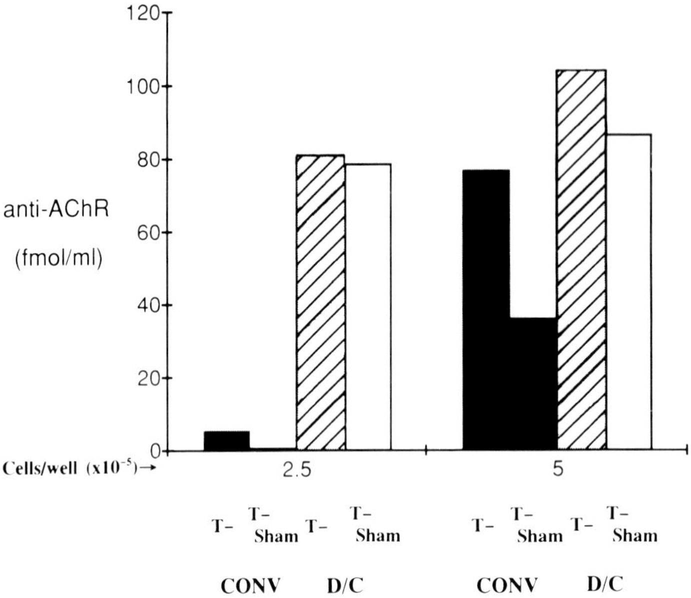

(a)

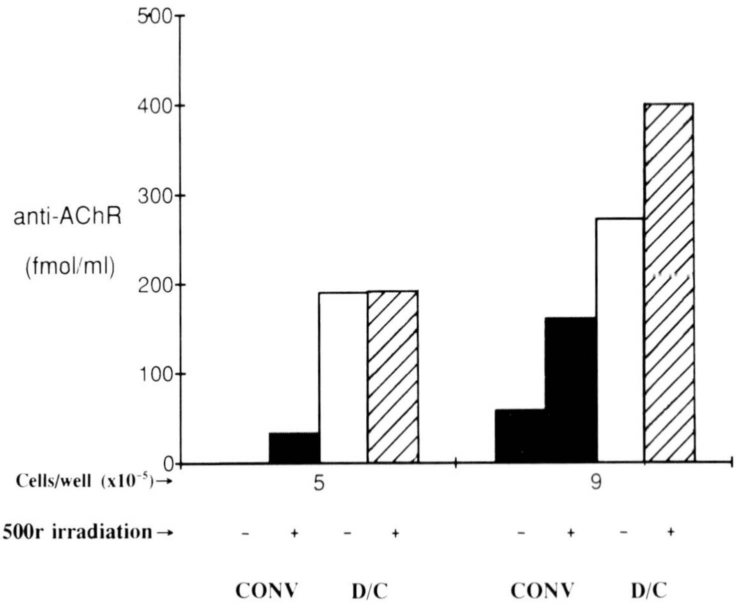

(b)

Figure 3 (a) Anti-AchR production after T-cell depletion of CONV and D/C spleen cells with an anti–Thy-1 (T-) or an irrelevant IgM MAb (sham T-) followed by rabbit complement before culturing. Mice primed as for Figure 2 were used 7 days after their fifth boost. (b) Anti-AchR production after 1500 rad irradiation of CONV and D/C spleen cells. Balb/c mice primed i.s. were used 7 days after their fifth boost.

Spleen D/C suspensions typically produced substantially more anti-AchR (and IgG) than CONV (Fig. 2)—especially at low cell densities, perhaps because they included more "feeder" macrophages and fibroblasts. Nevertheless, the optimum productivity/10^6 cells was at least 1.5 × higher with D/C cells in 17/22 experiments, the difference averaging 3.0 (±0.44)–fold overall. Parallel incubation of CONV cells with dispase and DNAase did not increase their anti-AchR productivity (7). Hence D/C cells are not activated by the enzymes but must instead be enriched in some crucial cell type(s) that we tried to identify next.

After depletion of T cells to <1% frequencies, the productivity of the residual cells was unaffected or slightly enriched, both with D/C and CONV suspensions (Fig. 3a). Equally strikingly, after 1500 rad irradiation of both CONV and D/C cells in vitro, much of the anti-AchR productivity persisted or was even enhanced (Fig. 3b). Overall it was least 40% radioresistant—perhaps an underestimate because of the death (by days 2–4) of almost all cells except macrophages and fibroblasts. Moreover, anti-AchR synthesis persisted through the second week in culture in the three experiments checked (35–69% radioresistant; cf. Refs. 1 and 4). While thus long lived in vitro, these autonomous radioresistant plasma cells nevertheless depended in the spleen on an in vivo boost within the previous 12 days; perhaps they emigrate to the bone marrow thereafter.

DISCUSSION

The immunogenicity of such low doses of *Torpedo* AchR is particularly remarkable, since its 4 chains are 35–80% identical in mammals. Moreover, as syngeneic mouse AchR is similarly immunogenic (A. C. Jermy and A. Vincent, unpublished), mice are evidently not naturally tolerant to it. Indeed, we propose that such proteins with multiple transmembrane domains bind very efficiently to antigen-presenting cells, especially after i.s. injection (when no adjuvant is needed, Fig. 3b), and that this may underlie the striking similarity of the present findings to those in MG patients. The early spontaneous in vitro anti-AchR productivity by spleen and bone marrow cells from immunized mice that is recovered better with dispase and correlates so strongly with the serum anti-AchR titer is typical of the so-called "ongoing" response pattern (8). It is dominated by autonomous plasma cells (8) whose activity is characteristically depressed by PWM (5), T-cell–independent and long-lived in vitro (1,4), and above all radioresistant (9). These features are all so similar in myasthenia gravis that its cellular basis must be almost identical. If so, it too must likewise depend on recurrent boosting—e.g., by AchR/antibody complexes from damaged endplates. Furthermore, if confirmed, the production of anti-AchR by thymus cells after immunizing mice with extraneous antigen argues against any special role for the thymus in initiating MG (2).

Finally, in mice immunized repeatedly with sheep erythrocytes, we have seen sharply contrasting cellular behavior (6,7,10): (a) plaque-forming cells never show any D/C:CONV difference in fresh suspensions; (b) spontaneous and antigen-driven B-memory responses detected in vitro are both about 10 times higher with D/C than CONV cells; and (c) memory responses on cell transfer in vivo show no D/C:CONV difference (6). These data suggest that specific germinal center B-memory cells may be greatly enriched in D/C suspensions and they imply, in turn, that the sessile AchR-specific plasma cells described here localize in a distinct extrafollicular microenvironment and are coenriched in the D/C fortuitously.

ACKNOWLEDGMENTS

Supported by the Science and Engineering and Medical Research Councils, and by invaluable consultations with Dr. G. G. B. Klaus.

This paper is affectionately dedicated to the memory of John Humphrey (1915–1987), who generously helped us in initiating this work.

REFERENCES

1. Willcox N, Vincent A. Myasthenia gravis as an example of organ-specific autoimmune disease. In: Bird G, Calvert JE (eds). *B Lymphocytes in Human Disease.* Oxford University Press, 1988, pp. 469–506.
2. Schluep M, Willcox N, Ritter MA, Newsom-Davis J, Larché M, Brown AN. Myasthenia gravis thymus: clinical, histological and culture correlations. J Autoimmun. 1988; 1:445–467.
3. Jermy AC, Fisher CA, Vincent A, Willcox NA, Newsom-Davis J. Experimental autoimmune myasthenia gravis without adjuvant: genetic susceptibility and adoptive transfer of weakness. J Autoimmun. 1989; 2:675–688.
4. Willcox N, Schluep M, Bofill M, Newsom-Davis J. Isolation of germinal centre (GC) cells is greatly improved by using the protease dispase to prepare cell suspensions. Adv Exp Med Biol 1985; 186:979–984.
5. Willcox HNA, Newsom-Davis J, Calder L. Greatly increased autoantibody production in myasthenia gravis by thymocyte suspensions prepared with proteolytic enzymes. Clin Exp Immunol 1983; 54:378–386.
6. Brown AN, Willcox HNA. Enrichment of germinal centre cells. Adv Exp Med Biol 1988; 237:227–232.
7. Brown AN. Enrichment of Antigen-Specific Memory Cells and Plasma Cells. PhD Thesis, University of London, 1989.
8. Okudaira H, Ishizaka K. Reaginic antibody formation in the mouse, XI. Participation of long-lived antibody forming cells in persistent antibody formation. Cell Immunol 1981; 58:188–201.
9. Makinodan T, Nettesheim P, Morita T, Chadwick CJ. Synthesis of antibody by spleen cells after exposure to kiloroentgen doses of ionising radiation. J Cell Physiol 1967; 69:355–366.
10. Brown AN, Willcox HNA. Greatly improved recovery of B memory function after enzymic dispersion of immunised mouse spleens. 1990; (in preparation).

104
Enrichment of Hybridoma-Forming Cells

A. N. Brown and H. N. A. Willcox
Royal Free Hospital, London, England

INTRODUCTION

When lymphoid tissues are disrupted mechanically some cell types from certain microenvironments are suspended incompletely, and tend to be discarded in residual clumps. After dispersal of these clumps with the neutral protease Dispase, there is consistently an approximately 10-fold better recovery of specific B memory cells from spleens of mice immunized with sheep erythrocytes (SRBCs), and they show properties expected of germinal center (GC) cells (1). Likewise, both with the thymus of young myasthenia gravis patients (2), and with spleens of mice immunized with acetylcholine receptor (AchR) from the electric fish *Torpedo* (see Chapter 103), there is a three- to four-fold higher yield of anti-AchR–producing plasma cells in these dispersed clumps (D/C) than in conventional (CONV) single-cell suspensions. To test whether hybridoma-forming cells are enriched concomitantly, we have performed fusions on D/C and CONV spleen cell suspensions prepared from mice immunized with SRBCs or AchR, and we now report a two to three times better yield of specific and total hybrids from D/C cells.

MATERIALS AND METHODS

Spleen cell suspensions were prepared from Balb/c mice immunized with 3 monthly i.v. injections of $2{\cdot}10^8$ washed SRBCs, or with 1 μg purified soluble AchR intrasplenically and then × 5 i.p. (see Chapter 103). These were fused with exponentially growing P3/NS-1/1-Ag4-1 cells at ratios (to NS-1 cells) from 1.0–2.5:1.0, in a mixture of 44.4% polyethylene glycol 1500 (BDH)/8.3% dimethyl sulfoxide/47.3% RPMI for 2 min at 37°C, followed by gradual dilution. The cells were plated at $2{\cdot}10^5$ per 200 μl Costar well plus $2{\cdot}10^5$ syngeneic "feeder" thymus cells in RPMI/HAT/10% fetal calf serum (FCS). Half of the medium was replaced after 5 days and more frequently thereafter. After day 14, aminopterin was omitted and after day 21, RPMI/10% FCS was used exclusively.

Supernatants (50 μl) were assayed for anti-AchR (2); for anti-SRBCs, we screened for hemagglutination of 10 μl of 0.2% SRBCs in veronal-buffered saline in the presence of rabbit antimouse immunoglobulin (Ig) (1/20) over 3–4 hr, and for hemolysis after a further 3–4 hr incubation with absorbed guinea pig serum (1/20).

RESULTS

When spleen cell suspensions from SRBC- and AchR-immunized mice were fused with NS-1 cells, total and rapidly growing hybrids were two to eight times more frequent with D/C than CONV cells; this difference was still two- to threefold on day 26, even though nearly all slowly growing colonies had appeared by then (Table 1).

The supernatants of all wells with good growth were assayed for specific antibodies at days 18–26 (Fig. 1; see Table 1). In experiments 1 and 2, 5–20% of all wells produced anti-SRBC antibodies. This percentage was 1.7–3.0-fold higher with D/C than CONV cells, mainly because of the higher number of wells with good growth (see Table 1). In all positive wells there was a high percentage of plaque-forming cells (PFCs). In experiment 3, no specific anti-AchR was detected, but total hybrids were again considerably commoner in the D/C.

DISCUSSION

In three of three experiments, there were substantially more rapidly growing hybrids (per 10^5 input cells) from D/C than CONV cells and, after SRBC immunization, that was mirrored by a considerably higher percentage of specific antibody-producing hybridomata. Since the total D/C cell yield is usually only 10–20% of the CONV yield, the majority of hybrids from an entire spleen is likely to come from the CONV cells. However, where specific hybrids or feasible assay numbers are limiting, it may be wise to include D/C cells in the fusions. The earlier appearance of the hybrids from D/C cells may be a contribution of feeder macrophages and fibroblasts.

Table 1 Hybridoma Formation by D/C and CONV Cells

			% of wells (at day 26) with	
Experiment/ immunogen		Total number of wells	Good growth	Specific antibody/PFC
1. SRBC	D/C	340	44	19.1
	CONV	340	18	5.9
2. SRBC	D/C	300	53	19.0
	CONV	300	32	11.3
3. AchR	D/C	113	40	0
	CONV	295	14	0

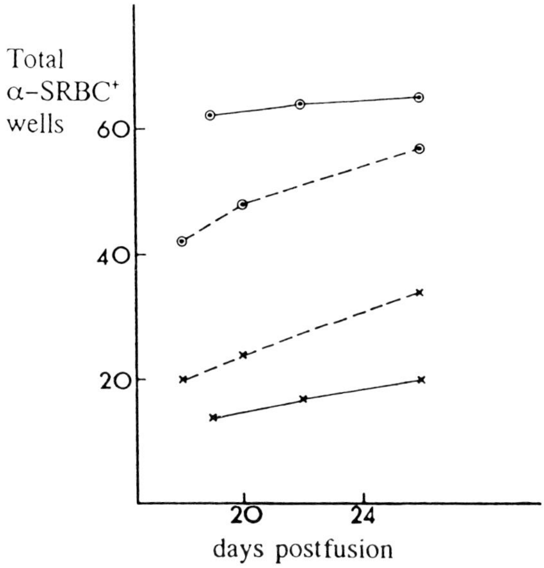

Figure 1 Total number of anti-SRBC antibody-producing wells at successive days of sampling after fusion of D/C (⊙) or CONV (x) spleen cells from mice immunized three times with SRBC. Experiments 1 (_____) and 2 (— — — —).

In many experiments with SRBC-immunized spleens we have consistently found an approximately 10-fold enrichment of GC memory B cells detected in culture (1), implying that fusions of D/C cells may prove valuable for studies on the mutations in antibody variable regions that apparently accumulate in GC cells as the response progresses (3). Varying the timing of the fusions reported here might have given similar 10-fold D/C:CONV differences in hybridoma yields. The ratios we actually observed were less dramatic, suggesting that these GC memory cells were outnumbered by other more ubiquitous cell types that are underestimated in the cultures. These probably also account for the very strong adoptive cell transfer responses that showed no consistent D/C:CONV difference at all (1).

Parallel cultures after immunization with AchR have shown an approximately threefold enrichment of specific autonomous plasma cells in D/C (2) (see Chapter 103). We reasoned that their precursors might coenrich with them, and, being more suitable fusion partners, might increase the yield of specific hybrids. However, these have proved elusive previously; as higher doses of immunogen and/or complete Freund's adjuvant (4) may be required, further work is needed to assess the value of D/C cells here.

ACKNOWLEDGMENTS

This work was supported by the Science and Engineering and Medical Research Councils, and by invaluable advice from Dr. J. R. F. Corvalan.

REFERENCES

1. Brown AN, Willcox HNA. Greatly improved recovery of B memory cell function after enzymic dispersion of immunised mouse spleens. 1990 (in preparation).
2. Willcox N, Schluep M, Bofill M, Newsom-Davis J. Isolation of germinal centre (GC) cells is greatly improved by using the protease Dispase to prepare cell suspensions. Adv Exp Med Biol 1985; 186:979–984.
3. Berek C, Milstein C. The dynamic nature of the antibody repertoire. Immunol Rev 1987; 96: 23–41.
4. Whiting PJ, Vincent A, Newsom-Davis J. Monoclonal antibodies to *Torpedo* acetylcholine receptor. Characterisation of antigenic determinants within the cholinergic binding site. Eur J Biochem 1985; 150:533–539.

105
Epidermal Cytokine Production in Rat Graft-vs-Host Disease

Milica Petrović, Stanislava Stosić-Grujicić, Marija Mostarica-Stojković, and Miodrag Lukić
University of Belgrade, Belgrade, Yugoslavia

INTRODUCTION

Graft-vs-host disease (GVHD) occurs when allogeneic T lymphocytes are introduced into a recipient which is incapable of rejecting them. It is encountered more often in the skin than in any other organ. Although a lot of data have been accumulated about the diverse clinical features, histological lesions, and phenotypic characteristics of cells involved in cutaneous GVHD (1), the precise nature of the effector cells and their targets is unknown. The primary event in the generation of skin pathology comprises recognition of allo–major histocompatibility complex (MHC) products by donor T lymphocytes, but host cells, besides being target, might also contribute to the development of GVHD. This could be achieved either directly (e.g., by expression of Ia antigens (2), or indirectly through production of variety of soluble factors. The purposes of this study was to analyze the capacity of epidermal cells to produce interleukin-1 (IL-1), as well as the molecules regulating IL-1 activity during the acute phase of GVHD.

Induction of GVHD

In this study, we established the model of rat GVHD in which (AOxDA)F_1 hybrid rats were sublethally irradiated (400 R) and injected i.v. with 5×10^7 spleen cells of either parental strain. Control F_1 rats were irradiated and injected with F_1 cells. Clinical signs of GVHD appeared in all F_1 rats 2 weeks after parental cell injection. They included diarrhea, raised fur, hunched posture, and erythroderma. After 21 days, rats displayed weight loss and partial alopecia, with dramatic skin alterations.

Skin Histology of GVHD Rats

The histological study in rats with GVHD revealed progressive skin architectural modifications (Fig. 1B), whereas in control F_1 rats, the general histological pattern remained normal

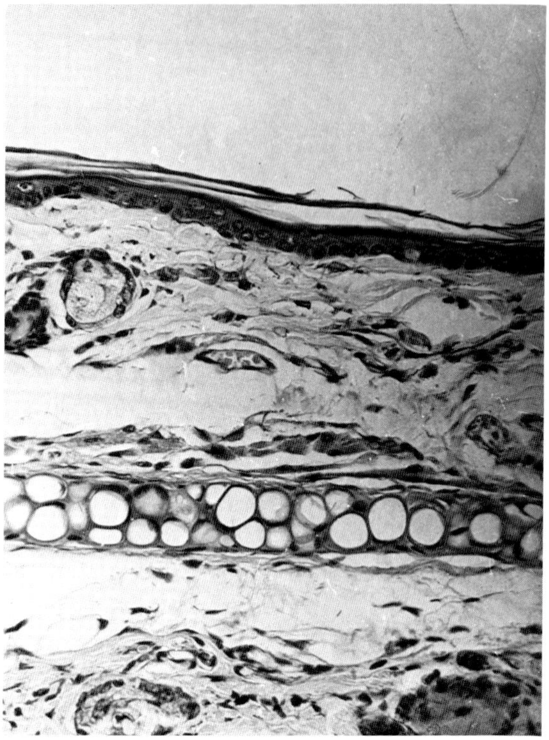

(A)

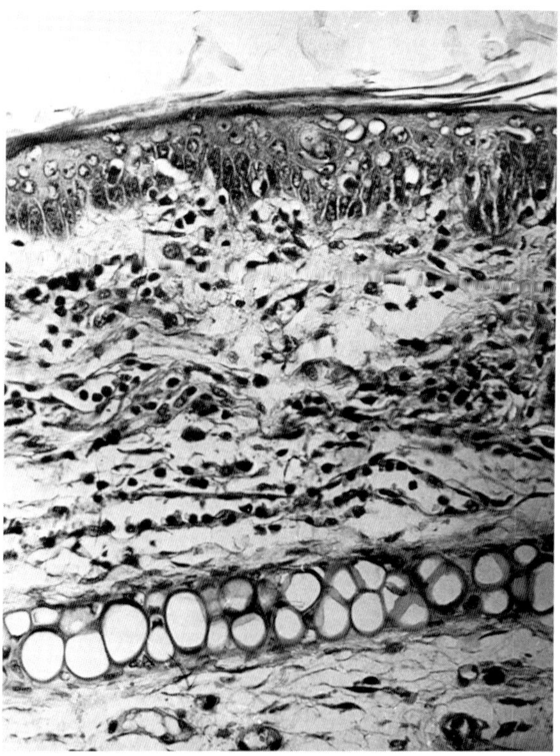

(B)

Figure 1 Histopathology of cutaneous acute GVHD. Skin sections from control F_1 rat (A), or from rat on the 13th day of GVHD. (Stained with hematoxylin and eosin; original magnification: ×400.)

(Fig. 1A). Characteristic alterations in the GVHD skin consisted of hyperplastic epidermal reaction, vasodilatation, hemostasis, infiltration of dermal mononuclear cells, acanthosis, and desquamation.

The Production of Epidermal Cytokines During the Course of GVHD

Epidermal cells (ECs) have been demonstrated to act as important immunoregulatory cells through secretion of various cytokines. In order to investigate the epidermal cytokine alterations associated with GVHD, the culture supernatants were prepared from ECs isolated from the ear skin at different time points after GVHD induction, as described earlier (3). The presence of IL-1 in the culture supernatant has been tested by measuring IL-1–dependent T-cell proliferation by comitogenic thymic T-cell assay (3), or by more specific T-cell subclone D10S bioassay (4) (D10S cells were kindly provided by C. A. Dinarello, Tufts University, Boston, Massachusetts). It was shown that in comparison to control animals the production of IL-1 was greatly enhanced in rats with GVHD (Fig. 2)

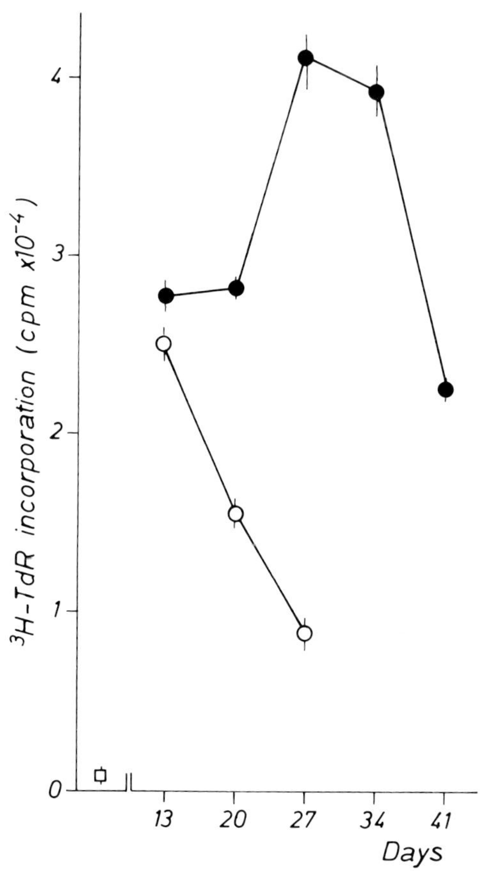

Figure 2 The production of IL-1 during the course of GVHD. IL-1-dependent T-cell proliferation in the presence of EC culture supernatant (10%, v/v) from rats with GVHD (●), or from control F_1 rats (○), taken at different time points after the induction of GVHD (mean ± SEM of triplicate cultures).

and correlated with the severity of the disease. Interleukin 1 and related proteins appear to be main factors contributing to epidermal proliferation through either direct or indirect effects on keratinocytes (5). Thus, IL-1–like cytokines released by ECs could explain the hyperproliferative epidermis found in GVHD.

Since IL-1 antagonists are often released along with IL-1 (6), next we analyzed the presence of the molecules regulating IL-1 activity. In order to detect putative inhibitors during titration of EC products, a standard preparation of human recombinant IL-1 (rIL-1) was added to either thymocytes or D10S cells. The results showed (Fig. 3) that during GVHD the inhibitor of IL-1 activity was produced. The inhibitory activity was dose dependent and was directly associated with the clinical signs of the disease. Thus, stimuli that augment release of IL-1 also induce the production of negative feedback regulators. However, by comparing the IL-1 production (see Fig. 2) with the production of IL-1 inhibitor (see Fig. 3), it can be seen that the inhibitory activity appeared somewhat later (day 20 of GVHD), while the IL-1 activity was already very high on day 13 of GVHD.

Finally, in order to assess whether ECs during GVHD release IL-2–like factors that stimulate T-cell blast proliferation, or transforming growth factor β–like cytokines, which block IL-2 activity, we tested EC supernatant on IL-2–dependent T-cell blasts or on the same cells, but supplemented with a standard preparation of human rIL-2. However, neither IL-2 nor IL-2–inhibitory activity were detected in EC supernatants during the course of the disease (data not shown).

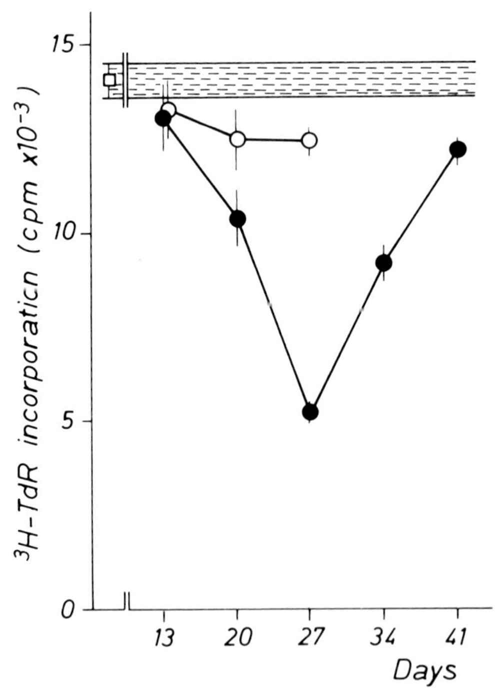

Figure 3 The production of IL-1 inhibitor during the course of GVHD. IL-1–dependent T-cell proliferation in the presence of exogenous human rIL-1β and EC culture supernatant (10%, v/v) from rats with GVHD (●), or from control F_1 rats (○), taken at different time points after the induction of GVHD (mean ± SEM of triplicate cultures).

Thus, presented data suggest that EC-derived immunoregulatory cytokines are complexly regulated in the epidermis. Under normal conditions, the release of IL-1 and IL-1 inhibitors plays a role in tissue homeostasis, while in GVHD the altered production of IL-1 and its antagonists might be important in the development of skin pathology and/or immune disfunction associated with the disease.

REFERENCES

1. Breathnach SM. Current understanding of the aetiology and clinical implications of cutaneous graft-versus-host disease. Br J Dermatol 1986; 114:139–43.
2. Breathnach SM, Katz SI. Keratinocytes synthesize Ia antigen in acute cutaneous graft-vs-host disease. J Immunol 1983; 131:2741–45.
3. Stosic-Grujicic S, Lalosevic Dj, Lukic ML. Modulatory effects of glucocorticoids on immunoregulatory functions of epidermal cells. Int J Immunopharmacol 1987; 9:577–85.
4. Orencole SF, Dinarello CA. Characterization of a subclone (D10S) of the D10.G4.1 helper T-cell line which proliferates to attomolar concentrations of interleukin-1 in the absence of mitogens. Cytokine 1989; 1:14–22.
5. Morhenn VB. Keratinocyte proliferation in wound healing and skin disease. Immunol Today 1988; 9:104–7.
6. Larrick JW. Native interleukin 1 inhibitors. Immunol Today 1989; 10:61–6.

106
Elimination of CD8-Positive T Cells Does Not Abrogate the Resistance to Experimental Allergic Encephalomyelitis in Rats

Marija Mostarica-Stojković,[1] Milica Radojković,[1]
Stanislav Vukmanović,[1] Zorica Ramić,[1] Slavica Vucković,[1]
Miroslav M. Simić,[1] and Miodrag L. Lukić[2]
[1]*University of Belgrade, Belgrade, Yugoslavia,*
and [2]*Kuwait University, Kuwait*

INTRODUCTION

Rats of the Albino Oxford (AO) strain do not exhibit signs of experimental allergic encephalomyelitis (EAE) after encephalitogenic challenge with BP-CFA (1). Although basic protein (BP)–reactive lymphocytes do exist in AO rats (1), their in vitro proliferation to BP is undetectable, which suggests the alterations in the inductive phase of the immune response to this self-antigen. In an attempt to analyze the cellular basis of this unresponsiveness, we have shown that the capacity of AO lymphocytes to produce interleukin-2 (IL-2) after appropriate stimuli is lower in comparison with EAE-susceptible Dark August (DA) rats (2). Further immunocytofluorometric analysis revealed that percentage of CD8-positive cells in the peripheral lymphoid tissues is higher in the AO strain when compared with DA rats (3). In several experimental models of induced autoimmunity, including EAE, the cells with CD8-positive phenotype were shown to suppress the activity of relevant autoreactive clones (4,5).

Although precise mechanisms whereby CD8-positive cells exert their inhibitory effect in the immune response are not completely understood, one which was clearly demonstrated in vitro is the inhibition of IL-2 production (6). The participation of CD8-positive cells in maintaining the natural resistance to EAE is assumed on the basis of the findings that low-dose cyclophosphamide pretreatment abrogates resistance to the disease, enhances IL-2 production, and decreases the percentage of CD8-positive cells in AO rats (3). Moreover, we have also observed that after encephalitogenic challenge symptom-free AO rats developed very mild central nervous system (CNS) mononuclear infiltrations, containing a higher percentage of CD8-positive cells compared to DA rats with full-blown EAE (7). In order to determine the role of CD8-positive cells in resistance of AO rats to the induction of EAE, we applied the method of in vivo selective depletion of CD8-positive cells and analyzed the effects of such procedure on IL-2 production and EAE induction. The results show that almost complete and long-lasting CD8$^+$ cell depletion had no influence upon both parameters which were tested.

MATERIALS AND METHODS

Animals, EAE Induction, and Evaluation

AO and DA rats, 5–6 weeks old, obtained from the Institute for Biological Research, Belgrade, Yugoslavia, were used in the experiments. Experimental allergic encephalomyelitis was induced and evaluated as described previously (1).

IL-2 Production and Assay

Interleukin-2 was produced according to the previously described method (2) and tested on IL-2–dependent T-cell line CTLL. Proliferation of CTLL cells was assessed by MTT cleavage assay as described elsewhere (8).

Depletion of CD8-Positive T Cells In Vivo

Depletion of CD8-positive cells was performed according to Sedgwick (9). Animals, aged 5–6 weeks, were thymectomized, left to recover for 4 weeks, and then treated with anti-CD8 monoclonal antibody (MAb). Each animal received i.p. 1 ml of MRC OX-8 (anti-CD8$^+$) hybridoma supernatant or 1 ml phosphate-buffered saline (PBS) for 7 consecutive days. Twelve days after completion of MAb administration, rats were used either for EAE induction or for testing of IL-2 production.

Cytofluorometric Analysis

Single-cell suspensions of spleen and lymph nodes (cervical and popliteal) were prepared and labeled with anti-CD8 (MRC OX-8) or anti-CD5 (MRC OX-19) MAbs and rabbit antimouse immunoglobulin (IgG) antiserum conjugated with fluorescein isothiocyanate (FITC) as previously described (8). Samples were analyzed on the EPICS C (Coulter, Hialeah, Florida).

RESULTS AND DISCUSSION

The depletion of CD8-positive cells was attempted by adult thymectomy and MRC OX-8 antibody. The effectiveness of this treatments is presented in Figure 1. Thymectomy alone resulted in a slight reduction of CD8-positive cells in the lymph nodes (Fig. 1) and spleen (data not shown). Additional treatment with MRC OX-8 antibodies almost completely depleted CD8-positive cells. The depletion was specific, since remaining CD5-positive cells were not affected. We have shown that immunization with antigen in CFA or CFA along expands CD8-positive cells in the draining lymph node (8). In order to assess the possible effects of encephalitogen plus adjuvant on the recruitment and/or selective expansion of the low number of CD8-positive cells that had survived thymectomy and MAb-treated animals as well as the duration of CD8-positive T-cell depletion, we repeated cytofluorografic analysis of lymphocytes obtained from popliteal (draining the site of antigen rejection) and cervical (nondraining) lymph node cells in animals after immunization. The same pattern of frequency distribution of CD8-positive and CD5-positive cells

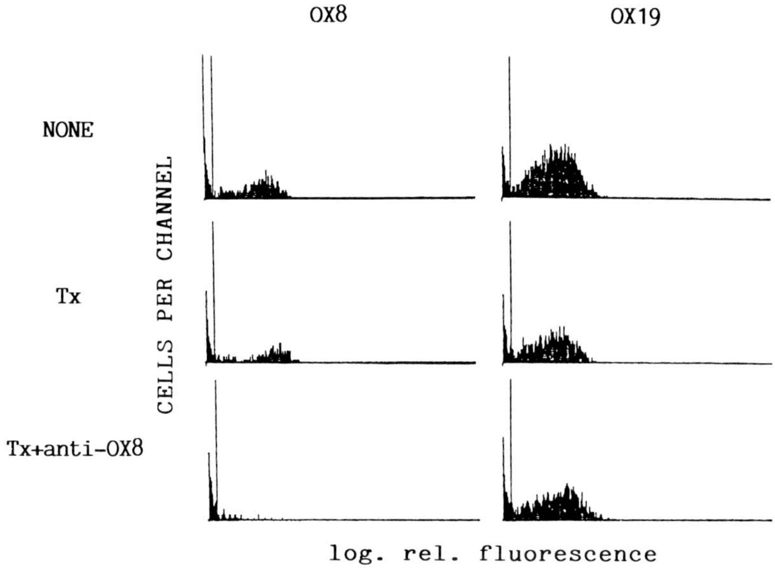

Figure 1 Depletion of CD8$^+$ cells in vivo. Phenotypes of lymph node cells from control, thymectomy (Tx), and Tx OX-8 MAb–treated rats taken 12 days after completion of MAb treatment were analyzed on the EPICS-C.

was obtained in both cervical and popliteal draining lymph node cells of immunized animals to those seen in animals before immunization. Therefore, we confirmed the efficacy of this regimen in establishing long-term CD8-positive T-cell depletion and excluded the possibility that immunization procedure led to any change in number or distribution of residual CD8-positive cells.

Cell suspensions from the same animals which were sampled for cytofluorografic analysis were stimulated with concanavalin A (Con A) for IL-2 production. Depletion of CD8-positive cells did not induce significantly reduction in the amount of IL-2. These results are in apparent contrast with previous findings (data not shown) that the rate of IL-2 synthesis and decrease in the number of CD8-positive cells run in parallel after cyclophosphamide pretreatment of AO rats, suggesting that the control over IL-2 production may be achieved by CD8-positive cells (3). Several explanations for observed phenomena should be considered. Differences in the amount of IL-2 produced by a single cell, number of IL-2–secreting CD4-positive cells, control mechanisms exerted by non–CD8-positive cells (e.g., suppressor CD4-positive cells), and preferential expansion of "EAE bystander CD8-positive cells might ultimately affect the quantity of IL-2 produced in bulk culture.

Finally, in order to find out whether natural resistance to EAE in AO rats is dependent on CD8-positive cells, we analyzed the incidence and severity of EAE after encephalitogenic challenge. The adult thymectomy without additional treatment with monoclonal antibodies had no effect on the outcome of immunization both in susceptible DA and resistant AO rats. The DA rats, either thymectomized or not, developed severe paralytic disease accompanied with intensive histological lesions in the CNS. On the contrary, both thymectomized and sham thymectomized AO rats did not exhibit any signs of disease, although mild infiltration in the CNS could be observed in some animals of both groups.

Table 1 Depletion of CD8$^+$ Does Not Affect Natural Resistance to EAE Induction in AO Rats

		Clinical EAE		
Strain	Treatment	Incidence[a]	Day[b]	Grade[c]
AO	—	0/5	—	—
AO	Thymectomy	0/6	—	—
AO	Thymectomy+OX-8	0/6	—	—
DA	—	5/5	9.6	3.0

[a]Number of rats with clinical signs at the time of sacrifice/total number of rats.
[b]Day after immunization with RSCH-CFA when animals were sacrificed.
[c]Average of grades 0–4.

When encephalitogenic challenge was applied to thymectomized AO rats, which were treated with anti-CD8 MAb, again none of the tested animals developed disease, whereas control DA rats developed paralytic disease (Table 1). Two major findings stem from the described experiments: (a) The elimination of CD8-positive cells do not significantly affect IL-2 production in a resistant strain; (b) CD8-positive cells do not play a role in IL-2– related strain-dependent resistance to EAE. The results presented here are compatible with the notion that the differences in CD4-positive cell subsets, ratios, and functions may be important for the outcome of the induction of experimental autoimmunity.

ACKNOWLEDGMENT

This work was supported by RSF, Belgrade, and KU Grant MI 064.

REFERENCES

1. Mostarica-Stojkovic M, Petrovic M, Lukic ML. Resistance to the induction of EAE in AO rats: Its prevention by the pretreatment with cyclophosphamide or low dose of irradiation. Clin Exp Immunol 1982; 50:311–317.
2. Mostarica-Stojkovic M, Ejdus-Konstantinovic L, Kostic M, Lukic ML. Resistance to the induction of T-cell mediated autoimmunity correlates with lower IL2 production. In: *Microenvironments in the Lymphoid System* GGB Klaus (ed). Plenum, New York, 1985, pp 713–720.
3. Mostarica-Stojkovic M, Vukmanovic S, Lukic ML. Correlation of IL2 production and lymphoid tissue make-up in two inbred strains of rats. Adv Exp Med Biol 1989; 237:407–411.
4. Kelly CJ, Silvers WK, Nelson EG. Tolerance to parenchimal self. Regulatory role of major histocompatibility complex-restricted, OX8$^+$ suppressor T cells specific for autologous renal tubular antigen in experimental intestitial nephritis. J Exp Med 1985; 162:1892–1903.
5. Sun D, Qin Y, Chluba J, Epplen JT, Wekerle H. Suppression of experimentally induced autoimmune encephalomyelitis by cytolytic T-T cell interactions. Nature 1988; 332: 843–845.
6. Chiba K, Nishimura T, Hashimoto Y. Stimulated rat T-cell derived inhibitory factor for cellular DNA synthesis (STIF). III. Effects on cell proliferation and immune responses. J Immunol 1985; 134:3172–3178.
7. Vukmanovic S, Mostarica-Stojkovic M, Lukic ML. Experimental autoimmune encephalomyelitis in "low" and "high" interleukin 2 producer rats. Cell Immunol 1989; 121:237–246.

8. Mosmann T. Rapid colorymetric essey for cellular growth and survival: Application to proliferation and cytotoxicity esseys. J Immunol Methods 1983; 65:55–61.
9. Sedgwick JD. Long-term depletion of $CD8^+$ T cells in vivo in the rat: no observed role for $CD8^+$ (cytotoxic/suppressor) cells in the immunoregulation of experimental allergic encephalomyelitis. Eur J Immunol 1988; 18:495–502.

107
Macrophages in Experimental Allergic Encephalomyelitis
Effect of Elimination and Strain Differences in the Expression of Activation Marker ED-3

Christine D. Dijkstra, Ingeborg Huitinga, and Jan G. M. C. Damoiseaux
Free University, Amsterdam, The Netherlands

INTRODUCTION

Experimental allergic encephalomyelitis (EAE) is a T-cell–mediated autoimmune disease that stands as a model for multiple sclerosis in humans (1). It can be induced in rats by inoculation of a homogenate of nervous tissue (or its constituents, like myelin basic protein), together with complete Freund's adjuvant. In strains which are susceptible (e.g., Lewis rats), the disease develops within about 10 days; paralysis of the tail and the hind limbs are the most important clinical features. In the central nervous system of these animals, mononuclear cell infiltrates are found. Apart from T lymphocytes, these infiltrates contain high numbers of macrophages (2). The role of macrophages in the pathogenesis of EAE is not fully understood; ultrastructural studies suggest that they are involved in the process of demyelination (3,4).

Macrophages display differences in the expression of membrane antigens, depending on their state of activation and/or their tissue localization. The monoclonal antibody (MAb) ED-3 recognizes an antigen that is in healthy adult rats only expressed by macrophages in lymphoid organs: In the spleen, the marginal zone macrophages and the marginal metallophils are ED-3 positive, and in the lymph nodes, the subsinusoidal and the medullary macrophages are positive (5). Nonlymphoid organs hardly contain any ED-3–positive macrophages. In several rat autoimmune models, such as arthritis (6,7) and nephritis (8), and also in EAE (2), many ED-3–positive macrophages are present in the affected tissue. ED-3 expression can be induced on macrophages derived from cultured bone marrow precursors by products of activated T cells; macrophages derived from cultured blood monocytes do not express the ED-3 antigen, at least not in Wistar rats (9).

In the present study, we investigate the role of macrophages in the pathogenesis of EAE by eliminating the macrophages just before the onset of clinical signs. The macrophages were eliminated by injecting liposomes containing dichloromethylene-diphosphonate (Cl_2MDP) intravenously (10). Special liposomes that are able to pass the blood-brain barrier were used (11). Furthermore, we compared the expression of ED-3 on cultured blood monocytes of rats that are susceptible to the induction of EAE (Lewis strain) with that of EAE-resistant rats (PVG strain).

MATERIALS AND METHODS

Animals

Wistar rats, PVG rats, F_1 (Lewis × PVG) rats were obtained from HSD/CPB, Zeist, The Netherlands; Lewis rats were obtained from ZFV, Hannover, West Germany.

Induction of EAE

Experimental allergic encephalomyelitis was induced by a single injection of 50 μl of an emulsion containing guinea pig spinal cord (GPSC) homogenate and complete Freund's adjuvant with 10 mg/ml extra *Mycobacterium tuberculosis* in one hind foot pad. Clinical signs were scored on a scale ranging from 1 to 4 depending on the severity of the paralysis (1: unsteady gait and loss of tail tonus; 2: paresis of the hind legs; 3: complete paralysis of hind legs or of the lower body half; 4: death in the course of EAE; sacrificing because of severity of symptoms. Cf. 12).

Immunohistochemistry

The mononuclear cell infiltrates in the central nervous system (CNS) were analyzed immunohistochemically by use of a two-step immunoperoxidase method on acetone fixed (10 min, RT) cryostat sections of 8–12 μm thickness. In the first step, mouse monoclonal antibodies (MAbs) recognizing macrophage subpopulations (ED-1 and ED-3) (5) and all T lymphocytes (OX19), which are all commmercially available (Serotec, Oxford, England), were used. In the second step, peroxidase-conjugated rabbit–antimouse immunoglobulin G (IgG) (Dakopatts, Tilburg, The Netherlands) was used.

Preparation of Liposomes

Liposomes were prepared as described previously (10): to enable the liposomes to pass the blood-brain barrier, mannose was incorporated in the lipid layer of the multilamellar liposomes (the molar ratio of phosphatidylcholine:cholesterol:mannoside was 7:2:1) according to Umezawa and Eto (11). Either Cl_2MDP or saline was incorporated in the aqueous compartment of the liposomes. Liposomes (2 ml) were injected i.v. on days 8 and 10 after inoculation of the GPSC, which is just before the onset of clinical signs.

Monocyte Culture

Monocytes were cultured as described previously (13). Briefly: Peripheral blood was obtained via cardiac punction, decoagulated with heparin, diluted, and centrifuged on Lymphoprep (density 1.077 g/ml; Nyegaard, Oslo, Norway). The interphase cells (monocytes and lymphocytes) were harvested, washed, and resuspended in culture medium. The cells were cultured in Teflon bags for 7 days in RPMI-1640 medium with 2 mM glutamine, 100 U/ml penicillin, 100 μg/ml streptomycin, and 20% (v/v) Hyclone serum (Greiner). Cytospin preparations were studied for positive immunocytochemical staining with the MAbs ED-1 and ED-3.

RESULTS

The Effect of Macrophage Elimination on EAE

When mannose-liposomes containing Cl_2MDP were injected i.v. on days 8 and 10 after inoculation of the encephalitogenic emulsion, no neurological signs developed. All control animals (treated with PBS-containing mannose-liposomes or with saline alone) developed neurological disorders (Fig. 1). No significant differences were observed in the loss of weight, which occurs in the initial phase of EAE, between the three experimental groups.

Immunohistochemical analysis of the CNS showed that in the treated animals only few macrophages were present in the perivascular infiltrates. In contrast, the CNS of the control animals contained many ED-1–positive and ED-3–positive macrophages (Fig. 2). This difference in the macrophage content of the perivascular infiltrates is not an absolute one. T cells were present in the CNS infiltrates of control animals as well as of liposome-treated animals in similar quantities.

Expression of ED-3–Activation Marker on Cultured Monocytes of Susceptible and Resistant Rat Strains

After 1 week culturing of monocytes, 50% of the total cell count consists of ED-1–positive macrophages. There were considerable differences in the ED-3 expression between the

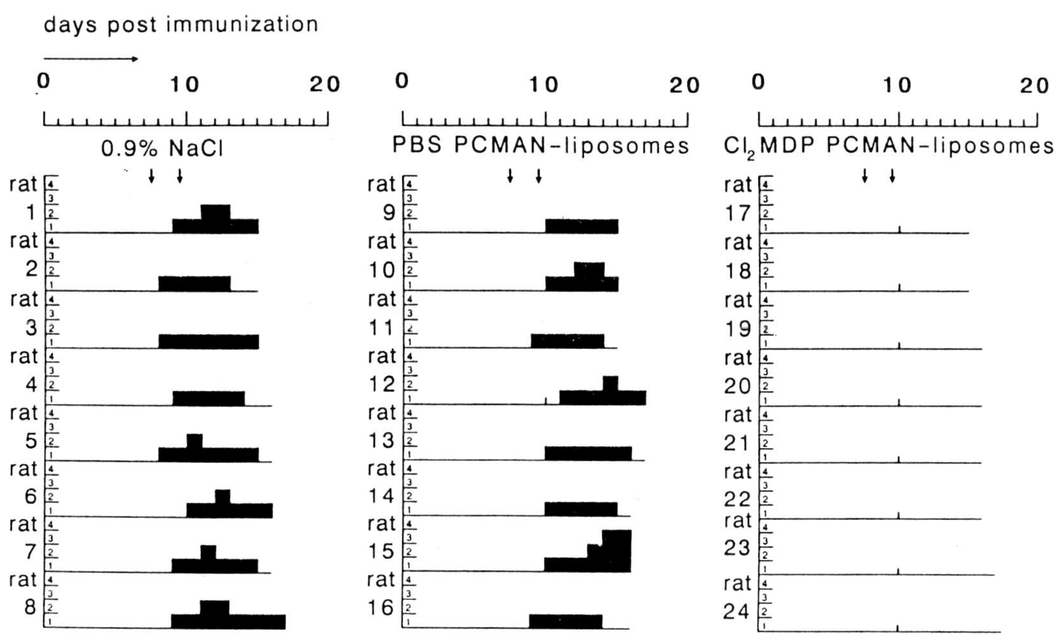

Figure 1 Diagram of the clinical course of EAE with and without elimination of macrophages. Horizontal axis: days after immunization; vertical axis: severity of clinical signs of eight rats per group, on a 1–4 scale. Rats 1–8: treatment with i.v. saline on days 8 and 10. Rats 9–16: treatment with PBS-containing mannose liposomes. Rats 17–24: treatment with Cl_2MDP-containing mannose liposomes.

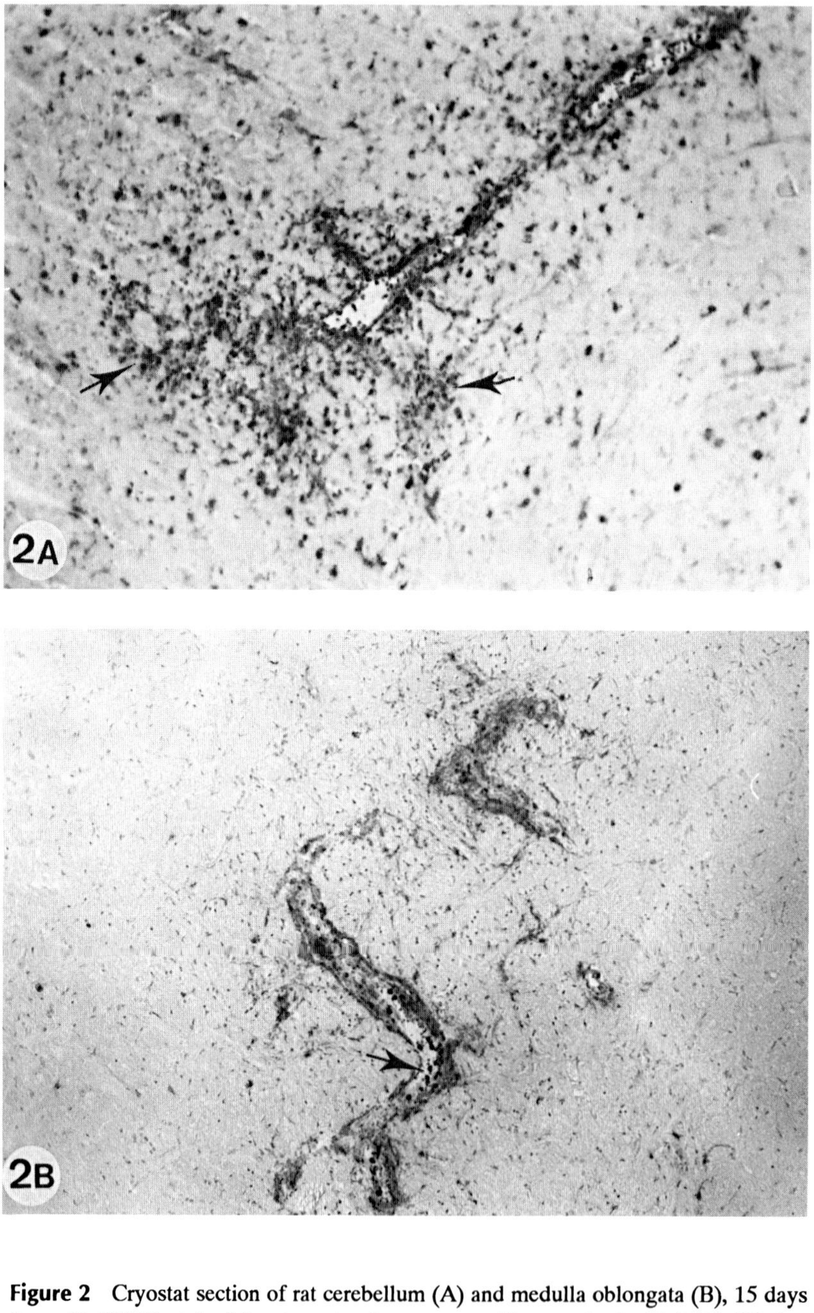

Figure 2 Cryostat section of rat cerebellum (A) and medulla oblongata (B), 15 days after inoculation with GPSC, stained in a two-step immunoperoxidase method with MAb ED-1, recognizing all monocytes and macrophages (magnification: ×80). (A) Control EAE rat: many ED-1–positive macrophages are present in the perivascular infiltrate (arrows). (B) EAE rat, injected i.v. with mannose Cl_2MDP liposomes on days 8 and 10 after inoculation: Hardly any ED-1–positive macrophages are present in the CNS parenchyma. In the blood vessel itself, some ED-1–positive monocytes are present (arrow), sometimes clustered against the blood vessel wall.

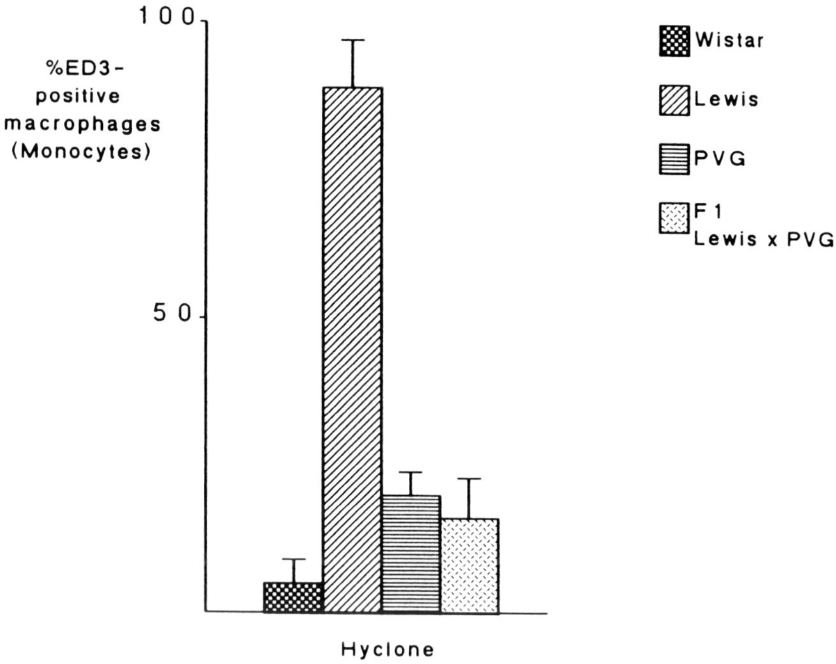

Figure 3 Expression of the macrophage-activation antigen, recognized by MAb ED-3, on monocyte-derived macrophages, 1 week after culture in Teflon bags, in different rat strains: EAE-susceptible Lewis rat and EAE-resistant PVG, F_1 (PVG x Lewis), and Wistar rats.

EAE-susceptible Lewis rats and the other tested strains (PVG, F_1 [PVG x Lewis], Wistar): A high percentage (85%) of the monocyte-derived macrophages of the Lewis rat expressed ED-3 strongly, whereas a *low* percentage (5–20%) of the monocyte-derived macrophages of the other strains expressed ED-3 only *weakly* (Fig. 3).

DISCUSSION

In the present study, we demonstrate that in actively induced EAE, macrophages play a crucial role in the initiation of clinical signs. Elimination of macrophages, infiltrating the CNS by means of mannosylated Cl_2MDP–containing liposomes, suppresses the occurrence of clinical signs almost completely.

This finding is in sharp contrast with the results of Sedgwick et al. (15), who showed that CD4-positive T lymphocytes alone are responsible for the development of EAE, since the transfer of CD4-positive, MBP-reactive T lymphocytes caused clinical signs in irradiated recipients. Hardly any macrophages were present in the CNS of these animals, as demonstrated by using MAbs W3/25 and OX-42 in immunohistochemistry. Several explanations are possible for the discrepancy between the findings of Sedgwick et al. (15) and those of the present study. One is that MAbs W3/25 and OX-42 do not recognize all macrophages, in contrast to the MAb ED-1 used in the present study. Another explanation is that macrophages only play a role in the generation of encephalitogenic, CD4-positive cells in actively induced EAE. When these CD4-positive cells are present or transferred, such a role for macrophages is not "requested" anymore.

Apart from revealing the pivotal role of macrophages in the pathogenesis of EAE, the method used for elimination of macrophages also opens new possibilities for targeting drugs toward the CNS. When conventional liposomes, with lipid composition of phosphatidylcholine:cholesterol = 6:1, were used, no effect on the clinical signs was observed (results not shown). Apparently the mannose incorporated in the lipid layers of the liposomes does not only allow the liposomes to pass the blood-brain barrier (11). Also the content of the liposomes (Cl_2MDP) reaches the CNS and is effective there (eliminating the brain macrophages). Further studies are needed to confirm the fact that the content of liposomes indeed reaches the CNS.

A role for macrophages in determining the susceptibility of different rat strains to the induction of EAE has been described in only few reports. Until now, predominantly differences in major histocompatibility complex (MHC) class II expression, in particular on glial cells (16) and endothelial cells (17), have accounted for the strain differences in susceptibility to induction of EAE. It appeared, however, that apart from the MHC class II–associated factor, another non–MHC-related factor also could play a role (18). The data that we present here suggest that this non–MHC-related gene might well be correlated to the expression of the ED-3 antigen on monocyte-derived macrophages, being high in susceptible Lewis rats and low in resistant other strains. The non–MHC-linked gene might either encode for the inducibility of ED-3 antigen on macrophages, or for the production of factors that influence the inducability of ED-3 expression on macrophages. Driscoll et al. (19) describe the nature of the non–MHC-linked factor that determines the resistance of a particular colony of Lewis rats (Le-R) as compared to susceptible normal Lewis rats. It appeared that the inability of Le-R rats to develop EAE after transfer of sensitized T cells could be corrected by the simultaneous transfer of lipopolysaccharide (LPS)–activated antigen nonspecific spleen cells. This antigen nonspecific cell type could well be a macrophage. With respect to the EAE resistance of Brown Norway rats, it has been suggested that antigen absorption, processing, and presentation are restrictive factors for the development of EAE (20). For both the above-mentioned studies (19,20) as well as for our present results, two possibilities exist for a non-MHC, macrophage-associated, genetic factor: The concerned gene encodes either for a property of the macrophage itself or for a product that strongly influences macrophage properties. The genetic variations in the neuroendocrine regulation of the immune response, in particular in the production of corticosterone, that can determine the susceptibility of different rat strains to EAE (21) might represent the second possibility.

CONCLUSIONS

We have shown that Cl_2MDP-containing mannose liposomes can be used to eliminate macrophages in the CNS of EAE animals and that macrophages, infiltrating in the CNS, play an essential role in the pathogenesis of EAE. Furthermore, we show that the susceptibility of Lewis rats to EAE correlates with a high inducibility of an activation marker on macrophages recognized by MAb ED-3. Whether this hyperinducibility is due to genetic properties of macrophages themselves or to those of other cells and/or products that influence ED-3 expression remains to be established.

REFERENCES

1. Raine CS. Experimental allergic encephalomyelitis and experimental allergic neuritis. In: Koetsier JC (ed). *Handbook of Clinical Neurology*. Vol 3. Amsterdam, Elsevier, 1985, pp. 47:229.

2. Polman CH, Dijkstra CD, Sminia T, Koetsier J. Immunohistological analysis of macrophages in the central nervous system of Lewis rats with acute experimental allergic encephalomyelitis. J Neuroimmunol 1986; 11:215–22.
3. Lampert PW. Demyelination and remyelination in experimental allergic encephalomyelitis—Further electron microscopical observations. J Neuropathol Exp Neurol 1965; 24:371–85.
4. Epstein LG, Prineas JW, Raine CS. Attachment of myelin to coated pits in macrophages in experimental allergic encephalomyelitis. J Neurol Sci 1983; 61:341–48.
5. Dijkstra CD, Döpp EA, Joling P, Kraal G. The heterogeneity of mononuclear phagocytes in lymphoid organs: distinct macrophage subpopulations in the rat recognized by monoclonal antibodies ED1, ED2 and ED3. Immunology 1985; 54:589–99.
6. Dijkstra CD, Döpp EA, Vogels ICM, Van Noorden CJF. Macrophages and dendritic cells in antigen induced arthritis: an immunohistochemical study using cryostat sections of the whole knee joint of rat. Scand J Immunol 1987; 26:513–23.
7. Verschure PJ, Van Noorden CJF, Dijkstra CD. Macrophages and dendritic cells during the early stages of antigen-induced arthritis in rats: immunohistochemical analysis of cryostat sections of the whole rat knee joint. Scand J Immunol 1989; 29:371–81.
8. Noble B, Ren K, Taverne J, DiPirro J, Van Liew J, Dijkstra C, Poulter LW. Mononuclear cells in glomeruli and cytokines in urine reflect the severity of experimental proliferative immune complex glomerulonephritis. Clin Exp Immunol 1990.
9. Damoiseaux JGMC, Döpp EA, Beelen RHJ, Dijkstra CD. Rat bone marrow and monocyte cultures: Influence of culture time and lymphokines on the expression of macrophage differentiation antigens. J Leucocyte Biol 1990; 46:246–53.
10. Van Rooijen N, Kors N, Van der Ende M, Dijkstra CD. Depletion and repopulation of macrophages in spleen and liver of rat after intravenous treatment with liposome encapsulated dichloromethylene diphosphonate. Cell Tissue Res 1990; 260:215–22.
11. Umezawa F, Eto Y. Liposome targeting to mouse brain: mannose as recognition marker. Biochem Biophys Res Commun 1988; 153:1038–44.
12. Matthaei I, Polman CH, De Groot CJA, Dijkstra CD, Koetsier JC, Sminia T. Observer agreement in the assessment of clinical signs in experimental allergic encephalomyelitis. J Neuroimmunol 1989; 23:25–8.
13. Damoiseaux JGMC, Döpp EA, Neefjes JJ, Beelen RHJ, Dijkstra CD. Heterogeneity of macrophages in the rat evidenced by variability in determinants: two new anti-rat macrophage antibodies against a heterodimer of 160 and 95 kd (CD11/CD18). J Leucocyte Biol 1989; 46:556–64.
14. Van Rooijen N, Claassen E. In vivo elimination of macrophages in spleen and liver, using liposome-encapsulated drugs: methods and applications. In: Gregoriadis G (ed) *Liposomes as Drug Carrier*. Wiley, London, 1988, pp 131–43.
15. Sedgwick J, Brostoff S, Mason D. Experimental allergic encephalomyelitis in the absence of classical delayed type hypersensitivity reaction. J Exp Med 1987; 165:1058–75.
16. Massa PT, Ter Meulen V, Fontana A. Hyperinducability of Ia antigen on astrocytes correlates with strain specific susceptibility to experimental allergic encephalomyelitis. Proc Natl Acad Sci USA 1987; 84:4219–23.
17. Male D, Pryce G. Induction of Ia molecules on brain endothelium is related to susceptibility to experimental allergic encephalomyelitis. J Neuroimmunol 1989; 21:87–90.
18. Happ MP, Wettstein P, Dietzschold B, Heber-Katz E. Genetic control of the development of experimental allergic encephalomyelitis in rats. J Immunol 1988; 141:1489–94.
19. Driscoll BF, Kies MW, Alvord EC. The nature of the defect in experimental allergic encephalomyelitis (EAE)-resistant (Le-R) rats. J Immunol 1985; 134:1567–70.
20. Levine S, Saltzman A. The role of antigen absorption in the resistance of Brown-Norway rats to experimental allergic encephalomyelitis. Immunol Lett 1988; 19:103–108.
21. Mason D, MacPhee I, Antoni F. The role of the neuroendocrine system in determining genetic susceptibility to experimental allergic encephalomyelitis in the rat. Immunology 1990; 70:1–5.

108

The Differential Anamnestic T-Cell Response to "Self" and "Foreign" Antigenic Determinants on Myelin Basic Protein

Paul V. Lehmann, Alexander Miller, Vatsala Bhardwaj, and Eli E. Sercarz

University of California at Los Angeles, Los Angeles, California

INTRODUCTION

When susceptible mouse strains are immunized with the self-constituent myelin basic protein (MBP), self-tolerance is broken, and activated autoreactive T cells are readily demonstrable in the lymph nodes draining the site of injection. However, the animals do not develop experimental allergic encephalomyelitis (EAE) unless they receive intravenous injections of pertussis toxin in addition. It is believed that pertussis affects the blood-brain barrier, permitting access of autoreactive T cells to the central nervous system.

Do the primed MBP-reactive T cells persist as dormant memory cells in the animals which have not been treated with pertussis? Furthermore, do these cells have the potential for inducing disease if they later gain access to the brain? Alternatively, are such autoreactive T cells, being "forbidden clones," inactivated by immunoregulatory mechanisms? To address these questions, we are following anamnestic T-cell responses specific for the "self" antigen, mouse MBP (mMBP), as well as to the partially cross-reactive antigen, guinea pig MBP (gpMBP), and to a foreign antigen, hen egg white lysozyme (HEL).

RESULTS

The Proliferative Response to Antigen Can Be Recalled in the Spleen and Blood over an Extended Period of Time

The proliferative recall response measured in an in vitro assay peaks in the draining lymph nodes 9–10 days after subcutaneous immunization with HEL, and then rapidly declines. When various lymphoid organs were tested 1 month later, the draining lymph nodes no longer responded (Table 1). However, significant antigen-specific proliferation could be induced in splenocytes and peripheral blood mononuclear cells. Splenic proliferation was detectable by day 8 after immunization and reactivity persisted for longer than 4 months

Table 1 Recall of Proliferative Responses in Blood and Spleen but Not in Lymph Nodes 1 Month After Immunization

	Proliferative response (cpm × 10^{-3}) to				
Organ tested	Medium	HEL	MBP	PPD	Con A
Draining LN[a]	3.5	5.4	3.2	18.9	170.1
Nondraining LN[a]	0.4	0.5	0.5	0.3	117.3
Mesenteric LN[a]	0.3	0.3	0.4	0.3	50.4
Spleen	1.6	53.6	2.1	65.3	76.1
Blood	1.4	8.3	0.9	12.5	ND

(B10.PL × SJL) F_1 mice were injected subcutaneously with HEL in CFA. Thirty days later, single-cell suspensions of the indicated lymphoid organs were tested at 4 × 10^5 cells/well. Representative data from one animal of 12 tested are shown.
[a]Lymph node

(data not shown). These data demonstrate that, in contrast to draining lymph nodes, responses can be recalled from the spleen and the blood over an extended period of time.

Splenic Proliferation Is Mediated by CD4-Positive T Cells

B10.A(4R) mice express a single major histocompatibility (MHC) class II product, 71-A^k. By blocking this molecule with the monoclonal antibody 10.2.16, inhibition of antigen-induced proliferation in splenocyte cultures was shown. Antibody GK1.5, specific for CD4, was similarly inhibitory (Fig. 1). Therefore, as in lymph node assays, the proliferation stimulated by antigen in splenocyte cultures appears to be induced by MHC class II–restricted T cells with the helper phenotype.

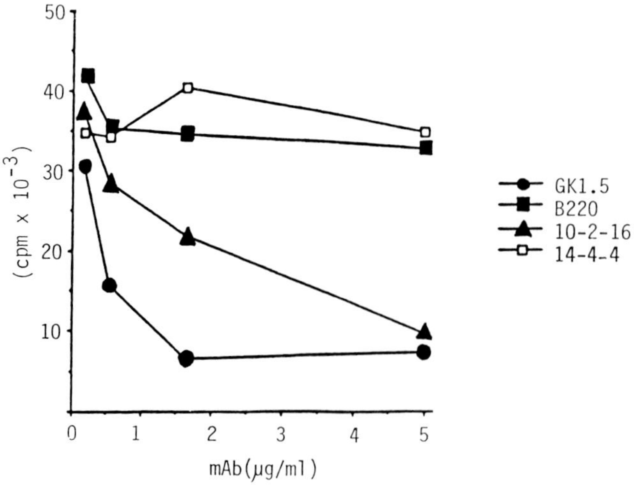

Figure 1 Splenic proliferation is T-cell mediated. The response of HEL-primed B10.A(4R) splenocytes to HEL was inhibited by anti-CD4 (GK1.5) and anti-I-A (10-2-16) mAbs. Monoclonal 14-4-4 is specific for I-E which is not expressed by B10.A(4R) mice. B220 is a marker for B cells.

Table 2 Recall of Proliferative Responses to Foreign and Self-Determinants After Immunization with gpMBP

Day of assay	i.v. pertussis	Organ tested	Proliferative response (cpm × 10^{-3}) to			
			Medium	gpMBP	mMBP	1–9 MBP
9	No	Draining LN	12.0	223.8	205.3	58.4
		Spleen	6.4	50.3	32.8	21.7
	Yes	Draining LN	6.4	125.0	101.1	17.5
		Spleen	2.7	175.8	119.0	130.2
70	No	Draining LN	0.4	6.8	0.2	ND[a]
		Spleen	2.1	96.4	2.3	ND[a]
	Yes	Draining LN	0.3	0.3	0.2	ND[a]
		Spleen	1.5	136.3	48.8	ND[a]

(B10.PL × SJL) F_1 mice were injected subcutaneously with gpMBP in CFA. Mice treated with pertussis received two i.v. injections of purified pertussis toxin on the day of immunization and 48 hr later. On days 9 and 70, proliferative responses were recalled in the draining lymph nodes and spleen with gpMBP, mouse MBP, or peptide 1–9 of MBP. Representative data obtained from a single animal are shown from one group of mice. The persistence of gpMBP reactivity but loss of responsiveness to mMBP was a consistent finding in splenocytes of each of six non-pertussis-treated mice tested individually in two experiments.
[a]Not determined.

Recall Responses to Foreign Determinants Persist in Mice, but the Reactivity to Self-Determinants is Lost

To study the fate of autoreactive T cells, (B10.PLxSJL)F_1 mice, which are highly susceptible to EAE, were immunized with gpMBP. One group of animals received two additional intravenous injections of pertussis (according to the protocol for induction of EAE), whereas the other group was injected with saline. As shown in Table 2, on day 9 of the experiment, a strong proliferative response was recalled by the autoantigen (mMBP) or peptide 1-9 of MBP, which is identical in murine and guinea pig MBP. When mice were tested 2 months later, a high level of reactivity to gpMBP was detected in spleens of both groups, but the reactivity to mMBP could be recalled only in animals treated with pertussis. The autoreactive component was not detectable in the mice which did not receive pertussis. Indeed, the proliferative response to the autoantigen was almost completely absent in the spleen by day 17 after immunization (data not shown).

DISCUSSION

It is unclear whether MBP is an immunologically sequestered autoantigen, since peripheral nerves, which are not within the blood-brain barrier, also contain myelin. The presence of autoreactive precursors in peripheral lymph nodes indicates that MBP is not available in a sufficient concentration in the thymus or in the peripheral lymphatic tissues to imprint tolerance by clonal deletion or anergy.

Given that MBP is sequestered from immunocompetent cells, autoreactive memory T cells should persist in the animal to the same extent as T cells which had been primed by a foreign antigen. Alternatively, if the primed MBP-reactive T cells have access to the autoantigen, continuous stimulation and clonal expansion can be expected which should lead to increased MBP reactivity. The data reported here reveal that while T-cell memory to foreign antigenic determinants persists in the animal, primed autoreactive T cells become undetectable. The following models could explain this finding: (a) The primed MBP-reactive T cells gain access to the nervous system and accumulate there. Thus, the pool of recirculating memory cells would be depleted of autoreactive clones. In order to maintain this model, it must be postulated that in spite of continuous T-cell stimulation and clonal expansion in the nervous system, no overt disease is induced in the absence of pertussis. (b) It is possible that primed autoreactive T cells are triggered by the encounter with endogenous MBP but that recognition of antigen inactivates rather than activates the T cells and imprints peripheral tolerance. Induction of unresponsiveness in T cells has been reported after recognition of antigen on "nonprofessional" antigen-presenting cells (1). (c) The autoreactive lymphocytes might be actively controlled by immunoregulatory mechanisms such as antigen- or idiotype-specific T-suppressor cells (2).

ACKNOWLEDGMENTS

PVL is a fellow of the Deutsch Forschungsgemeinschaft. This work is supported in part by grants from the Multiple Sclerosis Society RG 1755-B-2 and the National Institute of Health AI11183 and AI28419.

REFERENCES

1. Markmann, J., Lo, D., Naji, A., Palmiter, R.D., Brinster, R.L., Heber-Katz, E. Antigen presenting function of class II MHC expressing pancreatic beta cells. Nature 1988; 336:476.
2. Ellerman, K.E., Powers, J.M., Brostoff, S.W. A suppressor T-lymphocyte cell line for autoimmune encephalomyelitis. Nature 1988; 331:265.

109
Mimicry and Dominance in the T-Cell Response to Self-Proteins

Vatsala Bhardwaj,[1] Vipin Kumar,[2]
Paul V. Lehmann,[1] and Eli E. Sercarz[1]
[1]*University of California at Los Angeles, Los Angeles, California;*
[2]*California Institute of Technology, Pasadena, California*

INTRODUCTION

Immunological tolerance to self-components essentially monitors self-nonself discrimination, maintaining self-reactivity at a tolerable level. Whether immunological unresponsiveness to self of antibody-forming B cells or effector T cells is maintained by clonal deletion, clonal anergy, active suppression, regulation through the idiotypic network, or sequestration of self-antigens is still under investigation and a matter of wide speculation. However, it is believed that complete tolerance to a self-molecule rarely occurs (1), and certain determinants of the antigen never induce T-cell tolerance (2). If the mechanisms regulating self-tolerance break down, an excessive immune response against self-antigen begins which may culminate in autoimmune disease. Although in several autoimmune disease states there is a genetic linkage, the factors leading to initiation and maintenance of the autoimmune state remains to be elucidated.

One of the models for initiation of spontaneous autoimmune disease is based on immunological cross-reactivity, or "molecular mimicry," between microbial and host determinants (3). In this case, autoimmunity would occur if these determinants shared structural similarity or an amino acid sequence homology. Such cross-reactivities and associations have been implicated in several human autoimmune disease states. For example, ankylosing spondylitis and Reiter's syndrome (4), which have a strong correlation with the histocompatibility leukocyte antigen B27 (HLA-B27) haplotype, show a shared homology between antigens on HLA-B27 and components of *Klebsiella pneumoniae*. Similarly, in celiac disease (5) there is cross-reactivity between gliadin A and human adenovirus type 12 (Ad12). Furthermore, in rheumatoid arthritis (6) T-cell clones have been isolated from the synovium which recognize certain peptide sequences from a 65-kD mycobacterial protein which also is a member of the family of heat-shock proteins (7). A sequence homology between the 65-kD antigenic epitope implicated in adjuvant arthritis and the link protein of cartilage proteoglycan raises the possibility that 65-kD–specific T cells may cross-react with this antigen (8). Other such associations may account for viral encephalopathies following measles, mumps, herpes zoster, and Epstein-Barr or vaccinia infections may be associated with diseases such as myasthenia gravis, type I diabetes, primary Sjögren's syndrome, and Guillain-Barré syndrome.

MIMICRY IN THE MYELIN BASIC PROTEIN/EXPERIMENTAL ALLERGIC ENCEPHALOMYELITIS SYSTEM

Experimental models of molecular mimicry have primarily been focused on the identification of bacterial and viral protein sequences which bear identity with antigens capable of inducing disease in susceptible animals, and examining cross-reactivity at the polyclonal level (9–11). We have, however, in the experimental autoimmune encephalomyelitis (EAE) system, established a prototypic model of molecular mimicry which examines this phenomenon at the T-cell clonal level.

Results and Discussion

It has been shown previously that in B10.PL ($H\text{-}2^u$) mice immunized with myelin basic protein (MBP), the N-terminal nonapeptide elicits a dominant A^u-restricted response, whereas 35-47, an E^u-restricted determinant, is subdominant (12,13). A chimeric peptide consisting of Ac1-11 joined directly to 35-47 of mouse MBP by a peptide bond was prepared which proved to be immunologically active in vitro and in vivo (14; Bhardwaj et al., submitted). The chimeric peptide (CP) recalled a response following priming with the chimeric immunogen much better than either of its separate components. While defining the nature of the dominant chimeric determinant(s), it was noted that the hybrid peptides 7-11:35-44 and 7-11:35-47 could stimulate cell lines and clones specific for Ac1-9. Table 1 shows the response of a representative set of such T cells that had been induced with Ac1-9. There is no response at all by the Ac1-9–specific clones to 5-11:35-44 or 5-11:35-47 (Table 1) (data not shown), just like the negative response to 9-11:35-47. An identical pattern to the response of T-cell clones was obtained when groups of B10.PL mice were immunized subcutaneously with Ac1-9 and the chimeric peptides were used as recall antigens in vitro (unpublished data).

If the chimeric peptides could stimulate Ac1-9–specific T cells in vivo, this would resemble a prototype of molecular mimicry situations. We therefore determined whether the chimeric peptides (7-11:35-44 and 7-11:35-47) were capable of initiating a cross-reactive response in vivo in B10.PL mice. Ten days after immunization, the draining

Table 1 Proliferative Response of Ac1-9–Specific Lines and Clones

T-cell clones and lines	Origin	$[^3H]$Incorporation (CPM ± SD) × 10^{-3}					
		Medium	1–9	7–11:35–44	7–11:35–47	5–11:35–44	9–11:35–47
9.0(2)[a]	B10.PL	2.4	101	54.6	66.1	4.1	3.7
9.0(2.1)	B10.PL	4.3	146	72.0	71.6	ND[b]	ND[b]
9.0(2.2)	B10.PL	.42	102	0.82	91.1	.96	.66

[a]The data represents the arithmetic mean ± SD of duplicate wells. The final concentration of the antigen is 14 μM.
[b]Not determined.

popliteal lymph nodes were removed and tested for their ability to proliferate to a panel of antigens in vitro. Results indicate that the response to 7-11:35-44 and 7-11:35-47 could be recalled in vitro by Ac1-9, while this was not the case in other mice injected with 5-11:35-47 or 9-11:35-47 (Fig. 1A,B) (data not shown). Although the response was not enormous, it was very reproducible in different groups of mice. We have been successful in deriving Ac1-9 cross-reactive T cell clones from mice immunized with 7-11:35–47. It will be important to determine their T-cell receptor (TCR)V$_\beta$ usage and their fine specificities.

Collectively our results show that the hybrid peptides 7-11:35-44 and 7-11:35-47, which share a 3 amino acid homology with Ac1-9, can mimic effectively the conformation

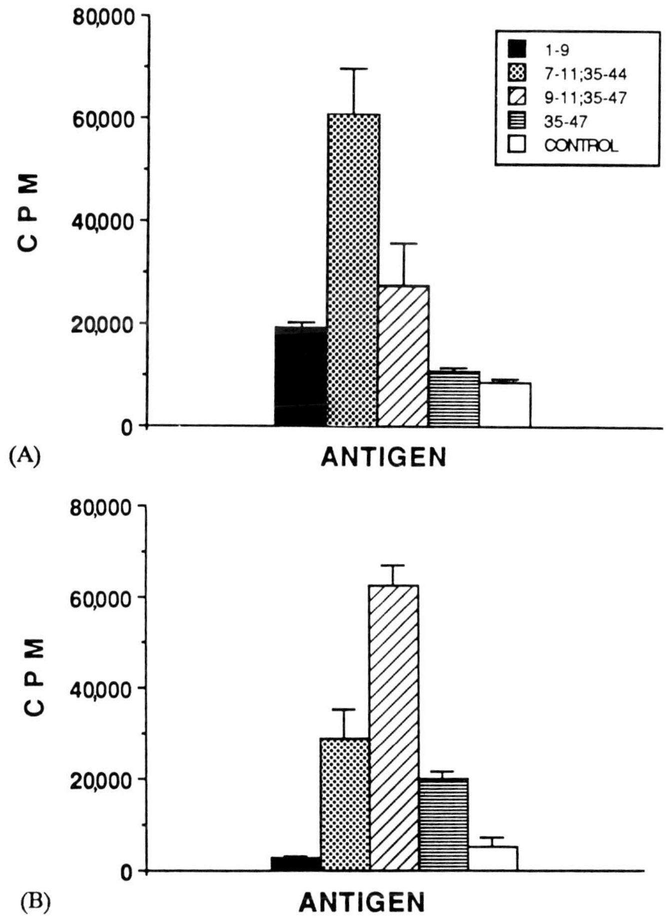

Figure 1 Response of lymphocytes from B10.PL mice immunized with (A) 7-11:35-44 (B) 9-11:35-47, to challenge with MBP peptides (■) Ac1-9, (▩) 7-11:35-44, (▨) 9-11:35-47, (▤) 35-47, (□) medium control. Four B10.PL mice were immunized subcutaneously with 14 nmol of 7-11:35-44 or 9-11:35-47 emulsified in complete Freund's adjuvant. Ten days later, cells from the draining lymph nodes were removed and stimulated with peptides (14 μM). Proliferation was measured by adding 1 μCi of [^{3}H]thymidine for the last 18 hr of a 5-day culture. Results represent means ± SD of triplicate cultures. Control responses to purified protein derivative (PPD) were (A) 110 and (B) 106 (cpm × 10^{-3}).

	1	2	3	4	5	6	7	8	9						
			TCR ↑		TCR ↑										
NAcl-9	AcA	S	Q	K	R	P	S	Q	R						
	↓ MHC			↓ MHC											
7-11:35-44		S	Q	R	S	K	I	L	D	S	I	G	R	F	F	S
		7	8	9	10	11	35	36	37	38	39	40	41	42	43	44

Figure 2 Amino acid sequences of synthetic mouse MBP peptides are given in the single letter code.

adopted by Ac1-9 in the groove. The N-terminal nonapeptide is very well defined in terms of its major histocompatibility complex (MHC) and TCR contact residues. A sequence comparison between NAc1-9 and 7-11:35-44 is shown in Figure 2, aligned for maximal homology. Ac1-6 (15) has been defined as the "core" residues of the determinant, whereas residues 7-9 (15) were designated nonspecific "tail" amino acids that provided some extra binding affinity for the MHC-binding site. Position 4 (lysine) (16) in very critical for MHC binding, whereas position 3 (glutamine) is a critical TCR residue. The important considerations that arise from these studies are that (a) sequence identity of two amino acids (SQ) and homology of a third (R instead of K) seem to be enough to permit stimulation of Ac1-9–specific T-cell clones; (2) the addition of two amino acids at the amino terminus (R and P) in 5-11:35-44 or 5-11:35-47 alters their confirmation and/or binding capacity to A^u or the TCR, so that they are no longer stimulatory for Ac1-9 clones; (3) sequence homology of one amino acid (R in 9-11:35-47) is not sufficient to stimulate cross-reactive T cells.

We believe that this model which seems to demonstrate intramolecular mimicry also has the promise of permitting the most detailed examination to date of the requirements for the cross-reactivity of T-cell determinants. The amino terminal determinant of MBP has been studied more extensively than any other protein determinant, both for its binding to class II molecules and to the TCR, and it should be possible to clearly define the limits of these interactions. Our results to date suggest that mimicry by foreign T-cell determinants, which can excite autoreactive clones, may be much more frequent than expected.

ACKNOWLEDGMENTS

This work was supported by National Institutes of Health Grants AI 11183 and AI-28419 and a grant from the Multiple Sclerosis Society, RG 1755-B-2, to ES. We thank Suzanna Horvath and Leroy Hood for providing the chimeric peptides.

REFERENCES

1. Gammon G, Sercarz E. How some T cells escape tolerance induction. Nature 1989. 342:183–185.
2. Benichou G, Takizawa PA, Ho PT, Killion CC, Olson CA, McMillan M, Sercarz EE. Immunogenicity and tolerogenicity of self-MHC peptides. J Exp Med 1990; 172:1341–1346.
3. Oldstone MBA. Molecular mimicry and autoimmune disease. Cell 1987. 50:819–820.
4. Schwimmbeck PL, Yu DTY, Oldstone MBA. Autoantibodies to HLA-B27 in the sera of HLA-B27 patients, ankylosing spondylitis and Reiter's syndrome. J Exp Med 1987, 166:173–181.

5. Kagnoff MF, Austin RK, Hubert JL, Bernardin JE, Kasarda DD. Possible role for a human adenovirus in the pathogenesis of celiac disease. J Exp Med 1984, 160:1544–1557.
6. Van Eden W, Thole JER, Zee R, Noordzij A, Van Embden JDA, Hensen EJ, Cohen IR. Cloning of the mycobacterial epitope recognized by T lymphocytes in adjuvant arthritis. Nature 1988, 331:171–173.
7. Young RA. Stress proteins and immunology. Ann Rev Immunol 1990, 8:401–420.
8. Van Eden W, Holoshitz J, Frenkel A, Klajman A, Cohen IR. Arthritis induced by a T lymphocyte clone that responds to Mycobacterium tuberculosis and to cartilage proteoglycans. Proc Natl Acad Sci USA 1985, 82:5064–5067.
9. Singh VK, Kalra HK, Yamaki K, Abe T, Donosa LA, Shinohara T. Molecular mimicry between a uveitopathogenic site of S-antigen and viral peptides. J Immunol 1990, 144:1282–1287.
10. Fujinami RS, Oldstone MBA. Amino acid homology between the encephalitogenic site of myelin basic protein and virus; mechanism for autoimmunity. Science 1985, 230:1043–1045.
11. Jahnke U, Fischer EC, Alvord EC. Sequence homology between certain viral proteins and proteins related to encephalomyelitis and neuritis. Science 1985, 229:282–284.
12. Zamvil SS, Mitchell DJ, Lee NE, Moore AC, Kitamura K, Steinman L, Rothbard JB. T cell epitope of the autoantigen myelin basic protein that induce encephalomyelitis. Nature 1986, 324:258–260.
13. Zamvil SS, Mitchell DJ, Powell MB, Sakai K, Rothbard JB, Steinman L. Multiple discrete encephalitogenic epitopes of the autoantigen myelin basic protein include a determinant for I-E class restricted T cells. J Exp Med 1988, 168:1181–1186.
14. Ria F, Chan BMC, Scherer MT, Smith JA, Gefter ML. Immunological activity of covalently linked T cell epitopes. Nature 1990, 343:381–383.
15. Urban JL, Horvath SJ, Hood LE. Autoimmune T cells; immune recognition of normal and variant peptide epitopes and peptide based therapy. Cell 1989, 59:257–271.
16. Kumar V, Urban JL, Horvath SJ, Hood L. Amino acid variations at a single residue in an autoimmune peptide profoundly affects its properties: T cell activation, MHC binding and ability to block experimental allergic encephalomyelitis. Proc. Natl. Acad. Sci USA 1990, 87:1337–1341.

110
Immunological Basis of the Strain Differences in Susceptibility to Low-Dose Streptozotocin-Induced Diabetes in Rats

Miodrag L. Lukić,[1,2] Rana Al-Sharif,[1] Marija Mostarica,[2] George Bahr,[1] and Kazem Behbehani[1]
[1]*Kuwait University, Safat, Kuwait;* [2]*University of Belgrade, Belgrade, Yugoslavia*

INTRODUCTION

Streptozotocin (STZ), a methylnitrosourea with a 2-substituted glucose, is a pancreatic β-cell toxin that has been widely used to induce experimental diabetes mellitus. Insulitis and diabetes can be induced in certain strains of inbred mice by the injection of multiple subdiabetogenic doses of STZ (1). It was found that the T-lymphocyte–dependent immune response is important to the development of multi–low-dose STZ-induced diabetes in mice (2). It had been also reported that persistent hyperglycemia could be induced in Lewis rats by administration of a nondiabetogenic dose of STZ in combination with complete Freund's adjuvant (3). This observation indicates that the exposure to STZ may induce an anti–beta-cell immune reaction in rats. In order to analyze the possible mechanisms by which the exposure to STZ may lead to autoimmune diabetes in rats, we used two strains of inbred rats for which we have previously shown the genetically determined differences in the level of interleukin-2 (IL-2) production (4) and susceptibility to antigen-induced organ-specific autoimmunity (5). In this report, evidence is provided showing that the susceptibility to low dose STZ-induced diabetes correlated with the level of IL-2 production, and that in the absence of insulitis T cells seem to play a role in low-dose STZ diabetes induction in the rats.

MATERIALS AND METHODS

Animals

Female AO and DA rats, 10–12 weeks old, were obtained from Olac. Rats were provided access to standard laboratory rat chow and water at libitum.

Induction of Diabetes

Several dose regimens of STZ were tested as indicated in the results. Streptozotocin (Sigma) was dissolved in cold 0.1 M sodium citrate buffer, pH 4.5, and immediately injected i.p. into rats in 0.2-ml volume.

Determination of Plasma Glucose

Blood was obtained from the retro-orbital sinus of nonfasting rats, between 9 and 11 a.m. The concentration of glucose was determined immediately by a glucose-oxidase method.

Monoclonal Antibodies

Monoclonal antibodies (MAbs) MRC-OX19, MRC-OX8, W3/25, and ED-1 were generously provided by Dr. D. Mason (Dunn School of Pathology, Oxford, England) or acquired from Serotec. Monoclonals produced by the herpes simplex virus type 1 (HSV-1)–specific glucoprotein D hybridoma was used as a control.

Immunohistochemistry

The pancreas and spleen were excised and snap-frozen in Tissue-Tek II OCT compound (Milles). Serial frozen sections were strained by immunoperoxidase as described previously by us (5).

RESULTS

Strain Differences in Susceptibility to STZ-Induced Diabetes

As in previous experiments (4), the spleen and lymph node cell culture supernatants obtained from DA rats exhibited significantly higher IL-2 activity when compared with those derived from the AO strain (data not shown). To test their susceptibility to diabetes induction, female rats of the DA and AO strains received a single injection of STZ, ranging from 20 to 200 mg/kg body weight. Both strains were completely resistant to the single low dose (20 mg), whereas high doses induced strong hyperglycemia in both strains. As illustrated in Figure 1 (upper panel), there were no significant differences in glycemia between the two s trains throughout the experiment. The weight loss was also similar; i.e., 13.1 and 12.5% after 1 week in DA and AO rats, respectively. To definite optimal conditions for analyzing the strain differences in response to multiple subdiabetogenic doses of STZ, different dose regimens were tested. When 20 mg/kg body weight of STZ was given for 4 consecutive days (Fig. 1 [lower panel]), AO rats had plasma glucose levels that were significantly lower than those of the DA rats.

Histochemistry

Preliminary histological and histochemical analysis of the pancreas of DA rats were performed by day 0 and on days 12 and 55 after low-dose STZ induction of diabetes. Histologically, the islets exhibited beta-cell degranulation and necrosis. It appeared that infiltrates of mononuclear cells were not present even at 55 days after diabetes induction. However, a significant number of macrophages were observed in DA rats in perivascular and periductal sites adjacent to the islets. Immunohistochemical analysis confirmed the

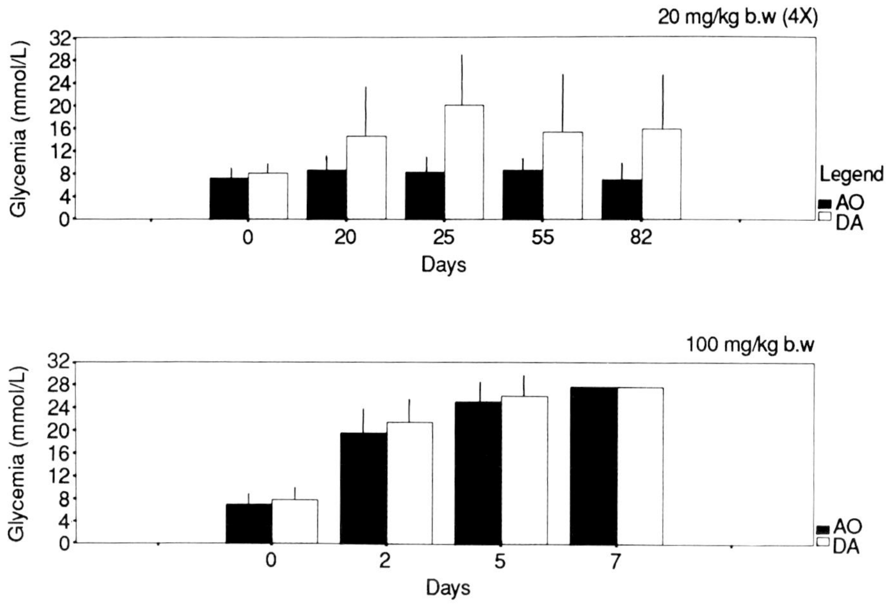

Figure 1 Upper panel: Single high-dose STZ-induced diabetes in AO and DA rats. In both strains all rats reached high glycemia level (about 27.7 mmol/l) by day 7 after the treatment. Lower panel: Multiple subdiabetogenic-dose STZ treatment in AO and DA rats. Results are presented as means values ± SD. The differences between the plasma glucose levels reached statistical significance (p 0.01) by day 20 after the disease induction.

lack of lymphocyte infiltrates in the damaged islets and revealed that recruited macrophages bore the ED-1 marker.

In contrast to results obtained in susceptible mouse strains, and in agreement with the previous finding of Wright and Lacy (6), we found no evidence of typical insulitis after the induction of diabetes with multiple low doses of STZ in rats. However, the presence of ED-1–positive macrophages appears to be a prominent feature in disease development. This finding supports the report of Walker et al. (7), and may be related to the assumption of Bone et al. (8) that treatment with cyclosporin prevented diabetes in BB/E rats by reducing the accumulation of ED-1–positive macrophages.

The Effect of Anti–T-Cell MAbs on Development of Low-Dose STZ-Induced Diabetes in Rats

Although insulitis appears not to be required for the development of low-dose STZ diabetes in rats, it cannot be excluded that the accumulation of ED-1–positive macrophages was T-cell dependent. Results summarized in Figure 2 strongly indicate that the treatment with anti-CD4 and -CD8 MAbs significantly affected the development of low-dose STZ-induced diabetes in susceptible DA rats.

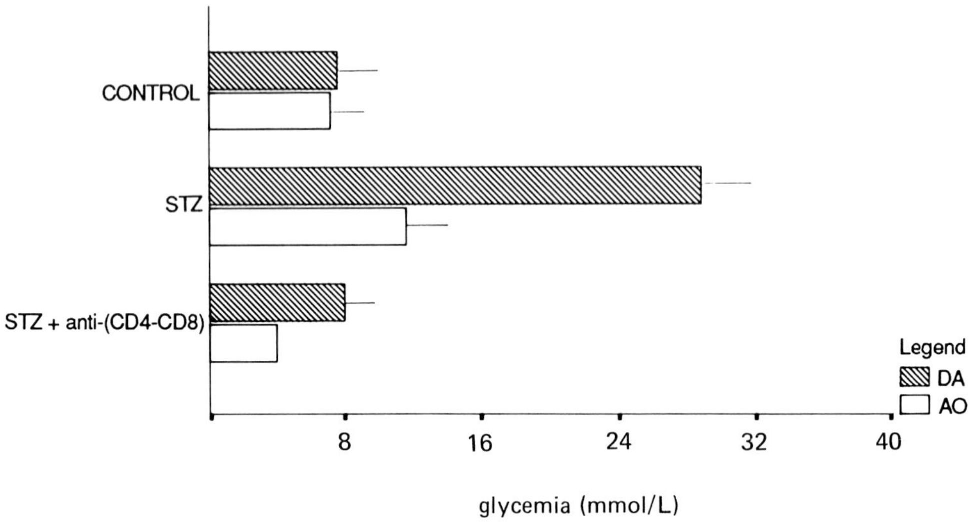

Figure 2 The effects of anti–T-cell MAbs on the development of low-dose STZ-induced diabetes in DA rats. The animals were treated with W3/25 and OX-8 or anti-gp D monoclonals (controls). Presented data (mean ± SD) were obtained by day 30 in an experiment still underway.

DISCUSSION

The experiments performed provided three new findings: the susceptibility of the induction of diabetes with multiple subdiabetogenic doses of STZ in rats; the differences in rat strains susceptibility to low-dose STZ diabetes; and T-cell dependence of the development of diabetes in susceptible strains despite the apparent absence of T-cell infiltrates in the target tissue. Previously, two groups reported the induction of low-dose streptozotocin diabetes in rats (3). However, in both studies an immunological adjuvant was required for the development of the disease; Kohnert et al. (3) used Wistar rats, whereas Wright and Lacy (6), after obtaining similar results in Lewis rats, assumed that susceptibility to low-dose STZ-induced diabetes is not strain dependent. Here we provided evidence that high IL-2–producer DA rats are susceptible to the induction of the disease with multiple low-dose STZ alone, whereas low IL-2–producer AO rats, similar to previously studied strains, are resistant. Although our preliminary analysis did not suggest significant involvement of T cells in pancreatic lesions, it could not be ruled out that T-cell products may be required for macrophage recruitment in this model. Additionally, it was found that IL-2 mainly produced by CD4-positive cells activated BB/W diabetic lymphoid cells cytotoxic to islet cells (9). Our results (see Fig. 2) indicated that although the insulitis is not observed in diabetic rats, T lymphocytes do play a role in the induction of the disease. The exact mechanism of this effect remain to be elucidated.

ACKNOWLEDGMENT

This work was supported by KU Grant MI 064 and Scientific Fund of Serbia (Belgrade).

REFERENCES

1. Rossini, A., Mordes, J., Like, A. Immunology of insulin-dependent diabetes mellitus. Annu Rev Immunol 3:289–320, 1985.
2. Herold, K.C., Montag, A.G., Fitch, F.W. Treatment with anti-T-lymphocyte antibodies prevents induction of insulins in mice given multiple doses of streptozocin. Diabetes 36:796–801, 1987.
3. Kohnert, K.D., Odselius, R., Falt, K., Ziegler, B., Ziegler, M., and Falkmer, A. Destruction of pancreatic beta cells in rats by complete Freund's adjuvant combined with non-diabetogenic doses of streptozotocin. Diabetes Res 5:1–11, 1987.
4. Lukic, M.L., Mostarica stojkovic, M., Kostic, M., Tucic, N. and Vukmanovic, S. Cellular and genetic basis of the strain differences in IL 2 production in rats. Transplant Proc 19:3137–3139, 1987.
5. Vukmanovic, S., Stojkovic, M.M., Zalud, I., Ramic, Z. and Lukic, M.L. Analysis of T cell subsets after EAE induction. J Neuroimmunol 27:63–59, 1990.
6. Wright, J.R. and Lacy, P.E. Synergistic effects of adjuvants, endotoxin, and fasting on induction of diabetes with multiple low doses of streptozocin in rats. Diabetes 37:112–118, 1988.
7. Walker, R., Bone A.J., Cooke, A., Baird J.D. Distinct macrophage subpopulations in pancreas of prediabetic BB/E rats: Possible role for macrophages in pathogensis of IDDM. Diabetes 37:301–304, 1988.
8. Bone, A., Walker, R., Varey, A., Cooke, A. and Baird, J.A. Effect of cyclosporin on pancreatic events and development of diabetes in BB/Edinburgh rats. Diabetes 39:509–517, 1990.
9. Pukel, C., Bagnezizo, H., Rabinovitch, H. Interleukin 2 activates BB/W diabetic rat lymphoid cell cytotoxic to islet cells. Diabetes 36:1217–1222, 1987.

111
In Vivo Treatment with Monoclonal Antibodies
A Probe for Studying Autoimmune Mechanisms in the NOD Mouse

P. Sempe, M. C. Villa, J. F. Bach, and C. Boitard
INSERM U 25, Hôpital Necker, Paris, France

INTRODUCTION

Monoclonal antibodies (MAbs) have long been used for studying autoimmune reactions in vivo in animals. By selectively aiming at membrane structures on lymphoid cells, they allow definition of the role of the different cell subsets involved in autoimmune reactions as well as cellular interactions mediated through selective membrane-recognition events.

Various monoclonal antibodies have been used to prevent diabetes in vivo in the nonobese diabetic (NOD) mouse. The NOD mouse disease is characterized by a large predominance in females, the occurrence of clinical diabetes after 10–12 weeks of age, and the development of a local lymphoid infiltrate around and within the islets of Langerhans several weeks prior to clinical diabetes (1). Both the low incidence and late onset of spontaneous diabetes in males have allowed for transferring diabetes by purified T (CD4-positive and CD8-positive) cells either in neonatal recipients (2) or preirradiated (>550 rad) male NOD recipients (3). Prevention of insulitis, spontaneous diabetes (particularly in females), and transfer of spleen cells from diabetic NOD mice have all been attempted following in vivo treatment with monoclonal antibodies.

A major issue in the understanding of anti-islet immunity is the biochemical characterization of target autoantigens on islet cells. Since circulating autoantibodies specific for islet cell antigens are detectable, they may allow defining autoantigens against which the anti-islet immune response is directed.

TREATMENT WITH ANTI–CLASS II MONOCLONAL ANTIBODIES

Antigens encoded within the major histocompatibility complex (MHC) are central to the development of immune responses. Class II MHC antigens complexed with peptides are directly involved in cellular cooperations between various lymphoid cells and by interacting with both CD4 molecules and the T-cell antigen receptor (TCR). They are encoded by genes located within the I region of the MHC, referred to as immune response genes in the mouse. Class II MHC antigens are essential to antigen presentation both in vitro and in vivo.

The role of class II MHC antigens is central to the development of autoimmune reactions. Genetic studies indicate a polygenic basis for susceptibility to autoimmunity in most experimental models. A clear association has been found between many autoimmune diseases and definite class II MHC alleles in human and experimental models (4).

The rationale for treating autoimmune diseases with monoclonal antibodies directed against class II antigen thus relies on both the role of class II genes in the genetic control of autoimmune response and the blockade of immune reactions against synthetic antigens in vivo and in vitro.

We have obtained evidence that autoimmune diabetes can be prevented in the NOD mouse by in vivo treatment with monoclonal antibodies directed against I-A encoded class II antigens (4). Susceptibility to insulin-dependent diabetes mellitus (IDDM) in this model has also a polygenic basis, one genetic component mapping to the MHC. The NOD mouse exclusively express I-A antigens which show a unique pattern characterized by five consecutive nucleotide changes on I-A β and two amino acid substitutions in positions 56 and 57 (6). The serine at position 57 differs from the aspartic acid present in nondiabetic inbred strains studied so far, including the nonobese normal (NON) strain. The NOD strain does not express I-E antigen. Expression of I-E antigens in (C57BL/6 × NOD)F_1 in which the parental C57/BL6 transgenic mouse was prepared by microinjection of $E\alpha^d$ gene sequence has been shown to prevent the development of insulitis (7). However (NOD × C57BL/10)F_1 chimeras reconstituted with T-cell–deprived NOD bone marrow cells exemplify insulitis and clinical diabetes, leaving open the interpretation of the role of I-E antigen in this model.

Further studies of the mechanisms of protection elicited by anti–class II monoclonal antibody treatment showed no protection against diabetes transfer into syngeneic adult recipients. By contrast, evidence was obtained that treatment of neonatal recipients with anti–class II MAbs did protect against the transfer of diabetes by spleen cells from diabetic mice. Irradiation of anti–class II–treated adult (3) recipients was opposed to the use of naive recipients in the neonatal period (2). Subsequently, it was hypothesized that anti–class II MAb treatment could only provide protection if administered to an immunocompetent host (e.g., nonirradiated recipients). In order to investigate the role of irradiation in abolishing the protection induced by anti–class II MAb injections, experiments were set up to test if protection could be restored by reconstituting irradiated recipients with lymphoid cells from anti–class II–treated syngeneic animals (5). Injection of irradiated male recipients with spleen cells from 8-week-old NOD mice treated from birth with anti–I-A^{NOD} MAbs prior to transfer of spleen cells from diabetic mice restored the protection elicited by anti–class II monoclonal antibody treatment.

Depletion experiments further showed that protection elicited by anti–class II monoclonal antibody treatment was mediated by CD4-positive suppressor T cells (4). We subsequently obtained evidence that induction of CD4-positive suppressor cells, which transfer protection in syngeneic nondiabetic irradiated recipients, was dependent on the presence of the thymus. CD4-positive suppressor T cells were short-lived cells, since no longer detected in NOD animals thymectomized at 3 weeks of age (8). Histological analysis of the pancreas of animals transferred with anti–class II–induced CD4-positive suppressor T cells or nonprotective T cells (from NOD animals treated with a control anti–class II antibody) prior to the injection of spleen cells from diabetic NOD animals showed in both cases "homing" of transferred cells around the islets of Langehans (peri-insulitis), although no destructive insulitis was seen in animal which received spleen cells from anti–I-A^{NOD} MAb-treated animals. These data bring histological evidence that non-specific homing of CD4-positive T cells was not sufficient to protect against the development of diabetes upon injection of spleen cells from diabetic animals.

Treatment with anti–I-A^{NOD} MAb was further used to define a therapeutic window which may allow for long-term protection against the development of autoimmune diabetes. Treatment with an anti–I-A^{NOD} antibody thus allowed for long-term protection against diabetes when applied between 3 and 8 weeks of age, although not between 8, 16, and 24 weeks. This may indicate that autoimmunization and ultimate activation of autoreactive T cells take place very early in the natural history of the NOD mouse disease, as indirectly suggested by the spontaneous appearance of insulitis at 3–4 weeks of age. Such therapeutic approaches indicate that immune effector mechanisms in autoimmune diseases are submitted to fine immunoregulation phenomena which may be elicited or increased by selective immunotherapy.

TREATMENT WITH ANTIBODY TO T-CELL RECEPTOR

Other therapeutic strategies have been developed in the NOD mouse aimed at defining the various T-cell subsets involved in the development of diabetes.

In order to test for the T-cell receptor used by autoreactive T cells involved in islet β-cell destruction, we used an MAb which is directed against a monomorphic part of the β chain associated with an α chain to form the αβ heterodimer which recognizes peptides in association with major histocompatibility antigens. Long-term treatment with anti–TCR αβ was shown to prevent the spontaneous development of diabetes in female NOD mice (P. Sempé et al., Eur. J. Immunol., in press). Interestingly, the protection was obtained in mice receiving the entire immunoglobulin (Ig) molecule as in mice treated with $F(ab')_2$ fragment of the same antibody. The protection was observed in mice treated late in the natural history of islet disease; e.g., starting at 3 months of age. This is strong evidence that the treatment was effective on effector T cells committed in islet β-cell destruction, and that such T cells used TCR αβ.

As anti–class II MAb, treatment with an anti–TCR MAb allows the emergence of suppressive T cells in treated animals (P. Sempé et al.). The use of an anti–TCR MAb allowed us to address two practical issues, referring to the feasibility of treating clinical diabetes. First, it was possible to transiently wipe out insulitis in 3 months old animals following a few i.p. injections of anti-TCR MAb. This opened new possibilities which could be applied in the treatment of human diabetes. Second, treatment of mice with ongoing clinical diabetes (e.g., mice which had been glycosuric for 4–7 days and demonstrating hyperglycemia over 250 g/dl at a 24-hr interval) reversed the disease in six of eight animals, three of which maintained normoglycemia for 2 months following treatment.

The efficacy on both insulitis and ongoing diabetes has direct implications on the human situation in which diabetes is diagnosed late in the natural history of the disease at a time when hyperglycemia is already present and up to 70–90% of the β cells are destroyed.

ANTI-CD4, ANTI-CD45RA, AND ANTI-CD8 MAb TREATMENT

As shown by several groups, anti-CD4 MAb treatment prevents spontaneous diabetes in female NOD mice (9). The transfer of NOD diabetes has been obtained in syngeneic recipients by purified T cells from diabetic animals, including both CD4 and CD8 cells. As previously developed, in vivo experiments showing the prevention of diabetes point to the central role of CD4 T cell/antigen-presenting cell interactions in the development of diabetes.

In order to define which CD4-positive subset is involved in activating the anti-islet immune response, we studied the role of $CD4^+CD45RA^+$ and $CD4^+CD45RA^-$ T cells in disease development. We used an anti-CD45RA MAb which defines two subsets within the CD4-positive T cells characterized by their lymphokine secretory pattern as well as suppressor/inducer function in vitro. This MAb very efficiently prevented spontaneous disease in NOD mice. We could observe a regression of insulitis in treated mice. The $CD4^+CD45RA^+$ T cells may thus be central to the activation of anti-islet autoimmunity in NOD mice.

In vitro experiments have shown the presence of cytotoxic CD8-positive T cells restricted by K-encoded class I MHC antigens on target β cells (10). The role of effector CD8-positive T cells in islet β-cell destruction was evidenced in vivo by treatment with anti-CD8 MAb. Female NOD mice treated from 12 weeks of age with anti-CD8 MAb showed a weak but significant protection against the development of spontaneous diabetes. By contrast there was no clear efficacy on insulitis prevention in treated mice.

ANTI–58 kD ANTIGEN ANTIBODY

Circulating autoantibodies were detected in the serum of diabetic mice using Western blot analysis. The autoantibodies reacted with a 58-kD antigen present in cell extracts prepared from Rin5F rat tumoral insulin-secreting cells (11). Anti–58-kD antibodies were detected neither in the serum of young NOD mice at weaning nor in the serum of other inbred mouse strains tested. The 58-kD antigen is expressed specifically in extracts prepared from normal rat islets. Importantly, the 58-kD islet antigen showed a cross-reactivity with class II major histocompatibility antigens, since it reacted in Western blot analysis with monoclonal antibodies specific for $I\text{-}A^{NOD}$. Various other possible target autoantigens have been defined in insulin-dependent diabetes mellitus, including a 64-kD protein on the basis of immunoprecipitation of labeled islets antigens using polyclonal sera from diabetic patients, BB rats, or NOD mice. Other antigens such as a glycolipid which may react with antibodies detected on human pancreatic sections using indirect immunofluorescence have been similarly characterized using monoclonal antibodies. In no case has the role of these antigens been defined with regard to their pathophysiological implications in the development of anti-islet autoimmunity.

The cross-reactivity between an islet autoantigen and $I\text{-}A^{NOD}$ class II MHC antigens opens new hypotheses with regard to a possible mechanism of defective tolerance to self-antigens in spontaneous autoimmune diseases. The definition of identified target antigens and the isolation of specific monoclonal autoantibodies may allow studying the role of corresponding structures in the development of autoimmunity. The purified target antigens will be used to either induce autoimmune response in naive animals or prevent the development of autoimmunity by inducing tolerance in disease-prone animals.

CONCLUSIONS

Monoclonal antibodies thus provide an adapted probe for studying immunological mechanisms involved in the development of autoimmunity in this model of diabetes. Our results contribute to a better understanding of the cellular components of the immune reactions leading to this disease, in particular the role of $CD4^+CD45RA^+$ T cells which may be central to the activation of anti-islet autoimmunity and the role of CD4-positive protective T cells. They also point out the importance of defining adequate therapeutic windows in MAb treatment which, without perturbing deeply the whole immune system of the animal, provides new interesting therapeutic approaches for the future. Moreover, characterization of circulating autoantibodies can also provide attractive strategy for defining putative autoantigens for which very little is actually known.

REFERENCES

1. Makino S., Kunimoto K., Muraoka U., Mizushima Y., Katagiri K., Tochino Y. Breeding a non-obese diabetic strain of mice. Exp. Anim. 1980;29:1–13.
2. Bendelac A., Carnaud C., Boitard C., Bach J.F. Syngenic transfer of autoimmune diabetes from diabetic NOD mice to healthy neonates. J. Exp. Med. 1980;166:823–832.
3. Miller B.J., Appel M.C., O'Neil J.J., Wicker L.S. Both the lyt-2^+ and the L3T4^+ T cell subsets are required for the transfer of diabetes in NOD mice. J. Immunol. 1988;140:52–58.
4. Todd J.A., Acha-Orbea H., Bell J.I., Chao J., Fronek Z., Jacob C.O., McDermott M., Sinha A.A., Timmerman L., Steinman, McDevitt H.O. A molecular basis for MHC class II-associated autoimmunity. Science 1988;240:1003–1009.
5. Boitard C., Bendelac A., Richard M.F., Carnaud C., Bach J.F. Prevention of diabetes in NOD mice by anti-IA monoclonal antibodies: transfer of protection by splenic T cells. Proc. Natl. Acad. Sci. U.S.A. 1988;85:9719–9723.
6. Acha-Orbéa H., McDevitt H.O. The first external domain of the non-obese diabetic mouse class-II I-Aβ is unique. Proc. Natl. Acad. Sci. U.S.A. 1987;84:2435–2439.
7. Nishimoto H., Kikutani H., Yamamura J., Kishimoto T. Prevention of autoimmune insulitis by expression of I-E molecules in NOD mice. Nature 1987;328:432–434.
8. Dardenne M., Lepault F., Bendelac A., Bach J.F. Acceleration of the onset of diabetes in NOD mice by thymectomy at weaning. Eur. J. Immunol. 1989;19:889–895.
9. Shizuru J.A., Taylor-Edwards S., Banks B.A., Gregory A.K., Fathman C.G. Immuno-therapy of the NOD mouse: treatment with an antibody to T-helper lymphocytes. Science 1988;240:659–661.
10. Nagata M., Yokono K., Hayakawa M., Kawase Y., Hatamori N., Ogawa W., Yonezawa K., Shii K., Baba S. Destruction of pancreatic islet cells by cytotoxic T lymphocytes in non obese diabetic mice. J. Immunol. 1989;143:1155–1162.
11. Boitard C., Villa M.C., Pham-Gia H., Sempé P., Bécourt C., Portier M.M., Bach J.F. Cross reactive epitopes on islet cells and class II MHC antigen in diabetes (1990) (submitted).

112

Susceptibility to Experimental T-Cell–Dependent Autoimmunity and Reactivity to Self–Major Histocompatibility Complex Antigens

Lota Ejdus, Jelena Mitić, Marija Mostarica-Stojković, Vera Pravica, Zorica Ramić, and Miroslav M. Simić
University of Belgrade, Belgrade, Yugoslavia

INTRODUCTION

The syngeneic mixed lymphocyte reaction (SMLR) represents the proliferative response of autoreactive T cells activated in the absence of any identifiable foreign antigen. There is ample evidence that the cells which proliferate in SMLR may play important immunoregulatory functions (1). This hypothesis is supported in part by the observation that the SMLR is impaired in a number of autoimmune diseases in man and animals (2,3). However, it is not established whether the impairment of SMLR precedes the development of autoimmunity, implicating its role in the pathogenesis of the disease, or represents a secondary phenomenon. The appearance of T cells reactive with class II major histocompatibility complex (MHC) products was shown to occur in some experimental models of drug-induced autoimmunity (4,5) and in animals immunized with various conventional antigens (6). In order to assess the possible role of anti–self-MHC–reactive T cells in the development of autoimmunity, we have analyzed the pattern of the SMLR response as well as the presence of autoreactive cells after immunization in the DA and AO strains of rats which differ in the susceptibility to the induction of organ-specific T-cell–dependent autoimmune diseases (7,8), the former being highly susceptible and the later resistant.

MATERIALS AND METHODS

Rats

Adult, female AO and DA rats were obtained from the Institute for Biological Research, Belgrade, Yugoslavia.

SMLR Culture

T lymphocytes obtained by passing cervical lymph node cells over a nylon wool column were used as SMLR responders. Irradiated (2000 R) thymic and splenic as well as epidermal and dendritic cells, prepared as described previously (9,10), were used as SMLR stimulators. T cells (5×10^5/well) were cultured with syngeneic stimulators (0.1–100×10^5/well) in U-bottom plates in 0.2 ml of RPMI 1640 medium supplemented with 2% fresh isologous serum. Proliferation was measured by [^{3}H]thymidine incorporation during the last 18 hr of 1- to 6-day cultures. Blocking of SMLR proliferation was studied by adding monoclonal antibodies (MAbs) MRC OX-6 (antirat IA), MRC OX-17 (antirat IE), or MRC OX-18 (antirat class I MHC) at the initiation of the cultures.

Immunization

Rats were i.d. injected with 0.1 ml of emulsion prepared by mixing equal amounts of complete Freund's adjuvant (CFA) and one of the following antigens: guinea pig basic protein (gpBP, 50 μg/rat), Herpes simplex virus type 1 (HSV-1, 2.5×10^6PFU/rat), or ABA-tyrosine (ABA-tyr, 100 μg/rat).

In Vitro Proliferative Response of Lymphocytes from Antigen-Primed Rats

Draining lymph node cells (4×10^5/well) 9–11 days after immunization were cultured in 0.2 ml of RPMI medium supplemented with 2% fresh isologous serum alone, with antigens or concanavalin (Con A). Proliferation was measured by [^{3}H]thymidine incorporation during the last 18 hr of 4-day cultures.

Establishment of T-Cell Lines

Autoreactive T-cell lines were generated from DA and AO rats immunized with HSV-CFA. Draining lymph node cells (5×10^6/ml) were cultured in RPMI medium without antigen. After 3 days of incubation, blast cells were recultured (2×10^5/ml) in interleukin-2 (IL-2)–containing (10%) medium. The lines were maintained on a basis of weekly restimulation with syngeneic dendritic cells followed by IL-2-dependent expansion. Specificity of T-cell lines was tested by stimulating the line cells (2×10^4/well) with syngeneic or allogenic dendritic cells (1-8×10^4/well) alone or in the presence of HSV-1. Proliferation was measured by [^{3}H]thymidine incorporation during the last 18 hr of a 3-day incubation.

RESULTS AND DISCUSSION

The comparative analysis of SMLR in DA and AO rats has shown that although T cells obtained from both strains proliferated in vitro upon stimulation with irradiated syngeneic cells, the response of DA lymphocytes was significantly larger (Fig. 1). In both strains, the proliferative response was dependent on stimulation with IA-positive cells as the addition of MAb OX-6 resulted in a dose-dependent inhibition of SMLR proliferation, whereas MAbs OX-17 and OX-18 added in the same dose range failed to exhibit any significant effect (data not shown). The difference in the magnitude of SMLR between AO and DA rats could not be ascribed to the different kinetics of the response because in both strains it had reached a peak on day 5 and declined thereafter (data not shown). This difference was

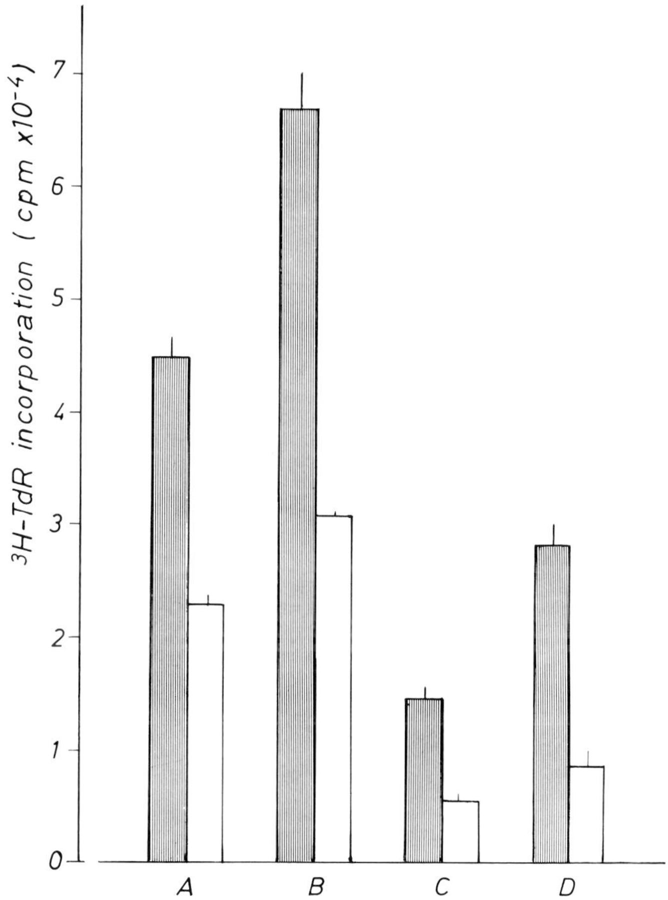

Figure 1 SMLR response of DA T cells to different sources of stimulators is higher than response of AO T cells. T cells ($5{\times}10^5$/well) from nonimmune DA (▥) or AO (□) rats were stimulated with: irradiated splenic ($5{\times}10^5$/well) (A), thymic ($5{\times}10^5$/well) (B), epidermal ($0.2{\times}10^5$/well) (C), and dendritic cells ($0.5{\times}10^5$/well) (D). Proliferation was measured by [^{3}H]thymidine incorporation during the last 18 hr of 5-day cultures.

consistently observed irrespectively of the source of stimulator cells (Fig. 1), the irradiated thymic cells being the most efficient in eliciting proliferation of syngeneic T cells of both strains.

As various observations have been made of anti-self response associated with conventional immune response, we compared the ability of lymphocytes derived from DA and AO rats immunized with different antigens to proliferate spontaneously in vitro. Although the rate of antigen- and mitogen-driven proliferation varied from experiment to experiment, the consistent finding was the significantly higher spontaneous proliferation of DA lymphocytes compared with AO cell proliferation (Fig. 2). This difference between AO and DA cells was observed irrespectively of the antigen used for immunization. In order to confirm that at least a number of lymphocytes proliferating without any antigen or mitogen are really autoreactive cells, we established T-cell lines from HSV-1–immunized AO and DA

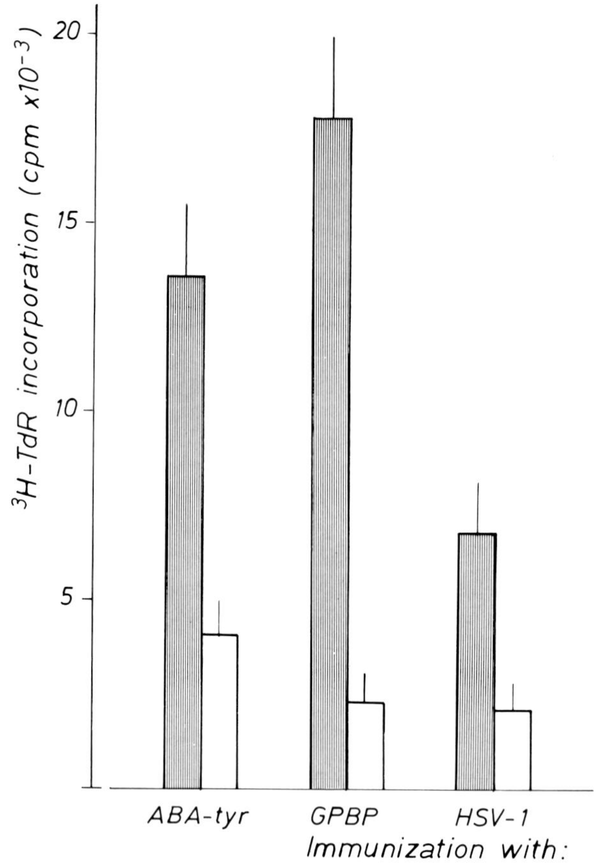

Figure 2 Spontaneous proliferation of lymphocytes from antigen-primed animals. Draining lymph node cells (5×10^4/well) from DA (▥) and AO (□) rats immunized with indicated antigens 9–12 days before were cultured for 4 days. Proliferation was measured by [^{3}H]thymidine incorporation during the last 18 hr of cultures.

rats by alternative cycles of stimulation with syngeneic dendritic cells and propagation of IL-2-containing medium. The initial capacity of both AO and DA cells to proliferate in response to HSV-1 was lost after a few cycles of in vitro selection without antigen (data not shown). However, the DA cell line quickly become strictly autoreactive and did not exhibit any alloreactivity in contrast to the AO cell line maintained under identical selection conditions (data not shown).

The data showing that lymphocytes from DA rats, both nonimmune and antigen-primed, exhibit high levels of autoreactivity confirm the hypothesis about the role of autoreactive cells in the amplification of the specific immune response to foreign and self–organ-specific antigens. It has been shown that a population of CD8-positive suppressor cells regulates autoreactive T cells in vitro and in vivo (11). The percentage of CD8-positive cells in the lymphoid tissues of DA rats is significantly lower than in AO rats (7). Thus, it could be assumed that susceptibility to the induction of T-dependent organ-specific autoimmune diseases in DA rats, at least in part, is determined by the level of reactivity to self-MHC antigens.

REFERENCES

1. Clauberger C, Dekruyff RH, Cantor H. Immunoregulatory activities of autoreactive T cells: An I-A specific T cell clone mediates both help and suppression of antibody response. J Immunol 1984; 132:2237–2243.
2. Sakane T, Steinberg AD, Green I. Failure of autologous mixed lymphocyte reaction between T and non-T cells in patients with systemic lupus erythematosus. Proc Natl Acad Sci USA 1978; 75:3414–3419.
3. Smith JB, Pasternak RD. Syngeneic mixed leukocyte reaction in mice: strain distribution, kinetics, participating cells and absence in NAB mice. J Immunol 1978; 121:1889–1892.
4. Pelletier L, Pasquier R, Hirsch F, Sapin C, Druet P. Autoreactive T cells in mercury-induced autoimmune disease: In vitro demonstration. J Immunol 1986; 137:2548–2554.
5. Tournade H, Pelletier L, Pasquier R, Vial M-C, Druet P. D-penicilamine-induced autoimmunity in Brown-Norway rats. Similarities with $HgCl_2$-induced autoimmunity. J Immunol 1990; 144:2985–2991.
6. DosReis GA, Sheavach EM. Analysis of autoreactive I region-restricted T cells colonies isolated from the guinea pig syngeneic mixed leukocyte reaction and from immune responses to conventional foreign antigens. Eur J Immunol 1985; 15:466–472.
7. Vukmanovic S, Mostarica-Stojkovic M, Lukic ML. Experimental autoimmune encephalomyelitis in "low" and "high" interleukin 2 producer rats. I. Cellular basis of induction. Cell Immunol 1989; 121:237–246.
8. Lalic NM, Latkovic ZV, Mostarica-Stojkovic M, Lukic ML. Experimental allergic uveitis in the rat: cellular characteristics and strain differences in the susceptibility to the induction. Period Biol 1983; 85:75–86.
9. Schuler G, Steinman RM. Murine epidermal Langerhans cells mature into potent immunostimulatory dendritic cells in vitro. J Exp Med 1985; 161:526–546.
10. Klinkert WFF, LaBadie JH, Bower WE. Accessory and stimulating properties of dendritic cells and macrophages isolated from various rat tissues. J Exp Med 1982; 156:1–19.
11. Nagakatti PS, Nagarkatti M, Mann LW, Jones LA, Kaplan AM. Characterization of an endogenous $Lyt2^+$ T-suppressor cell population regulating autoreactive T cells in vitro and in vivo. Cell Immunol 1988; 112:64–77.

113
A Non-Major Histocompatibility Complex-Associated Immune Response Gene Effect Is Determined by the Neuroendocrine System

Don Mason,[1] Ferenc Antoni,[2] and Iain MacPhee[3]
[1]*MRC Cellular Immunology Unit, Oxford, England;*
[2]*MRC Brain Metabolism Unit, Edinburgh, Scotland;*
[3]*University of Oxford Medical School, Oxford, England*

INTRODUCTION

The immune response to many antigens is subject to genetically determined variation but the mechanisms underlying these genetic effects are not well understood. The immune response genes that influence the magnitude of the responses to simple peptides and some proteins map to the major histocompatibility complex (MHC) (1,2), and in these instances it is probable that failure of presentation or recognition of the potential antigens is responsible for the lack of immunogenicity. Given the very limited repertoire of class I and class II MHC molecules possessed by any one individual, it is perhaps not surprising that, especially in the case of inbred homozygous experimental animals, some peptides fail to make stable interactions with these MHC molecules and are consequently not appropriately presented to T cells.

However, not all immune-response genes map to the MHC. This is particularly true for responses to complex antigens like bacteria (3) and protozoa (4) but also holds in the case of some simple peptides (see below). In these instances, failure of presentation is unlikely to be the underlying cause of the diminished immunogenicity, and it is possible that genetically determined variations in immunoregulation give rise to the immune-response gene effects that are observed.

GENETIC VARIATION IN SUSCEPTIBILILTY TO EXPERIMENTAL AUTOIMMUNE DISEASES IN THE RAT

The laboratory rat is used in the study of a number of experimentally induced autoimmune diseases. By appropriate choice of adjuvant and immunogen it is possible to induce diseases affecting joints (adjuvant arthritis, collagen-induced arthritis, streptococcal cell wall arthritis), the eye (experimental uveoretinitis), the peripheral nervous system (experimental allergic neuritis), and the central nervous system (experimental allergic encephalomyelitis). In all of these diseases the Lewis rat is the strain of choice. Given the widely diverse range of inducing antigens involved in these different diseases, one might anticipate that there must be some general, non–antigen-specific, characteristic of immunoregulation in Lewis strain rats that makes them more susceptible to these diseases than most other rat strains.

EXPERIMENTAL ALLERGIC ENCEPHALOMYELITIS IN RATS

Experimental allergic encephalomyelitis (EAE) can be induced in Lewis rats by the subcutaneous injection of guinea pig myelin basic protein in Freund's complete adjuvant (MBP/FCA) (5,6). The particular amino acid sequence of MBP that is responsible for its immunogenicity has been identified: EAE can be induced in the Lewis rat by using a peptide composed of residues 70–86 of the whole molecule (7). The disease starts 10–11 days after immunization, and there is an orderly progression of physical signs beginning with loss of ability to move the tail, progressing to hind-limb weakness followed by hind-limb paralysis and occasionally urinary incontinence. The signs reach their peak after 2–3 days and then subside with the sequence of recovery being the reverse of that of onset. Four to 5 days after the start of the disease recovery is virtually complete (8).

In contrast to Lewis rats, those of the PVG strain are resistant to EAE (9,10). However, failure of PVG rats to develop EAE cannot be attributed to failure of their T cells to recognize MBP as splenocytes from MBP/FCA–immunized PVGs respond in vitro to MBP as well as those obtained from similarly treated Lewis rats (10).

It has been shown that the spontaneous recovery of Lewis rats from EAE is a result of corticosterone released from the adrenal gland in response to the induction of the disease (8,11). The essential role of the hormone is demonstrated by the finding that adrenalectomized Lewis rats do not recover from EAE but instead develop a progressive paralysis which affects the upper as well as the lower parts of the body. Replacement therapy, using subcutaneous corticosterone pellets, allows adrenalectomized rats to recover normally, indicating that it is this product of the adrenal glands that mediates recovery in non-adrenalectomized animals.

Adrenalectomy of PVG rats up to 8 days after immunization with MBP/FCA renders them completely susceptible to progressive EAE and, as with the Lewis rat, replacement corticosterone therapy allows recovery (12). In adrenalectomized PVGs given a dose of corticosterone that produces serum levels similar to those developed by normal, immunized, Lewis rats, the course of EAE is very similar to that seen in the latter strain. Comparisons of ratios of adrenal weight to body weight and of serum corticosterone levels elicited by ether anesthesia have shown that PVG rats can make more vigorous stress responses than Lewis strain animals, and it is this difference that appears to determine the relative susceptibility of the two strains to EAE. Significantly PVG.RTI^1 rats, that have the same background genes as PVGs but have the MHC genes of Lewis rats are refractory to EAE unless the animals are adrenalectomized. This result maps the gene(s) responsible for resistance outside of the MHC. Consistent with this conclusion is the finding that in a variety of congeneic rat strains those that have their non-MHC genes derived from the PVG strain all have high adrenal weight/body weight ratios. However, adrenalectomy does not render all rat strains with PVG background genes susceptible to

EAE. In particular, PVG.RTI^u rats are resistant, indicating that MHC-associated Ir genes can also determine disease susceptibility (12).

CONCLUSION

Both MHC and non-MHC immune-response gene effects can be demonstrated to determine the susceptibility of different rat strains to EAE. The non–MHC-associated effects arise, at least in some instances, through variation in the levels of serum corticosterone that are generated in response to stress. The same mechanism has been shown to determine susceptibility to streptococcal cell wall arthritis in rats (13), and it is likely to play a part in the other experimental autoimmune diseases mentioned in the Introduction to this chapter. It is probable that genetically determined variations in the stress response occur in other species and may influence disease susceptibility (14).

REFERENCES

1. Benacerraf B, McDevitt HO. Histocompatibility-linked immune response genes. Science 1972; 175:273–279.
2. Günther E, Rüde E, Stark O. Antibody response in rats to synthetic polypeptide (TG)AL genetically linked to the major histocompatibility system. Eur J Immunol 1972;2:151–55.
3. Brown IN, Glynn AA, Plant J. Inbred mouse strain resistance to Mycobacterium lepraemurium follows the Ity/Lsh pattern. Immunology 1982;47:149–56.
4. Howard JG, Hale C, Ling Chan-Liew W. Immunological regulation of experimental cutaneous leishmaniasis. 1. Immunogenetic aspects of susceptibility to Leishmania tropica in mice. Parasite Immunol 1980;2:303–14.
5. McFarlin DE, Blank SE, Kibler RF. Recurrent experimental allergic encephalomyelitis in the Lewis rat. J Immunol 1974;113:712–15.
6. Willenborg DO. Experimental allergic encephalomyelitis in the Lewis rat: Studies on the mechanism of recovery from disease and acquired resistance to reintroduction. J Immunol 1979;123:1145–50.
7. Hashim GA. Myelin basic protein: Structure, function and antigenic determinants. Immunol Rev 1978;39:60–107.
8. MacPhee IAM, Antoni FA, Mason DW. Spontaneous recovery of rats from experimental allergic encephalomyelitis is dependent on regulation of the immune system by endogenous adrenal corticosteroids. J Exp Med 1989;169:431–45.
9. Hughes RAC, Stedronska J. The susceptibility of rat strains to experimental allergic encephalomyelitis. Immunology 1973;24:879–84.
10. Ben-Nun A, Einstein S, Cohen IR. Experimental allergic encephalomyelitis (EAE) in genetically resistant rats: PVG rats resist active induction of EAE but are susceptible to and can generate EAE effector T cells. J Immunol 1982;129:918–19.
11. Levine S, Sowinski R, Steinetz B. Effects of experimental allergic encephalomyelitis on thymus and adrenal. Relation to remission and relapse. Proc Soc Exp Biol Med 1980;165:218–24.
12. Mason D, MacPhee I, Antoni F. The role of the neuroendocrine system in determining genetic susceptibility to experimental allergic encephalomyelitis in the rat. Immunology 1990;70:1–5.
13. Sternberg EM, Hill JM, Chrousos GP, Kamilaris T, Listwak SJ, Gold PW, Wilder RL. Inflammatory mediator-induced hypothalamic-pituitary-adrenal axis activation is defective in streptococcal cell wall arthritis-susceptible rats. Proc Natl Acad Sci USA 1989;86:2374–78.
14. Mason DW. Genetic variation in the stress response and its effect on susceptibility to inflammatory diseases. Immunol Today 1991; 12:57–60.

114
Evidence of Abnormal Microenvironment in Mice with Autoimmune Diseases

Bernadette Nabarra and Mireille Dardenne
INSERM U 25, Hôpital Necker, Paris, France

INTRODUCTION

The pathogenesis of autoimmune disease in some inbred mouse strains has been the subject of functional studies for many years. Given the immunological dysfunction found in several earlier reports (1–8), and the primordial role played by the thymic microenvironment in the education of T cells, it appeared interesting to study the ultrastructural aspect of the thymus of these mice (9–10). Ultrastructural observation is the only technique that permits identification of the different cells forming the thymic reticulum and, therefore, and better knowledge of the thymic environment and, hence, it possible modifications. Three strains of mice with lupuslike disease (NZB, BXSB, MRL) having various common dysfunctions and some differences (1–4) and two strains of diabetic mice (db/db and nonobese diabetic [NOD]) considered as models of autoimmune diseases (5–8,11) were observed. These thymuses were studied by comparing their morphological aspect with that of the normal thymus described previously (12,13).

MATERIALS AND METHODS

Animals

For this study we used: (a) homozygous male MRL/1 and BXSB mice and male and female NZB mice, 15 days to 2 years of age; (b) homozygous db/db mice aged 15 days and 1, 4, and 6 months. (These strains of mice were purchased from C.S.A.L. Orléans-La Source, France.) (c) NOD female mice, aged from 1 to 10 months, bred in specific-pathogen free (SPF) conditions in our laboratory. Each experimental group included nine mice. Thymuses were removed immediately after sacrifice and prepared for electron microscopy.

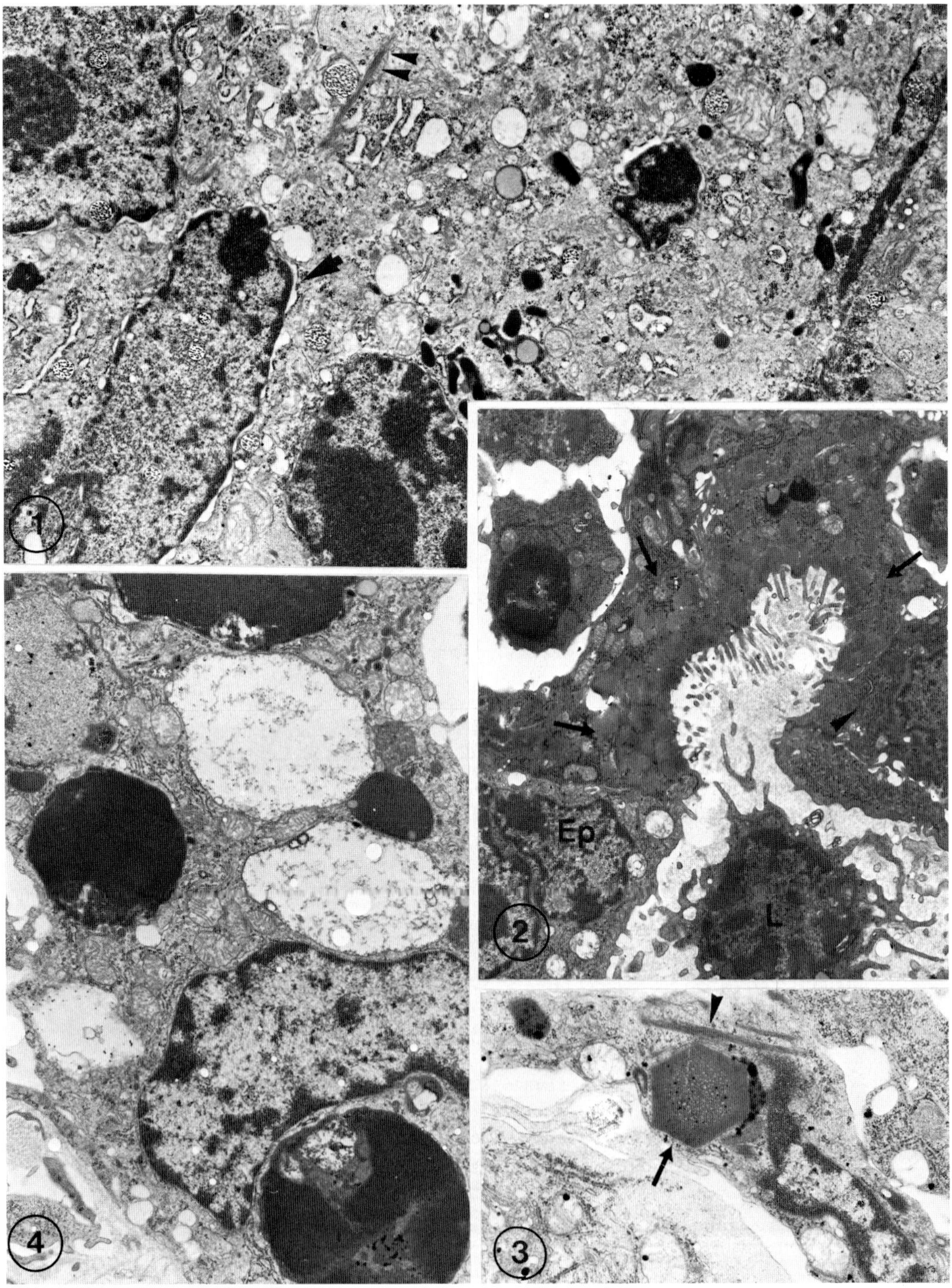
1
2
Ep
L
3
4

Preparation for Electron Microscopy

Thymus fragments were prepared according to a classic technique, more fully described previously (12,13). Briefly: The thymuses were fixed for 1 hr in 2% glutaraldehyde in phosphate buffer, pH 7.4, washed, postfixed for 1 hr in 1% osmium tetroxide, dehydrated, and then embedded in Epon. Ten blocks of each thymic area (cortex and medulla) were examined by electron microscopy for each mouse.

RESULTS

In these autoimmune thymuses we observed features present in all autoimmune mice, with various degrees of severity as well as some morphological differences among the strains observed. We first considered the premature aspect of involution of several areas of parenchyma present in all mice with various degrees of severity and extention. Second, we studied numerous cellular alterations in noninvoluted areas, which appear to be early lesions of involution in all mice.

Involuted Areas

General Aspect

An important finding was the presence of large zones of parenchyma showing a premature involuted appearance. Whereas in the normal thymus this morphological aspect is observed at about 8–10 months of life, in some autoimmune mice there coexisted early in life an involuted parenchyma and a more normal parenchyma forming an irregular patchwork. The involuted aspect extended with time. In these zones, the cells forming the microenvironment seems to have lost their limiting membranes and their cellular characteristics (Fig. 1). The cytoplasm was very clear, seemly to be empty, and completely disorganized with a few scattered cellular organites. In particular, the rough endoplasmic reticulum was often dilated. The characteristic cellular differentiation of these cells was missing but sometimes a few tonofilaments were present. Nevertheless, it was not possible to identify whether they were epithelial cells of the cortex or of the medulla, or another type of stroma cells. The number of lymphocytes was greatly decreased and only some of them were found

---

Figure 1 Five-month-old NZB mouse: Involuted aspect of the thymic reticulum with no clearly defined membrane between cells, giving an appearance of a large cytoplasmic layer (⯈ tonofilaments). The reticulum endoplasmic saccules in the cytoplasm and in perinuclear position were dilated. Impregnated with uranyl acetate and lead citrate (magnification: ±9500).

Figure 2 Three-month-old NOD mouse: Cystic cavity showing cells bordering the lumen containing moderately electron-dense inclusions (→), alternating with normal epithelial cells (Ep). (Lymphocytes: L). Impregnated with uranyl acetate and lead citrate (magnification: ±7000).

Figure 3 Three-month-old db/db mouse: Epithelial cell (► tonofilaments) containing a hexagonal crystalloid inclusion (→). Impregnation with uranyl acetate and lead citrate (magnification: ±7000).

Figure 4 Four-month-old NOD mouse: macrophages with numerous phagolysosomes containing damaged cells at various stage of lysis. Impregnated with uranyl acetate and lead citrate magnification: ±12000).

in these zones. In addition, numerous lipidic globules were present in this cellular layer and rapidly invaded the whole parenchyma.

These zones were little developed and occurred relatively later in NZB and BXSB mice, but early in comparison to the morphological aspect of normal involution, whereas they were very developed early in the life of MRL/1, db/db, and NOD mice.

Cystic Activities

Furthermore in these zones of parenchyma, we observed numerous, large cytic cavities. These formations existed in very small numbers in the young normal mouse, and their number and size increased with age. In autoimmune mice, early in life their number was very increased. They had a normal appearance in lupuslike mice; i.e., a large lumen bordered by epithelial cells, not surrounded by a basal membrane, in continuity with the reticulum. In some cases, a clear fine material was seen in the lumen and sometimes a small number of lymphocytes. In diabetic mice (db/db and NOD) a peculiar appearance was observed in the wall of these cystic cavities: two types of cells bordering the lumen, epithelial cells as in the normal thymus, and cells containing round and homogeneous, moderately electron-dense inclusions, occupying a large part of the cytoplasm and morphologically similar to what is observed in certain "mucoid" cells. Furthermore, these cavities were very dilated and extended and contained a great number of lymphocytes, blast cells, and macrophages (Fig. 2).

Noninvoluted Areas

Epithelial Cells

Severe and extensive vacuolization of type I epithelial cells (present in both the thymic cortex and medulla) was observed. This vacuolization was expressed by an increased number of "clear vacuoles," characteristic of this type of cell, and by considerable dilatation of the rough endoplasmic reticulum, which appeared empty. Contrary to the normal appearance, these clear vacuoles of type I epithelial cells contained no or only a few dense granulations. The other types of epithelial cells (types II and III in our classification, present only in the medullary area) occurred in almost normal numbers. Nevertheless, in lupuslike mice the alveolar cavity of type II cells contained numerous viral particles, more than that sometimes present in normal mice.

Crystalloid Inclusions

The three strains of mice with lupuslike disease and the strain of diabetic disease db/db showed peculiar crystalloid like inclusions in epithelial cells (Fig. 3), whereas these inclusions were absent in NOD mice. They were either hexagonal, diamond shaped, or rectangular in form and were strongly electron dense, with a more or less granular core. In NZB and BXSB mice, they were contained in the clear vacuoles of type I epithelial cells, occupying these vacuoles in totality or together with normal granular material. In MRL mice, they were present in epithelial cells of the cystic cavities, whatever the age of the mice. Furthermore, in BXSB mice, a second type of crystal-like inclusion with periodic striations was observed in the dilated reticulum endoplasmic saccules.

Macrophages and Interdigitated Cells

The number of macrophages with numerous phagolysosomes was slightly increased in NZB, MRL/1, and db/db mice, whereas in BXSB mice, it appeared normal. In NOD mice, the number and the phagocytic activity of macrophages was strongly increased. They showed enormous phagolysosomes containing phagocytized material. A macrophage might contain about six or more pyknotic nuclei of thymocytes, various types of cytoplasmic inclusions, and damaged lymphocytes cells at different stages of lysis (Fig. 4).

The number of interdigitating cells seemed to be higher in all three lupuslike strains, whereas in diabetic mice, they were normal in size and morphology.

Infiltrating Cells

In addition, we observed infiltrating cells of plasma cell type which more or less formed clusters NZB, BXSB, and db/db mice and were scattered in the reticulum in MRL and NOD mice. Furthermore, an increased number of mast cells forming small accumulations in NZB,BXSB, and NOD mice were noted in these thymuses.

DISCUSSION

Ultrastructural pathology revealed several features common to these different mouse strains. First, the thymus showed premature histological and cytological modifications similar to those observed in the aging involuted thymus, forming a patchwork with non-involuted zones. These alterations of the microenvironment showed cells without well-defined membranes, forming a large, no-limited cytoplasmic layer. They were observed in very young autoimmune mice, suggesting that a premature aging process occurred in these animals. Recently, Nakamura, studying BXSB mice (14), suggested that premature involution of the thymus in autoimmune mice may not be a genetically determined abnormality intrinsic to the thymus, but rather an abnormality secondary to other events occurring in these mice. This author affirmed that premature thymic involution was due to abnormal stem cells which migrate into the thymus.

We also observed in these involuted zones an increased number of cystics cavities. In normal mice, the cells bordering these cavities are chiefly epithelial and do not contain granulations. In diabetic (NOD and db/db) mice, several cells forming the wall bordering these cavities alternatively with epithelial cells show intracytoplasmic dense, homogeneous granules, which appear morphologically similar to mucoid granules of goblet intestinal cells, or according to the description of Pansky (15) to the granulation of pancreatic islets of Langerhans. This resemblance is also based upon embryological studies suggesting that both cell types arise from the endoderm. It seems that these cells produce a factor involved in the metabolism of carbohydrates, and which could be an insulinase inhibitor or a compound having an activity limiting insulin. In this regard, it is interesting to note that Eisenbarth et al. (16) have isolated two antipancreatic islet antibodies which react with subsets of thymic reticulum cells. For these authors, this observation could indicate that the autoimmunity of diabetes includes the thymus. We also observed a certain number of lymphocytes and several macrophages circulating in these cavities of diabetic mice. The accumulation of lymphocytes in these cavities can be compared with the observation of W. Savino (17), who showed in immunofluorescence technique a great accumulation of B and $CD4^+CD8^+$ T lymphocytes in the parenchyma of these thymuses.

In nonvoluted areas we observed a vacuolized aspect of the thymic epithelium and an increased number of macrophages. The vacuolization of type I epithelial cells was observed in all strains of mice. In normal mice, these cells are characterized by the presence in their cytoplasm of two or three vacuoles containing some granular material (12), which seems to be implicated in their secretory function (18). In autoimmune mice, "clear vacuoles" do not contain dense granular material as they normally do. The aspect of these cells with numerous vacuoles scattered in the cytoplasm is similar to that observed after blockage of the secretory function by monensin (18). This feature suggests an alteration of epithelial cell function. This hypothesis is confirmed by the fact that several authors (5,19,20) have described a premature decline in thymic hormone production in most autoimmune mice, as assessed by low hormonal levels in the serum and, at least for thymulin, decreased numbers of epithelial cells synthesizing the peptide, as assessed by immunofluorescence studies using monoclonal antibodies.

The other important fact observed is the presence of crystalloid-like inclusions in epithelial cells, which exist only in lupuslike mice and in db/db mice. Such crystalloid inclusions have already been observed in other autoimmune strains (21). These authors suggest that thymic hormone or its precursors could be stored in an abnormal form in some autoimmune diseases. This abnormal form could represent the inhibitory molecules detected in some lupus strains such as BXSB mice (5).

The relationship between the morphological abnormalities of thymic epithelial cells, the thymic dysfunction, and the development of the autoimmune disease is far from clear. However, the alterations that we observed could be considered as environmental factors inducing an acceleration of the autoimmune process, since the role of the thymus in differentiation of T cells and the perturbation of the microenvironment can lead to T- and B-cell dysfunction. In this way, the hypothesis of Ikehara (22) and Nakamura (14) of the existence in autoimmune mice of defective bone marrow stem cells suggests that these defective stem cells entering into abnormal thymus was differentiated in abnormal lymphocytes and macrophages, and thus involve a T-cell dysfunction.

REFERENCES

1. Talal N, Steinberg A. The pathogenesis of autoimmunity in NZB mice. Cur Top Microbiol Immunol 1974;64:79–103.
2. Andrew B, Eisenberg R, Theofilopoulos A, Izui S, Wilson C, Mc Conahey P, Murphy E, Roths J, Dixon F. Spontaneous murine lupus-like syndromes. Clinical and immunopathological manifestations in several strains. J Exp Med 1978;148:1198–1215.
3. Theofilopoulos A, Dixon F. Etiopathogenesis of murine SLE. Immunol Rev 1981;55:179–216.
4. Dardenne M, Savino W, Nabarra B, Bach JF. Male BXSB mice develop a thymic hormonal dysfunction: a serological and immunohistochemical study. Clin Exp Immunol 1989;52:392–397.
5. Dardenne M, Savino W, Gastinel L, Nabarra B, Bach JF. Thymic dysfunction in the mutant diabetic (db/db) mouse. J Immunol 1983;130:1195–1199.
6. Fernandes G, Handewerger B, Yunis E, Brown D. Immune responses in the mutant C57BL/db+ mouse. J Clin Invest 1978;61:243–247.
7. Tochino Y. The NOD mouse as a model of type I diabetes. C.R.C. Cirt. Rev. Immunol. 1987;8:49–81.
8. Katuoka S, Stoch J, Fujiya H, Toyota T, Suzuki R, Itoh K, Kumagai K. Immunologic aspect of the Non Obese Diabetic (NOD) mouse. Diabetes 1983;32:247–253.
9. Nabarra B, Andrianarison I. Thymic reticulum of autoimmune mice. I. Ultrastructural studies of the diabetic (db/db) mouse thymus. Exp Pathol 1986;29:45–53.
10. Nabarra B, Dardenne M, Bach JF. Thymic reticulum of autoimmune mice. II. Ultrastructural studies of mice with lupus-like syndrome (NAB, BXSB, MRL/1). J Autoimmune 1990;3:25–36.
11. Bendelac A, Carnaud C, Boitard C, Bach JF. Syngeneic transfer of autoimmune diabetes from diabetic NOD mice to healthy neonates. Requirement for both $L3T4^+$ and $Lyt2^+$ cells. J Exp Med 1987;166:823–828.
12. Nabarra B, Andrianarison I. Ultrastructural studies of thymic reticulum. I. Epithelial component. Thymus 1987;9:95–121.
13. Nabarra B, Andrianarison I. Ultrastructural studies of thymic reticulum. II. Non-epithelial component. Thymus (in press).

14. Nakamura T, Ikehara S, Good R, Iroe S, Sekita K, Furukawa F, Tanaka H, Maung O., Hamashima Y. Abnormal stem cells in autoimmune-prone mice are responsible for premature thymic involution. Thymus 1985;7:151–158.
15. Pansky B, House E. The granular reticulum cells of the thymus in the AKR mouse. Anat Rec 1965;152:451–456.
16. Eisenbarth G, Jackson E, Srikanta S, Powers A, Buse J, Mori H. Utilisation of monoclonal antibody techniques to study type I (insulin dependent) diabetes mellitus. In: *Immunology in Diabetes*, Adreani, Di Mairo, Federlin (eds.). Kripton Publications, London, 1984, p. 143.
17. Savino W, Boitard C, Bach JF, Dardenne M. Studies on the thymus in non obese diabetic (NOD) mouse. I. Changes in the microenvironmental compartments (submitted).
18. Nabarra B, Andrianarison I. Pattern of secretion in thymic epithelial cells: ultrastructural studies of the effect of blockage at various levels. Cell and Tissue Res 1987;249:171–175.
19. Savino W, Dardenne M, Bach JF. Thymic hormone containing cells. II. Evolution of cells containing the serum thymic factor (FTS or thymulin) in normal and autoimmune mice, as revealed by anti-FTS monoclonal antibodies. Relationship with Ia bearing cells. Clin Exp Immunol 1983;52:1–5.
20. Gershwin E, Steinberg A, Ahmed A, Derkay C. Study of thymic factors. II. Failure of thymosin to alter the natural history of NZB and NZB/NZW mice. Arthritis and Rheum. 1976;19:862–866.
21. Schmitt D, Monier JC. Possible reaction between (low thymosine-like activity in the serum of Swan mice (swiss antinuclear) and the formation of crystals in their thymic epithelial. Experientia, 1974;30:1349–1351.
22. Ikehara S., Tanaka H., Nakamura T., Furukawa F., Inone S., Sekita K., Shimuru I. Hamachina Y., Good R. The influence of thymic abnormalities on the development of autoimmune diseases. Thymus 1985;7:25–36.

ACCESSORY CELLS

115

Stromal Cells in the Lymphoid Organs

A Pivotal Role for Activation, Differentiation, and Selection

Martine Papiernik
Inserm U 25, Paris, France

Stromal cells of the lymphoid organs are obligatory partners for lymphocyte migration, activation, maturation, and selection. Indeed, precursors of lymphocytes as well as mature B and T cells need the cooperation of the so called "accessory cells" to pass through the different steps which lead them to differentiate and/or to become potent effector cells.

The organization of the vascular tree, which defines the initial cell circulation, the migration pathway within the organ, the nature of the stromal cells encountered by the migrating lymphocytes, the antigens they express, and the cytokines they produce are within the multiple elements which are involved in the partnership. This makes an incredibly complex network of influences to analyze in order to understand the role of the different cells involved. If we take the thymus as an example, one can measure how complex the system is and how far we are from understanding all the mechanisms which lead to T-cell maturation. At least four different types of stromal cells may be involved: the endothelial cells of the vessels which the precursors have to cross, the macrophages and the interdigitating cells (IDCs) which come from the bone marrow, the epithelial cells (ECs) which develop from the endoectodermic anlage, and finally the fibroblasts, which are usually forgotten, but which may intervene by the production of cytokines and the constitution of the extracellular matrix. Some arguments (1,2) strongly suggest that the precursors enter the thymus at the corticomedullary junction, at least in experimental in vivo models. At this location, the precursors may face all types of stromal cells, and their first activation signals may be driven by any of them. Nevertheless, the role of macrophages in vitro on $CD4^-8^-$ thymocyte activation (3), the local production of interleukin-1 (IL-1) (4) which may be involved in this activation, and the early formation of macrophage rosettes during reconstitution (2) argue that the first signals may be macrophage driven, although cooperative work cannot be excluded. While migrating through the cortex, the precursors will expand (in the subcapsular area), and go through the different steps of differentiation which lead them to rearrange the genes coding for the T-cell receptor (TCR) and to express both the TCR and the differentiation antigens CD4 and CD8. Selection of the repertoire will occur during this period, although the exact schedule of the selection is not known. Epithelial cells and a few macrophages are the stromal cells present in the cortex and involved in this process of maturation. Back to the corticomedullary junction, which is probably the last filter for selection, the maturing thymocytes may face all three types of stromal cells, macrophages, IDCs, and ECs. Mature T cells will then be exported to the periphery or stored in the medulla.

The intimate mechanisms of these processes are poorly understood. It is clear that none of the in vitro models which separate the precursors from their stromal partners is able to lead them through all the steps of the maturation. Cell-to-cell interactions between stromal cells expressing major histocompatibility (MHC) molecules and maturing thymocytes expressing the TCR molecules are needed, as shown by experiments which block this interaction (5,6). Adherence molecules are also probably involved (7). Cytokines are said to be major signals for maturation. And all types of cytokines have been shown to be produced by thymic cells either in vivo or in vitro, part of them being produced by stromal cells, such as colony-stimulating factor (CSF), IL-1, IL-6, IL-7, prostaglandins (PGs) and thymic hormones. But finally, the role of the cytokines in vivo is far from being clear and the models in vitro are usually biased, partly because the regulatory systems are missing.

In the peripheral lymphoid organs, the complexity of the systems is the same, although the epithelial cells are missing. Their stromal cells have to handle both B and T lymphocytes, and to process and present the antigens.

Stromal cells are more than accessory in all the processes which involve precursor maturation and B- or T-lymphocyte function. "Partner cell" would be a much better term.

REFERENCES

1. Penit C, Vasseur F. Sequential events in thymocytes differentiation and thymus regeneration revealed by a combination of bromodeoxyuridine DNA labelling and antimitotic drug treatment. J Immunol 1988;140:3315–23.
2. Kyewski BA, Rouse RV, Kaplan HS. Thymocyte rosettes: multicellular complexes of lymphocytes and bone marrow-derived stromal cells in the mouse thymus. Proc Natl Acad Sci USA 1982;79:5646–50.
3. Papiernik M, Penit C, El Rouby S. Control of prothymocyte proliferation by thymic accessory cells. Eur J Immunol 1987;17:1303–10.
4. Takacs L, Kovac EJ, Smith R, Yung HA, Durum SK. Detection of IL-1α and IL-1β gene expression by *in situ* hybridization. J Immunol 1988;141:3081–95.
5. McDuffie M, Born W, Marrack P, Kappler J. The role of the T cell receptor in thymocyte maturation effect in vivo of anti-receptor antibody. Proc Natl Acad Sci USA 1986;83:8728–32.
6. Kruisbeek AM, Mond JJ, Fowlkes BJ, Carmen JA, Bridges S, Longo DL. Absence of the Lyt-2, L3T4^{+} lineage of T cells in mice treated neonatally with anti-I-A correlates with absence of intrathymic I-A bearing antigen-presenting cell function. 1985; 161:1029–47.
7. El Rouby S, Papiernik M. Con A response and interleukin 2 receptor expression of thymocytes rosetting with phagocytic cells of the thymic reticulum. Thymus 1987;9:239–51.

116
Characterization of Human Follicular Dendritic Cells

Henk K. Parmentier, Dick van Wichen, Joke H. van der Linden, Andries C. Bloem, and Henk-Jan Schuurman
University Hospital, Utrecht, The Netherlands

INTRODUCTION

Follicular dendritic cells (FDCs) form the framework of primary and secondary follicles in lymphoid tissue (1,2). In situ, they are identified as large binucleated, DRC-1–positive (3) and Ki-M4–positive (4) cells with elongated cytoplasmic extensions, joined together by desmosomes, creating a complex three-dimensional network (2). In this matrix, predominantly B cells are localized (5,6). The FDCs probably do not phagocytose but trap and retain antigen on their protrusions, presumably in the form of immune complexes bound via receptors for the immunoglobulin (Ig) Fc fragment or for complement (7–10). Presentation of antigen in this form to B cells may contribute to the induction of antibody formation, and immunological memory within the B-lymphocyte population (11,12).

Data on the immunophenotype of FDCs are not consistent. We here describe a method to isolate FDCs from human tonsils, and present the evaluation of their immunophenotypical characteristics.

MATERIALS AND METHODS

Tonsils and Cells

Tonsils were obtained at tonsillectomy of young children. They were kept at 4°C in (transferrin-rich) Opti-MEM culture medium until initiation of FDC isolation. Epstein-Barr virus (EBV)–transformed B-cell lines kept and established at our hospital were used (13).

FDC Isolation

Tonsils were dissected free from surface epithelium and divided into 1-mm^3 cubes, which were rotated for 30 min at room temperature in 10 ml Opti-MEM containing 15 U/ml collagenase (type XI) (Sigma), 0.025 U/ml deoxyribonuclease (DNase) (Boehringer), and

0.5% bovine serum albumin (BSA, RIA-grade, Sigma) per tonsil. The supernatant was centrifuged for 10 min at 600 × G at 4°C. The pellet was resuspended in 3 ml Opti-MEM, and subjected to 1 G sedimentation in a discontinuous bovine serum albumin (BSA) gradient consisting of 1.5, 2.5, 5.0, and 7.5% BSA, respectively. Cells in the interphase between 2.5 and 5.0% BSA were collected, washed, and the suspension was layered in 2 ml on a Percoll (Pharmacia) gradient consisting of 1.5-ml layers with densities ranging from 1.070, 1.060, and 1.030, followed by 20 min centrifugation at 1200 × G. Cells with densities of 1.030 and 1.060 were collected and washed twice with Opti-MEM. This procedure yielded in between 5×10^6 and $1\text{-}2\times10^7$ cells per tonsil.

Characterization of FDCs

The expression of various cell markers (Table 1) in cytocentrifuge preparations of isolated FDCs was done by a three-step immunoperoxidase method. Air-dried preparations fixed in acetone (10 min at room temperature) were subsequently incubated with antibody diluted in 1% human serum albumin (HSA), rabbit antimouse Ig conjugated to horseradish peroxidase (RAM/PO, Dakopatts), and swine antirabbit Ig conjugated to horseradish peroxidase (SwAR/PO, Dakopatts). Conjugated antibodies were diluted in 10% AB serum. The preparations were developed with hydrogen peroxide using 3-amino-9-ethylcarbazole (AEC, Brunschwig) as substrate, and counterstained with hematoxylin. Surface IgG, IgM, and IgD and complement components C1q and C3b was analyzed by direct immunofluorescence using fluorescein isothiocyanate (FITC)–conjugated antibodies.

Table 1 Immunological Phenotype of Isolated FDCs

Positive expression	Reagent[c]	Negative expression	Reagent[c]
CD2 <[a]	[1]T11	CD1	[8]OKT6
CD4 <[a]	[2]Leu-3a	CD3	[2]Leu-4
CD22[b]	[3]DAKO panB	CD5	[2]Leu-1
CD37 <[a]	[4]IOB-1	CD8	[2]Leu-2a
DRC-1	[3]DAKO-DRC	CD25	[2]J0101
Ki-M4	[5]BMA 0340	CD30	[3]Ki-1
C3bR	[2]CR1	S-100	[3]RACow S-100
Macrophage	[3]EBM11		
sIgG	[3]RAH/IgG/FITC		
sIgM	[3]RAH/IgM/FITC		
sIgD	[4]RAH/IgD/FITC		
Clq	[6]RAH/Clq/FITC		
C3b	[6]RAH/C3b/FITC		
FcγR I	[7]32.2		
FcγR II	[7]IV.3		
FcγR III	[1]gran 1		

[a]Less than the percentage of DRC-1/Ki-M4 staining cells.
[b]It was not possible to discriminate unequivocally between FDCs and B-cell membranes.
[c]Reagents obtained from: [1]Central Laboratory of the Blood Transfusion Service, Amsterdam, The Netherlands; [2]Becton Dickinson, Mountain View, California; [3]Dakopatts, Glostrups, Denmark; [4]Serotec, Oxford, England; [5]Behringwerke, Marburg-Lahn, Germany; [6]Kallestad, Austin, Texas; [7]Dr. Guyre, Hannover, New Hampshire; [8]Ortho Diagnostic, Beerse, Belgium.

Two-color immunofluorescence for detection of DRC-1 and CD20 (B-cell) antigen was done by incubation of cells with DRC-1 and goat antimouse IgM/FITC, followed by B1(CD20)/biotine and an avidine/phycoerythrine conjugate. Cells were read by cytofluorography using a FACScan (Becton Dickinson).

RESULTS AND DISCUSSION

The FDCs isolated by BSA and Percoll density gradients were invariably labeled by DRC-1 and Ki-M4 monoclonal antibodies (MAbs) (Fig. 1), which revealed them as large binucleated cells with dendritic processes. The FDCs frequently formed clusters with B lymphocytes (determined by CD22 staining), which were enclosed by slender FDC protrusions. The relative proportion of the yielded DRC-1/Ki-M4–positive cells ranged from 30 to 70%, including clustered FDCs and small solitary mononuclear lymphocytic DRC-1/Ki-M4–positive cells.

The isolated FDCs were characterized for their immunophenotype (see Table 1). The FDCs were negative for CD1, CD3, CD5, CD8, CD30, and S-100. CD2 and CD37 were present on a minority of FDCs. Isolated FDCs expressed HLA-DR, and were weakly stained by the DAKO-macrophage antibody. Strong expression of CR1, surface IgG and IgM (7,8,9,14), and a weak expression of Fcγ receptors I, II, and III, and occasionally surface IgD was found. By immunochemistry, a weak CD4 expression was observed on approximately 20% of the FDCs (Fig. 2).

Follicular dendritic cell–specific surface markers were found on B cells. Cytofluorographic two-color analysis revealed that in several (CD20-positive) EBV-transformed

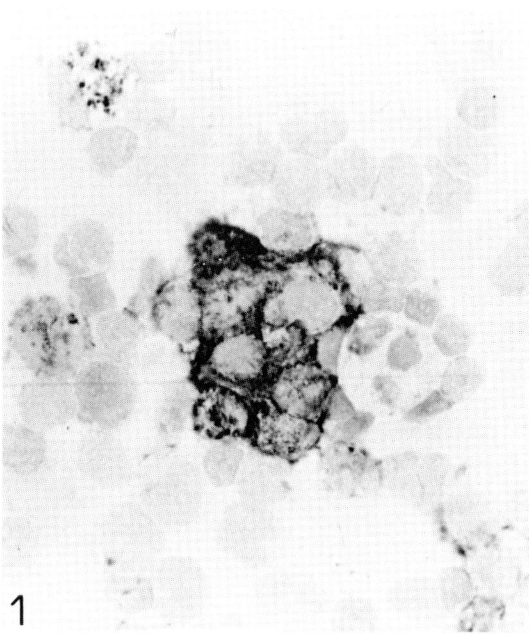

1

Figure 1 Immunolabeling of isolated FDC. Data of DRC-1. Three-step immunoperoxidase: RAM/PO, SwAR/PO, followed by AEC. Counterstaining by hematoxylin (magnification: ×610).

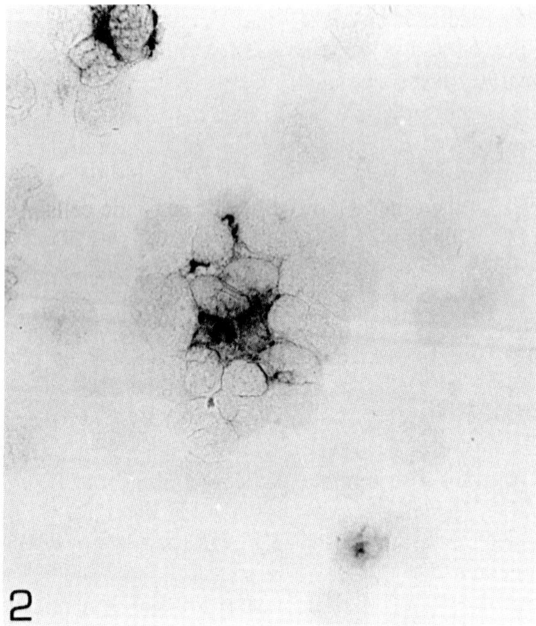
2

Figure 2 Immunolabeling of isolated FDC. Data of CD4. Three-step immunoperoxidase: RAM/PO, SwAR/PO, followed by AEC. Counterstaining by hematoxylin (magnification: ×610).

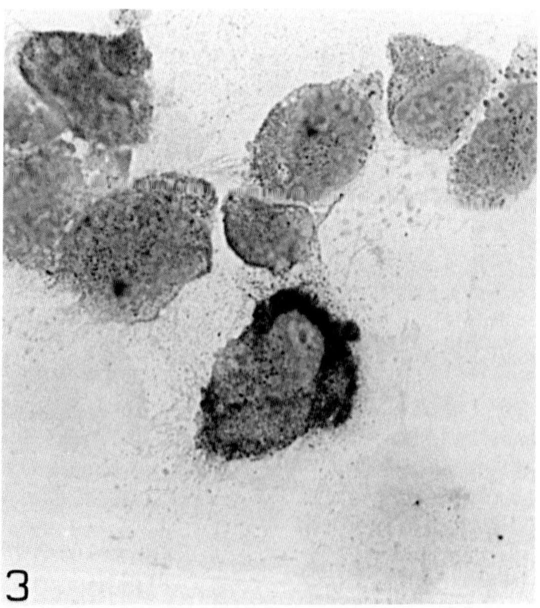
3

Figure 3 DRC-1 expressing EBV-B cell. Three-step immunoperoxidase: RAM/PO, SwAR/PO, AEC, with counterstaining by hematoxylin (magnification: ×1000). Similar staining was obtained with Ki-M4 antibody.

B-cell lines, approximately one-third of the cells expressed DRC-1 (Fig. 3). Positivity was also observed for approximately 90% of CD20-positive tonsillar cells irregardless of their surface immunoglobulin isotype expression, and 50% of peripheral CD20-positive cells. CD3 (T) cells were not stained by DRC-1 antibody. It has been claimed (3) that DRC-1 antibody may also stain mantle zone B cells. It is tempting to suggest that on one hand FDCs and B cells of different stages share a common marker, or the DRC-1 antigen may be derived from B cells and fixed by FDCs on the other hand. Follicular dendritic cells bear several B-cell–restricted antigens (15,16). This implies that the identification of FDCs or their precursor cells during in vitro culture may be hampered by the fact that B cells can express DRC-1 antigen.

ACKNOWLEDGMENT

This study was supported by the Dutch Ministry of Health, in the frame work of the National Program on AIDS Research, RGO/WVC nr. 88-79/89005.

REFERENCES

1. Nossal GJ, Abbot A, Mitchell J, Lummus Z. Antigens in immunity. XV. Ultrastructural features of antigen capture in primary and secondary follicles. J Exp Med 19876; 127:277–89.
2. Rademakers LHPM, Peters JPJ, van Unnik JAM. Histiocytic and dendritic reticulum cells in follicular structures of follicular lymphoma and reactive hyperplasia; a quantitative electron microscopic analysis. Virchows Arch 1983; 44:85–98.
3. Naiem M, Gerdes J, Abdulaziz Z, Stein H, Mason DY. Production of a monoclonal antibody reactive with human dendritic reticulum cells and its use in the immunohistochemical analysis of lymphoid tissue. J Clin Pathol 1983; 36:167–75.
4. Parwaresch MR, Radzun HJ, Hansmann ML, Peters KP. Monoclonal antibody Ki-M4 specifically recognizes human dendritic reticulum cells (follicular dendritic cells) and their possible precursor in blood. Blood 1983; 62:585–90.
5. Lilet-Leclerq C, Radoux D, Heinen E, Kinet-Denoël C, Defraigne JO, Houben-Defresne MP, Simar LJ. Isolation of follicular dendritic cells from human tonsils and adenoids. I. Procedures and morphological characterization. J Immunol Methods 1984; 66:235–44.
6. Heinen E, Kinet-Denoël C, Radoux D, Simar LJ. Mouse lymph node follicular dendritic cells: quantitative analysis and isolation. Adv Exp Med Biol 1985; 186:171–83.
7. Heinen E, Radoux D, Kinet-Denoël C, Moeremoins M, De Mey J, Simar LJ. Isolation of follicular dendritic cells from human tonsils and adenoids. III. Analysis of their Fc receptor. Immunology 1985; 54:777–84.
8. Gerdes J, Stein H. Complement (C3) receptors on dendritic reticulum cells of normal and malignant lymphoid tissue. Clin Exp Immunol 1982; 48:348–52.
9. Herd ZL, Ada GL. The retention of ^{125}I-immunoglobulin IgG subunits and antigen-antibody complexes in the rat food pads and draining lymph nodes. Aust J Exp Med Sci 1969; 47:63–77.
10. Radoux D, Kinet-Denoël C, Heinen E, Moeremans M, De Mey J, Simar LJ. Retention of immune complexes by Fc receptors on mouse follicular dendritic cells. Scand J Immunol 1985; 21:345–53.
11. Klaus GGB, Humphrey JH, Kunkl A, Dongworth W. The follicular dendritic cell: Its role on antigen presentation in the generation of immunological memory. Immunol Rev 1980; 53:3–28.
12. Tew JG, Kosco MH, Szakal AK. The alternative antigen pathway. Immunol Today 1989; 10:229–32.

13. Logtenberg T, Young FM, van Es J, Gmelig-Meyling FHJ, Berman JE, Alt FW. Frequency of V_H-gene utilization in human EBV-transformed B-cell lines: The most J_H-proximal V_H segment encodes autoantibodies. J Autoimmunity 1989 (suppl); 2:203–13.
14. Zwirner J, Felber E, Schmidt P, Riethmüller G, Feucht HE. Complement activation in human lymphoid germinal centers. Immunology 1989; 66:270–77.
15. Parwaresch MR, Radzun HJ, Feller AC, Peters KP, Hansman ML. Peroxidase-positive mononuclear precursors of human dendritic reticulum cells. J Immunol 1983; 131:2719–25.
16. Schriever F, Freedman AS, Messner E, Lee G, Daley JS, Nadler LM. Isolated human follicular dendritic cells display a unique antigenic phenotype. J Exp Med 1989; 169:2043–58.

117
Purification of Follicular Dendritic Cells

C. J. Marcoty, E. Heinen, A. L. Bosseloir, N. Cormann, C. Kinet-DeNoël, and L. J. Simar
University of Liège, Liège, Belgium

INTRODUCTION

Inside the germinal centers the follicular dendritic cells (FDCs) play an important role as accessory cells in the development of the humoral immune response. In 1984, our group developed a technique allowing the enrichment in FDCs of cell suspensions isolated from human tonsils (1). These FDCs appeared as spherical cellular complexes (FDC clusters) of 30–100 μm in diameter containing B lymphocytes retained by the long cytoplasmic extensions of the FDCs. These clusters represent in fact fragments of germinal centers (2). Their percentage ranged from 1 to 2% of the cell suspension.

We modified this technique in order to improve the efficiency of the cell isolation.

MATERIAL AND METHODS

Our enrichment technique is mainly based on the separation of cells by velocity sedimentation at unit gravity on bovine serum albumin (BSA) gradient which allows the separation of the cells according to their size. As defined by Miller (3), we respected the following parameters:

Low concentration of BSA: 0.2%
Low cell number in order to avoid the streaming effect
High sedimentation columns: 10 cm
Thick starting band of cells: 2 mm

Our isolation procedure is reported in Figure 1.

RESULTS

Our results are summarized in Table 1.

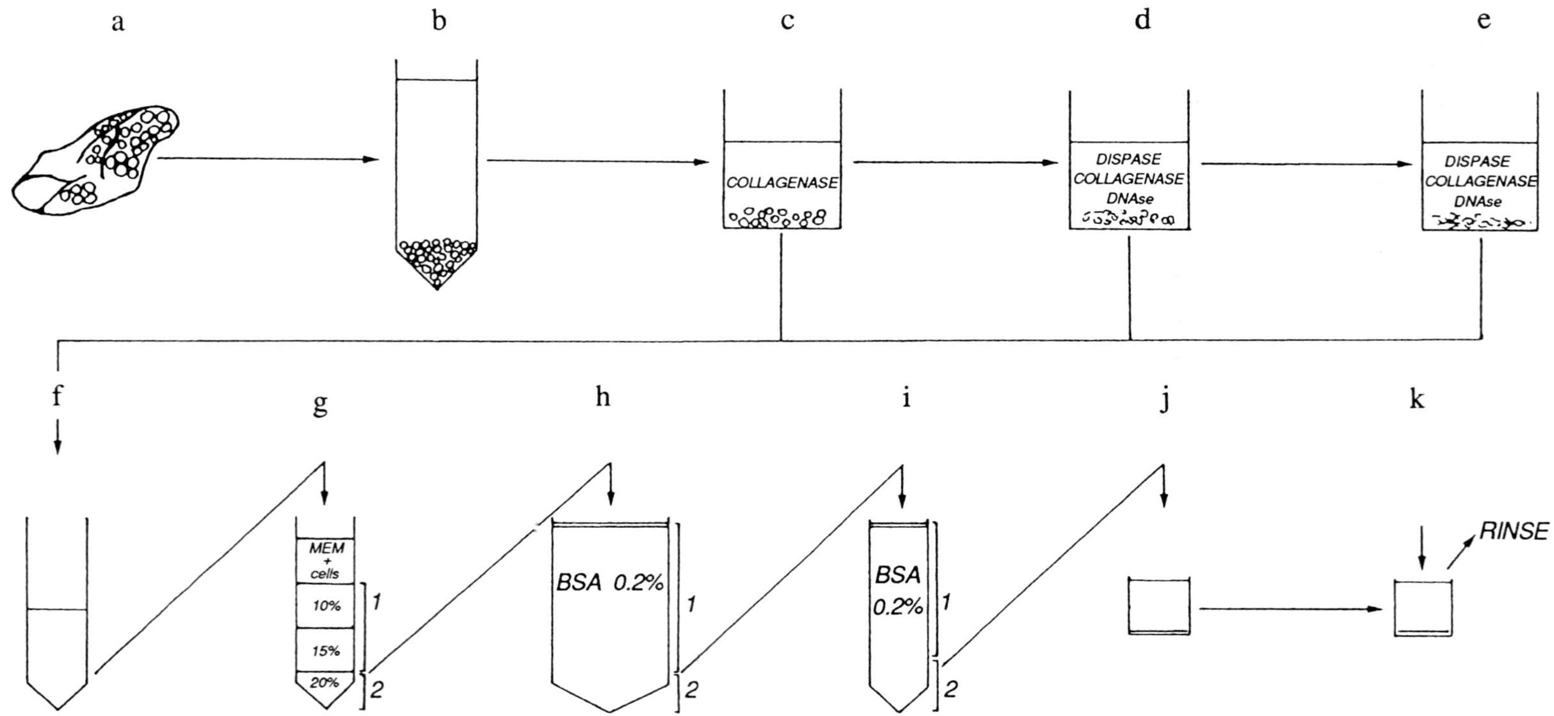

Figure 1 (a,b) The tonsils are cut in slices and the follicles are isolated under biomicroscopes. (c) Digestion of the follicles for 30 min at 20°C in collagenase (Boerhinger) 0.05% after which the freed cells are collected. (d) Digestion of the remaining follicles for 15 min at 37°C in collagenase 0.05%, Dispase (Boerhinger) 0.05% and DNase (Boerhinger) 0.004% after which the freed cells are collected. (e) The previous step is repeated one time. (f) The freed cells are gathered in MEM. (g) the cells are layered over a discontinuous BSA gradient (10, 15, and 20%) and centrifuged for 15 min at 25 G at 4°C. (1) The upper two phases are discarded; they contain lymphocytes and very rare small FDC clusters or free FDCs. (2) The lower phase, enriched in FDCs, is washed twice in MEM. (h) The FDC-enriched fraction is layered over tubes containing 50 ml of BSA 0.2% (height of the column: 10 cm); 5.10^6 cells in 1 ml of MEM per tube are allowed to sediment for 40 min at 1 G at 4°C. (1) The upper 43 ml is discarded. (2) The lower 7 ml is recovered; they contain the FDC clusters. (i) The previous step is repeated one time in 10-ml tubes ($1 \times 5 \times 10^6$ cells in 300 μl of MEM per tube). (1) The upper 7 ml is discarded. (2) The lower 3 ml is recovered; they are highly enriched in FDC clusters. (j) The FDC-enriched fraction is deposited in culture wells on glass cover slips and allowed to adhere for 3 hr in RPMI 1640 + 10% fetal calf serum at 27°C. (k) The cover slips are rinsed with the same medium in order to eliminate the nonadhering lymphocytes.

Table 1 Percentage of Recovered Cells and of FDC Clusters After Each Step of the Isolation Procedure (f, g, h, i, k)

	f	g		h	i	k
		10–15%	20%			
Recovered cells		60	40	6	2–4	?
FDC clusters	0.25–0.5	<0.04	0.6–2	4.5–20	25–50	80–95

We only used tonsils that provided us more than 0.25% of FDC clusters after the digestions (step f). The considered cells were trypan blue negative.

CONCLUSIONS

Our mild FDC isolation procedure allows us to obtain populations where most of the cells are DRC-1 positive, trypan blue negative. These cells are organized in clusters. They are useful for culture or immunohistochemical studies.

Tsunoda has been able to isolate FDC clusters and cultivate them for 150 days (4). However, these clusters rapidly dedifferenciate. In the future, in order to avoid this loss of surface antigens and morphological characters, we will cultivate them on different substrates and in conditioned media.

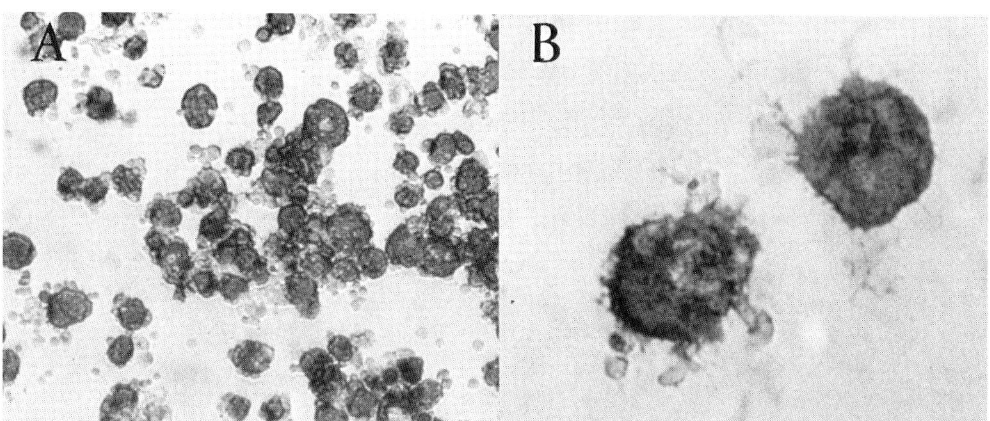

Figure 2 Peroxidase staining by DRC-1 antibody (DAKO, Dakopatts, Glostrup, Denmark) of our FDC-enriched suspensions. (A) After the two sedimentations (step i), (magnification: ×150). (B) After adherence (step k) (magnification: ×700).

ACKNOWLEDGMENTS

We gratefully acknowledge Drs. Evrard, Lepage, Daehl, Malaise, and Dr. Boniver for the supply of tonsils and Mmes. Jackers and Greimers for technical assistance. This work is supported by the Fonds de la Recherche Scientifique Médicale and by the Institut pour l'encouragement à la Recherche Scientifique dans l'Industrie et l'Agriculture.

REFERENCES

1. Lilet-Leclercq, C., Radoux, D., Heinen, E., Kinet-Denoel, C., Defraigne, J. O., Houben-Defresne, M.-P., and L. J. Simar. Isolation of follicular dendritic cells from human tonsils and adenoids. I-Procedures and morphological characterization, J. Immunol. Methods 66:235 (1984).
2. Tsunoda, R. and M. Kojima. A light microscopical study of isolated follicular dendritic cell clusters in human tonsils, Acta Pathol. Jpn. 37(4):575 (1987).
3. Miller, R. G., Separation of cells by velocity sedimentation, Methods Enzymol. 108:64 (1984).
4. Tsunoda, R., Virchows Arch. (in press).

118
Follicular Dendritic Cell–Dependent B-Cell Proliferation
An In Vitro "Germinal Center"

Marie H. Kosco, Rita Schmid, and David Gray
Basel Institute for Immunology, Basel, Switzerland

INTRODUCTION

The follicular dendritic cell (FDC) plays an essential role in the generation of the germinal center (GC) reaction and maintenance of immunoglobulin (Ig) levels (1–3). By retaining nonprocessed antigen, as immune complex on the plasma membrane of their dendritic processes, it appears that FDCs provide at least one component necessary to maintain a pool of circulating memory cell clones (4,5). To further dissect the role of FDCs in immune responses, we have attempted to produce a cellular microenvironment in culture similar to the germinal center in vivo. Using a method to isolate FDCs from immune mouse lymph nodes, a population of cells which form clusters within 24 hr of culture is obtained. These clusters consist of B cells, FDCs, and T cells which continue to proliferate for over 1 week. We propose that the in vitro system described here is representative of a germinal center, providing a means to study the role of FDCs in this reaction.

PRODUCTION OF PROLIFERATING CELLULAR CLUSTERS IN VITRO

Isolation and Enrichment for FDCs

Lymph nodes were obtained from immune mice primed and boosted with either dinitrophenylated-ovalbumin (DNP-OVA) or dinitrophenylated keyhold-limpet hemocyanin (DNP-KLH). Single cell suspensions were produced by the method reported by Schnizlein and colleagues (6). Following isolation, the cells were then resuspended in Iscove's modified Dulbecco's medium containing 5% fetal bovine serum, penicillin-streptomycin, and 2 mM mercaptoethanol for culturing in flat bottom 96-well plates at 37°C, 5% CO_2. 1–5 x 10^5 cells were added to each well. All groups were done in triplicate.

Cluster Formation and Phenotyping

Within hours of culturing, cellular clusters containing 10–50 lymphocytes formed. Immunoperoxidase staining of cytocentrifuge preparations revealed that these cultures were made up of 85–95% B cells, 5–10% FDCs, 1–10% CD4-positive T cells, and <1% macrophages (most were depleted by a 1 hr adherence step).

Proliferation and Autoradiography

By adding [^{3}H]thymidine during the last 4 hr of culture, a significant amount of proliferation could be demonstrated for at least 1 week (19,817 cpm after 1 day, 18,909 cpm after 4 days, 6,075 after 7 days, and 810 cpm after 11 days). Combining autoradiography with immunoperoxidase labeling of cytospin preparations demonstrated that >90% of the cells undergoing proliferation were B cells. Most of these cells expressed high levels of major histocompatibility complex (MHC) class II antigens and molecules labeled by the monoclonal antibody M1/69 (a heat-stable antigen, J11d equivalent), and were low for surface immunoglobulin and B220. In addition, most of the proliferating cells were associated with clusters and each cluster contained at least one FDC. An occasional CD4-positive cell was also observed and had incorporated [^{3}H]thymidine.

REQUIREMENTS FOR SPECIFIC CELL TYPES

To assess the effect of each cell type on cluster formation and proliferation, antibody-coated magnetic beads were used to deplete specific populations. For this sheep-antirat– or sheep-antimouse–conjugated magnetic Dynabeads (Dynal A.S., Oslo, Norway) (4) were coated with (a) the rat-antimouse FDC monoclonal antibody recently developed in our laboratory, designated 4C11 (a rat IgG_{2b}); (b) the rat-antimouse Thy 1 monoclonal antibody T24 (7); (c) the rat anti-B220 monoclonal antibody 14.8 (8); and (d) for irrelevant antibody control, a rat-antimouse monoclonal antibody, reactive with stromal cells (a rat IgG_{2b}). Coated Dynabeads were incubated with the isolated cells at a ratio of 40 beads per cell. The resulting cell populations were then assessed by flow cytometry to ensure depletion. By this method, it was determined that removing either FDCs or T cells significantly decreased the formation of clusters and the proliferation of B cells. Adding recombinant interleukin-1 to interleukin-6, individually or in combinations, or T-cell–conditioned supernatants to the FDC-depleted or T-cell–depleted populations did not restore cluster formation or proliferation levels. These data suggest that cell-cell contact is important to form a microenvironment which will support B-cell proliferation in vitro.

ANTIGEN SPECIFICITY

The ability to respond to a specific immunogen was assessed by adding either antigen to which the mice were primed or irrelevant antigen to the cultures. Mice were immunized with either DNP-OVA or DNP-KLH. The FDC-enriched preparations were then obtained from their lymph nodes 4–7 days after secondary immunization and placed in culture with DNP-KLH, KLH, DNP-OVA, or OVA. Cells from mice primed to DNP-KLH gave a twofold increase in [^{3}H]thymidine incorporation when 1 μg DNP-KLH or KLH was added per well but made no response to DNP-OVA or OVA. In contrast, cells from mice primed to DNP-OVA showed a twofold augmentation only to DNP-OVA and not the carrier alone or the irrelevant antigens. These results demonstrate that cells within the cultures are capable of responding only in an antigen-specific manner and that specific T-cell help is also required.

INHIBITION OF CLUSTER FORMATION AND PROLIFERATION

To determine which molecules were important for cluster formation and proliferation in vitro, cells were incubated with monoclonal antibodies directed against specific adhesion molecules in an attempt to block cellular interactions. The monoclonal antibodies YN1/1.7.4, which recognizes the mouse equivalent of the intercellular adhesion molecule, MALA-2 (9), and M17/4.2, which reacts with LFA-1 (10), the ligand for MALA-2, were added at the initiation of culture (at 1 μg of protein per well). [^{3}H]thymidine was added for the last 4 hr of a 24-hr culture period. Cluster formation decreased significantly when compared to wells with no added antibodies and proliferative levels decreased by one-third.

DISCUSSION

The results described here provide evidence that we can isolate cells necessary to maintain B-cell proliferation in vitro. The appearance of clusters and the necessity for FDCs and T cells to maintain these structures which give rise to centers of B-cell proliferation in vitro closely mimic the components present during germinal center formation in vivo. The fact that soluble factors could not restore the effect of depleting FDCs and T cells suggests that cell-contact is an essential part of the response. The system has also been shown to be antigen specific; augmentation of proliferation only occurs after addition of antigen to which the B cell was primed.

To maintain B-cell proliferation in vitro, the FDCs provide at least two important functions. They carry specific antigen on their plasma membrane and provide an elaborate network of dendritic processes that can facilitate cell-cell contact. Whether FDCs only provide these two components or additional signals through the other cell surface molecules they express is under investigation. Several groups, including ours, are interested in determining the role of CD23 and CD40 in B-cell activation, proliferation, and differentiation as well as to determine if FDCs produce their own cytokines. Currently, we are also extending our studies using these cellular clusters formed in culture to determine the molecules which play a role in the interaction of cells necessary for germinal center formation and maintenance of B-cell memory in vivo.

REFERENCES

1. Tew JG, Phipps RP, Mandel TE: The maintenance and regulation of the humoral immune response: Persisting antigen and the role of follicular antigen-binding dendritic cells as accessory cells. Immunol Rev 1980; 53:175–201.
2. Szakal AK, Kosco MH, Tew JG: A novel in vivo follicular dendritic cell dependent iccosome mediated mechanism for delivery of antigen to antigen processing cells. J Immunol 1988; 140:341–353.
3. Kosco MH, Szakal AK, Tew JG: In vivo obtained antigen presented by germinal center B cells to T cells in vitro. J Immunol 1988; 140:354–360.
4. Gray D, Skarvall H: Memory B cells are short lived in the absence of antigen. Nature (Lond) 1988; 336:70–73.

5. Gray D, Leanderson T: Expansion, selection and maintenance of memory B cell clones. Curr Top Microbiol Immunol 1990; 159:2–17.
6. Schnizlein CT, Kosco MH, Szakal AK, Tew JG: Follicular dendritic cells in suspension: Identification, enrichment, and initial characterization indicating immune complex trapping and lack of adherence and phagocytic activity. J Immunol 1985; 134:1360–1368.
7. Dennert G, Hyman R, Lesley J, Trowbridge, IS: Effects of cytotoxic monoclonal antibodies specific for T200 glycoprotein on functional lymphoid cell populations. Cell Immunol 1980; 53:350–364.
8. Kincade PW, Lee G, Watanabe T, Sun L, Scheid MP: Antigens displayed on murine B lymphocyte precursors. J Immunol 1981; 127:2262–2268.
9. Prieto J, Takei F, Gendelman R, Christenson B, Biberfeld, Patarroyo M: MALA-2, mouse homologue of human adhesion molecule ICAM-1 (CD54). Eur J Immunol. 1989; 19:1551–1557.
10. Sanchez-Madrid F, Simon P, Thompson S, Springer T: Mapping of antigenic and functional epitopes on the alpha and beta subunits of two related mouse glycoproteins involved in cell interactions, LFA-1 and Mac-1. J Exp Med 1983; 158:586–602.

119
Reconstitution of Follicular Dendritic Cell Defect in Scid Mice with Isogenic and Xenogeneic Bone Marrow and Lymphocytes

Andras K. Szakal,[1] Zoher F. Kapasi,[1] Leonard D. Shultz,[2] Gregory F. Burton,[1] Marie H. Kosco,[3] and John G. Tew[1]
[1]*Medical College of Virginia/Virginia Commonwealth University, Richmond, Virginia;*
[2]*The Jackson Laboratory, Bar Harbor, Maine;*
[3]*Basel Institute for Immunology, Basel, Switzerland*

INTRODUCTION

Antigen retention in lymphoid tissue follicles is one of the main properties of follicular dendritic cells (FDCs) (1–3). In the follicle, FDCs form a three-dimensional network, through interdigitation of dendrites of neighboring FDCs, called the antigen-retaining reticulum. Accumulating evidence indicates that FDCs and the retained antigen are important in the production of B-memory cells and the long-term maintenance of the secondary antibody response (2). Based on studies with athymic mice (4,5) and rats (6), follicular antigen localization is believed to be independent of T-cell–mediated mechanisms. Although antigen trapping by FDCs of thymus dysgenic animals is qualitatively normal, it appears to be quantitatively reduced (4,6).

Our recent studies revealed that old mice have a defective antigen transport and atrophic FDCs, resulting in the formation of defective FDC-reticula (3) and a nearly complete absence of germinal centers (7). Attempts to reconstitute the germinal center response in old mice with young bone marrow and thymus transplants showed that while bone marrow transfers increased germinal center size, germinal center numbers were increased only in the presence of thymus transplants (Kapasi et al., unpublished). Since the number of germinal centers appears to be dependent on the number of FDC-reticulum sites (7), these results implied that the thymus may be increasing germinal center numbers by increasing or regenerating the number of FDC-reticulum sites. This conclusion differs with previous results suggesting T-cell independence of FDC-reticulum development in athymic animals.

To reassess B- and T-cell requirements for antigen localization in the FDC-reticulum, we selected the severe combined immunodeficiency (Scid) mouse model which lacks functional B and T cells (8). The results of bone marrow and B and T cell transfers showed that while B cells are required for a functional FDC-reticulum, T cells markedly increased the frequency of FDC-reticula and the apparent rate of its development.

MATERIALS AND METHODS

Animals

Homozygous mutant C.B.17-scid/scid (Scid) and normal C.B.17 male mice (ages 6–8 weeks), nude mice (age 12–13 weeks), and Lewis rats (200–224 g) were housed in a virus-free environment and given water and food ad libitum. For 4 weeks after irradiation and cell transfers, recipient mice were given antibiotic-containing water (0.01% neomycin sulfate, Sigma, St. Louis, MO.).

Cell Transfers for Reconstitution

Prior to cell transfer, Scid mice were irradiated with 300 rad to facilitate reconstitution. Bone marrow (BM) cells were obtained from femurs and tibias of C.B.17 mice and Lewis rats. B cells were obtained from spleens of Balb/c nude mice. T cells were isolated by passing C.B.17 spleen cells through a 10-ml nylon wool column (2X) and by subsequent panning on anti-kappa– and anti-lambda–coated plates (purity: FACScan data, 97% mu-negative cells). For reconstitutions, mice received i.v. 10^7 BM, B or T cells, or 10^7 B plus 10^7 T cells.

Immunization

Animals were passively immunized i.p. with 0.75 ml of specific rabbit antiserum 1 day prior to footpad challenge with the histochemically detectable antigen, horseradish peroxidase (HRP; type VI, Sigma).

Histochemistry

For the histochemical localization of HRP, 24 hr after hind and fore footpad injection of HRP (5 μg/0.05 ml in saline), the animals were fixed by intracardiac perfusion as described previously (3). The lymph nodes (axillary, brachial, and popliteal) were serially sectioned at 50 μm thickness on a vibratome, treated with periodate, and developed for peroxidase activity of HRP in 0.1% diaminobenzidine hydrochloride (DAB)/0.01% H_2O_2 substrate (3). The sections were prepared for light and electron microscopy.

RESULTS

Our initial objective was to determine if Scid mouse lymph nodes had functional FDCs. (This information has not been reported before.) Once we determined that antigen was not localized in FDC-reticula, and FDCs were not detectable by anti-FDC monoclonal antibody (4C11), we attempted to reconstitute functional FDCs by adoptive transfer of BM cells and all combinations of B and T cells (Table 1). To evaluate the lymph nodes of recipients for antigen trapping by FDCs, the peroxidase activity of retained HRP was followed through serial sections and the numbers and sizes of FDC-reticula were recorded semiquantitatively on a scale of 0 to 5 (Table 1).

Unreconstituted, Scid mouse lymph nodes were very small and the antigen localized only in sinusoidal macrophages, primarily in the medulla (Fig. 1a). Control C.B.17 mice

Table 1 Results of Scid Mouse Reconstitutions

Group	Cell donors	Cells	Recipient	FDC-reticulum
1	None	—	C.B.17	+++++
2	None	—	Scid	—
3	C.B.17	B	Scid	++++
4	C.B.17	T	Scid	—
5	Nude (Balb)	B	Scid	+
6	Nude/C.B.17	B + T	Scid	++++
7	Lewis rat	BM	Scid	++

had normal lymph nodes with well-developed FDC-reticula (5+; Table 1, Fig. 1b). Reconstitution of Scid mice with C.B.17 bone marrow cells resulted in the development of FDC-reticula which in size and numbers approximated those of C.B.17 controls (4+; Table 1, Fig. 1c). While T-cell transfers increased lymph node size, T cells alone failed to reconstitute the FDC-reticulum (–; Table 1, Fig. 1d). On the other hand, B-cell transfers to Scid mice provided minimal support for FDC-reticulum development and only few, poorly developed FDC-reticula were seen which retained little antigen (1+, Table 1, Fig. 1e,f). In contrast, when B and T cells were transferred together, the addition of T cells provided nearly full support for FDC-reticulum development (4+, Table 1, Figs. 1g,h). Electron microscopy confirmed the morphological maturity of FDCs and showed that FDCs in B- and T-cell–reconstituted mice had comparable HRP-retaining dendrites to those of C.B.17 normal controls (not shown). Transfer of xenogeneic BM cells also resulted in reconstitution of FDC-reticula. These were seen in low numbers and were generally of mouse phenotype (4C11 positive and Ki M4R-negative). However, at least one FDC-reticulum of rat FDC phenotype was observed (4C11-negative, Ki M4R-positive).

DISCUSSION AND CONCLUSIONS

As shown by antigen localization and screening with anti-FDC antibodies, FDCs were not detectable in Scid lymph nodes. However, FDC function can be reconstituted with both isogenic and xenogeneic BM. To a degree, B cells can also initiate the development of FDC-reticulum, but the additional transfer of T cells promotes remarkably functional FDC development. We suggest that the demonstrated T-cell help may involve the potentiation of B- and/or T-cell cytokines.

The B-cell requirement for the development of FDC-reticula is in agreement with the studies of Cerny et al. (9) and MacLennan and Gray (10), who reported an absence of mature functional FDCs in lymph nodes of thymus dysgenic and normal mice and rats depleted of B cells. These studies demonstrated that after release of B-cell suppression the reappearance of B cells preceded the appearance of functional FDCs. In addition to this B-cell requirement of FDC development, the remarkable T-cell effects observed in this study agree with the noted thymus effects in old mice (see Introduction) and may also help explain the reported quantitative deficits observed in athymic animals (4,6).

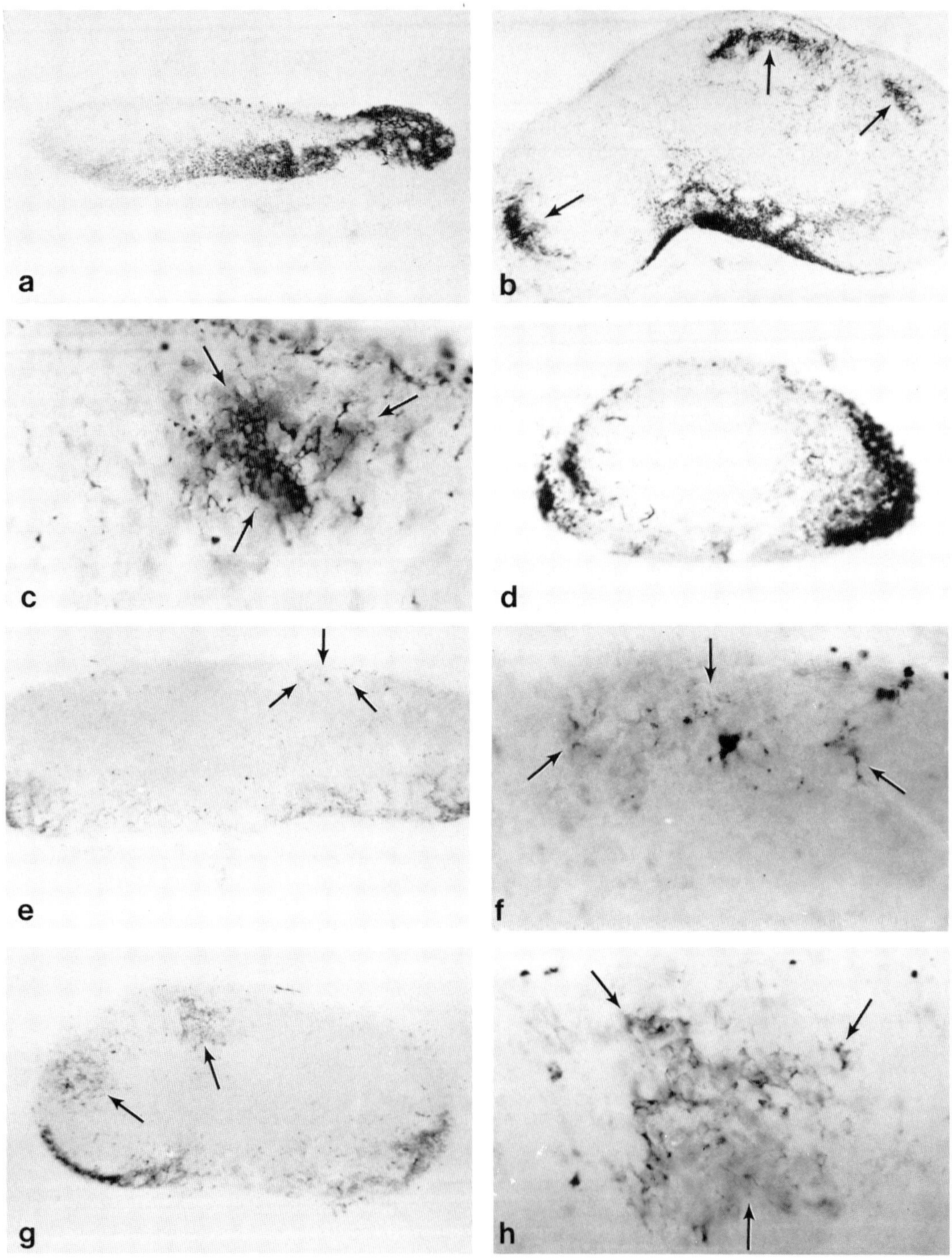

Figure 1 Representative micrographs of Scid and control mouse lymph node sections illustrating the localization of the antigen, HRP, in the FDC-reticulum before and after reconstitutions: (a) Scid (unreconstituted), antigen only in macrophages, no FDC-reticulum; (b) C.B.17 normal control with well-developed HRP positive FDC-reticula (arrows); (c) bone marrow–reconstituted Scid mouse FDC-reticulum (arrows); (d) T-cell–reconstituted Scid lymph node, no FDC-reticulum, HRP only in sinusoidal macrophages; (e,f) low and high power views of a poorly developed FDC-reticulum after B-cell reconstitution (arrows); (g,h) HRP-positive FDC-reticula in B- and T-cell–reconstituted Scid mouse lymph node (arrows). (Magnifications: a, b, e, ×45; c, f, h, ×230; d, ×72, g, ×60.)

REFERENCES

1. Szakal AK, Kosco MH, Tew JG. Microanatomy of lymphoid tissue during the induction and maintenance of humoral immune responses: Structure function relationships. Ann Rev Immunol 1989; 7:91–109.
2. Tew JG, Kosco MH, Burton GF, Szakal AK. Follicular dendritic cells as accessory cells. Immunol Rev 1990; 117:185-211.
3. Szakal AK, Taylor JK, Smith JP, Kosco MH, Burton GF, Tew JG. Morphometry and kinetics of antigen transport and developing antigen retaining reticulum of follicular dendritic cells in lymph nodes of aging immune mice. AGING: Immunol Infect Dis 1988; 1:7–22.
4. Mitchell J, Pye J, Hommes MC, Nossal GJV. Antigens in immunity. Antigen localization in congenitally athymic "nude" mice. AJEBAK 1972; 50:637–650.
5. Tew JG, Mandel TE, Miller GA. Immune retention: Immunological requirements for maintaining an easily degradable antigen in vivo. AJEBAK 1979; 57:401–414.
6. Mjaaland S, Fossum S. The localization of antigen in lymph node follicles of congenitally athymic nude rats. Scand J Immunol 1987; 26:141–147.
7. Szakal AK, Taylor JK, Smith JP, Kosco MH, Burton GF, Tew JG. Kinetics of germinal center development in lymph nodes of young and aging immune mice. Anat Rec 1990; 227:475–485.
8. Custer RP, Bosma GC, Bosma MJ. Severe combined immunodeficiency (SCID) in the mouse. Pathology, Reconstitution, Neoplasm. Am J Pathol 1985; 120:464–477.
9. Cerny A, Zinkernagel RM, Groscurth P. Development of follicular dendritic cells in lymph nodes of B-cell-depleted mice. Cell Tissue Res 1988; 254:449–454.
10. MacLennan ICM, Gray D. Antigen-driven selection of virgin and memory B cells. Immunol Rev 1986; 91:61–85.

120
Ultrastructural Aspects of Follicular Dendritic Cells in Germinal Centers of Lymph Nodes After HIV-1 Infection

L.H.P.M. Rademakers, H.-J. Schuurman, J.F. de Frankrijker, and A. Van Ooyen
University Hospital, Utrecht, The Netherlands

INTRODUCTION

Infection with the human immunodeficiency virus type 1 (HIV-1) can result in the development of a persistent generalized lymphadenopathy (PGL). Lymph nodes in PGL most commonly show a follicular hyperplasia (FH) in which regressive changes, such as loss of mantle zones and fragmentation of germinal centers may be observed (1–3). The destruction or fragmentation of the framework of follicular dendritic cells (FDCs) has been demonstrated by immunohistochemistry (2,4). After HIV-1 infection, intact HIV-1 virus particles are present between the extensions of FDCs (5–7). A cytopathic action of HIV-1 on FDCs has been suggested (7–9). Destruction of the FDC framework may contribute to the immunodeficiency by influencing the germinal center B cells as well. We analyzed germinal center B cells and FDCs simultaneously at the ultrastructural level in order to detect early alterations after HIV-1 infection.

METHODS

Twenty-five lymph nodes and 45 tonsils were processed for transmission electron microscopy. Fifteen lymph nodes were from HIV-1–infected patients (HIV-1). Eight lymph nodes with HIV-1–negative FH and tonsils served as a control group. Ultrastructural analysis of the cell composition of the lymph node germinal centers (GCs) and that of the dark and light zones of the tonsillar GCs, was followed by additional data analysis on germinal center cell types by means of pattern recognition methods. These procedures were performed as earlier described (10). The morphometric analysis of FDCs was done according to a point lattice method on samples of three GCs from each lymph node (11). The presence of ultrastructurally defined FDC subtypes was studied in dark and light zones of 32 tonsillar

GCs. The frequency distribution of FDC subtypes in lymph nodes was investigated using all FDCs present in sections three to six GCs.

RESULTS AND DISCUSSION

On the basis of the relative frequencies of lymphoid cells types (blast: i.e., cleaved blast, immunoblast, and centroblast; centrocyte, centroplasmacytoid cell, lymphocyte multilobated cell, and plasma cell; Fig. 1) and nonlymphoid cell types (i.e., histiocytic reticulum cell and follicular dendritic cells) two groups of lymph nodes were distinguished. Six HIV-1 lymph nodes as well as all FH lymph nodes clustered in group 1; the remaining nine HIV-1 lymph nodes were defined to group 2. In contrast to the GCs of the FH and HIV-1 lymph nodes, those of HIV-1 lymph nodes of group 2 were characterized (Table 1) by a predominance of lymphoid blasts and by decreased numbers of centrocytes resulting in a high centrocyte/blast ratio. The cell composition of the latter group was similar to that of

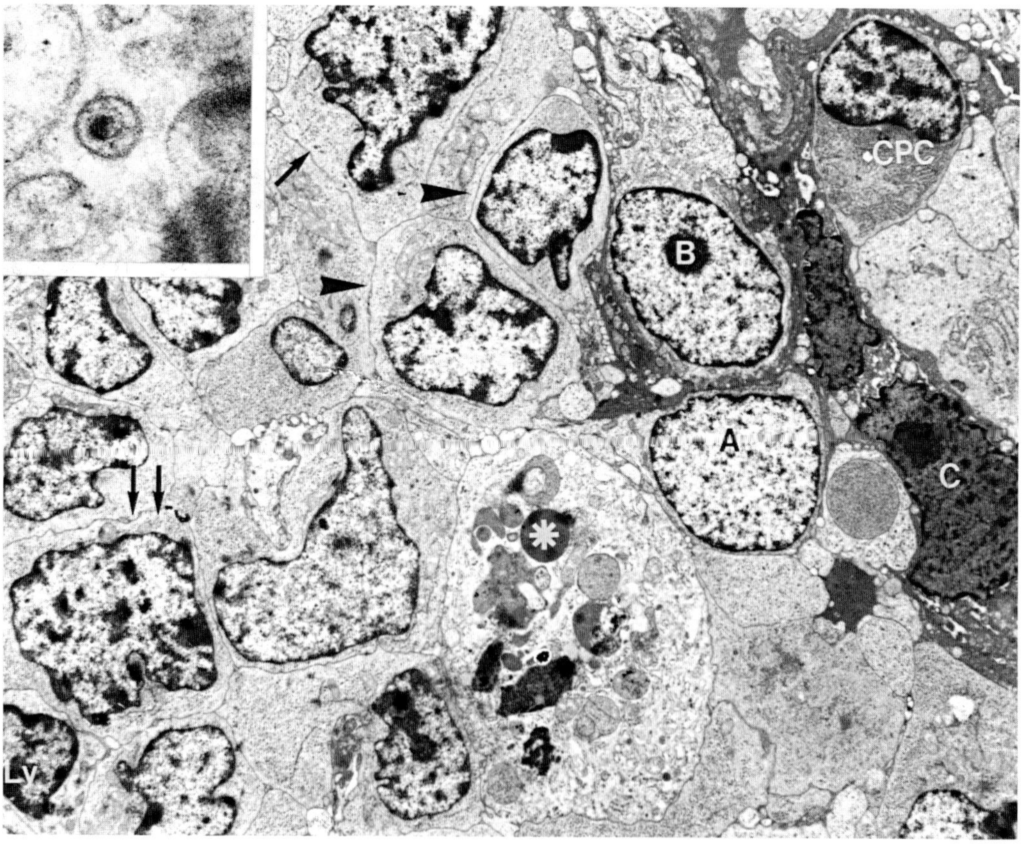

Figure 1 Electron micrograph of a GC of a HIV-1–infected patient (group 2), mainly composed of cleaved blasts (arrows) and centroblasts (arrowheads). Three types of FDCs are present: type 3 (A), type 4 (B), and type 7 (C). CPC: centroplasmacytoid cell; Ly: lymphocyte; asterisk: histiocytic reticulum cell (magnification: ×4000). Inset HIV-1 virion between FDC extensions (magnification: ×60,000).

Table 1 Mean Values of Ultrastructural Quantitative Data on Lymphoid Cells and FDCs Present in GCs of Hyperplastic Lymph Nodes of HIV-1–Infected Patients, Non–HIV-1–Infected Patients (FH), and Hyperplastic Tonsils

	Lymph node			Tonsil	
	FH group 1 (n=8)	HIV-1 group 1 (n=6)	HIV-1 group 2 (n=9)	Dark zone (n=10)	Light zone (n=10)
Lymphoid cells					
Blast*	$26.2^{a,c}$	$26.4^{b,d}$	$46.8^{a,b,f}$	$54.9^{c,d,e}$	$23.4^{e,f}$
Centrocyte*	$51.5^{a,c}$	$46.1^{b,d}$	$30.9^{a,b,f}$	$28.1^{c,d,e}$	$50.0^{e,f}$
Blast/centrocyte ratio	$0.52^{a,c}$	$0.58^{a,b,d}$	$1.60^{a,b,f}$	$2.3^{c,d,e}$	$0.50^{e,f}$
Mitosis*	$1.7^{a,d}$	1.8^{b}	$2.7^{c,e}$	$4.0^{a,b,c,f}$	$0.9^{e,f}$
FDCs	4.2^{a}	$6.1^{b,d}$	$4.2^{c,d}$	$2.5^{a,b,c,e}$	5.3^{e}
types*#				#	#
1	0.1	0.2	0.4	20.9	0
2	5.2	6.4	7.1	39.3	0.5
3	21.6	26.5	23.0	30.9	10.8
4	32.6^{a}	33.5^{b}	$20.1^{a,b}$	3.6	28.1
5	20.9^{a}	13.7	11.6^{b}	1.4	48.6
6	11.6	11.8^{a}	21.6^{a}	3.6	12.9
7	9.9	7.9^{a}	15.8^{a}	0	0
Relative volume FDCs (%)	10.7^{a}	16.2^{a}	13.0	—	—
Nucleus/cytoplasm ratio	$0.25^{a,b}$	0.15^{b}	0.15^{b}	—	—
Incidence of RER dilatation (%)	13.0	24.7	27.0	—	—
Incidence of lysosomal structures (%)	$4.6^{a,b}$	28.3^{a}	26.1^{b}	—	—

^{a,b,c,d,e,f} indicate significant differences ($P \leq 0.05$); *: relative frequencies; #: tonsil; relative frequencies of FDCs pooled from 32 germinal centers.

the dark zones of GCs of tonsils: the GC compartment having immature, proliferative properties. The cell composition of GCs in group 1 was similar to that of the light zones of GCs, which is a compartment of B-cell differentiation. After HIV-1 infection, the incidence of mitosis did not differ between GCs of groups 1 and 2. There was no difference in the blast counts in the GC dark zones and the GCs of group 2, but mitosis was lower in the latter GCs. This indicates that in lymph nodes of group 3, the differentiation of blasts into centrocytes is impaired. In contrast to dark and light zones of tonsils, the inversed blast/centrocyte ratio in group 2 is not related to differences in FDC numbers. This is suggestive of an altered FDC microclimate.

In GCs of tonsils, seven types of FDCs (see Fig. 1) could be recognized on the basis of the ultrastructural features of the nucleus, cytoplasm, and cell surface (Table 2). The frequency distribution pattern of these FDC types is characteristic of the distinct GC compartments (see Table 1). The undifferentiated FDC types 1, 2, and 3 are mainly present in the dark zone, whereas the differentiated types 4 and 5, showing morphological signs of cellular activity, populate the light zones. Lymph nodes do not show a polar structure of light and dark zones in their GCs. The distribution pattern in hyperplastic follicles was less marked with FDC types 4, 3, and 5 as main constituents. Germinal centers of group 1 and group 2 differed in frequency distribution patterns. In group 2, undifferentiated

Table 2 Ultrastructural Characteristics of the Distinct Types of FDCs Present in GCs of Human Lymph Nodes

FDC type	Cell shape	Extensions	Filaments	Ribosomes	RER	Golgi complex	Extracellular dense depositions
1	Rounded to elongated	Blunt, broad processes	Small bundles of microfilaments	Low numbers of polysomes	Short RER cisterns, scarce or absent	Mostly absent	Absent
2	Elongated	Elongated, broad	Small bundles of microfilaments	Preponderant ribosomes	Short, widened cisterns; scarce	Mostly absent	Absent
3	Rounded	Elongated, slender; broad villous extensions	Small bundles; submembranous condensations	Preponderant polysomes	Short, widened cisterns	Inconspicuous	Absent or inconspicuous
4	Rounded	Elongated, slender; fine villous extensions	Submembranous condensations	Free ribosomes; few polysomes	Well developed; short or elongated cisterns	Present; well developed	Present; moderate to heavy electron density
5	Rounded	Elongated, slender frequent villous extensions	Scarce; focal submembranous condensations	Mainly free ribosomes	Well developed; elongated cisterns	Extremely developed; several Golgi complexes present; numerous vesicles	Present; heavy electron density
6	Rounded; extensive cytoplasm	Retracted to cell body; villous extensions present	Absent	Mainly free ribosomes	Scarce elongated cisterns	Occasional Golgi complex; well developed	Present; moderate to heavy electron density
7	Elongated; dark cytoplasmic and nuclear matrix	Elongated, slender; villous extensions present or absent	Absent	Clusters of free ribosomes	Large widened cisterns	Not obvious; numerous lysosomal structures	Present

FDC type 3 predominated and there was a relative increase of the FDC types 6 and 7, whereas the relative frequencies of the differentiated FDC types 4 and 5 were lower. These FDC types show a regressive morphology as judged by the presence of lysosomes, distended cisterns of the rough endoplasmic reticulum (RER), and cell organelle organization. The FDC subtype distribution patterns of FH and HIV-1–infected lymph nodes of group 1 were similar. In HIV-1 lymph nodes, retroviral particles were regularly observed between the cellular extension of FDCs. Such particles were absent in FH lymph nodes and tonsils.

The FDCs in HIV-1 lymph nodes showed additional ultrastructural changes; e.g., a higher incidence of widened cisterns of the RER and of lysosomal structures, indicative of an altered cellular physiology.

We conclude that in nine out of 15 lymph nodes with HIV-1–related lymphadenopathy, early alterations in FDC morphology are observed suggestive of an immature and inactive state, without severe alterations in GC architecture. These alterations in FDCs coincide with an inverted blast/centrocyte ratio, without change in mitotic activity. The latter observation indicates impaired B-cell differentiation after HIV-1 infection. These changes may proceed the involution of GCs in stages of follicular degeneration and fragmentation. Apparently factors maintaining the FDC microclimate are involved. The participation of HIV-1 virus to this altered GC microenvironment is further supported by the finding that a proportion of FDCs can be infected by the HIV-1 virus (9) (see also Chapter 121).

REFERENCES

1. Schuurman HJ, Kluin PhM, Gmelig Meyling FHJ, Kater L. Lymphocyte status of lymph node and blood in acquired immunodeficiency syndrome (AIDS) and AIDS-related complex disease. J Pathol 1985; 147:269–80.
2. Burns BF, Wood GS, Dorfman RF. The varied histopathology of lymphadenopathy in the homosexual male. Am J Surg Pathol 1985; 9:287–97.
3. Porwit A, Bottiger B, Pallesen G, Bodner A, Biberfeld P. Follicular involution in HIV lymphadenopathy. A morphometric study. APMIS 1989; 97:153–65.
4. Janossy G, Pinching AJ, Bofill M, Weber J, McLaughlin JE, Ornstein M, Ivory K, Harris JR, Favrot M, Macdonald-Burns DC. An immunohistological approach to persistent lymphadenopathy and its relevance to AIDS. Clin Exp Immunol 1985; 59:257–66.
5. Armstrong JA, Horne R. Follicular dendritic cells and virus-like particles in AIDS-related lymphadenopathy. Lancet 1984; 2:370–2.
6. Tenner-Racz K, Racz P, Dietrich M, Kern P. Altered follicular dendritic cells and virus-like particles in AIDS and AIDS-related lymphadenopathy. Lancet 1985; 1:105–6.
7. Cameron PU, Dawkins RL, Armstrong JA, Bonifacio E. Western blot profiles, lymph node ultrastructure and viral expression in HIV-infected patients: a correlative study. Clin Exp Immunol 1987; 68:465–78.
8. Piris MA, Rivas C, Morente M, Rubio C, Martin C, Olivia H. Persistent and generalized lymphadenopathy: a lesion of follicular dendritic cells? An immunohistologic and ultrastructural study. Am J Clin Pathol 1987; 87:716–24.
9. Parmentier HK, van Wichen D, Sie-GO DMDS, Goudsmit J, Borleffs JCC, Schuurman HJ. HIV-1 infection and virus production in follicular dendritic cells in lymph nodes. A case report, with analysis of follicular dendritic cells. Am J Pathol 1990; 137:247–51.
10. Peters JPJ, Rademakers LHPM, De Boer RJ, Van Unnik JAM. Cellular composition of follicles of follicle centre cell lymphomas in relation to germinal centres of reactive lymph nodes. A morphometrical electron microscopic study. J Pathol 1987; 153:233–44.
11. Rademakers LHPM, Peters JPJ, Van Unnik JAM. Histiocytic and dendritic reticulum cells in follicular structures of follicular lymphoma and reactive hyperplasia. Virchows Arch (Cell Pathol) 1983; 44:85–98.

121
Follicular Dendritic Cells In Situ Are Infected by HIV-1

Henk K. Parmentier,[1] Dick van Wichen,[1] Jolanda Krijnen,[1] Jaap Goudsmit,[2] Louk H.P.M. Rademakers,[1] and Henk-Jan Schuurman[1]
[1]*University Hospital, Utrecht, The Netherlands;*
[2]*Academic Medical Center, Amsterdam, The Netherlands*

INTRODUCTION

The framework of lymphoid follicles consists of follicular dendritic cells (FDCs). The stage of persistent generalized lymphadenopathy (PGL) in individuals infected by the human immunodeficiency virus (HIV) is characterized by destruction of FDCs, as envisaged by fragmentation of GCs (1,2). In follicles, HIV-1 antigens (1–3) and HIV-1–like particles (4–7) are present but the intra- or intercellular location of these components has not been unequivocally demonstrated. By in situ-hybridization, HIV-1 messenger ribonucleic acid (mRNA)–positive elements have been demonstrated in follicles (1,4,8) but the identity of these infected cells is unknown. Thus, it is not possible to relate the destruction of FDCs to (a) a state of infection of FDCs resulting in viral production, (b) the presence of virus and viral components on these cells as the result of trapping during the "normal" immune response,and (c) mechanisms of virus entrance into FDCs.

The study of isolated FDCs from lymphoid tissue may facilitate such studies. We isolated FDCs from a lymph node of an HIV-1–infected patient and studied the presence of HIV by in situ hybridization and immunocytochemistry. Furthermore, binding of HIV components to FDCs isolated from a normal tonsil was studied. We present evidence that FDCs in vivo are infected by HIV-1.

MATERIALS AND METHODS

Lymph Node

The right axillary lymph node (measuring 2x1x1 cm) from a 28-year-old patient with acquired immune deficiency syndrome (AIDS) was studied. Parts of the node were processed for hybrido- and immunohistochemistry, and conventional light and electron microscopy. Half of the node was used for the isolation of FDCs. This was done by enzyme digestion, 1 G sedimentation on a discontinuous bovine serum albumin (BSA) gradient and

Percoll density gradient centrifugation (9). The 1×10^6 yield of isolated cells did not allow us to study these cells by electron microscopy.

Similarly, FDCs were isolated from tonsils obtained after tonsillectomy from young children (see Chapter 116). These cells were incubated for 1 hr at 37°C in 25% serum of the AIDS patient, washed, and either processed till cytocentrifuge preparations or for electron microscopy. The serum was obtained by routine blood collection 1 week before lymph node extirpation.

Determination of HIV-1

Cytocentrifuge preparations of isolated FDCs and frozen lymph node tissue sections were evaluated for the expression of HIV-1 proteins, CD4, and FDC markers using a three-step immunoperoxidase method after acetone fixation. Monoclonal antibodies applied were to FDC (DAKO-DRC-1, Dakopatts, Glostrup, Denmark; and Ki-M4, Behringwerke Marburg-Lahn, Germany); CD4 (Leu-3a, Becton Dickinson, Mountain View, California); and HIV-1 (31.42.19, anti-*gag* p15; 12.11.4, anti-*gag* p17; 31.89.8, anti-*gag* p24; 10.15.64, anti-*env* gp41; and 3A18-61, anti-*env* gp120; all from Abbott Laboratories). Immunoglobulin M (IgM) was detected by direct immunofluorescence with FITC- conjugated rabbit antihuman IgM (Dakopatts).

For detection of HIV-1 antigens/virions on FDCs incubated with patient's serum, cell pellets were fixed in 4% paraformaldehyde in 0.1 M phosphate-buffered saline (PBS) for 48 hr at 4°C, followed by twice washing in PBS/glycine (0.15% w/v), and embedding in 10% gelatin. After cooling at 4°C, small cubes of the pellet were impregnated overnight with 15% pyrrolidon with 2.3M sucrose, and frozen in liquid nitrogen. Ultrathin cryosections cut at –110°C were sequentially labeled with sheep anti-p24 antibody (Seromed), rabbit antisheep Ig, and protein A–gold complex (10). The cryosections (80 nm) were embedded in methylcellulose, and contrasted with 3% uranyl acetate. The sections were examined in a Jeol 1200 electron microscope.

In situ hybridization for HIV-1 *env* mRNA using a ^{35}S-labeled probe (NEP-200, Du Pont de Nemours, Biotechnology Systems Division, Den Bosch, The Netherlands) was performed according to previously described techniques (11) with minor modifications in the autoradiographic detection. On each slide 2.5×10^6 dpm was applied. The exposure time was 7 days.

RESULTS AND DISCUSSION

In frozen sections of the lymph node, anti-FDC antibodies identified germinal centers with fragmentation and indentations of the FDC network. Most T cells in the interfollicular zones were of CD8 phenotype; CD4-positive lymphocytes were almost absent. Expression of HIV-1 *gag* antigens p15, p17, and p24 was primarily found in germinal centers. In interfollicular areas, solitary cells with strong labeling intensity for gp41 were observed.

Cytocentrifuge preparations of isolated FDCs from the patient's lymph node revealed large dendritic binucleated cells labeled by DRC-1 and Ki-M4 (Fig. 1), frequently in clusters with lymphocytes (9,12). The clusters formed approximately 40% of the isolated cells, and expressed CD4 and surface IgM. HIV-1 core proteins p15, p17, p24 and envelope protein gp41 were determined on about two-thirds of the FDC-like cells. The antigens were present on the cytoplasmic extensions of FDCs (Fig. 2), but not on associated (B–) lymphocytes. The staining pattern for HIV antigens was similar to that for immunoglobulins, both on isolated FDCs and on FDCs in follicles in tissue sections (data not

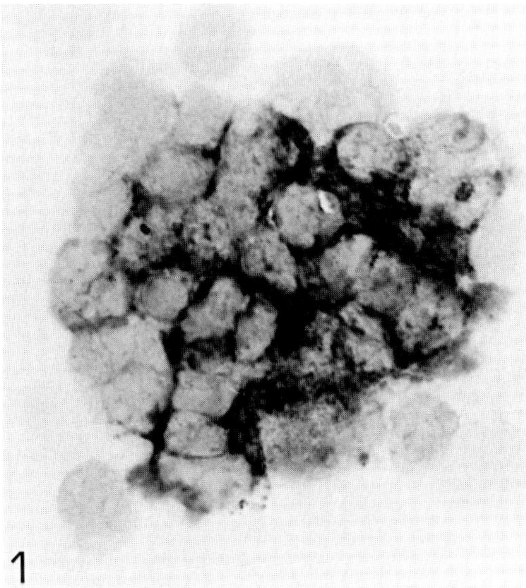

1

Figure 1 Isolated FDCs from the patient immunolabeled with Ki-M4 antibody (2). Similar labeling was found with DRC-1, anti-p15, anti-p24, and anti-gp41 antibodies. Omission of primary antibodies revealed no labeling. Three-step immunoperoxidase: RAM/PO, SwAR/PO, followed by AEC (3-amino-9-ethylcarbazole). Counterstaining by hematoxylin (magnification: ×520).

shown). This presumably reflects the in situ entrapment of antigen in the form of immune complex as part of the immune response to the virus.

In tissue sections, HIV-1 mRNA-positive cells were present in the follicles (1–2 per follicle). On cytocentrifuge preparations of isolated cells, we identified positive cells as FDCs (Fig. 3). The frequency of viral mRNA-positive FDCs in cytocentrifuge preparations was somewhat higher ($1/10^4$) than that reported for lymphocytes (13). The mRNA positivity of purified FDCs demonstrates that FDCs in vivo are in a state of infection by HIV-1 and actively produce mRNA.

Mechanisms of viral entry into FDCs have to be determined. Both CD4-negative and Fc receptor–mediated internalization of HIV-1 containing immune complexes are open for study, since FDCs express CD4 (9,14) and Fc receptors (12) (Parmentier et al.).

Serum from the HIV-infected patient contained high amounts of IgG and IgM immune complexes as determined by an indirect granulocyte-phagocytosis test. After incubation of normal FDCs with this serum, a thin membrane expression of *gag* antigens p15, p17, p24, and *env* antigens gp41 and gp120 (Fig. 4) was detected by immunocytochemistry. Ultramicroscopically, electron-dense material on the surface of FDCs was immunolabeled by sheep anti-p24 antibody (Fig. 5), indicating adherence of HIV-1–containing immune complexes to FDCs. Immunolabeling was not detected on FDC incubated with AB serum.

We conclude that the role of FDCs in HIV-1 infection is twofold: either as a target cell for HIV-1 cellular infection, or as an antigen-presenting cell after entrapment of exogenous HIV-1–containing immune complexes. The disruption of FDCs may be caused either by lytic infection of FDCs following viral replication, or by the lytic action of virions/viral antigens entrapped on the surface of these cells.

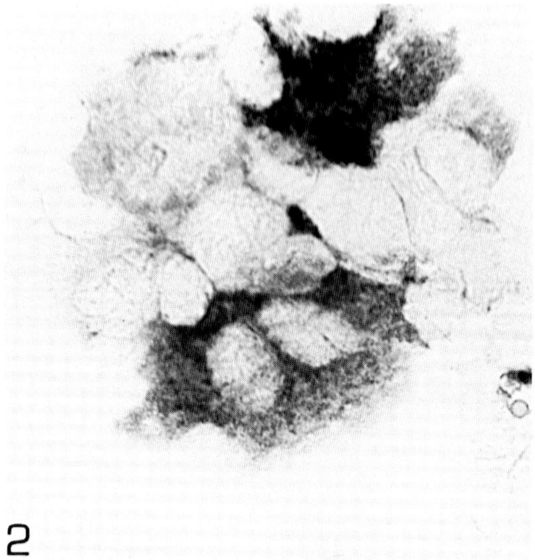

Figure 2 Isolated FDCs from the patient immunolabeled with anti-p17 antibody. Similar labeling was found with DRC-1, anti-p15, anti-p24, and anti-gp41 antibodies. Omission of primary antibodies revealed no labeling. Three-step immunoperoxidase: RAM/PO, SwAR/PO, followed by AEC (3-amino-9-ethylcarbazole). Counterstaining by hematoxylin (magnification: ×520).

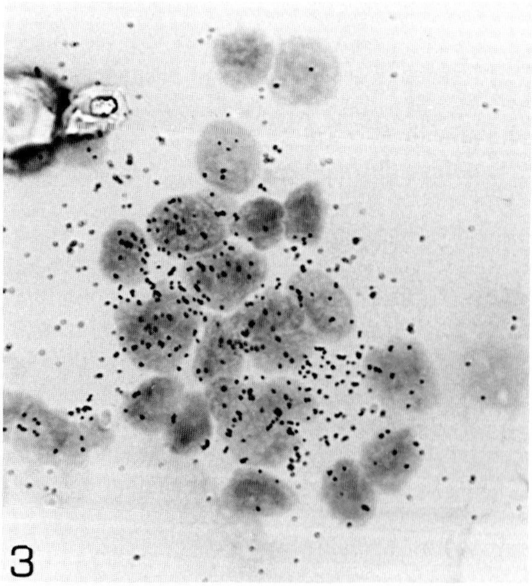

Figure 3 In situ hybridization with the ^{35}S-labeled probe for HIV-1 *env* mRNA (Du Pont NEP-200) on isolated FDCs from an HIV lymph node. Counterstaining by hematoxylin (magnification: ×520).

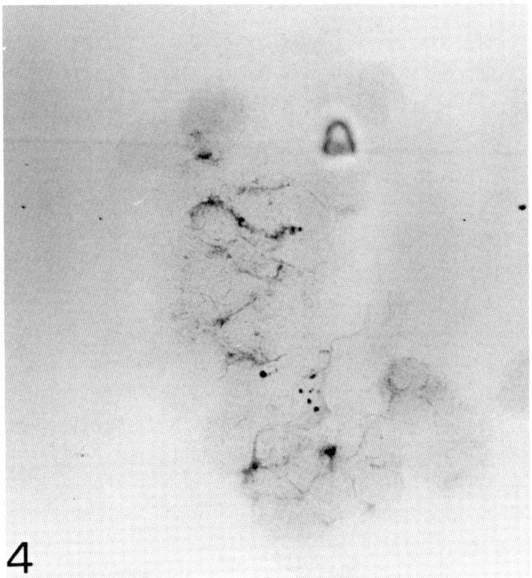

4

Figure 4 Isolated FDCs from a tonsil incubated with HIV-1–positive serum, and stained for gp120 expression. Similar labeling was found for p15, p17, p24, and gp41, respectively. Three-step immunoperoxidase: RAM/PO, SwAR/PO, followed by AEC. Counterstaining by haematoxylin (magnification: ×520).

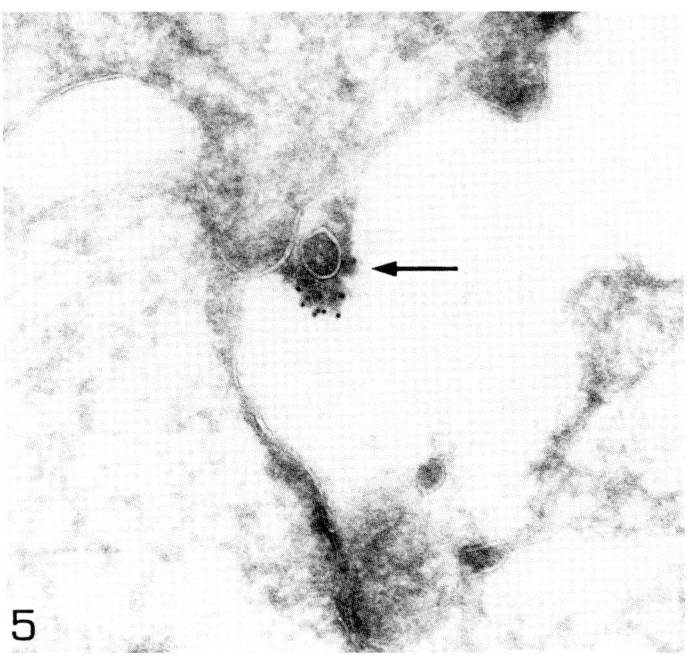

5

Figure 5 Immunoelectron microscopy; immunogold labeling (arrow) for HIV-1 p24 on the villous extension of an FDC, which had been incubated with HIV-1–positive serum. No labeling was observed without p24 antibody in the first incubation (magnification: ×60,000).

ACKNOWLEDGMENT

This study was supported by the Dutch Ministry of Health, in the framework of the National Program on AIDS Research, RGO/WVC nr. 88-79/89005.

REFERENCES

1. Schuurman HJ, Krone WJA, Broekhuizen R, Goudsmit J. Expression of RNA and antigens of human immunodeficiency virus type-1 (HIV-1) in lymph nodes from HIV-1 infected individuals. Am J Pathol 1988; 133:516–24.
2. Garcia CF, Lifson JD, Engleman EG, Schmidt DM, Warnke RA, Wood GS. The immunohistology of the persistent generalized lymphadenopathy syndrome (PGL). Am J Pathol 1986; 86:706–15.
3. Tenner-Racz K, Racz P, Bofill M, Schulz-Meyer A, Dietrich M, Kern P, Weber J, Pinching AJ, Veronese-Dimarzo F, Popovic M, Klatzmann D, Gluckman JC, Janossy G. HTLV-III/LAV viral antigens in lymph nodes of homosexual men with persistent generalized lymphadenopathy and AIDS. Am J Pathol 1986; 123:9–15.
4. Tenner-Racz K. Human immunodeficiency virus-associated changes in germinal centers of lymph nodes and relevance to impaired B-cell function. Lymphology 1988; 21:36–43.
5. O'Hara CJ, Groopman JE, Federman M. The ultrastructural and immunohistochemical demonstration of viral particles in lymph nodes from human immunodeficiency virus-related and non-human immunodeficiency virus-related lymphadenopathy syndromes. Human Pathol 1988; 19:545–9.
6. Armstrong JA, Horne R. Follicular dendritic cells and virus-like particles in AIDS-related lymphadenopathy. Lancet 1984; ii:370–2.
7. Le Tourneau A, Audouin J, Diebold J, Marche C, Tricottet V, Reynes M. LAV-like viral particles in lymph node germinal centers in patients with the persistent lymphadenopathy syndrome and the acquired immunodeficiency syndrome-related complex: an ultrastructural study of 30 cases. Human Pathol 1986; 17:1047–53.
8. Biberfeld P, Chayt KJ, Biberfeld G, Gallo RC, Harper ME. HTLV-III expression in infected lymph nodes and relevance to pathogenesis of lymphadenopathy. Am J Pathol 1986; 123:436–42.
9. Parmentier HK, van der Linden JA, Krujnen J, van Wichen D, Rademakers LHPM, Bloem A, Schuurman HJ. Human follicular dendritic cells: characteristics in situ and in suspension. Scand J Immunol (in press).
10. Slot JW, Geuze HJ. A new method of preparing gold probes for multiple-labeling cytochemistry. Eur J Cell Biol 1985; 38:87–93.
11. Denijn M, De Weger RA, Berends MJH, Compier-Spies PhI, Jansz H, Van Unnik JAM, Lips CJM. Detection of calcitonin-encoding mRNA by radioactive and non-radioactive in situ hybridization: improved colorimetric detection and cellular localization of mRNA in thyroid sections. J. Histochem Cytochem 1990; 38:351–8.
12. Heinen E, Radoux D, Kinet-Denoël C, Moeremans M, De Mey J, Simar LJ. Isolation of follicular dendritic cells from human tonsils and adenoids. III. Analysis of their Fc receptors. Immunology 1985; 54:777–84.
13. Harper ME, Marselle LM, Gallo RC, Wong-Staal F. Detection of lymphocytes expressing human T-lymphotrophic virus type III in lymph nodes and peripheral blood from infected individuals by in situ hybridization. Proc Natl Acad Sci USA 1986; 83:772–6.
14. Woods GS, Turner RR, Shiurba RA, Eng L, Warnke RA. Human dendritic cells and macrophages: In situ definition of subsets that exhibit specific and morphological characteristics. Am J Pathol 1985; 119:73–82.

122
Selective Inhibition of Immune Complex Trapping by a Monoclonal Antibody, ED11, Recognizing a Follicular Dendritic Cell–Associated Molecule

Timo K. Van den Berg, Ed A. Döpp, George Kraal, and Christine D. Dijkstra
Free University, Amsterdam, The Netherlands

INTRODUCTION

An important constituent of the microenvironment of lymphoid follicles is formed by follicular dendritic cells (FDCs). The FDCs have the characteristic ability to trap immune complexes (ICs) and retain them for long periods of time. Trapping of ICs has been suggested to be crucial to the generation of immunological memory (1,2) and to the affinity maturation of antibody responses (2), but direct evidence to support these ideas is lacking. Also, there is very limited information about the molecular mechanism underlying follicular trapping.

Most of the information on the role and the mechanism of trapping comes from experiments using various conditions that interfere with IC trapping, including lipopolysaccharides (LPS) (3–5) or cobra venom factor (CoVF) treatment (1,6), neonatal immunoglobulin M (IgM) or IgD treatment (7), or total body irradiation (8). However, none of these methods are suitable to study the role of follicular trapping selectively, since all of these treatments affect the normal humoral immune response considerably.

In vivo experiments using CoVF indicate that C3 is essential to the process (1,6), but it is not known whether the transportation of ICs to follicles or the actual binding to FDCs, or both, are C3 dependent. Other, mostly in vitro, evidence implicates that ICs are bound by some, as yet unidentified, Fc receptor (9).

Recently, we have described a panel of monoclonal antibodies recognizing reticular cells in the peripheral lymphoid organs of the rat (10). One of these antibodies, ED11, recognized FDCs as well as reticular cells in the T-cell compartments of lymphoid organs. Furthermore, a very restricted reactivity was found in nonlymphoid organs. In this chapter, we describe the involvement of the ED11 determinant in the process of follicular trapping.

METHODS

Animals

Male Wistar rats, between 7 and 10 weeks of age, were obtained from Harlan/Olac/CPB (The Netherlands). Animals were maintained under conventional laboratory conditions and were allowed free access to food and water.

Antibodies

The monoclonal antibodies used in this study were: ED11, recognizing FDCs and reticular cells in the T-cell compartments (10); ED5, directed against a subpopulation of FDCs (10,11); OX2 (Serotec), recognizing FDCs as well as certain blood vessel structures (12).

Immunohistochemistry

Tissues were frozen in liquid nitrogen and stored at –20°C. Cryostate sections (8–10 μm) were picked up on slides, air-dried, fixed in acetone for 10 min, and air dried again for at least 30 min. They were then incubated with optimal concentrations of primary antibodies in phosphate-buffered saline (PBS), containing 0.2% bovine serum albumin (BSA), for 1 hr at room temperature (RT). After several rinses in PBS, the slides were incubated for 1 hr with the appropriate enzyme conjugated diluted in PBS, containing 0.2% BSA and 1% normal rat serum. Normally, rabbit antimouse immunoglobulin (Ig) peroxidase (RAMPO Dakopatts, Glostrup, Denmark) was used as the enzyme conjugate, rabbit antimouse Ig alkaline phosphatase (RAMAF; Tago Inc., Burlingame, California) was used in case double staining with PAP complexes was done. After washing in PBS, peroxidase activity was demonstrated by incubation with 0.5 mg/ml 3,3′–diaminobenzidine tetrahydrochloride (DAB, Sigma, St. Louis, Missouri) in Tris-HCl, pH 7.6, containing 0.01% H2O2. Alkaline phosphatase activity was demonstrated according to Burstone (13) using fast blue BB salt (Sigma) and AS-BX phosphate as the substrate.

Dot-Blotting

The following protocol was used for dot-blotting. Spots were made on nitrocellulose sheets with 200 μl of normal rat serum. After a rinse in PBT (PBS, containing 0.1% Tween 20) the blots were incubated for 3 hr with ED11 1:2000, diluted in PBT at RT, washed in PBT, and incubated for 3 hr with 1:800 RAMPO at RT. The blots were stained in 0.5 mg/ml DAB, dissolved in Tris/HCl buffer pH 7.6 containing 0.01% H_2O_2.

LPS Treatment

Different doses of LPS (from *Escherichia coli*, Sigma) were injected i.v. into the tail vein 24 hr before sacrifice.

X-Irradiation

Animals received 1000 rad total body irradiation 48 hr before sacrifice.

CoVF Treatment

Cobra venom factor, *Naja naja* (Sigma), was purified as described by Ballow and Cochrane (14) on DEAE-cellulose followed by Sephadex G-200 gel filtration. Rats received two i.p. injections of 10 U CoVF in saline 72 and 48 hr before sacrifice.

Immune Complex Trapping In Vivo

Rats were injected i.v. with 200 µl of horseradish peroxidase rabbit anti–horseradish peroxidase (PAP) complexes (Dakopatts, Glostrup, Denmark) in the tail vein. Animals were killed after 24 hr and their spleens were removed and prepared for immunochemistry. The PAP complexes were visualized using the DAB/H_2O_2 method as described under Immunohistochemistry.

Immune Complex Binding to Cryostat Sections

This technique was performed as described previously (4) with minor modifications. Fresh cryostat sections were fixed in acetone for 10 min and air dried for at least 1 hr. Sections were preincubated with saturating concentrations of antibodies for 1 hr at RT. Subsequently they were incubated with 1:10 diluted PAP complexes for 30 min at RT. The PAP complexes were visualized as described above.

Antibody Injections

Animals were given a single i.p. injection of 1 ml of ED11 ascites (containing 3.75 mg/ml immunoglobulin) 2 hr before the injection of PAP complexes. Control animals were treated with equal doses of ED5 ascites or with an isotype-matched control ascites against penicillin, pen9, which has no known reactivity against rat tissue (15). Identical experiments were performed using purified ED11 antibodies or ED11 ($F(ab')_2$ fragments. ED11 immunoglobulins were purified from ascites by protein A–sepharose (Pharmacia). $F(ab')_2$ fragments were generated by pepsin digestion and isolated on a Superose-12 gel filtration column (Pharmacia). Purity was confirmed using SDS-PAGE. Both isolated ED11 antibodies and ED11 $F(ab')_2$ fragments were injected at a dose of 3.0 mg per animal. To check whether the antibodies indeed reached and covered the recognized tissue components, alternate sections of spleen were compared. One was incubated with RAMAF alone and the other with primary antibody followed by RAMAF (see above, under Immunohistochemistry).

RESULTS

Localization of ED11 Determinant in Tissues

Sections of lymphoid tissues were tested for ED11 reactivity. In spleen, a characteristic pattern was seen in both the PALS and the follicles. In the PALS, ED11 labeled the concentrically arranged reticular sheaths, surrounding the central arteriole. This pattern is very similar to the one observed after silver impregnation, which visualizes the reticular fibers. In the follicles, ED11 produces a weblike staining pattern characteristic for follicular cells (FDCs). The splenic capsule and trabeculae were also clearly positive, whereas no staining was observed in the marginal zone and the red pulp. To test the possibility that the follicular labeling actually represents binding to FDCs, we investigated the colocalization of ED11 and PAP complexes in the spleen. At 24 hr after PAP injection, the complexes were observed predominantly in the germinal center, and were located on ED11–positive cells exclusively. No PAP complexes were observed on reticular cells in other compartments. In follicles of lymph nodes and Peyer's patches, ED11 produced the same weblike staining observed in the spleen. Reticular cells (RCs) in the T-cell areas of these organs reacted weakly but significantly, whereas no staining was observed in the other compartments. Staining patterns in other organs have been described elsewhere (10).

Reactivity of ED11 with Serum Component(s)

To study a possible binding of our antibodies to serum components, tests were performed in a dot-blot assay. Assessment of the binding of ED11 to normal rat serum resulted in a positive reaction, whereas no significant binding could be detected using ED5 (results not shown).

Effect of ED11 Injection on Immune Complex Trapping In Vivo

To study a possible involvement of the ED11 determinant in the IC trapping process, animals were given a single injection of ED11 antibody and their ability to retain PAP complexes in vivo was tested. Control animals were treated with an irrelevant, isotype-matched, control antibody or with ED5. As shown in Figure 1, ED11 treatment completely blocked IC trapping by FDCs, whereas normal trapping occurred in control animals receiving ED5 or pen9 control antibody. Incubation of splenic sections with second-stage antibody alone in comparison to sections incubated with both primary, injected, and secondary antibody showed that (a) ED5 and ED11 were indeed present on their tissue determinants, and (b) that there was no difference between the alternate sections, demonstrating that the antibodies had been injected at more or less saturating doses. Purified ED11 and ED11 F(ab′)2 fragments inhibited IC trapping just as well as ascites fluid.

Effects of Antibodies on the Binding of Immune Complexes to Cryostat Sections

Incubation of cryostat sections with PAP complexes results in their binding to FDCs. For this in vitro binding of PAP complexes, no transport toward the follicle is required. Thus, the trapping of ICs on FDCs can be evaluated independently from their transport, unlike in vivo trapping. Although we were unable to establish the same level of labeling as we found after injection of PAP complexes, the typical FDC staining was observed. However, pre- or coincubation with ED11, ED5, or OX2 did not cause any obvious changes in binding capacity.

Effects of LPS on the Expression of FDC Determinants

In order to get a better understanding about the role of the ED11 determinant and other FDC determinants in the follicular trapping process, we studied their presence in follicles under different circumstances that are known to interfere with IC trapping. When animals were treated with LPS a dose-dependent inhibition of IC trapping was found (Table 1). Complete inhibition was observed when 50 μg LPS or more was given. A similar situation was found with respect to the expression of the FDC markers ED5 and ED11 (Fig. 2). On the other hand, very little or no effect was observed for OX2, indicating that FDCs are still present after LPS. In the case of ED11, the effect appeared to be specific for FDCs, since recognition of the reticular elements in the PALS by ED11 was not altered by LPS.

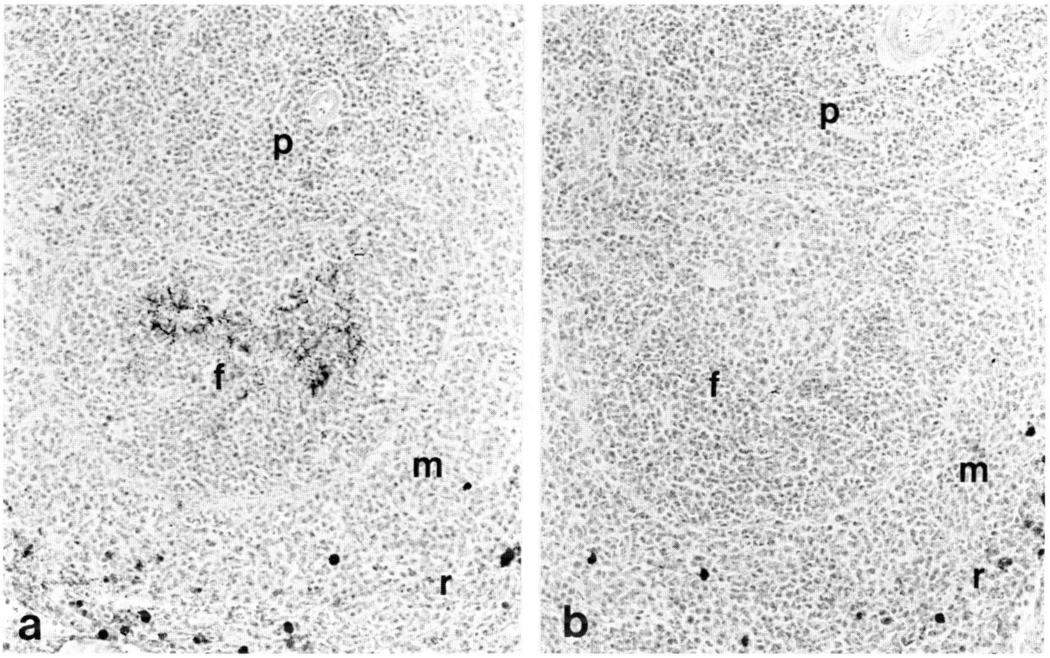

Figure 1 The effect of ED11 treatment on the in vivo trapping of immune complexes. Spleen sections of control-treated (a) or ED11-treated animals (b) stained for 24 hr previously injected PAP. f = follicle; m = marginal zone; p = periarteriolar lymphocyte sheath; r = red pulp.

Effect of Irradiation on the Expression of FDC Determinants

Animals which had been receiving sublethal irradiation did not show any follicular trapping of injected PAP complexes. On the other hand, the lymphocyte depleted follicles of these animals were strongly positive for ED5, ED11, and OX2. The weblike staining pattern was more compact in these animals than in unirradiated controls.

Effect of CoVF on the Expression of FDC Determinants

When animals were treated with CoVF a complete inhibition of trapping of injected PAP complexes was found. However, normal binding of PAP complexes by FDCs was observed

Table 1 Effect of LPS Treatment on the Trapping of Injected PAP Complexes and the Expression of the Markers ED5, ED11, and OX2 by FDCs.

	PAP	ED5	ED11	OX2
Control	++	++	++	++
5 μg LPS	++	+	+	++
15 μg LPS	+	+	+	++
50 μg LPS	–	–	–	++
150 μg LPS	–	–	–	+

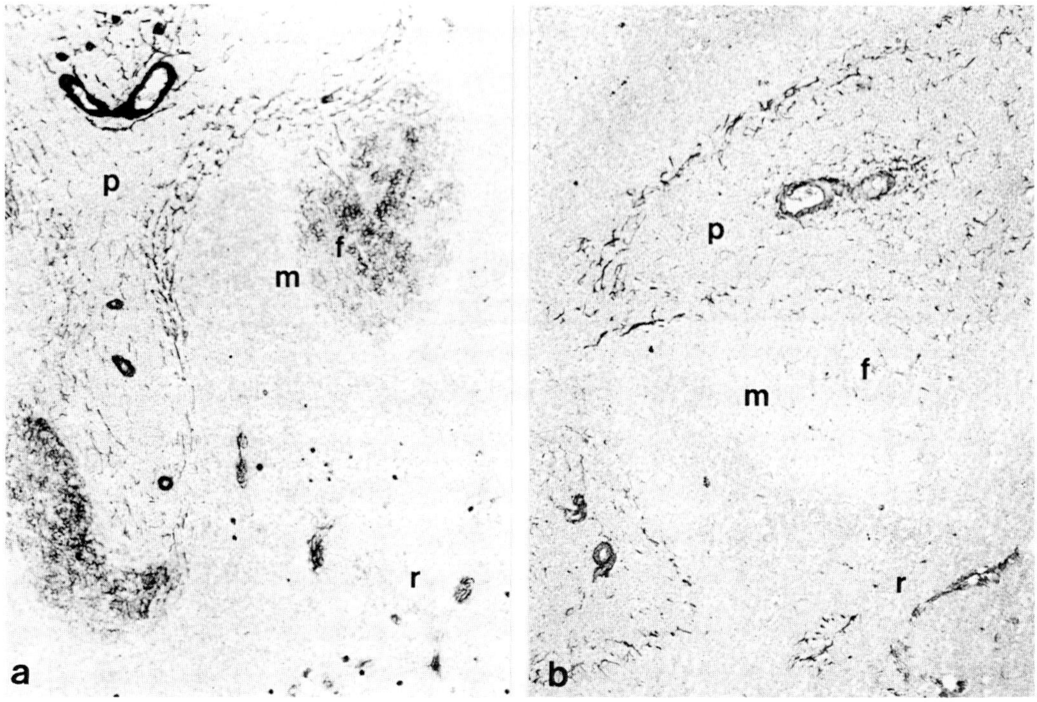

Figure 2 The effect of LPS treatment on the expression of the ED11 determinant. Spleen sections stained for ED11. (a) Control animal; (b) animal treated with 50 μg of LPS. Notice the absence of staining in the follicles in (b). f = follicle; m = marginal zone; p = periarteriolar lymphocyte sheath; r = red pulp.

in sections of spleens from CoVF-treated animals that had been incubated with PAP in vitro. Immunocytochemistry clearly demonstrated an unaltered distribution of the ED5, ED11, and OX2 determinants in the follicles of these animals. On the other hand, treatment with CoVF led to a complete loss of ED11 reactivity in serum.

DISCUSSION

In the present study we have investigated the involvement of an FDC determinant, recognized by the monoclonal antibody ED11, in the IC trapping process. In vivo treatment with ED11 completely inhibited the IC trapping in lymphoid follicles. Therefore, we conclude that the ED11 determinant is involved in the actual process of trapping.

To our knowledge, a method to selectively block the trapping of ICs, without severely affecting lymphoid and nonlymphoid cells, has not been described before. Treatment with LPS and irradiation both interfere with trapping, but also have major effects on B-cell function. The same holds true for anti-IgM or anti-IgD treatment. Therefore, these methods are not suitable to investigate the role of IC trapping in the humoral immune response.

Treatment of animals with LPS inhibits trapping (3,4). It appeared in our dose-response experiment with LPS that the (loss of) capacity to trap IC was correlated with (the loss of) ED11 expression. These results are also supportive for the fact that the antibody

ED11 recognizes a molecule with relevance for the trapping of ICs. The loss of expression of the ED11 determinant was not simply due to a toxic effect of LPS on FDCs, since, e.g., OX2 was found to be expressed by FDCs as usual. Moreover, experiments in the mouse have shown no morphological alterations of FDCs in response to LPS (5).

Our experiments provide evidence for a selective role of the ED11 determinant in the follicular trapping process, but it is unknown at what stage this antigen is involved. One explanation is that ED11 recognizes a receptor for ICs on FDCs and interferes with its binding of ICs. However, the fact that ED11 was unable to block IC binding to FDCs on frozen sections may indicate that this is not the case.

Alternatively, circulating ICs may bind the ED11 determinant in serum, which may in turn be involved in the transport of the complexes to the follicles and may also mediate binding to an appropriate receptor on FDCs. Such a mechanism was proposed earlier by Klaus (1), who suggested that C3 served as an intermediary molecule. Various complement components, including C3, can be detected within the FDC network (16). In the spleen, the distribution of ED11 is similar to that of C3 as reported in humans. Furthermore, like C3, the ED11 determinant is present in serum.

The experiments with CoVF, on the other hand, support the possibility that ED11 recognizes C3. Immune complex trapping as well as the ability to detect ED11 reactivity in serum is prevented by CoVF. Injection of CoVF results in the depletion of intact C3 and the generation of C3- and C5-derived split products. This indicates that ED11 may actually recognize C3, and/or a C3 derivative like C3b. The fact that C3 depletion does not cause disappearance of ED11 positivity in follicles does not exclude the possibility that ED11 recognizes C3. C3 (or C3b) containing ICs, already present on FDCs before depletion, can explain the persistence of C3 within the FDC network.

Biochemical evidence will be needed to establish the actual specificity of ED11, and functional assays will have to elucidate its putative effects on the complement system. It could be argued that another explanation for the observed inhibition of trapping by in vivo ED11 treatment is that the antibody forms ICs with the recognized ED11 molecule in serum. These ICs may then reach the follicles and compete with the injected PAP complexes for binding sites on FDCs via their Fc part. However, the fact that IC trapping was also blocked by injection of ED11 $F(ab')_2$ fragments excludes this possibility.

The role of the ED11–reactive component associated with reticular cells in the T-cell areas of peripheral lymphoid organs remains unknown. It seems unlikely that this determinant is also involved in IC binding, since these cells do not retain complexes after intravenous injection. At present, there is no definite proof concerning the origin of FDCs. Transitional forms between reticular cells and FDCs suggest that FDCs could be derived from RCs (17). The finding that the ED11 determinant is present on FDCs as well as on RCs in the T-cell areas adds further support to the idea that the FDCs actually represents a specialized type of RC.

In summary, our data provide direct evidence for a function of the ED11 determinant in the follicular trapping process. Treatment with ED11 antibodies appears to be a very useful method to interfere with IC trapping selectively. It provides the opportunity to study the role of IC trapping in the humoral immune response in vivo.

REFERENCES

1. Klaus GGB, Humphrey JH, Kunkl A, Dongworth DW. The follicular dendritic cell: Its role in antigen presentation in the generation of immunological memory. Immunol Rev 1980; 53:3–28.

2. Kunkl A, Klaus GGB. The generation of memory cells IV. Immunization with antigen-antibody complexes accelerates the development of B memory cells, the formation of germinal centres and the maturation of antibody affinity in the secondary response. Immunology 1981; 43:371.
3. Groeneveld PHP, Eikelenboom P, Van Rooijen N. Mechanism of trapping: Similarities and differences in trapping of antibody-complexed antigens and carbon particles in the follicles of the spleen. J Reticuloendothel Soc 1983; 33:109–17.
4. Dijkstra CD, Te Velde AA, Van Rooijen N. Localization of horseradish peroxidase (HRP)-anti-HRP complexes in cryostat sections: influence of endotoxin on trapping of immune complexes in the spleen of the rat. Cell Tissue Res 1983; 232:1–7.
5. Heinen E, Cormann N, Kinet-Denoël C, Simar LJ. Lipopolysaccharide suppresses immune complex retention by follicular dendritic cells without cytological alterations. Immunol Lett 1986; 13:323–7.
6. Papamichail M, Gutierrez C, Embling P, Johnson P, Holborow EJ, Pepys MB. Complement dependence of localization of aggregated IgG in germinal centers. Scand J Immunol 1975; 4:343–47.
7. Enriquez-Rincon F, Andrew E, Parkhouse RME, Klauss GGB. Suppression of follicular trapping of antigen-antibody complexes in mice treated with anti-IgM or anti-IgD antibodies from birth. Immunology 1984; 53:713–19.
8. Kroese FGM, Wubbena AS, Nieuwenhuis P. Germinal centre formation and follicular antigen trapping in the spleen of lethally X-irradiated and reconstituted rats. Immunology 1986; 57: 99–104.
9. Radoux D, Kinet-Denoel C, Heinen E, Moeremans M, De Mey J, Simar LJ. Retention of immune complexes by Fc receptors on mouse follicular dendritic cells. Scand J Immunol 1985; 21:345–53.
10. Van den Berg TK, Döpp EA, Breve JJP, Kraal G, Dijkstra CD. The heterogeneity of the reticulum of rat peripheral lymphoid organs identified by monoclonal antibodies. Eur J Immunol 1989; 19:1747–56.
11. Jeurissen SHM, Dijkstra CD. Characteristics and functional aspects of nonlymphoid cells in rat germinal centers, recognized by two monoclonal antibodies ED5 and ED6. Eur J Immunol 1986; 16:562–68.
12. Barclay AN. Different reticular elements in rat lymphoid tissue identified by localization of Ia, Thy-1 and MRC Ox2 antigens. Immunology 1981; 44:727–33.
13. Burstone MS. Histochemical comparison of naphta phosphates for the demonstration of phosphatases. J Natl Cancer Inst 1958; 20:601–16.
14. Ballow M, Cochane ChG. Two anticomplementary factors in cobra venom: haemolysis of guinea pig erythrocytes by one of them. J Immunol 1969; 103:944.
15. De Haan P, de Jonge AJR, Verbrugge T, Boorsma DM. Three epitope-specific monoclonal antibodies against the hapten penicillin. Int Archs Allergy Appl Immunol 1985; 76:42–6.
16. Halstensen TS, Mollnes TE, Brandtzaeg P. Terminal complement complex (TCC) and S-protein (vitronectin) on follicular dendritic cells in human lymphoid tissues. Immunol 1988; 65:193–7.
17. Dijkstra CD, Kamperdijk EWA, Döpp EA. The ontogenetic development of the follicular dendritic cell. Cell Tissue Res 1984; 236:203–6.

123
Immunohistochemical Analysis of Calcium-Binding Proteins Parvalbumin and Calbindin-D in Germinal Center Accessory Cells

Marco Chilosi,[1] Claudio Doglioni,[2] Aldo Mombello,[1] Licia Montagna,[1] Alice Benedetti,[1] Paola Pelosio,[2] Elena Piazzola,[1] Maurizio Lestani,[1] Giovanni Pizzolo,[1] and Fabio Menestrina[1]

[1]*University of Verona, Italy;* [2]*Ospedale di Feltre, Italy*

INTRODUCTION

Several reports suggest that in the thymus apoptosis can directly participate in the clonal deletion of autoreactive cells (1) as well as in the positive selection of T-cell clones on the basis of their affinity for self–major histocompatibility complex (MHC) antigens (2). A direct role of apoptosis has been also postulated in the antigen-driven postmutational selection of follicular B cells within the germinal center (GC) (3). It is widely accepted that in both the thymic and the germinal center microenvironments, the signals regulating cell proliferation and selection are delivered during the interaction of lymphocytes with accessory nonlymphoid cells (epithelial and interdigitating cells in the thymus and follicular dendritic cells [FDCs] in the lymphoid follicles). In the thymus, the first step of T-cell selection probably occurs within specialized "nurse" epithelial cells where clusters of thymocytes are completely secluded (4). In a similar fashion, multicellular aggregates formed by FDCs and B cells, resembling thymic nurse cells, can be isolated from human hyperplastic tonsils (5). Although FDCs are not of epithelial origin, they form desmosomal junctions, which contain desmoplakin immunoreactivity (5). It is possible to speculate that the formation of these structures can provide the molecular signals and the isolated milieu necessary for preventing the apoptosis of B cells.

Calcium ions are required for triggering the deoxyribonucleic acid (DNA) fragmentation observed during glucocorticoid-activated apoptosis of thymocytes (6). If calcium ions are also necessary for the activation of endonucleases in the programmed "suicide" of B cells in GCs is currently unknown, but if this is the case, the regulation of calcium concentration in the close vicinity of developing B cells could contribute to the control of apoptosis. In several biological systems, the spatial and temporal control of calcium concentration is mediated by a discrete number of small acidic proteins equipped with peculiar cavities which accept calcium ions with high selectivity (7). Some of these molecules, such as parvalbumin and calbindin-D (CB-D), do not interact with other structural proteins or enzymes, but are mainly involved in the transport or buffering of calcium.

A SUBSET OF FOLLICULAR DENDRITIC CELLS CONTAINS CALBINDIN-D

Monoclonal antibodies are available which specifically recognize CB-D on formalin-fixed tissue sections. We have analyzed reactive human lymphoid tissues (lymph node, spleen), demonstrating that the only CB-D immunoreactive cells in lymphoid tissues are FDCs within the pale zone of GCs (Fig. 1), and at the same, identifying the location where antigen in the form of immunocomplexes is entrapped (8). Interestingly, the expression of CB-D in other physiological systems such as intestinal cells is finely regulated by vitamin D (9). It is possible that in the GCs the expression of CB-D on FDCs can also be modulated by external signals; e.g., the interaction with B-cell products and/or immunocomplexes.

What can be the role of CB-D on FDCs? In intestinal cells this calcium-binding protein is directly involved in the transcellular movement of calcium ions (9). A similar role could be carried out by CB-D in FDCs. Recently we have been able to study the ultrastructure of FDC–multicellular complexes isolated from human tonsils showing that the lymphoid cells entrapped in these structures are completely secluded within the cytoplasmic processes of FDCs (5). Calbindin-D could significantly contribute to the regulation of calcium within

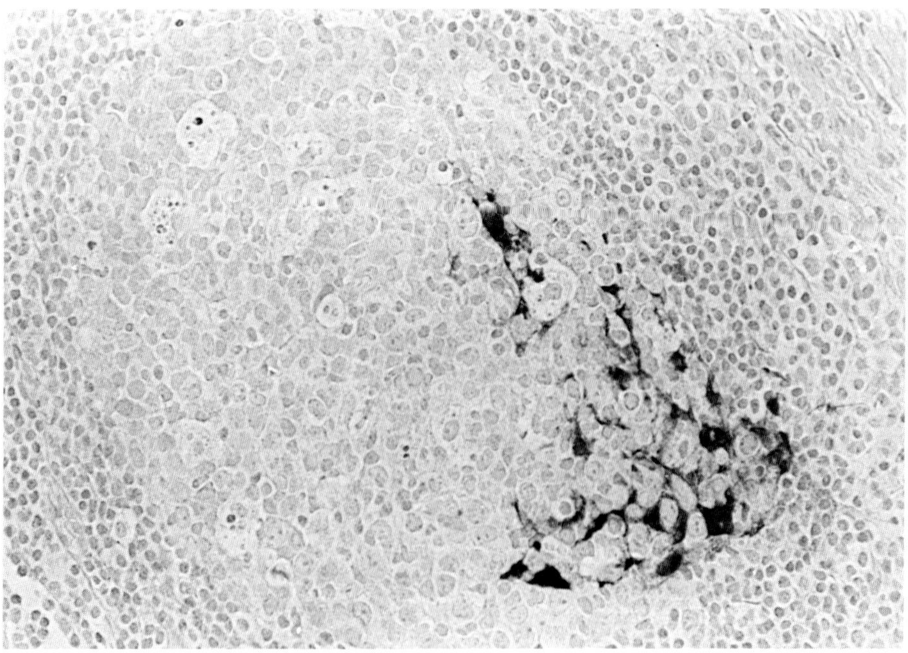

Figure 1 Calbindin-D immunostaining is restricted to the follicular dendritic cells homing the pale zone of a germinal center. Paraffin-embedded human reactive lymph node, immunoperoxidase.

these microenvironmental niches. At the same site a large amount of antigen and other molecular signals could be directly provided by FDCs to the B cells intended to survive. Interestingly, this model could be extended to thymocytes, since CB-D expression has also been demonstrated in cortical epithelial cells in the thymus of chick embryos (10).

A SUBSET OF GERMINAL CENTER LYMPHOCYTES CONTAINS PARVALBUMIN

When human lymphoid tissues are immunohistochemically analyzed using monoclonal antibody–recognizing parvalbumin (PV), a calcium-binding protein of the "buffer" type, a peculiar pattern is observed. A discrete population of strongly PV-positive lymphoid cells is present in all the follicles with GC compartmentalization, strikingly restricted to the pale zone (Fig. 2). Using double-marker immunohistochemical methods and phenotypical analysis of CD57-positive cells enriched with Dynabeads M-450, we could demonstrate that PV immunoreactivity is in fact restricted to the small but definite T-cell subpopulation homing within germinal centers and characterized by the peculiar $CD4^{+}CD3^{+}CD57^{+}$ phenotype (11). The function of this T-cell population is so far unknown. Although these T lymphocytes bear the CD4 determinant, they lack helper function on proliferation and differentiation of B lymphocytes (12). The demonstration of strong immunoreactivity for the calcium-binding parvalbumin could be of relevance for the assignment of a function, if

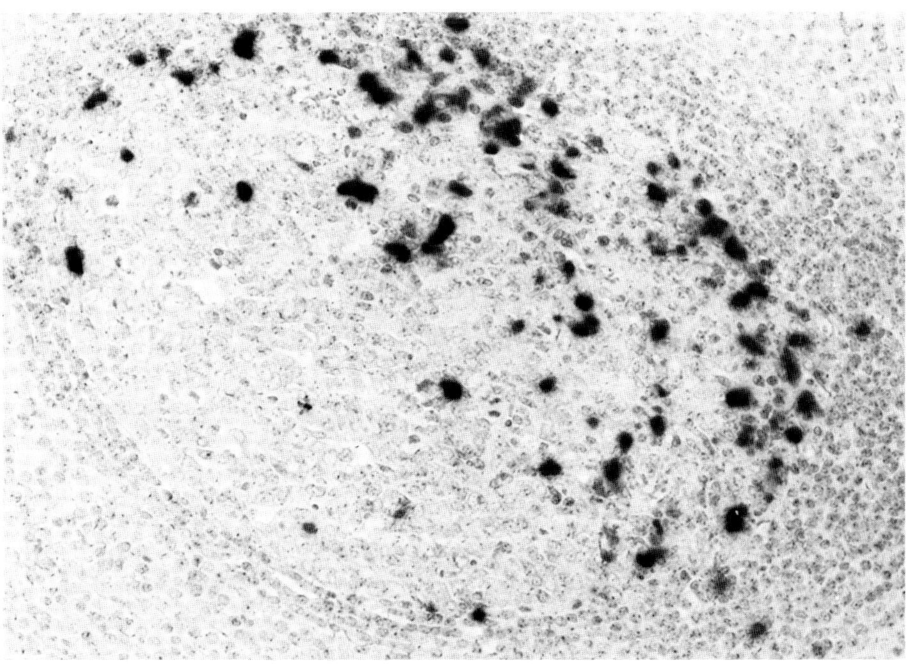

Figure 2 Parvalbumin immunostaining is restricted to a subset of lymphoid cells homing the pale zone of a germinal center. When immunohistochemically analyzed on serial sections and with double-staining techniques the same cells exhibited the peculiar $CD4^{+}CD3^{+}CD57^{+}$ phenotype (not shown). Paraffin-embedded human reactive lymph node, APAAP.

any, to this peculiar population. Detailed analysis of PV immunoreactivity compared with other phenotypical markers such as CD3 and CD21 in a variety of samples showed that PV-positive lymphocytes can only be demonstrated in the pale zone of GCs in reactive lymphoid tissues. This microenvironment must then have a specific role in the induction of PV gene expression in recruited CD4-positive lymphocytes.

What can be the role of PV in CD4-positive lymphocytes within the germinal center? Parvalbumin in fast-twitch muscles fibers functions as a calcium sink to facilitate rapid relaxation. A similar role in lowering of the concentration of free calcium ions could be hypothesized for PV-positive T lymphocytes included within the FDC cytoplasmic projections together with B cells.

ACKNOWLEDGMENTS

This work was supported in part by Ministero della Sanitá; Rome: IV Progetto AIDS.

REFERENCES

1. Smith CA, Williams GT, Kingston R, Jenkinson EJ, Owen JJT. Antibodies to CD3/T-cell receptor complex induce death by apoptosis in immature T cells in thymic cultures. Nature 1989;337:181–4.
2. Von Boehmer H. The selection of the alpha, beta heterodimeric T-cell receptor for antigen. Immunol Today 1986;7:333–36.
3. Liu YJ, Joshua DE, Williams Smith CA, Gordon J, MacLennan ICM. Mechanism of antigen-driven selection in germinal centers. Nature 1989;342:929–31.
4. Kyewski BA. Thymic cells: possible sites of T-cell selection. Immunol Today 1986;7:374–79.
5. Ennas MG, Chilosi M, Scarpa A, Lantini MS, Cadeddu G, Fiore-Donati L. Isolation of multicellular complexes of follicular dendritic cells and lymphocytes: Immunophenotypical characterization, electron microscopy and culture studies. Cell Tissue Res 1989;257:9–15.
6. McConkey DJ, Hartzell P, Nicotera P, Orrenius S. Calcium-activated DNA fragmentation kills immature thymocytes. FASEB J 1989;3:1843–49.
7. Heizmann CW, Berchtold MW. Expression of parvalbumin and other Ca2+ binding proteins in normal and tumor cells: A topical review. Cell Calcium 1987;8:1–41.
8. Chilosi M, Doglioni C, Pelosio P, Montagna L, Benedetti A, Mombello A, Piazzola E, Lestani M, Menestrina F, Scarpa A, Pizzolo G, Fiore-Donati L: Detection of calbindin-D immunoreactivity in follicular dendritic cells (submitted).
9. Wasserman RH, Fullmer CS. Calcium transport proteins, calcium absorption, and vitamin D. Ann Rev Physiol 1983;45:375–90.
10. Schreiner DS, Jande SS, Lawson DEM. Immunocytochemical localization of vitamin D-dependent calcium-binding protein in the growing chick lymphoid organs. Devel Comp Immunol 1986;10:365–76.
11. Chilosi M, Doglioni C, Montagna L, Benedetti A, Ennas MG, Mombello A, Piazzola E, Pelosio P, Lestani M, Menestrina F, Pizzolo G, Fiore-Donati L: $CD4^+/CD57^+$ T-cells of germinal center react with an antibody recognizing the calcium-binding protein parvalbumin (submitted).
12. Velardi A, Mingari MC, Moretta L, Grossi CE. Functional analysis of cloned germinal center $CD4^+$ cells with natural killer cell-related features. Divergence from typical T helper cells. J Immunol 1986;137:2808–13.

124
Immunohistochemical Localization of Intermediate Filament and Contractile Proteins in the Tonsil with Reference to Follicular Dendritic Cells

L. H. P. M. Rademakers, D. van Wychen, and R. A. de Weger
University Hospital, Utrecht, The Netherlands

INTRODUCTION

Follicular dendritic cells (FDCs) form a framework enclosing the lymphoid cells in germinal centers (GCs). Their origin is still a controversial issue. Ontogenic studies (1–2) suggest that FDCs transform from fibroblastic reticulum cells. Marker studies demonstrate that FDCs have antigens common to macrophages (3), myeloid, and B-cell lineages (4). However, chimera studies (5) excluded that FDCs originate from the bone marrow. A proportion of FDCs show alkaline phosphatase (AF) activity (6). The location of AF-positive FDCs around blood vessels, suggested that FDCs derive from perivascular cells; e.g., pericytelike mesenchymal cells. The latter cells have contractile properties (7), and we therefore studied the distribution of contractile and intermediate filament proteins in reticulum cells present in the human tonsil and, in particular, the GC.

METHODS

Fresh tonsils, obtained after tonsillectomy, were snap-frozen in liquid nitrogen. Cryosections (thickness 8μm) were allowed to dry overnight at room temperature. Prior to the immunohistochemical reactions, the sections were fixed in absolute acetone and subsequently rinsed with phosphate-buffered saline (PBS) supplemented with 0.05% Tween-20. Immunostaining reactions with monoclonal antibodies were done with a three-step reaction using a horseradish peroxidase (HRP)–labeled rabbit-antimouse immunoglobulin G (IgG)+IgM (Dakopatts, Glostrup, Denmark) antibody followed by HRP-labeled swine-antirabbit IgG. In the case of polyclonal rabbit antibodies, only HRP-labeled swine-antirabbit (Dakopatts) was used as second antibody. Double immunostaining reactions were performed with an indirect two-step reaction. The primary polyclonal antibody was demonstrated with HRP-labeled swine-antirabbit antibody; the second primary monoclonal antibody was demonstrated with the use of an AF-labeled goat-antimouse antibody (Kirkegaerd).

The HRP was developed with 3,3′-diaminobenzidine tetrahydrochloride (DAB) and hydrogen peroxide as substrate with or without ammonium nickel sulfate intensification. The AF development was performed using the Naphthol AS-MX method. Endogenous AF was inhibited by addition of levamisol. Histochemical localization of endogenous AF in combination with immunostaining was done with NBT/BCIP as substrate. The following polyclonal and monoclonal antibodies directed against vimentin and desmin (Eurodiagnostics), α-actin (1A4; Westburg), myosin, α-endotheel (Monosan), and DRC-1 (Dakopatts) were used.

RESULTS AND DISCUSSION

Vimentin was localized throughout the tonsillar tissue in a dense reticular pattern. In the GCs, this pattern varied in density. In large GCs, staining was restricted to large cells probably representing "starry sky" macrophages (8) and capillaries, whereas in small GCs, a distinct reticular vimentin reactivity was present.

Desmin staining was less frequent in comparison with vimentin. In tonsils which were composed of large GCs, reticular desmin staining was scarce and was only present

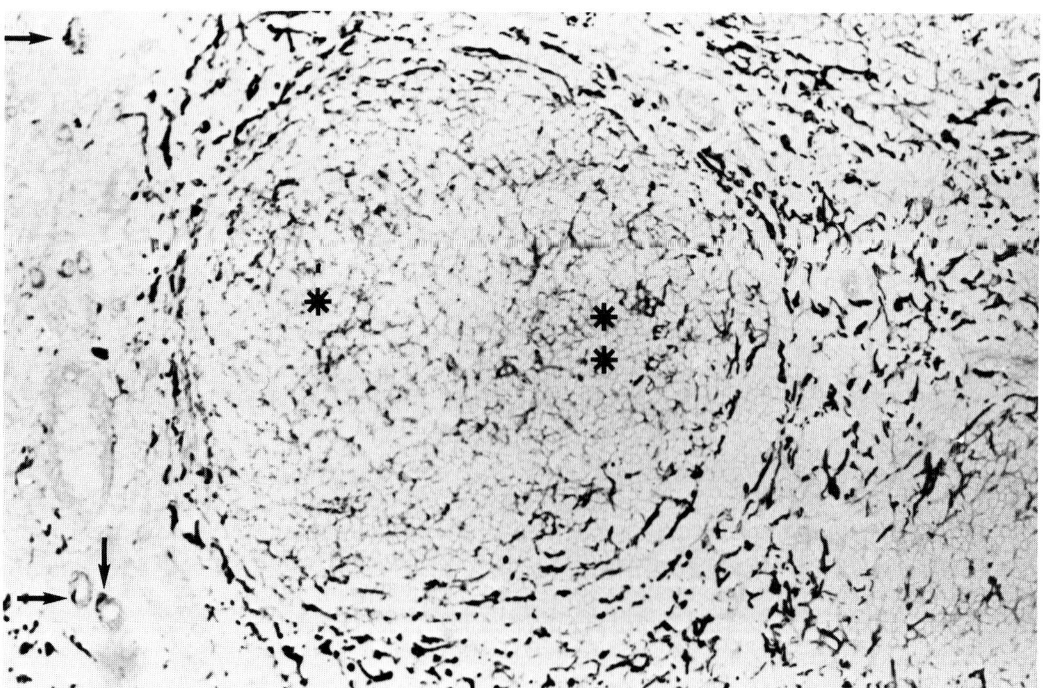

Figure 1 Small follicle in tonsillar tissue with localization of desmin-positive cells in the germinal centre (*) and in the mantle zone (**). The density of interfollicular desmin-positive cells is high; some (arrows) surround capillaries.

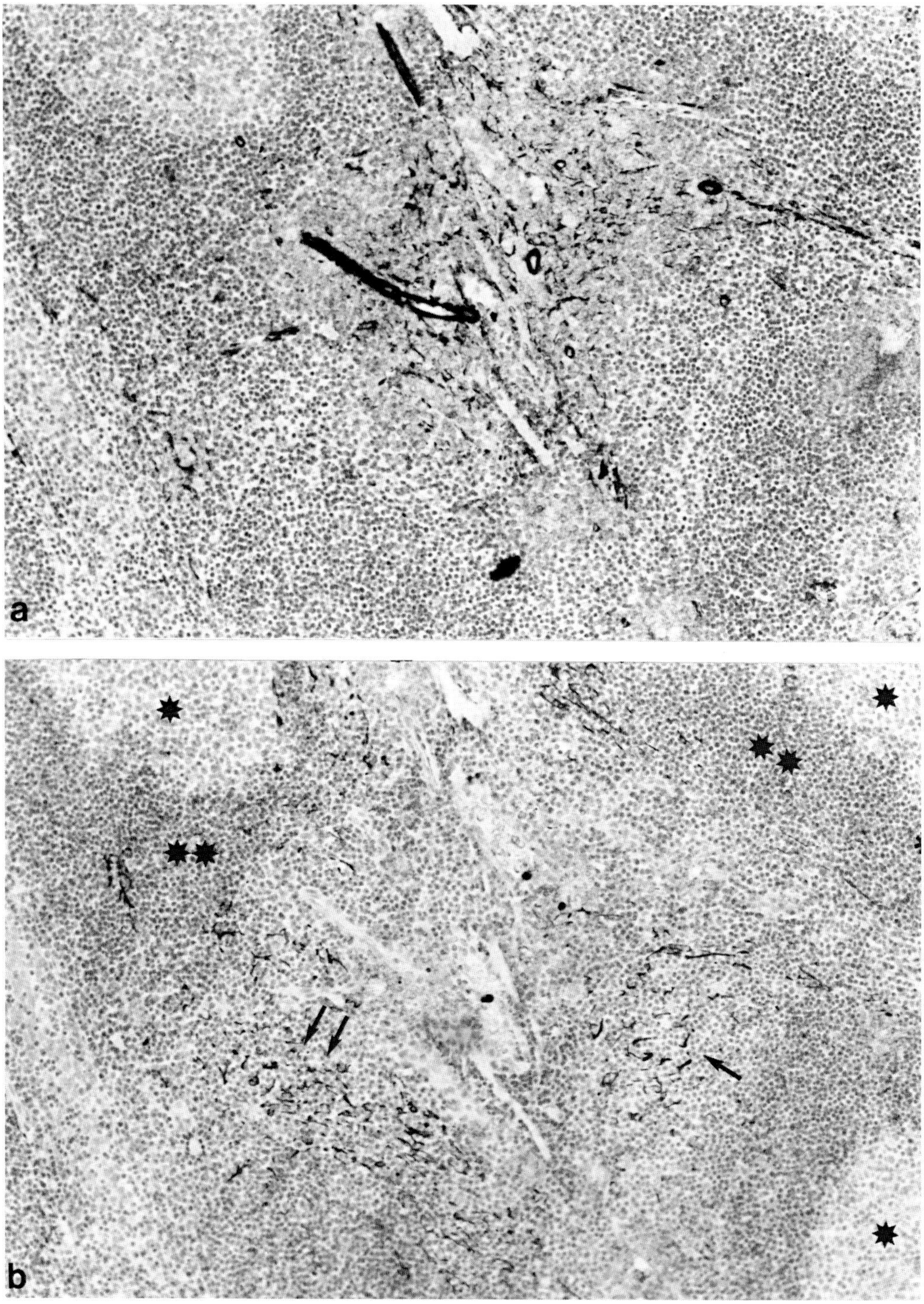

Figure 2 Serial sections of tonsil. (a) α-Actin reactivity in capillaries and reticular cells present in interfollicular areas. (b) Desmin reactivity of reticular cells in perifollicular location (arrows) and in mantle zones (**) of GCs (*)

scattered in interfollicular regions and peripherally in the mantle zone. In tonsils containing medium- and small-sized GCs, desmin reactivity was frequently present within these small GCs (Fig. 1), in interfollicular areas, and in rather dense patterns within the mantle zones (Fig. 1,2b). Double immunostaining showed colocalization of vimentin in all desmin-positive cells.

The localization of α-actin (Fig. 2a) reactivity was markedly different from desmin localization as observed in serial sections. It was present in endothelial cells and in elongated cells present in subepithelial location, in interfollicular areas, and at the outer border of mantle zones of, in particular, the large follicles. Double immunostaining for desmin and α-actin also demonstrated a different localization; colocalization of α-actin and myosin was present in few cells in interfollicular regions.

Myosin reactivity was only observed in elongated subepithelial cells and in large blood vessels. In contrast to observation with smooth muscle myosin antibodies (9), no myosin reactivity was observed within the GCs.

Immunostaining of FDCs by DRC-1 antibody was restricted to the GCs and, in a less intense pattern, to the mantle zones. After double immunostaining desmin reactivity could be demonstrated in DRC-1–positive cells, especially in small GCs, but no colocalization of α and DRC-1 reactivity was observed.

Endogenous AF reactivity was observed throughout the tonsilar tissue showing an intense staining pattern in the interfollicular areas and in mantle zones. In these areas scattered α-actin–positive and desmin-positive cells showed AF activity. Such a colocalization was also observed in perivascular cells in this location. Desmin-positive cells present in the mantle zones and GCs did not always express AF activity; occasionally colocalization was observed in solitary cells and in perivascular cells within the GCs. The latter cells also show DRC-1 activity (6).

These observations indicate that FDCs differentiate in primary follicles from AF-positive/vimentin-positive/desmin-positive α-actin–negative mesenchymal cells present in the lymphoid stroma. According to their ultrastructure and actin and myosin content, these mesenchymal cells in lymphoid tissue have been classified as myofibroblasts of myoid cells (10–11). Myofibroblasts appear in granulation tissues and diverse pathological conditions. Our observations, like others (12,13), suggest that myofibroblasts form a heterogeneous population with regard to the presence of contractile and intermediate filament proteins. Myofibroblasts may share properties with pericytes (12,14) and may be able to proliferate and differentiate quickly (14). As differentiated FDCs do not divide (15), the subpopulation of vimentin-positive/desmin-positive myofibroblasts might form a reserve pool for the generation of FDCs. Desmin-positive perivascular cells may transform in preexisting GCs and may be responsible for the increase in FDC numbers during GC expansion (16) (Chapter 120).

REFERENCES

1. Heusermann U, Zurborn K-H, Schroeder L, Stutte HJ. The origin of the dendritic reticulum cell. An experimental enzyme-histochemical and electron microscopic study on the rabbit spleen. Cell Tissue Res 1980, 209:279–94.
2. Dijkstra CD, Kamperdijk EWA, Döpp EA. The ontogenic development of the follicular dendritic cell. An ultrastructural study by means of intravenously injected horseradish peroxidase (HRP)-anti-HRP complexes as marker. Cell Tissue Res 1984, 236:203–06.

3. Gerdes J, Stein H, Mason DY, Ziegler A. Human dendritic reticulum cells of lymphoid follicles: Their antigenic profile and their identification as multi-nucleated giant cells. Virch Arch B 1983, 42:171–72.
4. Schriever F, Freedman AS, Freeman G, Messner E, Lee G, Daley J, Nadler LM. Isolated follicular dendritic cells display an unique antigenic phenotype. J Exp Med 1989, 169:2043–58.
5. Humphrey JH, Sundaram V. Origin and turnover of follicular dendritic cells and marginal zone macrophages in mouse spleen. Adv Exp Med Biol 1985; 186:167–72.
6. Rademakers LHPM, de Weger RA, Roholl PJM. Identification of alkaline phosphatase positive cells in human germinal centres as follicular dendritic cells. In: Histophysiology of the immune system. Fossum S and Rolstad S (eds). Plenum, London, Adv Exp Med Biol 1988; 191:165–69.
7. Herman IM, D'Amore PA. Microvascular pericytes contain muscle and non muscle actins. J Cell Biol 1985; 101:43–52.
8. Giorno R. Immunohistochemical analysis of the distribution of vimentin in human peripheral lymphoid tissues. Anat Rec 1985; 211:43–47.
9. Pinkus GS, Warhol MJ, O'connor EM, Etheridge CL, Fujiwara K. Immunohistochemical localization of smooth muscle myosin in human spleen, lymph node and other lymphoid tissues. Unique staining patterns in splenic white pulp and sinuses, lymphoid follicles and certain vasculature, with ultrastructural correlations. Am J Pathol 1986; 123:440–53.
10. Müller-Hermelink H-K, von Gaudecker B, Drenkhahn D, Jaworski K, Feldman C. Fibroblastic and dendritic reticulum cells of lymphoid tissue. Ultrastructural, Histochemical and ^{3}H-Thymidine labelling studies. J Cancer Res Clin Oncol 1981; 101:149–64.
11. Toccanier-Pelte MF, Skalli O, Kapanci Y, Gabbiani C. Characterization of stromal cells with myoid features in lymph nodes and spleen in normal and pathologic conditions. Am J Pathol 1987; 129:109–18.
12. Skalli O, Schürch W, Seemayer T, Lagacé R, Montandon D, Pittet B, Gabbiani C. Myofibroblasts from diverse pathologic settings are heterogenous in their content of actin isoforms and intermediate filament proteins. Lab Invest 1989; 60:275–85.
13. Franke WW, Moll R. Cytoskeletal components of lymphoid organs. I. Synthesis of cytokeratins 8 and 18 and desmin in subpopulations of extrafollicular reticulum cells of human lymph nodes, tonsils, and spleen. Differentiation 1987; 36:145–63.
14. Sims DE. The pericyte—A review. Tissue Cell 1986; 18:153–74.
15. Peters JPJ, Rademakers LHPM, Roelofs JJM, de Jong D, van Unnik JAM. Distribution of dendritic reticulum cells in follicular lymphoma and reactive hyperplasia. Light microscopical identification and general morphology. Virch Arch (Cell Pathol) 1984; 46:215–28.
16. Rademakers LHPM, Schuurman H-J, de Frankrïjker JF, Van Ooyen,A. Ultrastructural aspects of follicular dendritic cells in germinal centres of lymph nodes after HIV-1 infection. In: Lymphatic tissues and in vivo immune responses. Imhof et al. (eds.). Marcel Dekker, New York, 1991, pp. 697–702.

125
Induction of Dendritic Cells In Rat Peritoneal Cavity by Bacillus Calmette-Guérin

E. van Vugt, M. A. M. Verdaasdonk, R. H. J. Beelen, and E. W. A. Kamperdijk
Free University, Amsterdam, The Netherlands

INTRODUCTION

The antigen-presenting dendritic cells (DCs) (1) were first isolated by Steinman and Cohn (2) from the mouse spleen. Similar nonlymphoid cells have now been obtained from both lymphoid organs and nonlymphoid areas of other species, including man (3,4). These bone marrow–derived, nonphagocytic cells are dendritic in configuration, have low acid phosphatase (AP) activity, and lacked Fc receptor (FcR) by which they easily can be distinguished from macrophages. They appear to be related to the dendritic cells found in the blood (5), the Langerhans' cells in the epidermis, the veiled cells in the afferent lymph, and the interdigitating cells (IDCs) in the thymus-dependent areas of lymph nodes and spleen and in the medulla of the thymus (6,7).

All DCs strongly express major histocompatibility complex (MHC) class II antigens and are extremely potent accessory cells, particularly involved in the induction of a primary immune response. The DCs from rat lymphoid organs can be recognized by their irregular outline, AP activity centrally localized, and persistent Ia positivity (8). In contrast, macrophages show AP activity throughout the whole cytoplasm and only part of them express Ia antigens.

It has been shown that after antigenic stimulation rat lymph nodes in the induction phase of the provoked immune response contain an increased number of DCs (8). These cells have penetrated the nodes by way of the afferent lymphatics (6). It may be that the migration, differentiation, and/or activation of these cells (morphological and functional properties) are influenced by the local microenvironment in which they settle (i.e., a lymphoid microenvironment). In this respect, it is not clear if stimulation of a nonlymphoid area (i.e., the peritoneal cavity) also induces DCs. In this study, the kinetics of the accessory cells (DCs) and macrophages were studied after provoking an exudate in the rat peritoneal cavity by i.p. administration of bacillus Calmette-Guérin (BCG).

The cells were characterized on enzyme cytochemical, and immunocytochemical, and ultrastructural level.

MATERIALS AND METHODS

Animals

Male Wistar rats, 2 months of age, weighing 180–200 g were used. Enrichment experiments were performed using ACI/Mal rats. All animals were obtained from Harlan-CPB (Zeist, The Netherlands).

Immunization Procedures

Animals were given an i.p. injection of 5 ml BCG solvent containing 4×10^7 culturable particles (kindly provided by Dr. P. A. Steerenberg, RIVM, Bilthoven, The Netherlands). Three animals were killed by decapitation after 6, 12, 24, and 48 hr. Control animals did not receive BCG (0 hr). After decapitation, the peritoneal cells were obtained by peritoneal lavage. After washing, the cellular composition of the peritoneal lavages was determined on cytocentrifuge preparations (a minimum of 300 cells was counted).

Enzyme Cytochemistry and Immunocytochemistry

Acid phosphatase activity was demonstrated according to Burnstone (9). Detection of MHC Class II (Ia) antigen was done by an indirect immunoperoxidase method, using Ox6 (anti-Ia) described earlier (8). Double staining of Ia antigen and AP was performed by sequential incubation for Ia and AP. All preparations were stained with hematoxiline immediately after cytochemistry.

Enrichment of DCs

Enrichment of DCs from the peritoneal exudate, provoked by BCG (24 hr), was performed using a density gradient to remove the polymorphonuclear leukocytes (lymphoprep), adherence (1.5-hr culture in RPMI 1640 supplemented with 10% heat-inactivated fetal calf serum, 2 mM L-glutamine, 100 µg/ml penicillin, and 100 µg/ml streptomycin), and Nycodenz (14.5%; analytical grade, Nyegaard, Norway). The enriched fraction was studied both on the light and electron microscopical level.

Electron Microscopy

For electron microscopy the DC cell fraction was fixed in 1.5% glutaraldehyde in phosphate buffer (0.15 M, pH 7.4) at 4°C. After postfixation in 1% OsO_4 in phosphate buffer for 1 hr at 4°C, the cells were pelleted in 1% agar and subsequently dehydrated and embedded in an Epon/Araldite mixture. Ultrathin sections were stained with lead citrate and uranyl acetate.

RESULTS

Cellular Distribution of the Peritoneal Exudates

After i.p. BCG, an increase in the number of peritoneal cells was observed; a maximum was reached after 1 day (42×10^6 cells/rat; in controls 19×10^6 cells/rat).

Figure 1 shows the relative distribution of the different cell populations in the unstimulated and BCG-stimulated peritoneal cavities. In all peritoneal lavages cells conforming to DCs were present: They showed an irregular outline and ranged in size from 20 to 40 μm in diameter. Acid phosphatase activity was present in a central spot close to the eccentrically localized nucleus (Fig. 2a). However, the amount of reaction product and the spot size varied from cell to cell. Unstimulated cavities contained about 1% cells showing these characteristics, and 1 day after BCG a maximal number of these cells was visible (4%).

DC Enrichment

Enrichment for DCs finally resulted in a highly purified fraction (±70% DCs). The total number of cells decreased strongly during the enrichment procedure (about 3×10^4 cells/rat).

DC Ultrastructure

The plasma membrane of dendritic cells was always irregular (Fig. 3). They sometimes showed moderate smooth surface folds or veils; others possessed blunt pseudopodia of varying length. The nucleus/cytoplasm ratio ranged from 1:2 to 1:5. The nucleus commonly had an eccentric position and was irregularly shaped. The karyoplasm was euchromatic with some condensations against the nuclear envelope. Sometimes small smooth-surfaced vesicles and small and medium-sized (phago)lysosomes were centrally localized. However, distinct signs of phagocytic activity was not observed. Moreover, Birbeck granules, the characteristic cell organelle of the epidermal Langerhans' cell, were never seen.

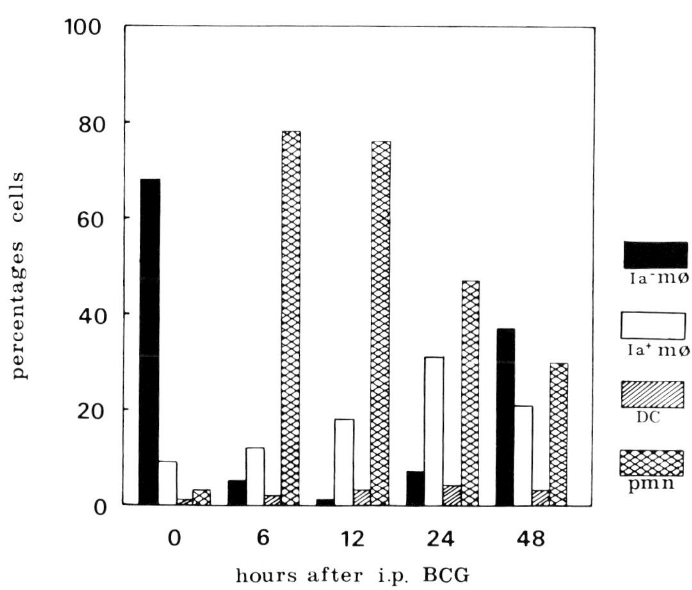

Figure 1 Cellular composition of rat peritoneal cavity at different time intervals after i.p. administration of BCG (4×10^7 c.p./5 ml solvent). mϕ = macrophage; pmn = polymorphonuclear cells.

2a

2b

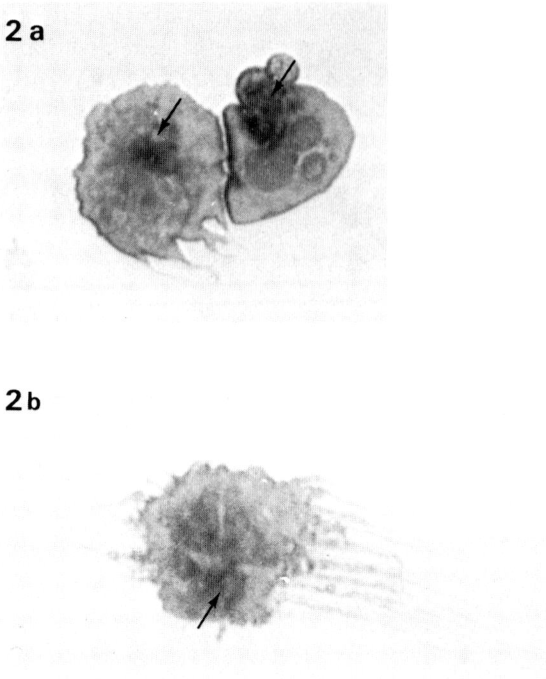

Figure 2 (a) Cytocentrifuge preparation of DCs from peritoneal cavity 24 hr after i.p. BCG. The cells have a dendritic outline and AP activity is localized in a central spot (arrows). The cells are Ia positive. (b) Cytocentrifuge preparation of a DCs isolated from rat lymph node. AP activity is present centrally (arrow).

DISCUSSION

In rat peritoneal lavages cells were identified which resemble DCs from lymphoid organs with respect to enzyme cytochemistry and immunocytochemistry and ultrastructure (Fig. 2a,b). These cells never showed Birbeck granules, which demonstrates again that they are not related to the epidermal Langerhans' cells (10). Injection of BCG resulted in an increase of DCs (both relative and absolute) in the peritoneal cavity during the first day. The same phenomenon was also observed at the same time intervals after antigenic stimulation of lymph nodes (8). This means that stimulation not only resulted in an increase of DCs in a lymphoid, but also in a nonlymphoid microenvironment.

In a previous study (11), the presentation of glutamine/tyrosine (GT) of lymph node DCs to GT-primed T cells from ACI/Mal rats was investigated. These animals are genetically defined as high responders for this copolymer in an Ia-dependent manner. In this study, a method is described to obtain a highly purified DC fraction from peritoneal lavages of ACI/Mal rats. This offers prospects to compare the antigen-presenting capacity of these DCs with DCs from lymphoid organs such as lymph nodes, spleen, and thymus.

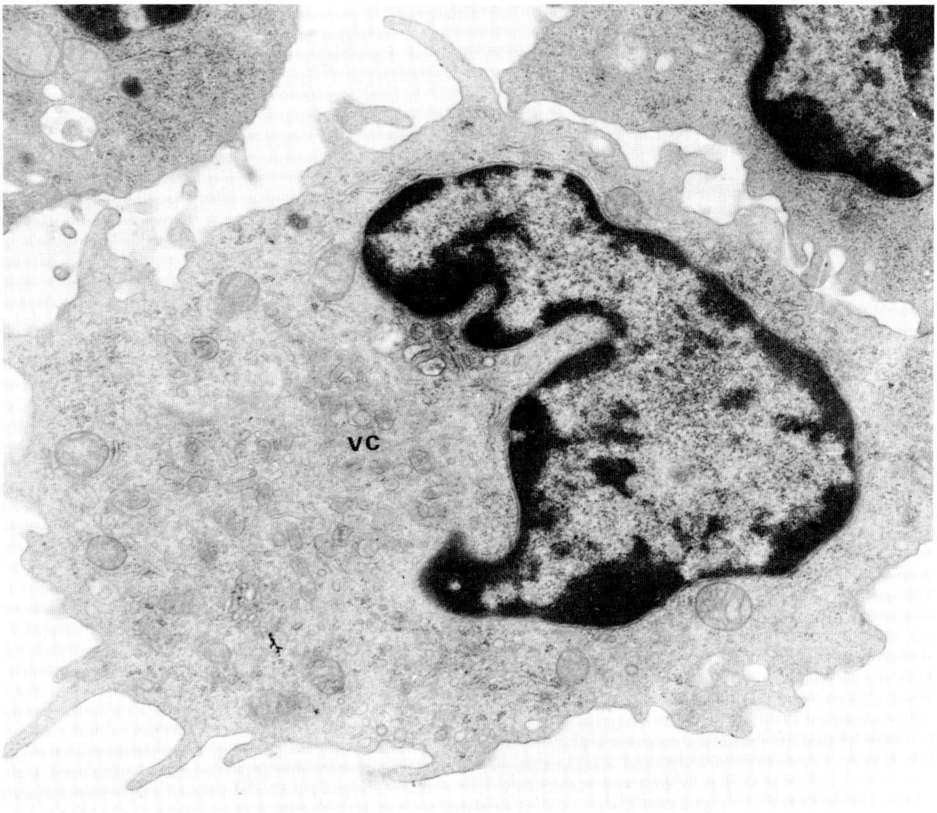

Figure 3 Ultrastructure of a DC from the peritoneal cavity 24 hr after BCG, showing an irregular outline. The nucleus is eccentrally situated. In the center, vesicles (vc) are present. Birbeck granules are not present.

REFERENCES

1. Tew JG, Thorbecke GJ, Steinman RM. Dendritic cells in the immune response. Characteristics and recommanded nomenclature. J Reticuloendothel Soc 1982, 31:371–80.
2. Steinman RM, Cohn ZA. Identification of a novel cell type in peripheral lymphoid organs of mice. J Exp Med 1973, 137:1142–62.
3. Klinkert WEF, La Badie JH, Bowers WE. Accessory and stimulating properties of dendritic cells and macrophages isolated from various rat tissues. J Exp Med 1982, 156:1–19.
4. Van Nieuwkerk EBJ, De Wolf CJM, Kamperdijk EWA, Van der Baan S. Lymphoid and non-lymphoid cells in the adenoid of children with otitis media with effusion: A comparative study. Clin Exp Immunol 1990, 79:233–9.
5. Knight SC, Farrant J, Bryant A, Edwarts AJ, Burman S, Lever A, Clarke J, Webster ADB. Non-adherent, low-density cells from human peripheral blood contain dendritic cells and monocytes, both with veiled morphology. Immunology 1986, 57:595–603.
6. Hoefsmit ECM, Duijvestijn AM, Kamperdijk EWA. Relation between Langerhans cells, veiled cells and interdigitating cells. Immunobiology 1982, 161:255–65.
7. Duijvestijn AM, Hoefsmit ECM. Ultrastructure of the rat thymus: the micro-environment of T lymphocyte maturation. Cell Tissue Res 1981, 218:279–92.

8. Kamperdijk EWA, Kapsenberg ML, Van den Berg M, Hoefsmit ECM. Characterization of dendritic cells, isolated from normal and stimulated lymph nodes of the rat. Cell Tissue Res 1985, 242:469–74.
9. Pearse AGE. *Histochemistry: Theoretical and Applied.* Vol. 1, 3rd ed. Edinburgh, Churchill Livingstone, 1968.
10. Kamperdijk EWA, Van den Berg M, Hoefsmit ECM. Lymph node accessory cells in the immune response. The primary response to paratyphoid vaccine in rat parathymic lymph nodes. Cell Tissue Res 1984, 39–42.
11. Kamperdijk EWA, Verdaasdonk MAM, Beelen RHJ. Visual and functional expression of Ia-antigen on macrophages and dendritic cells in ACI/Mal rats. Transplant Proc 1987, XIX:3024–8.

126
In Vitro Characterization of Rat Bone Marrow–Derived Thymic Stromal Cells

Raquel Navarro, Alfonso M.-Fontecha, Alberto Alvarez, Carlos Ardavin, and Agustin G. Zapata
Complutense University, Madrid, Spain

INTRODUCTION

Intrathymic T-cell development implies the induction of T-precursor cells to differentiate into mature T cells as well as the acquisition of restriction and tolerance for the self–major histocompatibility complex (MHC), considered to be mediated by thymic stromal cells through the establishment of stromal cell–thymocyte interactions. However, although epithelial cells seem to be involved in restriction induction, the role played by bone marrow–derived thymic stromal cells is controversial.

Dendritic thymic cells have been isolated and phenotypically characterized in humans and rodents (1–5), and are considered to be involved in tolerance induction by clonal deletion (6), intrathymic presentation of non-MHC antigens (7), and clonal amplification of mature medullary thymocytes (4).

Thymic macrophages have been classically related to the elimination of nonselected cortical thymocytes (6). However, their expression of MHC class II molecules (8), production of interleukin-1 (IL-1) (9), and establishment of interactions with thymocytes (10,11) suggest that they could be directly involved in T-cell differentiation.

In this regard, the present chapter analyses cytoplasmic and cell surface markers of isolated and cultured thymic macrophages and dendritic cells.

MATERIALS AND METHODS

Four- to six-week old Wistar rat thymus fragments were digested with 0.25% trypsin (Sigma) in 10% fetal calf serum (FCS) RPMI 1640 (Flow) for 15 min at 37°C; the cell suspension was filtered on a 150-mesh screen (E-C), and the low-density fraction (LDF) was obtained after centrifugation on Nycodenz (Nocymed A.S.) for 10 min at 650 G. Contaminating thymocytes were removed as nonadherent cells after adherence on 35-mm plastic Petri dishes (Costar) for 90 min at 37°C. Day 0 adherent dendritic cells (DCs) and macrophages were obtained after 4 min incubation at 37°C with a trypsin-EDTA solution (Gibco). Day 1 DCs were collected as they become nonadherent after 12–16 hr. Day 1 macrophages were removed using the trypsin-EDTA treatment. After 6 days of culture, non–adherent macrophages were obtained from culture supernatants.

Dendritic cells and macrophages were cultured in 35-mm Petri dishes in 10% FCS RPMI 1640 medium with 100 U/ml penicillin-streptomycin, at 37°C and 5% CO_2. Induction of MHC class II, Thy 1, IL-2R, and CR3 expression was tested after 72 hr incubation in RPMI 1640 supplemented with 13 U/ml of rIL-2 (Sigma) or 30% (Con A)-stimulated splenocyte-conditioned medium (SCM) containing 100–150 U/ml of IL-2.

Analysis of cell markers was achieved on cytospin preparations. Acid phosphatase (APM), nonspecific esterase (NSE), and peroxidase (PO) reactions were tested using naphthol AS-BI phosphate, alpha-naphthol acetate, and H_2O_2 as substrates. Cell surface and cytoplasmic antigens were detected with the monoclonal antibodies (MAbs) obtained from Serotec listed below, revealed with the avidin-biotin-peroxidase system (Vector).

MAb	Specificity	MAb	Specificity
OX18	MHC class I (RT1A)	OX39	IL-2R alpha chain (CD25)
OX17	MHC class II (RT1D)	OX48	T-cell activation antigen
OX6	MHC class II (RT1B)	OX8	CD8
OX7	Thy 1.1	W3/25	CD4
OX42	CR3 (C3bi receptor)	ED1	Rat macrophages
OX44	Rat myeloid cells (CD37)	ED2	Rat macrophages

RESULTS

Dendritic Cells

Thymic dendritic cells constitute 0.015% of total thymic cells. Isolated DCs display hairy stellated morphology with long narrow cell processes, an irregular indented nucleus excentrically located, and small cytoplasmic granules in the central area. Dendritic cells do not proliferate in culture, and die after 5–7 days.

Dendritic cell markers have been analyzed on day 0/1 isolated cells (Table 1). They are positive for MHC classes I and II antigens, Thy 1, CR3, OX48, CD37, acid phosphatase, and nonspecific esterase, but do not express IL-2R alpha chain, CD4, ED-1, and ED-2. Induction of CR3 and IL-2R expression cannot be achieved after incubation of day 1 DCs either with rIL-2 or SCM-supplemented medium.

Table 1 Dendritic Cell Markers (% of positive cells)

MHC class I	100	CD37	70–100
MHC class II	100	CD4	0
Thy 1	100	ED1	0
CR3	40–50	ED2	0
IL-2R	0	NSE/APH	50 low
OX48	100	PO	0

Table 2 Macrophage Markers (% of positive cells)

	Day 1	Day 30	Day 30 +rIL-2	Day 30 +SCM
MHC class I	100	100		
MHC class II	50–60	10–20	80–100	90–100
Thy 1	50–60	10–20	10–20	80–90
CR3	60–70	100		
IL-2R	0	0	80–100	30–50
OX48	0	100		
CD37	70–90	100		
CD4	ND	80–90		
ED-1	90–100	90–100		
ED-2	40–50	50–70		
AP/NSA	100	100		
PO	0	10–15		

Macrophages

Thymic macrophages constitute 0.005% of total thymic cells. After isolation (day 0), macrophages show a rounded cell shape with an oval nucleus and cytoplasmic vesicles.

Five to six days after adherence, macrophages begin to proliferate and most of them become nonadherent, and can be maintained in culture for more than 3 months. Macrophages in culture display the same morphological features as those isolated from the thymus, but show an increase in the number and size of cytoplasmic vesicles.

Macrophage markers have been analyzed after isolation (day 0/1) and from 6 to more than 30 days of culture (Table 2). Day 0/1 macrophages are positive for MHC classes I and II antigens, Thy 1, CR3, CD37, ED-1, ED-2, acid phosphatase, and nonspecific esterase, but do not express the IL-2R alpha chain nor the activation antigen recognized by MAb OX48. However, some macrophage markers change during culture: MHC class II and Thy 1 expression decreases, whereas CR3 and OX48 antigens are induced. The induction by rIL-2 or SCM of those antigens decreasing along the culture is shown in Table 2. Expression of MHC class II is increased with both rIL-2 and SCM, whereas Thy 1 induction is only obtained with SCM. Interleukin-2R, not expressed on day 0/1 or in cultured macrophages, can be induced either with SCM or rIL-2.

DISCUSSION

Rat thymic dendritic cell marker analysis is basically coincident with the existent data in humans and mice (3,5). However, our results indicate that DCs express Thy 1 and CR3 antigens in the rat thymus, whereas human DCs have been described as negative for both markers (3), and mouse DCs are Thy 1 negative but express CR3 (5). CR3 expression could be of great importance in T-cell development, since it has been demonstrated that in vitro rosette formation between mouse phagocytic cells of the thymic reticulum (PTRs) and cortical thymocytes is mediated by this molecule (12).

Rat thymic-isolated or long-term cultured macrophages display similar morphology and cell markers, which are essentially coincident with those characterizing PTRs described in mouse thymic cultures (13). Moreover, we have recently suggested (18) that PTRs obtained from rat thymic cultures could be the in vitro equivalent of thymic macrophages rather than the in vitro interdigitating cell counterpart, as indicated by Papiernik et al. (13). Expression of MHC class II decreases during the culture but can be induced with SCM, probably through its known interferon-γ (IFN-γ) activity. Decrease of MHC class II expression in culture, and its induction with rIFN-γ has also been described in mouse PTRs (14). Treatment with rIL-2 also induces MHC class II antigens as well as IL-2R alpha chain expression, according to Rocha et al. (15) on mouse PTRs. Thy 1 expression, not previously described in thymic macrophages or in PTRs, decreases during the culture, and as for MHC class II, can be induced with SCM.

Papiernik et al. have demonstrated mouse PTRs to produce IL-1 (13), and to induce thymocyte IL-2R expression (16) and prothymocyte proliferation (17). Moreover, Kyewski (10) has demonstrated that macrophage-thymocyte interactions are the earliest occurring during thymus development.

Taking all these data together, we suggest that thymic macrophages could be involved in T-precursor cell activation and proliferation through IL-1 production and thymocyte IL-2R induction.

REFERENCES

1. Wong TW, Klinkert WEF, Bowers WE. Immunological properties of thymic cells subpopulations: rat thymic dendritic cells are potent accessory cells and stimulators in a mixed leucocyte culture. Immunobiology 1982; 160:212.
2. Duijvestijn AM, Barclay AN. Identification of the bone marrow-derived Ia positive cells in the rat thymus: A morphological and cytochemical study. J Leukocyte Biol 1984; 36:561.
3. Landry D, Lafontaine M, Cossette M, Bathelemy H, Chartrand C, Montplaisir S, Pelletier M. Human thymic dendritic cells. Characterization, isolation and functional assays. Immunology 1988; 65:135.
4. Landry D, Doyon L, Poudrier J, Lafontaine M, Pelletier M, Montplaisir S. Accessory function of human thymic dendritic cells in Con A-induced proliferation of autologous thymocytes subsets. J Immunol 1990; 144:836.
5. Nabarra B, Papiernik M. Phenotype of thymic stromal cells. An immunoelectron microscopic study of anti-Ia, anti-MAC-1 and anti-MAC-2 antibodies. Lab Invest 1988; 58:524
6. Sprent J, Lo D, Gao EK, Ron Y. T cell selection in the thymus. Immunol Rev 1988; 101:173.
7. Kyewski BA, Fathman CG, Rouse RV. Intrathymic presentation of circulating non-MHC antigens by medullary dendritic cells. J Exp Med 1986; 163:231.
8. Beller DI, Unanue ER. Ia antigens and antigen presenting function of thymic macrophages. J Immunol 1980; 124:1433.
9. Howe RC, Lowenthal JW, MacDonald R. Role of interleukin 1 in early T cell development: Lyt2- L3T4- thymocytes bind and respond in vitro to recombinant IL-1. J Immunol 1986; 137:3195.
10. Kyewski BA. Seeding of thymic microenvironment defined by distinct thymocyte-stromal cell interactions is developmentally controlled. J Exp Med 1987; 166:520.
11. Shortman K, Vrenmec D, D'Amico A, Battye EF, Boyd DR. Nature of the thymocytes associated with dendritic cells and macrophages in thymic rosettes. Cell Immunol 1989; 119:85.
12. El Rouby S, Praz F, Halbwachs-Mecarelli L, Papiernik M. Thymic reticulum in mice. IV. The rosette formation between phagocytic cells of the thymic reticulum and cortical type thymocytes is mediated by complement receptor type III. J Immunol 1985; 134:3625.
13. Papiernik M, Nabarra B, Savino W, Pontoux C, Barbey S. Thymic reticulum in mice. II. Culture and characterization of non-epithelial phagocytic cells of the thymic reticulum: Their role in the syngeneic stimulation of thymic medullary lymphocytes. Eur J Immunol 1983; 13:147.

14. Papiernik M, Dombret S, Stephanos S, Wietserbin J. Control of Ia antigen expression on phagocytic cells of the thymic reticulum by interferon-gamma and prostaglandins. Eur J Immunol 1986; 16:296.
15. Rocha B, Lehuen A, Papiernik M. IL-2-dependent proliferation of thymic accessory cells. J Immunol 1988; 140:1076.
16. El Rouby S, Papiernik M. Con A response and interleukin 2 receptor expression of thymocytes rosetting with phagocytic cells of the thymic reticulum. Thymus 1987; 9:239.
17. Papiernik M, Penit C, El Rouby S. Control of prothymocyte proliferation by thymic accessory cells. Eur J Immunol 1987; 17:1303.
18. Fontecha AM, Alvarez A, Navarro R, Zapata A, Ardavin C. Rat thymic cultures: Morphological and phenotypical characterization. Immunology (in press).

127
Accessory Cells in Adenoids of Children with Otitis Media with Effusion

E. B. J. van Nieuwkerk, C. D. Richters, E. W. A. Kamperdijk, and S. van der Baan
Free University, Amsterdam, The Netherlands

INTRODUCTION

Otitis media with effusion (OME) is characterized by the presence of fluid in the middle ear without signs of an acute infection. It is a common disease among children and is the most frequent cause of hearing loss.

Although the exact pathogenesis of OME is still unclear, it has been suggested that the adenoid plays an important role in the pathogenesis of OME by functioning as a source of bacterial antigens owing to an inadequate handling of bacteria during upper respiratory tract infections (1–3). This inadequate handling of bacteria by the adenoid may lead to an inappropriate immune reaction, and so induce and/or maintain OME. Since it has been shown that nonlymphoid cells, i.e., dendritic cells (DCs) and macrophages, play a key role in the induction of immune responses against bacteria, we are interested in these cells.

In a previous study we showed that only very small numbers of DCs and macrophages are present in adenoids. Dendritic cells, the most potent antigen presenting cells, form less than 0.1% of the total cell population.

To study the role of these cells in the pathogenesis of OME, it is necessary to purify them from the adenoid cell suspensions.

In this chapter we describe a method to obtain enriched DC (and macrophage) fractions from adenoids of children with OME. These cells were identified using immunocytochemical and enzyme cytochemical, electron microscopy, and functional studies.

MATERIALS AND METHODS

Preparation of Different Cell Fractions

Suspensions of adenoids were made as described earlier (4). Removal of T lymphocytes from these suspensions was performed using a rosetting technique with AET-treated sheep erythrocytes. Erythrocyte rosette–positive (Er^+) and –negative (Er^-) fractions were obtained using a Ficoll-Paque gradient. The Er^- fraction was cultured for 24–48 hr in RPMI 1640, supplemented with 1 mM glutamine, penicillin (100 U/ml)–streptomycin (100 μg/ml), gentamycin (50 μg/ml), and 10% fetal calf serum (FCS) (heat inactivated for 30 min at 56°C). Culture was performed in Teflon beakers (2×10^6 cells/ml in 10 ml culture medium) to prevent monocyte/macrophage adherence. After culture, the Er^- fraction was washed in HBSS, resuspended, and brought at a concentration of 4×10^7 cells/ml in RPMI 1640 containing 10% FCS. The cells were layered over a continuous Percoll gradient and centrifuged at 3360 rpm for 25 min at 4°C. Hereafter a low-density (LD) and an high-density (HD) fraction were obtained.

The LD cells were subsequently panned for B lymphocytes using CD22 monoclonal antibody.

Immunocytochemistry and Enzymecytochemistry

Indirect immunoperoxidase procedures were carried out on cytocentrifuge preparations using standard methods. Enzyme cytochemistry for acid phosphatase (AP) was performed according to the method as described by Burnstone (5). Acid phosphatase staining was always preceded by major histocompatibility complex (MHC) class II immunoperoxidase staining.

Identification of Dendritic Cells

Dendritic cells were identified using criteria as described earlier: They have a dendritic configuration, are MHC class II positive, and show AP activity localized in a central spot in the vicinity of an eccentric localized nucleus (4).

Electronmicroscopy

Cells from the LD fractions were fixed in 1.5% glutaraldehyde in phosphate buffer (0.09 M, pH 7.4) at 4°C. After postfixation in 1% OSO_4 in 0.1 M cacodylate buffer for 1 h at 4°C, the cell suspensions were dehydrated and embedded in an Epon/Araldite mixture. Ultrathin sections were stained with lead citrate and uranyl acetate and examined in a Philips EM 301 electron microscope at 40 or 60 kV.

T-Cell Isolation from Peripheral Blood

For the functional analysis (mixed leukocyte reactions) of the different adenoid fractions, T cells were used from the blood of healthy persons as responder cells. Human blood was drawn by venipuncture into EDTA syringes and mononuclear peripheral blood cells were obtained by Ficoll-Paque centrifugation. These cells were adjusted to 5×10^6 cells/ml in culture medium and incubated at 37°C for 90 min in tissue culture–grade Petri dishes. The nonadherent cells were removed gently and subsequently panned for B lymphocytes using CD22 monoclonal antibody. Purification of the T cells was more than 99%.

Allogeneic Mixed Leukocyte Reaction

Allogeneic purified peripheral blood T lymphocytes (5×10^4) were cocultured with the different fractions (which were irradiated with 3000 rad) in 200 μl RPMI 1640 supplemented with 10% inactivated FCS, 1 mM glutamine, 100 U/ml penicillin, 100 μg/ml streptomycin, and 5×10^{-5} M 2-mercaptoethanol. The irradiated cells, stimulated with allogeneic T lymphocytes were cultured for 6 days in 96-well microtiter plates at 37°C in a 5% CO_2 atmosphere. Sixteen hours before cell harvesting, tritiated thymidine (0.5 μCi/well) was added. Incorporation of the isotope was measured by means of a liquid scintillation counter and expressed as mean counts per minute of triplicate cultures ± standard deviation.

RESULTS

Immunocytochemistry and Enzyme Cytochemistry of Cytocentrifuge Preparations

Using enzyme cytochemistry and immunocytochemistry, it was possible to identify both DCs and macrophages. The DCs were identified as described previously (see under Materials and Methods). They were positive for HLA-DR as well as HLA-DP and HLA-DQ. They contained an eccentric localized and often lobulated nucleus. The nucleo-cytoplasmic ratio ranged from 1:1 to 1:3 (Fig. 1). In contrast, macrophages showed AP activity in small granules which were randomly spread throughout the cytoplasm. About 50% of these cells were HLA-DR positive, whereas only a minority of these cells expressed HLA-DP or HLA-DQ antigens. The nucleocytoplasmic ratio ranged from 1:1 to 1:4. The distribution of these accessory cells (DCs and macrophages) in the different fractions are shown in Table 1.

Functional Properties of the Different Fractions

As shown in Table 2, cells with accessory capacity as measured in a mixed lymphocyte reaction (MLR) were predominantly present in the LD B-negative fraction. It appeared that these responses depended on the concentration of stimulator cells. Higher numbers of LD

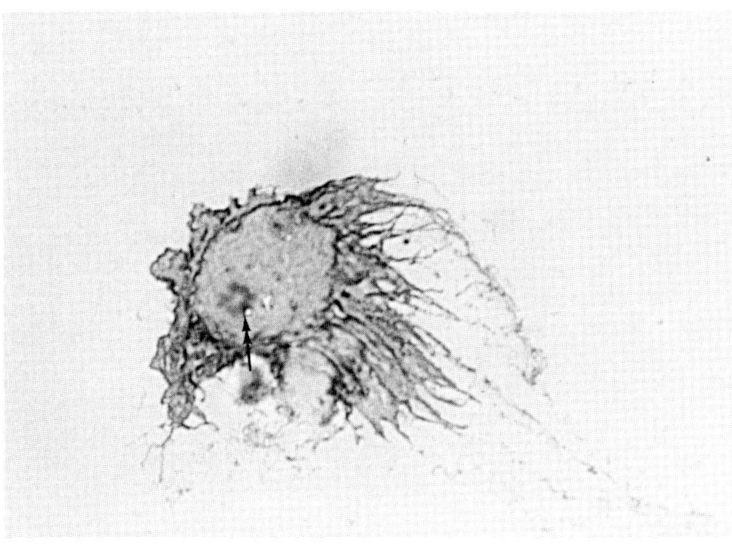

Figure 1 DC with AP localized in a spot (arrow), MHC class II positive, and cytoplasmatic extensions.

Table 1 Percentages of Macrophages and DCs as Determined by AP Pattern, MHC Class II Positivity, and Morphology

	Macrophages (%)	DCs (%)	No. of experiments
Unfract.	<1	<0.1	54
HD	<0.5	0.5–1	5
LD	1–4	4–14	5

cells corresponded with higher MLR responses. The responses could be blocked by anti HLA-DR/DQ monoclonal antibodies (MAbs) (data not shown). The HD fraction showed only minor stimulatory responses. It appeared that this HD fraction only contained B lymphocytes.

Electronmicroscopy

The LD fraction contained relative high numbers of cells with the ultrastructural characteristics of DCs (Fig. 2). They showed an irregular plasma membrane with smooth folds or veils. The nucleus had an eccentric position and was reniform with many identations. In some cells, (phago)lysosomes could be observed. They often contained one or more vacuoles; however, distinct signs of phagocytosis were not observed.

DISCUSSION

In this investigation, a new method is described to obtain a LD fraction containing high numbers of DCs (4–14%). These cells were characterized by (ultrastructural) morphology, enzyme cytochemistry, immunocytochemistry, and functional studies.

The percentages of DCs present in the LD fraction are comparable with percentages found in studies in which DCs were isolated from human tonsils using density gradients and FACS separation (5).

Table 2 Allogeneic T-Cell Responses[a] Induced by Fractionated Adenoid Cells[b]

Fraction	Allogeneic T cells	No T cells
Unfract.	390 ± 219	269 ± 47
Er^-	826 ± 267	662 ± 418
HD	439 ± 224	321 ± 123
LD	445 ± 117	363 ± 223
LD/B^-	39.764 ± 9960	919 ± 715

[a]Mean values (of representative experiment) of triplicate cultures are expressed as cpm ± SD.
[b]Five thousand cells of each fraction were cocultured with 50,000 T cells for 6 days. Sixteen hours before harvesting [^{3}H]thymidine was added.

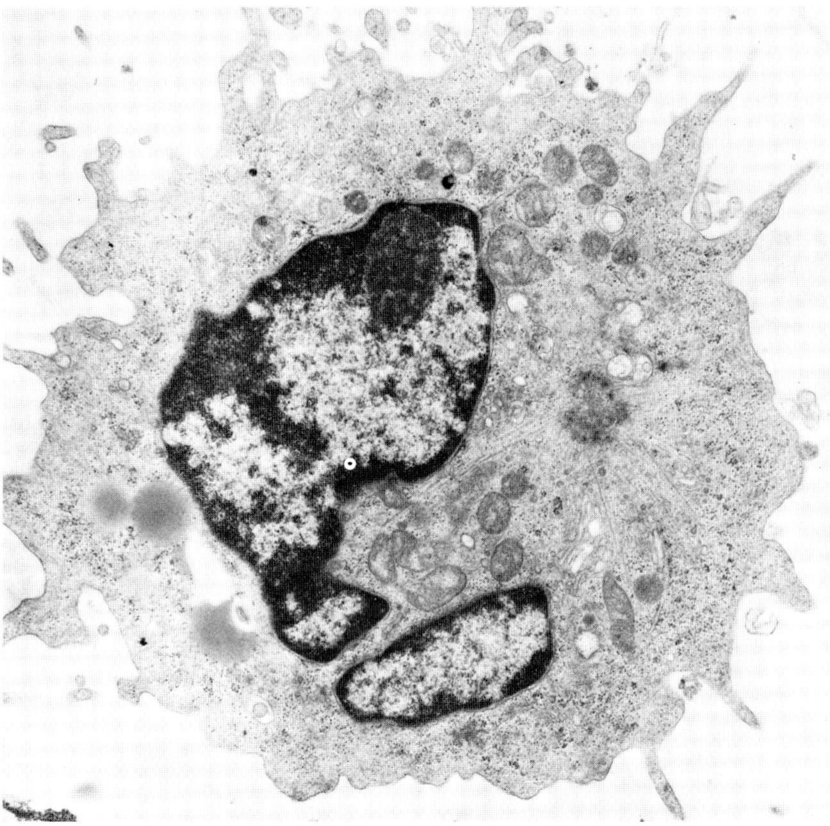

Figure 2 Ultrastructure of DC from LD fraction. The cell has an irregular outline and the nucleus is eccentrically localized.

In the literature, several studies are presented in which a much higher percentage of DCs, purified from human lymphoid organs, was claimed (6,7). However, it cannot be excluded that these fractions were contaminated with B lymphocytes, since these cells can assume a dendritic morphology in culture by which they are also MHC class II positive (8). This would mean that morphology and MHC class II positivity are not conclusive for the detection of DCs. For that reason, besides these criteria, we also used the characteristic AP spot in the vicinity of the nucleus of these cells. Moreover, we also used functional criteria (MLR responses).

Investigations are in progress to further clarify the functional properties of DCs and macrophages in OME.

ACKNOWLEDGMENTS

We thank Mr. S. Paniry for photographical and Mrs. M. Verdaasdonk for technical assistance.

REFERENCES

1. Bluestone CD Eustachian tube function, physiology, pathophysiology, and role of allergy in the pathogenesis of otitis media J Allergy Clin Immunol 1983; 72:242–7.
2. Gates GA, Avery CA, Prihoda TJ Effect of adenoidectomy upon children with chronic otitis media with effusion Laryngoscope 1988; 98:58–63.
3. Sprinkle PM, Veltri RW Pathophysiology of serious otitis media Am J Otol 1986; 7:113–8.
4. Van Nieuwkerk EBJ, De Wolf CJM, Kamperdijk EWA, Van der Baan S Lymphoid and non-lymphoid cells in the adenoid of children with otitis media with effusion: a comparative study Clin Exp Immunol 1990; 79:233–9.
5. Hart DNJ, McKenzie JL Isolation and characterization of human tonsil dendritic cells J Exp Med 1988; 168:157–70.
6. King PhD, Katz DR Human tonsillar dendritic cell induced T-cell responses: analysis of molecular mechanisms using monoclonal antibodies Eur J Immunol 1989; 19:581–7.
7. Le J, Yao JS, Knowles DM, Vilcek J Accessory function of thymic and tonsillar dendritic cells in interferon gamma production by T lymphocytes Lymphokine Res 1986; 5:205–13.
8. Corradi MP, Jelinek DF, Ramberg JE, Lipsky PE Development of a cell with dendritic morphology from a precursor of B lymphocyte lineage J Immunol 1987; 138:2075–81.

128
Dendritic Cell Function in Patients with Recurrent Upper Airway Infections

R. A. Scheeren,[1] E. W. A. Kamperdijk,[2] E. C. M. Hoefsmit,[2] S. T. Pals,[1] C. J. L. M. Meijer,[1] H. A. Drexhage,[3] and S. van der Baan[1]

[1]*Free University Hospital, Amsterdam, The Netherlands;*
[2]*Free University, Amsterdam, The Netherlands;*
[3]*Erasmus University, Rotterdam, The Netherlands*

INTRODUCTION

Sixty percent of patients with therapy-resistant chronic purulent rhinosinusitis have defects in their cell-mediated immunity (i.e., decreased monocyte polarization, defective delayed-type hypersensitivity [DTH] skin test reactivity, defective macrophage inhibitory factor [MIF] production upon certain antigen stimuli). These defects might be explained by the presence of a retroviral-like (p15E-like) low molecular weight factor (LMWF) in their serum (1).

Dendritic cells (DCs), the antigen-presenting cells par excellence, are important in the initiation of the immune response. Physical association between T lymphocytes and DCs is an early event in antigen presentation. This association can be measured in the cluster assay.

In this study, we examined the clustering properties of DCs isolated from the peripheral blood of three different patient groups with recurrent upper airway infections; i.e., chronic purulent rhinosinusitis, polyposis nasi, and primary ciliary dyskinesia. In addition, we investigated the influence of p15E-like serum factors on the DC–T-cell clustering.

MATERIAL AND METHODS

Patients

Chronic Purulent Rhinosinusitis (CPR)

Twenty-six patients (16 female, 10 male; mean age 32 years; range 7–71) with therapy-resistant rhinosinusitis not responding to adequate antibiotic treatment or surgical procedures and without nasal polyps present at endoscopic examination.

Polyposis Nasi (PPN)

Fourteen patients (seven female, 7 male; mean age 37 years; range 16–52) with recurrent upper airway infections and the presence of nasal polyps at the moment of surgery or endoscopic examination.

Primary Ciliary Dyskinesia (PCD)

Six patients (two female, four male; mean age 20 years; range 6–42) with evident primary ciliary dyskinesia based on abnormal ciliary motility (2) and abnormal ciliary ultrastructure (3).

Controls

Twenty-four healthy persons (nine female, 15 male; mean age 29; range 25–41) without known diseases.

DC Isolation

Dendritic cells were isolated according to Knight et al. (1986) (4). In brief, mononuclear cells were separated from heparinized blood via standard Ficoll gradients. From these mononuclear cells the adherent cells were removed on plastic for 90 min. The nonadherent cells were isolated using a 14.5% (w/v) hypertonic metrizamide gradient. The adherent cells and the pellet cells from the metrizamide gradient were incubated for a further 16 hr on plastic (37°C 5% CO_2). From the newly nonadherent populations the cells were again isolated on metrizamide. All low-density populations were pooled and these contained 60–80% with a dendritic morphology.

Cluster Assay

In this assay 50×10^3 (low-density) DCs were allowed to cluster (4 hr, 37°C, 5% CO_2) with 5×10^3 allogeneic lymphocytes (isolated via Ficoll gradients centrifugation of heparinized blood) in 250 μl flat-bottomed wells. Clusters (aggregates of more than five cells) were counted using an inverted microscope and expressed as the number of clusters per six microscopic fields, magnification ×200.

Retroviral-like Serum Factors

Serum fractions of molecular weight <25 kD were obtained by Amicon ultrafiltration. The capability of the serum fractions to inhibit the cluster capacity of normal DCs was determined by incubating DCs of healthy donors with allogeneic lymphocytes in the presence of these serum fractions from the three groups of patients. Control serum fractions were obtained from healthy individuals. To establish the p15E-like character of the serum fractions, adsorption experiments were carried out with a p15E-specific monoclonal antibody (MAb) (19F8) (5). Adsorbed serum fractions were next tested in the cluster assay using DCs of healthy individuals.

RESULTS

The clustering of DCs of patients with allogeneic lymphocytes was significantly ($p < 0.001$) reduced as compared to that of DCs of healthy controls (Fig. 1). This reduction was apparently independent of the underlying disease, since it was about equally strong in

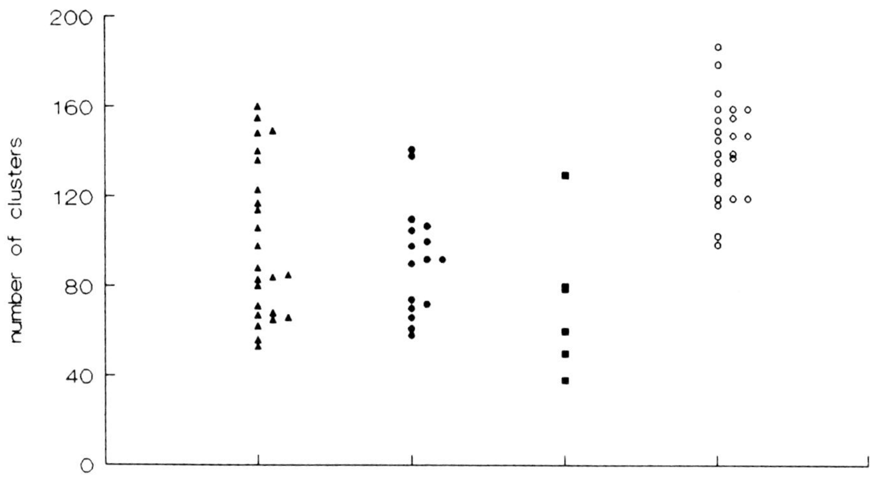

Figure 1 DC-lymphocyte clustering in patients with chronic purulent rhinosinusitis (▲), polyposis nasi (●), primary ciliary dyskinesia (■), and healthy controls (O). The number of clusters was counted using an inverted microscope, per six microscopic fields (magnification: ×200).

patients with chronic purulent rhinosinusitis (CPR), polyposis nasi (PPN), and primary ciliary dyskinesia (PCD).

Next, the influence of p15E-like LMWFs on the DC–T-cell clustering was investigated. Dendritic cells of healthy donors were incubated with allogeneic lymphocytes and LMWFs of patients, of healthy individuals or with medium. The LMWFs of all three patient groups caused a clear inhibition of the clustering capacity of DCs of healthy donors (CPR: 43% ± 6 inhibition; PPN: 40% ± 17 inhibition; PCD: 50% ± 6 inhibition). A significant difference ($p < 0.001$) with the influence of LMWFs of healthy donors on DCs, 9% ± 6 inhibition, was found (Fig. 2).

To establish the p15E-like character of the LMWFs, adsorption experiments were carried out (Fig. 3). The LMWFs of patients incubated with MAb anti-p15E (19F8, Cianciolo) showed a significantly decreased inhibitory capacity alone, 46% ± 7 inhibition or control MAb, 50% ± 6 inhibition.

DISCUSSION

Our findings show a decreased clustering capacity of blood DCs of patients with recurrent upper airway infections; i.e., chronic purulent rhinosinusitis, polyposis nasi, and primary ciliary dyskinesia. The influence of the p15E-like LMWFs, present in the patients' sera, on DC function (and the earlier reported influence on monocyte function [1]) suggest that these factors play a role in the immune defects in patients with recurrent upper airway infections. These retroviral-like factors might be of exogenous origin or might be endogenous products; i.e., immune-regulating peptides sharing structural homology with p15E. Studies to elucidate the mechanism via which p15E-like factors interact with the immune system to cause immune suppression, i.e., inhibition of clustering, are presently in progress.

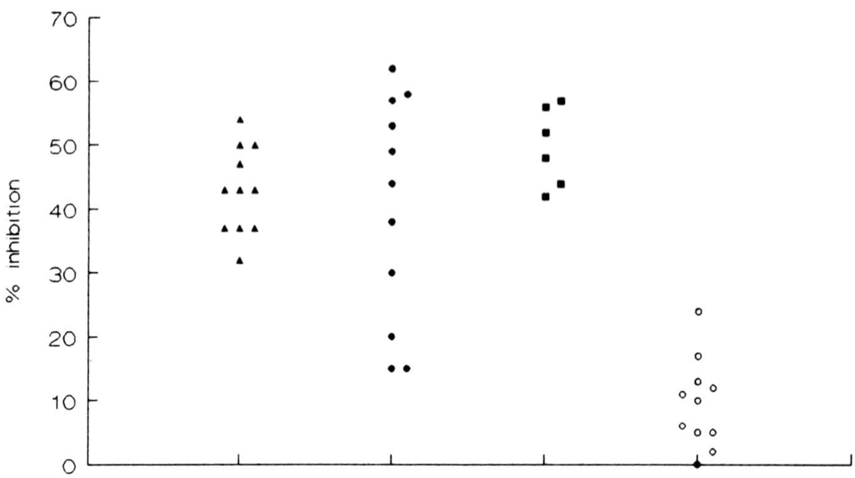

Figure 2 Inhibition of the clustering capacity of dendritic cells of healthy donors by LMWFs in the sera of patients with recurrent upper airway infections (chronic purulent rhinosinusitis (▲) n=11, polyposis nasi (●) n=11, primary ciliary dyskinesia (■) n=6, healthy controls (O) n=11. Dendritic cells were incubated with allogeneic lymphocytes in combination with the serum fractions. Results are expressed as % inhibition of the clustering of healthy donor DCs.

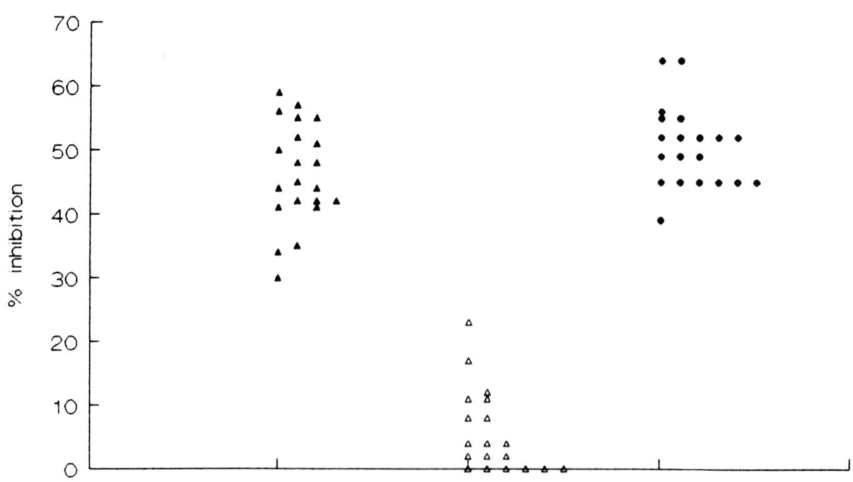

Figure 3 The p15E-like character of the low molecular weight serum factors. Serum fractions of patients diluted in medium (▲), and serum fractions after adsorption with the MAb anti-p15E (19F8) (Δ) and the control MAb antihuman immunoglobulin G (●) were tested. Results are expressed as % inhibition of the clustering of healthy donor DCs.

REFERENCES

1. Plassche-Boers EM van de, Tas M, Haan-Meulman M de, Kleingeld M, Drexhage HA. Abnormal monocyte chemotaxis in patients with chronic purulent rhinosinusitis: An effect of retroviral p15E-related factors in serum. Clin Exp Immunol 1988; 73:348–354.
2. Baan S van der, Veerman AJP, Wulffraat N, Feenstra L. Primary ciliary dyskinesia and ciliary activity. Acta Otolaryngol 1986; 102:274–281.
3. Baan S van der, Bezemer PD, Veerman AJP, Feenstra L. Primary ciliary dyskinesia. A quantitative investigation of the ciliary ultrastructure with statistical analysis. Ann Otol Laryngol 1987; 96:264–272.
4. Knight SC, Farrang J, Bryant A, Edwards AJ, Burman S, Lever A, Clarke J, Webster ADB. Non-adherent, low-density cells from human peripheral blood contain dendritic cells and monocytes, both with veiled morphology. contain dendritic cells and monocytes, both with veiled morphology. Immunology 1986; 57:595–603.
5. Lostrom ME, Stone MR, Tam M, Neal Burnette W, Pinter A, Nowinski RC. Monoclonal antibodies against murine leukemia viruses: Identification of six antigenic determinants on the p15(E) and gp70 envelope proteins. Virology 1979; 98:336–350.

129
Ultrastructural Localization of Human Leukocyte Antigen Class II Molecules in Human Blood–Derived Dendritic Cells and Monocytes

J. M. S. Arkema, D. M. Broekhuis-Fluitsma, and E. C. M. Hoefsmit
Free University, Amsterdam, The Netherlands

INTRODUCTION

Antigen-presenting cells (APCs) such as macrophages, B cells, and dendritic cells (DCs) present antigen, after intracellular processing, to T cells in the context of class II molecules (1). In contrast to macrophages, DCs are constitutionally and strongly class II positive, lack Fc receptors, and show little or no phagocytosis. Dendritic cells are unique APCs, especially for primary immune responses and in the mixed lymphocyte reaction (MLR) (2,3). It is still unknown what makes DCs such excellent APCs.

We isolated DCs from human peripheral blood and characterized them functionally (allogeneic mixed lymphocyte reaction [MLR]) and phenotypically (light microscopy [LM]).

We then studied to what extent these DCs are capable of endocytosis. Second, we studied the intracellular distribution of class II molecules in DCs in comparison to monocytes using cryoimmunoelectron microscopy. The results are discussed below.

MATERIALS AND METHODS

Cell Isolation

A DC-enriched population of cells (nonadherent low-density cells [NALDCs] that are Fc receptor [FcR] negative) was isolated from buffy coats derived from 500 ml human peripheral blood by the method according to Knight et al. (4). Briefly, this method is based upon an overnight adherence step to deplete monocytes and to obtain nonadherent cells (NACs), and a 14.5% metrizamide density gradient to remove lymphocytes and to obtain nonadherent low-density cells (NALDCs). Additionally, we performed Fc panning on

Petri dishes coated with human immunoglobulin G (IgG) to remove the rest of FcR-positive monocytes.

Preparation of Bovine Serum Albumin–Gold Complexes

Bovine serum albumin–gold complexes with a diameter of about 40 nm were prepared according to Frens (6) using the citrate method.

Mixed Lymphocyte Reactions

Allogeneic mixed lymphocyte reactions were performed in 20-μl hanging drops according to O'Brien et al. (5). Stimulator cells were irradiated (2000 rad) and added to responder T lymphocytes derived from healthy donors.

Light Microscopy

To identify DCs on cytospin preparations, we used RFD1, a monoclonal antibody (MAb) that is supposed to be specific for dendritic cells (7), and the anti-HLA-DR/DQ MAb 9.3F10 (8).

Cytospin preparations of NALDCFcR$^-$ were stained with RFD1 and 9.3F10 in combination with acid phosphatase (AP) cytochemistry according to Kamperdijk et al. (9).

Electron Microscopy

To study the internalization of BSA-gold we incubated NALDCFcR$^-$ for 60 min at 4°C and 15 min at 37°C in the presence of the BSA-gold conjugate. The cells were then washed three times before fixation in 1.5% glutaraldehyde and processed for electron microscopy (EM).

To study intracellular class II localization NALDCFcR$^-$ and monocytes were fixed in paraformaldehyde-lysine-periodate (PLP) for about 1 hr, 20 min fixed in PLP+0.25% glutaraldehyde, and put back in PLP for 30 min. After two washes in phosphate-buffered saline (PBS), the cells were peletted in 10% gelatin, immersed in 2.3 M sucrose for at least 30 min, and rapid frozen in liquid nitrogen. Ultrathin cryosections were stained with 9.3F10 (sup., undil.) and GAM-IgG-gold (10 nm) (1/10) according to Tokuyasu (10) and embedded in methylcellulose before examining.

RESULTS

Mixed Lymphocyte Reactions

The allogeneic MLR (Table 1) showed that the capacity to stimulate allogeneic lymphocytes in the different cell fractions obtained during enrichment of DCs increases. So we may conclude that NALDCFcR$^-$ contain most DCs; i.e., about 10-fold more than NACs. Highest responses are found with NALDCFcR$^-$ in a stimulator:responder ratio of 1:40.

Light Microscopy

Dendritic cells are RFD1 and class II positive, have many cell processes, and show AP in a spot near the nucleus. NALDCFcR$^-$ contained 30–55% DCs.

Table 1 Allogeneic MLR-Stimulating Capacity of Different Cell Fractions Performed in 20-μl Hanging Drops: [^{3}H]Thymidine Incorporation (cpm)

	Number of allogeneic lymphocytes			
	0	20,000	40,000	80,000
0	11.8 (2.8)	48.3 (6.3)	53.2 (3.4)	18.8 (5.9)
NAC	46.8 (27.8)	55.0 (34.8)	180.0 (80.1)	178.2 (45.8)
NALDC	32.8 (11.0)	256.5 (83.0)	437.8 (126.4)	1060.2 (115.0)
NALDCFcR$^-$	49.2 (22.0)	405.8 (97.2)	1457.0 (293.6)	1382.3 (242.8)

Allogeneic stimulator cells are irradiated (2000 rad) NACs, NALDCs, and NALDCFcR$^-$. Means and standard errors of triplicate cultures are shown in parentheses.

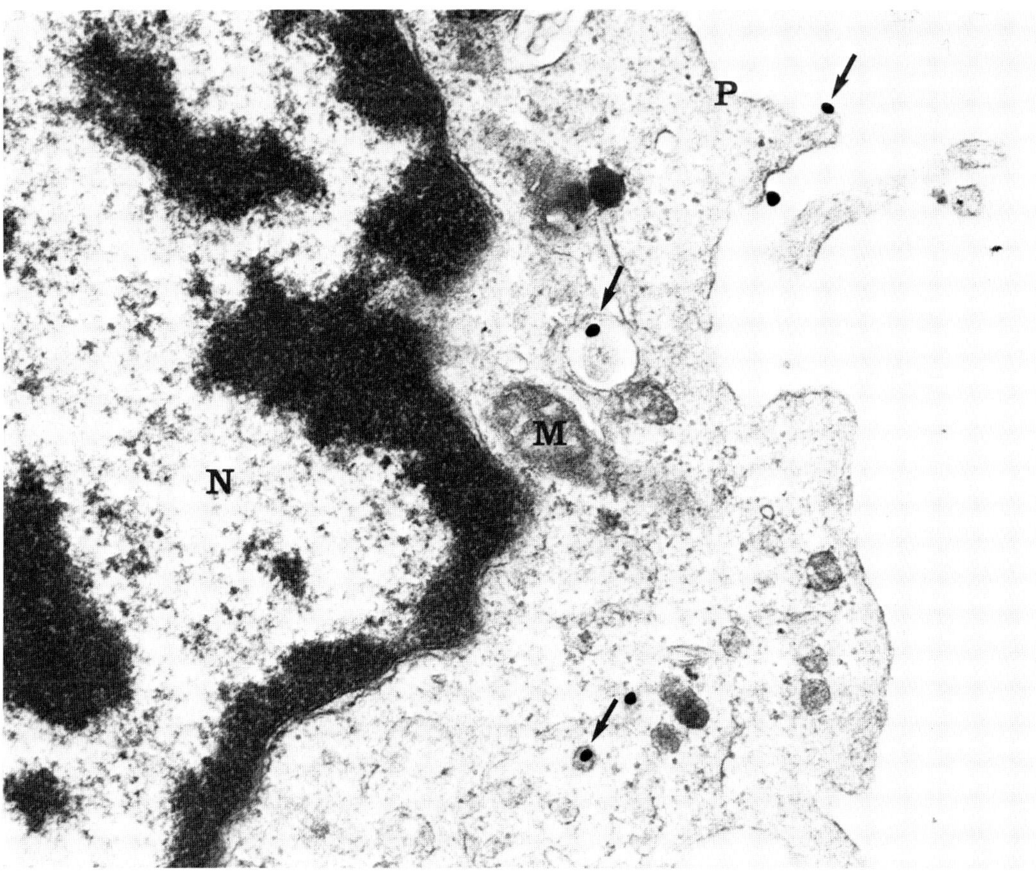

Figure 1 Dendritic cell incubated with the endocytotic marker BSA-gold (40 nm). A few gold particles are seen in vacuolar endosomes (arrows) and on the plasma membrane (P). N = nucleus, M = mitochrondrion (magnification: ×20,000).

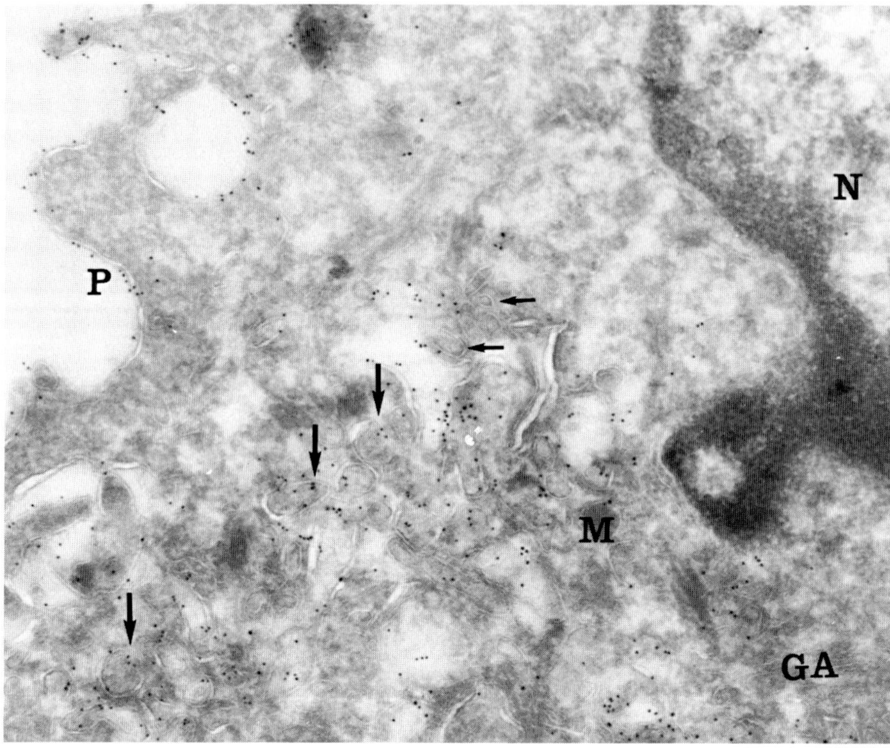

Figure 2 Ultrathin cryosection of a dendritic cell incubated with the anti–HLA-DR/DQ MAb 9.3F10 and GAM-IgG-gold (10 nm). The plasma membrane (P) and many intracellular vesicles are positive (large arrows). Nonlabeled vesicles are also present (small arrows). N = nucleus, M = mitochrondrion, GA = golgi apparatus (magnification: ×35,000).

Electron Microscopy

Endocytosis was studied using BSA-gold as an endocytotic marker. As shown in Figure 1, DCs show limited endocytosis. Ultrastructural cryoimmunoelectron microscopy revealed many class II–positive vesicles in the juxtanuclear area of DCs (Fig. 2). Mo, easily recognizable by the characteristic cytoplasmic granules (Fig. 3) showed little or no label for the anti–class II MAb.

DISCUSSION

We were able to enrich DCs for about 30–55% as shown by both functional and morphological criteria.

Our EM data lead us to the following considerations. The absolute level of endocytosis seems to be very low in comparison to monocytes/macrophages, cells that have phagocytic functions because they are mainly scavenger cells. So it is possible that endocytosis in DCs mainly plays a role in antigen processing.

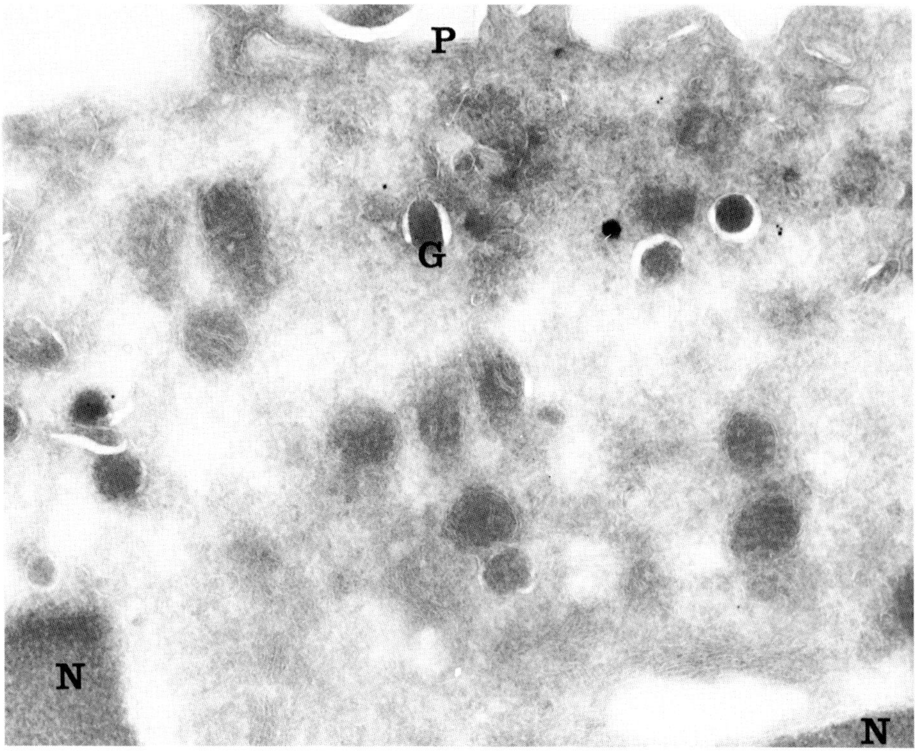

Figure 3 Ultrathin cryosection of a monocyte incubated with the anti–HLA-DR/DQ MAb 9.3F10 and GAM-IgG-gold (10 nm). No significant label is present. P = plasmamembrane, N = nucleus, G = cytoplasmic granule (magnification: ×40,000).

In this study, we were not yet able to determine whether class II–containing vesicles in juxtanuclear position belong either to the endocytotic or the biosynthetic route. Neefjes et al. (12) describes the intersection of biosynthetic (class II) and endocytotic route in B cells, so the presence of intracellular class II–containing vesicles in juxtanuclear position may play an important role in the processing of antigen. Rhodes et al. (11) also demonstrated the presence of antigen in this area, and we were able to demonstrate AP-containing vesicles in this area on the EM level (12).

CONCLUSIONS

Our results show that DCs endocytose BSA-gold and concentrate class II–containing vesicles and vesicles demonstrating APase activity in a juxtanuclear position. The interaction of these compartments may play a role during antigen processing.

REFERENCES

1. Unanue ER, Beller DI, Lu CY, Allen PM. Antigen presentation: comments on its regulation and mechanism. J. Immunol. 1984; 132:1–5.

2. Inaba K, Steinman RM. Accessory cell-T lymphocyte interactions. Antigen-dependent and -independent clustering. J. Exp. Med. 1986; 163:247–261.
3. Steinman RM, Nussenzweig M. Dendritic cells: Features and functions. Immunol. Rev. 1980; 53:127–147.
4. Knight SC, Farrant J, Bryant A, Edwards AJ, Burman S, Lever A, Clarke J, Webster ADB. Non-adherent, low-density cells from human peripheral blood contain dendritic cells and monocytes, both with veiled morphology. Immunology 1986; 57:595–603.
5. O'Brien JA, Knight SC, Quick NA, Moore AS, Platt AS. A simple technique for harvesting lymphocytes cultured in Terasaki plates. J. Immunol. Meth. 1979; 27:219–223.
6. Frens G. Controlled nucleation for the regulation of the particle size in monodisperse gold suspension. Nature 1973; 241:20–22.
7. Poulter LW, Campbell DA, Munro C, Janossy G. Discrimination of human macrophages and dendritic cells by means of monoclonal antibodies. Scand. J. Immunol. 1986; 24:351–357.
8. Van Voorhis WC, Steinman RM, Hair LS, Luban J, Witmer MD, Koide S, Cohn ZA. Specific anti-mononuclear phagocyte monoclonal antibodies: Application to the purification of dendritic cells and tissue localisation of macrophages. J. Exp. Med. 1983; 158:126–145.
9. Kamperdijk EWA, Kapsenberg ML, Van den Berg M, Hoefsmit ECM. Characterization of dendritic cells, isolated from normal and stimulated lymph nodes of the rat. Cell Tissue Res. 1985; 242:469–474.
10. Tokuyasu KT. *Cryosections for Immunohistochemistry*. Proc. XIth. Congr. EM, Kyoto, Japan, 1986, pp. 42–43.
11. Rhodes JM, Balfour BM, Blom BM, Agger A. Comparison of antigen uptake by peritoneal macrophages and veiled cells from the thoracic duct using isotype-, FITC-, or gold-labelled antigen. Immunology 1989; 68:403–409.
12. Arkema JMS, Schadee-Eestermans IL, Beelen RHJ, Hoefsmit ECM. A combined method for both endogenous myeloperoxidase and acid phosphatase cytochemistry as well as immunoperoxidase surface labelling discriminating human peripheral blood derived dendritic cells and monocytes. Histochemistry 1991 (in press).
13. Neefjes JJ, Stollorz V, Peters PJ, Geuze HJ, Ploegh HL. The biosynthetic pathway of MHC class II but not class I molecules intersects the endocytic route. Cell 1990; 61:171–183.

130
Antigen-Presenting Cells in Bronchoalveolar Lavages of Rats Intratracheally Inoculated with Bacillus Calmette-Guérin

C. E. G. Havenith, A. J. Breedijk, and E. C. M. Hoefsmit
Vrije University, Amsterdam, The Netherlands

INTRODUCTION

It has been shown that dendritic cells (DCs) are potent antigen-presenting cells which probably play a key role in primary immune responses (1). In normal lungs of the rat and mouse and also in the human lung, DCs can be found in airway epithelium, lung parenchyma, and visceral pleura (2–4). Alveolar macrophages (AMs) express a limited antigen-presenting capacity, depending on the species, and in some circumstances appear to suppress T-cell stimulation actively (5). It has been postulated that the interaction between Ia-positive antigen-presenting DCs and endogenous tissue macrophages play an important role in regulating T-cell activity in the respiratory tract (4,6,7).

Intravenous administration of bacillus Calmette-Guérin (BCG) to previously primed animals induced an increase of Ia-positive cells in the bronchoalveolar lavage (BAL) (8). Recently, we found that intraperitoneal administration of BCG to unprimed rats caused an increase of nonlymphoid mononuclear cells in the peritoneal fluid within 24 hr after administration. Dendritic cells, morphologically identified as Ia-positive cells with an acid phosphatase (AP) spot in the vicinity of the nucleus and dendritic processes, were present (9–11).

This study was undertaken to induce a change in the nonlymphoid mononuclear cells in the BAL in favor of potent antigen-presenting DCs. To cause this change we induced a nonspecific exudate in the lung by intratracheal inoculation of the BCG and tested the function of these BAL cells in vitro.

MATERIALS AND METHODS

Animals

Random bred male Wistar rats and inbred male ACI/Mal rats, weighing 180–200 g, were used. The animals were obtained from Centraal Proefdierenbedrijf (TNO, Zeist, The Netherlands). They were kept in Makrolon cages and allowed food and water ad libitum.

Immunization Procedures

Rats, lightly anesthetized with Hypnorm 0.1 ml intramuscularly, were intratracheally inoculated with 0.1 ml BCG suspension (kindly provided by Dr. P. A. Steerenberg, RIVM, The Netherlands).

Rats were immunized in both hind footpads with 50 μg of the copolymer glutamine tyrosine (GT) emulsified in Freund's complete adjuvant.

Cell Preparation

Free alveolar cells (BAL cells) were collected by repeated endobronchial lavage, as described by Holt (12). The BAL cells were separated into 5 density fractions on Percoll (1.062, 1.076, 1.083, 1.090, and ≥1.097 g/ml; Pharmacia Fine Chemicals, Sweden).

Pure DCs were isolated from the spleen according to the method of Knight et al. (13).

Isolation of T-cell–enriched lymph node cells (LNCs) of GT-primed rats 2 weeks after immunization was performed following a three-step procedure (adherence, nylon wool, and Sephadex G10). These LNCs were used as responder cells in the GT-primed proliferation assay.

Staining Procedures

Detection of antigens on cytocentrifuge preparations of BAL cells was done by an indirect immunoperoxidase method. Used were the monoclonal antibodies (MAbs) OX6 (αIa), His14 (B cells), OX19 and OX52 (T cells). Acid phosphatase activity was demonstrated according to Burstone (14).

Double staining of Ia antigens and AP was performed according to Duijvestijn et al. (9).

GT-Primed Proliferation Assay

Responder cells (2×10^5 cells/well) were plated into 96-well culture plates (culture medium: RPMI 1640, 10% heat-inactivated fetal calf serum [FCS], 20 mM L-glutamine, penicillin 50 U/ml, streptomycin 50 μg/ml, and 50 μM β-mercaptoethanol). GT was added at a final concentration of 100 μg/ml.

Different density fractions of BAL cells of control rats and of rats 48 hr after BCG were used as stimulator cells. They were irradiated with 3000 rad (^{60}Co) and added to the T cells in triplicate, into a final volume of 200 μl. The responses were compared with pure DCs isolated from the spleen used as stimulator cells.

The cultures were incubated for 3 days at 37°C in a humidified atmosphere of 5% CO_2 in air. Added was 1 μCi of [^{3}H]thymidine ([^{3}H]TdR), and the amount of [^{3}H]TdR uptake was determined 18 hr later using a cell harvester and liquid scintillation counter.

Table 1 Cell Yields and Cellular Composition of BAL After Intratracheal Inoculation of BCG

Hr after BCG	Cell yield ($\times 10^6$)	Different cell populations ($\times 10^6$)			
		Macrophages	Monocytes	Lymphocytes	Neutrophils
0	0.7	0.66	—	0.04	—
12	2.1	1.85	0.04	0.08	0.12
24	3.3	2.31	0.10	0.20	0.60
48	3.7	1.30	0.30	0.90	1.20

Mean absolute numbers are shown, derived from three Wistar rats.

RESULTS AND DISCUSSION

Induction of a Nonspecific Exudate in the Lung Using BCG

Intratracheal inoculation of BCG induced an increase in the absolute number of BAL cells recovered. The number of BAL cells 48 hr after inoculation was 5.3 times higher in comparison to normal control rats (Table 1). All the different cell populations, AMs, monocytes, lymphocytes, and neutrophils showed increasing absolute numbers in time after BCG (Table 1).

Rat AMs were morphologically characterized and are Ia-negative and have AP activity throughout the whole cytoplasm. Dendritic cells were defined as being Ia positive, having AP activity in a central spot in the vicinity of an eccentrically localized nucleus, and having dendritic processes. Monocytes have an eccentrically localized bean-shaped nucleus and hardly any AP activity in the cytoplasm (either Ia negative or positive).

Ia-positive monocytes and DCs (nonlymphoid mononuclear cells) were found in BAL of control rats, but in a very low percentage. After BCG, a sharp rise in the percentage of Ia-positive monocytes and DCs up to 7.5% at 48 hr after BCG was found (Table 2). Dendritic cells and DC precursors, with morphological features of both monocytes and large, mature DCs, were present (Fig. 1).

These results indicate that a change in the nonlymphoid mononuclear cells in favor of morphologically defined DCs can be induced. These cells were morphologically similar to those of the family of DCs (Langerhans' cells, veiled cells, and interdigitating cells), which are known to have potent antigen-presenting capacity (1,10). Also, morphologically described DC precursors were found, suggesting that maturation to DCs appears at the site of the exudate.

Table 2 Ia-Positive Cells in the BAL After Intratracheal Inoculation of BCG

HR after BCG	Ia^+ lymphoid cells	Ia+ nonlymphoid cells	Ia+/AP nonlymphoid cells
0	2.0%	<0.3%	<0.3%
12	0.7%	1.3%	<0.3%
24	1.6%	2.4%	0.5%
48	6.5%	7.5%	1.4%

Mean percentages are shown, derived from three Wistar rats.

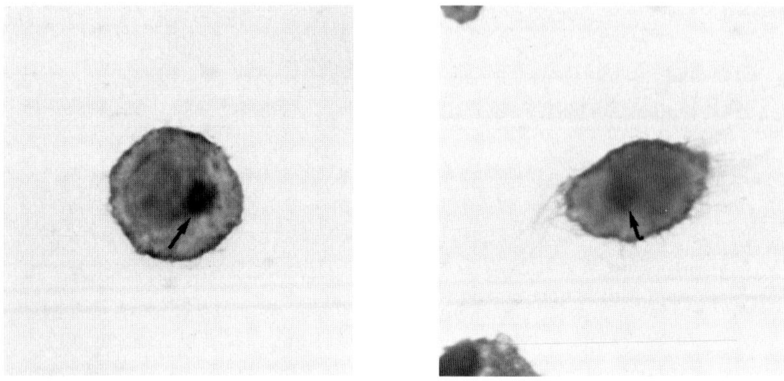

(a) (b)

Figure 1 Cytocentrifuge preparation of BAL 48 hr after intratracheal inoculation of BCG showing DC precursors: AP activity (arrow) in a central spot in the vicinity of an eccentrically localized nucleus and Ia-positive dark staining of the membrane.

Cell Composition of Density Fractions of BAL Cells

Figure 2 shows the percentage of Ia-positive monocytes (Mos) and DCs in the different density fractions of the BAL 48 hr after BCG. Also is given the ratio of Ia-positive monocytes and DCs (precursors included) to Ia-negative AMs. All the fractions contain more than 5% Ia-positive monocytes and DCs, going up to 43% in fraction 3. All the fractions of the normal rats contained less than 2% Ia-positive monocytes and DCs and the ratio of Ia-positive monocytes and DCs to Ia-negative AMs was smaller than 0.04 (data not shown).

A good purification of Ia-positive monocytes and DCs could be achieved by using a density gradient. Normally, adhesion and Fc rosetting or panning steps are used to purify DCs from blood and organs (1). However, with our method, without incubations steps at 37°C, we could obtain monocytes, DC precursors and more mature DCs.

Antigen-Presenting Capacity of Fractionated BAL Cells in Comparison to Pure DCs

Pure DCs isolated from the spleen of normal rats gave a high uptake of $[^3H]$TdR by GT-primed LNCs, up to 86.7×10^3 cpm if 2×10^3 cells were added. The LNCs (2×10^5 cells) gave background levels of incorporation of 3×10^3 cpm.

Addition of 8×10^4 BAL cells of the different fractions 48 hr after BCG gave low responses, except for fraction 5, which gave a considerable response (Fig. 3a). Although in fraction 5 the percentage of DCs is relatively low, the percentage of AMs is about 0.5%, which is at least a factor 16 less than in the other fractions (see Fig. 2).

If 2×10^4 BAL cells were added, fractions 1–4 gave moderate to high incorporation of $[^3H]$TdR and high responses for fraction 5 (Fig. 3b). Fractionated BAL cells of control animals, with mainly AMs, gave low responses in both concentrations (data not shown).

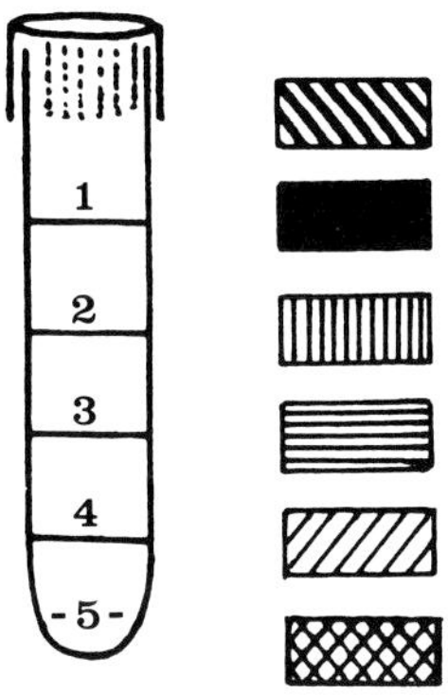

FRACTION	DENSITY (g/ml)	PERC. of Ia^+Mo/DC (%)	RATIO of $Ia^+Mo/DC : Ia^-AM$
	unfract.	15	0.83
	1.062	5	0.07
	1.076	13	0.18
	1.083	43	2.00
	1.090	27	3.33
	⩾1.097	5	10.00

Figure 2 Characteristics of density fractions of BAL cells 48 hr after BCG. BAL cells of 5 ACI/Mal rats were pooled and separated into fractions 1–5 as described in Materials and Methods.

Thus, DCs are present in all fractions of the BAL 48 hr after BCG and are capable of stimulating the response. The slightly higher response of fraction 5 and the higher responses of the other fractions at lower concentrations may indicate that the number of DCs does not limit the response, but AMs suppress the response. This is underlined by coculture of fractionated BAL cells with pure DCs which gave similar responses in both concentrations as BAL cells alone (Fig. 3c,d).

CONCLUSIONS

Fractions of BAL cells 48 hr after BCG, containing morphologically defined Ia-positive monocytes and DCs, are capable of in vitro antigen presentation to primed T cells. In agreement with the literature (5), the data also suggest that AMs are suppressive, and even suppress the T-cell responses to pure DCs of the spleen, which give maximal responses.

The balance between Ia-positive antigen-presenting DCs and AMs will play an important role in regulating T cells in the lower respiratory tract.

ACKNOWLEDGMENTS

This work was supported by a research grant from the Nederlands Astma Fonds. The authors thank Mr. S. Paniry for preparing the photographs.

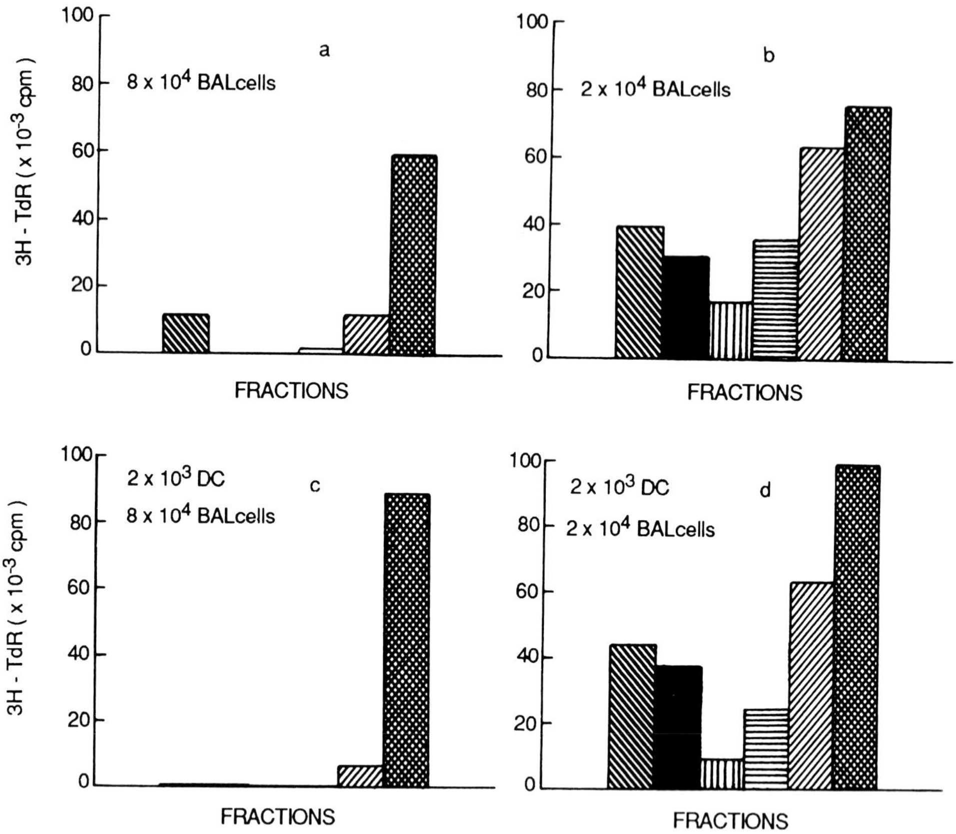

Figure 3 Antigen-presenting capacity of fractionated BAL cells 48 hr after BCG in comparison to pure DCs of the spleen. Data shown are mean uptake or $[^3H]$TdR from triplicate cultures. Cultures comprised 2×10^5 enriched GT-primed T cells, cocultured with 20 μg/ml GT and stimulator cells as follows: (a) 8×10^4 fractionated BAL cells per well; (b) 2×10^4 fractionated BAL cells per well; (c) 8×10^4 fractionated BAL cells and 2×10^3 pure spleen DCs per well; (d) 2×10^4 fractionated BAL cells and 2×10^3 pure spleen DCs per well; characteristics of the fractions and explanation of the bars are given in Figure 2.

REFERENCES

1. Steinman RM. Inaba K. Stimulation of the primary mixed leukocyte reaction. CRC Crit Rev Immunol 1985; 5:331–348.
2. Sertl K. Takemura T. Tschachler E. Ferrans VJ. Kaliner MA. Shevach EM. Dendritic cells with antigen-presenting capability reside in airway epithelium, lung parenchyma, and visceral pleura. J Exp Med 1986; 163:436–451.
3. Simecka JW. Davis JK. Cassell GH. Distribution of Ia antigens and T lymphocyte subpopulations in rat lungs. Immunology 1986; 57:93–98.
4. Holt PG. Schon-Hegrad MA. Oliver J. MHC class II antigen-bearing dendritic cells in pulmonary tissue of the rat. J Exp Med 1988; 167:262–274.
5. Holt PG. Down-regulation of immune responses of the lower respiratory tract: the role of alveolar macrophages. Clin Exp Immunol 1986; 63:261–270.

6. Rochester CL. Goodell EM. Stoltenborg JK. Bowers WE. Dendritic cells from rat lung are potent accessory cells. Am Rev Respir Dis 1988; 138:121–128.
7. Kradin RL. McCarthy KM. Gifford J. Schneeberger EE. Antigen-independent binding of T-cells by dendritic cells and alveolar macrophages in the rat. Am Rev Respir Dis 1989; 139:207–211.
8. Fuchs HJ. McDowell J, Shellito JE. Use of allophycocyanin allows quantitative description by flow cytometry of alveolar macrophage surface antigens present in low numbers of cells. Am Rev Respir Dis 1988; 138:1124–1126.
9. Duijvestijn AM. Schutte R. Köhler YG. Korn C. Hoefsmit ECM. Characterization of the population of phagocytic cells in thymic cell suspensions. A morphological and cytochemical study. Cell Tissue Res 1983; 231:313–323.
10. Kamperdijk EWA. Kapsenberg ML. van den Berg M. Hoefsmit ECM. Characterization of dendritic cells, isolated from normal and stimulated lymph nodes of the rat. Cell Tissue Res 1985; 242:469–474.
11. Kamperdijk EWA. Vugt van E. Verdaasdonk MAM. Beelen RHJ. Induction of dendritic cells in rat peritoneal cavity after Bacillus Calmette-Guérin (in press).
12. Holt PG. Alveolar macrophages. I. Simple technique for the preparation of high numbers of viable alveolar macrophages from small laboratory animals. J Immunol Methods 1979; 27:189–198.
13. Knight SC. Farrant J. Bryant A. Edwards AJ. Burman S. Lever S. Clarke J. Webster ADB. Non-adherent, low-density cells from human peripheral blood contain dendritic cells and monocytes, both with veiled morphology. Immunology 1986; 57:595–603.
14. Pearse AGE. *Histochemistry. Theoretical and Applied.* Vol. 1. 3rd ed. Edinburgh, Churchill Livingstone, 1968.

131
Synovial Antigen-Presenting Cells Have Potent Accessory Cell Function

N. J. Viner, J. S. H. Gaston, and P. A. Bacon
University of Birmingham, Birmingham, England

INTRODUCTION

Evidence for a Cell-Mediated Immune Response in Inflammatory Arthritis

In rheumatoid arthritis (RA), the most common and, therefore, best-studied form of inflammatory arthritis, there are several lines of evidence to suggest that a cell-mediated immune (CMI) response plays a significant pathological role. Histological examination of inflamed synovium reveals an extensive mononuclear cell (MC) infiltrate. Activated CD4-positive helper T cells are abundant and are found in association with strongly HLA-DR–positive antigen-presenting cells (APCs), an appearance which has been likened to that found in lymph node paracortex (1). Additional evidence for the role of CMI activity is derived both from the success of therapies such as thoracic duct drainage (2) or total lymphoid irradiation (3) in ameliorating established RA and from the association of the disease with HLA-DR (4).

Studies of the antigenic specificity of T cells in RA have been hampered by the lack of good candidates for the putative antigen(s) responsible either for the initial triggering or for the persistence of RA. Analyses of synovial T-cell receptor usage, which would be expected to show restriction in response to a dominant antigen, have produced conflicting results (5). Interest has recently been focused on heat-shock proteins (HSPs) as possible antigens in RA, prompted by their highly conserved nature. We and others have found that synovial fluid (SF) MC proliferative responses to *Mycobacterium leprae* 65-kD HSP are greater than those of peripheral blood (PB) MCs (6,7), but the role of HSPs remains to be elucidated.

In contrast, in reactive arthritis (ReA), sterile joint inflammation follows a defined gastrointestinal or genitourinary infection. We and others have shown that SF MCs from ReA patients proliferate when cultured with ReA-associated bacteria, the maximal response being to the triggering organism (8,9). Interestingly, we have also found significant responses to ReA-associated bacteria in >50% of RA patients (8); the reason for this is not known, but may be due to recognition of bacterial HSPs.

Evidence for a Role for APCs in Inflammatory Arthritis

Exogenous antigens must first be processed into immunogenic peptides and then presented on the surface of APCs combined with HLA molecules before they can be recognized by specific T cells. The evidence that implicates T cells in the pathogenesis of inflammatory arthritis, therefore, also implicates APCs. There is additional evidence from certain animal models of arthritis that synovial macrophage influx and activation may be the earliest cellular events (10). In human inflammatory arthritis, investigation of the cellular composition of SF reveals increased numbers of dendritic cells (11). These are recognized as potent immunostimulatory APCs and are also responsible for the transport of antigen to lymph nodes in CMI responses (12).

In patients whose SF MCs respond strongly to ReA-associated bacteria as described above, the corresponding PB MC response is much reduced or absent (8,9). It could be suggested that this is due to an accumulation of antigen-specific T cells within the joint, a hypothesis consistent with phenotypic studies demonstrating increased numbers of primed $CD45RO^+$ T cells in inflamed joints compared to PB (13). However, we have shown that PB MC hyporesponsiveness is not due to a lack of circulating antigen-specific T cells; purified PB T cells, which fail to proliferate when PB non-T cells are used as APCs, mount significant responses when the same antigens are presented by autologous synovial non-T cells (14). This suggests that enhanced SF APC function may play a significant part in this apparent synovial polarization of MC response.

CURRENT STUDY—AIMS AND METHODS

We wished to investigate whether or not the contrast in SF and PB APC function observed in previous experiments would be restricted either to patients preselected for their SF MC responsiveness or to the presentation of ReA-associated bacteria.

Eleven consecutive patients with seropositive, erosive RA presenting for therapeutic knee aspiration were studied. Mononuclear cells were obtained from PB and hyaluronidase-treated SF by Ficoll separation and divided into T- and non-T cell–enriched populations by sheep red cell rosetting. Non-T cells were irradiated (3000 rad) and used as APCs; PB T cells were depleted of adherent cells by incubation on plastic for 60 min. Proliferation assays were set up in triplicate in 200 μl wells with 5×10^4 of the following cell populations or combinations: SF MCs, PB MCs, PB T alone, PB T + PB APCs, PB T + SF APCs. In the latter two cases, the T:APC ratio used was 10:1. Assays were performed in medium alone or with optimal doses of either heat-killed *Salmonella*, influenza virus, or recombinant *M. leprae* 65-kD HSP as previously described (8). [^{3}H]Thymidine uptake was measured at day 6.

RESULTS

Modest responses to each antigen were found when either PB MCs, PB T cells alone, or PB T + PB APCs were the responding populations. In contrast, a significant enhancement of PB T-cell response was observed when the antigens were presented by autologous SF APCs (Fig. 1b–d). Increased background proliferation of PB T + SF APCs in the absence

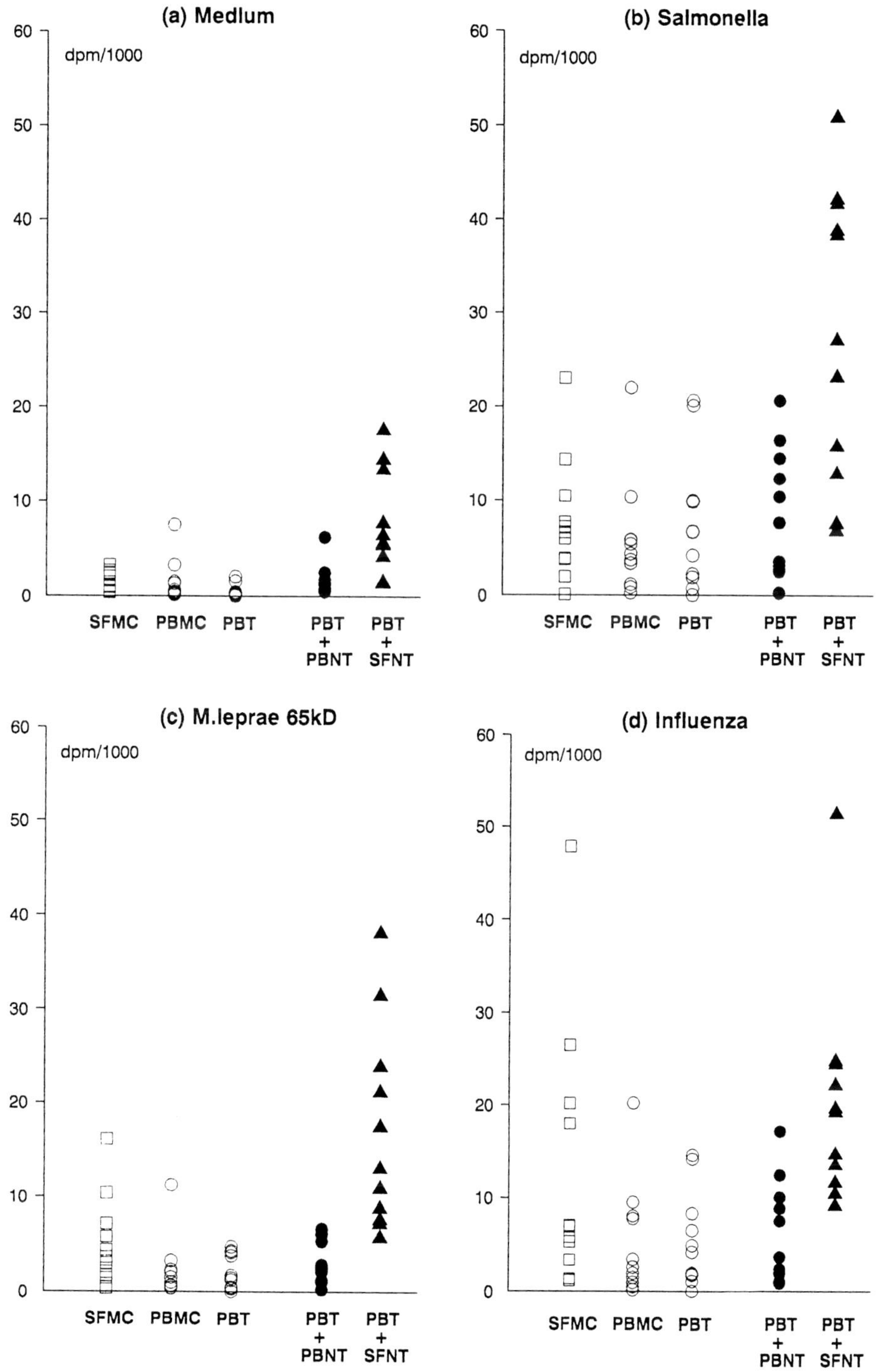

Figure 1 Responses to each antigen.

of antigen (Fig. 1a) was also observed, although this was by no means sufficient to account for the increased antigen-specific responses.

DISCUSSION

In this study, a direct comparison was made between the APC function of non-T cells derived from SF and PB of patients with RA. Markedly increased SF APC function relative to PB APCs was found for each antigen studied, demonstrating that this effect is not limited to patients with significant SF MC responses or to responses to ReA-associated bacteria. This disparity in APC function might have a qualitative or quantitative basis. Previous work in which T:APC ratios have been titrated over a wide range suggests that a numerical deficiency in a particular PB APC subset is an unlikely explanation (14), but does not completely exclude it. Although work is currently in progress to address this point, we would favor a qualitative basis for the observed results. It has been demonstrated in murine systems that in addition to an antigenic signal, an APCs must provide additional "co-stimulatory" signal(s) for T-cell activation (15), the nature of which are currently unknown. We speculate that SF APCs may have enhanced costimulatory activity compared to PB APCs which would be consistent with the activated phenotype of the former (16).

In the polyclonal T-cell responses in this study, there was an increased background proliferation to SF APCs in the absence of antigen. This might represent either recognition of xenoantigens introduced into the system (e.g., sheep red blood cells or fetal bovine serum) or an autologous mixed lymphocyte reaction. In the latter case, the naive $CD4/CD45RA^+$ T-cell subset would be expected to be the main responder population (17). Since this is also the main interleukin-2 (IL-2)–producing human T-cell subset (18), it is possible that such nonspecific T-cell activation could produce sufficient IL-2 to amplify an accompanying antigen-specific response; we are currently examining IL-2 production in the above assay system. The use of antigen-specific T-cell clones to standardize the responder population would circumvent these problems. In preliminary experiments, we have also found a similar disparity of SF and PB APC function using DR-compatible allogeneic T-cell clones as responders.

The potent accessory cell function of synovial APCs demonstrated here may play an important role in local T-cell activation, and thus maintenance of the synovial inflammatory response in inflammatory arthritis. In addition, the presence of such potent APCs within the synovium may be an important factor determining why in a systemic disease such as RA the inflammatory response is largely concentrated in the joints.

REFERENCES

1. Duke O, Panayi GS, Janossy G, Poulter LW. An immunohistological analysis of lymphocyte subpopulations and their microenvironments in the synovial membranes of patients with rheumatoid arthritis using monoclonal antibodies. Clin Exp Immunol 1982; 49:22–30.
2. Paulus HE, Machleder HI, Levine S, Yu DTY, MacDonald NS. Lymphocyte involvement in rheumatoid arthritis—studies during thoracic duct drainage. Arthritis Rheum 1977; 20: 1249–1262.
3. Zvaifler NJ. Fractionated total lymphoid irradiation: a promising new treatment for rheumatoid arthritis? Yes, no, maybe. Arthritis Rheum 1987; 30:109–114.
4. Statsny P. Association of the B cell alloantigen DRw4 with rheumatoid arthritis. N Engl J Med 1978; 298:869–871.

5. Dutz JP, Chan A, Mak T, Siminovitch KA, Rubin LA. T cell receptor genes in rheumatoid arthritis. Springer Semin Immunopathol 1989; 11:289–299.
6. Gaston JSH, Life PF, Bailey LC, Bacon PA. In vitro responses to a 65-kilodalton mycobacterial protein by synovial T cells from inflammatory arthritis patients. J Immunol 1989; 143:2494–2500.
7. Res PCM, Schaar CG, Breedveld FC, van Eden W, van Embden JDA, Cohen IR, de Vries RRP. Synovial fluid T cell reactivity against 65kD heat shock protein of Mycobacteria in early chronic arthritis. Lancet 1988; 2:478–480.
8. Gaston JSH, Life PF, Granfors K, Merilahti-Palo R, Bailey L, Consalvey S, Toivanen A, Bacon PA. Synovial T lymphocyte recognition or organisms which trigger reactive arthritis. Clin Exp Immunol 1989; 76:348–353.
9. Ford DK, da Roza DM, Schulzer M. Lymphocytes from the site of disease but not blood lymphocytes indicate the cause of arthritis. Ann Rheum Dis 1985; 44:701–710.
10. Vershure PJ, van Noorden CFJ, Dijkstra CD. Macrophages and dendritic cells during the early stages of antigen-induced arthritis in rats: immunohistochemical analysis of cryostat sections of the whole knee joint. Scand J Immunol 1989; 29:371–381.
11. Zvaifler NJ, Steinman RM, Kaplan G, Lau LL, Rivelis M. Identification of immunostimulatory dendritic cells in the synovial effusions of patients with rheumatoid arthritis. J Clin Invest 1985; 76:789–800.
12. Austyn JM. Lymphoid dendritic cells. Immunology 1987; 62:161–170.
13, Pitzalis C, Kingsley G, Murphy J, Panayi G. Abnormal distribution of the helper-inducer and suppressor-inducer T lymphocyte subsets in the rheumatoid joint. Clin Immunol Immunopathol 1987; 45:252–258.
14. Life PF, Viner NJ, Bacon PA, Gaston JSH. Synovial fluid antigen-presenting cells unmask peripheral blood T cell responses to bacterial antigens in inflammatory arthritis. Clin Exp Immunol 1990; 79:189–194.
15. Mueller DL, Jenkins MK, Schwartz RH. Clonal expansion versus functional clonal inactivation: A costimulatory signalling pathway determines the outcome of T cell antigen receptor occupancy. Annu Rev Immunol 1989; 7:445–480.
16. Hessian PA, Highton J, Palmer DG. Quantification of macrophage cell surface molecules in rheumatoid arthritis. Clin Exp J Immunol 1989; 77:47–51.
17. Morimoto C, Letvin NL, Rudd CE, Hagan M, Brown H, Takeguchi T, Schlossman SF. The role of the 2H4 molecule in the generation of suppressor function in Con A activated T cells. J Immunol 1986; 137:3247–3253.
18. Salmon M, Kitas GD, Gaston JSH, Bacon PA. Interleukin-2 production and responses by helper T cell subsets in man. Immunology 1988; 65:81–85.

132
Antigen Handling by Nonlymphoid Cells in the Chicken Spleen

Suzan H. M. Jeurissen, E. Marga Janse, and G. F. De Boer
Central Veterinary Institute, Lelystad, The Netherlands

INTRODUCTION

In the mammalian spleen, the white pulp is morphologically separated into periarteriolar lymphocyte sheaths (PALSs), follicles with corona and germinal centers, and the marginal zone. Each compartment contains its own characteristic populations of lymphoid and nonlymphoid cells. The PALSs contain T lymphocytes and interdigitating cells (IDCs); the follicles contain B lymphocytes, tingible body macrophages, and follicular dendritic cells (FDCs); and the marginal zone contains B lymphocytes, marginal metallophils, and marginal zone macrophages. In mammals, IDCs and macrophages are generally considered part of the mononuclear phagocyte system and are thought to originate from bone marrow precursors (1), whereas FDCs probably originate from fibroblastic reticulum cells, which are not derived from bone marrow (2,3). After mice are intravenously injected with immunologically different antigens such as particulate colloidal carbon, immune complexes, and thymus-independent type 2 FITC-Ficoll, the various nonlymphoid cells can be classified according to their function. After some hours, carbon localizes in the red pulp macrophages, FITC-Ficoll in marginal zone macrophages (4), and immune complexes on the FDCs (5).

The white pulp of the chicken spleen differs considerably from its mammalian counterpart. The former also has morphologically distinct PALSs containing T cells and follicles with germinal centers containing B cells. In addition to the mammalian compartments, periellipsoid lymphocyte sheaths (PELSs) containing B cells exist. The corona and marginal zone, however, can not be distinguished. Also, the nonlymphoid cell system in chickens is often considered to be completely different from that of mammals. This hypothesis is based on electron microscopical observations of cell populations (6) and on the localization of immune complexes (7). Blood-derived precursor cells are supposed to mature into splenic ellipsoid-associated dendritic cells (EADCs) under the influence of bursal secretory cells (6). The EADCs, which absorb immune complexes, are thought to migrate into T-cell areas to mature into IDCs, which in turn migrate to germinal centers to mature into FDCs (6,7).

Recently, we developed monoclonal antibodies CVI-ChNL-68.1 and CVI-ChNL-68.2 (8,9). CVI-ChNL-68.1 is specific for mononuclear phagocytes, including monocytes in bone marrow and blood, IDCs, and classic macrophages in the red pulp of the spleen (8). In the spleen, CVI-ChNL-68.2 is specific for EADCs. The specifities of both monoclonal antibodies indicate that as in mammals, chicken mononuclear phagocytes are separated from ellipsoid- and follicle-associated dendritic cells.

Three immunologically different antigens—colloidal carbon, FITC-Ficoll, and immune complexes—were intravenously injected into chickens to investigate the function of EADCs, IDCs, FDCs, and macrophages in the chicken spleen.

MATERIALS AND METHODS

Animals

White Leghorn strain A chickens were bred and kept under specific-pathogen free conditions in Horsefall-Bauer isolators. Adult chickens were injected intravenously with one antigen or a combination of two antigens. After 2, 24, and 48 hr, spleens were removed, frozen in liquid nitrogen, and stored at –20°C.

Antigens

A solution of 500 μl colloidal carbon (Pelican Ink c11/1413a, Günther Wagner, West Germany) diluted twofold in 0.9% NaCl was used to trace particulate antigens.

An amount of 500 μg fluoresceinated Ficoll (FITC-Ficoll) was used to trace thymus-independent type 2 antigen. For double staining, mouse monoclonal antibodies were visualized with TRITC-conjugated rabbit antimouse immunoglobulin (Ig) (Dakopatts, Glostrup, Denmark). The sections were examined with a Zeiss microscope equipped with excitation/barrier filters for FITC and TRITC.

An amount of 500 μl rabbit anti–peroxidase-peroxidase (PAP; Sigma, St. Louis, Missouri) was used to trace immune complexes. For double staining, PAP was visualized with goat antirabbit Ig peroxidase conjugate (Institute Pasteur, Paris, France) and peroxidase activity was developed with DAB (see below). Then, mouse monoclonal antibodies were visualized with rabbit antimouse Ig peroxidase conjugate (Dakopatts) and peroxidase activity was developed with AEC (see below). For simultaneous detection with FITC-Ficoll, PAP was visualized with TRITC-conjugated swine antirabbit Ig (Dakopatts).

Immunohistochemistry and Enzyme Histochemistry

Cryostat sections of 8 μ thickness were picked up on slides, air dried, and fixed in pure acetone for 10 min. Sections were incubated with monoclonal antibodies and conjugates (see below) in an appropriate dilution for 60 min. Between incubations, slides were rinsed in phosphate-buffered saline. Peroxidase activity was developed with 0.01% H_2O_2 in a solution of either 0.5 mg 3,3′-diaminobenzidine-tetrahydrochloride (DAB, Sigma) per ml Tris-HCl buffer (0.05 M, pH 7.6) or of 0.5 mg 3-amino-9-ethylcarbazole (AEC; Sigma) per ml Na-acetate buffer (0.5 M, pH 5).

Monoclonal Antibodies

Monoclonal antibodies with the following specificities were used: HIS-C7, leukocytes (10); HIS-C1, B lymphocytes (10); CVI-ChNL-68.1, mononuclear phagocytes (8); CVI-ChNL-68.2, ellipsoid-associated dendritic cells (9).

RESULTS AND DISCUSSION

Three immunologically different antigens were investigated for their localization in the spleen. The localization of the antigens at various time points is summarized in Table 1. With monoclonal antibodies, nonlymphoid cells that absorbed antigens, were recognized. CVI-ChNL-68.1 was used as marker for IDCs and macrophages in the PALSs and red pulp, and ChNL-68.2 was used as marker for EADCs in the PELSs. Because none of the antigens induced a new staining pattern by ChNL-68.1 or -68.2, we were able to deduce the relationship between the various nonlymphoid cell population and to compare these cells with nonlymphoid cells in the mammalian spleen.

Colloidal Carbon

Two hours after injection, colloidal carbon was located in the ellipsoid in and between ChNL-68.2–positive EADCs. The absorption resembled pinocytosis because tiny grains of carbon were distributed very finely. At 24 and 48 hr, mostly large grains of carbon were detected in ChNL-68.1–positive red pulp macrophages, although some carbon was still situated in the ellipsoid just as it was at the 2-hr time point.

These results agree with the results of Eikelenboom et al. (11), which were obtained, however, at different time points (5 min, 6 days, and 12 days after intravenous injection of carbon).

PAP Immune Complexes

The PAP localized first in the ellipsoid and then in the germinal center. This finding was identical to results of others (7,11,12). By examining the localization of PAP at briefer time intervals and by using monoclonal antibodies, however, we obtained new results. At 2 hr, PAP localized exactly at the same site in the ellipsoid that was the stained by ChNL-68.2, though more intensely at the inner part than at the outer border. At 24 hr, some PAP was

Table 1 Distribution of Intravenously Injected Antigens

	Amount of antigen detected in (hr)											
	Ellipsoid			PALS			Germinal center			Red pulp		
Antigen	2	24	48	2	24	48	2	24	48	2	24	48
Carbon	++	+	+/–	–	–	–	–	–	–	–	++	++
PAP	++	+/–	–	–	++	+	–	–	+	–	–	–
FITC-Ficoll	++	++	++	–	–	–	–	–	–	–	–	–

++ = large amount of antigen detected; + = some antigen detected; +/– = little antigen detected; – = no antigen detected.

still situated at ChNL-68.2–positive EADCs at the outer border of the ellipsoid. Most PAP, however, was detected in the T-cell areas on large cells with minor cell protrusions; these cells were not recognized by ChNL-68.2 nor ChNL-68.1. This finding indicates that PAP was not located on EADCs or IDCs. At 48 hr, PAP was detected in germinal centers on dendritic cells. In addition, some PAP was still located in T-cell areas, but it was no longer detected in the ellipsoids. After injection of PAP, ChNL-68.2 did not stain other cells outside the ellipsoids at any time point. At 6 and 12 days after injection, PAP is detected only in germinal centers in the chicken spleen (11,12); this finding is comparable to results obtained with mouse spleens. Therefore, PAP localizes in the PELSs and PALSs before localizing in the germinal center.

FITC-Ficoll

Two hours after intravenous injection, FITC-Ficoll localized exactly at the same site in the ellipsoid that was stained by ChNL-68.2. In contrast to carbon and PAP, FITC-Ficoll continued to be detected on ChNL-68.2–positive EADCs at all later timepoints. FITC-Ficoll, therefore, finally localizes in the EADCs of the ellipsoid. In the mammalian spleen, FITC-Ficoll selectively localizes in the marginal zone and its macrophages (4). The EADCs, therefore, resemble mammalian macrophages of the marginal zone.

We showed in this experiment that in addition to carbon particles and immune complexes even an antigen as specific as FITC-Ficoll localized in the ellipsoid on EADCs immediately after intravenous injection. Functionally, the ellipsoid capillary resembles the marginal sinus of the mammalian spleen. This result underscores the opinion of Eikelenboom et al. (11) that the segregation of antigen in the ellipsoid is a nonspecific process that is followed by diffusion of the antigen through the splenic compartments. On the other hand, the hypothesis of Glick et al. (6) that EADCs migrate with antigen through the PALSs to the germinal center can not be completely excluded. The population of ChNL-68.2–positive EADCs may in fact be two or even more subpopulations each with its own antigen specificity. In addition, cells may loose their markers, recognized by monoclonal antibodies, in the process of migration and differentiation. To investigate whether PAP and FITC-Ficoll localize in different subpopulations of EADCs, we injected both antigens simultaneously and studied where they localized at 2 and 24 hr.

Simultaneous Injection of FITC-Ficoll and PAP Immune Complexes

After 2 hr, the green fluorescence of FITC-Ficoll coincided completely with the red fluorescence of the TRITC-conjugate bound to the PAP immune complexes. Probably because the amount of each injected antigen differed, PAP immune complexes stained more intensely than FITC-Ficoll. At 24 hr, FITC-Ficoll was still situated in the same sites in the ellipsoids. In contrast, most PAP immune complexes had diffused from the ellipsoids, and only small amounts were detected at the outer border.

CONCLUSIONS

Various antigens were found to localize in the ellipsoid directly after intravenous injection. Immune complexes and FITC-Ficoll localized in the same EADCs, but FITC-Ficoll remained longer in these cells. PAP immune complexes migrated via the PALSs to the germinal centers. We concluded that depending on their immunological characteristics, antigens may migrate from EADCs to other nonlymphoid cells, but that EADCs themselves do not migrate. This conclusion implies that IDCs do not develop from EADCs and that

FDCs probably do not develop from IDCs. Chicken nonlymphoid cells, therefore, like mammal nonlymphoid cells, separate into mononuclear phagocytes and FDCs.

REFERENCES

1. Steinman RM, Nussenzweig MC. Dendritic cells: Features and functions. Immunol Rev 1980; 53:127–32.
2. Humphrey JH, Grennan D, Sundaram V. The origin of follicular dendritic cells in the mouse and the mechanism of trapping of immune complexes on them. Eur J Immunol 1984; 14:859–64.
3. Dijkstra CD, Kamperdijk EWA, Döpp E. The ontogenetic development of the follicular dendritic cell. An ultrastructural study by means of intravenously injected horseradish peroxidase (HRP)-anti-HRP complexes as marker. Cell Tissue Res 1984; 236:203–6.
4. Humphrey JH, Grennan D. Different macrophage populations distinguished by means of fluorescent polysaccharides. Recognition and properties of marginal zone macrophages, Eur J Immunol 1981; 11:221–8.
5. Nossal GJV, Abbot A, Mitchell J, Lummus Z. Antigens in immunity. XV. Ultrastructural features of antigen capture in primary and secondary lymphoid follicles. J Exp Med 1968; 127:277–90.
6. Glick B, Olah I. A continuum of cells leading to an *in vivo* humoral response. Immunol Today 1984; 5:162–5.
7. White RG, French VI, Stark JM. A study of the localization of a protein antigen in the chicken spleen and its relation to the formation of germinal centers. J Med Microbiol 1970; 3:65–83.
8. Jeurissen SHM, Janse EM, Koch G, De Boer GF. The monoclonal antibody CVI-ChNL-68.1 recognizes cells of the monocyte-macrophage lineage in chickens. Dev Comp Immunol 1988; 12:855–64.
9. Jeurissen SHM, Janse EM, Kok GL, De Boer GF. Distribution and function of non-lymphoid cells positive for monoclonal antibody CVI-ChNL-68.2 in healthy chickens and those infected with Marek's disease virus. Vet Immunol Immunopathol 1989; 22:123–33.
10. Jeurissen SHM, Janse EM, Ekino S, Nieuwenhuis P, Koch G, De Boer GF. Monoclonal antibodies as probes for defining cellular subsets in the bone marrow, thymus, bursa of Fabricius, and spleen of the chicken. Vet Immunol Immunopathol 1988; 19:225–38.
11. Eikelenboom P , Kroese FGM, Van Rooyen N. Immune complex-trapping cells in the spleen of the chicken. Cell Tissue Res 1983; 231:377–86.
12. Kroese FGM, Eikelenboom P, Van Rooyen N. Electronmicroscopical and enzymehistochemical characterization of immune complex trapping cells in the spleen of different vertebrate species. Dev Comp Immunol 1982; Suppl 2:69–74.

133
Sensitization of Allogeneic T Cells In Vivo
Donor or Host Antigen-Presenting Cell Function?

M. A. Ibrahim, B. M. Chain, and D. R. Katz
University College and Middlesex School of Medicine, London, England

INTRODUCTION

T lymphocytes do not respond directly to most antigens unless accessory or antigen-presenting cells (APCs) expressing major histocompatibility complex (MHC) class II products are present (1). Antigen-specific T lymphocytes are generally believed to recognize a peptide antigen fragment bound to MHC class II molecules on the surface of APCs. However, the mechanism of T-cell recognition of foreign MHC, a crucial factor in transplantation immunobiology, is less well understood (2). Previous reports have shown that immunogenicity of organ grafts declines following depletion of donor strain dendritic cells (DCs) and is restored following their readministration (3). Therefore, it was suggested that sensitization to alloantigens may be achieved in two ways: (a) direct presentation by donor APCs, or (b) acquisition of alloantigens by host APCs and their subsequent presentation to T cells. Earlier work, however, had shown that rejection of nonvascularized grafts was dependent on intact lymphatics (4), suggesting a role for the lymphoid tissues as the site for T-cell sensitization to alloantigens.

In this study, we have examined the role of APCs directly introduced in the peripheral subcutaneous tissues of allogeneic hosts in sensitizing T cells in the draining lymph nodes.

METHODS AND RESULTS

Antigen-presenting cells used in this study were murine peritoneal and splenic macrophages, splenic dendritic cells, and B cells. The APCs were purified according to standard protocols and injected subcutaneously into both hind footpads of syngeneic and allogeneic mice. To investigate their potential traffic from peripheral subcutaneous tissues to draining lymph nodes, the presumed site for T-cell priming, APCs were prelabelled with [^{3}H]uridine, [^{111}In]oxine, FITC, or DiI and cell migration was monitored for up to 7 days.

For the first 24 hr: (a) There was a sharp fall in the radioactivity detectable in the hindfeet of injected animals in the first hour; i.e., to 57% of the radioactivity detectable within 5 min of injection; (b) after the first hour the level of hindfeet radioactivity did not show any significant change for up to 24 hr after injection (Fig. 1a); and (c) there was a minimal but significant increase in the level of radioactivity in the popliteal but not the inguinal lymph nodes throughout the first 24 hr following injection (Table 1).

Radioactivity detectable in the hindfeet of injected animals on the third day following injection was 54% of the radioactivity detectable at the same site 1 day following injection. After the third day, no significant change in hindfeet radioactivity levels was observed

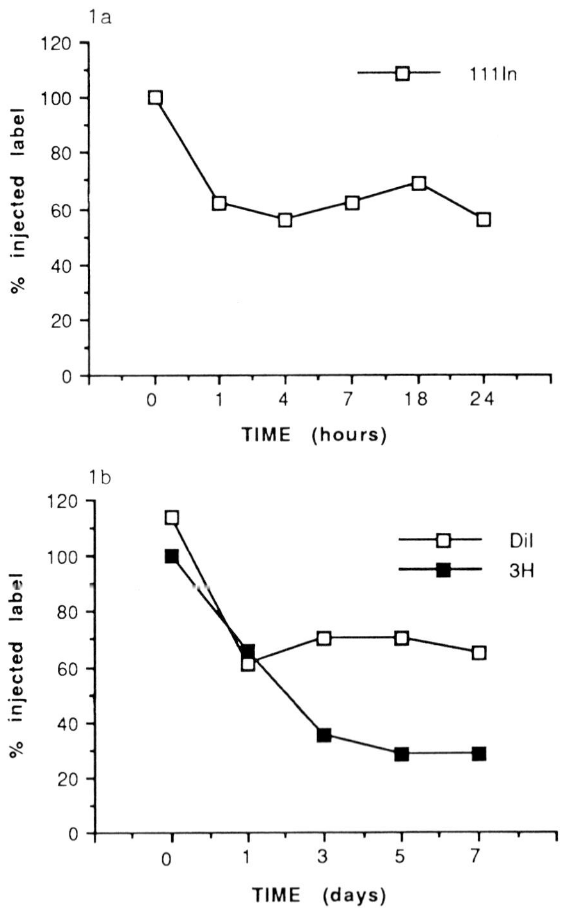

Figure 1 Mice received subcutaneous hind footpad injections of labeled APCs, hindfeet were excised at different time points, and their label content was measured (when the label was ^{111}In by gamma counting, when ^{3}H by scintillation counting of hindfeet extracts, and when DiI by chloroform/methanol extraction then fluorometry). Data were expressed as percentage of the injected dose of the label, after correction for extraction efficiency and label decay if necessary. ^{111}In was used for short time course experiments (up to 1 day) and ^{3}H and DiI were used for longer time course experiments (up to 7 days).

Table 1 A Small Increase in the Level of Radioactivity in the Popliteal Lymph Nodes in the First 24 hr Following the Injection of [^{111}In]oxine-labeled DCs in Hindfeet

Time (hr)	Counts/min
Saline injected	114/13
0	155/16
1	187/18
4	263/31
7	235/36
18	324/54
24	274/42

Popliteal lymph nodes were directly measured for radioactivity by gamma counting at the time points shown. No radioactivity above background was detectable in inguinal lymph nodes.

(Fig. 1b). However, in contrast to the findings during the first 24 hr, there was no significant change in the radioactivity seen in either the popliteal or the inguinal lymph nodes between 1 and 7 days following injection. A similar pattern was observed when DCs were labeled with the hydrophobic fluorescent compound DiI, and the lipid-associated fluorescence was measured following chloroform/methanol extraction. The mean fluorescence intensity extractable from the hindfeet steadily declined with time, reaching on the seventh day 64% of that originally injected (Fig. 1b). However, no label could be extracted from the popliteal lymph nodes at any time point.

Subcutaneous hind footpad injection of soluble isotope (either ^{3}H or ^{111}In) produced the same transient increase in popliteal radioactivity in the first 24 hr as had been observed following labeled APC injection (data not shown). Furthermore, no detectable cell-associated fluorescence was observed in the popliteal nodes for 24 hr following the injection of FITC-labeled APCs as analyzed by FACS (data not shown). The latter two experiments favor soluble isotope drainage as an explanation for the transient popliteal radioactivity rather than APC migration.

Further evidence against active cellular migration of footpad-injected radiolabeled APCs was derived from experiments comparing labeled glutaraldehyde fixed APCs with labeled unfixed APCs. Both fixed and unfixed cells allowed a similar increase in popliteal radioactivity, arguing against active cell migration (data not shown). Likewise, the same pattern of reduced footpad radioactivity was observed with both fixed and unfixed cells.

In allopriming experiments, both fixed and unfixed DC primed alloreactive T cells effectively in vivo as measured by a secondary in vitro mixed lymphocyte reaction (MLR) (data not shown), but in vitro fixed APCs failed to stimulate allogeneic T cells. Furthermore, frozen sections of draining lymph nodes following injection of DiI-labeled DCs were monitored over a 7-day period. Red fluorescence persisted in the subcapsular sinus from day 1 to day 7 (Fig. 2). The pattern seen is consistent with the notion that the hydrophobic label is not cell associated and is trapped at that site.

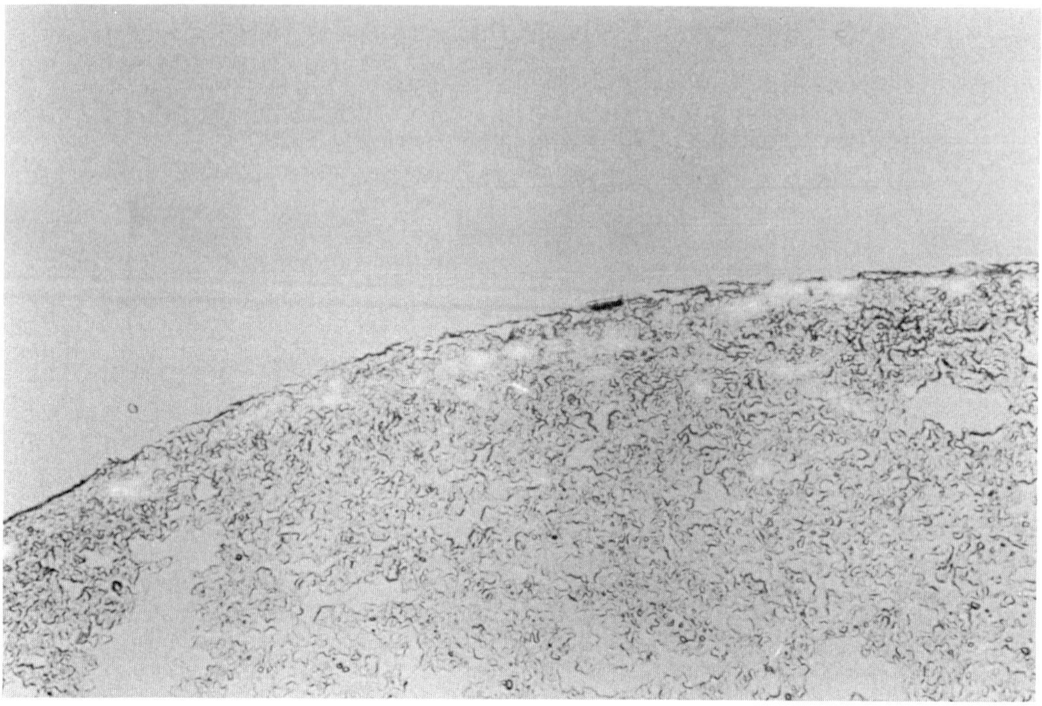

(a)

Figure 2 Light microscopical appearance of frozen sections of popliteal lymph nodes (a) by phase contrast, and (b) by fluorescence microscopy using the filter set for rhodamine) from CBA/Ca mice 1 day after subcutaneous injection in hind footpads of DiI-labeled DCs. Red fluorescence is predominantly present in the subcapsular sinus.

DISCUSSION

We have established the cell migration system to investigate whether APCs migrate from peripheral tissues to draining lymph nodes during allopriming. It is clear from our data that effective sensitization of T cells to alloantigens can be achieved without migration of the allogeneic APCs to draining lymph nodes.

Evidence against cell migration includes: (a) Soluble isotope produces a similar decline in hindfeet radioactivity with time compared to the decline seen following injection of labeled APCs; (b) the lack of cell-associated fluorescence in draining lymph nodes by FACS analysis; and (c) the absence of any difference in kinetics of label between fixed and unfixed cells. On the other hand, evidence for a role of host APCs in allopriming includes: (a) effective priming without detectable migration of allogeneic APC to draining lymph nodes; (b) effective priming by fixed allogeneic APCs; and (c) the lack of cell-associated fluorescence in lymph node sections (Fig. 2). Our data are consistent with a previous report (5) that host APCs play an important role in this type of T-cell sensitization.

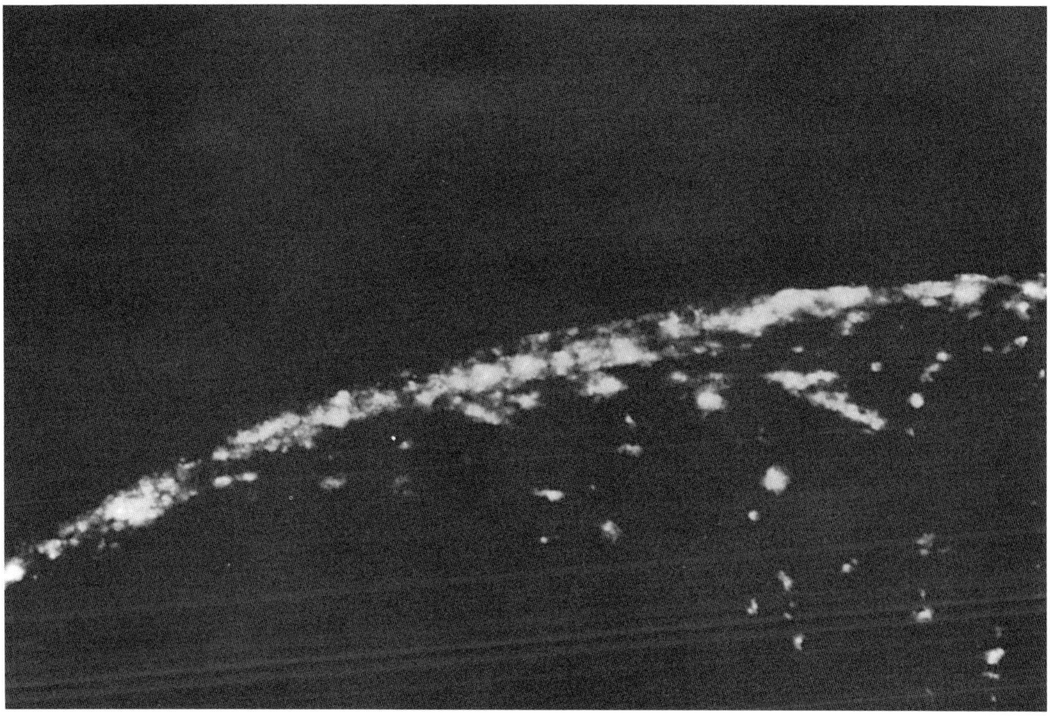

(b)

Figure 2 (Continued)

CONCLUSIONS

We suggest that during allopriming of lymph node T cells, the majority of injected APCs do not migrate to the lymph nodes. Other mechanisms operate to achieve effective priming, and we believe that the most likely possibility is that there is transfer of alloantigens to the draining lymph nodes predominantly in a "noncellular" form.

REFERENCES

1. Unanue ER. The regulatory role of macrophages in antigenic stimulation Part two: symbiotic relationship between lymphocytes and macrophages. Adv Immunol 1981; 31:1–136.
2. Lechler RI, Lombardi G, Batchelor JR, Reinsmoen N, Bach FH. The molecular basis of alloreactivity. Immunol Today 1990; 11:83–88.
3. Lechler RI, Batchelor JR. Restoration of immunogenicity to passenger cell-depleted kidney allografts by the addition of donor strain dendritic cells. J Exp Med 1982; 155:31–41.
4. Barker CF, Billingham RE. The role of afferent lymphatics in the rejection of skin homografts. J Exp Med 1968; 128:197–207.
5. Sherwood RA, Brent L, Rayfield LS. Presentation of alloantigens by host cells. Eur J Immunol 1986; 16:569–574.

134

Immunocytochemical Detection of Human Immune Deficiency Virus Epitope–Specific Antibody-Forming Cells

Comparisons of Antigens in the Mouse Model

Jon D. Laman, Marianne J. Fasbender, Wim J. A. Boersma, and Eric Claassen
TNO Medical Biological Laboratory, Rijswijk, The Netherlands

INTRODUCTION

Infection by human immune deficiency virus type 1 (HIV-1) evokes enormous changes in the organization and function of the microenvironment of lymph nodes and spleen. In three progressive stages, ranging from follicular hyperplasia to lymphoid depletion, the lymph nodes degenerate. In the terminal phase of the disease, the architecture of the lymph node is lost, lymphoid depletion has occurred, and the network of follicular dendritic cells (FDCs) is destroyed (2). The disruption of germinal centers and FDCs (2,3) may be the basis for the development of B-cell disorders (4) in the acquired immune deficiency syndrome (AIDS). Little is known about the mechanisms that govern the progressive damage to the lymphoid organs during the development of AIDS, although they may be the key to HIV-induced immunopathogenesis. Especially, the role of B cells and immune complexes (ICs) during development of histopathogenesis has received little attention. We, therefore, developed an immunocytochemical method to study epitope specificity, isotype and anatomical localization of HIV-specific antigen-forming cells (AFCs) and ICs. By incubation of tissue sections of lymphoid material with synthetic peptides (SP) coupled to detector enzymes, epitope specificity of locally present antibody can be demonstrated. Anti-isotype sera allow double staining for the detection of the isotype (1). In the present study, we determined if recombinant (rec) gp120 could also be used in these techniques, and we compared SP and rec gp120 with HIV- and SIV-infected cell lines as an antigen source.

MATERIALS AND METHODS

Animals

Female Balb/c mice were bred at the TNO breeding facility under specific-pathogen free (SPF) conditions and maintained in Makrolon cages with free access to acidified water (pH 3) and pelleted food. Animals were used for immunization at the age of 12–20 weeks.

Antigens

SP 68, a 21-mer homologous to the cleavage site of HIV-1 gp120 and 41 (amino acids 506–525), was synthesized and purified as described before (1). Rgp120, SIVmac251-infected HUT78 and HIV-1 (HTLV-IIIB)–infected Sup-T1 were a kind gift of Dr. P. Bentvelzen and coworkers (ITRI-TNO, Rijswijk, The Netherlands).

Immunizations

Synthetic peptides: three mice were immunized twice with a 3-week interval in both hind footpads with 25 μg of the SP suspended in Specol, a water and oil adjuvant, in a volume of 50 μl. Rgp120: Two mice were immunized as described for the synthetic peptides but two additional groups were immunized with 50 and 100 μg, respectively. Virus-infected cells were killed by fixation with ethanol (final concentration 70%) and stored at –20°C. Before use, they were washed three times with phosphate-buffered saline (PBS). SIVmac251–infected HUT78: 5 mice were immunized twice with a 3-week interval in both hind footpads with 0, 5×10^2, 5×10^3, 5×10^4 or 5×10^5 cells suspended in Specol in a volume of 50 μl. HIV-1–infected Sup-T1: Four mice were immunized twice with a 3-week interval in both hind footpads with 0, 5×10^3, 5×10^4 or 5×10^5 cells suspended in Specol in a total volume of 50 μl. A second group of four mice received the same doses suspended in Specol in a volume of 200 μl intraperitoneally.

ELISA and Immunocytochemistry

Five days after the booster immunization, serum was taken and tested in ELISA as described previously (5), with a goat-antimouse total immunoglobulin G (IgG) alkaline phosphatase (AP) (KPL). The spleen and popliteal lymph nodes were taken and snapfrozen in liquid nitrogen. Eight-micrometer cryostat sections were fixed for 10 min in fresh acetone, containing 0.02% H_2O_2. After air drying for 10 min, sections were incubated for 16 hr with antigen-AP conjugates or antigen–horseradish peroxidase (HRP) conjugates (10 μg/ml) at 4°C in 0.1% bovine serum albumin (BSA) in PBS. Conjugates were produced as described previously (1,6). Sections were washed three times with PBS and stained for AP or HRP as previously described (6) and mounted in glycerol/gelatin. Double staining was performed for mice immunized with SP 68 by simultaneous incubation of tissue sections with SP 68–AP and polyclonal rabbit–antimouse isotype–HRP antisera (Miles), specific for IgM and IgG_1. Subsequently, sections were stained for AP and for HRP after washing once with PBS.

RESULTS AND DISCUSSION

The aim of this study was to compare the ability of different types of HIV antigens (i.e., synthetic peptides, rgp120, and virus-infected cells) to evoke antibody responses and to be

Table 1 Application of Different Antigens in Immunization and Detection of Specific B Cells

Antigen	Evokes serum titers	Use as detector ligand
SP 68	Yes	Yes
rgp120	Yes	Yes
SIVmac251–HUT	No	NT
HIV-SuPt1	No	NT

NT = not tested.

used as detector molecules for immunocytochemical detection of AFCs in tissue sections. The results (summarized in Table 1) show that both synthetic peptides and rgp120 give rise to circulating antibodies, and that they can be used as detector molecules in immunocytochemistry. In the dose range used, SIV- and HIV-infected cells do not give rise to anti-gp120 or anti-SP titers.

Figure 1 shows ELISA data of sera tested on coatings of SP and rgp120. It is clear that rgp120 is a potent antigen with the adjuvant Specol (Fig. 1A). The SP 68 is also able to induce specific antibodies (Fig. 1B). Virus-infected cells are not able to evoke responses against either SP or rgp120 (Fig. 1A and 1B). Three alternatives may explain this finding: (a) The quantity of the antigen in the cell preparations is too low. (b) Ethanol fixation has disrupted the antigenic structure of the determinants. (c) Cross reactivity between rgp120 and SIVmac251 glycoproteins is low. The fact that cell preparations in a strong adjuvant are poor inducers of humoral responses may be relevant for vaccination strategies with recombinant prokaryotic organisms which express HIV protein. This problem may be overcome by the use of recombinants expressing high levels of antigen, immunization with higher doses of cells, the use of recombinants replicating in the host, or a combination of these options.

Immunocytochemical staining with rgp120-HRP and SP 68–AP allowed detection of specific AFCs and immune complexes. Figure 2 shows a group of specific AFCs in a lymph node section of a mouse immunized with SP 68. Double staining with SP 68–AP and polyclonal rabbit-antimouse Ig sera coupled to HRP allowed discrimination between (a) antigen-specific AFCs of unknown isotype; (b) AFCs producing antibodies of the isotype under investigation, of unknown specificity; and (c) AFCs specific for the SP, producing antibodies of the isotype under investigation (results not shown). Mice immunized with the adjuvant only showed few or no cross-reactive cells.

CONCLUSIONS

This study shows that both recombinant HIV proteins and synthetic peptides can be used to induce humoral responses in mice. Furthermore, these reagents can be used in immunohistochemistry to detect specific AFCs and ICs in tissue sections of patient and animal material. Such studies will help to elucidate the mechanisms involved in lymphoid histopathogenesis, B-cell (dys)function, and fluctuations of antibody titers. Recently, we showed that both protein-enzyme and peptide-enzyme conjugates can be used successfully for the detection of HIV-specific B-cells in human lymph nodes (7).

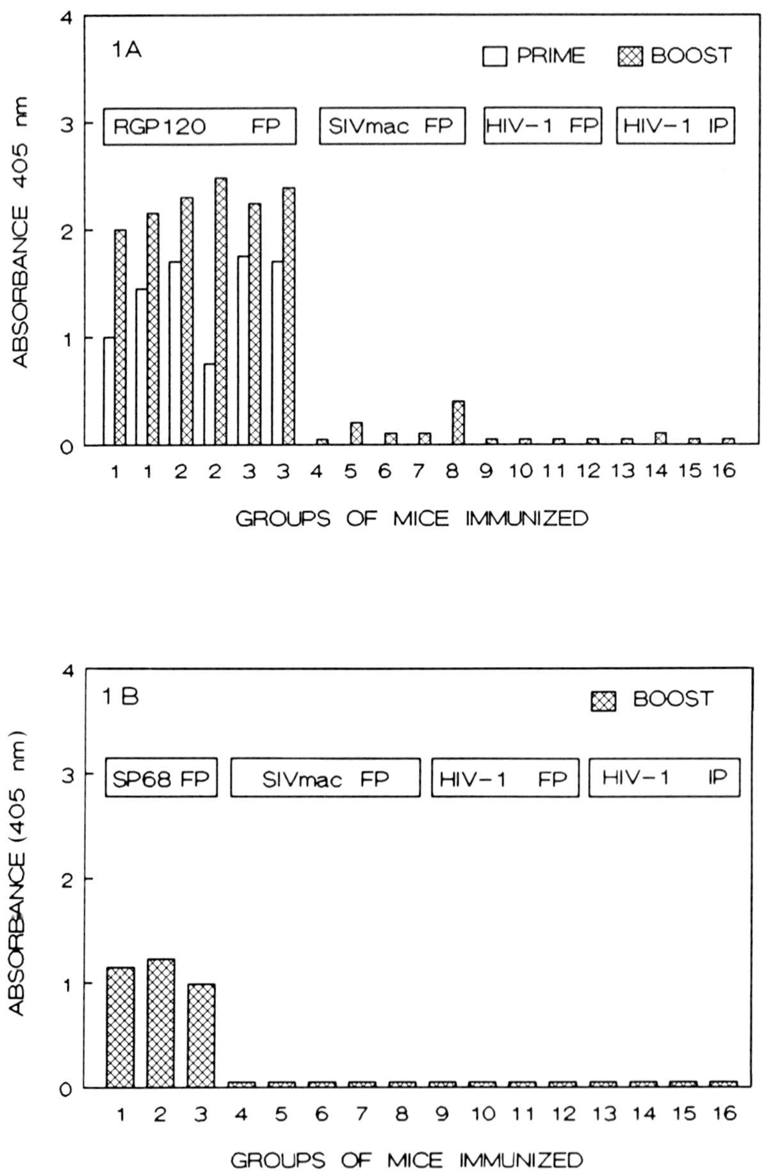

Figure 1 Responses in ELISA of mouse sera after immunization with different HIV/SIV–antigens. 1:100 dilutions of sera are shown. Each bar represents an individual mouse. FP = footpad immunization, IP = intraperitoneal immunization. (A) Evaluation on a rgp120 coat shows that rgp120 induces good responses, whereas HIV-1 and SIVmac–infected cells are ineffective. 1, 2, and 3 represent mice injected with 25, 50, and 100 μg rgp120 per injection, respectively. For rgp120, reactivity of sera three weeks after priming is also shown. 4–8, 9–12 and 13–16 represent increasing doses of virus-infected cells as indicated in the Materials and Methods section. (B) Evaluation on a SP 68 coat shows that the SP induces specific responses, whereas the infected cells induce no antibodies cross reactive with this epitope. 1–3 represent the mice immunized with the SP 68. 4–16 represent the same sera as shown in (A).

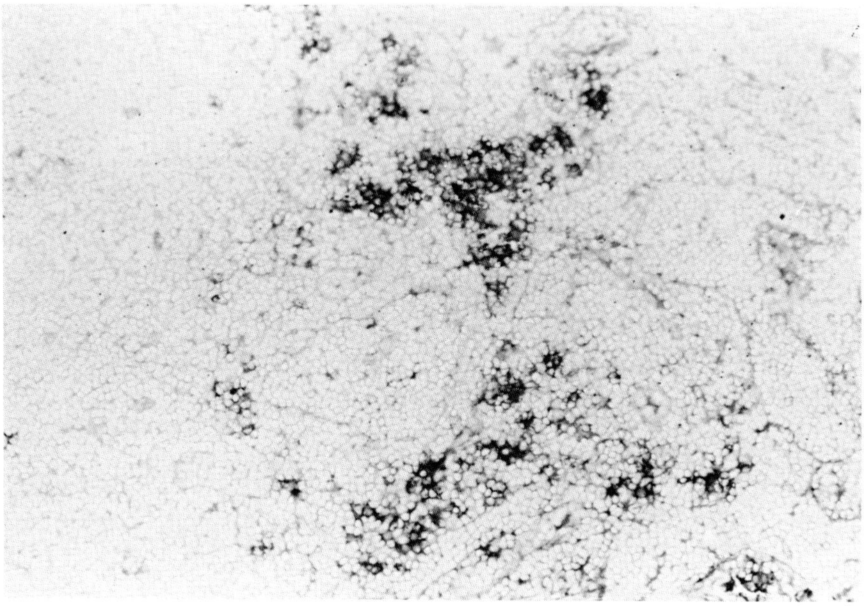

Figure 2 Photomicrograph of a lymph node section of a mouse immunized with SP 68 and stained with SP 68–AP. Darkly stained SP 68–specific AFCs surround a lymphoid follicle.

REFERENCES

1. Laman JD, Gerritse K, Fasbender MJ, Boersma WJA, van Rooijen N, Claassen E. Double immunocytochemical staining for the in vivo detection of epitope specificity and isotype of antibody forming cells against synthetic peptides homologous to human immunodeficiency virus type 1. J Histochem Cytochem 1990; 38:457–462.
2. Rácz P, Tenner-Rácz K, Kahl C, Feller AC, Kern P, Dietrich M. Spectrum of morphological changes of lymph nodes from patients with AIDS or AIDS-related complexes. Prog Allergy 1986; 37:81–181.
3. Laman JD, Claassen E, van Rooijen N, Boersma WJA. Immune complexes on follicular dendritic cells as a target for cytolytic cells in AIDS. AIDS 1989; 3:543–544.
4. Spickett GP, Dalgleish AG. Cellular immunology of HIV-1 infection. Clin Exp Immunol 1988; 71:1–7.
5. Boersma WJA, Claassen E, Deen C, Gerritse K, Haaijman JJ, Zegers ND. Antibodies to short synthetic peptides preferably recognize partly denatured protein. Analyt Chim Acta 1988; 213:187–197.
6. Claassen E, Adler LT, Adler FL. Double immunocytochemical staining for the in situ study of allotype distribution during an anti-TNP immune response in chimeric rabbits. J Histochem Cytochem 1986; 34:989–994.
7. Laman JD, Rácz P, Tenner-Rácz K, Klasmeier M, Fasbender MJ, Neelen C, Zegers ND, Dietrich M, Boersman WJA, Claassen E. Immunocytochemical determination of antigen- and epitope-specificity of HIV-1 specific B-cells in lymph node biopsies from HIV-infected individuals. AIDS 1991 (in press).

135
Cytochemical Analysis of Mast Cell Phenotypes in the Lymph Nodes of Allogeneic Tumor–Grafted Mice and in the Thymus of Preleukemic Mice

Robert Courtoy, Marie-Paule Defresne, and Jacques Boniver
Liege University Hospital, Liege, Belgium

INTRODUCTION

Variations in mast cell (MC) phenotype have been investigated from morphological, biochemical, immunological, and functional points of view (1). Histologically, the MC heterogeneity is easily shown by use of the sequential staining of Alcian blue followed by safranin. This allow to currently discriminate between the alcianophilic (blue) mucosal mast cells (MMCs) and the safraninophilic (red) connective tissue–type mast cells (CTMCs). This staining reaction has been used to study the MC response to fibrosarcoma graft in mice (2). It was shown that MC number was increased in the graft-draining lymph nodes (LNs). However, most of the MCs appeared red in syngeneic tumor-draining LNs, whereas they were blue in allogeneic tumor-draining LNs. To define the phenotypes of these MC subpopulations, we have compared their tinctorial properties to those of peritoneal MCs (CTMCs) and of intestinal MCs (MMCs) by use of several cytochemical reactions. We have also studied the thymus MCs in irradiated mice (lymphoma induction) as in irradiated and bone marrow–grafted mice (lymphoma inhibition).

MATERIALS AND METHODS

C57BL/6 and CBA mice from our breeding colony were used at 3 months of age.

Tissues

The cells of the peritoneal cavity of several mice were harvested by gently washing with cold culture medium (RPMI 1640 Gibco) without serum. Some cell suspensions were incubated for 30 min at 37°C in a solution of 0.5 μg/ml of poly-L-lysine in RPMI in order to induce MC secretion (3).

Pieces of intestine of normal mice were resected.

Tumor pieces of about 10.6 living tumor cells were implanted s.c. in CBA or C57BL/6 mice. The tumor was the transplantable fibrosarcoma T2, originally induced in C57BL/6 mice by MCA and maintained by serial s.c. transplantation of solid tumor fragments. The allogeneic or syngeneic tumor-draining lymph nodes were removed from CBA or C57BL/6 mice every 2 days during 10 days after the graft. Control lymph nodes were removed from normal mice.

C57BL/6 mice were irradiated with four doses of 1.75 Gy applied at weekly intervals. Some of them were grafted with 10.10^6 bone marrow cells immediately after the last irradiation. Mice were sacrificed at days 13 and 20 after the last irradiation and their thymuses were resected.

Histology

The different tissues were fixed for 60 min at 4°C in Carnoy's fluid, in 10% formaldehyde in water, or in 4% glutaraldehyde in phosphate buffer. They were dehydrated in ethanol and embedded in paraffin. Sections of 5 μ were performed.

Histochemistry

Enzymatic Digestion

The sections were incubated for 90 min at 37°C in a solution of trypsin (0.1 mg/ml) in phosphate buffer in order to remove the protein fraction of the mast cell granules.

Biebrich Scarlet Reaction

The sections were stained for 60 min in the staining solution at pH 9.5. This anionic dye is known to selectively demonstrate histones and other basis proteins (4).

Silver Methenamine Reaction

The sections were stained for 90 min at 60°C in the silver basic solution; in these conditions, the silver is known to form mercaptides with the sulfhydryl groups of basic proteins (5).

Alcian Blue–Safranin Reaction

The sections were stained for 60 min in 3% Alcian blue in sulfuric solution (2N), pH 0.2 and counterstained for 5 min in 0.1% safranin O solution in water, pH 6.5 Alcian blue stains sulfate groups ionized at very low pH, whereas safranin strains most of the acid groups ionized at pH near the neutrality (6).

Berberine Sulfate Reaction

The sections were stained for 20 min in 0.02% berberine sulfate solution in 1% citric solution, pH 4. This cationic dye forms strongly fluorescent complexes with heparin. This yellow fluorescence is contrasting with green fluorescence of the nucleoproteins (7).

RESULTS

The results are summarized in Table 1.

Table 1 Tinctorial Properties of Different Mast Cell Subsets

Histochemical reactions	Intestinal MCs	Peritoneal MCs		Lymph node MCs	
		Normal	Post-secretion	Syngeneic tumor graft	Allogeneic tumor graft
Basic protein demonstration					
Biebrich Scarlet (BS)	Orange-red	Orange-red	—	Orange-red	—
Trypsin BS	—	—	—	—	—
Silver methenamine	—	Black	—	Black	—
Acid polysaccharide demonstration					
Alcian blue–safranin (ABS)	Blue	Red	Blue	Red	Blue
Trypsin ABS	Blue	Blue	Blue	Blue	Blue
Berberine sulfate	—	Yellow (fluo)	Yellow (fluo)	Yellow (fluo)	Yellow (fluo)

Intestinal Mast Cells

Glutaraldehyde fixation inhibited the staining of those MCs that appeared alcianophilic after the other fixations. They contained basic proteins demonstrated by the Biebrich Scarlet (BS) but no sulfhydryl groups (silver methenamine negativity); the polyanions were different from heparin, since they were unstained by the berberine sulfate (BbS) reaction.

Peritoneal Mast Cells

Whatever the fixation was, these MCs exhibited the tinctorial properties of the CTMCs. They contained basic proteins (BS^+), they were silver methenamine (SM) positive; the polyanions were heparinlike (BbS^+). They were safraninophilic (red) but became blue (alcianophilic) after a trypsin digestion. Poly-L-lysine treated MC (secretion induced) became BS^-, SM^-, and alcionophilic but remained berberine sulfate positive.

Lymph Node Mast Cells

Syngeneic tumor graft–draining LNs contained numerous MCs that appeared BS positive and SM positive (SH-rich basic proteins). They contained heparin (BbS^+) and were safraninophilic but became blue (alcianophilic) after trypsin digestion. Allogeneic tumor graft–draining LNs contained also numerous MCs that were BS negative, SM negative, contained heparin (BbS^+) but were alcianophilic. Control LNs contained few MCs; some were alcianophilic, other were safraninophilic.

Thymus Mast Cells

Normal mouse thymus sections contained few MCs, generally located outside the capsula. These MCs were safraninophilic or alcianophilic. Irradiated mouse thymuses were infiltrated with red (safraninophilic) MCs, located in the septa. Irradiated and bone marrow–grafted mouse thymuses contained MCs in their septa; most of these MCs were alcianophilic (blue).

DISCUSSION AND CONCLUSIONS

The mast cells appeared safraninophilic as far as they contained SH-rich basic protein, in normal peritoneal cell suspensions, in syngeneic tumor–draining lymph nodes, or in irradiated thymus.

The mast cells appeared alcianophilic as far as they do not contain SH-rich protein, in secretagogue-treated peritoneal cells, in allogeneic tumor-draining LNs, or in irradiated and bone marrow (BM)–grafted mouse thymus. The blue intestinal MCs do not contained heparin (BbS$^-$), and were thus different from the other MC subsets studied.

The mast cells in lymph node and thymus would thus be of the connective tissue type.

The s.c. implantation of tumor induced an increase of MCs in the subcapsular space and around the germinal centers in the draining LNs. As the tumor was syngeneic and grew, the MCs contained their usual heparin–basic protein complexes. As the tumor was allogeneic and would be rejected, the MCs did not contain basic proteins anymore but conserved heparin.

Irradiation and irradiation followed by a BM graft induced MC infiltration of the thymus septa. In preleukemic mice (irradiation), the MCs contained basic protein, whereas in nonpreleukemic mice (irradiation + BM) they contained only heparin.

In lymph nodes and in thymus, alcianophilic MCs would thus herald, respectively, allogeneic tumor rejection and thymic lymphoma inhibition. Most probably, this mast cell alcianophily could reflect a previous secreting activity. However, it cannot be excluded that this could represent an early stage in the maturation/differentiation process of CTMCs (8).

REFERENCES

1. Kitamura Y. Heterogeneity of mast cells and phenotypic change between subpopulations. Ann. Rev. Immunol. 1989; 7:59–76.
2. Courtoy R. Degraef-Lovens D; Dupont K. Schaaf-Lafontaine N. Boniver J. Mast cell response to tumor graft. Histophysiology of the immune system. S Fossum and B Rolstad (eds). Plenum, New York, 1988, pp. 427–32.
3. Courtoy R. Boniver J. Simar L.J. Cytochemistry of mouse mast cell reaction to polylysine. Histochemistry 1980; 66:49–58.
4. Enerbäck L. Mast cells. Histochemistry in pathologic diagnosis. SS Spicer (ed). Dekker, New York, 1987, pp. 695–728.
5. Courtoy R. Simar L.J. Importance of controls for the demonstration of carbohydrates in electron microscopy with the silver methenamine or the thocarbohydrazide-silver proteinate methods. J. Microscopy 1974; 100:199–211.
6. Spicer S.S. A correlative study of the histochemical properties of rodent acid mucopolysaccharides. J. Histochem. Cytochem. 1960; 8:18–35.
7. Enerbäck L. Berberine sulphate binding to mast cell polyanions: a cytofluorometric method for the quantitation of heparin. Histochemistry 1972; 42:301–13.
8. Combs J.W. Lagunoff D. Benditt E.P. Differentiation and proliferation of embryonic mast cells of the rat. J. Cell Biol. 1965; 25:577–92.

136

Histological Study of Germinal Center Macrophages in Peripheral Lymphoid Organs of the Rat

A Reinvestigation

N. M. Milićević,[1] Ž. Milićević,[1] and M. Čolić[2]
[1]*Institute of Histology; Belgrade, Yugoslavia;*
[2]*Military Medical Academy, Belgrade, Yugoslavia*

INTRODUCTION

For a long time it has been known that macrophages are present in the germinal centers (GCs) of secondary lymphoid nodules (1). It is believed that their role is to phagocytose dead lymphocytes, which originate from rapidly proliferating GC centroblasts (2) and plasma cells. Electron microscopical studies have confirmed such a viewpoint (3).

During our earlier studies of the rat thymus we described a type of macrophage with distinct morphological features in the corticomedullary zone (CMZ), different from both cortical macrophages (containing dead lymphocytes) and medullary interdigitating cells (IDCs) (4,5). The prominent feature of CMZ macrophages is the aldehyde fuchsin (AF)–positive reaction of their cytoplasmic content (4).

Considering that some GC macrophages also show an AF-positive reaction (6), we believed that it would be interesting to reinvestigate the histological features of GC macrophages, in particular to try to identify AF-positive macrophages by electron microscopy because there are no data in the literature about these cells.

Our results demonstrate the morphological dichotomy of GC macrophages in lymphatic organs of the rat. Besides macrophages containing dead cells, another population of GC macrophages, with hitherto undescribed morphological features which suggest the specific functional role, is seen.

MATERIALS AND METHODS

Eight-week-old Wistar rats were used. The pieces of parathymic, mesenteric, and inguinal lymph nodes as well as pieces of spleen were taken and fixed in neutral buffered formalin or in Bouin's solution, processed to paraffin, and stained with hematoxylin-eosin and AF (4). Activity of SD was demonstrated in cryostat sections (4). For electron microscopy tissues were fixed in glutaraldehyde, postfixed in OsO_4, and embedded in Epon 812. Semithin sections were stained with methylene blue. Ultrathin sections were contrasted with uranyl acetate and lead citrate or treated by thiocarbohydrazide–silver proteinate (TCH-SP) method for detection of polysaccharides (5).

RESULTS

Light Microscopy

Aldehyde fuchsin–positive macrophages are located in GCs of secondary follicles in lymph nodes and spleen (Fig. 1a). These cells contain AF-positive granules of varying size (Fig. 1b). In semithin sections conspicuous inclusions of blue-green color are seen (Fig. 1c). SD-positive cells are distributed within GCs in an identical manner to the AF-positive macrophages (Fig. 1d; cf Fig. 1a). SD-positive cells are confined to GCs of secondary follicles (Fig. 1e).

Electron Microscopy

Macrophages containing cellular debris, similar to those described in the literature (3), are readily detected in GCs (not shown).

A second type of macrophages contains cytoplasmic inclusions of characteristic morphology. Vacuolar inclusions filled with fine, flocculent, electron-lucent material are seen in these cells (Fig. 2a–d). These vacuoles vary greatly in size (Fig. 2b,c), ranging from very small ones, which still have the characteristic appearance (Fig. 2c) to giant vacuolar inclusions, which make up the large part of the cytoplasm (Fig. 2b). Dense bodies are often seen at the inner aspect of the vacuolar membrane (Fig. 2a,b,d) and show the positive TCH-SP reaction (Fig. 2a). Membrane profiles can be observed within the vacuolar content in varying amount (Fig. 2b,d). Very rarely phagocytosed dead lymphocytes are seen. The nucleus is very euchromatic with prominent nucleoli. The cytoplasm also has a very active appearance with dilated cisternae of rough endoplasmic reticulum and an abundance of polyribosomes (Fig. 2c).

DISCUSSION

Our results show that besides macrophages already described in the literature (which contain phagocytosed cellular debris in the cytoplasm) (3), in GCs there are macrophages with specific histological characteristics, which qualify them as a hitherto undescribed cellular component of the GC microenvironment.

In addition to specific histochemical features (aldehyde fuchsinophilia), these cells have a specific enzyme capacity (strong activity of SD and increased activity of AcP and NSE) that is suggestive of activated functional state (7), and particular ultrastructural characteristics (cytoplasmic inclusions) which are similar to those of macrophages stimulated to produce increased amounts of arachidonic acid metabolites in vitro (8).

The type of macrophages which we describe here has histological features very similar to those of CMZ macrophages in the thymus (4,5). However, in contrast to CMZ macrophages (9), this type of GC macrophage does not show any chloroacetate esterase activity (not shown here).

If it is true that this type of GC macrophage is involved in arachidonic acid metabolism rather than in phagocytosis of cellular debris (as suggested by their morphological features), then these cells could represent one of the most significant regulators of GC activity.

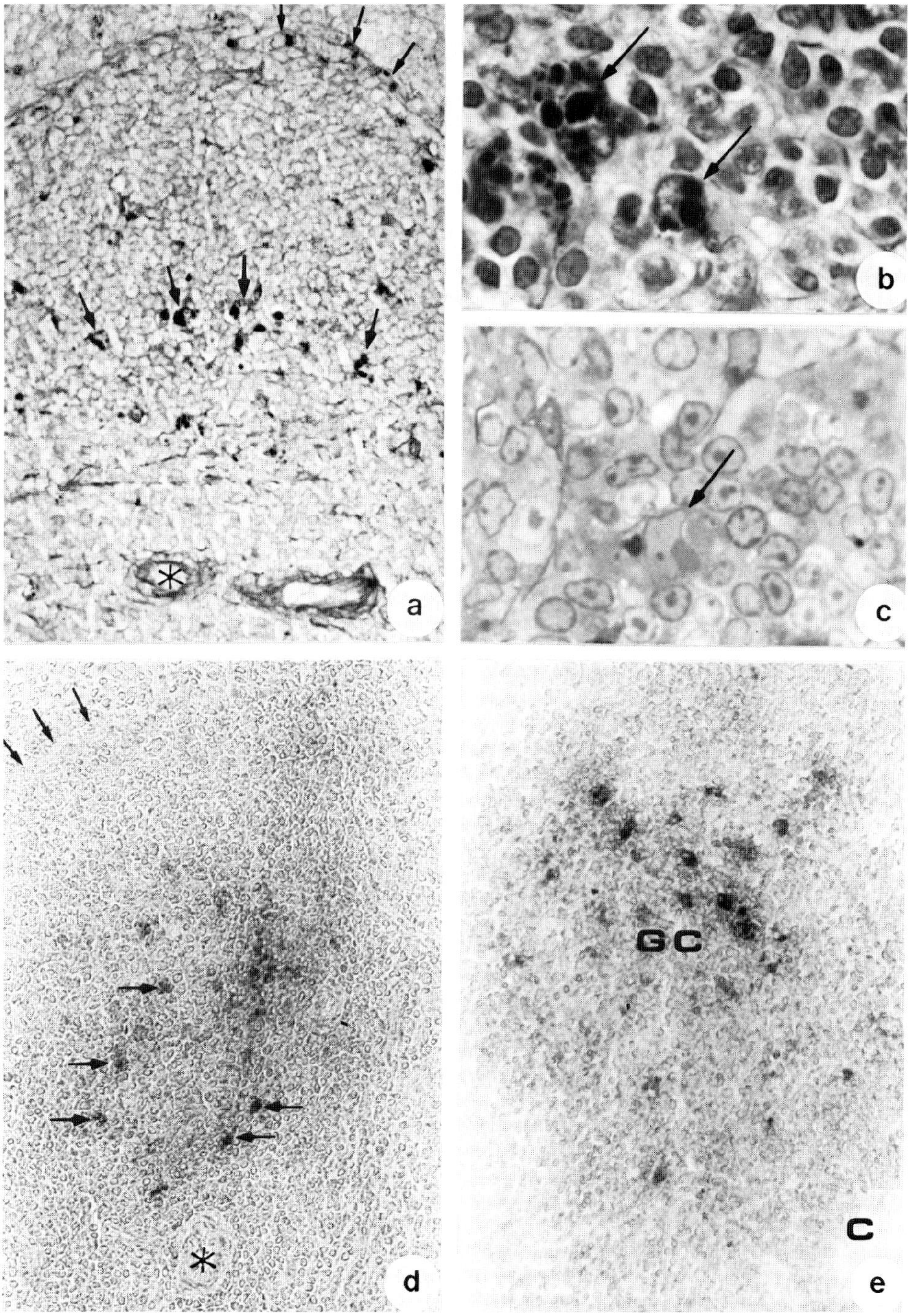

Figure 1 (a) AF$^+$ macrophages in splenic follicle (large arrows). Marginal metallophils are also AF$^+$ (small arrows). Central artery=asterisk (magnification: ×280). (b) AF$^+$ granules in macrophages of splenic follicle GC (arrows) (magnification: ×1380). (c) CG macrophage in splenic follicle (arrow) with cytoplasmic inclusion. Semithin section (magnification: ×1380). (d) SD$^+$ macrophages in splenic follicle (large arrows). Central artery=asterisk, marginal sinus=small arrows (magnification: ×350). (e) SD$^+$ macrophages in GC of parathymic lymph node. C = capsule (magnification: ×350). (Partly from Milićević NM et al. Anatomischer Anzeiger 170:39–47, 1990; used with permission.)

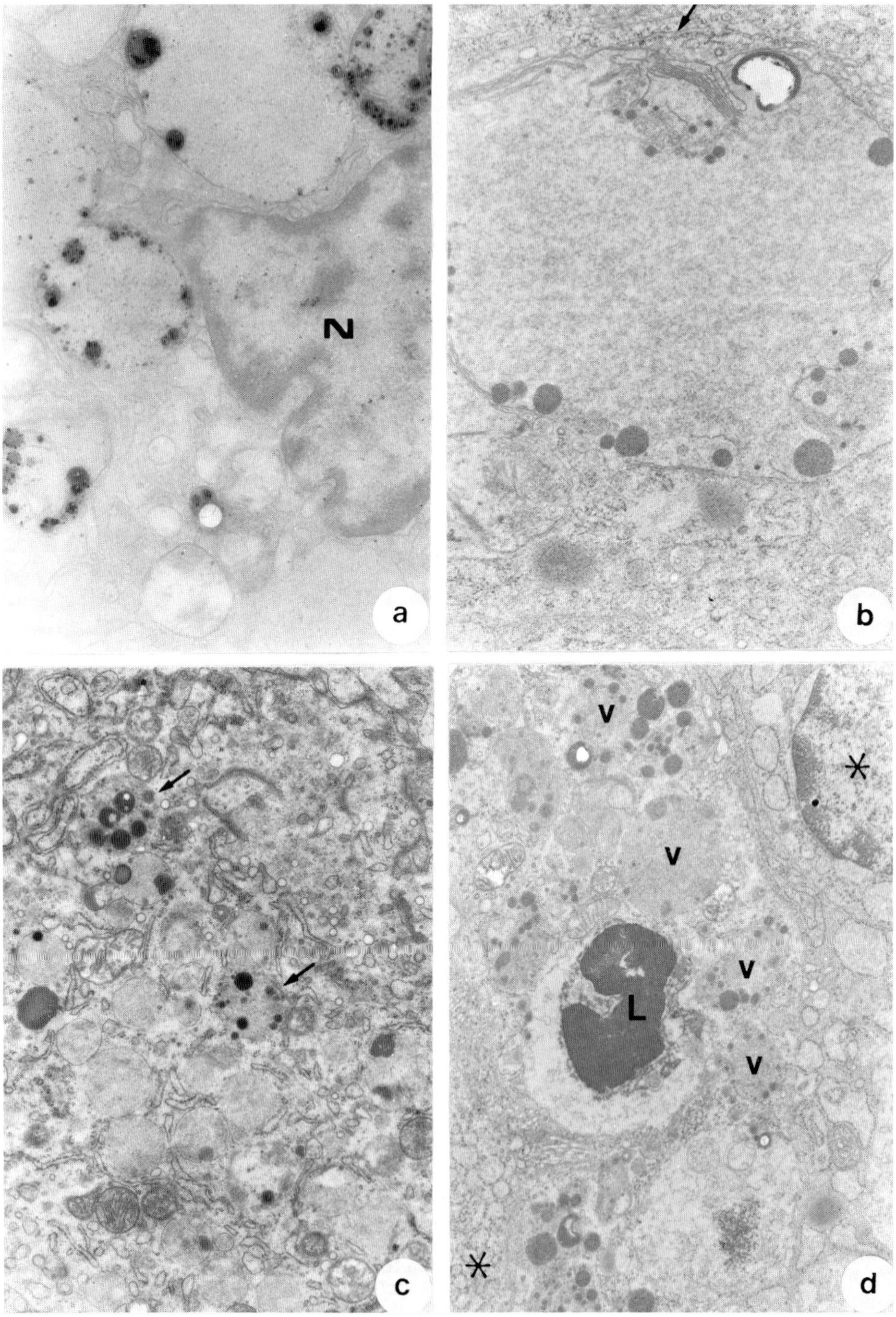

Figure 2 (a) Numerous vacuolar inclusions in GC macrophage. Dense bodies contain polysaccharides. N = nucleus. TCH-SP (magnification: ×12000). (b) Giant vacuolar inclusion filled with electronuclent content. Dense bodies at its inner side. Rough endoplasmic reticulum (arrow) near membrane profiles (magnification: ×12000). (c) Numerous very small, typical inclusions (arrows). Very active appearance of cytoplasm (magnification: ×18500). (d) Phagocytosed lymphocyte (L) is easily distinguished from cytoplasmic vacuoles (v). Ab cells=asterisks (magnification: ×6350). (Adapted from Milićević NM et al. Anatomischer Anzeiger 170:39–47, 1990; used with permission.)

REFERENCES

1. Flemming W. Studien über Regeneration der Gewebe. Arch mikr Anat 1885; 24:50–91.
2. Odartchenko N, Lewerenz M, Sordat B, Roos B, Cottier H. Kinetics of cellular death in germinal centers of mouse spleen. In: Cottier H, Odartchenko N, Shindler R, Congdon CC (eds). *Germinal Centers in Immune Response*. Berlin, Springer-Verlag, 1966, pp. 212–17.
3. Swartzendruber DC, Congdon CC. Electron microscope observations on tingible body macrophages in mouse spleen. J Cell Biol 1963; 19:641–46.
4. Milićević NM, Milićević Ž. Enzyme-histochemical characterization of macrophages in the rat thymus, with special reference to metallophilic cells of the cortico-medullary zone. J Leukocyte Biol 1984; 36:761–69.
5. Milićević NM, Milićević Ž, Čolić M, Mujović S. Ultrastructural study of macrophages in the rat thymus, with special reference to the corticomedullary zone. J Anat 1987; 150:89–98.
6. Eikelenboom P. Dendritic cells in the rat spleen follicles. A combined immuno- and enzyme histochemical study. Cell Tissue Res 1978; 190:79–87.
7. Poulter LW, Turk JL. Studies on the effect of soluble lymphocyte products (lymphokines) on macrophage physiology. II. Cytochemical changes associated with activation. Cell Immunol 1975; 20:25–32.
8. Brune K, Glatt M, Kälin H, Peskar BA. Pharmacological control of prostaglandin and thromboxane release from macrophages. Nature 1978; 274:261–63.
9. Milićević NM, Milićević Ž. Naphthol AS D chloroacetate esterase-positive macrophages in the cortico-medullary zone of the normal rat thymus. Virchows Arch (Cell Pathol) 1985; 50:193–8.

137

Induction of Coexpression of Major Histocompatibility Complex Class II Protein and Forssman Glycolipid on Murine Macrophages by Interleukin-4 and Interleukin-6

Peter F. Mühlradt and R. von Kleist
Society for Biotechnology Research, Braunschweig, Germany

INTRODUCTION

Forssman antigen (Fo) is a typical example of a glycolipid-differentiation antigen; in this case, for murine macrophages which reside in the red pulp of the spleen (1,2). Resident peritoneal macrophages from healthy mice are double negative for Fo and Ia (major histocompatibility complex [MHC] class II antigen), whereas inflammatory stimuli lead to the appearance of double-positive macrophages in the peritoneum (3). We have now performed in vitro studies to clarify whether these effects were due to migration of Fo-positive and Ia-positive macrophages into the peritoneal cavity, or whether the expression of Fo and Ia antigen might be the result of an in situ modulation by cytokines.

METHODS

Preparation of Peritoneal Macrophages

CBA/J mice at the age of 12 weeks were asphyxiated with CO_2. Where indicated, mice were pretreated 4 days previously by i.p. injection with 1 ml 3% proteose peptone. Peritoneal cells were obtained immediately after killing by injecting i.p. 3 ml ice-cold RPMI 1640 medium with 7.5% fetal calf serum (FCS), and withdrawing the liquid after gently massaging of the abdomen. 5×10^5 cells/ml of the above medium were seeded into LAB-TEK four-chamber tissue culture glass slides, and left to adhere for 4 hr. Nonadherent cells were rinsed off with warm medium, the remaining cells left overnight, rinsed again, and cultured for 4 days in the presence of cytokines or other additions. These preparations consisted of >95% macrophages.

Immunostaining

Before staining, cells were fixed with 3.7% formaldehyde in phosphate-buffered saline (PBS). Rat α-Fo immunoglobulin G_{2c} (IgG_{2c}), purified over protein G Sepharose, was used at 4 μg/ml; mouse α-Ia^k monoclonal antibody (MAb) was bought from Biotest (Frankfurt, West Germany); rat α-mouse $Ia^{b,d,k}$ MAb from Hybritech. Incubations were for 30 min in the cold in 2% FCS, 0.02% azide, followed by three washes with cold PBS. The percentage of positive cells were enumerated from 400 cells by double fluorescence microscopy.

Cytokines

Murine recombinant interleukin-5 (recIL-4) was a generous gift from R. Devos, LaRoche Research, Ghent, Belgium; natural murine IL-4 was produced as described previously (5). Murine IL-6 was produced in stimulated macrophage cultures, ammonium sulfate precipitated, and enriched by Sephadex G100 chromatography. Human recIL-6 was a kind gift of W. Fiers, Rijksuniversiteit Ghent, Belgium; murine (recIFN-γ) was generously supplied by Dr. Adolf, Boehringer Institute, Vienna, Austria; neutralizing IL-4 (F128a MAb (4) was a kind gift from W. E. Paul.

RESULTS

In an early experiment, kindly performed by Dr. J. Westermann, Med. Hochschule Hannover, West Germany, it was shown that the lipopolysaccharide (LPS)–induced appearance of Fo, Ia, double-positive macrophages in the peritoneal cavity could not be prevented by splenectomy, making immigration of double-positive macrophages from this organ unlikely (6). We sought, therefore, to induce modulation of these antigens by LPS in vitro. Within 4 days, 0.1 μg/ml phenol-extracted smooth-type *Salmonella typhimurium* LPS caused a moderate increase in Fo, Ia double-positive macrophages (Fig. 1). Pretreatment of mice with proteose peptone (PP) increased this number considerably. Since LPS is a known stimulator of the release of several monokines, such as tumor necrosing factor (TNF), IL-1, and IL-6, these substances were tried in our in vitro system for the capacity to induce Fo and/or Ia expression. Whereas neither TNF (50–1000 U/ml) nor IL-1 (50 U/ml) had any effects, IL-6, in a dose-dependent manner, induced Fo/Ia double-positive macrophages (Fig. 2). Because LPS as well as IL-6 induced both Fo and Ia on the same cells, we next assayed IFN-τ and IL-4 as known inducers of Ia. Although IFN-γ induced Ia on 90% of the macrophages, no Fo was expressed. In contrast, IL-4 coinduced both antigens (Fig. 3). The IL-4 and IL-6 effects were always more pronounced when macrophages from PP-primed animals were used.

SUMMARY AND CONCLUSIONS

Two different cytokines, IL-4 and IL-6, were able to induce expression of Fo and Ia antigen on the same macrophages. Since more pronounced effects required priming of the animals, we assume the responsive population within the newly arrived macrophages. This is the first example for the modulation of a glycolipid differentiation antigen by defined cytokines. Although coexpression of Fo and MHC class II protein suggests a role of Fo for the interaction of IL-4 and IL-6 activated macrophages with T cells, its role is as yet unknown.

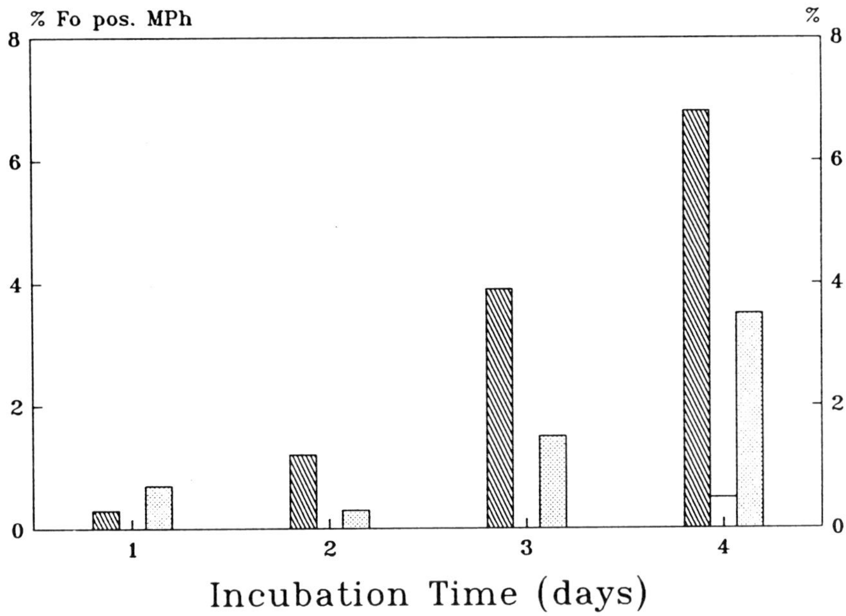

Figure 1 In vitro induction of Fo on peritoneal macrophages by LPS. Macrophages were cultured for 4 days in the presence of 0.1 μg LPS/ml. Cross-hatched bars: macrophages from PP-treated animals; stipled bars: macrophages from sham-treated (saline) animals; empty bar: macrophages from PP-treated animals cultured without LPS.

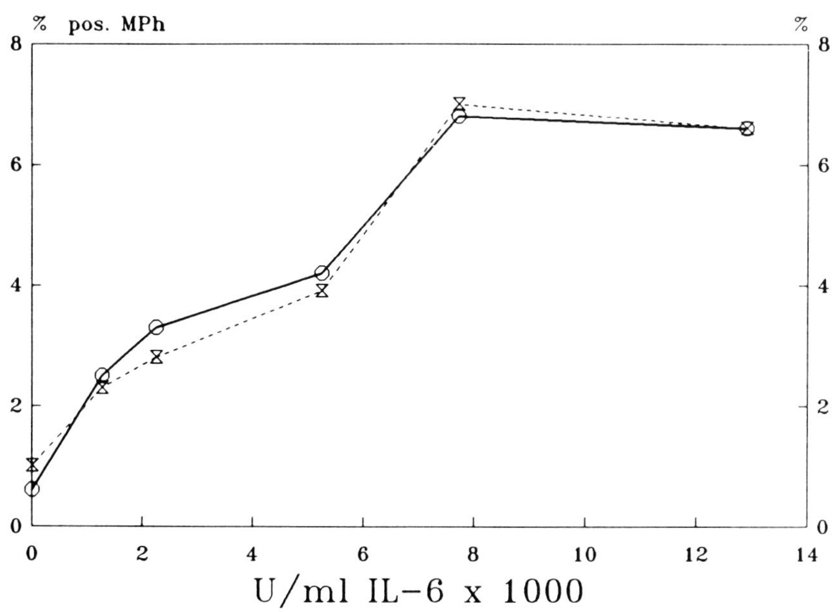

Figure 2 In vitro induction of Fo and Ia antigen on peritoneal macrophages by IL-6. Macrophages from PP-treated animals were cultured for 4 days in the presence of the indicated activities of IL-6. o–o: Forssman, x . . . x: Ia positive macrophages.

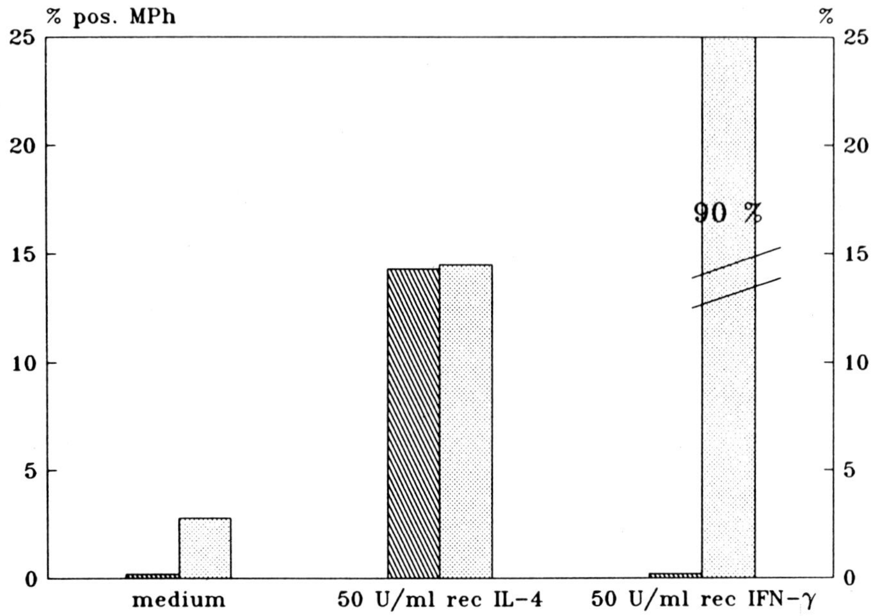

Figure 3 Effects of IL-4 and IFN-γ on expression of Fo and Ia antigen by peritoneal macrophages. Macrophages from PP-treated animals were cultured for 4 days in the presence of the indicated activities of the lymphokines. Cross-hatched bars: Fo, stipled bars: Ia-positive macrophages.

REFERENCES

1. Bethke U, Kniep B, Mühlradt PF. Forssman glycolipid, an antigenic marker for a major subpopulation of macrophages from murine spleen and peripheral lymph nodes. J Immunol 1987; 138:4329–4335.
2. Mühlradt PF, Monner DA, Dijkstra CC. Immunohistochemical localization of Forssman glycosphingolipid positive macrophages and reticular cells in murine lymphoid tissue. Immunobiology 1989; 179:259–270.
3. Conradt P, von Kleist R, Mühlradt PF. Tissue localization and migration of murine spleen macrophages carrying the Forssman glycolipid antigen. In: Fossum S, Rolstad B (eds). *Histology of the Immune System: The Life History, Organization, and Interactions of Its Cell Population.* New York, Plenum, 1988, pp. 577–582.
4. Schmitt E, Fassbender B, Beyreuther K, Spaeth E, Schwarzkopf R, Rüde E. Characterization of a T cell derived lymphokine that acts synergistically with IL 3 on the growth of murine mast cells and is identical with IL 4. Immunobiology 1987; 174:406–419.
5. Ohara J, Paul WE. Production of a monoclonal antibody to and molecular characterization of B-cell stimulatory factor-1. Nature 1985; 315:333–336.
6. von Kleist R, Schmitt E, Westermann J, Mühlradt PF. Modulation of Forssman glycolipid expression by murine macrophages: Coinduction with class II MHC antigen by the lymphokines IL4, IL6. Immunobiology 1990; 180:405–418.

138
Expression of Interleukin-2R on Rat Thymic Macrophages in Culture

Dubravka Drabek and Miodrag Čolić
Military Medical Academy, Belgrade, Yugoslavia

INTRODUCTION

The interactions between thymic accessory cells (epithelial cells, macrophages, dendritic cells) and thymocytes are of crucial importance in T-cell development (1). Thymic macrophages and dendritic cells belonging to the monocyte/macrophage cell lineage express a number of functional and differentiation antigens by which they communicate with surrounding thymocytes. Recent results (2) showed that one of these antigens, interleukin-2 receptor (IL-2R), initially found on activated T cells, was also present on phagocytic cells of the thymic reticulum in mice continuously produced in long-term thymic stroma cultures. We present here new data concerning IL-2R expression on macrophages/dendritic cells in rat thymic cultures and interrelationship between IL-2R on these cells with other subset-specific macrophage markers.

MATERIALS AND METHODS

Animals

AO rats, 4–6 weeks old, both sexes, bred at the Farm for Experimental Animals, MMA Belgrade, Yugoslavia, were used.

Primary Culture of Thymic Nonlymphoid Cells

Small fragments of thymic tissues were cultivated onto glass Petri dishes or on coverslips placed into Petri dishes using serum-free medium (Biorich 2, Flow, Irving, Scotland) containing 2 mM glutamine, 1% gentamicin, and 30% L conditioned medium (supernatant of L929 fibroblast cell line) as a source of macrophage colony-stimulating factor. This medium inhibited the proliferation of fibroblasts and epithelial cells and favored the growth of macrophage colonies. Adherent macrophages were detached from dishes at various intervals after cultivation using phosphate-buffered saline (PBS) and 0.02% EDTA. Alternatively, some coverslips with adherent macrophage colonies were fixed and stained in situ. Simultaneously, nonadherent cells (NACs) released in culture medium were collected and further analyzed.

Macrophage-Thymocyte Rosettes

Rosettes were performed by mixing detached adherent macrophages from cultures or NACs with syngeneic thymocytes (ratio 1:100) and incubated 3 hr at +4°C.

Antibodies and Reagents

Monoclonal antibody (MAb) OX39, specific for rat IL-2R, was obtained from Serotec, U.K., while K.8.13 MAb, recognizing various cytokeratin-polypeptides, was purchased from ICN-Farmakos, Belgrade, Yugoslavia. ED-1 MAb specific for cells of monocyte/macrophage lineage was a generous gift of Dr. C. Dijkstra. The R-MC series of MAbs were produced in our laboratory. A panel of secondary whole or isotype-specific antibodies and streptavidin conjugated with peroxidase or Texas Red were purchased from Amersham International, U.K.

Immunohistochemistry

Monolayers or cytospins of adherent macrophages and NACs were fixed in acetone, incubated with MAbs for 60 min, followed by blocking of endogenous peroxidase activity in methanol containing 0.3% H_2O_2. After that slides were incubated with goat-antimouse immunoglobulin (Ig) biotinylated antibodies and subsequent streptavidin peroxidase. Revelation of the peroxidase activity was performed using 0.06% 3,3′-diaminobenzidine (DAB) and 0.01% H_2O_2. Double immunofluorescence was used to compare the phenotype of IL-2R–positive cells with other markers. In all combinations MAbs mutually differed in isotype specificity. The sequence of incubation was as follows: First MAb, goat-antimouse Ig isotype-specific biotinylated antibody, streptavidin Texas Red; second MAb, sheep-antimouse Ig isotype specific antibody coupled with fluorescein isothiocyanate (FITC). All controls consisting of an irrelevant MAb of the same isotype instead of first or second MAbs gave negative results.

RESULTS

Our previous results showed that the majority of adherent cells growing in serum-free medium, which is also used in this study, belongs to cells of the monocyte/macrophage lineage (defined by ED-1 MAb) (3). In addition, 85–95% NACs released into medium during cultivation were ED-1 positive (Čolić et al., Thymus, in press). In this work, we tested the expression of IL-2R on these cells and found (Table 1) a high percentage of IL-2–positive cells in the NAC population, whereas a relatively small percentage of IL-2R–positive cells were detected among adherent cells (ACs) (Table 1; Fig. 1). In both cell populations, the expression of IL-2R considerably decreased during cultivation.

We further confirmed that the expression of IL-2R is associated with cells belonging to the monocyte/macrophage system by their round or dendritic morphology, simultaneous expression of ED-1 and R-MC 38 MAbs (both reactive with rat macrophages and interdigitating cells) and nonreactivity with K8.13 MAbs specific for keratin-positive epithelial

Table 1 Expression on IL-2R on Rat Macrophages/Dendritic Cells

	Exp. I		Exp. II		Exp. III	
Days in culture	NACs (%)	ACs (%)	NACs (%)	ACs (%)	NACs (%)	ACs (%)
3	63	—	—	—	—	—
7	82	8	94	—	—	—
8	—	—	54	—	64	16
10	89	—	—	—	—	—
13	—	—	42	0.5	38	3
14	56	14	—	—	—	—

The percentages of positive cells are given on the basis of 400 calculated cells.

cells (not shown). A number of NACs in culture (5–25%) coexpressed IL-2R and R-MC 40 antigen present on cortical macrophages in the rat thymus (Fig. 2a,b).

A high percentage of IL-2R–positive NACs form rosettes with thymocytes (Table 2; Fig. 3). Their percentages also decreased after cultivation. A considerably percentage of ED-1–positive rosettes (41%) freshly isolated from collagenase-treated thymuses were also IL-2R positive (Table 2). Much less IL-2R positivity was detected in rosettes consisting of adherent macrophages and thymocytes.

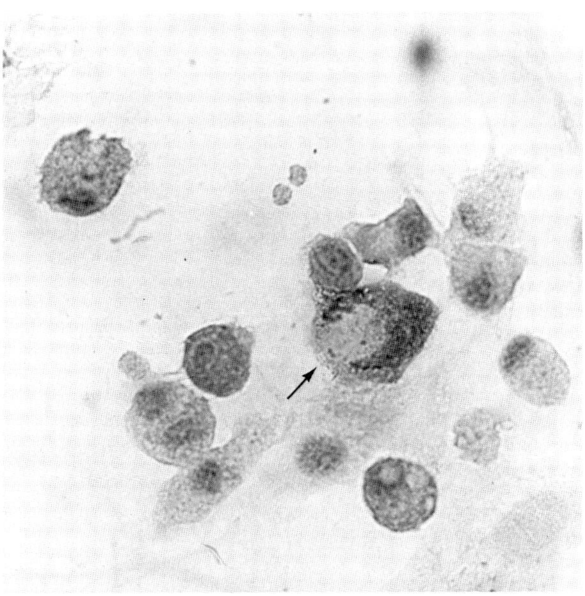

Figure 1 Streptavidin-biotin immunoperoxidase staining of adherent macrophages from 7-day-old rat thymic culture with OX39 MAb. An IL-2R^{+} cell is arrowed (magnification: ×500).

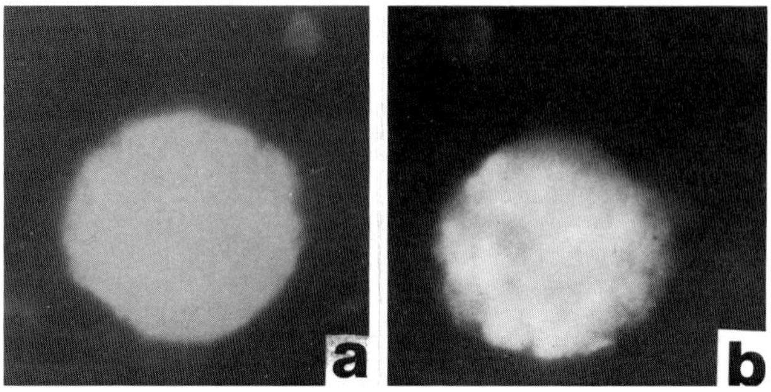

Figure 2 Double immunofluorescence staining of NACs from 7-day-old rat thymic culture with OX39 MAb (a) and R-MC 40 MAb (b). Note simultaneous expression of IL-2R on a R-MC 40^{+} cortical macrophage (magnification: ×500).

DISCUSSION

The results of our previous studies (Čolić et al., Thymus, in press) demonstrated that adherent macrophages in thymic explant cultures were an heterogeneous cell population, consisting predominantly of highly differentiated macrophages of cortical phenotype. The NACs were enriched in cells with hairy morphology, but they also contained a considerable proportion of cortical macrophages. The main difference between these two cell populations was observed in class II (MHC) antigen expression. While almost all NACs were strongly MHC class II positive, adherent cells progressively lost these antigens during cultivation. We found in this work the same difference between adherent cells and NACs in IL-2R expression.

A question resulting from this study is the nature and origin of IL-2R–positive accessory cells in thymic cultures. Based on the results that IL-2R is present on a small subset of thymocytes and on interdigitating cells (IDCs) (4), which were also confirmed in our study (not shown), and that NACs, significantly expressing IL-2R, were enriched in cells with hairy (dendritic) morphology, it can be hypothesized that a large proportion of IL-2R–positive cells in culture are dendritic cells as an in vitro equivalent of IDCs in vivo. Our

Table 2 Expression on IL-2R on Rat Thymic Rosette-Forming Cells

Days in culture	Exp. I NACs (%)	Exp. I ACs (%)	Exp. II NACs (%)	Exp. II ACs (%)	Exp. III (%)
a					41
3	80	—	87	—	
7	57	—	71	—	
13	—	23	—	7	

The percentage of positive cells forming rosettes with thymocytes is given on the basis of 200–400 calculated cells.

[a]The percentage of positive rosettes obtained from collagenase-treated thymuses.

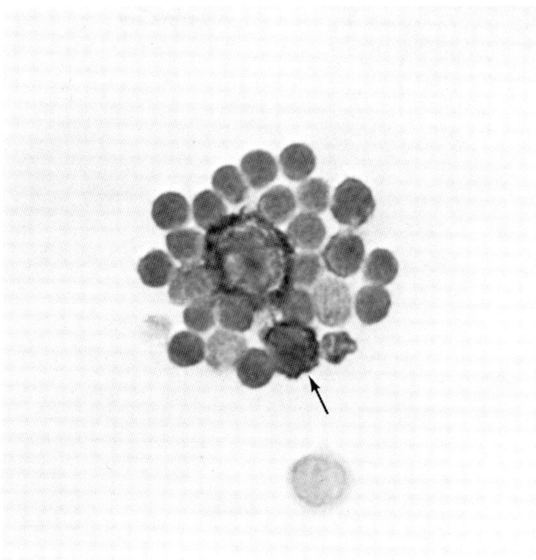

Figure 3 Streptavidin-biotin immunoperoxidase staining of rat thymic NACs forming rosettes with syngeneic thymocytes with OX39 MAb. Note IL-2R$^+$ central (rosette-forming cell) and an IL-2R$^+$ thymocyte (arrow) (magnification: ×500).

results are in accordance with those published in mice (2) that phagocytic cells produced in long-term thymic stroma cultures (P-TRs) as well as splenic accessory cells produced in vitro by the same technique are IL-2R positive. Although P-TRs share morphological and phenotypic properties with thymic macrophages, the authors (5) favor the hypothesis that P-TRs rather represent dendritic cells than classic macrophages. MacPherson (6) also found highly inducible expression from rat thoracic duct cells. Using MAbs discriminating between macrophages and interdigitating cells in rat thymus (7), we clearly demonstrated that a proportion of classic thymic macrophages bearing cortical phenotype (R-MC 40–positive cells) (7) also expressed IL-2R during cultivation. Although it was found that IL-2R is present on some macrophages (8), no such data have been published concerning thymic macrophages.

The significance of IL-2R expression on accessory, cells of the immune system (monocytes, macrophages, Langerhans' cells, IDCs), including thymic macrophages/ dendritic cells, is not sufficiently known. Hermann et al. (9) demonstrated that the function of IL-2R on monocytes is very different from the roles of these receptors on activated T and B cells. Monocytes do not appear to proliferate in response to IL-2 but sequential treatment of monocytes with interferon-γ which induced their IL-2R expression in combination with IL-2 stimulate IL-1 secretion by these cells. These results indicate that the expression of IL-2R on monocytes could be involved in amplification of the immune response.

Recent studies by Rocha et al. (2) clearly showed that IL-2R–positive P-TRs in mice, in contrast to other IL-2R–positive accessory cells, have the unique property of proliferating in the presence of recombinant IL-2, but it is not still clear whether IL-2R on these cells is a proliferating or differentiating marker. Based on our results that all IL-2R–positive cells both in adherent and the NAC population form rosettes with thymocytes, it can be concluded that IL-2R–positive macrophages/dendritic cells are functionally very active and involved in interactions with thymocytes by close contacts. The possible role of IL-2R in these processes is very attractive for further studies.

REFERENCES

1. Lobach DF, Haynes BF. Ontogeny of human thymus during fetal development. J Clin Immunol 1987; 7:81–97.
2. Rocsha B, Lehuen A, Papiernik M. IL-2-dependent proliferation of thymic accessory cells. J Immunol 1988; 140:1076–80.
3. Dijkstra CD, Dopp EA, Joling P, Kraal G. The heterogeneity of mononuclear phagocytes in lymphoid organs: Distinct macrophage populations in the rat recognized by monoclonal antibodies ED1, ED2, ED3. Immunology 1985; 54:589–99.
4. Peterson DJ, Jefferies WA, Green JR, Brandon MR, Corthesy P, Puklavec M et al. Antigens of activated rat T lymphocytes including a molecule of 50 000 Mr detected only on CD4 positive T blasts. Mol Immunol 1987; 24:1281–90.
5. Papiernik M, and Homo-Delarche F. Thymic reticulum in mice. III. Phagocytic cells of the thymic reticulum in culture secrete both prostaglandins E_2 and interleukin 1 which regulate thymocyte proliferation. Eur J Immunol 1983; 13:689–92.
6. MacPherson GG. Phenotypic changes in cultured rat dendritic cells: expression of IL-2 receptor, Thy-1 and other antigens. Adv Exp Biol Med 1988; 237:765–70.
7. Čolić M, Popović Lj, Gašić S, Dragojević-Simić V, Milićević NM, Matanović D et al. Immunohistochemical characterization of rat thymic non-lymphoid cells. II. Macrophages and granulocytes defined by monoclonal antibodies. Immunology 1990; 69:416–22.
8. Hancock WW, Muller WA, Cotran RS. Interleukin-2 receptors are expressed by alveolar macrophages during pulmonary sarcoidosis and are inducible by lymphokine treatment of normal human lung macrophages, blood monocytes and monocyte cell lines. J Immunol 1987; 138: 185–91.
9. Herrmann F, Cannistra SA, Lindemann A, Blohm D, Rambaldi A, Mertelsmann RH et al. Functional consequences of monocyte IL-2 receptor expression. J Immunol 1989; 142:139–43.

139

Interferon-γ Treatment Alters Distribution and Phenotype of Monocytes, Macrophages, and B Lymphocytes in Rats

Birte Steiniger,[1] Detlev Schröder,[1]
Hans-Heinrich Wacker,[2] and Peter H. van der Meide[3]
[1]*Medical School, Hannover, Germany;* [2]*University of Kiel, Germany;*
[3]*TNO Institute of Radiobiology and Immunology, Rijswijk, The Netherlands*

INTRODUCTION

Interferon-γ is a pleiotropic mediator with multiple effects on the immune system. It activates monocytes and macrophages (1) and induces these and many other cells to express class II major histocompatibility complex (MHC) antigens in vivo (2) and in vitro (3). Interferon-γ leads to new or increased synthesis of certain membrane proteins such as adhesion molecules (4) and influences T- and B-lymphocyte functions in vitro (5,6).

In clinical medicine, interferon-γ is applied as a therapeutic agent in certain malignancies and other conditions. We were thus interested in studying the systemic effects of the mediator on phenotype and distribution of immunocompetent cells in a rat model.

MATERIALS AND METHODS

Animals and Treatment

Male adult LEW rats (n=50) were continuously infused with recombinant rat interferon-γ at a dose of 50,000 U/hr (=0.5 mg/kg/day) for 3 or 6 (n=3) days via a catheter placed into the inferior vena cava through the femoral vein. This regimen yields interferon serum levels of about 200–300 U/ml. Three animals were coinfused with 25 mg/day bromodeoxyuridine (BrdUrd) and interferon-γ for 3 days. Another three rats received 25 mg BrdUrd intravenously for 30 min on day 3 of interferon treatment. At the end of the infusion period specimens of all major organs were frozen in liquid nitrogen or embedded in paraffin. Intravascular cells were recovered by partial perfusion of the vasculature with 800 ml PBS/EDTA in six animals. The cells recovered after discarding the first 100 ml of perfusate were characterized phenotypically in cytospin preparations. Organ sections and perfusates of the treated animals were compared to those of control rats having received a 3-day infusion of buffer and normal serum only (n=6) and to those of untreated LEW rats (n=6).

Antibodies

Antibodies are listed in Table 1. The reagents and anti-kappa chain reagent Ox12 (7) were obtained from Serotec, Oxford, England; Anti–B cell antibody HIS 14 (8) was bought from Bissendorf/Bachem Biochemicals, Hannover, West Germany. Ki-M2R and Ki-M9R were produced by H. H. Wacker. Anti-BrdUrd was bought from Becton Dickinson, Heidelberg, West Germany.

Immunohistology and Immunocytology

Single and double staining procedures for ED-1 and Ox6 or ED-1 and BrdUrd on frozen sections and cytospins have been described previously (9).

RESULTS

After 3 days of continuous intravenous infusion of recombinant rat interferon-γ, major histological alterations occurred in the spleens and submandibular lymph nodes of all rats.

Spleen

All treated rats exhibited a marked splenomegaly with expansion of the red pulp. In paraffin sections, the white pulp appeared reduced owing to substantial loss of cells from the marginal zones, collapse of the follicles, and moderate narrowing of the periarteriolar lymphocyte sheath (PALS). The marginal zones appeared empty and were sometimes

Table 1 Monoclonal Antibodies Used

Code	Specificity
Ox6	MHC class II, I-A like
Ox8	Rat CD8
Ox19	Rat CD5
Ox12	Rat immunoglobulin kappa light chains
Ox33	B-cell form of leukocyte common antigen (gp240)
His14	Presumably B-cell form of leukocyte common antigen (gp205), not identical to Ox33
W3/25	Rat CD4
W3/13	Rat CD43 (leukosialin)
ED-1	Intracellular antigen of all rat macrophages and monocytes, molecule unknown
ED-2	Antigen of rat macrophage subset, molecule unknown
ED-3	Antigen of rat macrophage subset, molecule unknown
Ki-M2R	Antigen of rat tissue macrophages, molecule unknown (tissue distribution identical to ED-2)
Ki-M9R	Antigen of rat macrophage subset, molecule unknown

For references see Materials and Methods section and see Ref. 9.

indistinguishable from the red pulp. All these alterations were found exaggerated after 6 days of treatment. The spleens of control-treated rats did not differ from normal.

White Pulp

Phenotyping for T- and B-lymphocytes and macrophage subsets showed that Ox33- and His 14-positive B-cells were nearly totally lost from the marginal zones. Only remnants of the His 14-positive follicles were left. The T cells in the PALS were also reduced in number. However, the PALS still remained a well detectable compartment with substantial cellularity. In the outer PALS W3/13-positive plasmablasts and plasma cells had accumulated. Instead of B lymphocytes, ED-3–positive and Ki-M9R–positive macrophages filled a large portion of the marginal zones (Fig. 1). These cells were only weakly reactive or negative with ED-1. They did also not react with ED-2. After pulse labeling with BrdUrd for 30 min on day 3, about 15% of the Ki-M9R–positive marginal zone cells had incorporated the nuclear label.

Red Pulp

In comparison to control rats, immunohistology showed that the splenomegaly was caused by two phenomena. First, patchy accumulations of W3/13-positive plasmablasts and plasma cells were scattered all over the red pulp. The vast majority of these cells incorporated BrdUrd during 30 min on day 3. Many cells in the patches stained for intracellular immunoglobulin kappa light chains in paraffin sections. Second, the red pulp macrophages detected by ED-1 and ED-2 appeared enlarged and increased in number. In addition, ED-3 was induced in red pulp macrophages, especially near the marginal zone. All macrophages and the majority of cells in the red pulp expressed class II MHC antigens.

Submandibular Lymph Nodes

Follicles and B-cell areas were also very much reduced in the lymph nodes. A moderate reduction of the T-cell areas was found. The medulla was enlarged with W3/13-positive plasmablasts and plasma cells, which moderately expressed class II MHC antigens. ED-3–positive and Ki-M9R–positive macrophages were increased.

Intravascular Monocytes

Intensely class II MHC and ED-1–positive aggregates of large leukocytes were observed occluding medium-sized veins in all organs. Phenotyping in situ and in cytospin preparations obtained by partial perfusion of the vasculature revealed the cells to be activated monocytes (9). After pulse labeling on day 3, about 10% of the ED-1–positive intravascular cells incorporated BrdUrd, whereas only <0.1% did so in control rats. Metaphase figures were also observed in the intravascular monocytes.

CONCLUSIONS

We show that intravenously administered interferon-γ has two major impacts on lymphatic organs of rats. It leads to a generalized activation and proliferation of monocytes and macrophages. In addition, it reduces the number of B lymphocytes in favor of terminally differentiating plasmablasts and plasma cells. These phenomena will contribute to interferon-γ–associated pathology.

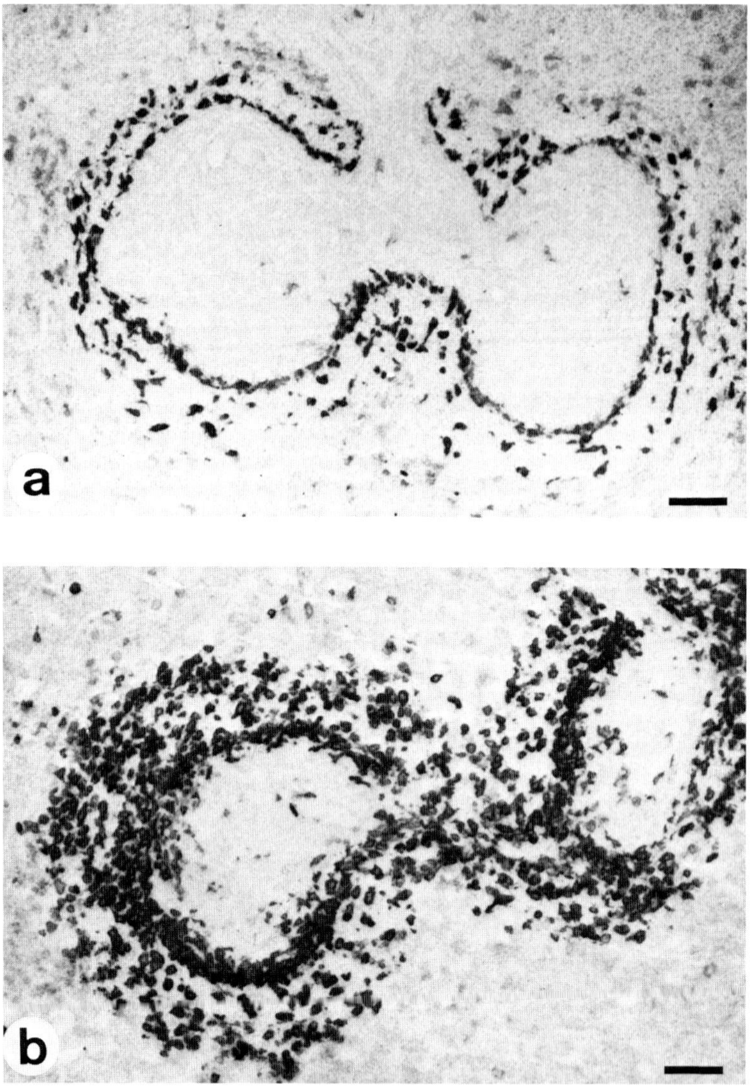

Figure 1 (a) Ki-M9R–positive cells in the marginal zone of a control-treated LEW rat. Only a small rim of marginal metallophilic macrophages and scattered cells in the marginal zone are stained. (b) Ki-M9R–positive cells after 3 days of continuous infusion of recombinant interferon-γ. The rim of marginal metallophilic macrophages is enlarged and many Ki-M9R–positive cells are present throughout the marginal zone. Indirect immunoperoxidase staining with hemalum counterstain (original magnification: ×75). (bar = 100 μm)

ACKNOWLEDGMENT

This work was supported by grant Ste 360/2-3 of the Deutsche Forschungsgemeinschaft.

REFERENCES

1. Murray HW, Spitalny GL, Nathan CF: Activation of mouse peritoneal macrophages in vitro and in vivo by interferon-γ. J Immunol 1985; 134:1619–1622.
2. Steiniger B, Falk P, van der Meide PH: Interferon-γ in vivo. Induction and loss of class II MHC antigens and immature myelomonocytic cells in rat organs. Eur J Immunol 1988, 18:661–669.
3. Wong GHW, Clark-Lewis I, Harris AW, Schrader JW: Effect of cloned interferon-γ on expression of H-2 and Ia antigens on cell lines of hemopoietic, lymphoid, epithelial, fibroblastic and neuronal origin. Eur J Immunol 1984, 14:52–56.
4. Dustin ML, Rothlein R, Bhan AK, Dinarello CA and Springer TA: Induction by IL1 and interferon-γ: Tissue distribution, biochemistry and function of a natural adherence molecule (ICAM-1). J Immunol 1986, 137:245–254.
5. Simon MM, Landolfo S, Diamantstein T and Hochgeschwender U: Antigen- and lectin-sensitized murine cytolytic T-lymphocyte-precursors require both interleukin 2 and endogenously produced immune (γ) interferon for their growth and differentiation into effector cells. Curr Top Microbiol Immunol 1986; 126:173–185.
6. Jurado A, Carballido J, Griffel H, Hochkeppel HK and Wetzel GD: The immunomodulatory effects of interferon-gamma on mature B-lymphocyte responses. Experientia 1989, 45:521–526.
7. Hunt S V; Fowler M H: A repopulation assay for B- and T-lymphocyte stem cells employing radiation chimeras. Cell Tissue Kinet 1981, 14:445–464.
8. Kroese FGM, Wubbena AS, Opstelten D, Deenen GJ, Schwander EH, de Leij L, Vos H, Poppema S, Volberda J and Nieuwenhuis P: B-lymphocyte differentiation in the rat: Production and characterization of monoclonal antibodies to B lineage-associated antigens. Eur J Immunol 1987, 17:921–928.
9. Steiniger B, Schröder D, Lück R, Luciano L and van der Meide PH: Gamma interferon treatment in vivo provokes accumulation of activated monocytes in the venous circulation of rats. Am J Pathol 1990, 136:967–978.

140
Clonal Expansion of Bone Marrow–Derived Macrophage Cell Lines, Which Can Be Repopulated In Vivo

Josien F. A. M. Wijffels, Zegerine de Rover, Nico van Rooijen, George Kraal, and Rob H. J. Beelen
Vrije University, Amsterdam, The Netherlands

INTRODUCTION

Macrophages can show phenotypic and functional heterogeneity in situ. The variation in their appearance suggests that macrophage subsets, originating from the pluripotent hemopoietic stem cell in the bone marrow, represent different lineages.

Identification of macrophage precursors in the bone marrow has been severely hampered by the lack of suitable monoclonal antibodies (MAbs) and the fact that the precursor cells occur at a very low frequency. However well-defined colony-stimulating factors (CSFs) can regulate the proliferation and differentiation of bone marrow macrophages (precursors) in vivo and in vitro (1). Bone marrow–derived macrophages obtained from cultures supplemented with CSF-1 are a heterogeneic cell population that consists of diversely differentiated cells (2). Different macrophage cell lines have been generated by transfection (3) or somatic cell hybridization with tumor cell lines (4).

However, to investigate whether macrophage subsets in situ originate from different precursors in the bone marrow, cloning of bone marrow cells is essential. Cloning of bone marrow cells enriched for macrophage precursors in the presence of CSF-1 has been described (5) to investigate the colony-forming potention of these cells.

The aim of our study is to investigate whether phenotypic heterogeneity between bone marrow–derived macrophages can be detected on clonal level. Therefore, cloning of bone marrow cells, enriched for macrophage precursors, was performed in the presence of M-CSF. We report here the continuous proliferation of cloned macrophage precursors in liquid culture for more than 1 year, without immortalization. Furthermore, we investigated the influence of the microenvironment in vitro, but also after repopulation in vivo, on the phenotype and function of our cell lines.

MATERIALS AND METHODS

Soft agar cloning of bone marrow–derived macrophage precursors from C57Bl/6 or C3H mice has been performed as described by Johnson (5). Colonies appeared within 2 weeks and were picked from the agar and resuspended in 1 ml complete growth medium plated in 24 wellsplates as one colony/well. The medium was replaced each week when cell proliferation was observed. Confluent cultures were treated with trypsin and expanded in a greater culture volume. Samples of the macrophage cell lines were frozen in liquid nitrogen. After thawing, the macrophage cell lines survive and proliferate in liquid culture.

Tissue Culture Medium

The complete growth medium for cloning in soft agar and subsequent propagation in liquid culture was Dulbecco's modified Eagle's medium supplemented with 100 U/ml penicillin, 100 μg/ml streptomycin, and 2 mM glutamine, 20% (v/v) bovine calf serum (BCS), 20% (v/v) L-cell–conditioned medium of the L929 fibroblast cell line, as the source of CSF-1.

RESULTS

Soft Agar Cloning

Soft agar cloning was performed with a cloning efficiency of 2% (1–5 colonies/250 cloned cells) after 2 weeks. The cells within the colonies showed a round morphology (Fig. 1). However, propagation of the picked macrophage colonies in liquid culture altered their morphology: The cells became adherent and showed a more flat morphology. We have observed that not all cloned cells show the same growth rate. Variation in colony size could be found after 2 weeks of culture and differences in doubling time during propagation in

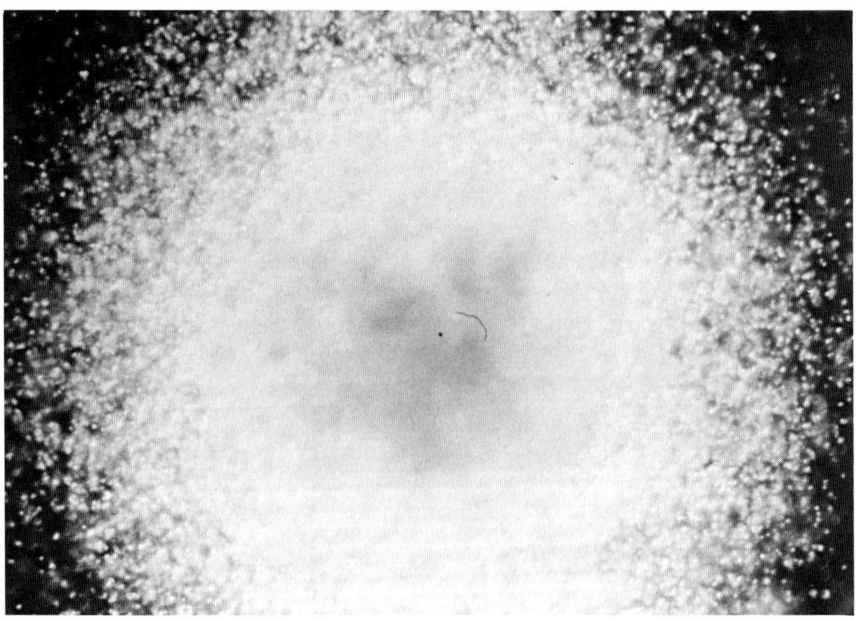

Figure 1 Soft agar colony of 3 days nonadherent bone marrow–derived cells.

liquid culture were observed between different cell lines. We have isolated up to 50 cell lines. All of them show the same morphology in liquid culture and grow loosely adherent as a confluent monolayer (Fig. 2), so that transfer could take place after treatment with trypsin. However, when cultured in Teflon bags large cell clusters were formed.

Some of our cell lines were found to be CSF-1 dependent and died upon withdrawal. But factor-independent cell lines also were found.

Phenotypic Characteristics of Our Cell Lines

By comparing the phenotype of our macrophage cell lines (100% positive staining for Moma-2, Mac-2, Mac-3, and acid phosphatase) with 3 days cultured nonadherent cells enriched for macrophage precursors we can conclude that the cell lines have lost some macrophage antigens as M5/114 and F4/80 during prolonged proliferation in vitro.

Electronmicroscopic studies have confirmed the macrophage characteristics of the cell lines, and showed negative staining for endogenous peroxidase (Fig. 3). The established phenotype of the cell lines were shown to be stable after 1 year of culture. In addition to macrophage markers, we found positive staining for the B220 and GR-1 antigen, but not for T-cell markers.

Functional Characterization of Our Cell Lines

Although our cell lines have phenotypic characteristics of a mature macrophage, they show weak to negative staining for Fc receptor (FcR) and could not perform FcR-dependent phagocytosis. However, ingestion of latex beads was performed by almost all cells. The capacity to ingest latex seems to decrease after a prolonged period of growth in liquid culture.

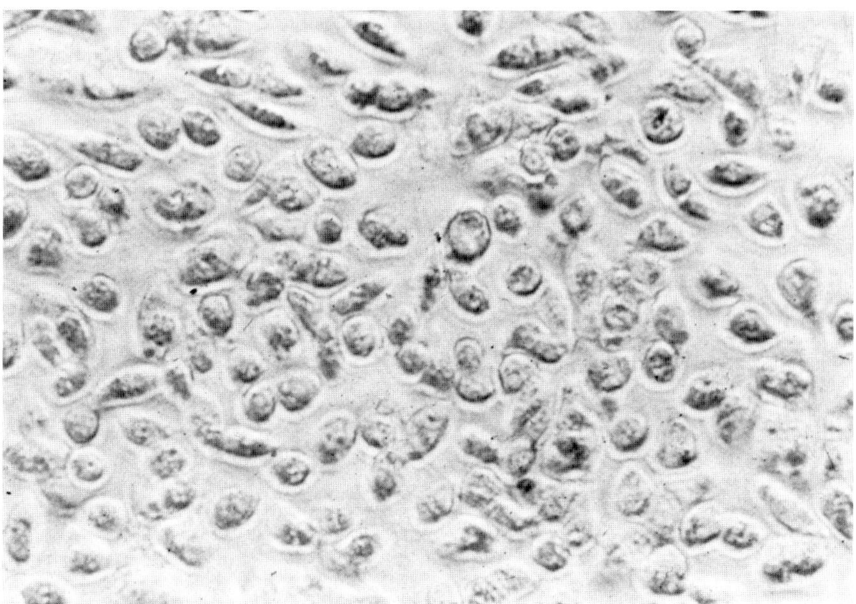

Figure 2 Light microscopic study of one of the macrophage cell lines.

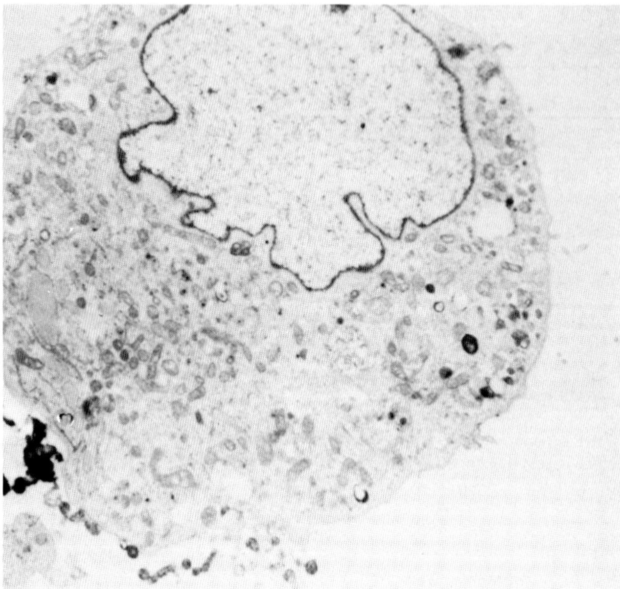

Figure 3 Ultrastructural study of one of the macrophage cell lines.

Repopulation studies in vivo in macrophage-depleted animals were performed (6). Injection of our cell lines i.v. was done to investigate the influence of the microenvironment on the phenotypic and functional behavior of our cell lines in vivo. Macrophages could be detected as well in the white as the red pulp of the spleen within 1 week, proving that at least macrophages can be repopulated in vivo.

DISCUSSION

In this study, we have shown in contrast to others the continuous proliferation, for more than 1 year, of freshly isolated bone marrow–derived macrophages in vitro. The normal macrophage cell lines generated in vitro in the presence of CSF-1 have the potention to repopulate the spleen in vivo. By injecting i.v. macrophages, we can investigate the role of the in vivo microenvironment on the phenotypic and functional behavior of our cell lines.

The observed minor phenotypic heterogeneity between our macrophage cell lines can be explained in the following ways: (a) We have not used the right MAbs to observe phenotypic heterogeneity between our cell lines because the most monoclonal antibodies are directed against antigens on mature tissue macrophages. (b) On the other hand, we can not exclude that CSF-1 selects a special macrophage precursor population in the bone marrow to survive and proliferate in vitro; or (c) that CSF-1 induces progenitor cells to a certain maturation or differentiation stage. Therefore, it is interesting to investigate whether clonal heterogeneity can be detected between macrophage colonies generated by other CSFs. Furthermore, the expression of diverse antigens can disappear after prolonged culture as described for immortalizated macrophage cell lines (3). In vivo repopulation of bone marrow–derived macrophage cell lines will show the importance of the microenvironment in situ by generation of phenotypic and functional macrophage heterogeneity.

Table 1 Rat-Antimouse MAbs Directed Against Different Macrophage-Associated Antigens

Hybridoma	Specificity	Refs.
Moma-2	General macrophage marker	7
F4/80	Macrophage differentiation antigen	8
M1/70	Mac-1: CR3 α chain	12
M18/2a8	Mac-1: CR3 β chain	10
M3/38	Mac-2	11
M3/84	Mac-3	11
M5/114	Anti–I-Abdg, I-Edk	9

REFERENCES

1. Metcalf D. 1984. *The Hemopoietic Colony Stimulating Factor.* Elsevier, Amsterdam.
2. Neumann, C., C. Sorg. 1980. Sequential expression of functions during macrophage differentiation in murine bone marrow liquid culture. Eur. J. Immunol. 10:834.
3. Gandino L., L. Varesio 1990. Immortalization of macrophages from mouse bone marrow and fetal liver. Exp. Cell. Res. 188:192.
4. Leenen P. J. M., W. A. T. Slieker, M. Melis, W. van Ewijk. 1989. Murine macrophage precursors, characterization. I. Production, phenotype and differentiation of macrophage precursor hybrids. Eur. J. Immunol. 20:15.
5. Johnson, C. R., D. Kitz, J. R. Little. 1983. A method for the derivation and continuous propagation of cloned murine bone marrow macrophages. J. Immunol. Methods. 65:319.
6. van Rooijen N., N. Kors, G. Kraal. 1989. Macrophage subset repopulation in the spleen: differential kinetics after liposome-mediated elimination. J. Leukocyte Biol. 45:97.
7. Kraal G, M. Rep, M. Janse. 1987. Macrophages in the T and B Cell compartments and other tissue macrophages recognized by monoclonal antibody MOMA-2. Scand. J. Immunol. 26:653.
8. Austyn J. M., S. Gordon. 1981. F4/80, a monoclonal antibody directed specifically against the mouse macrophage. Eur. J. Immunol. 11:805.
9. Bhattacharya A., M. E. Dorf, T. A. Springer T. 1981. A shared alloantigenic determinant on Ia antigens encoded by the I-A and I-E subregion: Evidence for I region gen duplication. J. Immunol. 17:2488.
10. Sanchez-Madrid F., P. Simon, S. Thompson, T. A. Springer. 1983. Mapping of antigenic and functional epitopes on the α- and β-subunits of two related glycoproteins involved in cell interactions, LFA-1 and MAC-1. J. Exp. Med. 158:586.
11. Springer T.A. 1981. Monoclonal antibody analysis of complex biological systems: combinations of cell hybridization and immunoadsorbents in a novel cascade procedure and its application to the macrophage cell surface. J. Biol. Chem. 256:3833.
12. Springer T. A ., G. Galfre, D. S. Secher, C. Milstein. 1979. MAC-1 a macrophage differentiation antigen identified by monoclonal antibody. Eur. J. Immunol. 9:301.

141
Effect of Cytokines In Vitro on $CD4^-CD8^-$ Thymocytes
An Ultrastructural Study

B. Nabarra and M. Papiernik
INSERM U25, Hôpital Necker, Paris, France

INTRODUCTION

The lymphocyte precursors within the thymus are part of a subset of cells which lack CD4 and CD8 differentiation antigens. These $CD4^-CD8^-$ cells (double-negative or DN) can momentarily repopulate the thymus of an irradiated animal and give rise to all lymphocyte subsets (1). Double-negative cells also contain precursors of accessory cells which may be induced to mature Ia-positive and/or Mac-1–positive cells when cultured with colony/stimulating factors (CSFs) (2). We have also shown that the presence of accessory cells may potentiate the response of DN thymocytes to interleukin 2 (IL-2) (3). The same proliferation would be obtained if accessory cells were generated from their precursors by CSFs; also, in this system, IL-1 associated with IL-2 gives the same result (2). Cell interactions through membrane antigen recognition and the production of factors are probably the essential mechanisms which lead to thymocyte activation and maturation. It was interesting to identify the cells which were involved in the potentiation of the response when GM-CSF or IL-2 were added. Characterization of membrane antigen expression was not sufficient to discriminate macrophages from interdigitating cells within accessory cells, as they both express Ia and Mac-1, although at different levels (4–5). Electron microscopy was the only technique able to clearly characterize both types of cells. In this chapter, we show that DN cells stimulated by GM-CSF and IL-2 contain both macrophages and interdigitating cells associated with lymphocytes, while IL-1 and IL-2 only contain interdigitating cells and lymphocytes. Interleukin-1 may directly induce maturation and activation of interdigitating cells, whereas GM-CSF first induces macrophage maturation, which in turn produces IL-1, the cytokine necessary to induce maturation of interdigitating cell.

MATERIALS AND METHODS

DN Cell Preparation

$CD4^-CD8^-Ia^-Mac^-$ thymic cells of DBA/2, H-2d, 4- to 5-week-old females, were prepared by negative selection using anti-CD4, anti-CD8, anti-Ia, anti–Mac-1 antibodies, in the presence of complement. Three successive cytotoxicity treatments were done, and purification of DN cells was >97% as assessed by using directly labeled antibodies or a second layer only. Selected cells were termed $CD4^-CD8^-$ or DN cells.

DN Thymic Cell Culture

Double-negative thymic cells were cultured in 24-well plastic culture plates. 5×10^5 cells were seeded in 1 ml culture medium. RPMI 1640 supplemented with 1% Na pyruvate, 100 U/ml penicillin and streptomycin, containing 10% fetal calf serum (FCS) and 10^{-5} M 2-ME. The following reagents were added: recombinant IL-2 (rIL-2) (100 U/ml); rIL-1 (5 U/ml); rGM-CSF (100 U/ml) (Genzyme, Boston, Massachusetts). Cultures were set up in a CO_2 humidified atmosphere at 37°C for 3 days.

Electron Microscopy

Day zero DN cells and cultures of DN cells plus rGM-CSF and rIL-2, or rIL-1 plus rIL-2 at day 3 were fixed in 2% glutaraldehyde in phosphate buffer pH 7.4 for 1 hr, postfixed 1 hr in 2% osmium tetraoxyde, dehydrated in alcohol series, and embedded in Epon. Between each step, cells were centrifuged at 1200 rpm. Ultrathin sections were impregnated with uranyl acetate and lead citrate. Observations were made with a EM 300 Philips electron microscope. Analyses were made on microphotographs systematically taken in the left quarter of the grid to randomize the observations. The different types of cells were analyzed and counted on these microphotographs (3600, 9000, and 12,000 magnification).

RESULTS

We have already shown that DN cells are induced to proliferate when rIL-2 is associated to rGM-CSF or to rIL-1. Kinetic studies indicate that maximum proliferation was obtained at day 4 in these two groups. Recombinant IL-1 and rGM-CSF alone never induced substantial proliferation, and IL-2 alone gave poor proliferation (2). Clusters of cells developed in cultures with GM-CSF plus IL-2 and IL-1 plus IL-2 which were maximum at day 3.

Electron microscopic study was performed on fresh DN cells just after purification. At this time, two types of cells were observed: blastlike cells and medium-sized immature lymphocytes (mature small lymphocytes were less than 1%) (Fig. 1). Blastlike cells were large cells with an immature nucleus (clear chromatin and few clumps of heterochromatin) and an extended clear cytoplasm with numerous ribosomes. Medium-sized immature lymphocytes had a large nucleus with coarse chromatin and often a prominent nucleolus. Most of the nuclei were round, but some had a more convoluted shape. The cytoplasm formed a clear rim around the nucleus, with very few cellular organelles. Neither macrophages nor interdigitatinglike cells or epithelial cells were found. However, very rare granulocytes were isolated by our technique (0.5%). We observe that 30.0% of the cells were immature lymphocytes and 69.5% were blastlike cells.

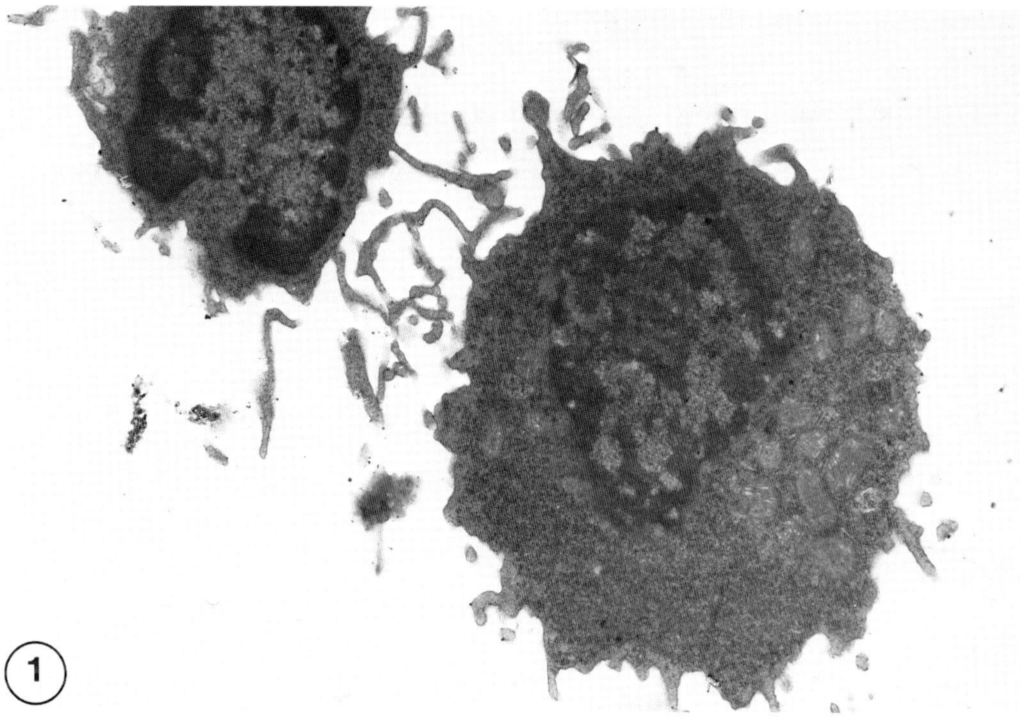

1

Figure 1 DN cells at day 0: medium-sized immature lymphocyte and blast cell were observed. Impregnated with uranyl acetate and lead citrate (magnification: ×10000).

After 3 days in culture, cell populations were deeply modified, and clusters of cells appeared. The distribution of cells was a function of the cytokine used in culture. In cultures with GM-CSF + IL-2 less immature medium-sized lymphocytes (12%) and more large blastlike cells (65%) were found with the same morphology as at day 0. Some of the blast cells had small, irregular, dense granules, which suggested that they may be already committed to the myelomonocytic lineage. Mature small lymphocytes were very rare (<1%). In this culture, two types of accessory cells were found: typical macrophages with phagolysosomes (8.7%), and large cells with an indented mature nucleus, a clear cytoplasm with large and long pseudopods, and fingerlike thin processes on their surface, which were identified as interdigitating-like cells (9.3%). The most striking difference with IL-1 + IL-2 culture was the composition of accessory cells. In culture with IL-1 + IL-2, we never observed macrophages, and interdigitating-like cells were the only accessory cells present in addition to cells of the lymphocyte lineage.

Another important finding in this culture was the presence of aggregated cells, the central cell of which was exclusively of an interdigitating-like type (Fig. 2). All these clusters were formed by immature lymphocytes and/or blast cells centered by interdigitating-like cells. In this case, numerous interdigitations and microvilli were closely linked to the lymphocyte membrane. Thus, it appears that lymphoid or blast cells were closely attached to the central cell or its pseudopods with a broad area of contact. It is noteworthy that in the junctional zones, there was clarification of the cytoplasm, with a loss of cellular organelles and ribosomes.

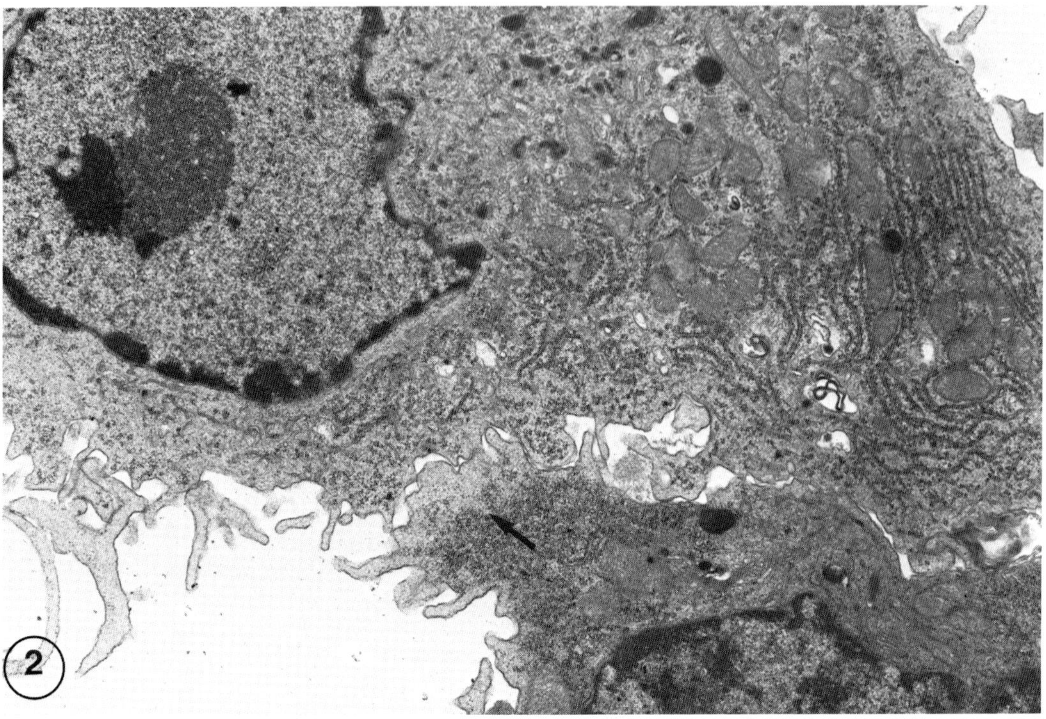

Figure 2 Aspect of interdigitating cell/blast cell interrelationship in a cluster formed at 3 days of culture with IL-1 + IL-2. Large zones of the membrane of both cells were in contact (→). Part of the cytoplasm of the blast cell in contact is clear, without ribosomes or other cellular organelles. Impregnated with uranyl acetate and lead citrate (magnification: ×45000).

DISCUSSION

In the thymus, production of cytokines by different types of stromal cells and lymphocytes is part of the system needed for precursor maturation. We have already shown, using in vitro systems, that IL-1, IL-2, IL-3, and GM-CSF are included in a cytokine network which induces thymic accessory cell maturation and thymocyte activation (2–6). Accessory cells expressing the third receptor of complement and/or class II major histocompatibility complex (MHC) antigens were generated in such cultures (2), but they were not characterized. In the present chapter, we have compared the effect of two different combinations of cytokines on $CD4^-CD8^-$ thymic cells and analyzed their morphological aspect at the electron microscopical level. Both IL-1 plus IL-2 and CM-CSF + IL-2 in vitro give rise to the same type of lymphocytes which are mainly blastlike cells, with a small percentage of immature lymphocytes (these later being reduced, compared to the initial freshly isolated population). The initial cell population was depleted of mature accessory cells. After 3 days in culture, accessory cells were generated and were different according to the type of cytokines used. Interleukin-1 plus IL-2 induced the appearance of interdigitating cells but not of macrophages. This is in agreement with the results of Inaba et al. (7), showing that $CD4^-CD8^-$ thymocytes contain a small number of Ia-negative dendritic cell precursors which may give rise to Ia-positive cells in the presence of IL-2. GM-CSF + IL-2 induces the maturation of both macrophages and dendritic-like cells, with an enhanced proportion of granulocytes (3.5% compared to 0.5% in the initial population). It is obvious that GM-CSF is able to act directly on macrophage precursors. Whether or not it acts directly on interdigitating cell precursors is a matter of discussion. Maturation of interdigitating cells may be the result of IL-1 production by macrophages which are induced to mature under the influence of GM-CSF. Interleukin-2 may also intervene in accessory cell maturation and activation, as we have already shown that phagocytic cells of the thymic reticulum in vitro express IL-2 receptors, and are able to proliferate in the presence of IL-2 (8). In both culture conditions, clusters of cells are formed after three days in culture. These clusters are shown to be organized around interdigitating cells, and never around macrophages. Multicellular complexes have been shown to occur in the thymus with epithelial cells (9), interdigitating cells, and macrophages (9–11). These cellular complexes are probably the functional units where the different steps of T-cell maturation occur. We show in the present chapter that activation of $CD4^-CD8^-$ thymocytes is associated with the constitution of interdigitating cell clusters which provide the needed microenvironments.

REFERENCES

1. Fowlkes BJ, Edison L, Mathieson BJ, Chused TM. Early T lymphocytes differentiation in vivo of adult intrathymic precursor cells. J. Exp. Med. 162:802–822, 1985.
2. Papiernik, L., Lepault, F., Pontoux, C. Synergistic effect of colony stimulating factors and IL-2 on prothymocyte proliferation linked to the maturation of macrophage/dendritic cells within $L3T4^-Lyt\text{-}2^-Ia^-Mac^-$ cells. J. Immunol., 240:1431–1433, 1988.
3. Papiernik, M., Penit C., El Rouby S. Control of prothymocyte proliferation by thymic accessory cells. Eur. J. Immunol. 17:1303–1310, 1987.
4. Schuler G, Steinman RM. Murine epidermal Langerhans cells mature into potent immunostimulatory dendritic cells in vitro. J. Exp. Med. 161:526–546, 1985.
5. Nabarra, B, Papiernik M. Phenotype of thymic stromal cells: An immunoelectron microscopic study with anti-Ia, anti-Mac-1, anti-Mac-2 antibodies. Lab. Invest., 58:524–531, 1988.
6. Papiernik M. Thymic accessory cells, cytokines and thymocyte activation. Res. Immunol., 191:275–280, 1990.
7. Inaba K, Witmer-Pack MD, Inaba M, Muramatsu S, Steinman RM. The function of Ia^+ dendritic cells and Ia^- dendritic cell precursors in thymocyte mitogenesis to lectin and lectin plus interleukin 1. J. Exp. Med., 167:149–162, 1988.
8. Rocha B, Lehuen, A, Papiernik M. IL-2 dependent proliferation of thymic accessory cells. J. Immunol., 140:1076–1080, 1988.
9. Wekerle H, Ketelsen UP, Ernst M. Thymic nurse cells. Lympho-epithelial cell complexes in murine thymuses: Morphological and serological characterization. J. Exp. Med., 151:925–944, 1980.
10. Kyewski BA. Seeding of thymic microenvironments defined by distinct thymocyte-stromal cell interactions is developmentally controlled. J. Exp. Med., 166:520–538, 1987.
11. El Rouby S, Praz F, Halbwachs-Mecarelli L, Papiernik M. Thymic reticulum in mice. IV. The rosette formation between phagocytic cells of the thymic reticulum and cortical type thymocytes is mediated by complement receptor type three. J. Immunol. 134:3625–3631, 1985.

142
Exudate Macrophages Can Express Dendritic Cell Markers In Vitro

Josien F. A. M. Wijffels, Zegerine de Rover, Nico van Rooijen, Georg Kraal, and Robert H. J. Beelen
Vrije University, Amsterdam, The Netherlands

INTRODUCTION

Macrophages in situ show phenotypic and functional heterogeneity. Such heterogeneity can not only be found between populations at different locations such as alveolar and peritoneal macrophages (1), but also heterogeneity within one overall-population of macrophages has been described (2). Induction of heterogeneity may result from the cellular and mineral composition of the microenvironment, as has been suggested by several studies (3,4). In this study, we investigated the influence of an inflammatory microenvironment on macrophage heterogeneity in situ. Therefore, peritoneal (exudate) macrophages were phenotypically characterized directly or after culturing, using a panel of monoclonal antibodies. Functional analysis was performed in the mixed lymphocyte reaction (MLR) to study the antigen-presenting capacity of peritoneal exudate cells. Antigen presentation was tested, since the marker NLDC-145, normally only present on dendritic cells, could be upregulated on cultured thioglycollate-induced exudate macrophages.

MATERIALS AND METHODS

Peritoneal cells (PCs) were elicited by i.p. injection of 1 ml NBCS (Greiner), 1 ml Brewer's thioglycollate broth (TG) (Difco, Detroit, Michigan), or 1 ml paraffin-oil (paraffinum liquidum, Brocacef). Pooled peritoneal exudate cells (PECs), from two to four mice, were harvested 1 day after NBCS injection and 4 days after injection with TG or paraffin-oil.

The PECs were cultured for 2–48 hr under nonadherent conditions in Teflon bags (10^6/ml) or on glass coverslips (2×10^5/well, 24-wells plates (Greiner) in RPMI 1640 culture medium supplemented with 2 mM glutamine, 100 U/ml penicillin, 100 µg/ml streptomycin, and 10% (v/v) fetal calf serum (FCS) (Greiner). Immunohistochemistry and enzyme histochemistry of Cytospin preparations or glass coverslides were performed with

Table 1 Rat-Antimouse Monoclonal Antibodies Used to Characterize Peritoneal Exudate Cells

Hybridoma	Antigen	Isotype	Source	Refs.
Moma-2	Moma-2	$IgG2^b$		9
F4/80	F4/80	$IgG2^b$	S. Gordon	10
2.4G2	FcRII	IgG		11
NLDC-145	NLDC-145	$IgG2^a$		12
M5/114	$I\text{-}A^{bdq}$	$IgG2^b$	ATCC	13

a panel of monoclonal antibodies (Table 1) and compared with fluor cytofluorometric analysis of cell suspensions.

The antigen-presenting capacity of PECs was compared with dendritic cells (DCs) isolated from the spleen according to Breel (5) and tested in the allo-MLR.

RESULTS

Phenotypic analysis with Moma-2 in comparison with May Grunwald Giemsa of the peritoneal (exudate) cells showed that 50–60% of the cells in the steady state were macrophages. However, after stimulation, especially with TG, an increase in the amount of macrophages was found, to more than 95% of the exudate cells (Fig. 1). Staining for F4/80 showed phenotypic heterogeneity between the freshly isolated peritoneal (exudate) cells. F4/80 could not be detected on TG macrophages, but stained all or most of the macrophages in the steady-state situation and after NBCS stimulation. Some of the paraffin oil–elicited macrophages showed a very weak staining for F4/80 (Fig. 1).

To select for macrophages, peritoneal (exudate) cells were cultured on glass coverslides for 2 hr. Culture of these PECs showed that exudate macrophages can further differentiate in vitro. Moreover, in contrast to 2–48 hr cultured steady-state macrophages or NBCS exudate macrophages, we found that the expression of the dendritic cell marker NLDC-145 was acquired by cultured TG exudate macrophages and to a lesser extent by cultured oil-induced exudate macrophages (Fig. 1). The expression of NLDC-145 could not be found on freshly isolated peritoneal steady-state or exudate cells. The immunohistochemical staining was confirmed by FACScan analysis. In addition to the induction of NLDC-145, we studied whether TG macrophages showed other phenotypic characteristics of DCs as high Ia membrane expression and acid phosphatase in a spot near the nucleus of the cell. All freshly isolated TG macrophages showed strong cytoplasmic acid phosphatase staining and less Ia positivity (Fig. 1), but Ia expression could be induced by recombinant rat interferon-γ (IFN-γ).

To study whether TG exudate cells, which acquire NLDC-145 during culture, had other characteristics of NLDC-145–positive DCs, freshly isolated TG exudate cells were tested in an allo-MLR and compared with the antigen-presenting capacity of isolated DCs. We found that TG exudate cells as well as other exudate cell populations (NBCS, paraffin oil–induced) could not stimulate the T-cell proliferation as DCs do (Fig. 2). However, the small response induced by the different exudate populations is Ia dependent because inhibition of the response was found in the presence of anti-Ia. Interferon-γ–treated NLDC-$145^{+}Ia^{+}$ TG exudate cells did not result in an increased antigen-presenting capacity. Our

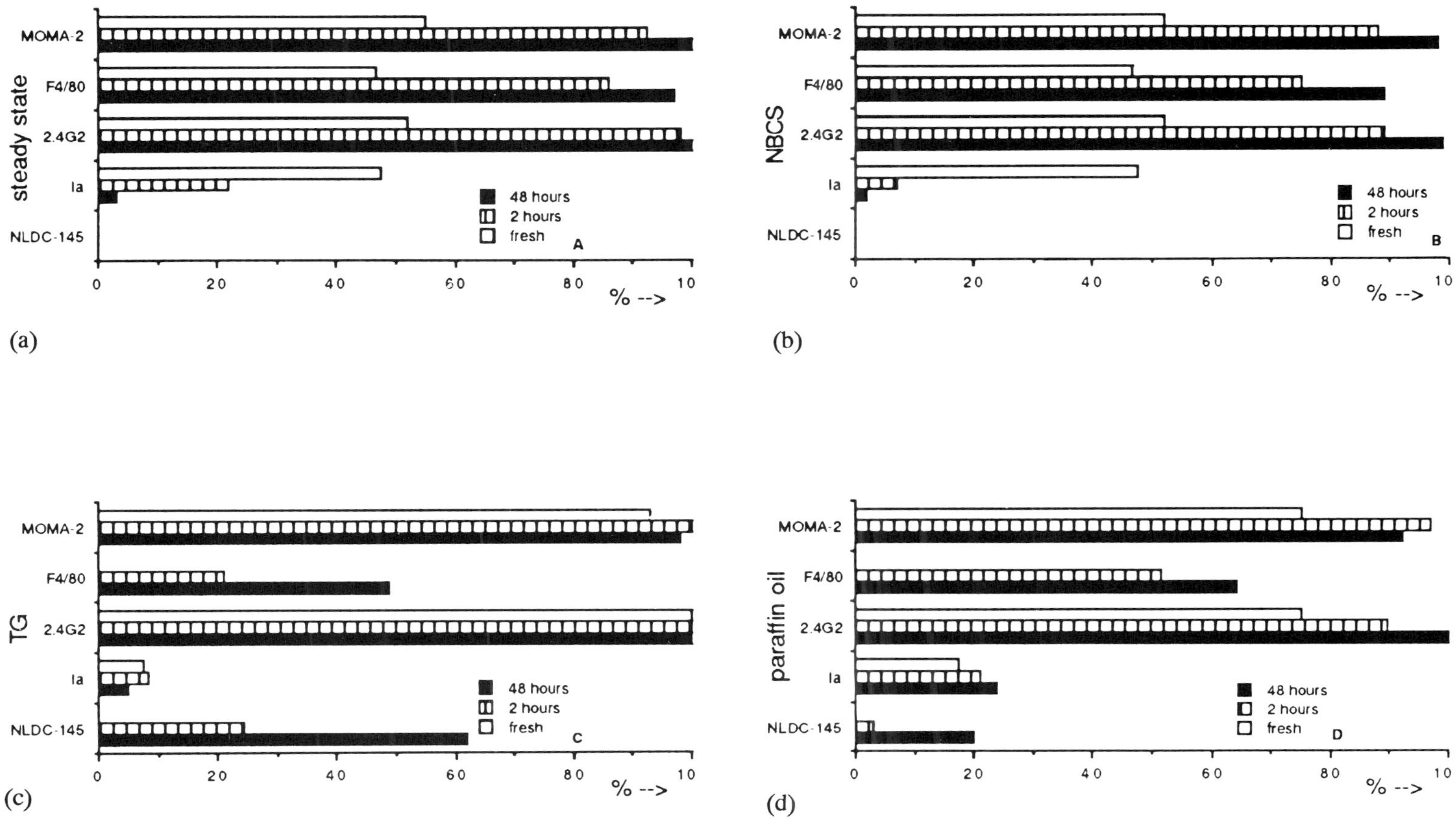

Figure 1 Immunoperoxidase staining of freshly isolated or cultured steady-state macrophages (a), 1-day NBCS-stimulated (b), 4-days TG-stimulated (c), and 4-day paraffin oil–stimulated (d) peritoneal (exudate) cells. Note the presence of the dendritic cell marker NLDC-145 on cultured TG exudate macrophages.

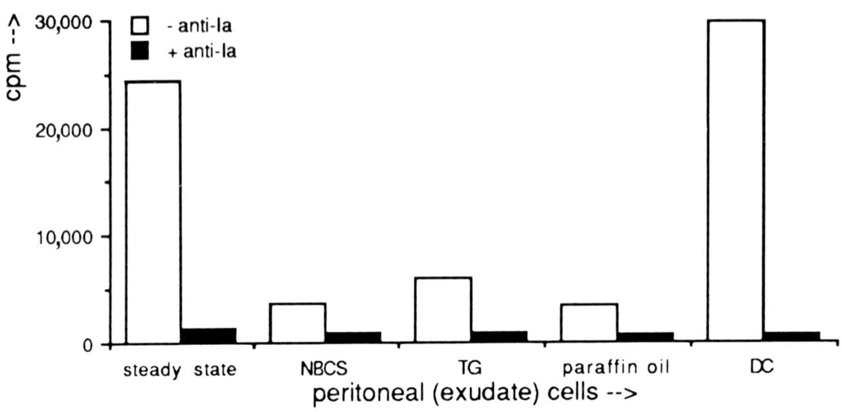

Figure 2 TG-elicited cells (2×10^4/well) were compared with DCs (2×10^3/well), steady-state peritoneal cells (4×10^4/well), or other acute (NBCS) and chronic (paraffin oil) peritoneal exudate cells (2×10^4/well) in their antigen-presenting capacity in an allo-MLR. Despite the presence of NLDC-145 on TG-elicited cells, they do not support antigen presentation in the allo-MLR.

data show that TG exudate cells are incapable of stimulating the T-cell proliferation in an allo-MLR, despite the presence of the dendritic cell marker NLDC-145.

DISCUSSION

In our study, we found differences in F4/80 and Ia staining on peritoneal (exudate) cells induced by different inflammatory reagents, which show phenotypic heterogeneity. Furthermore, we showed that TG exudate cells were not a homogeneous population of elicited cells, but rather a complex population, consisting of a subpopulation, which acquired NLDC-145 during culture. The induction of NLDC-145 antigen on a subpopulation of TG exudate cells during culture suggests that we have detected maturation of exudate cells or clonal variation in antigen expression. However, there will be also an influence of the microenvironment in situ because NBCS exudate cells did not acquire NLDC-145 on their cell membrane. We can not exclude that the detection of NLDC-145 on a subpopulation of exudate cells is caused by a variation in NLDC-145 expression during macrophage cell cycling as, for instance, has been shown for the Fc receptor in the rat (6).

The fact that in addition to TG exudate macrophages NLDC-145 positivity has also been described on alveolar macrophages (7) suggests that the chronic excitated microenvironments in lung and peritoneum are comparable and suitable for the induction of NLDC-145 antigen on macrophages.

Furthermore, Moma-2^+NLDC-145^+ double-positive TG exudate cells showed suppressive activity comparable to double-positive alveolar macrophages (7) in the allo-MLR. The role of NLDC-145 in antigen presentation is still unclear. In agreement with our results, Poulter (8) has shown that $RFD1^+RFD7^+$ double-positive cells are also suppressive in the mixed lymphocyte reaction.

CONCLUSION

It seems that double-positive macrophages in some way exert a suppressive influence on antigen presentation. The mechanism of this suppressive activity is still unclear.

REFERENCES

1. Gordon S., S. Keshav, L.P. Chung. 1988. Mononuclear phagocytes: tissue distribution and functional heterogeneity. Curr. Opin. Immunol. 1:26.
2. Beelen R.H.J., W.S. Walker. 1983. Dynamics of cytochemically distinct subpopulations of macrophages in the elicited rat peritoneal exudates. Cell. Immunol. 82:246.
3. Beller, D.I., J. Kiely, E.R. Unanue. 1980. Regulations of macrophages populations. I. Preferential induction of Ia-rich peritoneal exudates by immunologic stimuli. J. Immunol. 124:1426.
4. Morse S.S., P.B. Moore. 1988. Expression of 67000 MW calcimedin and its binding protein in resident and thioglycollate-elicited macrophages. Immunology 65:537.
5. Breel M., R.E. Mebius, G. Kraal. 1987. Dendritic cells of the mouse recognized by two monoclonal antibodies. Eur. J. Immunol. 17:1555.
6. Walker, W.S., Beelen R.H.J. 1988. Macrophage cell cycling: Influence of proliferation state on the antibody mediated activities of rat resident peritoneal macrophages. Cell. Immunol. 11:992.
7. Breel M., M. van der Ende, T. Sminia, G. Kraal. 1988. Subpopulations of lymphoid and non-lymphoid cells in bronchus associated lymphoid tissue (BALT) of the mouse. Immunology 63:657.
8. Poulter L.W. 1988. Immune aspects of sarcoidosis. Postgrad. Med. J. 64:536.
9. Kraal G, M. Rep, M. Janse. 1987. Macrophages in the T and B Cell compartiments and other tissue macrophages recognized by monoclonal antibody MOMA-2. Scand. J. Immunol. 26:653.
10. Austyn J.M., S. Gordon. 1981. F4/80, a monoclonal antibody directed specifically against the mouse macrophage. Eur. J. Immunol. 11:805.
11. Unkeless J.C. 1979. Characterisation of a monoclonal antibody directed against mouse macrophage and lymfocyte Fc receptors. J. Exp. Med. 150:580.
12. Kraal G., M. Breel, M. Janse, G. Bruin. 1986. Langerhans' cells, veiled cells, and interdigitating cells in the mouse recognized by a monoclonal antibody. J. Exp. Med. 163:981.
13. Bhattacharya A., M.E. Dorf, T.A. Springer T. 1981. A shared alloantigenic determinant on Ia antigens encoded by the I-A and I-E subregion: Evidence for I region gen duplication. J. Immunol. 17:2488.

143
A Subpopulation of Macrophages with a Migratory Capacity in the Rat Liver

Kenjiro Matsuno, Kazuhisa Miyakawa, Taichi Ezaki, and Masahiko Kotani
Kumamoto University Medical School, Kumamoto, Japan

INTRODUCTION

Recently, we have found that in rats, only the celiac nodes draining the liver, but not other lymph nodes, turn back 12 hr after intravenous injection of carbon particles. And it has been demonstrated that this blackening is due to the accumulation in the nodes of heavily carbon-laden (HC) macrophages that have migrated from the liver sinusoids via the two lymphatic pathways (1). The aim of this study is to characterize both morphology and phenotype of the migrating HC macrophages in the celiac nodes. Macrophage populations locating in the sinusoidal site after carbon injection are also examined by the liver perfusion (3). These two macrophage populations are compared with Kupffer cells in the liver. The significance as well as the origin of these migrating macrophages are discussed.

MATERIALS AND METHODS

Experimental Protocol

Male DA rats were injected i.v. with carbon particles (Pelikan ink, 25 mg/100 g body weight). They were killed at 9 and 12 hr after the injection and tissues were either fixed in Carnoy's fluid and embedded in paraffin or fresh frozen in liquid nitrogen. Paraffin sections were stained with methyl green–pyronin and cell size was measured as described previously (2). Perfusion of the liver (3) was performed at 1, 6, 14, 24, and 48 hr after carbon injection.

Immunohistochemistry

Cryosections or smears were stained for monoclonal antibodies using the indirect immuno-alkaline phosphatase method as described previously (4). Monoclonal antibodies used were to rat macrophage subpopulations (ED1 and ED2) and to MHC class II molecules (Ia antigen) (OX6). The Fast Red reaction product of alkaline phosphatase emits stable orange fluorescence which enables the specific staining to be readily observable even after ingestion of carbon particles (2).

RESULTS AND DISCUSSION

Migrating Macrophages Form a Unique Subpopulation Distinct from Kupffer Cells

Migrating heavily carbon-laden (HC) macrophages in the celiac nodes showed a morphological homogeneity. They were ovoid or spherical in shape with a mean diameter of 7.5 μm in paraffin sections (Fig. 1a). While in the liver two types of HC macrophages were recognized. The first type, forming the majority of macrophages, was very large and polygonal with a mean diameter of 15 μm (Fig. 1b). They correspond to so-called Kupffer cells. The second type was small and oval (mean diameter of 6 μm) with a morphological similarity to the migrating HC macrophages in the celiac nodes. Immunostaining (Table 1) revealed that most of the HC macrophages in the celiac nodes were $ED1^+$,$ED2^-$ (Fig. 1c) and $OX6^+$. While typical Kupffer cells were $ED1^+$,$ED2^+$ (Fig. 1d) and $OX6^+$ or $OX6^-$. Thus, the migrating macrophages in the present study has been shown to be different from Kupffer cells, though there is a report suggesting the migration of Kupffer cells into the hepatic nodes (5). We have demonstrated the presence of a macrophage subpopulation in the rat spleen that actively migrates into the white pulp (2). This subpopulation shows similar morphology and phenotype to those of the HC macrophages in this study. It is, therefore, speculated that the migrating HC macrophages both in the liver and the spleen may belong to one unique subpopulation in the rat mononuclear phagocyte system. Comparison to the other subpopulations such as blood monocytes and dendritic cells is now under study.

Possible Origin of Migrating Macrophages

Perfusion study revealed that various types of HC macrophages were yielded from the sinusoid, though the perfusate contained only few numbers of large Kupffer-type cells. Migratory-type HC macrophages could be obtained in the order of 10^6 already 1 hr after carbon injection and the cell yield reached its peak (about 1×10^7 cells/rat) at 24 hr. Their phenotype was $ED1^+$,$ED2^-$, and $OX6^+$ or $OX6^-$ (see Table 1). A preliminary study showed that HC macrophages of migratory type did not appear in the spleen, lung, bone marrow, and blood until 3 hr or later after carbon injection. Together it is suggested that the migrating HC macrophages first appear in the liver sinusoid and later in other tissues after carbon injection. We do not know whether they are resident cells in the liver or recruited cells from other parts of the body after carbon injection. They may take up carbon particles in the liver sinusoids before starting their migration.

HC Macrophages May Also Migrate Hematogenously

Heavily carbon-laden macrophages are easily collected by the simple perfusion technique, which suggests they are loosely attached to the sinusoidal wall. Hence, in addition to the lymph-borne migration, we speculate a possibility that these HC macrophages migrate hematogenously. Time kinetic distribution of this macrophage subpopulation in the body after carbon injection are now under study.

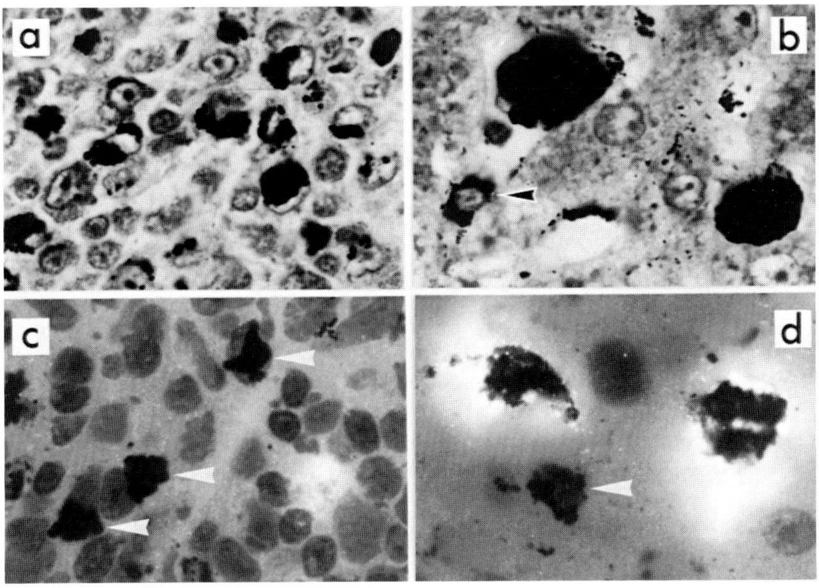

Figure 1 Paraffin section of the celiac lymph nodes at 12 hr (a) and the liver at 9 hr (b) after carbon injection. The migrating HC macrophages in the celiac nodes are homogeneous in size and shape. Note a similar type of cell in the liver (arrowhead) among typical Kupffer cells (large HC macrophages). Methyl green–pyronin staining (magnification: ×960). ED2 immunostaining of the celiac lymph nodes at 12 hr (c) and the liver at 9 hr (d) after carbon injection. The migrating macrophages in the celiac nodes and small macrophages in the liver (arrowheads) are negative for ED2, whereas Kupffer cells are clearly positive (brightly fluorescent) (magnification: ×960).

CONCLUSIONS

It has been demonstrated that a distinct subpopulation of macrophages ($ED1^+2^-$ and $OX6^+$) with a migratory capacity appear in the liver sinusoids after i.v. injection of carbon. They carry out lymph-borne migration into the celiac nodes and possibly blood-borne migration into the other part of the body. It is plausible to speculate that their migratory capacity and the high expression of MHC class II molecule (Ia antigen) may represent their function as messengers of antigenic informations and/or antigen-presenting cells. An antigen-presenting function of the migratory macrophages is now under investigation.

Table 1 Phenotype of HC Macrophages and Kupffer Cells

Markers (%)	HC macrophages in celiac nodes	HC macrophages in perfusate	Kupffer cells[a] in liver
$ED1^+$	73 ± 4[b]	91 ± 1	94 ± 2
$ED2^+$	1 ± 1	2 ± 1	96 ± 3
$OX6^+$	89 ± 8	46 ± 2	37 ± 6

[a]Large HC macrophages with a diameter of the longest axis of more than 20 μm were designated as so-called Kupffer cells.
[b]Mean ± standard errors of three rats.

ACKNOWLEDGMENT

This work was partly supported by the Inoue Foundation for Science.

REFERENCES

1. Matsuno K, Miyakawa K, Ezaki T, Kotani M. The liver lymphatics as a migratory pathway of macrophages from the sinusoids to the celiac lymph nodes in the rat. Arch Histol Cytol 1990; 53 Suppl:179–87.
2. Miyakawa K, Matsuno K, Ohmori J, Kotani M. Localization in the rat spleen of carbon-laden macrophages introduced into the splenic artery: A subpopulation of macrophages entering the white pulp. Anat Rec 1990; 227:464–74.
3. Bouwens L, Remels L, Baekeland M, Van Bossuyt H, Wisse E. Large granular lymphocytes or "Pit cells" from rat liver: isolation, ultrastructural characterization and natural killer activity. Eur J Immunol 1987;17:37–42.
4. Matsuno K, Ezaki T, Kotani M. Splenic outer periarterial lymphoid sheath (PALS): An immunoproliferative microenvironment constituted by antigen-laden marginal metallophils and ED2-positive macrophages in the rat. Cell Tissue Res 1989;257:459–70.
5. Hardonk MJ, Dijkhuis FWJ, Grond J, Koudstaal J, Poppema S. Evidence for a migratory capability of rat Kupffer cells to portal tracts and hepatic lymph nodes. Virchows Arch Cell Pathol 1986;51:429–42.

144

Peritoneal Macrophages of Patients Treated with Continuous Ambulant Peritoneal Dialysis Are Very Potent Stimulators of an Allogeneic Mixed Leukocyte Reaction

M. G. H. Betjes,[1] C. W. Tuk,[1] L. Arisz,[2] and R. H. J. Beelen[1]
[1]*Free University, Amsterdam, The Netherlands;*
[2]*Academical Medical Center, Amsterdam, The Netherlands*

INTRODUCTION

Presentation of antigen to T cells in a suitable form is essential for the initiation of a primary immunoresponse. Stimulatory capacity in an allogenic mixed leukocyte reaction (aMLR) correlates well with the antigen-presenting capacities of the stimulator cell in vitro as in vivo (1). Dendritic cells (DCs) are especially potent stimulator cells in an aMLR (2). They can be separated since they are nonadherent, Fc receptor–negative cells and have a low buoyant density on a hypertonic gradient of metrizamide (2,3). The allogeneic T-cell proliferative response is major histocompatibility complex (MHC) class II dependent and can be partially blocked by addition of anti-MHC class II monoclonal antibodies (MAbs) (4).

We investigated the stimulatory capacity in an one-way aMLR of peritoneal cells isolated from patients treated with continuous ambulatory peritoneal dialysis (CAPD). The peritoneal cells were separated in macrophage. B-cell, T-cell, and DC-enriched fractions and the stimulatory capacities of these fractions were compared with autologous peripheral blood mononuclear cells (PBMCs).

MATERIALS AND METHODS

Isolation of Different Cell Fractions

Culture Medium and Serum

Culture medium was RPMI 1640 supplemented with 10% heat-inactivated fetal calf serum, 2 mM L-glutamine, 50 U/ml penicillin, 50 μg/ml streptomycin, and 50 μM β-mercaptoethanol.

Peritoneal Cells and PBMC

Peritoneal cells were harvested from a single overnight peritoneal dialysis effluent (dwell time 8–10 hr), by centrifugation (300 G, 10 min, 4°C of the complete dialysate (1.0–2.5 L). All patients were free of peritonitis at the time of investigation. The yield of peritoneal cells per effluent varied greatly (ranging from 1 to 30 × 10^6 cells) and characteristically contained 60–80% macrophages with less than 5% granulocytes. Peripheral blood (10 ml) was taken from these CAPD patients by venipuncture into sterile heparin-containing glass tubes. The PBMCs were isolated on a Ficoll-Pacque density gradient. After isolating part of the peritoneal cells, the PBMCs were reserved for later use by culturing in 60-ml Teflon beakers which prevent macrophages to adhere. The remaining cells were cultured on plastic tissue culture Petri dishes at 37°C in 5% CO_2. After 16 hr the nonadherent cells were washed off and the adherent cells were removed with a rubber policeman.

Enrichment of DCs (Fig. 1)

First, the nonadherent peritoneal cells were depleted of T cells by rosetting with neuraminidase-treated sheep erythrocytes. Second, the contaminating macrophages (Fc receptor [FcR] positive) were removed by panning on immunoglobulin G (IgG)–coated Petri dishes. Finally, the FcR-negative cells were separated on a metrizamide gradient into a low-density fraction (LoD; DC enriched) and a high-density fraction (HiD; B cell enriched).

Isolation of T Cells for the MLR

T cells were isolated from the buffy coats by E rosetting of nonadherent cells after 16 hr culture on plastic tissue culture Petri dishes. They were cryopreserved in medium-containing 50% culture medium, 20% dimethylsulfoxide (DMSO), and 30% fetal calf serum at –70°C until use.

Function as Stimulator Cells in aMLRs

Allogeneic MLRs were set up as described by Mottolese et al. (5). The different cell fractions after irridiation (3000 Ci, ^{60}Co) served as stimulator cells and 5 × 10^4 cryopreserved T cells as responder cells. After pulsing for 16 hr with 1 μCi [^{3}H]thymidine ([^{3}H]TdR) cells were harvested at day 6. For blocking studies MAb SPVL3 (mouse anti-HLA-DQ,) and MAb 3B3 (mouse anti-HLA-DR) were used (both a kind gift from Dr. K. Figdor, The Netherlands Cancer Institute, Amsterdam) in a concentration of 5 μg/ml per well. Experiments were done in triplicate in a final volume of 200 μl culture medium per well.

Phenotypical Analysis

For phenotypical analysis of lymphocytes we used MAbs recognizing CD22 (pan–B-cell marker; Dakopatts, Glostrup, Denmark) and CD2 (pan–T-cell marker; CLB, Amsterdam).

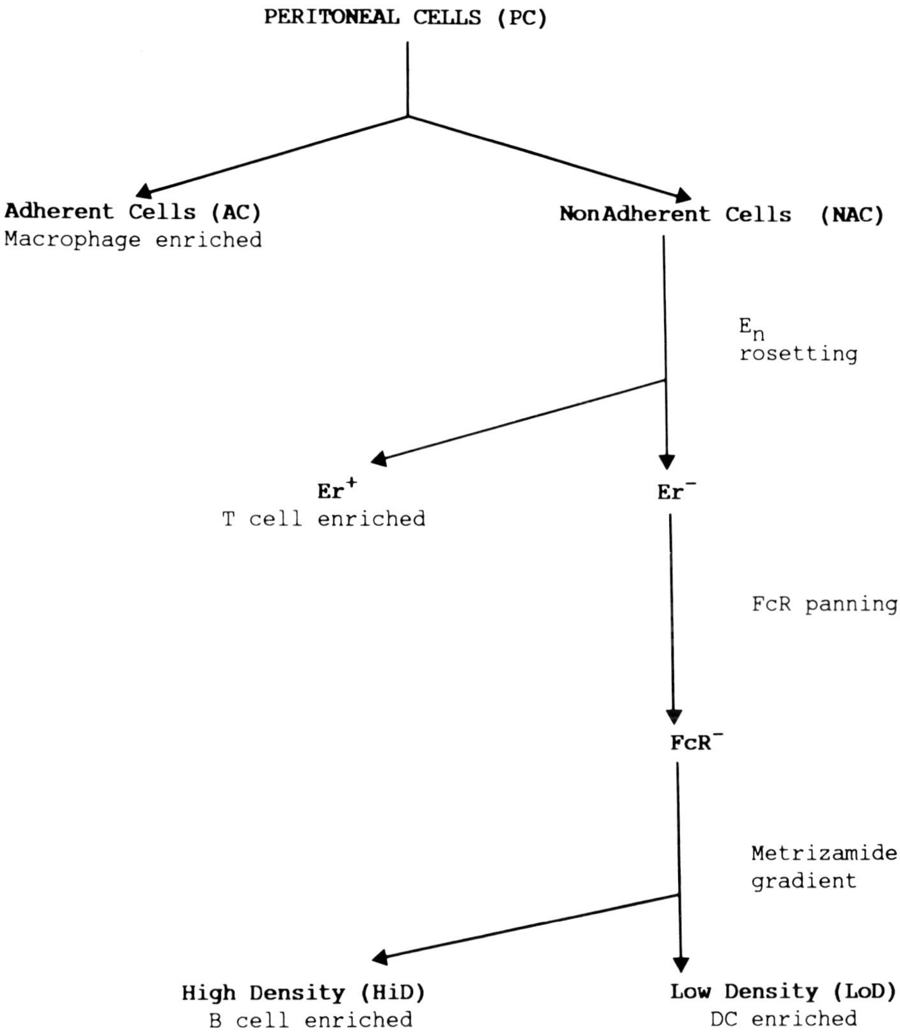

Figure 1 Enrichment procedure of dendritic cells from the non-adherent peritoneal cells of CAPD patients.

For recognition of monocytes and macrophages EBM11 (Dakopatts, Denmark) was used. Dendritic cells (DCs) were identified as large cells with an irregular outline, eccentric nucleus, acid phosphatase staining in a paranuclear spot and strong HLA class II expression on their cell surface. Monoclonal antibody 9.3F10 (ATCC) was used to detect MHC class II–positive cells. The MAbs were used on cytocentrifuge preparations in combinating with a routine immunoperoxidase procedure.

RESULTS AND DISCUSSION

Peritoneal cells from CAPD patients were potent stimulator cells in aMLRs as compared to autologous PBMCs (Fig. 2A). The adherent peritoneal cells (±90% macrophages)

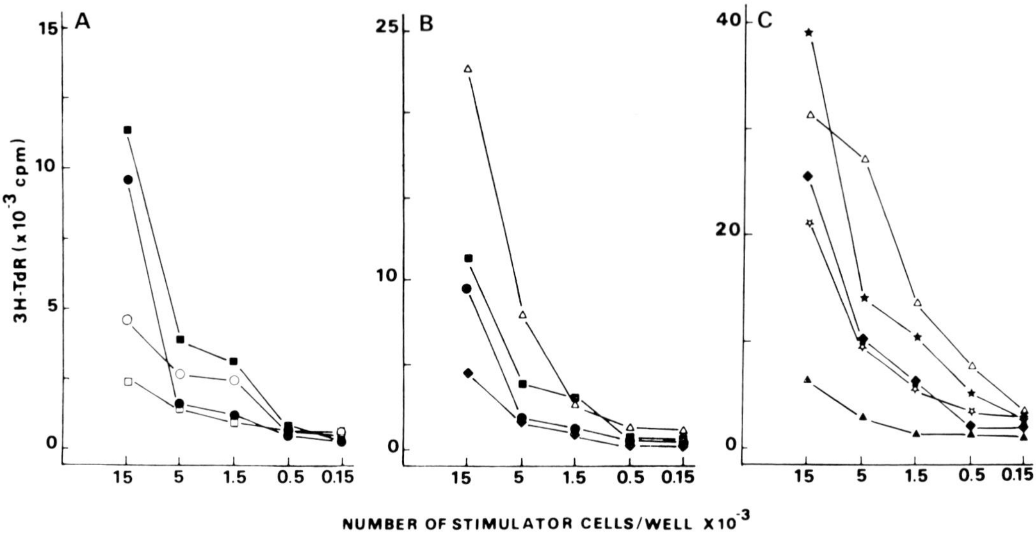

Figure 2 Representative aMLRs with the different peritoneal cell fractions and autologous PBMCs as stimulator cells. Stimulator cells were added to 5×10^4 cryopreserved T cells in a total volume of 200 μl/well. After pulsing for 16 hr with 1 μCi [^{3}H]thymidine, cells were harvested at day six. Responder T cells without stimulator cells gave responses <500 cpm. (A) The stimulator capacity of the adherent cell fractions of the peritoneal cells (—■—) and of the PBMCs (—□—) as compared to the unfractionated peritoneal cells (—●—) and PBMCs (—○—) is shown. (B) Data of the same patient as in (a) are used, and it shows the nonadherent cell fraction (—◆—) and the DC-enriched fraction (—Δ—) as compared to the unfractionated peritoneal cells and the adherent cell fraction. (C) The stimulatory capacity of the successive cell fractions in the enrichment of DC is shown; Er$^-$ (—★—), FcR$^-$ (—☆—), LoD (—Δ—), HiD (—▲—). Note that removal of macrophages from the Er$^-$ results in a sharp decrease of stimulatory capacity.

accounted largely for this stimulatory capacity, although the nonadherent peritoneal cells contained a higher percentage of DCs (Fig. 2B). In contrast, the adherent cells of the PBMCs were less potent stimulators in aMLRs than the unfractionated PBMCs (Fig. 2A). Dendritic cells could be enriched up to 40% purity and were three to four times better stimulator cells than the adherent peritoneal cells. Depletion of macrophages always diminished the stimulatory capacity of the remaining cell fraction, unless the simultaneous enrichment of DCs could compensate for this loss (Figs. 2C and 3). The T- and B-cell–enriched fractions had a poor stimulating capacity (Fig. 2C).

Human monocytes and peritoneal macrophages are normally poor stimulator cells in an aMLR (2–5). Our findings strongly suggest that macrophages when they are elicited like in CAPD patients (6) can acquire a potent stimulating capacity in aMLRs.

Addition of anti–HLA-DR blocked the aMLR better than anti–HLA-DQ. The highest blocking percentages were observed when we added both MAbs (Fig. 4). These findings are in accordance with those from Waalen et al. (4), and suggest that although DCs and peritoneal macrophages are strongly HLA-DQ positive (4,5), this only plays a minor role in antigen presentation.

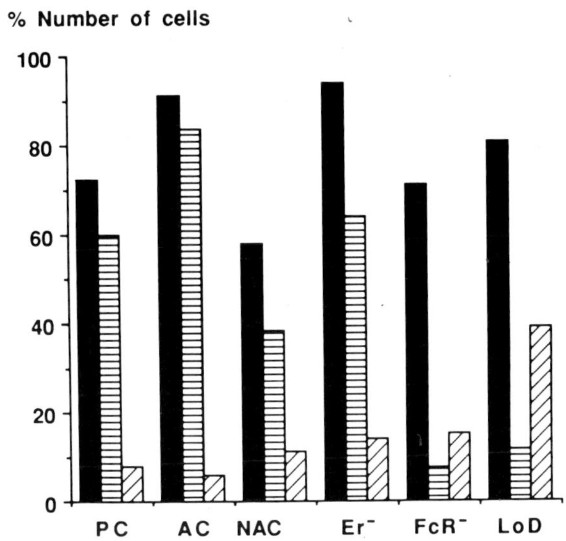

Figure 3 A representative enrichment of DC (▨) from the nonadherent peritoneal cells of a CAPD patient. The percentage of MHC class II–positive cells (■) as determined with MAb 9.3F10 and the percentage of macrophages (▤) as determined with MAb EBM11 are also shown.

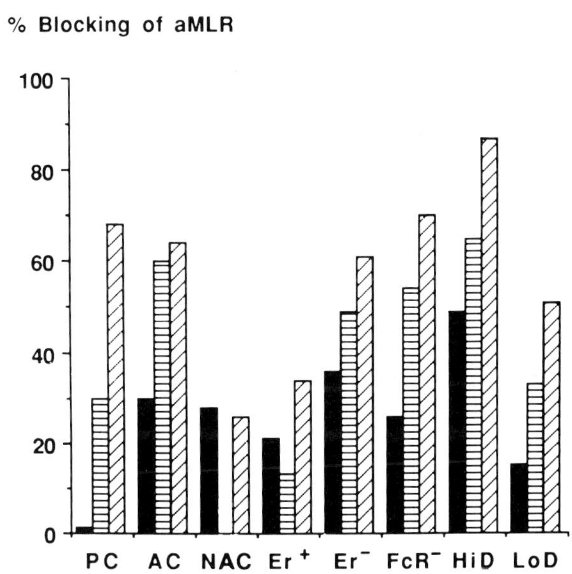

Figure 4 A representative aMLR blocking study of all peritoneal cell fractions. 5 μg/ml MAb was added to 5×10^4 irradiated stimulator cells and 5×10^4 cryopreserved T cells in a total volume of 200 μl/well. Anti–HLA-DQ (SPVL3; ■) and anti–HLA-DR (3B3; ▤) monoclonal antibodies were used solely and in combination (▨). Note that there is a similar pattern throughout all fractions. Additional experiments showed that the blocking percentage of a cell fraction varied greatly with no marked differences between fractions.

REFERENCES

1. Steinman RM, Inaba K. Stimulation of the primary mixed leukocyte reaction. CRC Crit Rev Immunol 1985; 5:331–348.
2. Young JW, Steinman RM. Accessory cell requirements for the mixed leukocyte reaction and polyclonal mitogens, as studied with a new technique for enriching blood dendritic cells. Cell Immunol 1988; 111:167–182.
3. Knight SC, Farrant J, Bryant A, Edwards AJ, Burman S, Lever A, Clarke J, Webster ADB. Non adherent, low-density cells from human peripheral blood contain dendritic cells and monocytes, both with veiled morphology. Immunology 1986; 57:595–603.
4. Voorhis van WC, Valinsky J, Hoffman E, Luban J, Hair LS, Steinman RM. Relative efficacy of human monocytes and dendritic cells as accessory cells for T cell replication. J Exp Med 1983; 158:174–191.
5. Mottolese M, Natali PG, Atlanta G, Cavallari A, DiFilippo F, Ferrone S. Antigenic profile and functional characterization of human peritoneal macrophages. J Immunol 1985; 135:200–206.
6. Waalen, Forre O, Teigland J, Natvig JB. Human rheumatoid synovial and normal blood dendritic cells as antigen presenting cells; comparison with autologous monocytes. Clin Exp Immunol 1987; 70:1–9.
7. Bos HJ, Bronswijk van H, Helmerhorst ThJM, Oe PL, Hoefsmit ECM, Beelen RHJ. Distinct subpopulations of elicited human macrophages in peritoneal dialysis patients and women undergoing laparoscopy: a study on peroxidatic activity. J Leukocyte Biol 1988; 43:172–178.

145
The Role of Spleen and of Lymph Node Macrophages in the Immune Response to Particulate Antigens

Frans G. A. Delemarre, Nel Kors, and Nico van Rooijen
Free University, Amsterdam, The Netherlands

INTRODUCTION

To evoke an immune response to thymus-dependent (TD) antigens, presentation of these antigens to T cells is required. Different cell types, like macrophages (2), dendritic cells (2), B cells (3), intestinal villus enterocytes (4), and even liposomes (5) bearing the appropriate major histocompatibility complex (MHC) class II molecules, may stimulate T cells in vitro. Although these in vitro studies contribute considerably to our understanding of the mechanism of antigen presentation, in vitro studies cannot answer the question of which cells actually are involved in the induction of an immune response in vivo.

Recently, a hypothesis was presented as to the cooperation between lymphoid and nonlymphoid cells in the inductive phase of an antibody response in the spleen (6). It was postulated that in the spleen B cells encounter the antigen in the marginal zone and migrate into the outer part of periarteriolar lymphocyte sheaths (PALSs). Here, these B cells present processed antigen to the appropriate T cells and with their help they differentiate into antibody-forming cells. As B cells have a less prominent phagocytic and lysosomal function than macrophages, it was speculated that macrophages in the marginal zone process large particulate antigens and transfer the processed antigens to the B cells in the marginal zone (6).

It was the purpose of the present experiments to study the role of splenic macrophages in the immune response to particulate antigens. Therefore, the development of antibody-forming cells (AFCs) to the TD particulate antigen trinitrophenylated sheep red blood cells (TNP-SRBCs) was investigated after liposome-mediated depletion of splenic macrophages (7). The in situ immune response to TNP-SRBCs was also studied in popliteal lymph nodes (PLNs). Here, macrophage lining the subcapsular sinus (SCS) which are eliminated together with medullary macrophages after treatment with Cl_2MDP-liposomes (8) might be involved in the induction of an immune response because of a strategic location comparable to that of the marginal zone macrophages in the spleen.

MATERIALS AND METHODS

Female mice (C57Bl/6xDBA/2)F1 (Bomholtgard, Ry, Denmark) were subcutaneously (s.c.) injected in the hind footpads with 50 μl of a solution of Cl_2MDP-liposomes (7). After 5 days, mice were injected s.c. in the same footpads with 10^8 TNP-SRBCs. Mice were sacrificed 3, 5, 7, and 10 days after immunization. In other experiments mice were intravenously (i.v.) injected with 0.2 ml of a solution of Cl_2MDP-liposomes, followed by intravenous immunization with 0.2 ml of 10^8 TNP-SRBCs in 0.9% NaCl the next day. These mice were sacrificed 3, 6, 7, and 10 days after immunization. Control animals received phosphate-buffered saline (PBS)–containing liposomes. Mice were killed by cervical dislocation and spleen and PLNs were removed for the enumeration of antibody-forming cells (AFCs) on 8-μm cryostat sections as described by Claassen et al. (9) and for enumeration of antibody-secreting cells (ASCs) in a spot enzyme–linked immunosorbent assay (spot-ELISA) as described by Sedgwick and Holt (10). Cryostat sections of spleen and PLNs were checked for the absence of macrophages after Cl_2MDP-liposome treatment by staining for acid phosphatase (11).

RESULTS

Anti-TNP Response After Intravenous Immunization

Antibody-forming cells were present in the spleen on day 3, and the peak of the anti-TNP response was found on day 5 in the control mice after immunization with TNP-SRBCs (Table 1). After treatment with Cl_2MDP-liposomes, the number of AFCs was strongly depressed on day 5 after immunization (Table 1). This was also demonstrated in the spot-ELISA (Table 2): Five days after immunization with TNP-SRBCs, the number of AFCs in the spleen of Cl_2MDP-liposome–treated mice decreased by 82%. Especially, the number of anti–TNP-AFC of the immunoglobulin (IgG)–isotype were strongly reduced (Table 2).

Anti-TNP Response After Subcutaneous Immunization

Three days after s.c. immunization with TNP-SRBCs, no AFCs were observed in PLNs of control mice. The first AFCs were found on day 5 in high numbers, and the anti-TNP response showed a decrease on days 7 and 10 (see Table 1). Treatment with Cl_2MDP-liposomes before immunization with TNP-SRBCs had no effect on the number of AFCs

Table 1 Number of Antibody-Forming Cells per Tissue Section of Spleen and PLNs After Immunization with TNP-SRBCs.

Organ	Antigen	Route of injection	Liposomes	Days after immunization[a] 3	5	7	10
Spleen	SRBC	i.v.	PBS	+	+++	+	±
			Cl_2,MDP	+	+	+	±
PLN	SRBC	s.c.	PBS	–	++	+	±
			Cl_2MDP	–	++	+	±

[a]AFCs absent = – ,1–10 = ±, 10–50 = +, 50–100 = ++, 100–250 = +++.

Table 2 Number of IgM and IgG Antibody-Secreting Cells in Spleen and PLNS After Immunization with TNP-SRBCs

Organ	Route of injection	Cl_2MDP-liposomes	Days after immunization: number of ASCs/10^6 cells 5 IgM	IgG
Spleen	i.v.	No	165 ± 25	180 ± 32
		Yes	55 ± 11	10 ± 5
PLN	s.c.	No	28 ± 15	9 ± 9
		Yes	29 ± 14	3 ± 1

and the kinetics of the anti-TNP response (see Table 1). Neither in the spot-ELISA did we observe a difference in the number of AFCs in PLNs of control and Cl_2MDP-liposome–treated mice on day 5 after immunization, although the number of anti–TNP–IgG–forming cells had slightly decreased (see Table 2).

DISCUSSION

In this study, splenic macrophages were depleted by i.v. injection of Cl_2MDP-liposomes. Intravenous immunization of the treated animals with TNP-SRBCs resulted in a strong decrease in the number of AFCs in the spleen. Elimination of macrophages lining the SCS and in the medulla of PLNs after subcutaneous injection of Cl_2MDP-liposomes, followed by s.c. immunization with TNP-SRBCs, had no effect on the number of AFCs and the kinetics of the anti-TNP response in the PLNs. These results suggest that the macrophages of the PLNs are not essential for the antibody response to TD particulate antigens, but those of the spleen are involved in the "in vivo" processing of the TD particulate antigen TNP-SRBCs.

Similar findings on the role of splenic macrophages in the immune response were described by Su and Van Rooijen (12). Liposome-mediated elimination of macrophages in the spleen resulted in a reduction in antibody-serum titers to intravenously injected liposome-associated human serum albumin. Also, in other studies, it has been demonstrated that macrophages are vital for the processing of particulate antigens (13–15).

Earlier experiments showed that elimination of macrophages in the spleen did not affect the immune response after i.v. immunization with TNP-coupled antigens such as lipopolysaccharide (LPS), Ficoll, and keyhole limpet hemocyanin (KLH) (16,17). Lipopolysaccharide and Ficoll are thymus-independent (TI) antigens and presentation to T cells is not an obligatory step for the induction of an immune response to these antigens. Although macrophages could be involved in the presentation of TI antigens to B cells, elimination of macrophages was not expected to inhibit the TI antibody response. The TD antigen KLH, which was administered in a soluble form, may also be taken up, processed, and presented to T cells by other accessory cells like interdigitating cells (IDCs) and B cells, with a less prominent phagocytic and lysosomal function than macrophages. In the PLNs, macrophage elimination had no effect on the immune response to TNP-LPS and TNP-Ficoll either, whereas the number of AFCs strongly increased after s.c. immunization with TNP-KLH (18). Similar findings have been reported for the lung-associated lymph node after intratracheal Cl_2MDP-liposome treatment followed by immunization with TNP-KLH (19). Janeway et al. (20), who studied B cells as antigen-presenting cells, found no T-cell proliferation in the PLNs of mice immunized with KLH after elimination of B cells, in spite of the presence of macrophages. It was suggested that the B cells were critical antigen-presenting cells in peripheral lymph nodes of mice. All these studies illustrated that macrophages of spleen and lymph nodes are not essential for the induction of an immune response to soluble antigens.

In contrast to the spleen, the number of AFCs in the macrophage-depleted PLNs was not decreased after immunization with the TD particulate antigen TNP-SRBCs. In the immune response to particulate antigens, B cells or IDCs are not likely to act as antigen-presenting cells, which means that in the Cl_2MDP-liposome–treated PLNs, macrophages other than those lining the SCS and in the medulla are involved in the processing of TNP-SRBCs. The influx of macrophages in an area below the deep cortex, above the hilus, and flanked by the medulla in the normal and macrophage-depleted PLNs after immunization with TNP-SRBC (data not shown) is suggestive of a role of these newcomer macrophages in the processing of particulate antigens.

The data on the differential role of splenic macrophages in the immune response to soluble and particulate antigens fit into a recently presented hypothesis on cellular interactions in the early phase of an antibody response in the spleen (6). It was postulated that B cells meet antigens in the marginal zone of the spleen, migrate into the outer part of the PALS, and present processed antigen to T cells. Although B cells may process small and soluble antigens, processing of particular antigens requires macrophages, and especially the marginal zone macrophages are believed to play a prominent role herein. These macrophages with cell processes between the B cells in the marginal zone may transfer the processed antigen to the latter cells. Recent experiments, using the elimination-repopulation model as described by Van Rooijen (21), strongly indicate that indeed the marginal zone macrophages are involved in the processing of the particulate antigen TNP-SRBCs (Delemarre, academic thesis, Free University, Amsterdam).

REFERENCES

1. Unanue ER. Antigen-presenting function of the macrophage. Ann. Rev. Immunol. 1984; 132:1.
2. Inaba K, Steinman RM, Van Voorhis WC, Muramatsu S. Dendritic cells are critical accessory cells for thymus-dependent antibody responses in mouse and man. Proc. Natl. Acad. Sci. U.S.A. 1983; 80:6041.
3. Ashwell JD. Are B lymphocytes the principal antigen-presenting cells in vivo? J. Immunol. 1988; 140:3697.
4. Bland PW, Whiting CV. Antigen processing by isolated rat intestinal villus enterocytes. Immunology 1989; 68:497.
5. Walden P, Nagy ZA, Klein J. Induction of regulatory T-lymphocytes response by liposomes carrying major histocompatibility complex molecules and foreign antigen. Nature 1985; 315:327.
6. Van Rooijen N. Antigen processing and presentation in vivo. The microenvironment as a crucial factor. Immunol. Today 1990; 11:436.
7. Van Rooijen N. The liposome-mediated macrophage 'suicide' technique. J. Immunol. Methods 1989: 124:1.
8. Delemarre FGA, Kors N, Kraal G, Van Rooijen N. Repopulation of macrophages in popliteal lymph nodes of mice after liposome mediated depletion. J. Leukocyte Biol. 1990; 47:251.
9. Claassen E, Van Rooijen N. TNP-enzyme conjugates for the detection of anti-TNP antibody containing cells in vivo. J. Immunol. Methods 1984; 75:181.

10. Segdwick JD, Holt PG. A solid-phase immunoenzymatic technique for the enumeration of specific antibody-secreting cells. J. Immunol. Methods 1983; 57:301.
11. Burstone MS. Histochemical comparison of naphthol-phosphates for the demonstration of phosphatase. J. Natl. Cancer Inst. 1958; 20:601.
12. Su D, Van Rooijen N. The role of macrophages in the immunoadjuvant action of liposomes: Effect of splenic macrophages on the immune response against intravenously injected liposome associated albumin antigen. Immunology 1989; 66:466.
13. Kapsenberg ML, Teunissen MBM, Stiekema FEM, Keizer H. Antigen-presenting cell function of dendritic cells and macrophages in proliferative T cell responses to soluble and particular antigens. Eur. J. Immunol. 1986; 16:345.
14. Ziegler HK, Orlin CA, Cluff CW. Differential requirements for the processing of soluble and particulate bacterial antigens by macrophages. Eur. J. Immunol. 1987; 17:1287.
15. Wright MD, Wood PR, Coia G, Cheers C. Particulate antigens may be reprocessed after initial phagocytosis for presentation to T cells in vivo. Immunol. Cell Biol. 1987; 65:505.
16. Claassen E, Kors N, Van Rooijen N. Influence of carriers on the development and localization of anti-2,4,6-trinitrophenyl (TNP) antibody-forming cells in the murine spleen. II. Suppressed antibody response to TNP-Ficoll after elimination of marginal zone cells. Eur. J. Immunol. 1986; 16:492.
17. Kraal G, Ter Hart H, Meelhuizen C, Venneker G, Claassen E. Marginal zone macrophages and their role in the immune response against T-independent type 2 antigens: Modulation of the cells with specific antibody. Eur. J. Immunol., 1989; 19:675.
18. Delemarre FGA, Kors N, Van Rooijen N. The in situ immune response in popliteal lymph nodes of mice after macrophage depletion. Differential effects of macrophages on thymus-dependent and thymus-independent immune responses. Immunobiology 1990; 180:395.
19. Thepen Th, Van Rooijen N, Kraal G. Alveolar macrophages elimination in vivo causes a severe increase in pulmonary immune response in mice. J. Exp. Med. 1989; 170:499.
20. Janeway Jr. CA, Ron J, Katz ME. The B cell is the initiating antigen-presenting cell in peripheral lymph nodes. J. Immunol. 1987; 138:1051.
21. Van Rooijen N, Kors N, Kraal G. Macrophage subset repopulation in the spleen: Differential kinetics after liposome-mediated elimination. J. Leukocyte Biol. 1989; 45:97.

146

Cellular Binding Mechanism on Rat Macrophages with Specificity for Sialylyated Glycoconjugates Recognized by the Monoclonal Antibody ED-3

Jan G. M. C. Damoiseaux, Ed A. Döpp, and Christine D. Dijkstra
Free University, Amsterdam, The Netherlands

INTRODUCTION

The marginal zone macrophages (MZMs) and the marginal metallophilic macrophages (MMMs) belong to a subpopulation of the splenic white pulp macrophages in the rat and can be identified by their capacity to ingest fluorescein isothiocyanate (FITC)–conjugated Ficoll (1). In the mouse, these macrophage subpopulations also express the sheep erythrocyte receptor (SER), binding unopsonized erythrocytes of several species (2,3). This receptor has been characterized as a lectinlike hemagglutinin with specificity for sialylated glycoconjugates (2,4). In the rat, both macrophage populations (MZMs and MMMs) are recognized by the monoclonal antibody (MAb) ED-3 (5,6). Expression of the ED-3 antigen in the spleen is normally restricted to the MZMs, surrounded by the marginal zone B cells, and to the MMMs, located on the border of the periarteriolar lymphocyte sheath and the marginal zone, where the differentiation of antibody-forming cells takes place. In the lymph nodes, ED-3 is expressed on macrophages in the subsinus, the marginal zone equivalent of the lymph node, and on macrophages in the medulla, the place of differentiation of antibody-forming cells (5). The expression of the ED-3 antigen can strongly be upregulated on bone marrow–derived macrophages in vitro by factors produced by activated lymphoid cells (7). These characteristics of the ED-3 antigen are very similar to SER.

The functional significance of the ED-3–positive macrophage populations is still obscure. MZMs are supposed to play a part in presenting thymus-independent type-2 antigens to the marginal zone B cells (8), although recently there has been discussion about this function (9,10). Nevertheless, strong macrophage–B-cell interactions have been observed in the splenic marginal zone as well as in lymph nodes (8,11).

The aim of the present study was to determine the relation between SER and the ED-3 antigen in the rat and the involvement of this receptor in macrophage–B-cell interactions.

MATERIALS AND METHODS

SER Assay

The tissue agglutination assay with SRBCs was performed according to Stejskal and Fitch (12). Fresh cryostat sections of rat spleen and lymph node (from Wistar rats, HSD/CPB, Zeist, The Netherlands) were incubated with a 1% solution of SRBCs during 15 min at room temperature. Afterward the sections were gently washed with saline. In the case of blocking studies with MAb ED-3 (5), MAb ED-9 (6), or rabbit-antimouse SER polyclonal (kindly provided by Dr. P. R. Crocker, Institute Pasteur, Paris, France), the sections were first incubated with the appropriate antibody.

To identify the receptor mechanism as SER, differentially 1 mM EDTA was added, SRBCs were treated with *Vibrio cholerae* neuraminidase (Behringwerke AG, Marburg, West Germany), or cryostat sections were treated with trypsin (type IX, 15.100 BAEE U/mg protein; Sigma, St. Louis, Missouri) in a concentration of 0.2 μg/ml for 60 min at 37°C.

Macrophage–B-Cell Clusters

Clusters between macrophages and B cells were isolated from lymph node suspensions according to Chao and MacPherson (11). After enzymatic digestion the macrophage clusters were allowed to adhere to glass coverslips for 3 hr. To determine the involvement of the ED-3 antigen, MAb ED-3 was added prior to adherence. To study if MAb ED-3 was able to desintegrate already established clusters, lymph node suspensions were incubated with SRBCs and after 1 hr of adherence the MAb ED-3 was added.

After the adherence step, the coverslips were immunohistochemically stained with MAb ED-3 (5) and MAb His-14 (13) as described previously (6).

RESULTS

SER Assay

Sheep red blood cells bound to the MMMs and MZMs in the spleen and the subsinusoidal and medullary macrophages in the lymph node. Incubation of rat tissue with MAb ED-3 resulted in complete blocking of the binding to macrophages. The MAb ED-9, which also recognizes rat MMMs and MZMs, or the polyclonal SER antiserum did not affect SRBC binding.

Neuraminidase treatment of the erythrocytes inhibited the binding to the macrophage subpopulations, whereas EDTA did not affect this binding. Although trypsin treatment of tissue sections completely inhibited SRBC binding, the immunocytochemical staining with MAb ED-3 was not affected (Table 1).

Macrophage–B-Cell Clusters

On the basis of morphology two types of macrophages could be identified after adherence to the coverslips; small round macrophages and large well-spread macrophages. In contrast to the small round macrophages, only the large well-spread ones stained positive for ED-3,

Table 1 SER and ED-3 Reactivity on Cryostat Sections

	Spleen	Lymph node
ED-3[a]	++	++
SRBC[b]	++	++
SRBC + ED-3[b]	–	–
SRBC + ED-9[b]	++	++
SRBC + polySER[b]	++	++
SRBC + neuraminidase[b]	–	–
SRBC + EDTA[b]	++	++
SRBC + trypsine[b]	–	–
ED-3 + trypsine[a]	++	++

Reactivity was restricted to MMMs and MZMs in the spleen and to subsinusoidal and medullary macrophages in the lymph node.
[a]Immunocytochemical staining.
[b]SER assay.

showed SER activity, and were associated with several small round cells. These small round cells could be identified as B cells with MAb His-14 (Fig. 1).

In case MAb ED-3 was added during macrophage adherence, the large macrophages were still associated with B cells to the same extent. To determine whether already established clusters could be dissolved by the MAb, the lymph node suspension was incubated with SRBCs during adhesion and after 1 hr when the macrophage-SRBC rosettes had been formed, MAb ED-3 was added. In control experiments in which no MAb was added, the large macrophages clustered with B cells as well as enormous numbers of SRBCs (Fig. 2). Addition of MAb ED-3 only dissolved the binding of SRBCs, but not that of B cells (Fig. 3).

1

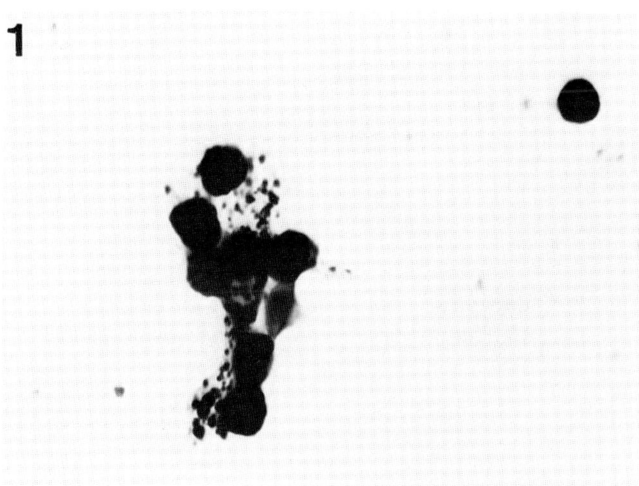

Figure 1 Cluster of macrophages and several B cells isolated out of lymph node cell suspension by adhesion and immunoperoxidase stained with MAb His-14 (magnification: ×1000).

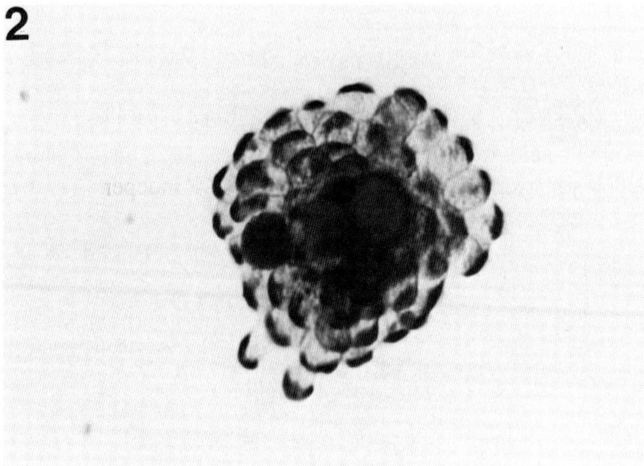

Figure 2 Macrophages clustered with lymphocytes form rosettes with SRBCs; immunoperoxidase stained with MAb ED-3 (magnification: ×1000).

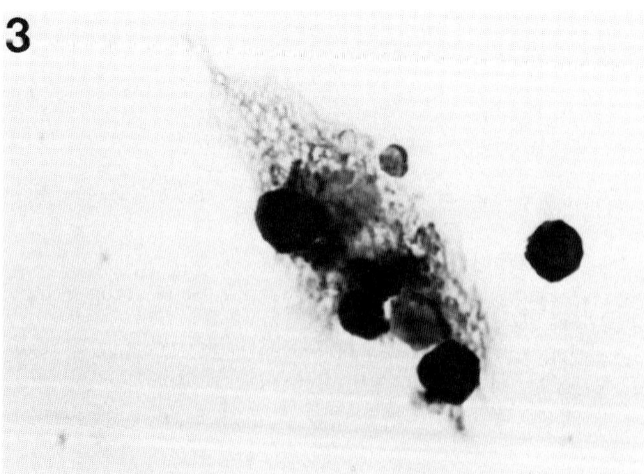

Figure 3 Addition of MAb ED-3 after establishment of clusters between macrophages, B cells, and SRBCs results in loss of binding of SRBCs but not of B cells; immunoperoxidase stained with MAb His-14 (magnification: ×1000).

DISCUSSION

In this study, we have identified the antigen, recognized by the anti-rat macrophage MAb ED-3, as the rat equivalent of SER in the mouse by binding inhibition experiments. In the rat, as in the mouse, the binding mechanism is divalent cation independent, SER is trypsin sensitive, and the ligand is a sialic acid–containing glycoconjugate. Also, the in vitro regulation of the ED-3 and SER expression are similar; both are M-CSF independent and are strongly downregulated with interferon-γ (IFN-γ) (7,14).

The tissue distribution of SER in the lymphoid organs of the rat and the mouse is rather comparable (3,5). The only difference is that resident bone marrow macrophages in the mouse have a high SER expression, whereas resident bone marrow macrophages in the rat have undetectable levels of ED-3 (3,6). This underlines the fact that SER is not related to the receptor which is responsible for the formation of hematopoietic cell clusters (15).

The localization of ED-3–positive macrophages in the spleen and lymph nodes is restricted to the marginal zone and its equivalent in the lymph nodes as well as to places where the differentiation of the antibody forming cells takes place. Strong interactions of MZMs and MMMs with B cells have been noticed in mouse and rat (1,8). Also, in lymph nodes of the rat, the ED-3–positive macrophages preferentially interact with B cells in vitro and in situ (11). These macrophages in spleen and lymph nodes fail to express MHC class II antigen Ia, which eliminates a function that requires CD4-positive T cells (8,11). On the contrary, they themselves express the CD4 antigen as well as the CD2 antigen, suggesting an interaction between these macrophages and Ia-positive B cells (16). In this study, we excluded that SER, recognized by MAb ED-3, is involved in this macrophage–B-cell interaction in lymph nodes. This implies that the immunological function of SER still remains obscure.

REFERENCES

1. Matsuno, K., H. Fujii, and M. Kotani. 1986. Splenic marginal-zone macrophages and marginal metallophils in rats and mice. Cell Tissue Res. 246:263.
2. Radaszkiewicz, T., E. Weirich, and H. Denk. 1979. Erythrocyte adherence to the marginal zone of mouse spleen follicle mediated by receptor(s) for neuraminic acid. Z. Immun.-Forsch. 155:319.
3. Crocker, P. R. and S. Gordon. 1986. Properties and distribution of a lectin-like hemagglutinin differentially expressed by murine stromal tissue macrophages. J. Exp. Med. 164:1862.
4. Crocker, P. R. and S. Gordon. 1989. Mouse macrophage hemagglutinin (sheep erythrocyte receptor) with specificity for sialylated glycoconjugates characterized by a monoclonal antibody. J. Exp. Med. 169:1333.
5. Dijkstra, C. D., E. A. Döpp, P. Joling, and G. Kraal. 1985. The heterogeneity of mononuclear phagocytes in lymphoid organs: Distinct macrophage subpopulations in the rat recognized by monoclonal antibodies ED1, ED2 and ED3. Immunology 54:589.
6. Damoiseaux, J. G. M. C., E. A. Döpp, J. J. Neefjes, R. H. J. Beelen, and C. D. Dijkstra. 1989. Heterogeneity of macrophages in the rat evidenced by variability in determinants: Two new anti-rat macrophage antibodies against a heterodimer of 160 and 95 kd (CD11/CD18). J. Leukocyte Biol. 46:556.
7. Damoiseaux, J. G. M. C., E. A. Döpp, R. H. J. Beelen, and C. D. Dijkstra. 1989. Rat bone marrow and monocyte cultures: Influence of culture time and lymphokines on the expression of macrophage differentiation antigens. J. Leukocyte Biol. 46:246.
8. Humphrey, J. H. and D. Grennan. 1981. Different macrophage populations distinguished by means of fluorescent polysaccharides. Recognition and properties of marginal-zone macrophages. Eur. J. Immunol. 11:221.

9. Claassen, E., A. Ott, W. J. A. Boersma, C. Deen, M. M. Schellekens, C. D. Dijkstra, N. Kors, and N. Van Rooijen. 1989. Marginal zone of the murine spleen in autotransplants: Functional and histological observations in the response against a thymus-independent type 2 antigen. Clin. Exp. Immunol. 77:445.
10. Kraal, G., H. Ter Hart, C. Meelhuizen, G. Venneker, and E. Claassen. 1989. Marginal zone macrophages and their role in the immune response against T-independent type 2 antigens: Modulation of the cells with specific antibody. Eur. J. Immunol. 19:675.
11. Chao, D. and G. Gordon MacPherson. 1989. Lymph node macrophage heterogeneity: The phenotypic and functional characterization of two distinct populations of macrophages from rat lymph node. Eur. J. Immunol. 19:1273.
12. Stejskal, R. and F. W. Fitch. 1970. Tissue agglutination reaction with normal rat spleen. J. Ret. Soc. 7:121.
13. Kroese, F. G. M., D. Opstelten, A. S. Wubbema, G. J. Deenen, J. Aten, E. H. Schwander, L. De Ley, and P. Nieuwenhuis. 1985. Monoclonal antibodies to rat B lymphocyte (sub-)populations. Adv. Exp. Med. Biol. 186:81.
14. Crocker, P. R., M. Hill, and S. Gordon. 1988. Regulation of a murine macrophage haemagglutinin (sheep erythrocyte receptor) by a species-restricted serum factor. Immunology 65:515.
15. Crocker, P. R., L. Morris, and S. Gordon. 1988. Novel cell-surface adhesion receptors involved in interactions between stromal macrophages and hematopoietic cells. J. Cell Sci. (S) 9:185.
16. Williams, A. F., A. N. Barclay, S. J. Clar, D. J. Paterson, and A. C. Willis. 1987. Similarities in sequences and cellular expression between rat CD2 and CD4 antigens. J. Exp. Med. 165:368.

147

Role of the Splenic Marginal Zone in the Removal of, and Immune Response Against, Neutral Polysaccharides

Eric Claassen,[1] Quirijn Vos,[2] Alewijn Ott,[1] Marc M. Schellekens,[1] and Wim J. A. Boersma[1]
[1]*TNO Medical Biological Laboratory, The Netherlands;*
[2]*Erasmus University, Rotterdam, The Netherlands*

INTRODUCTION

The spleen plays an important role in the protection against overwhelming postsplenectomy infections (OPSIs) (1). Protective antibodies against OPSIs eliciting microorganisms are mainly directed against the neutral polysaccharide component (thymus-independent type-2 antigen, TI-2) of the bacterial capsule (2). Both marginal zone macrophages (MZMs), which specifically take up and retain TI-2 antigens (3), and MZ B cells (4) have been suggested as being responsible for the splenic dependency of the TI-2 response. Splenectomy in adult animals results in a marked depression of the anti–TI-2 response, which can not be restored by administration of splenic cell suspensions (1,5). In a previous study, we have shown that after splenectomy normal antibody responses against a TI-2 antigen, trinitrophenylated-Ficoll (TNP-Ficoll), can be restored by autotransplantation of splenic tissues (6,7). Furthermore, we showed that normal response speed and peak titers of anti-TNP serum antibodies could be obtained in the absence of MZ macrophages, and that anti-TNP antibody-forming cells (AFCs) can be demonstrated (after immunization with TNP-Ficoll) in the autotransplants. In a previous study, we observed a similar splenectomylike decrease in the anti–TI-2 response after elimination of most MZ cells with dichloromethylene diphosphonate (DMDP)–liposomes (8). In this study, we investigated the role of MZMs in the TI-2 response in two experimental models in which these cells were eliminated in vivo, whereas leaving all other cell types and the normal splenic architecture intact.

MATERIALS AND METHODS

Experimental Design for Autotransplantation

Sixty mice, 14 weeks of age, were divided into three groups: splenectomized (n = 15 mice), autotransplanted (n = 30), and sham-operated (n = 15) animals. All animals were operated on the same day. Each of the three groups was subdivided in five equally sized groups (Fig. 1). All animals in these subgroups were immunized with TNP-Ficoll (↓ at either 0, 1, 2, 4, or 8 weeks after surgery. Venous tail blood was taken 0, 3, 6, 12, 24, and 34 days (▼) after immunization. In parallel groups, animals were killed 5 days after immunization (↑) and spleen or autotransplants removed and snap-frozen in liquid nitrogen for immunohistochemistry.

Experimental Design for MZM Elimination with DMDP-Liposomes

Mice were pretreated by intravenous injection of phosphatidylcholine/cholesterol liposome encapsulated: DMDP, liposome encapsulated phosphate-buffered saline (PBS), or PBS. Two days after pretreatment, mice were immunized (doses as in Fig. 4) with TNP-Ficoll or TNP–keyhole limpet hemocyanin (TNP-KLH) (8). Five days later animals were sacrificed, spleens were frozen for immunohistochemistry and blood was taken for determination of anti-TNP serum titers.

Preparation of Liposomes

Liposomes were prepared as described in detail previously (9), and mice were injected with 200 μl (4.7 mg lipid) of the suspension.

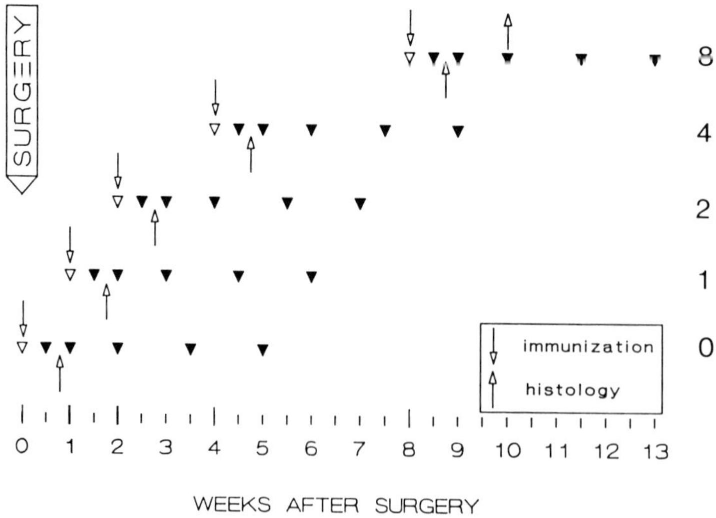

Figure 1 Operating, immunization, and bleeding schedule for autotransplantation groups. Triangles indicate pre- (open) and postimmunization (closed) sera. Groups are indicated as 8, 4, 2, 1, and 0 weeks, from top to bottom rows.

ELISA

Anti-TNP serum titers were determined according to a modification of the anti-insulin ELISA described by Vos et al. (10). Briefly, 96 well plates (titertek 77-172-05) were coated with 100 μl of a solution containing 10 μg/ml GAM–IgG + IgM or $IgG_{1,2a,2b,3}$ (Southern Biotechnology, Birmingham, Alabama). Serum samples were prediluted 1:500 in eightfold. After incubation and washing with PBS, TNP–alkaline phosphatase (AP) (11) was added in 1:100, 1:500, 1:2500, and 1:12500 in duplicate. After incubation and washing with PBS, the AP activity was revealed with PNP and determined spectrophotometrically at 405 nm. All duplicates were obtained within 10% confidence limits.

Immunohistochemistry

Stainings on 8-μm cryostat sections were performed as described in detail previously (6). ERTR-9 was a kind gift of Dr. W. Van Ewijk (EUR, Rotterdam, The Netherlands). Moma-1, antimouse IgM and Thy-1 were a kind gift of Dr. G. Kraal (VUA, Amsterdam, The Netherlands). Image analysis was performed with automated quantitation of the total stained surface, on an Artek Counter (model 880, Farmingdale, New York) as described in detail previously (12).

RESULTS

Regeneration of Autotransplants

As we described previously (6) and as is summarized in Table 1, the cell types we investigated disappeared almost completely owing to necrosis after transplantation. However, they were back to normal numbers and to their proper localization at 4–8 weeks after transplantation. One notable exception, also shown in Figure 2, were the ERTR-9^{+ve} MZMs which were not found in normal numbers in the MZ until 10 weeks after surgery (data not shown).

Table 1 Qualitative and Image Analysis Data of Histochemical Stainings for Different Splenic Cell Types of Mice Sacrificed at 5 Days After TNP-Ficoll Immunization

	Autotransplantation (weeks after surgery)				Liposomal elimination	
	1	2	4	8	PBS	DMDP
B cells	+	++	++	++	95 ± 10	76 ± 13
T cells	+	++	++	++	102 ± 20	95 ± 12
MZ Macrophages	–	–	–	±	97 ± 16	0 ± 3
MZ Metallophils	–	+	+	++	92 ± 15	0 ± 9

Qualitative results expressed as – not present; ± weakly positive; + positive but subnormal numbers; ++ similar as control. Quantitative data expressed as percentage of staining determined against untreated controls (100%), see also section Materials and Methods.

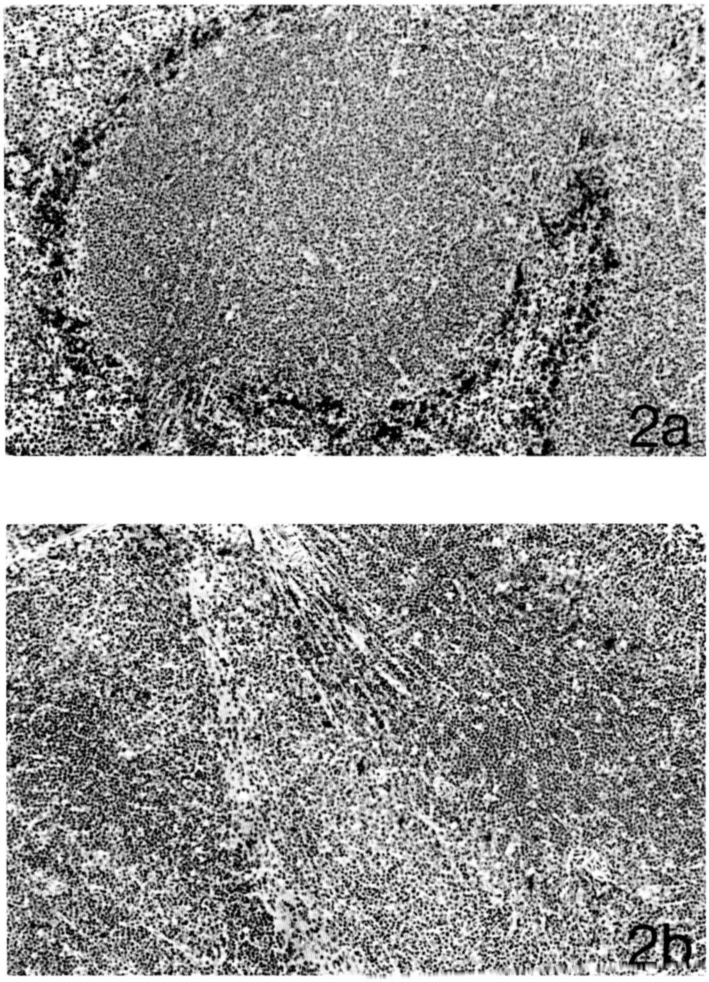

Figure 2 Immunocytochemical detection of MZMs with ERTR-9 in cryostat sections of a sham-operated spleen (a) and splenic autotransplant (b) 8 weeks after surgery.

Anti-TNP Response After Splenectomy and Autotransplantation

In splenectomized animals, a drastic increase in the total amount of anti-TNP antibodies (IgM and IgG) was observed as compared to sham-operated animals (Fig. 3a). Animals immunized 1 and 2 weeks after autotransplantation showed significantly ($p < 0.05$) lower titers than sham-operated animals. At 4 and 8 weeks, when MZMs were not yet present, these titers were again significantly the same as in sham-operated animals. All sera were also investigated for specific anti-TNP antibodies of the IgG isotypes 1, 2a, 2b, and 3. Essentially no other findings than those described above were found for $IgG2_{2a,2b,3}$. However, as Figure 3b clearly shows, anti-TNP titers of the IgG_1 isotype were decreased to less than 10% of their values in control animals. Only at 8 weeks after autotransplantation,

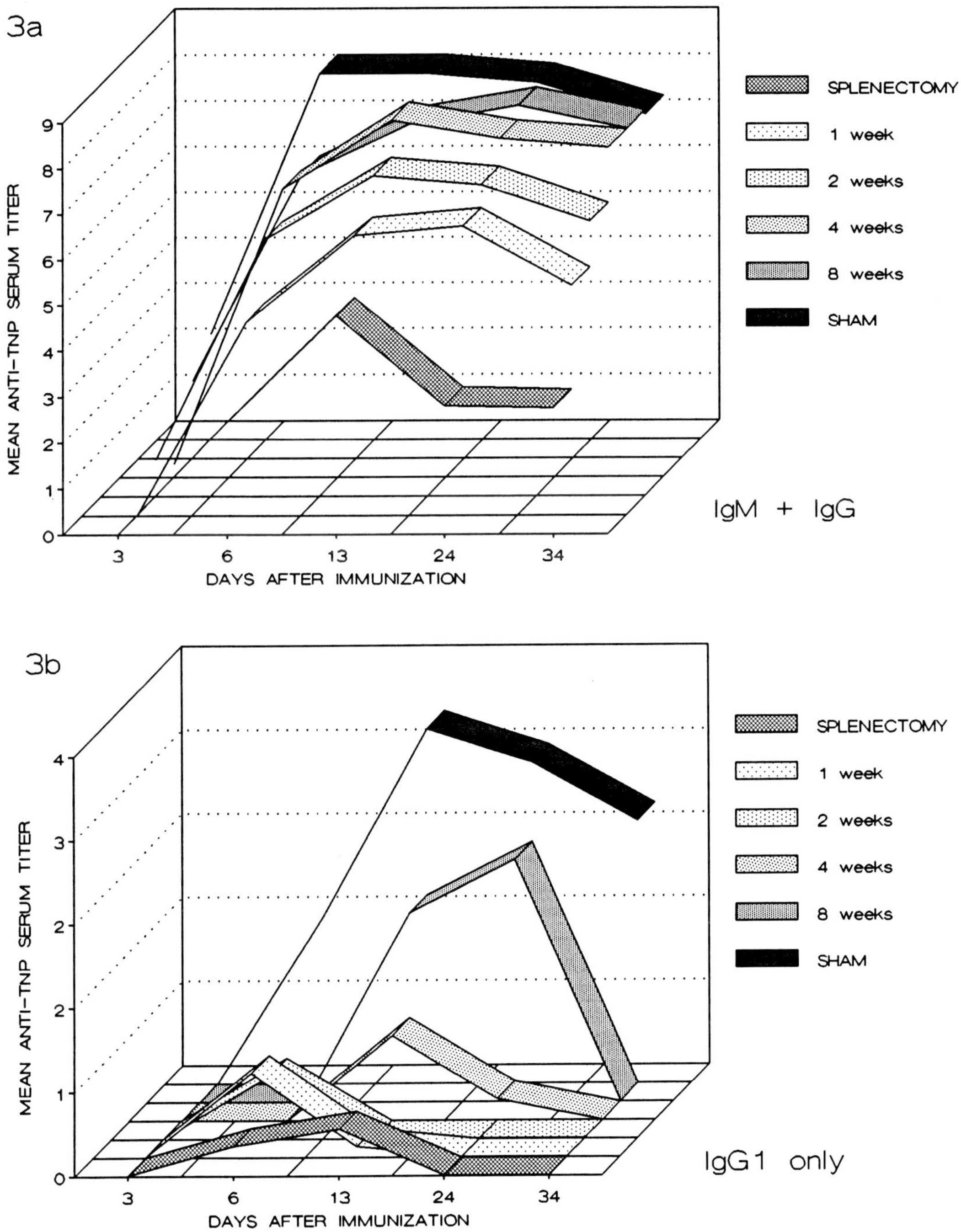

Figure 3 Anti-TNP serum titers after immunization of sham-operated (mean of weeks 0–8; 30 mice/point), weeks 1, 2, 4, and 8 autotransplanted (n = 12/point/week) and splenectomized (mean of weeks 0–8; n = 30/point) mice. Values are expressed as $^{-2}$log of the serum titers as detected in an anti-TNP ELISA for all anti-TNP antibodies (a) or IgG1 isotype and anti-TNP antibodies only (b).

simultaneously with the recurrence of the first MZMs, were they rising to higher levels (±30% of control).

Elimination of Macrophages by DMDP-Liposomes

By using a single dose of DMDP-liposomes we were able to eliminate all splenic macrophages while leaving the splenic architecture and the number of T and B cells essentially intact (see Table 1; elimination of red pulp macrophages complete but not shown). This was an important feat, since in previous macrophage-elimination studies we used two doses of liposomes, thereby also eliminating up to 80% of all B cells (8).

Effect of Macrophage Elimination on the Anti-TNP Immune Response

Figure 4 shows anti-TNP serum titers after immunization of mice pretreated with PBS, PBS-liposomes, or DMDP-liposomes with TNP-KLH (a thymus-dependent antigen [TD]) and TNP-Ficoll in decreasing doses. The response against TNP-KLH in macrophage-depleted animals did not differ at any dose from that seen in control animals. However, a drastic increase of the specific immune response against the TI-2 antigen TNP-Ficoll was observed in macrophage-depleted animals as compared to controls. Significant ($p < 0.01$) differences were observed from 0.3–8.0 μg/mouse.

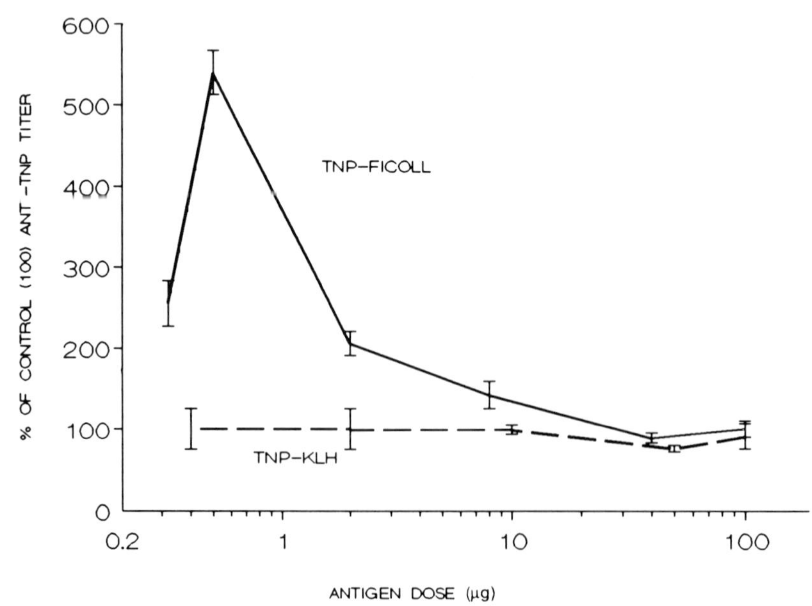

Figure 4 Anti-TNP serum titers of macrophage-depleted mice (DMDP-liposomes at day –2) 5 days after TNP-Ficoll immunization (day 0). Data are mean of six animals in two experiments and expressed as percentage of the titer of untreated and PBS-liposome control animals (100%); bars indicate standard deviation.

DISCUSSION

In this study, we show that MZ B cells, and not MZMs, are essential for antigen presentation of TI-2 antigens and a specific immune response. Furthermore, we demonstrate that elimination of MZMs only, whereas leaving all other cell types and the splenic architecture intact results in an (unexpected) increase of the specific immune response against TNP-Ficoll.

Taking these and previous data (6) together, this means that although MZMs are not essential for a normal anti–TI-2 response in terms of peak antibody titers and kinetics (speed), they can influence the isotype of the specific antibodies produced. No specific anti–TI-2 antibodies of IgG_1 isotype were produced as long as the MZMs were absent from the spleen (up to 10 weeks after autotransplantation). This IgG_1 deficiency was compensated by a slight increase of other isotypes (never more than 20%; data not shown). The IgG:IgM ratio of anti-TNP antibodies after immunization with TNP-Ficoll is 4:6 (±10%), IgG_1 made up 40–50% of the IgG isotypes we found. Consequently, the decrease of specific IgG_1 antibodies is maximal 20% of the total amount of antibodies produced. The physiological role of IgG_1 and IgG_3, which are the predominant IgG isotypes in a typical TI-2 immune response, is still a matter of discussion, but the selective reduction of IgG_1 after splenectomy is clearly related to MZMs.

A striking finding in this study was the increase in a specific anti–TI-2 response at lower doses of TNP-Ficoll and not of TNP-KLH) once the macrophages have been removed. The data shown in Figure 4 pertain to immunization 2 days after liposome treatment, but similar results were found at 19 days after treatment (data not shown). At this time, all B cells and marginal metallophils were back to normal numbers (see also Ref. 13). Together with our earlier observations on uptake and presentation of TI-2 antigens by MZMs after elimination with immunotoxins, these data indicate that the cell responsible for this increase was the MZM. Since TI-2 antigens are not degraded or presented by MZMs, these antigens are obscured from the immune system once they are taken up by MZMs. We suggest that postsplenectomy OPSI is facilitated not so much because of a deficient humoral response, but mainly by the decreased phagocytosis of TI-2 antigens in OPSI patients. Elimination of macrophages facilitates a better anti–TI-2 response. This fact might be used in vaccination with TI-2 antigens (cf. Ref. 15) where temporary blocking of macrophages could give better responses. Detrimental effects of macrophage elimination on the anti-TD response per se are not to be expected in view of the current findings with TNP-KLH, but further study on side effects and memory induction after macrophage elimination (cf. Ref. 16) are needed.

CONCLUSION

We conclude that IgM-positive IgD-negative B cells in a marginal zone architecture are necessary for a normal anti–TI-2 response, for which marginal zone macrophages are dispensable. We suggest that the role of local concentration of TI-2 antigens, as described in the literature, by marginal zone macrophages is not primarily antigen presentation but antigen removal, and that a negative effect of this concentration is a decrease of the anti–TI-2 response.

REFERENCES

1. Amlot PL and Hayes AE. Impaired human antibody response to the thymus-independent antigen, DNP-Ficoll, after splenectomy. Implications for post-splenectomy infections. Lancet 1985; 1:1008–1009.

2. Rijkers GT and Mosier DE. Pneumococcal polysaccharides induce antibody formation by human B lymphocytes in vitro. J Immunol 1985; 135:1–9.
3. Humphrey JH. Splenic macrophages: Antigen presenting cells for TI-2 antigens. Immunol Lett 1985; 11:149–154.
4. Gray D, Chassoux D, MacLennan ICM and Bazin H. Selective depression of thymus independent anti-DNP antibody responses induced by adult but not neonatal splenectomy. Clin Exp J Immunol 1985; 60:378–386.
5. Goud SN, Muthusamy N and Subbarao B. Differential responses of B-cells from the spleen and lymph node to TNP-Ficoll. J Immunol 1988; 140:2925–2930.
6. Claassen E, Ott A, Dijkstra CD, Boersma WJA, Deen C, Kors N, Schellekens M and Van Rooijen N. Marginal zone of the murine spleen in autotransplants: Functional and histological observations in the response against a thymus independent type-2 antigen. Clin Exp Immunol 1989; 77: 445–451.
7. Bohnsack JF and Brown EJ. The role of the spleen in resistance to infection. Ann Rev Med 1986; 37:49–58.
8. Claassen E, Kors N and Van Rooijen N. Influence of carriers on the development and localization of anti-2,4,6-trinitrophenyl (TNP) antibody-forming cells in the murine spleen. II. Suppressed antibody response to TNP-Ficoll after elimination of marginal zone cells. Eur J Immunol 1986; 16:492–497.
9. Claassen E and Van Rooijen N. Preparation and characteristics of dichloromethylene disphosphonate-containing liposomes. J Microencapsul 1986; 3:109–114.
10. Vos Q, Claassen E and Benner R. Enumeration of anti-insulin antibody-secreting cells using an improved spot-ELISA. J Immunol Methods 1990; 126:89–94.
11. Claassen E and Van Rooijen N. A trinitrophenyl-poly-L-lysine-horseradish peroxidase conjugate for the detection of anti-TNP antibodies in vivo. J Histochem Cytochem 1985; 33:840–844.
12. Claassen E, Westerhof Y, Versluis B, Kors N, Schellekens M and Van Rooijen N. Effects of chronic injection of sphingomyelin containing liposomes on lymphoid and non-lymphoid cells in the spleeen. Transient suppression of marginal zone macrophages. Br J Exp Pathol 1988; 69:865–875.
13. Laman JD, Kors N, Van Rooijen N and Claassen E. Mechanisms of follicular trapping: Localization of immune complexes and cell remnants after elimination and repopulation of different spleen cell populations. Immunology 1990; 71:57–62.
14. Kraal G, TerHart H, Meelhuysen C, Venneker G and Claassen E. Marginal zone macrophages and their role in the immune response against TI-2 antigens. Modulation of the cells with specific antibody. Eur J Immunol 1989; 19:675–680.
15. Austrian R, Douglas RM, Schiffman G, Coetzee AM, Koornhof HJ, Hayden-Smith S and Reid RDW. Prevention of pneumococcal pneumonia by vaccination. Trans Assoc Am Physicians 1976; 89:184–193.
16. Claassen E, Kors N and Van Rooijen N. Immunomodulation with liposomes: The immune response elicited by liposomes with entrapped dichloromethylenediphosphonate and surface associated antigen or hapten. Immunology 1987; 60:509–515.

148
Immunotoxic Effects of the Food Additive Ammonia Caramel

Geert F. Houben,[1,2,3] Marga H. M. Kuijpers,[2] Bert W. Lam,[1] Henk van Loveren,[3] and André H. Penninks[1,2]
[1]*Research Institute of Toxicology, University of Utrecht, The Netherlands;*
[2]*TNO-CIVO Toxicology and Nutrition Institute, Zeist, The Netherlands;*
[3]*National Institute of Public Health and Environmental Protection (RIVM), Bilthoven, The Netherlands*

INTRODUCTION

The term caramel (E150) refers to a large number of poorly defined and very complex products used as colorants in human foodstuffs and beverages. It has been demonstrated that oral administration of ammonia caramel (AC; Class III caramel colour) can cause a reduction in total white blood cell counts in rats, owing to reduced lymphocyte counts (1,2,4). This lymphopenic effect was found to occur only when the animals were fed a diet low in pyridoxine (vitamin B_6) (4).

2-Acetyl-4(5)-(1,2,3,4-tetrahydroxybutyl)imidazole (THI) has been isolated from AC (3) and this compound has been identified as the major, if not the only, component responsible for the reduction in the number of lymphocytes (4). In this chapter, the results of two studies, which were conducted to compare and to characterize the effects of AC and THI on the various lymphoid organs in dependence of the vitamin B_6 content of the diet, are presented and discussed. Besides, some data with respect to ex vivo effects of THI are presented.

MATERIALS AND METHODS

Materials

Class III caramel food colour (AC) was manufactured by Cerestar (Vilvoorde, Belgium). The batch of AC was specified as HT2207 and had a THI content of 143 mg/kg. (Today, Class III caramel colour manufacturers are meeting the proposed specifications of the EC for no more than 25 mg THI/kg.) The 2-acetyl-4(5)-(1,2,3,4-tetrahydroxybutyl)imidazole

(THI) used in these studies was kindly provided by The International Technical Caramel Association, Washington, D.C.

Experimental Design of the In Vivo Studies

Young male Wistar-derived rats (RIV-TOX) from a specific pathogen free colony (RIVM, Bilthoven, The Netherlands), weighing 35–60 g, were used in these studies. The animals were housed in groups of four in wire-mesh floored cages in an animal room maintained at 23 ± 1°C, with a light/dark cycle of 12 hr and a relative humidity of 50 ± 10%. The animals were fed a semipurified casein diet prepared by TNO-CIVO (Zeist, The Netherlands). The vitamin B_6 content of the diet was 2–3 ppm (low) or 12 ppm (high). The vitamin was supplemented as pyridoxine·HCl. The AC and THI were administered in the drinking water. Demineralized water (pH 3), whether or not supplemented with AC or THI, was freely available. Two studies were conducted: a low vitamin B_6 diet study in which rats were fed a diet containing 2–3 ppm pyridoxine and a high vitamin B_6 diet study with a 12 ppm pyridoxine diet. In each study, three groups of 12 rats were provided with a different drinking solution: control water; a 4% (w/w) AC solution, equal to a 5.72 ppm (w/w) THI solution; or a 5.72 ppm (w/w) THI solution. The AC and THI exposure was started immediately after weaning the animals and was continued during 28 days. Prior to each of the studies, the rats were allocated in groups with approximately equal mean body weights.

Body weights of the individual rats and the food intake per cage were recorded weekly. Fluid intake was determined by weighing water bottles daily. At the termination of the experiments the rats were bled by aorta puncture under ether anesthesia. Total white and red blood cell numbers were counted. An estimation of the different types of leukocytes was obtained by counting 100 cells in a smear made from blood samples after Pappenheim staining. From the total and the differential leukocyte counts, the absolute number of lymphocytes, neutrophils, eosinophils, basophils, and monocytes were calculated.

At necropsy, weights of thymus, spleen, liver, kidneys, and adrenals were recorded. Cell suspensions in phosphate-buffered saline (PBS) were prepared from thymus, spleen, femoral bone marrow, and mesenterial and popliteal lymph nodes by passing the tissue through a nylon sieve (pore diameter 250 μm). To remove cell clumps, the suspensions were passed through a 25-gauge needle. The cells were counted and the total numbers of nucleated cells per organ were calculated. Cell numbers in blood and tissue suspensions were counted using a Coulter counter model ZF (Coulter Electronics Ltd, Harpender, Herts, United Kingdom). Sera, blood plasma, and organs were stored for further investigations.

Conduct of the Ex Vivo Studies

Groups of eight male Wistar rats, weighing 150–250 g, were fed a diet low in vitamin B_6 (1.5–2.0 ppm pyridoxine) during and at least for 7 days prior to the experiments. Four animals were exposed to 11.44 ppm THI in drinking water for 13 days. Four control animals received normal drinking water. At the termination of the exposure period, the rats were killed by decapitation and splenic cell suspensions were prepared in cooled (4°C) PBS containing 40 mg D-glucose/100 ml by passing the tissue through a nylon sieve (pore diameter 250 μm). To remove cell clumps, the suspensions were passed through a 25-gauge needle and subsequently the cells were washed three times. Finally, suspensions of 5×10^6 cells/ml RPMI 1640 culture medium were prepared and were used in mitogenic-stimulation assays. Samples of 100 μl of the cell suspensions were mixed with 50 μl of RPMI 1640 culture medium containing graded amounts of mitogen or without mitogen. The mitogens used were phytohemagglutinin (PHA: 0, 15, and 25 μg/well), concanavalin A (Con A: 0, 0.2, and 0.5 μg/well) and lipopolysaccharide (LPS: 0, 15, and 25 μg/well). The cells were incubated at 37°C for 40 hr. After this incubation period, 25 μl of a [^{3}H]thymidine solution was added, leading to a final thymidine concentration of 0.5 nmol/ml and an activity of 2.5 μCi/ml. After an additional incubation period of 8 hr, the cells were harvested onto glass fiber filters using a cell culture harvester. The filters were dried at 70°C for 16 hr and were transferred into a sample bag containing 10 ml of Beta Plate scintillation fluid. The amount of label incorporated was measured in a flat bed liquid scintillation counter for 1 min. All incubations were performed in fourfold.

RESULTS

Results of In Vivo Studies

Food and Water Intake, Body Weight Gain

Water intake, food intake, and body weight gain of the control animals, the AC-treated animals, and the THI-treated animals did not differ significantly in either the low (2–3 ppm) or the high (12 ppm) vitamin B_6 diet study. The equal water intake in the treatment groups indicated that AC- and THI-treated rats were exposed to equivalent amounts of THI.

Relative Organ Weights

Of the lymphoid organs weighed, relative spleen weights of AC- and THI-treated animals were significantly decreased by about 25% in the low vitamin B_6 diet study. The relative spleen weights in the high vitamin B_6 diet study were decreased significantly (8%) in the THI-treated animals only. No significant differences in the relative thymus weights and the relative adrenal weights were observed. Relative kidney weights were significantly increased by about 10% in both the low and high vitamin B_6 diet study in AC-exposed rats. Neither AC nor THI exposure clearly affected relative liver weights. Only in the case of AC treatment in the high vitamin B_6 diet study, the relative liver weights were slightly increased.

Total Cell Numbers Isolated from Lymphoid Organs

Total cell numbers of spleen were decreased by about 55% in both the AC- and THI-treated animals in the low vitamin B_6 diet study. In the case of the high vitamin B_6 diet study, a significant reduction in spleen cell numbers was observed in the THI-treated animals only (32%). In the low vitamin B_6 diet study, thymus cell numbers were significantly decreased (by 22%) in AC-treated animals, whereas THI exposure did not affect the cell numbers in thymus. In the high vitamin B_6 diet study, no significant differences were observed in the cell numbers isolated from thymus. Total cell numbers isolated from popliteal lymph nodes of AC- and THI-treated animals were decreased by about 50% in the low vitamin B_6 diet study. No statistically significant differences were observed in cell numbers of lymph nodes in the high vitamin B_6 diet study. The total cell numbers isolated from bone marrow did not differ in the AC- or THI-treated animals when compared to the corresponding control animals.

Blood Cell Numbers

Total white blood cell numbers of AC- and THI-exposed animals were significantly decreased by about 67% in the low vitamin B_6 diet study when compared to the corresponding control animals. These decreased numbers were caused by a significant reduction in the number of blood lymphocytes by about 74%. A tendency toward a reduction in blood leukocyte and lymphocyte counts was also observed in the high vitamin B_6 diet study. No clear differences were observed in red blood cell numbers, monocyte numbers, and blood neutrophil, eosinophil, and basophil numbers in either of the two studies.

Results of Ex Vivo Studies

Results of ex vivo studies with THI indicate that splenic cells of THI-exposed rats show a reduced in vitro incorporation of labeled thymidine when compared to cells of control animals. This effect is most obvious after mitogenic stimulation of the cells. From two representative experiments it was calculated that in the absence of a mitogen, cells of THI-exposed rats incorporate only 44% of the amount of label compared to cells of control rats. In the presence of graded amounts of the mitogens, these percentages were 28 and 18 (PHA), 22 and 24 (Con A), and 19 and 18 (LPS). Statistical analysis of the results demonstrated that the cells of THI-exposed rats did not show an appropriate response upon mitogenic stimulation.

DISCUSSION

Results obtained in these studies indicate that THI and AC (containing 143 mg THI/kg) cause a strong and comparable decrease in total white blood cell counts in male rats owing to reduced lymphocyte counts. Besides in blood, reduced cell numbers were observed in spleen and lymph nodes. There were no marked differences in the effects on lymphoid organs of equivalent amounts of THI and THI in AC. The lymphopenic effects of THI and AC were found to be reduced by pyridoxine to the same degree.

The mechanism underlying the lymphopenic effect of AC and THI is not known so far. Lymphocyte subset determinations by means of flow cytometric analysis indicated that a comparable decrease in the number of lymphocytes in various subsets (B cells and T cells) was induced (Houben, unpublished results). There were no indications for a shift in lymphocytes from blood into other tissue compartments or for a bone marrow involvement.

Thymus cell numbers of AC-exposed rats in the low vitamin B_6 diet study appeared to be decreased. However, other studies have indicated that thymus weight and cell numbers in general are not markedly affected by AC or THI. But nevertheless, (immuno)histological examinations indicate that thymus function may be disturbed (Houben, unpublished results). A strong decrease in the thymic cortex/medulla area ratios of AC- and THI-exposed rats was observed and the increased medullary area showed a strong increase in the number of thymocytes with a mature phenotype. Beside these changes in thymus, a very strong decrease in the number of macrophages positive for the differentiation antigen recognized by the MAb ED-2 (5) was observed in the cortex of thymus, in spleen, and in liver.

The ex vivo studies with THI demonstrated that splenic cells of THI-exposed rats did not show an appropriate response upon mitogenic stimulation with PHA, Con A, or LPS. It was remarkable that without mitogenic stimulation the incorporation of labeled thymidine by splenic cells of THI-exposed rats was already clearly reduced.

More detailed studies to investigate the possible relationship between this ex vivo effect and the reduction in the number of lymphocytes in vivo are being conducted. Since in vivo, this batch of AC and THI have been found to influence the number of lymphocytes as well as the number of macrophages positive for the MAb ED-2, and accessory cells are known to be of importance in mitogenic stimulation assays, it will have to be investigated whether the observed in vivo and ex vivo effects result from an effect on lymphocytes, accessory cells, or both types of cells. Because the expression of the differentiation antigen recognized by ED-2 has not been associated clearly with functional characteristics of the cells, THI might provide an interesting tool in investigating the role of this type of macrophage in the immune system.

ACKNOWLEDGMENTS

The ex vivo studies with THI were financially supported by the International Technical Caramel Association. The studies presented are part of a project subsidized by the Utrecht Toxicology Centre (UTOX), a research cooperation program of the Research Institute of Toxicology, University of Utrecht, the TNO-CIVO Toxicology and Nutrition Institute, Zeist, and the National Institute of Public Health and Environmental Protection, Bilthoven, The Netherlands.

REFERENCES

1. Evans JG, Butterworth KR, Gaunt IF, Grasso P (1977): Long-term toxicology study in the rat on a caramel produced by the "half open-half closed pan" ammonia process. Food Cosmet Toxicol 15:523–531.
2. Gaunt IF, Lloyd AG, Grasso P, Gangolli SD, Butterworth KR (1977): Short-term study in the rat on two caramels produced by variations of the "ammonia process." Food Cosmet Toxicol 15:509–521.
3. Kröplien U, Rosdorfer J, Greef van der J, Long RC, Goldstein JH (1985): 2-Acetyl-4(5)-(1,2,3,4-tetrahydroxybutyl)imidazole: Detection in commercial caramel color III and preparation by a model browning reaction. J Org Chem 50:1131.
4. Sinkeldam EJ, Groot de AP, Berg van den H, Chappel CI (1988): The effect of pyridoxine on the number of lymphocytes in the blood of rats fed caramel colour (III). Food Chem Toxicol 26:195–203.
5. Dijkstra CD, Döpp EA, Joling P, Kraal G (1985): The heterogeneity of mononuclear phagocytes in lymphoid organs: Distinct macrophage subpopulations in the rat recognized by monoclonal antibodies ED1, ED2 and ED3. Immunology 45:589–599.

LYMPHOCYTE MIGRATION AND HOMING

149
Lymphocyte Migration and Homing: Introduction

Eugene Butcher
Stanford University School of Medicine, Stanford, California, and Center for Molecular Biology and Medicine, Veterans Administration Medical Center, Palo Alto, California

The molecular mechanisms of lymphocyte–high endothelial venule (HEV) recognition first became experimentally approachable with the development of an in vitro assay of lymphocyte binding to HEV in frozen sections by Stamper and Woodruff in the late 1970s. At that time, it seemed reasonable to assume that lymphocyte-HEV binding would be mediated by a single receptor/ligand pair wherever such interactions occurred in the body. Although selective trafficking of lymphoblasts to the gut or to cutaneous sites of inflammation had been described, we and many others assumed that the specificity of such migration would be conferred by chemoattractants rather than selective recognition of vascular endothelium.

It is now clear that the trafficking of lymphocytes displays a more refined specificity than initially thought, with unique populations of memory cells and immunoblasts targeted to mucosal, peripheral lymph nodes, skin, and potentially other sites. Furthermore, although chemoattractants are undoubtedly involved as well (which remains to be fully explored), tissue-selective lymphocyte–endothelial cell recognition mechanisms play a dominant role in targeting unique lymphocyte populations to organized lymphoid tissues, to the skin, the mucosal lamina propria of the small intestine, and potentially the joints and pulmonary lymphoid tissues. Distinct vascular addressins, providing tissue "address" signals for circulating lymphocytes, have been identified in peripheral lymph nodes, in mucosal Peyer's patches and lamina propria, and in inflamed skin. In some cases, complementary lymphocyte "homing receptors" have been defined. The vascular addressins are tissue-specific endothelial cell adhesion molecules for lymphocytes, with each addressin binding a defined subset of circulating virgin and/or memory and presumably blast cells whose prior history of antigen-independent or antigen-dependent differentiation has resulted in the expression of one or more homing receptors permitting recognition of the addressin. Adhesion molecules have been recruited from a number of distinct gene families to mediate these tissue-specific lymphocyte–endothelial cell recognition events. Vascular addressins of endothelial cells and adhesion molecules on lymphocytes include lectins, carbohydrate ligands whose cell distribution is regulated by glycosyltransferases, and members of the immunoglobulin, hyaluronate-binding, and integrin families of cell adhesion receptors.

The abstracts presented in this session not only illustrate the level of our understanding (or in some cases, the level of our confusion) regarding the molecular and physiological mechanisms of lymphocyte trafficking, they also define many important issues and questions that remain to be answered, and that represent areas of ongoing and future investigation. What are the molecular mechanisms and physiological parameters of lymphocyte trafficking to and from the bursa of Fabricius, the thymus, the inflamed synovium in rheumatoid arthritis, and other sites? Is the tissue-specific expression of vascular addressins regulated by the local tissue microenvironment, and/or by developmental predetermination? Are lymphocyte homing receptors and vascular addressins merely adhesion molecules, or are they receptor/counter-receptor pairs that mediate not only adhesion, but also signal transduction events that alter the phenotype and behavior of interacting lymphocytes and endothelial cells? How is the specificity of lymphocyte homing regulated during lymphocyte differentiation, and what subsets of virgin and/or memory cells traffic through lymphoid vs extralymphoid tissues? Finally, as our understanding of the molecular nature and patterns of expression of homing receptors and vascular addressins improves, it is now becoming clear that these alone cannot explain completely the selectivity of lymphocyte/leukocyte extravasation observed in vivo. Thus, it is appropriate that we see in addition a renewed interest in the role of chemoattractants in regulating the diapedesis and tissue targeting of lymphocytes.

150

Very Late Antigen-4–Dependent Adhesion of Lymphocytic Cell Lines to Cultured Human Endothelium

Robert H. Vonderheide and Timothy A. Springer
The Center for Blood Research, Harvard Medical School, Boston, Massachusetts

INTRODUCTION

Lymphocyte adhesion to cultured endothelium has recently been shown to involve two members of the integrin family of cell surface heterodimers; namely, lymphocyte function–associated antigen 1 (LFA-1) and very late antigen-4 (VLA-4) (1,2). Several endothelial cell counterreceptors for these two molecules have also been identified: LFA-1 can bind to intercellular adhesion molecule 1 (ICAM-1) or to ICAM-2 (1,3), whereas VLA-4 can bind to vascular cell adhesion molecule 1 (VCAM-1) (2,4,5).

To determine whether there might exist counterreceptors for VLA-4 other than VCAM-1, we have compared the ability of anti–VLA-4 vs anti–VCAM-1 monoclonal antibodies (MAbs) to block adhesion of human lymphocytic cell lines to stimulated and unstimulated cultured human endothelium. Results reported here suggest that VLA-4–dependent lymphocyte-endothelial interactions may involve inducible counterreceptors distinct from VCAM-1.

MATERIALS AND METHODS

Cell Culture

Human umbilical vein endothelial cells (HUVECs) were purchased from Clonetics (San Diego, California) and maintained for up to 20 doublings in RPMI 1640 with 20% fetal bovine serum, 100 μg/ml bovine endothelial cell growth supplement (Biomedical Technologies, Stoughton, Massachusetts), 100 μg/ml heparin, 20 mM HEPES (N-2-hydroxyethylpoperazine-N-2-ethanesulfonic acid), 5 mM glutamine, and 50 μg/ml gentamicin. Tissue culture surfaces were pretreated with 1 μg/cm^2 of human plasma fibronectin in Hank's balanced salt solution. For binding assays, HUVECs were grown to confluence in 96-well tissue culture plates.

Human lymphocytic cell lines were maintained in complete media (i.e., RPMI 1640 with 10% fetal bovine serum, 5 mM glutamine, and 50 μg/ml gentamicin).

Monoclonal Antibodies

The MAbs used were TS1/22 (anti–LFA-1); HP2/1 (anti–VLA-4; a gift of Dr. F. Sanchez-Madrid, Universidad Autonoma de Madrid, Spain); E1/6 (anti–VCAM-1; a gift of Dr. G. E. Rice, Brigham and Women's Hospital, Boston, Massachusetts); and 4B9 (anti–VCAM-1; a gift of Dr. J. Harlan, University of Washington, Seattle, Washington).

HUVEC Stimulation

Recombinant human tumor necrosis factor α (TNFα) (Genzyme, Boston, Massachusetts) was used at 25 ng/ml for 24 hr to stimulate HUVECs in culture.

Adhesion Assay

Lymphoid tumor cells were labeled with the carboxyfluorescein compound BCECF-AM (Molecular Probes Inc., Eugene, Oregon) and resuspended in complete media with 20 mM HEPES. Cells were preincubated with control media or with MAb TS1/22 and/or HP2/1 for 30 min at 37°C. The HUVEC monolayers in 96-well plates were preincubated with MAbs E1/6 or 4B9 for 30 min at 37°C. Without removal of excess MAbs, lymphoid cells (10^5/well) were overlayed on HUVECs and allowed to settle and adhere for 30 min at 37°C. Nonadherent cells were removed by washing five times with complete media and 20 mM HEPES. Percent binding was determined using a fluorescence concentration analyzer (Pandex Laboratories, Inc., Mundelein, Illinois).

Results

A function-blocking anti–VLA-4 MAb, HP2/1, and two blocking anti–VCAM-1 MAbs, E1/6 and 4B9, were compared for their ability to inhibit the adhesion of four lymphocytic cell lines to TNF-stimulated and unstimulated HUVECs. To block any simultaneous interactions between LFA-1 and endothelial ICAM-1 or ICAM-2, cell line binding to HUVECs was assessed in all experiments in the presence of the anti–LFA-1 MAb TS1/22. For the four cell lines examined—T lymphocytic lines Jurkat and SKW3 and B lymphocytic cell lines Raji and Ramos—preincubation with TS1/22 MAb alone blocked adhesion to stimulated or unstimulated HUVECs by <10% compared to preincubation with control media, the control MAb X63, or the anti-CD44 MAb F10442 (Fig. 1). As a control, TS1/22 was observed to block completely the adhesion of the lymphoblastoid cell line JY to TNF-stimulated HUVECs.

Additionally preincubating each of the four cell lines with the anti–VLA-4 MAb HP2/1 significantly blocked adhesion to TNF-stimulated HUVECs (shown in Fig. 1 for one of at least three representative experiments per cell line), as expected from results of a previous study (2). Adhesion of Ramos and Raji cells was blocked by >80%, SKW3 cells by about 70%, and Jurkat cells by 30%. In contrast, preincubation of TNF-stimulated HUVECs with either of two MAb against VCAM-1, a ligand of VLA-4 (2), inhibited cell line adhesion by only a fraction of that observed following preincubation with the anti–VLA-4 MAb (see Fig. 1).

For all cell lines, percent binding following preincubation with anti–VLA-4 MAb *plus* anti–VCAM-1 MAb was the same as that following pretreatment with anti–VLA-4 MAb alone. Neither anti–VLA-4 MAb nor anti–VCAM-1 MAbs affected the basal cell line binding to unstimulated HUVECs, with the possible exception of SKW3 cells.

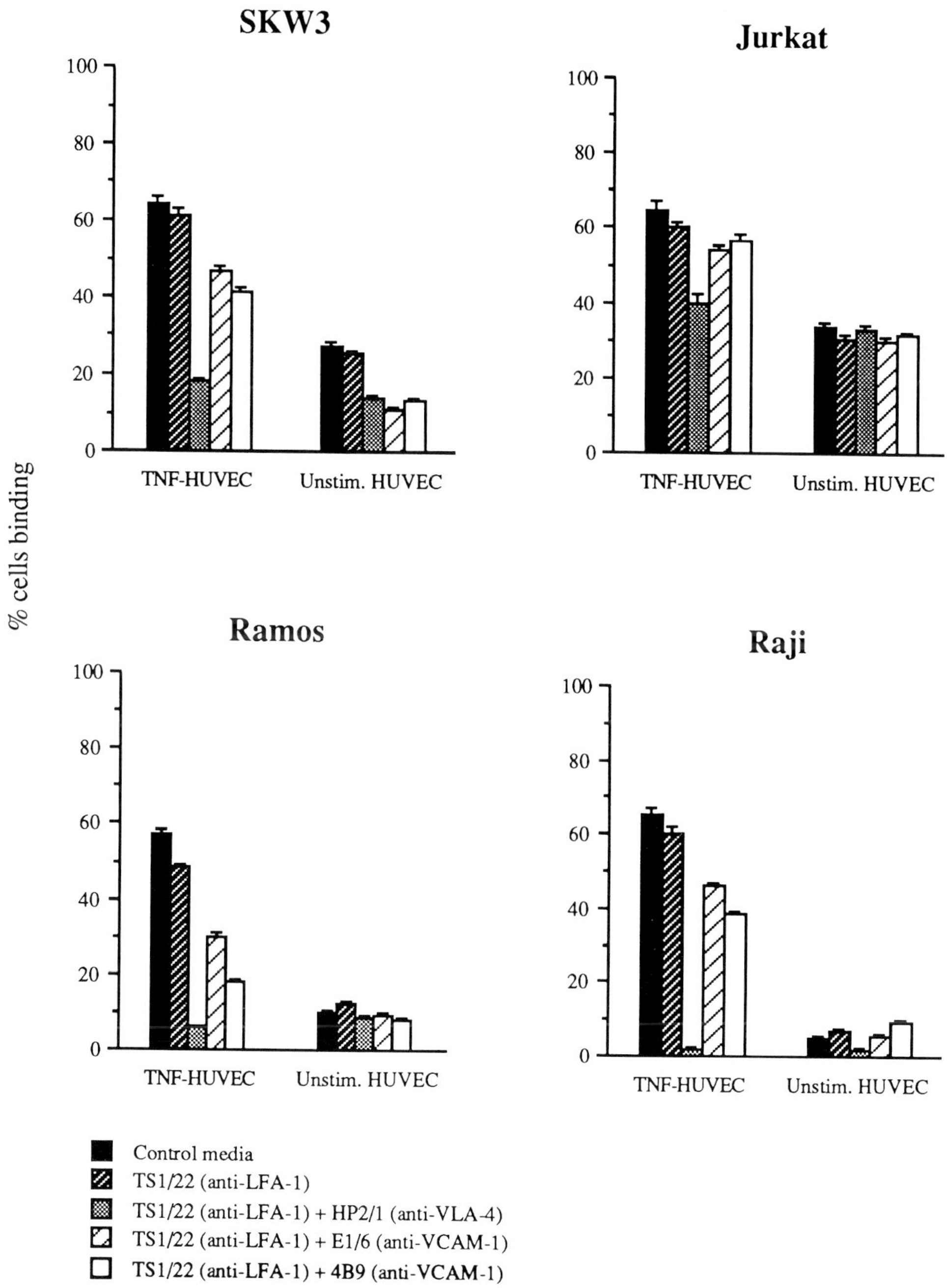

Figure 1 Lymphocytic cell line binding to 24-hr TNF-stimulated or unstimulated human umbilical vein endothelial cells.

DISCUSSION

Preincubation with the anti–VLA-4 MAb HP2/1 blocked adhesion of lymphocytic cell lines to TNF-stimulated HUVECs much greater than preincubation with either of two blocking anti–VCAM-1 MAbs. This observation suggests both a VLA-4–dependent/VCAM-1–independent adhesion pathway as well as a VLA-4–dependent/VCAM-1–dependent pathway mediating lymphocyte-endothelial interactions. Furthermore, comparison of cell line binding to both stimulated and unstimulated HUVECs suggests that the expression of potential VLA-4 counterreceptors distinct from VCAM-1 is cytokine inducible.

Whether such a counterreceptor(s) includes novel inducible surface antigens on endothelial cells and/or extracellular matrix components, such as fibronectin which does interact with VLA-4 (6), is currently being investigated. Preliminary evidence indicates that cell line binding to TNF-stimulated HUVECs is not inhibited further by preincubating HUVECs with an antihuman fibronectin antisera in addition to anti–LFA-1, anti–VLA-4, and anti–VCAM-1 MAbs.

REFERENCES

1. Dustin ML, Springer TA. Lymphocyte function-associated antigen-1 (LFA-1) interaction with intercellular adhesion molecule-1 (ICAM-1) is one of at least three mechanisms for lymphocyte adhesion to cultured endothelial cells. J. Cell Biol. 1988; 107:321–31.
2. Elices MJ, Osborn L, Takada Y, Crouse C, Luhowsky S, Hemler ME, Lobb RR. VCAM-1 on activated endothelium interacts with the leukocyte integrin VLA-4 at a site distinct from the VLA-4/fibronectin binding site. Cell 1990; 60:577–84.
3. deFougerolles T, Springer TA. J. Exp. Med. (in press).
4. Carlos TM, Schwartz BR, Kovach NL, Yee E, Rosso M, Osborn L, Chi-Rosso G, Newman B, Lobb R, Harlan J. Vascular cell adhesion molecule-1 (VCAM-1) mediates lymphocyte adherence to cytokine-activated cultured human endothelial cells. Blood 1990; 76:965–70 .
5. Rice GE, Munro JM, Bevilacqua MP. Inducible cell adhesion molecule 110 (INCAM-110) is an endothelial receptor for lymphocytes. A CD11/CD18-independent adhesion mechanism. J. Exp. Med. 1990; 171:1369–74.
6. Wayner EA, Garcia-Pardo A, Humphries MJ, McDonald JA, Carter WG. Identification and characterization of the lymphocyte adhesion receptor for an alternative cell attachment domain in plasma fibronectin. J. Cell. Biol. 1989. 109:1321–30.

151

Immunoelectron Microscopic Demonstration of Increased Intercellular Adhesion Molecule 1 Expression on High Endothelial Venules in Human Palatine Tonsils

M. E. Perry,[1] B. von Gaudecker,[2] W. Sterry,[2] and V. Mielke,[2]
[1]*Guy's Hospital, London, England;* [2]*University of Kiel, Kiel, Germany*

INTRODUCTION

The palatine tonsils are lymphoepithelial organs strategically positioned in the oropharynx, and continuously exposed to both airborne and alimentary antigens. The human tonsil is divided into two main structural compartments: the tonsillar epithelium and the subepithelial lymphoid tissue. This structural arrangement is closely related to the immunological function of the organ (1–3).

Many lymphocytes recirculate through the palatine tonsils and their extravasation into this lymphoid tissue is due to recognition of the high endothelial venules (HEVs) (4,5). Considerable evidence suggests that this selective interaction is mediated by lymphocyte function-associated antigen-1 (LFA-1), expressed on the surface of lymphocytes, binding to its ligand intercellular adhesion molecule 1 (ICAM-1) on the endothelium of HEVs (4–6).

We have previously identified the HEVs within palatine tonsils using light microscopy (LM), scanning (SEM), and transmission (TEM) electron microscopy (1,3). The purpose of the present study was to determine the distribution of ICAM-1 on the endothelium of the tonsillar vasculature by using gold-coupled reagents in immunoelectron microscopy.

MATERIALS AND METHODS

Material was obtained from children undergoing tonsillectomy. Dissected pieces of tissues were fixed, cryoprotected, and frozen in liquid nitrogen. 30-μm cryostat sections were incubated with one of the three following monoclonal antibodies (MAbs): anti–factor VIII–related antigen (Dakopatts, Denmark); anti-human endothelium, IV 9-1-20 (a gift of Dr. Radzun, Kiel, Germany); and anti–ICAM-1 (a gift of Dr. Springer, Boston,

Massachusetts). The first antibody was followed by an incubation with goat-antimouse immunoglobulin (IgG) coupled with 5-nm gold particles (Janssen Life Science Products, Holland). After postfixation, the sections were silver enhanced (Janssen Life Science Products, Holland), osmicated, dehydrated, and flat embedded in Araldite or TAAB-resin. The 30-μm sections were examined using LM, and subsequently ultrathin sections were cut and viewed in TEM. In addition to the above procedure, the remaining tonsillar tissue was used for routine light microscopy.

RESULTS

In all the examined specimens the vascular network of the parafollicular areas, which contained many transected arterioles, venules, HEVs (Fig. 1), and lymphatics, was denser than that of the adjacent lymphoid follicles. Many small vessels were also present in the reticulated crypt epithelium, and HEVs were seen in some of the lower border regions of this epithelium. The cobblestone appearance of the endothelial cells lining these HEVs was clearly visible in SEM (Fig. 2).

After incubation of tonsillar sections with the MAb to factor VIII–related antigen, both LM and the TEM revealed a positive reaction on the endothelium lining all vessels, hence demarcating the profuse vasculature of the palatine tonsil.

The arterioles and the lymphatics were only weakly stained by the MAbs to ICAM-1 and IV 9-1-20, whereas the venules, and in particular the HEVs, exhibited a strong reactivity to

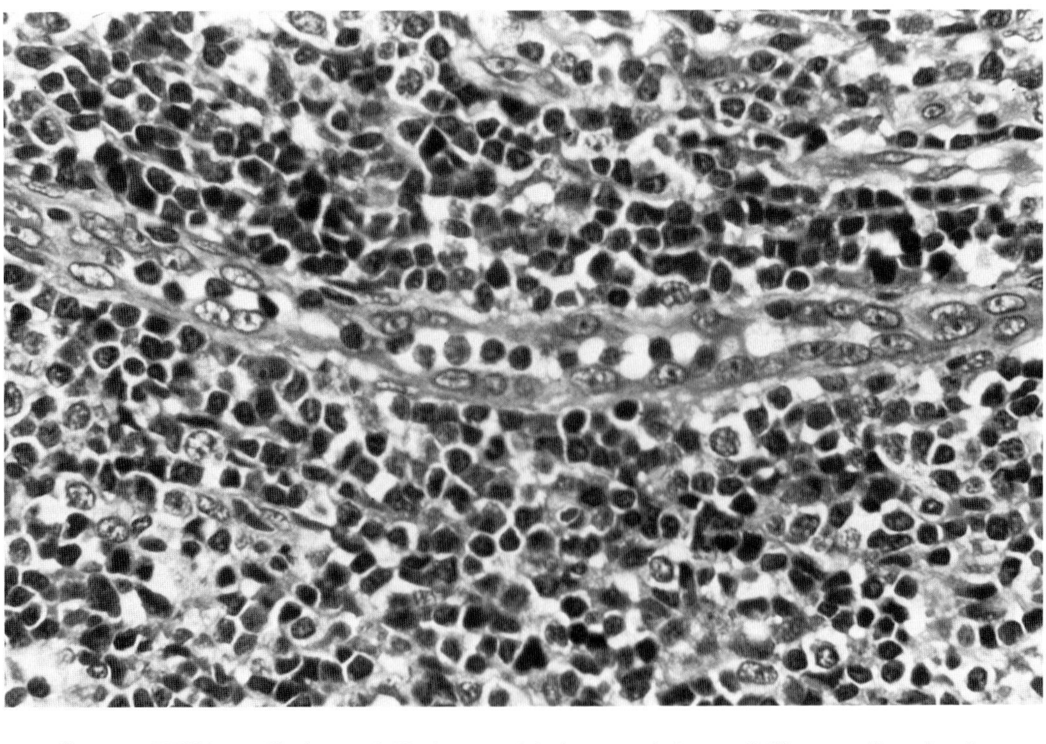

Figure 1 HEV located in the parafollicular area of the human palatine tonsil. Hematoxylin and eosin (magnification: ×640).

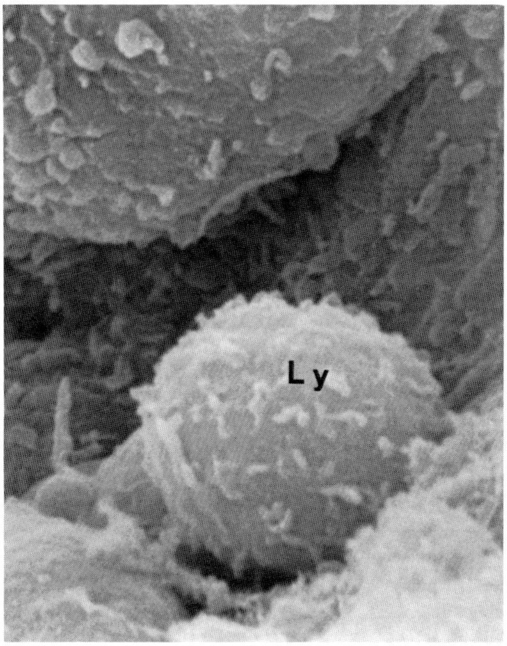

Figure 2 Lumen of a tonsillar HEV showing the typical appearance of the high endothelium. Ly = lymphocyte. SEM (magnification: ×10,000).

both antibodies. However, the endothelium lining the HEVs showed a stronger staining with the anti–ICAM-1 antibody than with the IV 9-1-20 (Figs. 3 and 4). It was also found that the higher the endothelium, the greater the expression of ICAM-1. In all examined sections, ICAM-1 label was seen to be uniformly distributed on the luminal surfaces of the high endothelial cells, including their blebs and microvillous processes (see Figs. 3 and 4).

DISCUSSION

The present study has shown that ICAM-1 is preferentially expressed on the HEVs of the palatine tonsils in contrast to its distribution on the arterioles, low endothelial venules, and lymphatics. As ICAM-1 is the ligand for LFA-1, its preferential expression on the HEVs suggests that it may play an important—if only accessory (4,6)—role in promoting and strengthening the binding of lymphocytes to these particular sites (4,7).

Several reports indicate that lymphocytes recirculate through the palatine tonsils by their initial recognition of HEVs (7–11), which are located in both the parafollicular T-cell regions and in the lower border regions of the crypt epithelium (1,2,8). The anti–ICAM-1–labeled HEVs in the latter location suggest that some of the recirculating lymphocytes may home directly into the crypt epithelium, and thus contribute to its infiltration by lymphoid cells. The present report indicates that the increased expression of ICAM-1 on the tonsillar HEVs mediates the homing of lymphocytes to this lymphoid organ.

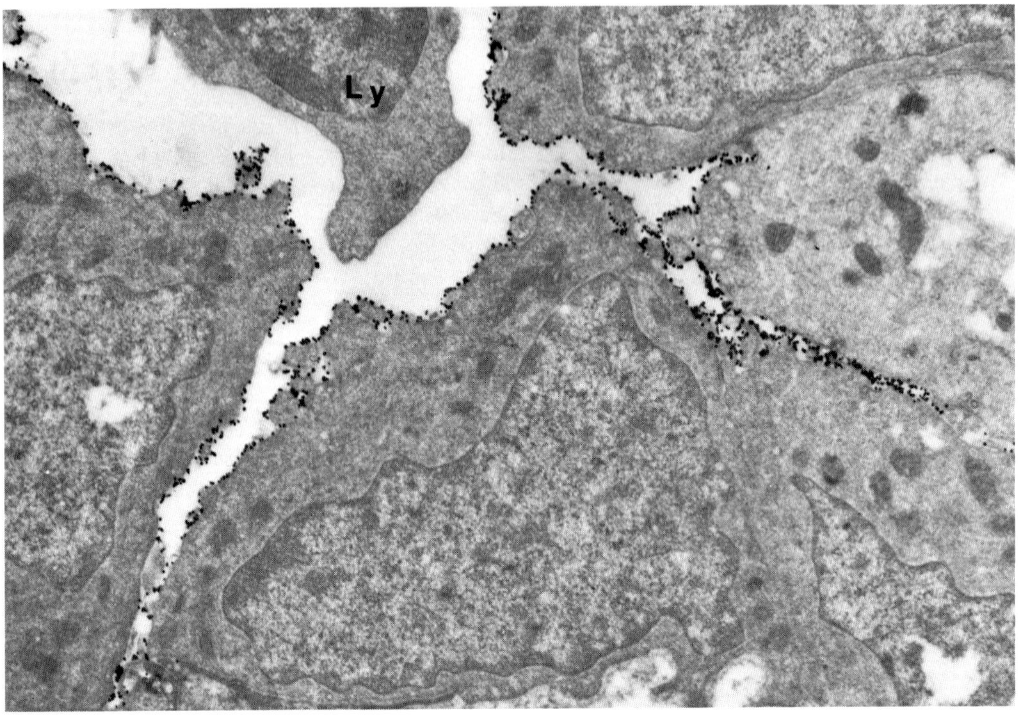

Figure 3 Immunogold-electron microscopy, MAb to ICAM-1. Surface label on luminal aspect of endothelial cells in an HEV. Ly = lymphocyte. TEM (magnification: ×11,250).

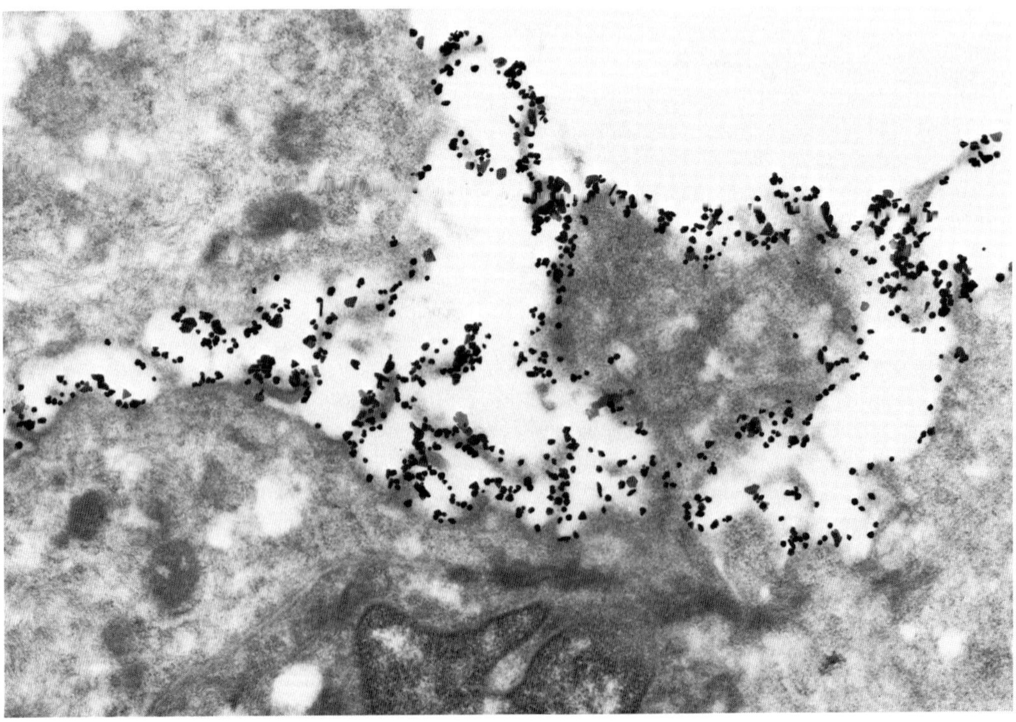

Figure 4 Immunogold-electron microscopy, MAb to ICAM-1. Surface label on high endothelium. Note the labeled luminal blebs and microvillous processes. TEM (magnification: ×20,250).

ACKNOWLEDGMENTS

This investigation was supported by grants from the Special Trustees of Guy's Hospital and from the Deutsche Forschungsgemeinschaft. The authors appreciate the excellent technical assistance of Mmes. W. Müller, K. Schlender, and Waluk, Messrs. Y. Mustafa, K. Brady, and K. Fitzpatrick, and Mrs. S. Bishop who typed this manuscript.

REFERENCES

1. Perry ME. A Study of the Microscopical Structure of the Human Palatine Tonsil with Special Reference to the Epithelium. PhD thesis, University of London, England, 1989.
2. Perry ME, Jones MM, Mustafa Y. Structure of the crypt epithelium in human palatine tonsils. Acta Otolaryngol (Stockh) 1988; Suppl 454:53–59.
3. Von Gaudecker B, Müller-Hermelink HK. The development of the human tonsillar palatina. Cell Tissue Res 1982; 224(3):579–600.
4. Yednock TA, Rosen SD. Lymphocyte homing. Adv Immunol 1989; 44:313–378.
5. Kieran MW, Blank V, Le Bail O, Israel A. Lymphocyte homing. Res Immunol 1989; 140: 399–450.
6. Duijvestijn A, Hamann A. Mechanisms and regulation of lymphocyte migration. Immunol Today 1989; 10(1):23–28.
7. Berg EL, Goldstein LA, Jutila MA, Nakache M, Picker LJ, Streeter PR, Wu NW, Zhou D, Butcher EC. Homing receptors and vascular addressins. Immunol Rev 1989; 108(2):5–18.
8. Butcher EC, Kraal G, Stevens SK, Weissman IL. A recognition function of endothelial cells: Directing lymphocyte traffic. In *Pathobiology of the Endothelial Cell.* London, Academic Press, pp. 409–424, 1982.
9. Nakache M, Berg EL, Streeter PR, Butcher EC. The mucosal vascular addressin is a tissue-specific endothelial cell adhesion molecule for circulating lymphocytes. Nature 1989; 337:179–181.
10. Umetani Y. Postcapillar venule in rabbit tonsil and entry of lymphocytes into its endothelium. Arch Histol Jpn 1977; 49(2):77–94.
11. Schmedtje JF, Batts AF. Immunoglobulins and blood vessels in the tonsillar crypt epithelium. Ann Otol Rhinol Laryngol 1973; 82(3):359–369.

152

Lymphocyte Penetration Through Endothelial Monolayers Is Augmented by Interleukin-1 via Cyclic Adenosine Monophosphate as a Second Messenger

Juha Pekka Turunen, Jarkko Ustinov, Pirkko Mattila, Pekka Häyry, and Risto Renkonen
University of Helsinki, Helsinki, Finland

INTRODUCTION

The circulation and distribution of lymphocytes (i.e., lymphocyte homing) from blood to the tissues is regulated in many levels. In inflammatory conditions there is a broad spectrum of substances mediating the body's responses to foreign antigens. Interleukin-1 (IL-1) is a potent cytokine produced by many cell types, especially by mononuclcar phagocytes and endothelial cells (1). The cffects of IL-1 are various: Among other things, it inducts several ligands taking part in the leukocyte homing (endothelial leukocyte adhesion molecule 1 [ELAM-1], intercellular adhesion molecule 1 [ICAM-1], vascular cell adhesion molecule 1 [VCAM-1]). It also regulates the production of chemotactic factors and inhibitors of leukocyte adhesion and chemotaxis. Since the interaction between lymphocytes and endothelial cells (ECs) is essential in the initiation of one subclass of inflammation, we studied this phenomenon and the role of IL-1 in our filter model.

We were able to show that IL-1 induced a transient increase in the number of lymphocytes penetrating through the endothelial monolayer into the filter. This was both a time- and a dose-dependent process. The same effect was achieved by increasing the cytosolic cyclic adenosine monophosphate (cAMP) levels by forskolin or dibutyryl-cAMP. Correspondingly, we were able to show that IL-1 increased the cytosolic cAMP levels in ECs. An inhibitor of adenylate cyclase, 2′,5′-dideoxyadenosine (DDADO), diminished both the IL-1–induced cAMP ascent and lymphocyte penetration. These findings show that cAMP is a second messenger for IL-1 in endothelial cells.

MATERIALS AND METHODS

Inbred DA rat heart endothelial cells were isolated, purified, and cultured as previously described (2). Lymphocytes were isolated mechanically from mesenteric lymph nodes of 10- 12-week-old DA rats. The lymphocyte penetration assay was performed at +37°C as previously described (3). The filters were stained with Papanicolau technique and mounted with Aquamount Gurr (BDH, Limited Poole, England). The number of lymphocytes penetrated through the endothelial monolayers was calculated with light microscopy with a magnification of ×1000. Only the lymphocytes which had penetrated under the endothelial monolayer into the filter were taken into account. The average number of penetrated lymphocytes per sample was calculated from 20 high-power fields per sample and the number of lymphocytes penetrated through endothelial cell monolayer per square millimeter was calculated. For measuring the cytosolic cAMP levels a commercial radioimmunoassay (RIA) kit (RPA.509; Amersham, Arlington Heights, Illinois) was used according to the manufacture's instructions. The histone phosphorylation assay was determined by a method developed by Iwasa et al. (4). The reagents used are previously described (5).

RESULTS

The endothelial cells were grown on filters for 24 hr before application of reagents and the monolayer structure was confirmed by electron microscopy. The lymphocyte concentration was 3×10^6 cells/500 μl per one glass cylinder which formed a lymphocyte monolayer on the top of the EC monolayer. About 20% of these lymphocytes bound to the EC monolayers in this experiment model and IL-1 increased this lymphocyte binding. Normally an intact EC monolayer permits only a small amount of lymphocytes to penetrate through it. In our experiments, only <1% of the bound lymphocytes could penetrate through EC monolayers. In nonstimulated intact ECs, the number of penetrated lymphocytes was 1312±230/mm^2 of EC monolayer in a 3-hr assay.

Pretreatment of ECs with IL-1 increased the penetration up to 5851+1324 lymphocytes/mm^2 of ECs corresponding to 4.26-fold increase (Fig. 1A). This effect was both time and dose dependent. The increase of penetration induced by IL-1 began in 1–2 hr, reaching the maximum in 4 hr (Fig. 1B). In 24 hr, this effect was abolished, although IL-1 was continuously present. The maximal effect was achieved with IL-1 concentration of 1–10 U/ml, which represents concentration values that have been measured in inflammational conditions in situ.

To analyze the second messenger pathway of IL-1 effect, we incubated ECs with various second messenger analogue stimulators. Incubation with dibutyryl-cAMP (1 μM) increased the penetration up to 2.5±0.35-fold compared to control values. Also, an adenylate cyclase activator, forskolin (0.1 μM), increased the penetration 2.3± over the control values. A cGMP-analogue, dibutyryl-cGMP, had no effect. Calcium ionophore A23187, which rapidly increases the intracellular Ca^{2+} concentration, was also ineffective (Fig. 2).

We analyzed further the possible role of cAMP as a second messenger for IL-1 in the endothelial cells. After a 0- to 60-min incubation with IL-1, the ECs were lysed with perchloric acid, vortexed, and the cytosolic cAMP levels were measured with RIA. Already after 2-min incubation of IL-1 (10 U/ml), the cAMP levels were 1.5-fold over the control values and the maximal effect was reached in 15 min, leading up to a 2.7-fold increase (from 0.15±0.03 to 0.41±0.035 pM of cAMP/10^6 cells). This IL-1–induced effect declined

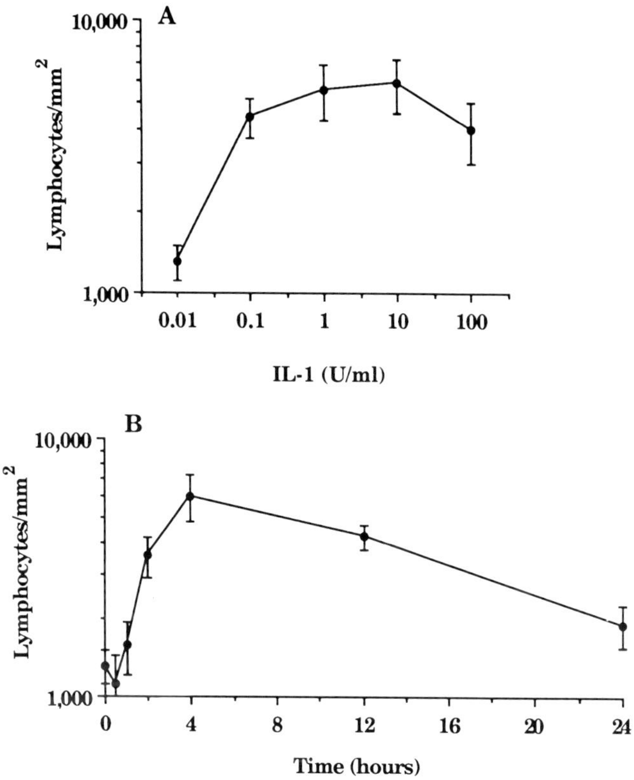

Figure 1 IL-1 induced a dose- and a time-dependent (A and B) increase in the number of lymphocytes that penetrate through intact endothelial monolayers. Endothelial monolayers were incubated with various concentrations of IL-1 for 4 hr before the lymphocytes were placed on top of the monolayer inside the glass cylinder. After a 3-hr incubation, the cylinder and loose lymphocytes were removed and the filters were washed and stained. From these preparations it was possible to determine the number of lymphocytes that had penetrated through the endothelial monolayer into the filter. Note the logarithmic scale on the Y-axis.

to the control levels in 60 min, although IL-1 was continuously present. This effect was also dose dependent and the maximal response was achieved with 1 U/ml of IL-1.

2′,5′-Dideoxyadenosine is an competitive inhibitor of adenylate cyclase. One millimole of DDADO inhibits both the increase of lymphocyte penetration and of cystolic cAMP (Table 1).

We also analyzed the role of some kinase inhibitors in this assay. Although these inhibitors do have a variety of functions, they had different effects. Only a protein kinase A inhibitor, HA 1004, could inhibit the IL-1 effect at a concentration of 10 mM (reduction of penetration in relative numbers from 4.2±0.7 to 1.5±0.2). Neither a protein kinase C inhibitor, H7, nor a calcium calmodulin antagonist, W7, had any effect at studied concentrations (relative penetration 3.8±0.4 and 3.9±0.5, respectively). Finally, we were able to show that IL-1 did not induce protein kinase C translocation to EC cell membrane in a histone phosphorylation assay.

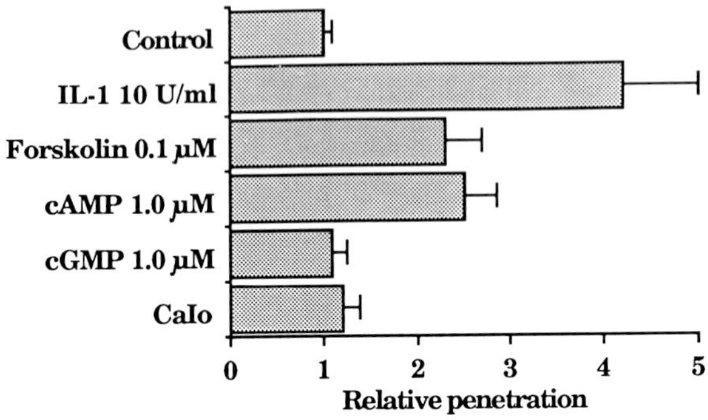

Figure 2 The role of various second messengers in the IL-1–induced lymphocyte penetration were analyzed. Endothelial cells were treated with IL-1 (10 U/ml) or with various second messenger stimulators for 4 hr and the penetration assay was carried out as described in the legend to Figure 1.

DISCUSSION

Lymphocyte homing is crucial in the initiation of acute inflammation (6). In such a condition, many cytokines mediate the immunological response against foreign antigens. Interleukin-1 is an important cytokine with many functions. It is a 17-kD peptide produced in two forms, α and β, by many cell types, such as monocytes and endothelial cells (1). Recently it has been documented that there are at least two types of receptors mediating the IL-1 response. Murine T cells, epithelial cells, and fibroblasts have and IL-1 receptor (IL-1R) which differs from the IL-1R of macrophages and B cells (7,8). These two types of IL-1Rs which do have different gene products might explain the various effects of IL-1 in different cell types. So far, nothing is known about the IL-1R of endothelial cells.

In analyzing the lymphocyte penetration in vitro we have developed further a model recently described by Oppenheimer Marks and Ziff (9). The ECs were grown on filters to confluency and the lymphocytes were placed on the top of the filters. Various agents, including IL-1, were added to ECs cultured prior to the penetration assay. Only about 1%

Table 1 Role of DDADO on the IL-1–Induced Binding of Lymphocytes to Endothelial Cells and cAMP Production

Pretreatment	No. of penetrated lymphocytes/mm^2	cAMP (pM/10^6 EC)
Control	1728 ± 768	0.15 ± 0.03
IL-1 (10 U/ml)	5632 ± 896	0.45 ± 0.035
IL-1 + DDADO (1 mM)	2304 ± 869	0.18 ± 0.02

Endothelial cells were treated with IL-1 with or without DDADO for 4 hr, then the lymphocytes were placed on the top on the EC monolayer, and after 3 hr the number of penetrated lymphocytes were analyzed from the filter. Concomitantly the production of cAMP by endothelial cells after a 15-min incubation with IL-1 in the presence or absence of DDADO was measured with RIA.

of the bound lymphocytes could penetrate through EC molecules. How an IL-1–induced signal is transduced in ECs is not clear. In T cells, both protein kinase C (PKC) and cAMP have been candidates as second messengers alone or together (10,11). The explanation for this can be the different development of cells, possible variation of IL-1R cytoplasmic region, or possible IL-1R accessory binding proteins.

The increased lymphocyte penetration by IL-1 could be mimicked by increasing the cAMP levels in endothelial cells either by dibutyryl-cAMP or forskolin. We were also able to show that IL-1 induced a rise in cytosolic cAMP in ECs. An inhibitor of adenylate cyclase, DDADO, decreased both the IL-1–induced cAMP elevation and the lymphocyte penetration. The inhibition of IL-1–induced penetration increase could be achieved by protein kinase A inhibitor HA 1004, although the specificity of the commercial protein kinase inhibitors is questionable. The other protein kinase inhibitors, H7 or W7, could not inhibit this phenomenon. Though PMA, a protein kinase C activator could stimulate the IL-1 effect and a PKC inhibitor H7 could decrease this effect, H7 could not inhibit the IL-1 effect. Neither did IL-1 cause PKC translocation in the histone phosphorylation assay.

Interleukin-1 induced a rapid rise of cytosolic cAMP within 5–15 min. However, 2–4 hr of IL-1 incubation were needed until the maximal response in lymphocyte penetration was detectable. Also dibutyryl-cAMP needed 2–4 hr for the maximal response that increased cAMP levels.

ACKNOWLEDGMENTS

This study was supported by grants from The Duodecim Society, Helsinki, Finnish Academy, Sigrid Juselius Foundation, Helsinki, and by a research grant from the University of Helsinki, Finland.

REFERENCES

1. Dinarello C.A. Biology of interleukin-1. FASEB J. 1988; 2:108.
2. Renkonen R., Mattila P., Leszczynski D, Häyry P. Leukotriene B4 increases the lymphocyte binding to endothelial cells. Febs. Lett. 1988; 235:67.
3. Renkonen R, Mattila P, Turunen J.P, Häyry P. Lymphocyte binding to and penetration through vascular endothelium is stimulated by platelet-activating factor. Scand. J. Immunol. 1989; 30:673–678.
4. Iwasa T, Takai Y, Nishizuka Y. Phosphorylation of calf thymus H1 histone by calcium-activated phospholipid dependent protein kinase. Biochem. Biophys. Res. Commun. 1980; 96:180.
5. Renkonen R, Mattila P , Häyry P, Ustinov J. Interleukin-1 induced lymphocyte binding to endothelial cells. Eur. J. Immunol. 1990; 20:1563.
6. Duijvestijn A, Hamann A. Mechanisms and regulation of lymphocyte migration. Immunol. Today 1989; 10:23.
7. Chizzonite R, Truitti T, Kilian P.I., Stern a.S., Nunes P, Parker K.P., Kaffka K.L., Chua A.O., Lugg D.K., Gubler U. Two high affinity interleukin-1 receptors represent separate gene products. Proc. Natl. Acad. Sci. U.S.A. 1989; 86:8029.
8. Bomsztyk K, Sims J.E., Stanton T.H., Slack J., McMahan C.J., Valentine M.A., Dower S.K. Evidence for different interleukin-1 receptors on murine B and T cell lines. Proc. Natl. Acad. Sci. U.S.A. 1989; 86:8034.
9. Oppenheimer-Marks N, Ziff M. Migration of lymphocytes through endothelial cell monolayers: augmentation by interferon-gamma. Cell Immunol. 1988; 114:307.

10. Shirakawa F, Yamashita U, Chedid M, Mizel S.B. Cyclic AMP an intracellular second messenger for interleukin 1. Proc. Natl. Acad. Sci. U.S.A. 1988; 85:8201.
11. Didier M, Aussel C, Pelassy C, Fehlmann M. IL-1 signaling for IL-2 production in T cells involves a rise in phosphatidylserine synthesis. J. Immunol. 1988; 141:3078.

153
Lymph Node Nondendritic Reticular Cells Modulate Lymphocyte Function

Jenny J. Li and Steven G. Bramlet
Shriners Burns Institute; Massachusetts General Hospital, Boston, Massachusetts; Harvard Medical School, Cambridge, Massachusetts

INTRODUCTION

Circulating lymphocytes transverse the postcapillary high endothelial venules (HEVs) to the lymph node; during their short stay in the lymph node (up to 18 hr) (1), cells are located in close vicinity of antigen-presenting cells and stromal cells. In contrast to the well-documented interactions between lymphocytes and antigen-presenting cells, the impact of stromal nondendritic reticular cells (NDRCs) on the host immune system has not been clearly defined. Bidirectional interactions may exist between the immunological and stromal NDRC components of the lymph node and may be essential to the regulation of lymphocyte activity.

METHODOLOGY

Animal

Pathogen-free male Sprague-Dawley rats (Taconic Farms, Germantown, New York), weighing 200–225 g, were used in our studies.

Preparation of Lymph NDRCs

Rat axillary and inguinal lymph nodes were minced and digested repeatedly in a mixture of collagenase (50 U/ml), trypsin (0.1%), and 1% chicken serum at 37°C for 20 min. The single cell suspension was centrifuged, and the pellet was resuspended in the RPMI 1640 containing 10% fetal calf serum (complete medium). Cells were then plated in tissue culture dishes and incubated at 37°C for 24 hr. At the end of incubation, nonadherent cells were discarded, and the adherent cells were incubated in the complete medium for an additional 3 days.

At the end of incubation, adherent cells were trypsinized, and a 1-hr differential attachment protocol was applied to these detached cells. At the end of 1 hr, nonattached cells were discarded, and the adherent cells were cultured in the complete medium. The characteristics of the isolated cells were examined using immunoperoxidase staining techniques.

Isolated NDRCs (5×10^4) were incubated in chamber/slide at 37°C overnight. At the end of incubation, cells were then fixed in formalin, and a battery of antibodies (antidendritic cell [R4/23], antihistiocyte [Mac-387], antirat class II major histocompatibility complex [MHC] antigen, anti–factor VIII, and anticytokeratin antibodies [Dako, Carpenteria, California]) were used on the fixed NDRCs. The ABC staining protocol was used (Vector, Burlingame, California), and slides were then developed in the 0.02% H_2O_2 phosphate-buffered saline containing 0.1% diaminobenzidine. Cells were then counterstained with hematoxylin.

Preparation of NDRC-Conditioned Medium

Subconfluent stromal cells (NDRCs) in the complete medium were incubated in the absence or presence of 10 μg lipopolysaccharide (LPS)/ml (List BioLab, Campbell, California) at 37°C for 6 hr. At the end of incubation, cells were washed extensively; cells were then incubated in the medium RPMI 1640 containing 2% fetal calf serum for another 24 hr. Medium controls (no cells) were also prepared and collected accordingly.

Lymphocyte Binding to Lymph Node HEVs

Lymphocyte single cell suspension was prepared from the rat axillary and inguinal lymph nodes. Thirty-one million lymphocytes were incubated in medium RPMI 1640 containing 2% fetal calf serum or in the NDRC-conditioned medium at 37°C overnight. At the end of incubation, cells were resuspended in Hanks' balanced salt solution containing 5% fetal calf serum. Lymphocytes (0.15 ml of 21×10^6 cells/ml) were pipetted onto freshly prepared 8-μ thick frozen lymph node sections. The slides were then agitated at 75–80 rpm on an orbital shaker at 4°C for 40 min. At the end of incubation, excess lymphocytes were removed, and the slides were then placed in 1% glutaraldehyde solution. For the controls (i.e., nonspecific bindings), 0.15 ml of lymphocytes were first incubated with 3 μg fucoidin at 4°C for 10 min and then incubated with frozen lymph node sections accordingly.

Quantitation of HEV-Bound Lymphocytes

The HEV-bound lymphocytes were counted a ×200 magnification using a grid in the eyepiece of a microscope; 4–6 lymph node sections were analyzed for each treatment group. Lymphocytes bound to the HEV were expressed as lymphocytes bound per 100 mm^2 area (mean ± SEM).

Effects of NDRC-Conditioned Medium on Lymphocyte Deoxyribonucleic Acid and Protein Synthesis

Two hundred and fifty thousand lymphocytes were incubated in the presence or absence of NDRC-conditioned medium in 96-well microtiter plates at 37°C for 3 days. Tritiated thymidine (1 μCi/well) (Amersham, Arlington Heights, Illinois) was added to the cells 24 hr after starting the culture, and cells were incubated for an additional 48 hr. At the end of 3 days, lymphocytes were harvested using a PhD Cell Harvester (Cambridge Technology

Inc.); the amount of [^{3}H]thymidine incorporated was quantitated after samples were counted in the scintillation counter.

The incorporation of [^{14}C]leucine by cells was also analyzed: 24 hr after starting the lymphocyte culture, 0.25 μCi [^{14}C]leucine was added to the cells and incubated for an additional 48 hr. Cellular proteins were precipitated by 10% trichloroacetic acid, then dissolved in 20% sodium dodecylsulfate (SDS) and counted in the scintillation counter.

Statistics

The unpaired Student's t-test was used to analyze the binding of lymphocytes to HEVs.

RESULTS

Using an immunoperoxidase staining technique, we show that the isolated NDRCs are not of a dendritic or histiocyte origin and do not contain interleukin-1 α or interleukin-1 β, or stain with anti–factor VIII antibody (data not shown). Isolated NDRCs (Fig. 1), however, does stain positive with antipancytokeratin antibody.

Previously we showed that overnight incubation in the complete medium was necessary for freshly isolated lymphocytes of the peripheral lymph node to interact with the HEVs (3). The protein synthesis inhibitor cycloheximide abolishes the overnight incubation-enhanced lymphocyte binding to the HEVs. We then proceed to examine the effects of the NDRC microenvironment on lymphocyte-HEV interactions.

The NDRC-conditioned medium was obtained according to the methods described. Using an ex vivo lymph node lymphocyte binding study (2,3), we show that lymphocytes, when incubated at 37°C for 18 hr in the supernatant of the conditioned medium, had a greater ability to bind to the HEVs. The number of lymphocytes bound to the HEVs in a randomly chosen field (100 mm^2) was (83.6 ± 38.4), which is significantly greater than that of controls (62.4 ± 30.9) ($p < 0.01$) (Fig. 2).

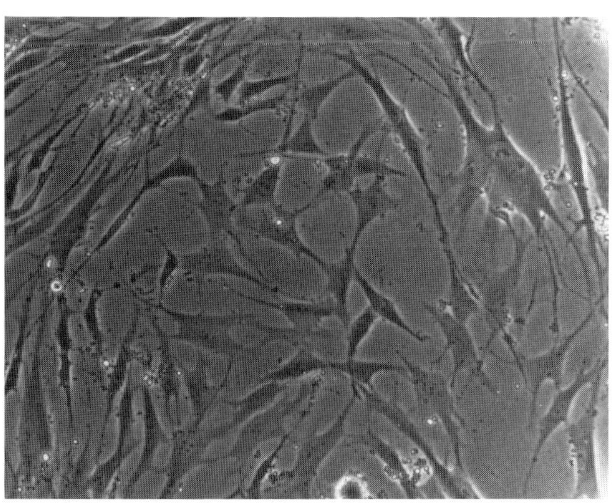

Figure 1 The morphology of isolated NDRCs.

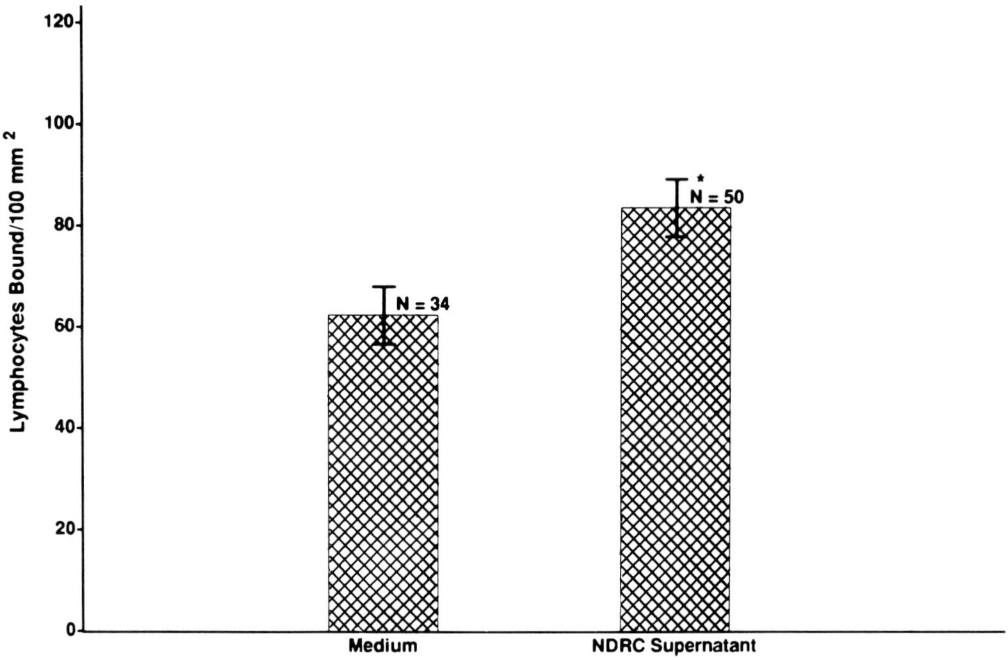

Figure 2 Effect of NDRC supernatant on lymphocyte-HEV interaction.

These results suggest that the stromal NDRCs might secrete a factor(s) that enhances the interactions between lymphocytes and HEVs, consequently priming the latter cells for the next cycle of trafficking.

The NDRC-conditioned medium also increases the incorporation of [^{3}H]thymidine and [^{14}C]leucine into lymphocyte deoxyribonucleic acid (DNA) (Fig. 3) and protein (Fig. 4), respectively, and treating NDRCs with endotoxin (LPS) provides no additional stimulating effect on lymphocytes.

DISCUSSION

After migrating into the lymph node, the individual lymphocyte stays in the collagenous framework of reticular cells and fibers. It has been shown that the stromal cells of thymus produce lymphokine(s) that subsequently modulate the growth/differentiation of immature lymphocytes. The effects of peripheral lymph node stromal cells on mature lymphocytes are still unclear.

Franke et al. have identified a subpopulation of stromal reticular cells located in the paracortical area of lymph nodes that are of neither dendritic nor interdigitating origin (4). Together with their findings, our results suggest that stromal NDRCs seem to represent an important nonimmunological component that may modulate lymphocyte function in a lymph node.

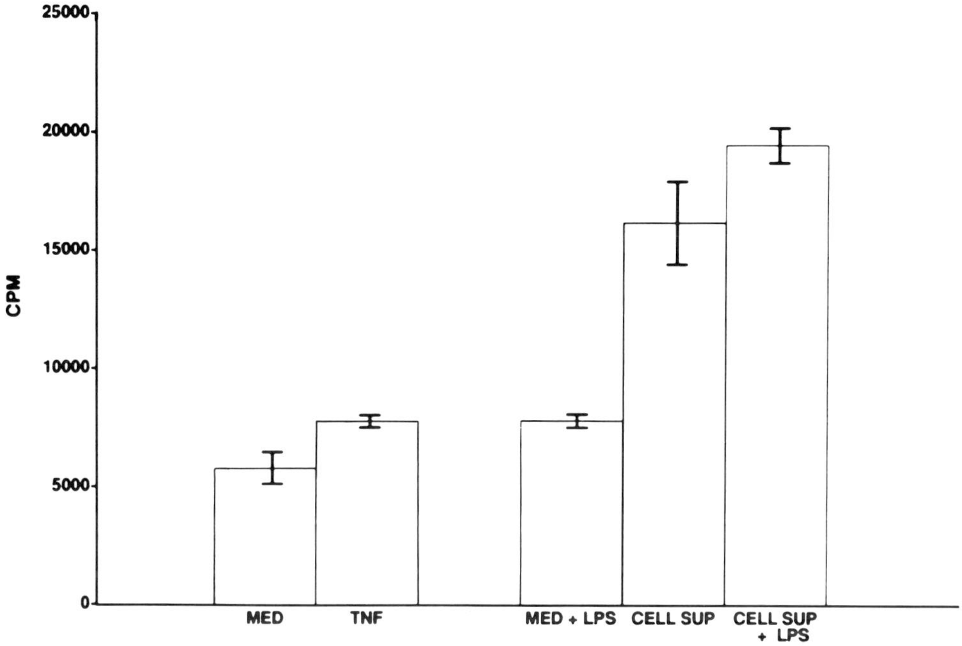

Figure 3 [^{3}H]Thymidine incorporation by lymphocytes incubated with NDRC-conditioned medium.

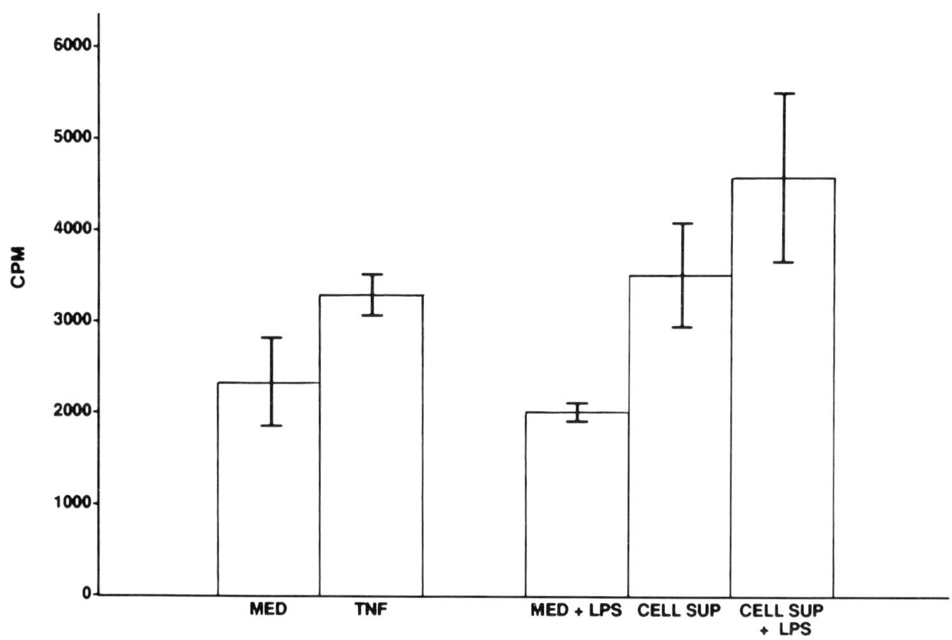

Figure 4 [^{14}C]Leucine incorporation by lymphocytes incubated with NDRC-conditioned medium.

CONCLUSION

In summary, our results strongly suggest that interactions between lymphocytes and stromal reticular cells occur in the lymph node microenvironment. Further studies are required to understand the interaction under both normal and abnormal immunosuppressive conditions.

REFERENCES

1. Smith ME, Ford WL. The recirculating lymphocyte pool of the rat: a systemic description of the migratory behavior of circulating lymphocytes. Immunology 1983; 49:83.
2. Woodruff JJ, Clarke LM. Specific cell-adhesion mechanisms determining migration pathways of recirculating lymphocytes. Ann Rev Immunol 1987; 5:201.
3. Li JJ, Sellers, Jr. JR. Inflammation enhances lymphocytes and peripheral lymph node interaction. [Abstract] Clin Res 1989; 37:414A.
4. Franke WW, Moll R. Cytoskeletal components of lymphoid organs. I. Synthesis of cytokeratins 8 and 18 and desmin in subpopulations of extrafollicular reticulum cells of human lymph nodes. tonsils, and spleen. Differentiation 1987; 36:145.

154
The Microenvironment of the Lymph Node and the Expression of Vascular Addressins

Reina E. Mebius,[1] Philip R. Streeter,[2] John Brevé,[1] and Georg Kraal[1]
[1]*Free University, Amsterdam, The Netherlands;* [2]*SyStemix Inc., Palo Alto, California*

INTRODUCTION

Circulating blood delivers lymphocytes to all regions of the body. Lymphocytes can leave the blood stream and enter lymphoid tissue by specific recognition of and adherence to specialized high endothelial venules (HEVs[2]) (1). Specific cell surface receptors on lymphocytes, called homing receptors, and their putative ligands on HEV, the tissue-specific vascular addressins, are involved in extravasation of lymphocytes (2–4). In the mouse, two different subsets of HEVs can be discriminated by means of monoclonal antibodies (MAbs): (a) HEVs in peripheral lymph nodes (PLNs) expressing the peripheral vascular addressin recognized by MAb MECA-79 (4); and (b) HEVs in mucosal lymphoid tissue, such as Peyer's patches, expressing the mucosal addressin defined by MAb MECA-367 (3). Both vascular addressins are expressed in mesenteric lymph nodes (MLN). Antibodies MECA-79 as well as MECA-367 are able to interfere with binding of lymphocytes to HEVs.

From previous studies in the rat it has become clear that cells or factors in the afferent lymph of the lymph nodes have an important role in the regulation of HEVs (5,6) and may contribute to the microenvironmental factors, unique at a certain location, that direct the specificity of HEVs in vivo.

Here we have studied what effect the interruption of afferent lymphatics to popliteal lymph nodes would have on the expression of vascular addressins. The effect of local environmental factors on vascular addressin expression was studied in lymph nodes after transplantation into an ectopic site.

AFFERENT LYMPH SUPPLY

Interruption of the afferent lymph supply to murine popliteal lymph nodes, performed as described earlier for rats (7), resulted in an impaired HEV function within 7 days. The

HEV-specific MAb MECA-325 was weakly expressed at 4 days after deafferentization and had totally disappeared at day 7. Although a function of MECA-325 in the adherence process of lymphocytes to HEV has never been attributed to this antigen, the transmigration of lymphocytes across the venular wall here is very well correlated with the expression of MECA-325 because staining with MECA-79, which recognizes the peripheral vascular addressin, showed flat-walled vessels at day 7. The expression of the peripheral addressin could mostly be observed at the abluminal aspect of the vessel. At this time point, the entrance of i.v.-injected fluorescein isothiocyanate (FITC)–labeled cells into operated lymph nodes was minimal. Remarkable is the observation of an increased expression of MECA-367, recognizing the mucosal vascular addressin, at 4 days after deafferentization. At 7 days after operation, no expression of MECA-367 could be observed. The binding capacity of HEVs decreased during the days after deafferentization and could hardly be measured at day 7.

The observed alterations in morphology and function of HEVs might be caused by depletion of chemotactic factors presumably present in afferent lymph (8–11). These chemotactic factors might cause migration of lymphocytes from the blood stream into lymph nodes along a chemotactic gradient, which will be disturbed by interruption of afferent lymphatic vessels to the lymph node. Lymphocytes in the blood will, therefore, be less well attracted to the luminal aspects of the HEVs, resulting in a decreased lymphocyte migration across the wall of the HEVs. The flat-walled endothelial cells that we could observe is probably a result of the diminished migration of lymphocytes across the venular wall. Other studies have shown that decreased migration of lymphocytes across HEVs can cause flattening of HEVs, which will become high walled again by restoration of the cell population in the blood that is responsible for migration across HEVs (12,13). The increased expression of MECA-367 at day 4 might be seen as an alternative way to establish lymphocyte migration across the venular wall caused by an impaired afferent lymph flow.

The adherence capacity of normal endothelial cells for leukocytes can be induced by interferon-γ (IFN-γ) (15–17), whereas the expression of the HEV-specific marker MECA-325 can be induced by IFN-γ in endothelial cell lines derived from mouse lung or bone marrow cells (18). However, when we tried to restore the binding capacity of HEVs in operated lymph nodes by intranodal injections of cytokines such as IFN-γ or tumor necrosis factor (TNF), we could never confirm a role for these cytokines in controlling the function and maintenance of HEVs (14). This is suggestive for the existence of a mechanism that controls the activity of high endothelial cells distinct from the mechanism that directs the activity of normal endothelial cells.

After deafferentization a relative decrease of lymphocytes with a migratory phenotype could be observed. A decreased percentage of Mel-14–positive B cells in operated lymph nodes at day 4 preceded the decreased percentage of Mel-14–positive T cells in the lymph node observed at day 7 after deafferentization. Interdigitating cells in the paracortical area, defined with MAb NLDC-145, also decreased and the MOMA-1–positive macrophages in the subcapsular sinus had completely disappeared.

LOCAL MICROENVIRONMENT AND VASCULAR ADDRESSIN EXPRESSION

These data show that lymph-borne cells or factors are centrally involved in maintaining the homeostasis of PLNs. Are they also responsible for the tissue-specific expression of vascular addressins? Are microenvironmental factors of PLNs different from these of mesenteric lymph nodes (MLN) and, if so, are these factors directing the differentiation of HEV?

Studies in which we transferred lymph nodes from their original peripheral location into a mucosal site and vice versa, showed a fixed expression of the vascular addressins and no changes in binding specificity of HEVs. When adult PLNs were transplanted into the mesentery for 8 weeks, HEVs showed high expression of the peripheral addressin and lacked mucosal addressin expression. Additionally, binding of T cells vs B cells pointed to HEVs of the peripheral phenotype. This conservation of vascular addressin expression and binding specificity could also be observed in adult MLNs when transplanted into a peripheral site for 8 weeks. These data show a fixed expression of the vascular addressins, which could not be changed during implantation at another local microenvironment.

These experiments were all performed with adult organs into an adult environment. The imprint of the HEV specificity may have been fixed during ontogeny. We, therefore, started experiments in which neonatal LNs were transplanted. In the first 2 days of postnatal development HEVs appear to consist of three cell layers. The innermost is formed by endothelial cells, surrounded by the basal lamina which contains a few pericytes. The outermost cell layer consists of sinus-lining cells (8). The development of organelles such as the Golgi apparatus, ribosomes, endoplasmic reticulum covered with ribosomes, and mitochondria takes place at the third day of neonatal life (8) but the expression of the peripheral vascular addressin does not start until 1–2 days after birth. In contrast, vessels in MLNs as well as in PLNs express high levels of the mucosal vascular addressin at birth (19). Expression of the mucosal addressin in PLNs disappears over 4 weeks.

Transplantation studies of lymph nodes taken at day of birth showed a role for the local microenvironment of the lymph node in induction of the HEV phenotype. Peripheral lymph nodes transplanted into the mucosal site showed vessels with high levels of the peripheral addressin or vessels which were partly negative for MAb MECA-79. All these vessels lacked expression of MECA-367. These results show that already at their early development HEVs in PLNs are different from HE cells in MLNs. Transplantation of MLNs into a peripheral site, however, showed either vessels which expressed the mucosal addressin as normally seen in MLNs or vessels which were negative for MECA-367. All these vessels showed a high expression of the peripheral vascular addressin. These data reveal that further induction of the peripheral addressin and a concomitant loss of the mucosal addressin is possible in MLNs when transplanted into a peripheral site at the time that expression of the addressins is regulated.

Development of normal fetal endothelium has been studied extensively, in contrast to the fetal development of high endothelium,which is poorly understood. Rat intestinal capillaries showed endothelial cells without a basal lamina at days 14–17 of gestation, which was prominent at approximately 2 days post partum (20). In vitro studies showed that differentiation of endothelial cells was influenced by the substrate, the so-called extracellular matrix (ECM), on which the endothelial cells were grown (21–23). During the early days of life the basement membrane of HE cells might be formed, which directs the specificity of HEVs during ongoing life. It has been postulated by Murphy et al. that deposition of the ECM may be critical to the final differentiation of the vessel wall (24). This ECM is probably produced by the pericytes surrounding the layer of HE cells and by the HE cells themselves. The local environment of the lymph node during late fetal and early neonatal life might have a function in controlling the composition of the ECM and thus in the permanent HEV phenotype. However, once HEVs are established and function normally the phenotype seems to be fixed, and cannot be affected by another local microenvironment.

ANTIGENIC STIMULATION AND HEV FUNCTION

The previous results showed the unmutable character of adult HEVs concerning their binding specificity and addressin expression. The only way to interfere with HEV function is by interruption of afferent lymphatics to PLNs: A decreased binding capacity of HEV upon deafferentization could be observed. Would it be possible to induce HEVs in supporting more lymphocyte traffic from the blood into lymph nodes by antigenic stimulation? Studies in which lymph nodes were stimulated with the contact allergen oxazolone revealed that lymph nodes were increasing in size and so were the number of HEVs in these lymph nodes (25). However, the new forming of HEVs lagged behind the increase in size. At all time points after antigenic stimulation it was found that the entrance of cells, determined by FITC labeling, was perfectly reflected by the ability to enter the lymph node; namely, the amount of HEVs per T-cell area, measured by means of morphometric analysis. No differences in binding capacity of HEVs in stimulated LNs vs control LNs could be observed. These data showed that HEVs work constantly, unaffected by antigen stimulation.

CONCLUSIONS

The interaction of lymphocytes and HEVs in lymphoid tissue exhibits a very specific process, which seems to be region specific. However, the long-established idea that local microenvironmental factors direct the differentiation of HEVs in vivo is only true during the early time of HEV development. During late fetal and early neonatal life the differentiation of HEVs is locally regulated and terminated. After this period the vascular addressins are unmutably expressed, irrespective of the local environment. Only interruption of afferent lymph supply can downregulate the capacity of HEVs to bind lymphocytes and to support lymphocyte traffic from the blood-stream in vivo. Cytokines such as IFN-γ or TNF cannot restore this impaired function. Antigenic stimulation of control lymph nodes could not affect the function of HEVs either. All these results taken together show that the function of the HEVs is tightly regulated, and that the afferent lymph plays an important role in the maintenance of their function.

ACKNOWLEDGMENT

This work was supported by the Netherlands Organization for Scientific Research (Grant: 900-505-211).

REFERENCES

1. Gowans JL, Knight EJ. The route of recirculation of lymphocytes in rat. Proc R Soc Lond Ser B 1964; 159:257–82.
2. Gallatin WM, Weissman IL, Butcher EC. A cell-surface molecule involved in organ-specific homing of lymphocytes. Nature 1983; 304:30–4.
3. Streeter PR, Berg EL, Rouse BTN, Bargatze RF, Butcher EC. A tissue-specific endothelial cell molecule involved in lymphocyte homing. Nature 1988; 331:41–6.
4. Streeter PR, Rouse BTN, Butcher EC. Immunohistologic and functional characterization of a vascular addressin involved in lymphocyte homing into peripheral lymph nodes. J Cell Biol 1988; 107:1853–62.

5. Hendriks HR, Duijvestijn AM, Kraal G. Rapid decrease in lymphocyte adherence to high endothelial venules in lymph nodes deprived of afferent lymphatic vessels. Eur J Immunol 1987; 17:1619–5.
6. Drayson MT, Ford WL. Afferent lymph and lymph borne cells: Their influence on lymph node function. Immunobiol 1984; 168:362–79.
7. Hendriks HR. Occlusion of the lymph flow to rat popliteal lymph nodes for protracted periods. Z Versuchtierkd 1978; 20:105–12.
8. Van Deurs B, Röpke C. The postnatal development of high-endothelial venules in lymph nodes of mice. Anat Rec 1974; 181:659–77.
9. Miranda JL, Rocha B, Freitas AA. Lymphocyte migration into membrane filters: divergent effects of syngeneic mouse serum and lymph. Ann Immunol (Inst. Pasteur) 1984; 135D:271–81.
10. Rocha B, Haston WS, Freitas AA. 1984. Lymphocyte migration into collagen gels: Role of lymph. Scand J Immunol 1984; 19:297–305.
11. Rocha B, Freitas AA. The effects of lymph on lymphocyte migration in vivo. Ann Immunol (Inst. Pasteur) 1986; 137C:105–16.
12. Goldschneider I, McGregor DD. Migration of lymphocytes and thymocytes in the rat. I. The route of migration from blood to spleen and lymph nodes. J Exp Med 1967; 127:155.
13. Syrjänen KJ. Post-capillary venules of the lymphatic tissues in mice with special reference to the depletion of T-lymphocyte population. Exp Mol Pathol 1978; 29:291–302.
14. Mebius RE, Hendriks HR, Brevé J, Kraal G. Macrophages and the activity of high endothelial venules. The effect of interferon gamma. Eur J Immunol 1990; 20:1615–8.
15. Pober JS, Collins T, Gimbrone Jr. MA, Cotran RS, Gitlin JD, Fiers W, Clayberger C, Krensky AM, Burakoff SJ, Reiss CS. Lymphocytes recognize human vascular endothelial and dermal fibroblast Ia antigens induced by recombinant immune interferon. Nature 1983; 305:726–9.
16. Masuyama J, Minato N, Kano S. Mechanisms of lymphocyte adhesion to human vascular endothelial cells in culture. J Clin Invest 1986; 77:1596–605.
17. Hughes CCW, Male DK, Lantos PL. Adhesion of lymphocytes to cerebral microvascular cells: effects of interferon-γ, tumour necrosis factor and interleukin-1. Immunology 1988; 64:677–81.
18. Duijvestijn AM, Schreiber AB, Butcher EC. Interferon-γ regulates an antigen specific for endothelial cells involved in lymphocyte traffic. Proc Natl Acad Sci USA 1986; 83:9114–8.
19. Butcher EC. Cellular and molecular mechanisms that direct leukocyte traffic. Am J Pathol 1990; 136:3–11.
20. Milici AJ, Bankston PW. Fetal and neonatal rat intestinal capillaries: a TEM study of changes in the mural structure. Am J Anat 1981; 160:435–48.
21. Milici AJ, Furie MB, Carley WW. The formation of fenestrations and channels by capillary endothelium in vitro. Proc Natl Acad Sci USA 1985; 82:6181–5.
22. Kubota Y, Kleinman HK, Martin GR, Lawley TJ. Role of laminin and basement membrane in the morphological differentiation of human endothelial cells into capillary-like structures. J Cell Biol 1988; 107:1589–98.
23. Lawley TJ, Kubato Y. Induction of morphologic differentiation of endothelial cells in culture. J Invest Dermatol 1989; 93:59S–61S.
24. Murphy ME, Carlson EC. An ultrastructural study of developing extra cellular matrix in vitelline blood vessels of the early chick embryo. Am J Anat 1978; 151:345–75.
25. Mebius RE, Brevé J, Duijvestijn AM, Kraal G. The function of high endothelial venules in mouse lymph nodes stimulated by oxazolone. Immunology 1990; 71:423–7.

155

Differences Between the Homing Patterns of Lymphocytes and Lymphoblasts from the Blood and of Splenic and Lung Emigrants

Reinhard Pabst,[1] Steve T. Licence,[2] and Richard M. Binns[2]
[1]*Medical School of Hannover, Hannover, Germany;*
[2]*AFRC Institute of Animal Physiology and Genetics Research, Babraham, Cambridge, England*

INTRODUCTION

Many lymphoid cells continuously migrate from one lymphoid organ to another using the lymphatics and the blood as traffic routes. Nonlymphoid organs are also included in this system, and it has been concluded that lymphocyte homing is either mediated by high endothelial venules (HEVs) as in lymph nodes, Peyer's patches (PPs), and tonsils, whereby this traffic is protease-sensitive; or directed to organs without HEVs, having a huge marginal pool, a short transit time, and not being influenced by previous trypsin incubation; i.e., the protease-sensitive receptor mechanism is not involved (1,2). Thus, lymphocyte migration is not only regulated by binding and transit through HEVs, but also by the homing receptors and with addressins being involved, on which many studies have focused recently (3–5). The marginal pool of the lung vascular bed has recently been found to be much larger than was thought, and to be of physiological relevance and not an artifact (6). Nothing is known so far about which organs lymphocytes migrate to after leaving this pulmonary pool. The first aim was, therefore, to define the organ distribution of ^{51}Cr-labeled lymphocytes washed out of the lung vascular bed and to compare this migration pattern to that of lymphocytes from the blood and splenic emigrants. Much less is known about the migration of lymphoblasts (7,8) in comparison to lymphocytes, potential homing receptors, and regulatory processes. Therefore, the second aim was to compare lymphoblasts from the same three sources to lymphocytes in their organ distribution. The pig with its interesting structural and functional aspects of the immune system (1) was used as an experimental animal. The data from many studies are difficult to compare, as different cell sources (lymph cells, blood lymphocytes, or cell suspensions from different lymphoid organs) have been used in different species and with variable labels. These drawbacks were avoided by using both labels simultaneously and comparing the homing pattern in the same animals in a large number of lymphoid and nonlymphoid organs. Mainly data concerning lymph nodes and the gut will be documented here. Further details on the other organs will be published elsewhere (9).

MATERIALS AND METHODS

Large Whites of a closed major histocompatibility complex (MHC) homozygous herd were used as donor (~4 months of age) and recipient pigs (5–8 weeks old). These animals accept allogeneic lymphocytes. Blood was collected and lymphocytes separated (1). The isolated lungs and spleens of the same animals were perfused in vitro with a tissue culture medium at 37°C (9,10) and the venous effluent collected and lymphocytes separated. The cells were incubated with ^{51}Cr (10 μCi/ml) or 0.5 μCi ^{125}IdUrd/ml for 30 min at 37°C (9). For clarity, cells incorporating the deoxyribonucleic acid (DNA) precursor ^{125}IdUr were called lymphoblasts, as small lymphocytes are not proliferating cells and do not incorporate DNA precursors. Some large lymphocytes will be included in the population of lymphoblasts. The labeled lymphoid cells from a single donor were injected i.v. into two recipients. About 1 day later, the animals were exsanguinated and weighed samples of several organs were used for counting. Most data were expressed as the cell concentration factor (CCF) (CPM/g organ divided by cpm/body weight) or the percentage of injected and recovered labeled cells, and the spillover of each isotope was corrected.

RESULTS AND DISCUSSION

Interesting differences between the three cell sources were seen in the uptake of the isotypes. For ^{51}Cr the mean uptake per 10^6 cells was: peripheral blood 1190 cpm, spleen emigrants 670 cpm, and lung emigrants 820 cpm; and for ^{125}I: 177 cpm, 98 cpm, and 292 cpm, respectively. Thus, there were about three times more blasts among the lung emigrants than among the splenic cells. Blood lymphocytes outnumbered lymphoblasts in lymph nodes and Peyer's patches. Slightly more lymphoblasts than lymphocytes homed to the intestinal wall excluding PPs (Fig. 1).

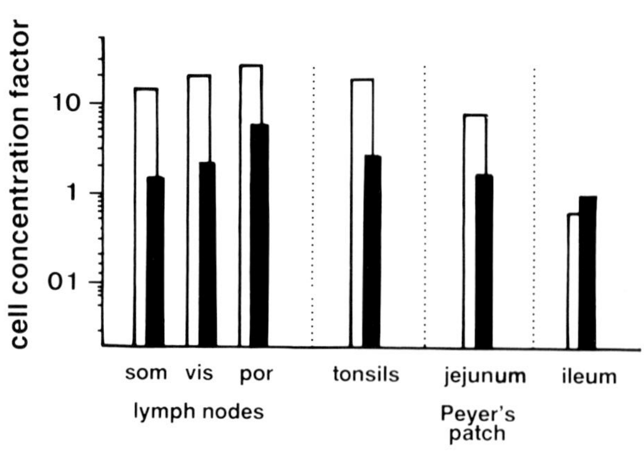

Figure 1 Comparison of the cell concentration factors for blood lymphocytes (open bars) with blood lymphoblasts (black bars) to different lymph nodes (som = somatic, vis = visceral, por = portal), Peyer's patch in the jejunum, and ileal wall not containing a Peyer's patch. Note the logarithmic scale.

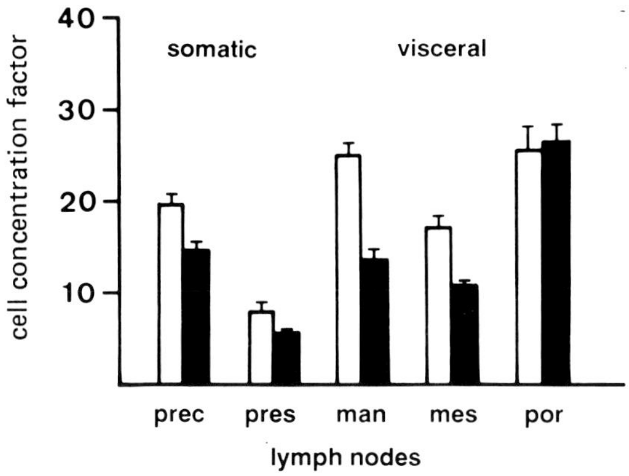

Figure 2 Comparison of the homing of blood lymphocytes (open bars) to lymphocytes from the lung (black bars) to different lymph nodes (prec = precrural, pres = prescapular, man = mandibular, mes = mesenteric, por = portal).

When the homing pattern of lymphocytes from the blood to different lymph nodes was compared to that of lymphocytes from the lung, interesting differences became obvious (Fig. 2). There was no difference in the homing to the portal lymph node but many more blood lymphocytes entered the other lymph nodes. A further important aspect was that for lung lymphocytes the difference in the CCF between the precapsular and portal lymph nodes was about fivefold, which means the entry into different lymph nodes showed a great variation with more lymphocyte homing to visceral than to peripheral lymph nodes.

A similar variation in the homing of blood and lung lymphocytes became obvious when the ratio of $^{51}Cr/^{125}IdUrd$ was plotted. When the ratio was 1, comparable numbers of cells had entered the organ irrespective of the absolute numbers. In organs such as the gut wall no difference was found, but for lymph nodes a great difference was found (Fig. 3), with

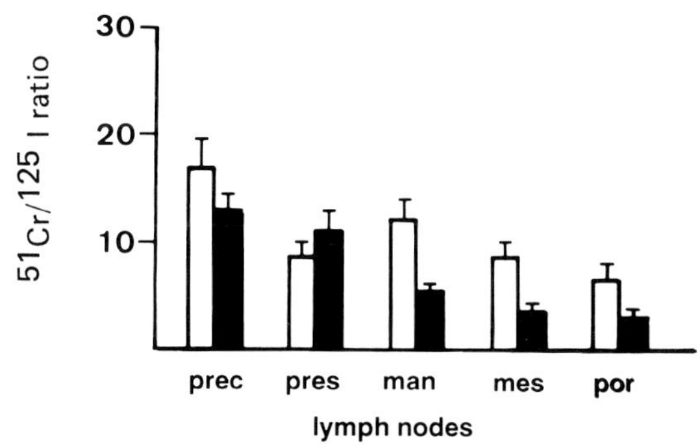

Figure 3 Ratio of lymphocyte to lymphoblast from the blood (open bars) and from the lung vascular bed (black bars) indicating the homing differences to different lymph nodes (prec = precrural, pres = prescapular, man = mandibular, mes = mesenteric, por = portal).

little or no differences in surface lymph nodes but huge differences in mandibular, mesenteric, and portal lymph nodes. The preference of blood lymphocytes for the spleen, lung, and liver was much more pronounced than for lung emigrants.

In plotting the percentage recovery of the three blast types it became obvious that they all showed very high levels of migration to the bone marrow (~25%) and very low levels to the spleen and lymph nodes. Lung blasts had a preference for lung, spleen blasts for muscle and skin, and blood blasts for the peripheral blood.

CONCLUSION

Great differences were seen in the migration pattern of lymphocytes and lymphoblasts of different physiological compartments. The mucosa-containing organs were outnumbered in lymphoblast migration by non-lymphoid organs. The regulatory factors for these migration patterns remain to be studied.

ACKNOWLEDGMENTS

These studies were partly supported by the Deutsche Forschungsgemeinschaft and the German Federal Ministry of Research (O1KE88141).

REFERENCES

1. Binns RM, Pabst R. Lymphoid cell migration and homing in the young pig: alternative immune mechanisms in action. In Husband AJ (ed). *Migration and Homing of Lymphoid Cells.* Vol II. Boca Raton, Florida, CRC Press, 1988, pp. 137–74.
2. Pabst R, Binns RM. Heterogeneity of lymphocyte homing physiology: several mechanisms operate in the control of migration to lymphoid and non-lymphoid organs in vivo. Immunol Rev 1989; 108:83–109.
3. Jalkanen S, Reichert RA, Gallatin WM, Bargatze RF, Weissman IL, Butcher EC. Homing receptors and the control of lymphocyte migration. Immunol Rev 1986; 91:39–60.
4. Yednock TA, Rosen SD. Lymphocyte homing. Adv Immunol 1989; 44:313–78.
5. Kieran MW, Blank V, le Bail O, Israel A. Lymphocyte homing. Res Immunol 1989; 140:399–450.
6. Pabst R, Binns RM, Licence ST, Peter M. The selective major vascular marginal pool of lymphocytes in the lung. Am Rev Respir Dis 1987; 136:1213–8.
7. Rannie GH, Donald KJ. Estimation of migration of thoracic duct lymphocytes to non-lymphoid tissues. Cell Tissue Kinet 1977; 10:523–541.
8. Smith ME, Ford WL. The recirculating lymphocyte pool of the rat. A systematic description of the migration of recirculating lymphocytes. Immunology 1983; 49:83–94.
9. Binns RM, Licence ST, Pabst R. Homing of blood, splenic and lung emigrant lymphoblasts: Comparison with the behaviour of lymphocytes from these sources. 1991 (submitted).
10. Binns RM, Pabst R, Licence ST. Classification of lymphocytes recirculating in the spleen. Immunology 1981; 44:273–9.

156

The Binding of CD8-Positive Thoracic Duct and Blood Lymphocytes to High Endothelial Venules Is Influenced by the Spleen

J. Westermann, K. U. Willführ, G. Zimmermann, and R. Pabst
Medical School of Hannover, Hannover, Germany

INTRODUCTION

The number of lymphocytes in the blood is regulated by their migration properties (1). Since the spleen plays an important role in lymphocyte migration (2), removal of the spleen leads to alterations in the number of blood lymphocytes in both man and animals (3). Thus, after splenectomy the number of CD8-positive lymphocytes in the blood is increased (3). To investigate whether this is caused by decreasing the *exit* of lymphocytes from the blood, the lymphocyte adherence assay was used. In this test, lymphocytes are added to cryostat sections of organs containing high endothelium venules (HEVs) and the binding of these cells to the HEVs is measured (4,5). Thoracic duct lymphocytes (TDLs) or blood lymphocytes were used because these cells represent migrating populations. Sections of mesenteric lymph nodes (MLNs) from normal rats were overlaid with lymphocytes of normal and splenectomized animals, and after binding and fixation the sections were stained for CD8-positive lymphocytes (6). Thus, the aim of the present study was to investigate whether the loss of the spleen influences the adherence of CD8-positive lymphocytes to HEVs and whether this depends on the source of the cells.

MATERIAL AND METHODS

Animals and Operations

Adult male Lewis rats (n = 18; mean body weight 340 g) were either sham splenectomized (n = 12) or splenectomized (n = 6) as previously described (3). At least 6 weeks after the operation, either cell suspensions (n = 12) or cryostat sections were made (n = 6).

Cell Suspensions

Blood Lymphocytes

Heparinized arterial blood was obtained, red cells were removed by ammonium chloride (15 min at room temperature), and the cells resuspended in RPMI 1640 containing 2% bovine serum albumin (BSA). Since platelets interfere with the binding of lymphocytes to HEVs, their concentration was reduced by counterflow centrifugation (100 min, 2000 rpm, 4°C, 4.5 ml/min). Then the lymphocytes were suspended in medium (Earle's medium containing 0.1% BSA and 0.5% HEPES [N-2-hydroxyethylpeperazine-N-2-ethanesulfonic acid]), washed once and adjusted to 15×10^6 cells/ml.

Thoracic Duct Lymphocytes

Thoracic duct lymphocytes were collected as described previously (7). After centrifugation (800 g, 15 min) the red cells were removed and then the TDs were either resuspended in medium at 15×10^6 cells/ml or subjected to counterflow centrifugation.

Standard Lymphocytes

Standard lymphocytes were obtained from MLNs of female rats (n = 18; mean body weight 200 g), incubated with fluorescein isothiocyanate (FITC), resuspended in medium, and adjusted to a concentration of 15×10^6 cells/ml (6).

Cryostat Sections

Normal MLNs were excised, snap-frozen in liquid nitrogen, and stored at –70°C. Cryostat sections (10 μm) were cut from the frozen organs and stored at –20°C.

In Vitro Assay of Lymphocyte Binding

The assay was modified in such a way that it was possible to observe FITC-positive and CD8-positive lymphocytes using light microscopy (6). Briefly: Standard lymphocytes and either TDLs or blood lymphocytes were mixed 1:1, put on rotating lymph node sections, and after 20 min carefully washed and fixed. Then FITC-positive and CD8-positive lymphocytes were detected using antibodies and standard immunocytochemical staining techniques. At least 200 FITC-positive and 80 CD8-positive lymphocytes adherent to HEVs were scored. Mean and standard deviations are given. Differences were regarded as significant when they reached $p < 0.05$ in Student's t-test.

RESULTS

Using this modified HEV assay, the binding of lymphocytes to HEVs is highly specific, and FITC-positive and CD8-positive lymphocytes can be clearly seen (Fig. 1A).

After splenectomy the *percentage* of CD8-positive blood lymphocytes adhering to HEVs increases, whereas no change is seen for TDLs (Fig. 1B). However, the percentage of CD8-positive lymphocytes in the inoculum may differ owing to a different source (blood and TD), owing to the animals or to splenectomy. Therefore, the *adherence index* (ADI; percentage of lymphocytes bound to the HEVs divided by the respective percentage of inoculum) is a better indicator of the effects of splenectomy. Using the ADI, after removal of the spleen a significantly better adherence is seen for both CD8-positive TDLs and blood lymphocytes (Fig. 1C).

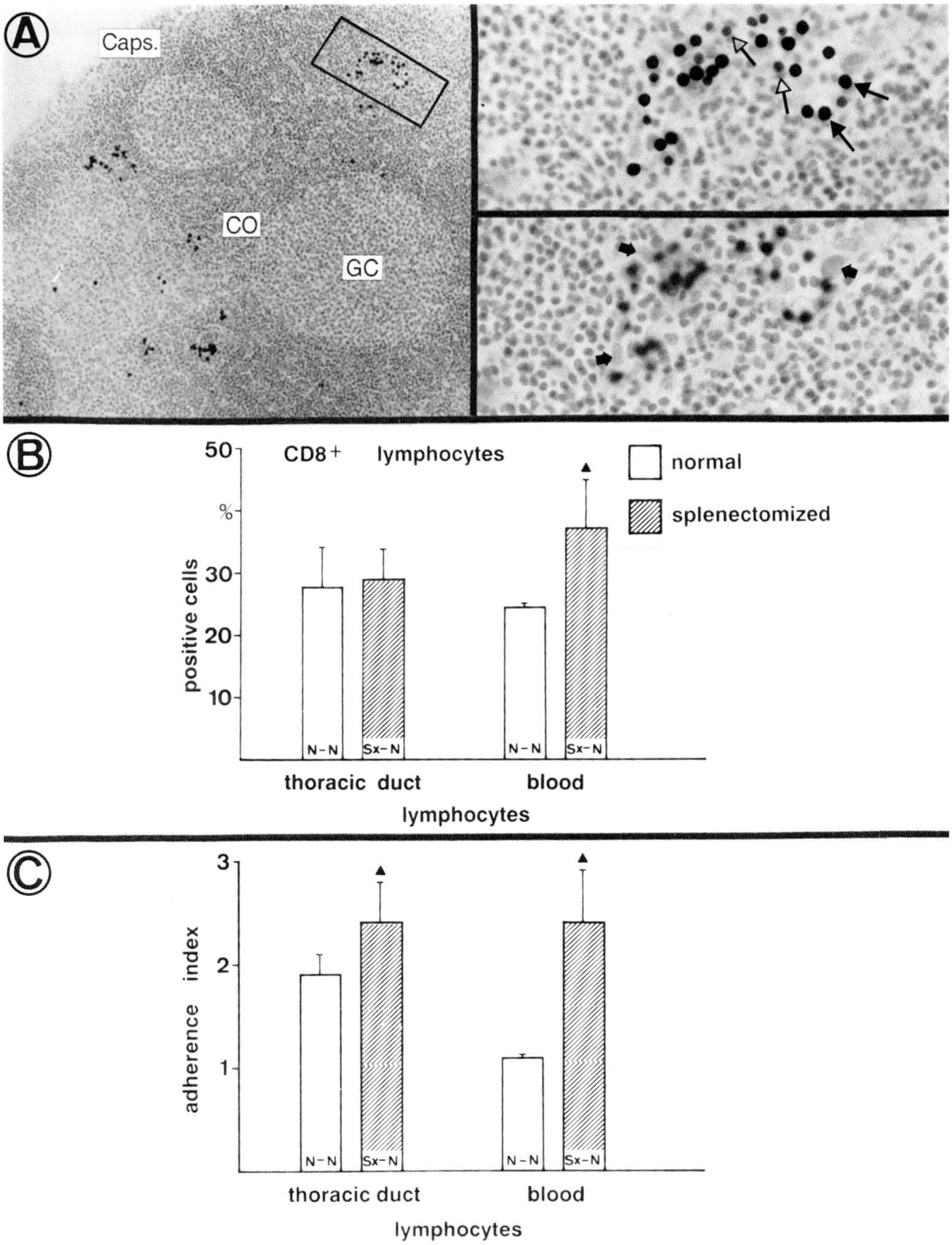

Figure 1 (A) HEV preparation of a rat MLN stained for $FITC^+$ lymphocytes. The HEV in the enclosed area is shown at a higher magnification on the right. Upper right: lymphocytes are focused. Open arrows indicate $FITC^-$ lymphocytes, closed arrows indicate $FITC^+$ lymphocytes. Lower right: HEVs are focused. Arrows indicate high endothelium. Caps: capsule, CO: corona, GC: germinal center (×50, ×330). (B) Percentage of $CD8^+$ lymphocytes bound to the HEVs of normal MLN. TDLs or blood lymphocytes of either normal or splenectomized rats were used. N-N: normal lymphocytes on normal sections; Sx-N: lymphocytes of splenectomized rats on normal sections. ▲ = $p<0.05$. (C) The ADI of $CD8^+$ lymphocytes is given, which is calculated by dividing the percentage of $CD8^+$ lymphocytes bound to the HEV by the respective percentage in the inoculum, in order to account for the variations in the cellular composition of the inoculum. ▲ = $p<0.05$.

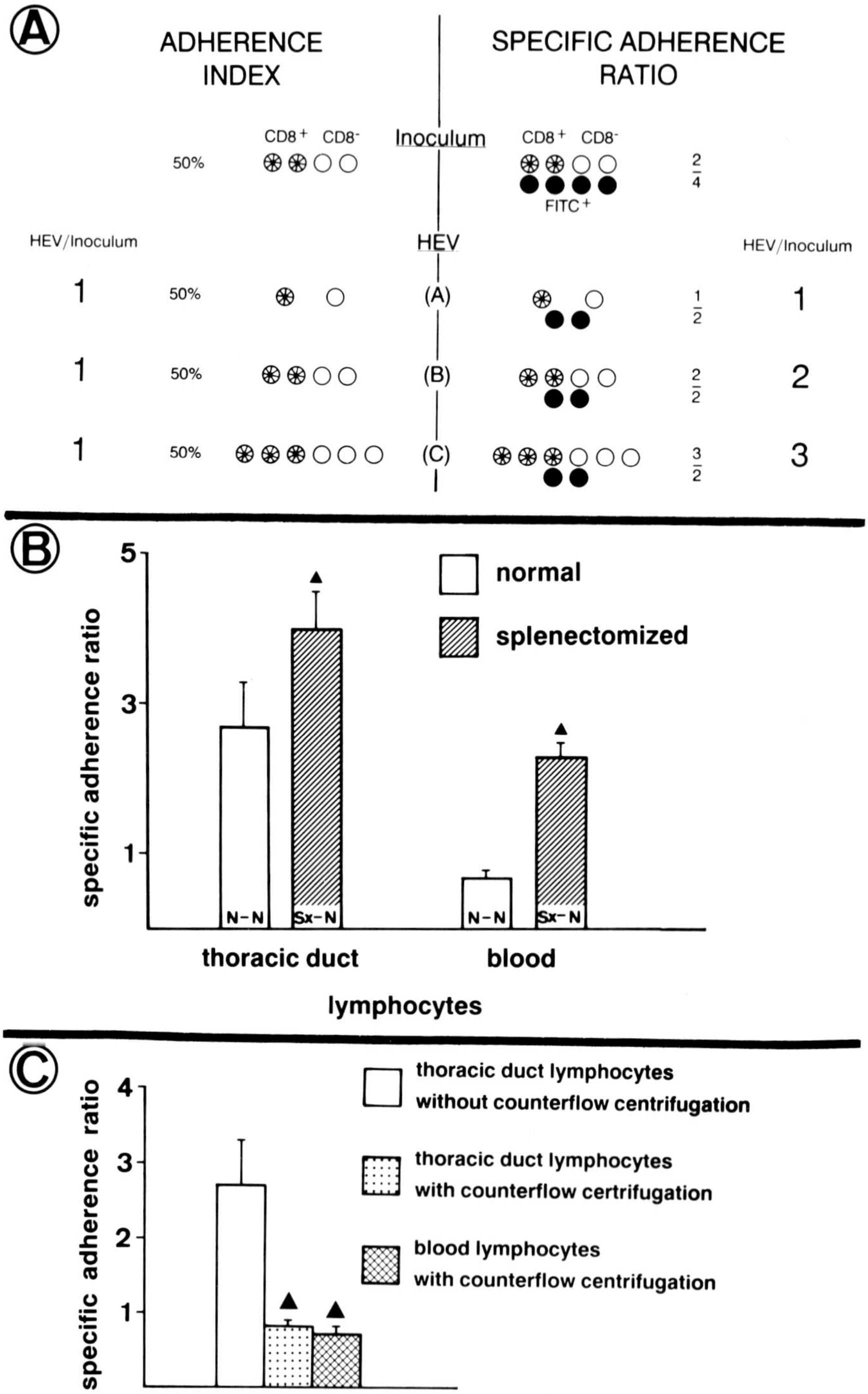

Figure 2 (A) Schematic drawing illustrating the function of the SAR. The different binding of the $CD8^+$ lymphocytes in the three assays (A, B, C) is not detected by the ADI. However, relating the binding of these lymphocytes to the constant binding of standard lymphocytes (e.g., $FITC^+$ MLN cells) reveals a different binding behavior (SAR = $CD8^+$ cells per $FITC^+$ cells on the HEV divided by $CD8^+$ cells per $FITC^+$ cells of the inoculum). (B) SAR of $CD8^+$ TDLs and blood lymphocytes showing for both populations an increase in bound $CD8^+$ lymphocytes after splenectomy, however, for blood lymphocytes on a reduced level. ▲: $p<0.05$. (C) SAR of $CD8^+$ TDLs and blood lymphocytes demonstrating the effect of counterflow centrifugation on the binding behavior. ▲: $p<0.05$.

In order to investigate the binding of lymphocytes in an absolute rather than relative fashion, the binding of CD8-positive lymphocytes can be related to the binding of FITC-positive standard lymphocytes (specific adherence ratio, SAR; Fig. 2A). The SAR reveals that splenectomy still leads to an increase in the binding of both CD8-positive TDLs and blood lymphocytes (Fig. 2b). However, compared to the standard lymphocytes, TDLs bind significantly better than blood lymphocytes (Fig. 2B). Subjecting TDLs to the counterflow centrifugation procedure (as carried out on the blood lymphocytes) decreases their binding to exactly the same low level as seen in CD8-positive blood lymphocytes (Fig. 2C). Neither the percentage (28 ± 7% vs 25 ± 4%) nor the ADI (1.9 ± 0.2 vs 1.5 ± 0.3) of bound CD8-positive TDLs are affected by this procedure.

DISCUSSION

Splenectomy clearly leads to a relative increase in the binding of both CD8-positive TDLs and blood lymphocytes to HEVs of MLN. This is in agreement with short-term in vivo migration experiments demonstrating an increased localization in CD8-positive TDLs within the MLN after splenectomy (7). However, these data do not explain the increased number of CD8-positive lymphocytes in the blood after splenectomy (3). Whether removal of the spleen influences the immigration into or the transit through other organs, or whether it alters the receptors on the surface of the lymphocytes or of the epithelium is unknown.

The SAR is often used to compare the binding of different cell populations in an absolute rather than relative fashion (8). This has to be done with great care for several reasons. First, a "harmless" procedure such as counterflow centrifugation dramatically alters the SAR (see Fig. 2c), whereas the ADI is not affected. Second, the SAR does not recognize whether different procedures, e.g., splenectomy or treatment with cytokines, influence the absolute number of HEVs within a lymph node. For example, when the number of HEVs is decreased, a reduced number of bound lymphocytes may lead to an increased SAR. Thus, quantitative comparisons can only be made in combination with other techniques, such as morphometry to determine the HEV area and the binding density of the lymphocytes, or detection of radioactive-labeled lymphocytes as the amount of radioactivity within a lymph node correlates with the number of lymphocytes in the region of the HEV up to 15 min after injection. Last, using only the SAR the binding of the same lymphocyte population to HEVs of different organs cannot be compared, which would be important in order to decide whether increased binding is due to the lymphocytes or due to the endothelium. The SAR relates the adherence of "test" lymphocytes to the adherence of FITC-positive standard lymphocytes. These lymphocytes can only be considered standard when they always come from the same source and overlay the section of the same organ, thus resulting in constant binding behavior. If the cryostat section were cut from another organ, the binding of the standard lymphocytes might be altered, and therefore could no longer be taken as standard.

CONCLUSION

Splenectomy induces an increase in the binding of both CD8-positive TDLs and blood lymphocytes to the HEVs of MLNs by mechanisms so far unknown. Since the lymphocyte adherence assay detects relative rather than absolute changes in the binding of lymphocytes, the magnitude of the increase after splenectomy remains to be investigated.

ACKNOWLEDGMENTS

This work was supported by the Deutsche Forschungsgemeinschaft SFB 244,A7. The authors wish to thank U. Hirschfeld, I. Dressendörfer, and P. Schwarz for their technical assistance and S. Fryk for editing the manuscript.

REFERENCES

1. Westermann, J, Pabst, R. Lymphocyte subsets in the blood: A diagnostic window on the lymphoid system? Immunol Today 1990; 11:406–410.
2. Pabst, R. The spleen in lymphocyte migration. Immunol Today 1988; 9:43–45.
3. Westermann, J, Schwinzer, R, Jecker, P, Pabst R. The influence of splenectomy, splenic autotransplantation, ageing, and the site of blood sampling on the number of B, T, CD4+ and CD8+ lymphocytes in the rat. Scand J Immunol 1990; 31:327–334.
4. Stamper, HB, Woodruff, JJ. Lymphocyte homing into lymph nodes: In vitro demonstration of the selective affinity of recirculating lymphocytes for high-endothelial venules. J Exp Med 1976; 144:828–833.
5. Butcher, EC, Scollay, RG, Weissman, IL. Lymphocyte adherence to high endothelial venules: Characterization of a modified in vitro assay, and examination of the binding of syngeneic and allogeneic lymphocyte populations. J Immunol 1979; 123:1996–2003.
6. Willführ, KU, Hirschfeld, U, Westermann, J, Pabst, R. The in vitro lymphocyte/endothelium binding assay: An improved method employing light microscopy. J Immunol Meth 1990; 130:201–207.
7. Westermann, J, Willführ, KU, Rothkötter, HJ, Fritz, FJ, Pabst, R. Migration pattern of lymphocyte subsets in the normal rat and the influence of splenic tissue. Scand J Immunol 1989; 29:193–201.
8. Stevens, SK, Weissman, IL, Butcher, EC. Differences in the migration of B and T lymphocytes: Organ-selective localization in vivo and the role of lymphocyte-endothelial cell recognition. J Immunol 1982; 128:844–851.

157

Low Frequency of Adherence In Vivo of Lymphocytes from Gut- and Bronchus-Associated Lymphoid Tissues to High Endothelial Venules of Peyer's Patches and Peripheral Lymph Nodes

Jeenan Tseng and Jack Komisar
Walter Reed Army Institute of Research, Washington, D.C.

INTRODUCTION

Lymphocytes of the Peyer's patches (PPs), bronchus-associated lymphoid tissue (BALT), and peripheral lymph nodes (PLNs) each have a unique migration and homing route. These migration-homing routes appear to be critically defined by the specific interactions between homing receptors on lymphocytes and the tissue-specific ligand on high endothelial venules (HEVs) of lymphoid tissues. The idea of this organ-specific migration is mainly derived from studies using monoclonal antibodies in passive transfers in animals of lymphocytes labeled with isotopes or fluorescein or tetramethyl rhodamine isothiocyanate and in studies using the in vitro assay of lymphocyte adherence to HEV of freshly cut lymph node sections (1–4). However, the former studies generally encountered technical pitfalls inherent in the use of isotopes; in the latter studies, lymphocytes adhered to HEVs best in the cold (7–9°C) and worst at 37°C. Fluorescein and tetramethyl rhodamine isothiocyanate labels in lymphocytes are relatively weak in fluorescence; the dyes also conjugate to the proteins on cell membranes, which may alter their homing properties. To avoid these problems, Brenan et al. (5) have successfully developed a labeling technique using a deoxyribonucleic acid (DNA)–binding fluorescent dye for lymphocyte migration studies. We have also been successful in using carboxyfluorescein diacetate, a fluorescent dye that only crosses the membranes of living cells, in lymphocyte homing studies. We have now further improved the technique by using carboxyfluorescein diacetate succinimidyl ester (CFDSE), which covalently binds to the proteins in the cytoplasm of living cells but does not diminish viability. This chapter summarizes our studies.

IN VIVO ADHERENCE TO HEV OF PP AND PLN

When lymphocytes from PPs and BALT were labeled with CFDSE and passively transferred into syngeneic mice (Balb/c to Balb/c), they showed a remarkably low frequency of adherence and localization to HEVs of PPs and PLNs. A vast majority of the PP cells and a substantial portion of BALT cells were unable to adhere to and localize in HEVs. In contrast, PLN cells showed a high frequency of adherence and localization to HEVs of not only the PLNs but also the PPs. When lymphoid cells from PPs, BALT, and PLNs were separated into T and B cells, they showed essentially the same pattern of adherence and localization as the unseparated cells, although B cells tended to adhere and localize better to HEVs of PPs than to those of PLNs. These results coupled with those reported in earlier studies (6) suggest that PLN cells have the capability to migrate to all the secondary lymphoid tissues, whereas PP cells have the tendency to migrate to the gut lamina propria and other mucosal tissues and differentiate into effector cells when they mature to a certain stage. Because of the fact that most PP lymphoid cells are antigen-committed cells well stimulated by intestinal ligands, whereas PLN cells are virgin, mature lymphocytes inaccessible to antigens in normal animals (7), the differential migration pattern in our study is consistent with the recent proposal that virgin lymphocytes possess a variety of homing receptors and hence no tissue specificity, whereas antigen-stimulated cells possess only limited numbers of homing receptors, and hence a tissue specificity (4). However, the differential migration pattern in our study is inconsistent with the current lymphocyte migration model, which suggests an organ-specific homing pattern for lymphocytes. Lymphoid cells from PPs migrate and recirculate in the gut tissues, whereas the PLN cells migrate and recirculate among peripheral lymph nodes (1–3).

MEL-14 HOMING RECEPTOR

We went further to characterize the molecular basis of lymphocyte adherence to HEVs in our study. As shown in published reports, the MEL-14 antigen constitutes the primary homing receptor for PLN cells to adhere to HEVs of the PLNs (1). We used phorbol myristate acetate (PMA) to remove the MEL-14 antigen in culture (8) and studied the HEV adherence and localization by passive transfer of the cultured cells. Lymphocytes from PLNs, BALT and PPs cultured with PMA lost the ability to adhere and localize to the HEVs of either the PPs or PLNs. Since PMA activates protein kinase C and indirectly eliminates MEL-14 antigen (8), further study using lymphoid cells depleted of MEL-14–positive cells was conducted, and the result of which confirmed that MEL-14 homing receptor is indeed involved in the in vivo adherence of lymphocytes to HEVs of both the PLNs and PPs.

MEL-14–POSITIVE CELLS IN PPs

When PPs and BALT cells were examined, they possessed a relatively large population of MEL-14–positive cells (30% for PP cells and 45% for BALT cells). The possession of this large number of MEL-14–positive cells is inconsistent with the low frequency of adherence and localization to the HEVs of both PLNs and PPs. The reason is unknown. Two possibilities are plausible. First, most MEL-14–positive cells in PPs and BALT may be masked by the mucins and/or carbohydrates that are transported from the lumen of the bronchus or gut tract. Supporting this possibility are the findings that adherence of lymphocytes to HEVs of PLNs can be inhibited by carbohydrate, which reacts with MEL-14 antigen and/or which possesses negative charges (4,5). Another possibility is that PP lymphocytes are heavily bombarded by the intestinal ligands and are undergoing differentiation to gain gut-specific homing receptors. MEL-14 antigen somehow is inactivated during the process.

INHIBITION BY HEPARIN

To test if negative charges and carbohydrates were involved in our study, heparin, a negatively charged carbohydrate, was investigated for its effect. When lymphocytes were incubated with heparin, washed, and transferred, essentially no effect on the HEV adherence and localization was seen. However, when the lymphocytes were combined with heparin in the transfer, a remarkable degree of inhibition was seen. This result suggests that heparin acts on HEVs rather than on the lymphocytes, and that negative charges and carbohydrates are also involved in HEV adherence.

EFFECT OF SENSITIZATION WITH DINITROPHENOL–KEYHOLE LIMPET HEMOCYANIN

To study if the loss of capability of PP lymphocytes to adhere to HEVs of PPs and PLNs was due to heavy bombardment by antigens, we injected mice with dinitrophenol–keyhole limpet hemocyanin (DNP-KLH) emulsified in complete Freund's adjuvant (CFA) in the area of the right inguinal lymph nodes and studied the adherence of lymphocytes from the stimulated inguinal nodes and other unstimulated lymph nodes. Preliminary results showed that 2 weeks after DNP-KLH stimulation, the right inguinal lymph nodes of DNP-KLH–stimulated mice have three times more cells than the left inguinal nodes and other nodes. However, lymphocytes from both right and left inguinal nodes as well as other lymph nodes of these DNP-KLH–sensitized mice adhered equally well to the HEVs of PPs and of all the PLNs of either the DNP-KLH–sensitized and nonsensitized mice. Furthermore, cells from DNP-KLH–sensitized mice adhered four to five times more than cells from CFA-sensitized mice to PP HEVs of either the DNP-sensitized and CFA-sensitized mice. Thus, DNP-KLH combined with CFA, instead of stimulating PLN cells to a stage similar to PP cells of losing HEV adherence capability, enhances the ability of PLN cells to adhere to HEVs of both the PPs and PLNs. Since DNP-KLH and CFA are the only antigen and stimulant used in the study, the role of antigens in lymphocyte migration remains to be determined.

CONCLUSIONS

Using the in vivo assay of lymphocyte adherence to HEVs, a differential migration pattern of lymphoid cells was seen in the present study. The PLN cells adhere and localize efficiently to HEVs of both the PPs and PLNs, whereas PP and BALT lymphocytes do poorly. This differential migration pattern, although consistent with published reports, is different from the current organ-specific homing model in migration route. Nevertheless, consistent with the organ-specific migration model are the findings that lymphocyte adherence to HEVs involves the MEL-14 antigen (the homing receptor), carbohydrates, and negative charges. The DNP-KLH stimulation of PLN cells resulted in an increase, instead of a decrease, of adherence to HEVs of PPs. Nevertheless, the mechanism by which lymphocytes differentially migrate in the body remains to be investigated.

REFERENCES

1. Gallatin WM, Weissman IL, Butcher EC. A cell-surface molecule involved in organ-specific homing of lymphocytes. Nature 1983, 304:30–34.
2. Woodruff JJ, Clarke LM, Chin YH. Specific cell-adhesion mechanisms determining migration pathways of recirculating lymphocytes. Ann Rev Immunol 1987, 5:201–222.
3. Berg EL, Goldstein LA, Jutila MA, Nakache M, Picker LJ, Streeter PR, Wu NW, Zhou D, Butcher EC. Homing receptors and vascular addressins: Cell adhesion molecules that direct lymphocyte traffic. Immunol Rev 1989, 108:5–18.
4. Yednock TA, Rosen SD. Lymphocyte homing. Adv Immunol 1989, 44:313–378.
5. Brenan M, Parish CR. Modification of lymphocyte migration by sulfated polysaccharides. Eur J Immunol 1986, 16:423–430.
6. Tseng J. Migration and differentiation of IgA precursor cells in the gut associated lymphoid tissues. In Husband AJ (ed). *Migration and Homing of Lymphoid cells.* Vol II. Boca Raton, Florida, CRC Press, 1988, Chap. 13.
7. Cebra JJ, Gearhart PJ, Kamat R, Robertson SM, Tseng J. Origin and differentiation of lymphocytes involved in the secretory IgA response. Cold Spring Harbor Symp Quant Biol 1977, XLI:201–215.
8. Jung TM, Dailey MO. Rapid modulation of homing receptors ($gp90^{MEL-14}$) induced by activators of protein kinase C. Receptor shedding due to accelerated proteolytic cleavage at the cell surface. J Immunol 1990, 144:3130–3136.

158
Regulation of Adhesion Molecule Expression by Antigen-Specific T Cells In Vivo

James L. Mobley and Morris O. Dailey
University of Iowa College of Medicine, Iowa City, Iowa

INTRODUCTION

The tissue-specific homing of lymphocytes from the blood stream into peripheral lymphoid tissues depends upon the interaction of lymphocyte homing receptors with their ligands on organ-specific postcapillary high endothelial venules (HEVs) (1). In mice, the expression of the lymph node homing receptor $gp90^{MEL\text{-}14}$ (gp90), recognized by the monoclonal antibody (MAb) MEL-14, is required for binding to lymph node (LN) HEVs and subsequent entry into LN (2). T lymphocytes activated in vitro by mitogen or alloantigen downregulate expression of gp90 and consequently lose the ability to bind to HEVs in frozen sections (3) and home to LN in vivo (4). Although the tissue specificity of lymphocyte homing is governed by the lymphocyte homing receptors, other adhesion molecules, such as Pgp-1 (CD44) and lymphocyte function–associated antigen 1 (LFA-1) (CD11a/18), play accessory roles in the binding of lymphocytes to endothelium. The expression of these molecules has also been reported to change upon T-cell activation (5,6).

In this study, we examined LN lymphocytes for the expression of gp90 as well as Pgp-1 and LFA-1 following activation in vivo by an allogeneic skin graft. In addition, we also employed sponge-matrix allografts as an in vivo stimulus. Sponge grafts, unlike skin grafts, permit the recovery of large numbers of graft-infiltrating lymphocytes for analysis. The graft-infiltrating T cells were also examined for the surface expression of gp90, Pgp-1, and LFA-1. We report the appearance of a population of lymphocytes with the phenotype $CD8^{+}gp90^{-}Pgp\text{-}1^{high}LFA\text{-}1^{high}$ in the LN draining skin allografts that is rare or undetectable in LNs from isografted or ungrafted animals. These cells are highly activated effector cells that contain all of the allospecific cytolytic activity detectable in those LNs. This phenotype is shared by the CD8-positive T cells recovered from sponge allografts. Taken together, these results indicate that in vivo activation is associated with a change in homing receptor/adhesion molecule expression concomitant with the acquisition of effector function. These findings suggest a mechanism by which antigen-activated lymphocytes can be removed from the recirculating pool, and can be targeted to the site of inflammation and/or antigenic challenge.

MATERIALS AND METHODS

Skin Grafting

Adult C57BL/6 or BALB/c mice (Jackson Laboratories, Bar Harbor, Maine) were grafted with tail skin as previously described (7).

Sponge-Matrix Grafting

Sponge-matrix allografting is a modification of that of Roberts and Hayry (8). Briefly: Extensively cleansed 1.5 × 1.0 cm polyurethane sponges were loaded with approximately 20 million allogeneic spleen cells by soaking for 30 min in a single cell suspension of allogeneic spleen cells. Two of these sponges were inserted subcutaneously into an anesthetized recipient as previously described (8). After 10 days, the mice were sacrificed, the sponges removed, and the infiltrating leukocytes recovered by the gentle squeezing of the sponge. The recovered cells were passed over a nylon wool column to enrich for T cells.

Flow Cytometry

In this study, 1×10^6 lymphocytes from lymph nodes draining skin grafts or recovered from sponge grafts were stained for FACS analysis as previously described (3) using phycoerythrin-conjugated MEL-14, fluorescein-conjugated MAb to Pgp-1 (9F3) or LFA-1 (M17/4.2), biotinylated MAb to Lyt-2 (53-6.7), and Texas Red–conjugated avidin (Vector). The cells were analyzed on a FACS 440 (Becton Dickinson) using the FACS/DESK computer program for data collection and analysis.

Cell-Mediated Cytotoxicity Assay

Lymphocytes from LN draining 9-10–day skin grafts were incubated with MAb to CD4 (GK1.5) and B220 (RA3 6B2) and panned on anti-rat Ig-coated plates to enrich for CD8 T cells. The panned cells were stained for FACS analysis as above and sorted on a FACS 440 (Becton Dickinson) into the three populations listed below. ^{51}Cr-labeled P815 target cells were placed into V-bottom 96 well plates (Costar) and the sorted effector cells were added at various E/T ratios in a total volume of 250 μl. The plates were incubated and harvested, and the samples counted as previously described (9).

RESULTS

Draining LN Contain New Population of CD8 T Cells

Nine to ten days postgraft, draining LN were greatly enlarged, containing more than six times the number of lymphocytes found in LN from ungrafted controls. Upon FACS analysis, T cells from these draining LN were found to be greater than 85% $gp90^+$, only a slight change from the 90–95% $gp90^+$ T cells from normal, unstimulated LN. However, three-color FACS analysis of the $CD8^+$ T cells from the activated LN demonstrated the appearance of a population of $CD8^+$ $gp90^-Pgp\text{-}1^{hi}$ T cells that is rare or undetectable in isografted or ungrafted control mice (Fig. 1). T cells with this phenotype also show increased surface expression of LFA-1 (Fig. 1) as well as the activation antigens IL-2 R and

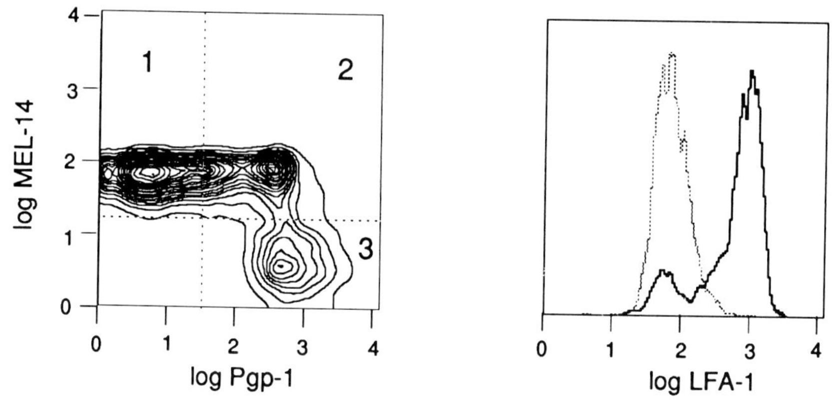

Figure 1 Three-color FACS analysis of the lymphocytes from LN draining a 10-day skin allograft. Left: The correlated expression of Pgp-1 and gp90^{MEL-14} is shown only on those cells expressing Lyt-2 (CD8). Dotted lines divide the cells into three populations based upon surface expression of gp90^{MEL-14} and Pgp-1. Population 3 cells are rare or nonexistent in isografted and ungrafted controls. Right: Expression of LFA-1 on gp90$^+$ (dotted line) or gp90$^-$ (solid line) CD8 T cells. LFA-1 expression is higher on those CD8$^+$ T cells which do not express gp90^{MEL-14}.

Transferrin R (data not shown). The CD8$^+$ lymphocytes from the draining LN will be referred to as populations 1, 2, and 3 based on their surface expression of gp90, Pgp-1, and LFA-1 as follows: population 1: gp90$^+$Pgp-1$^-$LFA-1^{lo}; population 2: gp90$^+$Pgp-1$^+$ LFA-1^{lo}; population 3: gp90$^-$Pgp-1^{hi}LFA-1^{hi}.

Population 3 Contains Allospecific Effector Cells

Because relatively few lymphocytes from draining LN were found to be gp90$^-$, we tested these cells for their antigen-specific effector activity by 4-hr ^{51}Cr release assay. Populations 1, 2, and 3 from C57BL/6 LN draining a BALB/c graft were purified by using a fluorescence-activated cell sorter (FACS) and assayed for their ability to lyse target cells

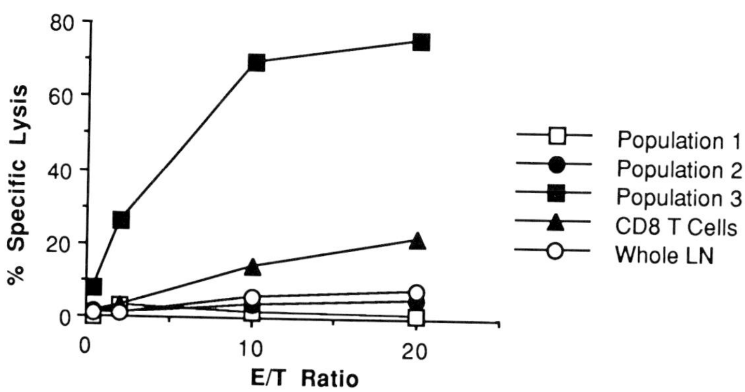

Figure 2 Allospecific cytolytic activity of sorted populations 1, 2, and 3. Lymphocytes from LN draining a 10-day allograft were purified on a FACS into the three populations indicated in Figure 1. Only population 3 (CD8$^+$Pgp-1$^+$gp90$^-$) possessed potent allospecific lytic ability in a ^{51}Cr-release assay.

with the same H-2 haplotype as the stimulating graft. As shown in Figure 2, population 3 lymphocytes were highly effective at lysing allogeneic targets whereas population 1 and 2 had virtually no cytolytic activity against these targets. Population 3 did not lyse the syngeneic target EL-4 or the NK-sensitive YAC-1 target (data not shown). A similar result was seen when cells of the population 3 phenotype were isolated from BALB/c LN draining C57BL/6 skin grafts in that these cells efficiently lysed allogeneic but not syngeneic targets (data not shown).

Sponge Graft-Infiltrating T Cells Are of the Population 3 Phenotype

Skin grafts are an excellent device for stimulating a response in a local lymph node, but unfortunately, they are not ideal for recovering graft-infiltrating lymphocytes, the cells responsible for graft rejection. Sponge matrix allografts, on the other hand, are well suited for this purpose. We therefore examined the homing receptor/adhesion molecule phenotype of $CD8^+$ T lymphocytes infiltrating a day 10 sponge allograft. Figure 3 shows that greater than 90% of the $CD8^+$ T cells infiltrating a sponge allograft are of the $gp90^-Pgp\text{-}1^{hi}$ (population 3) phenotype.

DISCUSSION

The activation of lymphocytes in vivo results in the altered expression of a series of cell surface adhesion molecules involved in the binding of lymphocytes to vascular endothelium. The complete cessation of expression of the lymphocyte homing receptor, $gp90^{MEL\text{-}14}$, on CD8 T cells appears to be concomitant with the acquisition of cytotoxic T lymphocyte (CTL) effector function. This is consistent with the observation that effector CTL infiltrating sponge allografts are gp90-negative. In order to fit the loss of gp90 into the overall scheme of regulation of lymphocyte migration, we examined the correlated

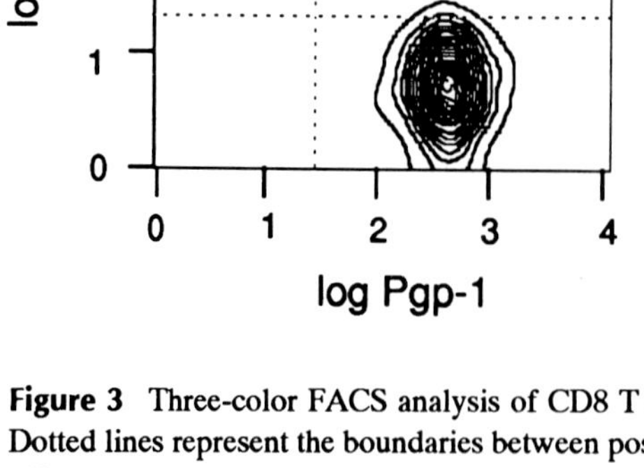

Figure 3 Three-color FACS analysis of CD8 T cells infiltrating a 10-day sponge-matrix allograft. Dotted lines represent the boundaries between positive and negative staining. These graft-infiltrating effector cells, which express high levels of Pgp-1, but do not express surface $gp90^{MEL\text{-}14}$, are the same phenotype as population 3 cells in LN.

expression of two other adhesion molecules which appear to have a role in leukocyte-endothelial interactions. Pgp-1 (CD44) expression increases following antigenic stimulation of T cells, and its levels remain high throughout the life of the activated cell, prompting some to call Pgp-1 a "memory T-cell" marker (5). In man, CD44 (HERMES-1, 515, ECMR III) is reported to function as an adhesion molecule for endothelium (10) or for extracellular matrix proteins (11). The broad tissue distribution of CD44 in both man and mouse makes it likely that CD44 serves an important adhesive function. Expression of LFA-1 (CD11a/18) also increases on activated T cells. The ligand for LFA-1, intracellular adhesion molecule 1 (ICAM-1), is a molecule found on T cells and endothelium. Interestingly, the levels of ICAM-1 increase dramatically on cytokine-activated endothelium such as that present at inflammatory sites in vivo (12). The regulation of LFA-1–mediated adhesion after cell activation occurs not only by modulating the level of surface LFA-1 protein, but also by inducing a change in its conformation which increases its binding affinity for ICAM-1 (13).

Figure 4 illustrates a model suggesting a mechanism by these activation-induced changes in adhesion molecule expression would redirect lymphocyte traffic. A T cell encountering antigen, in this case within the confines of a LN draining an antigenic site, begins to express surface Pgp-1, changing from a population 1 to a population 2 phenotype. Further differentiation of antigen-specific precursors into effector T cells is associated with downregulation of $gp90^{MEL\text{-}14}$, similar to that seen in models of T-cell activation in vitro (3). Acquisition of lytic activity also correlates with increased expression of LFA-1. These cells, once released into the circulation, would then have an increased ability to migrate to the peripheral antigenic site. That is, the loss of gp90 expression would prevent bloodborne effector cells from homing back to LNs, which otherwise would tend to clear them from the

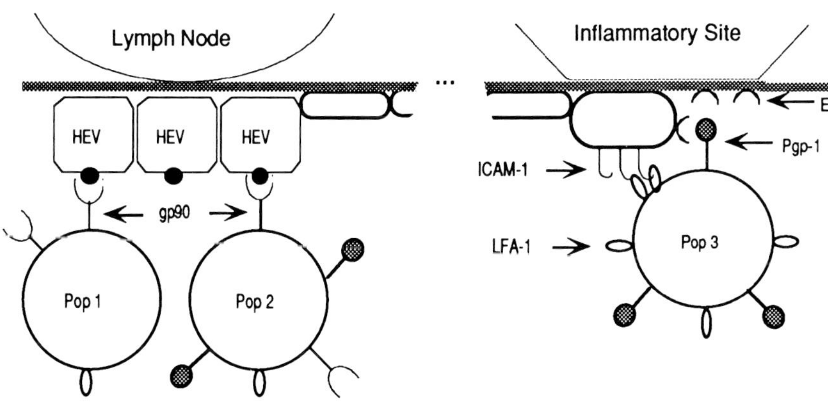

Figure 4 Model depicting the regulation of lymphocyte migration due to differential expression of an array of adhesion molecules. Lymphocytes from populations 1 and 2 preferentially home to LN HEVs owing to the expression of gp90 on the lymphocyte surface. Population 3 lymphocytes are highly activated cells that do not express gp90, and therefore do not bind HEVs or recirculate through LNs. These cells, therefore, remain in the circulation longer, enhancing their opportunity to interact with endothelium at an inflammatory site. The increased level of LFA-1 on population 3 cells augments lymphocyte adherence to this endothelium, which expresses high levels of ICAM-1. The upregulation of Pgp-1 on population 3 cells would also increase endothelial adherence, by binding to its ligand on the endothelium or on the extracellular matrix (ECM). Thus, the down regulation of gp90 and the increase in LFA-1 and Pgp-1 would block lymphocyte homing to LNs and enhance delivery of effecteor cells to inflammatory sites.

circulation. At the site of antigenic challenge, the nascent inflammatory response causes increased expression of ICAM-1, the ligand for LFA-1. There may also be exposed extracellular matrix proteins due to local tissue injury. The activated T cells, expressing LFA-1 and Pgp-1, would bind to these areas with high avidity, thereby enhancing migration of the effector cells into the inflammatory site.

Recent evidence suggests that the affinity of certain VLA molecules for their ligands increases on activated T cells, and that one VLA ligand, VCAM-1, increases on cytokine-activated endothelium, lends support to our hypothesis (14). There are several unanswered questions that are currently being addressed. One deals with the subject of T-cell memory. There is good evidence that memory T cells are found among the Pgp-1–positive cells, suggesting that memory T cells could be population 2 cells that did not differentiate into population 3, or alternatively they could result from the reexpression of gp90 by population 3 T cells. We are currently investigating alteration of adhesion molecule expression on CD4 T cells following in vivo activation in order to determine if there are lymphocyte subset differences in adhesion molecule expression before and after activation.

REFERENCES

1. Streeter, P. R., E. L. Berg, B. T. N. Rouse, R. F. Bargatze and E. C. Butcher. A tissue-specific endothelial cell molecule involved in lymphocyte homing. Nature 331:41 (1988).
2. Gallatin, W. M., I. L. Weissman and E. C. Butcher. A cell surface molecule involved in organ-specific homing of lymphocytes. Nature 304:30 (1983).
3. Jung, T. M., W. M. Gallatin, I. L. Weissman and M. O. Dailey. Down-regulation of homing receptors after T cell activation. J. Immunol. 141:4110 (1988).
4. Dailey, M. O., W. M. Gallatin and I. L. Weissman. The in vivo behavior of T cell clones: Altered migration due to loss of the lymphocyte surface homing receptor. J. Mol. Cell. Immunol. 2:27 (1985).
5. Budd, R. C., J. C. Cerottini, C. Horvath, C. Bron, T. Pedrazzizi, R. C. Howe and H. R. MacDonald. Distinction of virgin and memory T lymphocytes. J. Immunol. 138:3120 (1987).
6. Springer, T. A., M. L. Dustin, T. K. Kishimoto and S. D. Marlin. The lymphocyte function associated LFA 1, CD2, and LFA-3 molecules: Cell adhesion receptors of the immune system. Annu. Rev. Immunol. 5:223 (1987).
7. Steinmuller, D. S. Skin grafting. In: *Methods in Enzymology* Vol. 108 (Sabato, Langore and Vunakis, eds.). New York, Academic Press, 1984.
8. Roberts, P. J. and P. Hayry. Sponge matrix allografts: a model for analysis of killer cells infiltrating mouse allografts. Transplantation 21:437 (1976).
9. Brunner, K. T., J. Mavel, J. C. Cerottini and B. Chapuis. Quantitative assay of the lytic action of immune lymphoid cells on 51C4-labeled allogeneic target cells in vitro: Inhibition by isoantibody and by drugs. Immunology 14:181 (1968).
10. Jalkanen, S. T., R. F. Bargatze, L. R. Herron and E. C. Butcher. A lymphoid cell surface glycoprotein involved in endothelial cell recognition and lymphocyte homing in man. Eur. J. Immunol. 16:195 (1986).
11. Gallatin, W. M., E. A. Wayner, P. A. Hoffman, T. St.John, E. C. Butcher and W. G. Carter. Structural homology between lymphocyte receptors for high endothelium and class III extracellular matrix receptor. Proc. Natl. Acad. Sci. U.S.A. 86:4654 (1989).
12. Dustin, M. L. and T. A. Springer. Lymphocyte-function associated antigen-1 (LFA-1) interaction with intercellular adhesion molecule-1 (ICAM-1) is one of at least three mechanisms for lymphocyte adhesion to cultured endothelial cells. J. Cell Biol. 107:321 (1988).
13. Springer, T. A. and M. L. Dustin. T-cell receptor cross-linking transiently stimulates adhesiveness through LFA-1. Nature 341:619 (1989).
14. Shimizu, Y., G. A. Van Seventer, K. J. Horgan and S. Shaw. Regulated expression and binding of three VLA (B1) integrin receptors on T cells. Nature 345:250 (1990).

159
Sera from Patients with Multiple Sclerosis Enhances Lymphocyte Adhesion to Inflammatory Endothelium In Vitro

K. A. Brown,[1] A. Vora,[1] D. Perkin,[2] A. Forti,[3] R. Jenkins,[1] and D. C. Dumonde[1]
[1]*St. Thomas' Hospital Campus, London, England;*
[2]*Charing Cross Hospital, London, England;*
[3]*Central Middlesex Hospital, London, England*

INTRODUCTION

Multiple sclerosis (MS) is an inflammatory disease affecting the white matter of the central nervous system (CNS), and is characterized by perivascular infiltrates of lymphocytes and macrophages within focal zones of demyelination. T lymphocytes are reported to move rapidly from the blood into the cerebral spinal fluid of patients with MS (1), and it is likely that the extravasation of blood mononuclear cells (MNCs) into the CNS constitutes an important pathological event of this disease. Since a specific "target" antigen has yet to be associated with MS, we suggest that a disorder of leukocyte-endothelial interaction in the microvascular environment of the CNS could initiate the onset or relapse of the disease in susceptible subjects (2). Such an abnormality may stem from the altered behavior of subpopulations of MNCs, the local endothelium, a modification of the milieu (plasma) in which MNC:endothelial interaction is taking place, or combination of these.

We have recently demonstrated that blood MNCs isolated from patients with MS are more adherent than control cells to cultured endothelium pretreated with the inflammatory cytokine, tumor necrosis factor (TNF) (3). To determine if this effect was related in part to the action of soluble circulating factors, the present study investigated if MS sera modified the attachment of MNCs to endothelial cells.

MATERIALS AND METHODS

Patients and Controls

Sera were collected from healthy subjects (controls) and patients with MS. Mononuclear leukocytes (purity >98%) were prepared from the blood of healthy subjects by centrifugation on Lymphoprep (4). Enriched lymphocytes (purity >90%) were obtained following the centrifugation of blood MNCs on Percoll gradients.

Culture of Endothelial Cells

Endothelial cells were obtained from the veins of human umbilical cords by a modification of the method of Jaffe et al. (5). Briefly: Each vein was treated with 1 mg/ml collagenase solution for 15 min at 37°C. Thereafter, the collagenase solution was centrifuged so as to produce an endothelial cell pellet. The cells were resuspended in RPMI 1640 medium supplemented with 20% human AB serum and cultured in a 10% CO_2-humidified atmosphere at 37°C. When the endothelial cells had formed a confluent monolayer the cells were disrupted by treatment with 0.05% trypsin and 0.025% EDTA and transferred into wells of a gelatin-coated 96-well microtiter plate. Confluent monolayers of endothelial cells were obtained after 4 days' culture at 37°C. Identification of the endothelial cells was confirmed by immunofluorescent staining with an antihuman factor VIII antiserum. Prior to the adherence assay, most of the endothelial monolayers were pretreated for 4 hr with 0.1–50.0 U/ml of recombinant TNF.

Adherence Assay

Endothelial monolayers were washed twice with RPMI without serum at 37°C to remove any contaminating serum. To each well was added 200 μl of ^{51}Cr-labeled MNCs (0.2×10^6 cells/well) suspended in RPMI medium. Prior to the assay, MNCs or lymphocytes were incubated for 2 hr in RPMI medium containing 50% control or patient serum. Each test was performed in quadruplicate. After incubation at 37°C for 1 hr, the nonadherent MNCs were aspirated and the endothelial monolayers washed with RPMI without serum at 37°C to remove any loosely adherent cells. The endothelium was osmotically disrupted, and the lysate collected and counted in a Packard auto-gamma scintillation counter. The percentage of MNCs adhering to endothelium was calculated as follows:

$$\%\ \text{adherence} = \frac{\text{cpm in 200 μl lysate} - \text{cpm background}}{\text{cpm in 200 μl original MNC suspension} - \text{cpm background}} \times 100$$

RESULTS

There was no difference in the adhesive properties of blood MNCs from normal subjects and patients with MS to untreated endothelium. When endothelial cells had been pretreated with 1 U/ml of TNF the blood MNCs of the patients were significantly more adherent than those of controls (33% increase; $p < 0.005$) (Fig. 1). To determine if this effect was related to adherence enhancing factors present in patients' sera, blood MNCs from normal subjects were incubated in control and MS sera for 2 hr prior to transfer to endothelial cultures that were either untreated or pretreated with TNF. The attachment of MNCs to untreated endothelium was not modified by MS sera. Although MNCs pretreated with MS or control serum demonstrated a maximum 22 ± 13% and 23 ± 8% increase to TNF-treated endothelium, respectively, there was no difference in the activity of sera from the two groups of subjects.

Similar experiments were also performed using enriched populations of normal blood lymphocytes. From Figure 2b it can be seen that pretreatment of lymphocytes with MS sera produced a greater increase in adhesion to endothelium pretreated with 10 and 50 U/ml

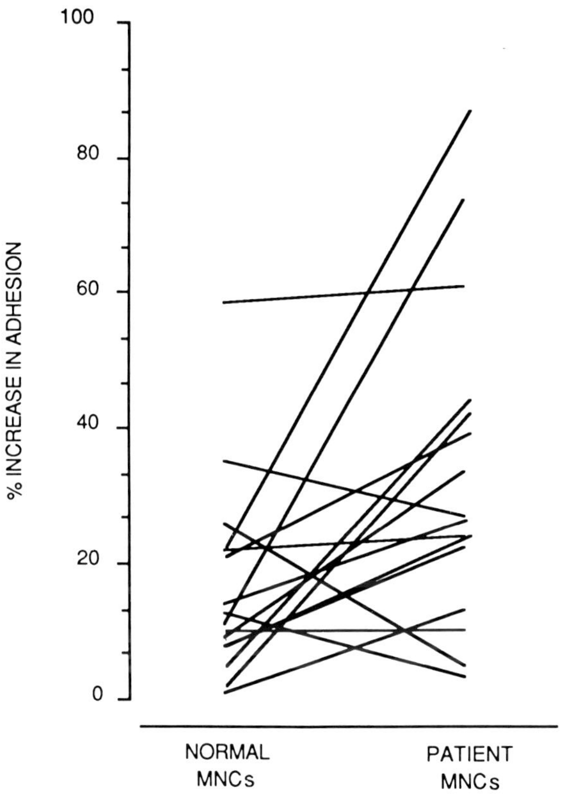

Figure 1 Increased adherence of blood mononuclear cells (MNCs) from patients with MS to endothelium pretreated with TNF. Each line represents one experiment in which MNCs from one control subject and one patient were incubated with endothelial monolayers prepared from the same umbilical cord.

TNF (61 and 91% increase, respectively) from that seen with normal sera. This augmented responsiveness by the MS sera was not apparent when using endothelium that was untreated or pretreated with lower concentrations of TNF (0.1 and 1.0 U/ml).

All lymphocyte preparations demonstrated a significant increased attachment ($p < 0.001$) to endothelium pretreated with 1–50 U/ml TNF. Moreover, Figure 2 illustrates that irrespective of the serum used, lymphocyte preparations exhibit a greater increased adherence to TNF-treated endothelium than mononuclear cells.

DISCUSSION

This study has shown that MS sera is more active than normal sera in increasing the adhesion of blood lymphocytes to TNF-pretreated endothelium. Such an enhancing effect did not occur with blood MNCs, implying that monocytes may be abrogating the effect of MS sera on lymphocytes. The nature of these enhancing factors remains to be identified. Cytokines enhance the adhesion of leukocytes to endothelium (6), and although a plasma abnormality has been described in MS (7), we are unaware of reports describing elevated

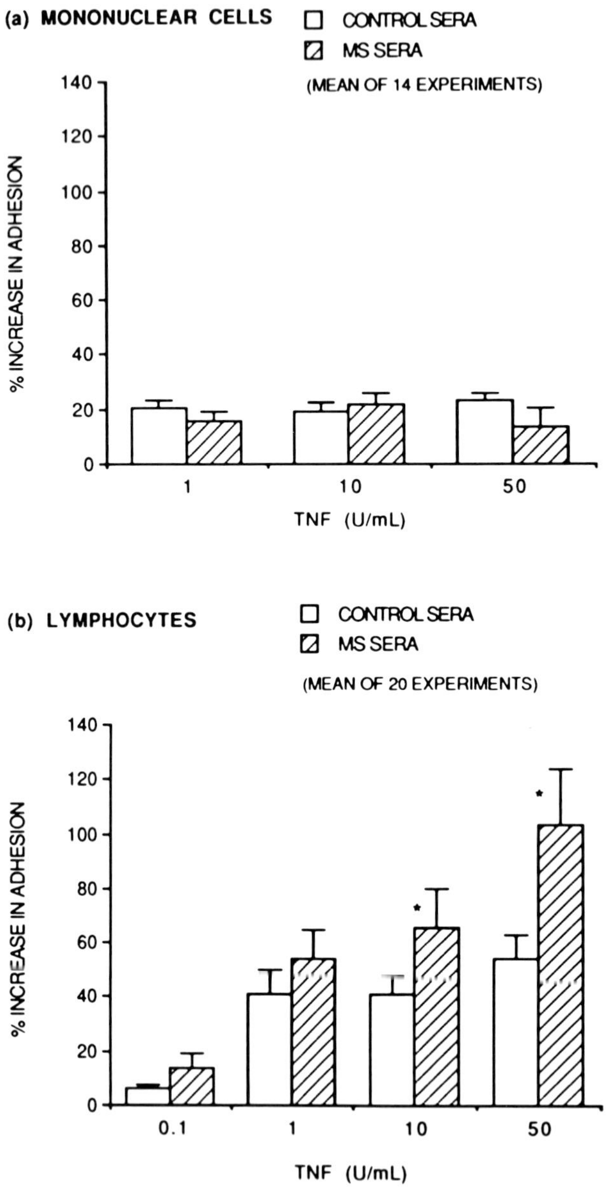

Figure 2 Adhesion to TNF-treated endothelium of normal blood (a) mononuclear cells, and (b) lymphocytes following pretreatment with sera from patients with MS. Mononuclear leukocytes and lymphocytes were pretreated with sera for 2 hr prior to the adherence assay. $^*p < 0.02$.

levels of cytokines in MS serum. During the relapse phase of MS disease there is a reduction in the number of CD8-positive lymphocytes (8) and of the suppressor-inducer T-cell population in patients with progressive disease (9). It is likely that the exacerbation phases of MS may be related to the extravasation of a particular subpopulation of lymphocytes into the CNS. In order to identify those cells which are most likely to adhere to inflammatory endothelium, experiments are in progress to investigate the activity of serum from patients during distinct phases of disease activity on the adhesion of isolated subpopulations of lymphocytes to cytokine-treated endothelium.

That the serum-enhancing activity on lymphocytes was only seen when using TNF-treated endothelium suggests that MS serum may modify the lymphocyte surface so as to facilitate recognition of those endothelial determinants that are induced by inflammatory cytokines such as TNF. Cytokines act on endothelial cells to increase the expression of the intercellular adhesion molecule-1 (ICAM-1), which is the ligand for lymphocyte function antigen-1 (LFA-1) (10). In view that ICAM-1 is upregulated on blood vessels in the CNS of animals with experimental allergic encephalomyelitis (11), it is possible that factors present in MS serum enhance the expression of receptors on the lymphocyte surface that bind ICAM-1 and other ligands. Such mechanisms could mediate the homing of blood lymphocytes to CNS-related endothelium in patients with MS and bring about the characteristic lymphocyte infiltration into the perivascular region and lesion edge.

ACKNOWLEDGMENT

This work was supported by Action for Research into Multiple Sclerosis.

REFERENCES

1. Hafler DA and Weiner HL (1987). Ann. Neurol., 21:89–93.
2. Brown KA and Dumonde DC (1987). In: *Multiple Sclerosis* (ed. F Clifford-Rose). John Libley, pp. 3–10.
3. Vora A, Perkin D, Forti A, Dumonde DC and Brown KA (1990). Adherence characteristics of blood mononuclear cells from patients with multiple sclerosis to cytokine treated endothelium (submitted).
4. Brown KA, Emblin PH, Perry JD and Holborow EJ (1979). Clin. Exp. Immunol., 36:272–278.
5. Jaffe EA, Nachman RL, Becker CG and Minick CR (1978). J. Clin. Invest., 52:2745.
6. Cavender D, Saegusa Y and Ziff M. J. Immunol., 139:1855–1860.
7. Swark RL, Peetoom F, Tamblyn CH, Daley ML and Seaman GVF (1983). Plasma Ther. Transfus. Technol., 4:301–311.
8. Reinherz EL, Weiner HL, Hauser SL, Cohen JA, Distaso JA and Schlossman SF (1980). N. Engl. J. Med., 303:125–129.
9. Morimoto C, Halfer DA, Weiner HL, Letvin NL, Hagan M, Daley J and Schlossman SF (1987). N. Engl. J. Med., 316:67–72.
10. Pober JS, Lapierre LA, Stolpen AM, Brock TA, Springer TA, Fiers W, Bevilacqua MP, Mendrick DL and Gimbrone MA Jr (1987). J. Immunol., 18:543–552.
11. Wilcox CE, Ward AMV, Brown KA, Baker D, Rothlein R and Turk TL (1990). J. Neuroimmunol. 30: 43–51.

160
Mononuclear Cells Affect Proteins Synthesized by Endothelial Cells

S. E. Bergström and K. G. Sundqvist
Huddinge University Hospital, Huddinge, Sweden

INTRODUCTION

The adhesion of lymphocytes to vascular endothelium is the first event in the passage of lymphocytes into a chronic inflammatory reaction. This adhesion is dependent on several endothelial proteins (intercellular adhesion molecule [ICAM] and vascular cell adhesion molecule [VCAM]) the expression of which is regulated by various cytokines (1–3). These structures belonging to the immunoglobulin superfamily (4) interact with integrins on the lymphocytes. An important aspect of the presence of integrin receptors on lymphocytes is that these cells may be interpreted to interact extensively with components of the extracellular matrix such as fibronectin. In this chapter, we present evidence suggesting that lymphocytes can cause degradation of fibronectin produced by endothelial cells.

METHODS

Mononuclear cells were obtained from healthy adults, isolated by Ficoll-Paque centrifugation, and depleted of phagocytic cells by iron and a magnet. The cells were cultured together with allogeneic mononuclear cells in order to be stimulated.

Endothelial cells were obtained from umbilical veins. Mononuclear cells were cultured at a density of $5–13\times10^6$ per 60-mm plastic Petri dish, whereas endothelial cells were used when grown to confluence.

Biosynthetic labeling of polypeptides synthesized during the coculture period was carried out with 35S-methionine for 4 hr in medium without methionine or serum. Components in the culture medium which had incorporated 35S-methionine were separated on SDS-PAGE gels (5) and finally visualized by fluorography (6). Immunoblotting was carried out after transfer of SDS-PAGE separated proteins from gels to nitrocellulose.

RESULTS

Mononuclear Cells Affect Proteins Synthesized by Endothelial Cells

Human mononuclear cells, depleted of phagocytic cells, were allowed to settle on monolayers of endothelial cells. After coculture for 4 hr, the synthesis of secreted proteins by the endothelial cells as measured using 35S-methionine incorporation and SDS-PAGE was studied. The synthesis of secreted proteins in media of mononuclear cells and endothelial cells cultured alone were used as controls.

The presence of activated mononuclear cells changed the pattern of medium proteins synthesized by endothelial cells. In comparison with endothelial cells not exposed to mononuclear cells, proteins with a molecular weight of 250–500 kD had disappeared or were present in reduced amounts. Instead several biosynthetically labeled components with a lower molecular weight appeared (Fig. 1, lanes a–c). This effect was more pronounced when using higher numbers of mononuclear cells (Fig. 2, lanes a–c). In contrast to "lymphocyte-enriched mononuclear cells" a cell population which had not been depleted of phagocytic cells did not affect high molecular weight biosynthetically labeled endothelial proteins in the culture medium (Fig. 2, lane k).

When endothelial cells were cultured in the presence of monensin and cycloheximide the appearance of labeled material in the medium was almost completely inhibited (Fig. 2, lanes d and e). The labeled proteins, therefore, most likely represented secreted synthesized material and are unlikely to reflect cell lysis.

Conditioned medium from mononuclear cells or different cytokines (interleukin-1, -2, and -4; T-cell growth factor β; tumor necrosing factor; and interferon-γ) added to endothelial cell cultures did not affect the synthesis of the high molecular weight biosynthetically

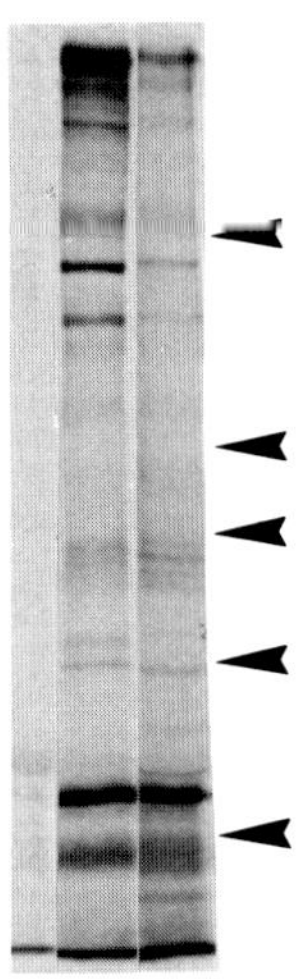

Figure 1 Fluorography of biosynthetically labeled proteins in culture media of mononuclear cells (a) depleted of phagocytic cells, endothelial cells alone (b), and from coculture of endothelial cells and mononuclear cells (c). The density of mononuclear cells was 2×10^5 cells/cm^2. Molecular weights markers 200, 116, 92, 66, and 45 kD are denoted by arrows.

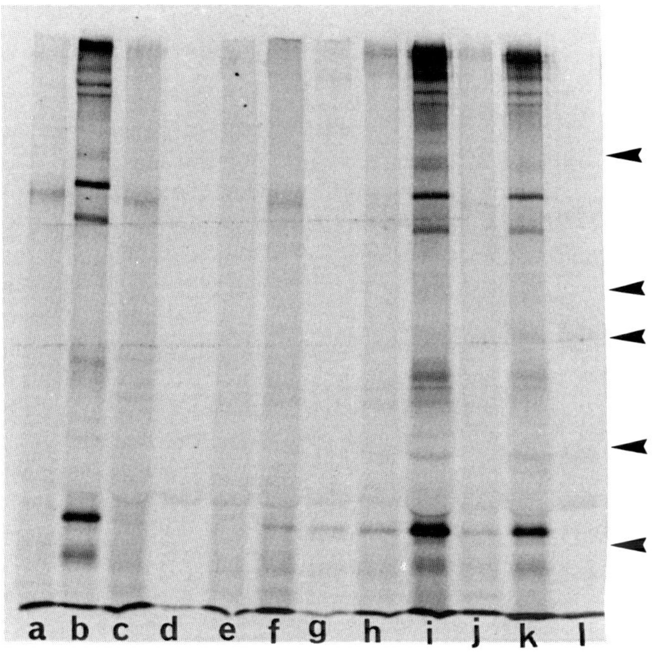

Figure 2 Fluorography of biosythetically labeled proteins in endothelial cell culture media after culture for 4 hr in the absence (b) and presence of mononuclear cells depleted of phagocytic cells (c–h,j) and not depleted of phagocytic cells (k). (a) shows mononuclear cell depleted and (l) shows mononuclear cells not depleted of phagocytic cells. (d–h,j) shows endothelial cells cocultured with mononuclear cells depleted of phagocytic cells in presence of cycloheximide 10 μg/ml (d), monensine $0{,}5\times10^{-7}$M (e), trasylol 0,5% (f), 1:10 phenantroline 0.3 mM (g), PMSF 1 mM (h), and $ZnCl_2$ 200 μM (j). (i) shows endothelial cells cultured in presence of conditioned medium from mononuclear cells. The concentration of mononuclear cells was $3{,}5\times10^5$ cells/cm^2 when depleted of phagocytic cells and 4×10^5 when not depleted of phagoacytic cells.

labeled endothelial proteins (Fig. 2, lane i). These results indicated that the reduction of these proteins was dependent on direct cell contact between mononuclear and endothelial cells.

To examine whether the disappearance of high molecular weight proteins synthesized by endothelial cells when exposed to mononuclear cells reflects enzymatic degradation, the coculture experiments described in Figures 1 and 2, lanes a–c, were performed in the presence of protease inhibitors. As can be seen in Figure 2, lanes f and h, trasylol and PMSF exerted a partial inhibitory effect on the changes in protein pattern.

Identification of the 250- to 500-kD Proteins Affected by Mononuclear Cells as Fibronectin

The high molecular weight endothelial cell protein which disappeared during co-culture with mononuclear cells comigrated with iodinated plasma fibronectin (Fig. 3B).

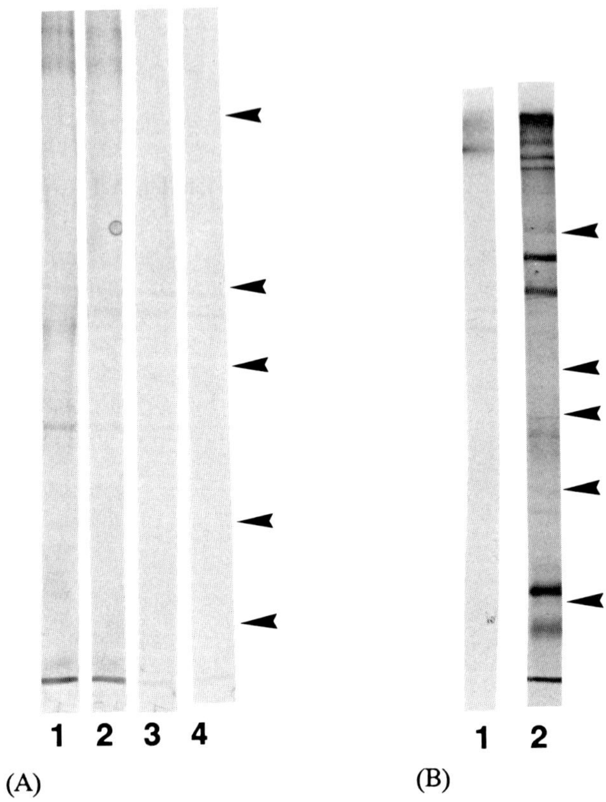

Figure 3 (A) Immunoblotting of endothelial cell medium proteins using two monoclonal anti-fibronectin antibodies (1,2) (Ist = 1 and 0 37 from Sera Lab), anti–Leu-4 (3) (Becton Dickinson), and PBS (4) as detected by a biotin-avidin peroxidase system. (B) Comigration of iodinated fibronectin (1) and high molecular weight biosynthetically labeled endothelial medium proteins (2).

Immunoblotting of the same material also demonstrated reactivity with antifibronectin antibodies (Fig. 3A). The high molecular weight protein, therefore, probably represents fibronectin.

DISCUSSION

These results indicate that mononuclear cells change the pattern of secreted proteins synthesized by endothelial cells and provoke disappearance of a high molecular weight protein which seems to be identical to fibronectin. Since the presence of monocytes rather counteracted the change in protein synthesis induced by the mononuclear cells, it appears likely that lymphocytes are responsible for the effect. The proteins detected in the endothelial cell medium probably represented secreted synthesized material because monensin (inhibitor of secretion) and cycloheximide (inhibitor of protein synthesis) prevented their appearance.

CONCLUSIONS

The present results suggest that lymphocytes have a fibronectin-degrading enzymatic function. Further investigations are required to elucidate whether this putative enzyme is related to previously characterized proteinases such as granzyme/TSP or perforine (7–10). However, TSP and perforine are released into the extracellular environment, whereas the activity responsible for disappearance of the high molecular weight endothelial protein from the present study is not.

ACKNOWLEDGMENT

This work was supported by the Swedish Heart and Lung Foundation, the Swedish Medical Research Council (project nr 16X-08295), and the Swedish Cancer Society (project nr 1940-B90).

REFERENCES

1. Marlin SD. Springer TA. Purified intercellular adhesion molecule-1 (ICAM-1) is a ligand for lymphocyte function-associated antigen 1 (LFA-1). Cell 1987. 51:813–19.
2. Makgoba MW. Sanders ME. Luce GEG. Dustin ML. Springer TA. Clark EA. Mannoni P. Shaw S. ICAM-1 a ligand for LFA-1 dependent adhesion of B, T and myeloid cells. Nature 1988. 331:86–88.
3. Elices JE. Osborn L. Takada Y. Crouse C. Luhowskyj S. Hemler ME. Lobb RR. VCAM-1 on activated endothelium interacts with the leucocyte integrin VLA-4 at a site distinct from the VLA-2/fibronectin binding site. Cell 1990. 60:577–84.
4. Osborne L. Hession C. Tizard R. Vassalo C. Luhowskyj S. Chi-Rosso G. Lobb R. Direct cloning of vascular cell adhesion molecule 1, a cytokine-induced endothelial protein that binds to lymphocytes. Cell 1989 59:1203–11.
5. Laemmli UK. Cleavage of structural proteins during the assembly of the head of bacteriophage T4. Nature 1970. 227:680-85.
6. Laskey RA. Mills AD. Quantitative film detection of 3H and 14C in polyacrylamide gels by fluorography. Eur J Biochem 1975. 56:335–41.
7. Simon MM. Hoschützky H. Simon HG. Kramer MD. Purification and characterization of a T-cell specific serine proteinase (TSP-1) from cloned cytolytic T-lymphocytes. EMBO J 1986. 5:3267–74.
8. Young JDE. Leong LG. Liu CC. Damiano A. Cohn ZA. Extracellulare release of lymphocyte cytolytic pore forming protein (perforin) after ionophore stimulation. Proc Natl Acad Sci USA 1986. 83:5668–72.
9. Held W. MacDonald HR. Mueller C. Expression of genes encoding cytotoxic cell-associated serine proteases in thymocytes. Int Immunol 1990. 2:57–62.
10. Masson P. Tschopp J. A family of serine esterases in lytic granules of cytolytic T-lymphocytes. Cell 1987. 49:679–85.

161
Lymphocyte Components with Fibronectin-like Properties

Dan Hauzenberger and Karl-Gösta Sundqvist
Huddinge University Hospital, Huddinge, Sweden

INTRODUCTION

T-Lymphocytes recirculate between an intravascular and an extravascular state in blood/lymph and lymphoid and nonlymphoid organs, respectively (1–4). Although lymphocytes in their extravascular state are surrounded by extracellular matrix (ECM) components, relatively little is known concerning lymphocyte interaction with these components. In support of the hypothesis that lymphocytes may interact with ECM, surface receptors for fibronectin (FN) and collagen have been demonstrated on certain cell lines and on circulating T cells (5–10). It has further been shown that lymphocytes have components, detectable by anti-FN antibodies, which have been implicated as playing a role in delayed hypersensitivity and motility (10–13). Taken together with the fact that denatured collagen, to which FN displays high-affinity binding, binds some of the anti-FN antigenicity and triggers motile behavior in lymphocytes, this points to the existence of a FN-like molecule in T lymphocytes. The present study is an analysis of the possible presence in and synthesis of FN or FN-like molecules by peripheral blood lymphocytes.

MATERIALS AND METHODS

Cell Preparations and Culture Conditions

Mononuclear cells were obtained from normal adult volunteers by centrifuging heparinized venous blood on a Lymphoprep gradient (Nycomed A/S, Oslo, Norway). Recovered cells in the interface were extensively washed, remaining erythrocytes were lysed with a buffer containing 0.15 M NH4Cl, 0.01 M KHCO3, and 0.1 M EDTA. Subsequently the remaining mononuclear cells were treated with carbonyl iron and phagocytic cells removed by a magnet. Recovered cell populations were resuspended in RPMI 1640 (Gibco Ltd., Paisley, Scotland) supplemented with 2 mM L-glutamine, 0.16% sodium bicarbonate, 100 IU benzyl penicillin, 100 μg streptomycin, and 10% fetal calf serum (FCS), if not otherwise stated. The cells were set up in a mixed lymphocyte culture (MLC) in Nunclon bottles. Cell viability as measured by trypan blue exclusion was >90% in all experiments.

35S-Methionine Labeling of Lymphocytes

The MLC-activated lymphocytes (5–7 days) were cultured under methionine-free conditions for 3 hr, whereas 10 μCi/ml culture medium L-35S-Methionine (>1000 Ci/mmol, Amersham Int., Bucks, England) was supplemented for 3 hr. After pulsing, the cells were lysed and centrifuged as described. The supernatant was immunoprecipitated with gelatin Sepharose. The methionine-labeled material was then separated on 6% SDS-PAGE gel. The slab gel was before drying enlighted, using EN3HANCE (Dupont Biotech. Systems, Boston, Massachusetts) for 30 min. Kodak X-Omat AR X-ray film was used for the fluorography.

Immunoprecipitation

Lymphocytes were radioiodinated with NA125 I (Amersham Int., Bucks, England) using the lactoperoxidase method as described (14). After iodination, the cells were lysed in an ice bath using a lysis buffer (0.5% NP 40, 50 mM TRIS, 5 mM EDTA, and 1 mM PMSF, pH 7.6) for 15 min. The lysed cells were then centrifuged at 3500 rpm, 25 min, 4°C. The lysed supernatant was immunoprecipitated with insolubilized collagen (Cytodex 3, Pharmacia Fine Chem., Uppsala, Sweden), gelatin Sepharose 4B (Pharmacia, Sweden) or monoclonal antibodies (037 and Ist-1 from Sera Lab. and anti–Leu-4 from Becton Dickinson); 75 μl of beads were incubated with 1 ml supernatant in conic centrifuge tubes for 13 hr at 4°C, whereafter the beads were extensively washed and transferred to sample buffer and boiled for 7 min.

Electrophoresis and Autoradiography

SDS-PAGE was carried out on vertical 6% slab gels according to the Laemmli procedure under nonreducing conditions (15). Reference proteins (Bio Rad) with molecular weights of 200, 116, 92, 66, and 45 kD were run simultaneously with the samples. Autoradiography of iodine labeled material separated using SDS-PAGE, was carried out after the gels were dried. Kodak X-Omat AR X-ray film was used for the autoradiography.

Immunoblotting

Lysed human lymphocytes (<1% monocytes, generally >90% T cells) were precipitated with gelatin Sepharose as described above. The material was then separated using 6% slab gels and transferred electrophoretically from the gel to nitrocellulose paper (0.45 μm, Kabi AB, Stockholm, Sweden). The transfer conditions, using the Bio Rad transblot apparatus, were similar to those described in the addendum to transblot cell operating instructions. Transfer was performed at 160 mA for 18 hr. The reactivity of monoclonal antibodies with the transferred proteins was determined by biotin-avidin-peroxidase staining.

RESULTS

Detection of Lymphocyte Surface Components with Insolubilized Collagen and Anti-FN Antibodies

The autoradiograms in Figure 1 show that immunoprecipitation with anti-FN antibodies (A) and insolubilized collagen (B) bound iodinated lymphocyte components with molecular weights of 200–250 and 400–500 kD, whereas the controls did not. Insolubilized collagen and the anti-FN antibody also bound iodinated 130- and 55-kD lymphocyte components. These lymphocyte surface components could be detected in freshly purified cells as well as in MLC-activated lymphocytes. Furthermore, insolubilized collagen inconstantly bound 90- and 150-kD bands. In order to show identity between the components precipitated with insolubilized collagen and anti-FN antibodies, Western immunoblotting of lymphocyte components precipitated with collagen (Fig. 2) was performed. It can be seen in Figure 2 that the anti-FN antibodies stained collagen binding components with molecular weights of 400 and 200–250 kD, whereas anti–Leu-4 and phosphate-buffered saline (PBS) did not. In other Western blot experiments the anti-FN antibodies stained the 55 and 130 kD components as well (not shown).

Biosynthesis of Collagen Binding Lymphocyte Molecules

In order to investigate the origin of the collagen binding molecules with fibronectin epitopes detected on lymphocytes, the possibility of lymphocytes synthesizing these components was tested. Figure 3 shows a fluorogram of collagen binding material from

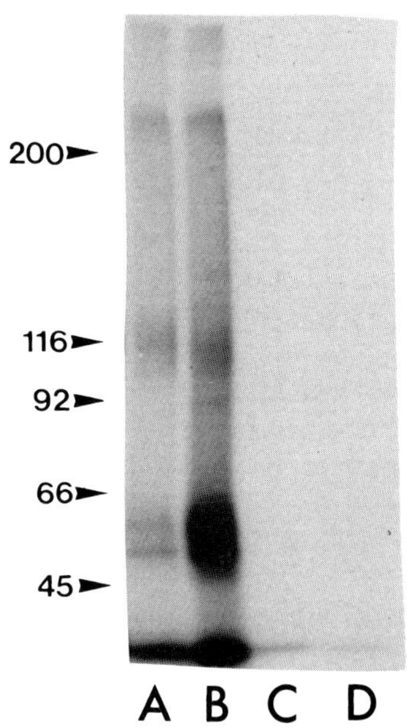

Figure 1 Autoradiogram of iodinated lymphocytes precipitated by the anti-FN antibody 037 (A), insolubilized collagen (B), anti–Leu-4 (C), and PBS (D).

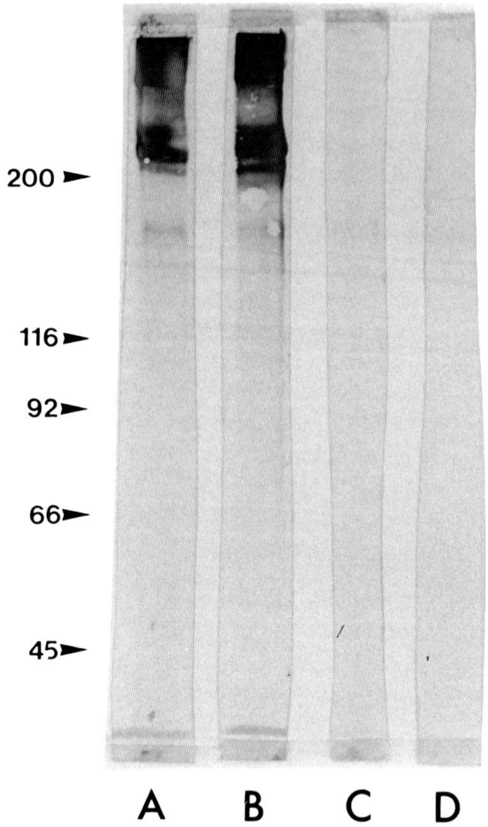

Figure 2 Western immunoblotting of collagen binding lymphocyte components. The collagen-precipitated material was transferred onto nitrocellulose and stained with anti-FN antibodies 037 (A) and Ist-1 (B) as well as with anti–Leu-4 (C) and PBS (D).

lymphocytes, which had been cultured in the presence of 35S-methionine for 3 hr. After separation of collagen binding lymphocyte components using 6% SDS-PAGE, the gel was dried and enlighted as described above. The fluorogram shows a major high molecular weight (MW 400–500 kD) and a minor 200–250 kD band (arrow), which both comigrate with two high molecular weight collagen binding lymphocyte components in a Western blot.

In the pulse chase experiment in Figure 4, lymphocytes were 35S-methionine labeled for 3 hr, whereafter unlabeled methionine (15 mg/L) was added. After harvesting portions of the cells at different times (see figure legend), the cells were precipitated with gelatin and separated using 6% SDS-PAGE. It can be seen that initially a high molecular weight band could be detected and that new bands appeared (arrows) during the 24-hr culture period as compared to the cells harvested directly after ending the pulse (A). Since the protein synthesis after ending the pulse was performed with unlabeled methionine, this result suggests processing or degradation of the high molecular weight gelatin binding components.

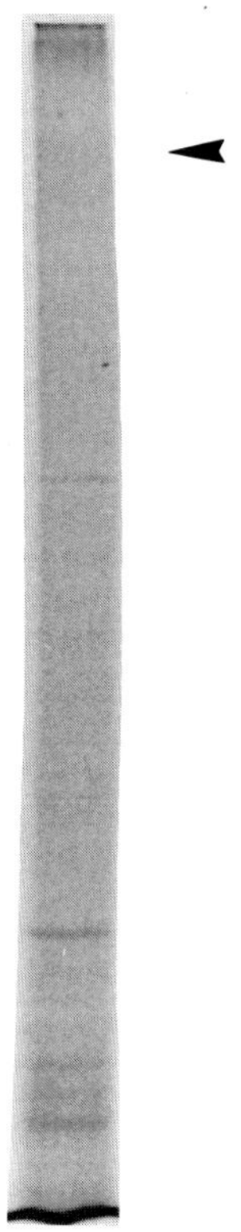

Figure 3 Fluorogram of 35S-methionine–labeled collagen binding lymphocyte material separated on 6% SDS-PAGE.

DISCUSSION

The present study demonstrates that peripheral lymphocytes have high molecular collagen binding components with a molecular weight of 200–250 and 400–500 kD which also react with anti-FN antibodies. These data may be compatible with the presence of FN or a related molecule in lymphocytes. Fluorograms of 35S-methionine–labeled lymphocyte components revealed that at least a portion of the high molecular weight fibronectinlike molecules detected in lymphocytes are synthesized by the cells.

The finding that lymphocytes have and also probably synthesize fibronectinlike molecules should be considered in the light of the fact that lymphocytes during part of their recirculation are tissue-bound cells and, therefore, are very likely to interact with ECM components. The fact that lymphocytes are recirculating cells assumes that the cells have to limit the time and extent of their interaction with the ECM. One possible mechanism for this limitation might be via proteolytic degradation of the receptor for ECM components or of the ligand for this receptor. One explanation for the appearance of new bands in the pulse chase experiment after ending the pulse period may be that lymphocytes degrade or process an endogenous high molecular weight collagen binding component into fragments with lower molecular weight. The regular appearance of gelatin binding components also

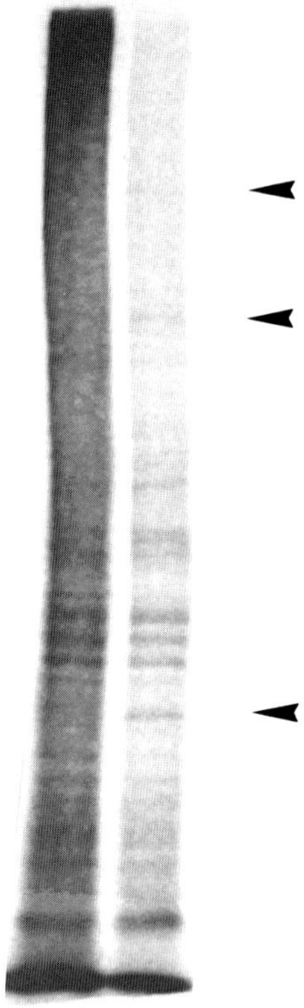

Figure 4 Pulse chase experiment of 35S-methionine–labeled lymphocytes. Lane A represents collagen binding lymphocyte components harvested 3 hr after ending the pulse, and lane B collagen binding lymphocyte material 24 hr after ending the pulse.

reacting with anti-FN antibodies may reflect the existence of a protease mechanism for rapid degradation of fibronectin or a related molecule.

ACKNOWLEDGMENTS

This work was supported by grants from the Swedish Cancer Society (1940-B90), the Swedish Medical Research Council (16X-08925), and the Foundation of King Gustav V.

REFERENCES

1. Ford W.L., Smith M.E. and Andrews P. Cell-cell recognition. *Symposia of the Society for Experimental Biology*. Cambridge University Press, London 1978 32:359.
2. De Dousa, M. *Lymphocyte Recirculation: Experimental and Clinical Aspects*. Wiley, New York, 1981.

3. Parrot, D.M.V., and Wilkinson P.C., Lymphocyte locomotion and migration. Prog. Allergy 1981 28:193.
4. Jalkanen, S., Reichert R.A., Gallatin W.M., Bargatze R.F., Weissman I.L., and Butcher E.C. Homing receptors and the control of lymphocyte migration. Immunol. Rev. 1986 91:39.
5. Bernardi P., Patel V.P., and Lodfish H.F., Lymphoid precursor cells adhere to two different sites on fibronectin. J. Cell. Biol. 1987 105:489.
6. Cardarelli P.M. and Pierschbacher M.D. Identification of fibronectin receptors on T lymphocytes. J. Cell. Biol. 1987 105:499.
7. Kurki P., Vartio T. and Virtanen I. Mitogen stimulation promotes human T lymphocyte adhesion to fibronectin. Scand. J. Immunol. 1987 26:645.
8. Liao N.S., St-John J., Du Z.J., and Cheung H.T. Adhesion of lymphoid cell lines to fibronectin-coated substratum: Biochemical and physiological characterization and the identification of a 140 kD fibronectin receptor. Exp. Cell Res. 1987 171:306.
9. Wayner E.A., Garcia-Pardo A., Humphries M.J., McDonald J.A. and Carter W.G. Identification and characterization of the T lymphocyte adhesion receptor for an alternative cell attachement domain (CS-1) in plasma fibronectin. J. Cell Biol. 1989 109:1321.
10. Arencibia I. and Sundqvist K.G. Collagen receptor on T lymphocytes and the control of lymphocyte motility. Eur. J. Immunol. 1989 19:929.
11. Godfrey H.P., Canfield L.S., Kindler H.L., Angadi C.V., Tomasek J.J., and Goodman J.W. Production of a fibronectin-associated lymphokine by cloned mouse T cells. J. Immunol. 1988 141:1506.
12. Godfrey H.P., Canfield L.S., Haak-Frendscho M., Melancon-Kaplan J., Brown E.J., and Kaplan A.P. Relationship of human macrophage agglutination factor to other fibronectins. Immunology 1989 57:1508.
13. Sundqvist, K.G. and Otteskog P. A labile antigen complex at the lymphocyte surface: The effect of the substratum on its expression. J. Immunol. 1987 138:825.
14. Haustein D. Effective radioiodination by lactoperoxidase and solubilization of cell surface proteins of cultured murine T lymphoma cells. J. Immunol. Methods 1975 7:25.
15. Laemmli U.K. Cleavage of structural proteins during the assembly of the head of bacteriophage T4. Nature 1970. 227:680.

162
Adhesion Between Hemopoietic Cell Lines and Human "Normal" and "Leukemic" Long-Term Bone Marrow Cultures

I. A. M. Denkers, R. H. J. Beelen, G. J. Ossenkoppele, A. J. M. de Jong, and M. M. A. C. Langenhuijsen
Free University, Amsterdam, The Netherlands

INTRODUCTION

Bone marrow stromal cells are critical for the proliferation and differentiation of hemopoietic stem cells (1–3). In order to describe the relation between hemopoietic cells and their local microenvironment in situ, we have studied the cellular composition of human long-term bone marrow cultures (HLTBMCs) and the adhesion of hemopoietic cells to these stromal cells. We are specially interested in the microenvironment of patients with acute myeloid leukemia. Therefore, we studied HLTBMCs established from bone marrow aspirates of healthy volunteers and untreated patients suffering from acute myeloid leukemia. These long-term bone marrow cultures (LTBMCs) were cultured for up to 6 weeks, and every week the stromal cells were stained with MGG and several defined antibodies (4).

Bone marrow stromal monolayers consist of fibroblasts, macrophages, fat cells, and other cells (endothelial cells, hemopoietic cells, and undefined cells) (5).

To study the adhesion of hemopoietic cells to stromal cells, hemopoietic cell lines were labeled with chromium-51 (6,7). The adhesion of hemopoietic cell lines to stromal cells was obtained by incubating them on 3-week HLTBMCs and their extracellular matrices (ECMs) for 2 hr.

MATERIALS AND METHODS

HLTBMCs and Their Cellular Composition

Bone marrow aspirates from eight healthy volunteers and 15 untreated adult patients with acute myeloid leukemia were obtained by aspiration from the posterior iliac crest and cultured as described by Gartner and Kaplan (8). Every week one stromal monolayer was trypsinized and cytocentrifuge preparations were made and stained with MGG and three monoclonal antibodies (TE7, CD14, EN4). Three main categories of cells could be distinguished: fibroblasts, macrophages, and other cells (endothelial cells, hemopoietic cells, and undefined cells). Fat cells were lost after trypsinization.

Chromium-51 Adhesion Assay

The HLTBMCs were established from the bone marrow (BM) of healthy volunteers and a patient with acute myeloid leukemia in 96-well plates. The ECMs of the stromas were prepared by incubation with 0.5% Triton–phosphate-buffered saline (PBS). Three hemopoietic cell lines were labeled with chromium-51: KG1 cell line, a myeloblastic cell line; HL60 cell line, a promyelocytic cell line, and HL60 cells stimulated with vitamin A, differentiated into a granulocytic direction. After labeling, 0.1×10^6 hemopoietic cells per well were layered onto the monolayer for 2 hr. The adherent cell fraction was measured by gamma counting.

RESULTS AND DISCUSSION

"Normal" HLTBMCs show during 6 weeks of culturing an increase of fibroblasts and a decrease of macrophages and other cells (Fig. 1). The results demonstrate that normal stromal cells consist of 58% fibroblasts and 29% macrophages in the first week. Both cell types reach a steady state and show a consistent development to 70 and 25% after 3 weeks of culture. Endothelial cells, hemopoietic cells, and undefined cells show a decline during 6 weeks toward 5%.

"Leukemic" stromas demonstrate a different pattern in the development of the cellular composition (Fig. 2). Leukemic HLTBMCs consist of 35% fibroblasts and 37% macrophages. Both cell types do not reach an equilibrium and show an inconsistent development. Endothelial cells, hemopoietic cells and undefined cells show also a decline during 6 weeks toward 5%.

These differences and the results of the chromium-51 adhesion assay may indicate that there are also differences in the adherence of hemopoietic cells to normal or leukemic stromal cells and their ECMs (Table 1). The adhesion experiment shows that 26.9% of the KG1 cell line attach to the normal HLTBMC and 1.2% of the cells to the ECM of the HLTBMC. Adherence of the KG1 cell line to a leukemic stroma is 27.7%, and 2.6% to the ECM. Adhesion of HL60 cells to normal stroma is 7%, and 1.3% to the ECM.

HL60 cells adhere 9.4% to leukemic stroma, and 1.9% to the ECM. HL60 cells stimulated with vitamin A show 4.8% adhesion to normal LTBMC, 1.2% to ECM, and 5.4% to leukemic HLTBMC, and 1.7% to the ECM. Immature cells (KG1) show more adherence than mature cells (HL60 and HL60 with vitamin A). There is a little difference between

Table 1 Adherence of Hemopoietic Cell Lines to Stromal Monolayers and ECM

	Normal stroma (%)	ECM (%)	Leukemic stroma (%)	ECM (%)
KG1	26.9	1.2	27.7	2.6
HL60	7.0	1.3	9.4	1.9
HL60 + vitamin A	4.8	1.2	5.4	1.7

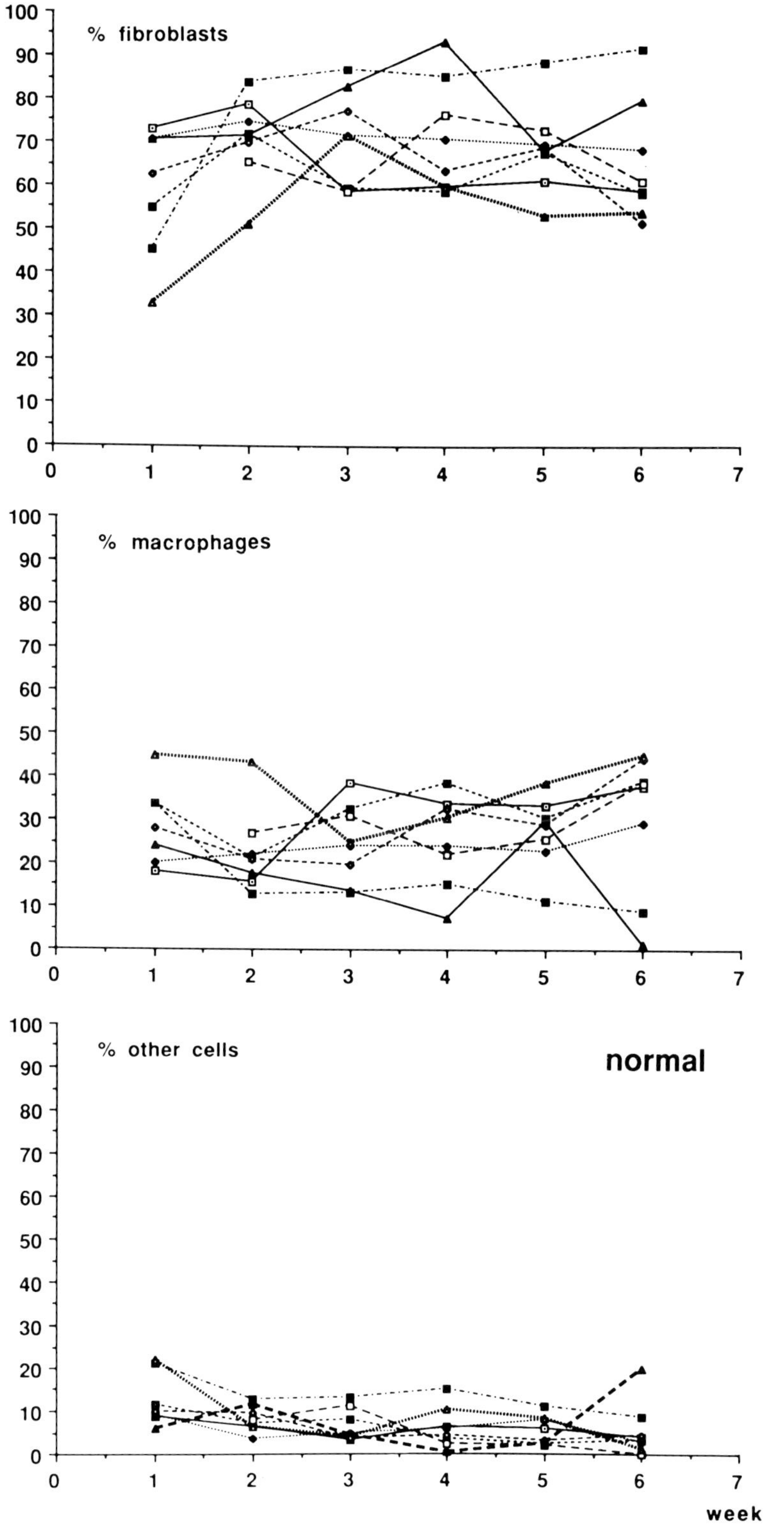

Figure 1 Each line represents the percentage of fibroblasts/macrophages/other cells in HLTBMCs of one healthy volunteer.

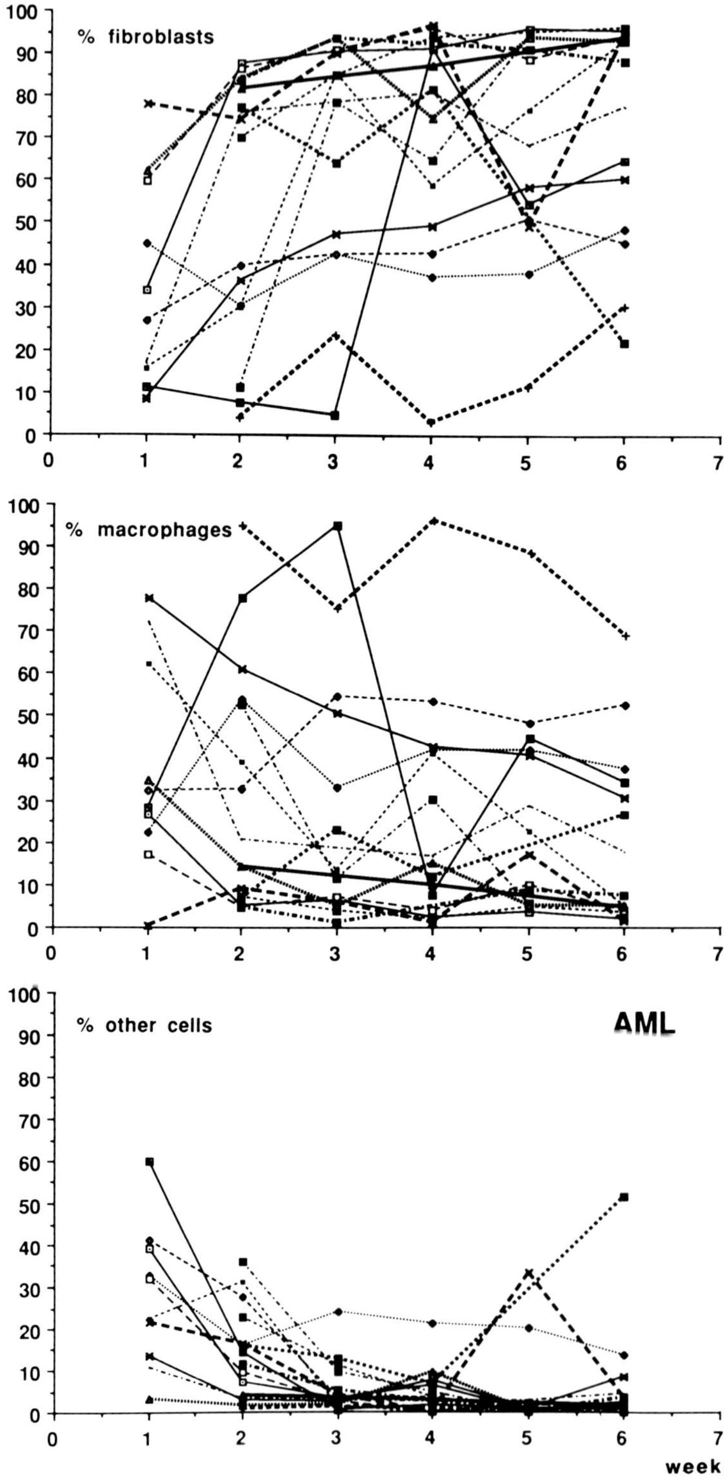

Figure 2 Each line represents the percentage of fibroblasts/macrophages/other cells in HLTBMCs of one patient with acute myeloid leukemia.

normal vs leukemic stromas. These results indicate a cell-cell interaction between the immature cell line and the stromal cells. Adhesion between hemopoietic cells and HLTBMC as also the mechanism by which this adhesion can be blocked are presently under study.

CONCLUSIONS

There is remarkable difference in the development of the cellular composition between normal and leukemic HLTBMCs, and there is also a remarkable difference in adhesion between stromal cells and their ECMs. Immature cells demonstrate more adhesion capacity than mature cells.

REFERENCES

1. Schölzel C, Löwenberg B. Stimulation of proliferation and differentiation of acute myeloid leukemia cells on a bone marrow stroma in culture. Exp. Hematol. 1985;13:664.
2. Iland HJ, Croaker GM, Repka E, Radloff TJ, Vincent PC. Long term bone marrow culture induces terminal differentiation of human myeloid leukemic cells. Exp. Hematol. 1987;15:1109.
3. Coulombel L, Eaves C, Kalousek D, Gupta C, Eaves A. Long term marrow culture of cells from patients with acute myelogenous leukemia. J. Clin. Invest. 1985;75:961.
4. Schiro R., Couthinho LH, Testa NG, Dexter TM. Effects of exogenous growth factors on stromal cells from human LTBMC. Tissue Antigens 1989;3:229.
5. Allen TD, Dexter TM. The essential cells of the hemopoietic microenvironment. Exp. Hematol. 1984;12:517.
6. Hocking WG, Golde DW. Long term human bone marrow cultures. Blood 1980;56:118.
7. Gordon MY. Adhesive properties of haemopoietic stem cells. Brit. J. Haematol. 1988;68:149.
8. Gartner S, Kaplan HS. Long-term culture of human bone marrow cells. Proc. Natl. Acad. Sci. U.S.A. 1980;8:4756.

163 Lymphocyte Homing in Mammary Neoplasia

Diana M. Lopez, Daniela Cideciyan, Krishna Rao, and Yee-Hon Chin
University of Miami School of Medicine, Miami, Florida

INTRODUCTION

Systemic changes in the phenotype and functions of lymphoreticular cells have been shown to occur in hosts with developing tumors. Profound alterations in the composition of the various lymphoid organs such as the lymph nodes, spleen, thymus, and bone marrow can be observed in mammary tumor–bearing mice (1,2). Furthermore, the tumors are infiltrated by immune-related cells that differ in their lineage representation of those in the peripheral organs (3). Lymphocyte migration from the blood into lymph nodes and other organs is not a random process. Rather, they depend on the specific interaction of lymphocyte adhesion molecules with specialized high endothelial cells lining postcapillary venules in secondary lymphoid organs (4). The specificity of these events could account for the selective homing of distinct lymphocyte subsets into the draining lymph nodes and neoplastic tissue in tumor bearers (3,5). The studies presented herein demonstrate alterations in the lymphocyte binding capacity of high endothelial venules (HEVs) from mucosal lymph nodes of mammary tumor–bearing mice. Furthermore, within the tumor mass itself there are specialized endothelial structures to which lymphocytes bind specifically. These findings indicate that lymphocyte traffic into mammary tumors and into lymphoid tissues may be regulated through similar lymphocyte-endothelial interactions.

BINDING OF LYMPHOCYTES FROM NORMAL AND TUMOR-BEARING MICE TO LYMPH NODE HEVs

Using an in vitro adherence assay we studied the effects of mammary tumor growth on lymphocyte binding to the endothelial cells lining the postcapillary venules of mesenteric and cervical lymph nodes, the first step for lymphocyte migration into these organs. Initial studies examined the adherence of splenic lymphocytes from normal and tumor-bearing mice to cervical lymph nodes (CLNs). No changes were observed in the level of binding of normal spleen lymphocytes to frozen sections of CLNs from normal mice as compared to those of tumor-bearing mice. Likewise, a kinetic analysis of the binding of tumor bearers' spleen lymphocytes to the same types of tissue revealed no differences in this parameter when contrasted with the binding of lymphocytes from control Balb/c mice. In sharp contrast were the results obtained when frozen sections of mesenteric lymph nodes (MLNs) were utilized in the assays (Table 1). Whereas spleen lymphocytes from both normal mice and tumor bearers were capable of binding efficiently to MLNs of control mice, there was a significant decrease in the adherence of tumor spleen cells to the MLNs of tumor-bearing animals when compared to the level of binding exhibited by splenocytes from normal mice. In kinetics studies (data not shown) it was found that the capacity of the MLNs to mediate tumor lymphocyte adherence was altered as early as 7 days post–tumor implantation and continued to be depressed until the animal's death.

A study of the expression of the MEL-14 antigen in the surface of normal and tumor-bearing mice showed no major alterations of the percentages of cells positive for this marker in the spleens of tumor bearers. Thus, these results indicate that the lymphocytes from mammary tumor–bearing animals may have a defect of some accessory adhesion molecule(s), which could be obscured by the strong binding with the major mucosal homing receptor, allowing for apparent normal binding to normal MLNs. However, the ligands of HEVs of the mucosal lymph nodes may have been modified by the tumor presence, thereby causing the selectivity altered autologous lymphocyte adhesion to MLNs without affecting their adherence to cervical lymph nodes.

SPECIALIZED ENDOTHELIAL STRUCTURES WITHIN MAMMARY TUMORS

We have previously shown a selective infiltration by certain lymphocyte subsets in mammary tumors (3). Histological examinations of cryostat sections of these tumors revealed the presence of vessels lined by flat endothelial tissue to which mononuclear cells bind. To investigate this adhesion phenomenon, frozen cryostat sections of line 410.4, a mammary tumor syngeneic to Balb/c mice, were tested for capacity to support lymphocyte binding using an in vitro assay. Splenic lymphocytes from both normal Balb/c mice, as well as 410.4 mammary tumor bearers, adhered to discrete areas within the tumor mass, albeit at

Table 1 Altered Binding Capacity of Splenic Lymphocytes from Tumor-Bearing Mice to HEVs from Tumor Bearers' Mesenteric Lymph Nodes

MLN sections	Lymphocyte source	Number of positive HEV[a]
Normal mice	Normal mice	20 ± 5
	Tumor bearers[b]	17 ± 4
Tumor bearers	Normal mice	25 ± 6
	Tumor bearers	4 ± 2

[a]Quantitation of positive HEvs in frozen sections of MLNs was accomplished by overlaying 0.2 ml aliquot of 3 ± 10^6 cells/ml per tissue section.
[b]The spleens of tumor bearers were removed 4 weeks after tumor implantation.

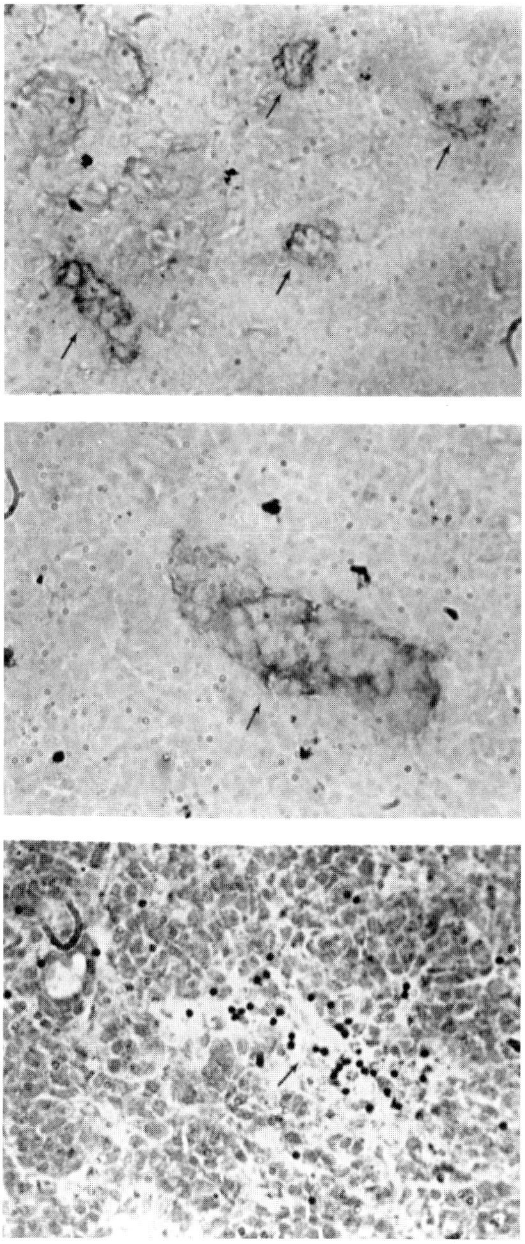

Figure 1 (Top) Adherence of splenic lymphocytes from normal Balb/c mice to frozen sections of tumors from the 410.4 tumor line. Note the pattern of lymphocyte adherence (arrows) to discrete areas. (Middle) Immunoperoxidase staining with rat antimouse HEV antibody of a frozen section from the 410.4 tumor line with arrows indicating the presence of positive venularlike structures. (Bottom) Lymphocyte binding to an adjacent frozen section to the one presented above. Lymphocytes adhered to discrete areas stained by the anti-HEV reagent.

different levels. To analyze the structures in the tumor mass that are binding the lymphoid cells, we utilized immunoperoxidase staining. We utilized an antibody developed in our laboratory obtained after repeated immunization of mouse mesenteric lymph node stromal tissue into Lewis rats. This reagent was shown to specifically stain mouse HEVs from cervical and mesenteric lymph nodes without reacting with other cells in the parenchyma. This antibody was found to stain discrete areas in the tumor frozen sections (Fig. 1, top panel). However, these tumor endothelial structures do not display the tall, columnar morphology characteristic of cells in HEVs. Interestingly, using sequential tissue sections in parallel immunoperoxidase staining and lymphocyte binding studies, it was found that the lymphoid cells bound to endothelial structures capable of reacting with the anti-HEV antibody (Fig. 7, middle and bottom panels). In addition, we have found evidence that the specialized structures react in immunoperoxidase assays with MECA-325 (a generous gift from Dr. Eugene Butcher), which is a monoclonal antibody previously shown to react with HEV antigens (6).

A further study, using three other types of mammary tumors, revealed that although these neoplasms supported adherence of lymphocytes, no discrete binding to specialized structures could be detected. However, when sequential immunoperoxidase and lymphocyte adhesion studies were performed, positive staining with the anti-HEV antibody was observed in the same tumor areas to which lymphocytes were bound. In all cases, the lymphocytes from normal mice were capable of binding in higher numbers to all four types of mammary tumors than spleen lymphocytes from tumor-bearing mice. These results indicate that the tumor lymphocyte adhesion phenomenon is not predicated in a previous priming of the lymphoid cells.

CONCLUSIONS AND SPECULATIONS

Our data indicate that mammary tumor development selectively alters tumor bearers' lymphocyte adhesion to their autologous MLNs without affecting their adherence to CLNs. Since the numbers of MEL-14–positive cells are not changed during tumorigenesis, it is tempting to speculate that two types of changes may have occurred: (a) the accessory adhesion molecules in lymphocytes of tumor bearers have been altered, and (b) the ligands on MLNs are likewise changed by the tumor development. Based on our discovery of specialized endothelial structures within the tumor capable of supporting lymphocytes adherence, we propose that initiation of extravasation of cells into nonlymphoid solid neoplasms is mediated by interactions between lymphocyte adhesion molecules and specific ligands present within the tumors. Such a mechanism could explain the observed regulation of tumor infiltration by lymphocytes which in turn would profoundly influence the final outcome of the host-tumor interactions.

ACKNOWLEDGMENT

This work was supported by NIH grant CA-25583.

REFERENCES

1. Lopez DM, Paul RD. Analysis of the lymphoid cells responding to viral and tumor associated antigens in spleen of syngeneic mouse mammary tumor systems with low and high oncogenic potentials. J. Natl. Cancer Inst. 1982 69:1403–1409.

2. Fu YX, Paul RD, Wang Y, Lopez DM. Thymic involution and thymocyte phenotypic alterations induced by murine mammary adenocarcinomas. J. Immunol. 1989, 143:4300–4307.
3. Buessow SC, Paul RD, Lopez DM. Influence of mammary tumor progression on phenotype and function of spleen and *in situ* lymphocytes in mice. J. Natl. Cancer Inst. 1984, 73:249–255.
4. Woodruff JJ, Clarke LM, Chin YH. Specific cell-adhesion mechanisms determining migration pathway of recirculating lymphocytes. Ann. Rev. Immunol. 1987, 5:201–222.
5. Farzad Z, Cochran AJ, McBride WH, Gray JD, Wong V, Morton DC. Lymphocyte subset alterations in nodes regional to human melanoma. Cancer Res 1990, 50:3585–3588.
6. Duijvestijn AD, Schreiber A, Butcher EC. Interferon-gamma induces an antigen specific for endothelium involved in lymphocyte homing. Proc. Natl. Acad. Sci. U.S.A. 1986, 83:9114–9118.

164

Migration of Hemopoietic Precursors Toward β_2-Microglobulin Is Involved in Thymus Colonization of Chicken Embryos

Dominique Dunon and Beat A. Imhof
Basel Institute for Immunology, Basel, Switzerland

INTRODUCTION

Colonization implies multiple events that occur en route from the location of hemopoietic precursor emergence to the thymic target tissue. In birds, the thymus is colonized in three waves during embryogenesis and the first days following hatching (Le Douarin et al., 1984; Coltey et al., 1987). For each wave, the first step is the accumulation of basophilic cells in the jugular vein, in capillaries, and in the mesenchyme surrounding the thymus. Cell surface homing receptors might be responsible for adhesion of these hemopoietic cells to the endothelium of thymic capillaries. Precursors extravasate into the perivascular space enriched with mesenchymal cells embedded in extracellular matrix. Integrins on the plasma membrane of precursors may be involved in the subsequent cell migration toward the thymic epithelial cells. These events might be governed by chemotactic molecules secreted by thymic stroma (Le Douarin, 1978). Evidence for chemotaxis of avian hemopoietic precursors from embryonic bone marrow was obtained initially by observing individual cells migrating in a Zigmond chamber (Ben Slimane et al., 1983). Bone marrow cells from 11.5-day-old quail embryos migrated toward a soluble gradient created by the secretory activity of an embryonic thymus. Locomotion of single cells was found to be oriented (chemotactically) when the cells were exposed to medium conditioned by a thymus explanted during its first colonization period. Chemotactic migration was not observed when the thymic rudiment was taken during the refractory state with respect to its colonization.

Chemotaxis was also suggested to be involved in mammalian thymic colonization (Imhof et al., 1989). Using an epithelial cell line from rat thymus (IT-45 RI), we purified a peptide exerting a chemotactic effect on rat hemopoietic precursors (Imhof et al., 1988). Recently, this peptide was identified as β_2-microglobulin (β_2m) (Dargemont et al., 1989). Rat hemopoietic cells responding to β_2m were resting cells and could acquire T-cell markers in coculture experiments (Deugnier et al., 1989).

In this chapter we correlate the β2m chemotactic activity with the second wave of thymus colonization in chicken embryos.

RESULTS AND DISCUSSION

Bone Marrow Cells Migrating Toward β2-Microglobulin Are Enriched in Pre–T Cells

It had already been shown that avian bone marrow cells from 13.5-day-old embryos (during the second wave of thymus colonization) were able to migrate toward a thymus (Jotereau et al., 1980; Ben Slimane et al., 1983; Champion et al., 1986). These cells responded with a maximal chemotactic effect when the chicken β2m concentration was 3×10^{-11} M in the lower compartment of the migration chamber (Dunon et al., 1990a).

Cells attracted by β2m and embryonic bone marrow cells at this stage have been found to be negative for T- and B-cell differentiation markers (CD4, CD8, T3, and immunoglobulin M [IgM]) confirming their immature phenotype. Since antigens present solely on prethymic cells have not yet been described, a functional differentiation assay was used to show that these cells were truly lymphoid precursors. In vivo differentiation was tested in chickens congenic for the antigen of expressed on thymocytes and mature T cells (H.B19ov-positive, H.B19ov-negative). Bone marrow cells from 13.5-day-old H.B19-positive embryos were injected, after chemotactic migration toward chicken β2m, into 13-day-old H.B19ov-negative embryos (second wave of thymus colonization). The advantage of such studies is that host embryos can be taken without irradiation or drug treatment, and that injected donor precursors compete with endogenous cells for thymus homing. The thymus of injected H.B19ov-negative animals was subsequently analyzed for of-positive cells 5 or 7 days after hatching (Table 1). Bone marrow cells that migrated toward β2m colonized the thymus and expressed the T-cell marker CD8, whereas control cells did not.

Moreover, hemopoietic precursors were prepared from embryonic bone marrow at different stages of embryogenesis and submitted to the chemotactic activity of β2m. Interestingly, the number of β2m-responsive cells in our assay presented a peak during the second wave of thymus colonization (Fig. 1).

Analysis of β2-Microglobulin Expression During Thymus Colonization

Northern blot experiments revealed that the first organ to express large amounts of β2m messenger ribonucleic acid (mRNA) was the thymus. The peak of β2m transcription revealed by the scanning of the autoradiography coincided in time with the start of the second wave of thymus colonization (see Fig. 1). During this period, only low levels of β2m transcripts were observed in all other studied organs.

Staining of frozen sections with A4G2, an antibody which binds only the free β2m form, showed that only the thymus and to a lesser extent the bursa are positive for this antigen during embryogenesis. In concordance with the northern blot experiments, a peak of free β2m is also detected at the beginning of the second period of thymus colonization (see Fig. 1). Although major histocompatibility complex (MHC) class I antigens were detected in the thymus by day 10 of embryogenesis (Dunon et al., 1990b), double-staining experiments showed that a large subset of free β2m-positive cells was MHC class I heavy chain negative. This result suggests that this subset secretes really β2m in its free form.

Table 1 Competitive Thymus Colonization by β2-Microglobulin Responding Cells from Congenic Embryos

	Time after hatching	Control animals		H.B19ov$^+$ cells injected into H.B19ov$^-$ animals			
				Total bone marrow	Precursors enriched bone marrow	After migration toward	
		H.B19ov$^-$	H.B19ov$^+$			β^2m	Control medium
Gated for immature thymocytes	5 days	3	45	2	5.4	27.5	1.7
	7 days	2.5	66	2.9	2.8	16	3
Gated for mature thymocytes	5 days	5.5	43	3.7	5	9	3.3
	7 days	6.5	61	1.5	2.4	17	1.8

H.B19ov$^+$ (expressing ov antigen) and H.B19ov$^-$ (deficient for expression of ov antigen) are of two congenic strains. Total bone marrow cells, precursors enriched bone marrow on BSA gradient, and precursors selected by chemotactic migration toward β2-microglobulin from 13.5-day-old H.B19ov$^+$ embryos were injected in H.B19ov$^-$ embryos. Each embryo received 5 ± 10^4 cells. Animals were sacrificed at day 5 or 7 after hatching and cell surface expression of ov antigen on their thymocytes were studied by flow fluorometry. The results are expressed as percentage of ov$^+$ thymocytes. This table corresponded to one representative experiment based on 24 animals. Four independent experiments were performed and provided similar results.

β$_2$m-Microglobulin Chemotactic Activity Could Be One of Several Redundant Mechanisms Supporting Thymus Colonization

Figure 1 shows that the timing of the second wave of thymus colonization is correlated to expression of β2m and to a peak of β2m-responsive cells in our chemotactic assay. We have also shown that high amounts of β2m transcripts and free β2m are present only in the thymus of chicken embryos during the second wave of colonization. We conclude that chemotactic activity of β2m plays a role in the second wave of colonization.

However, the step of colonization involving the β2m chemotactic activity appears to be supported by different molecular processes. Recently, two groups obtained mice which totally lack β2m using homologous recombination in stem cells, and such mice have a normal-sized thymus (Ziljstra et al., 1990; Koller et al., 1990). If the chemotactic activity of β2m plays the same role in chicken and mouse thymus colonization, then the work of these two groups implies that at least two redundant mechanisms support the migration of hemopoietic precursors. Several clues are in agreement with this hypothesis. It has already been shown that during embryogenesis chicken thymus secretes different chemotactic molecules attracting hemopoietic precursors (Ben Slimane et al., 1983; Champion et al., 1986). In addition, extracellular matrix molecules are used as tracks during migration of hemopoietic precursors, and homing molecules are also probably present on the vascular endothelium. Thus, these different molecules should be involved in different processes supporting the colonization of thymus.

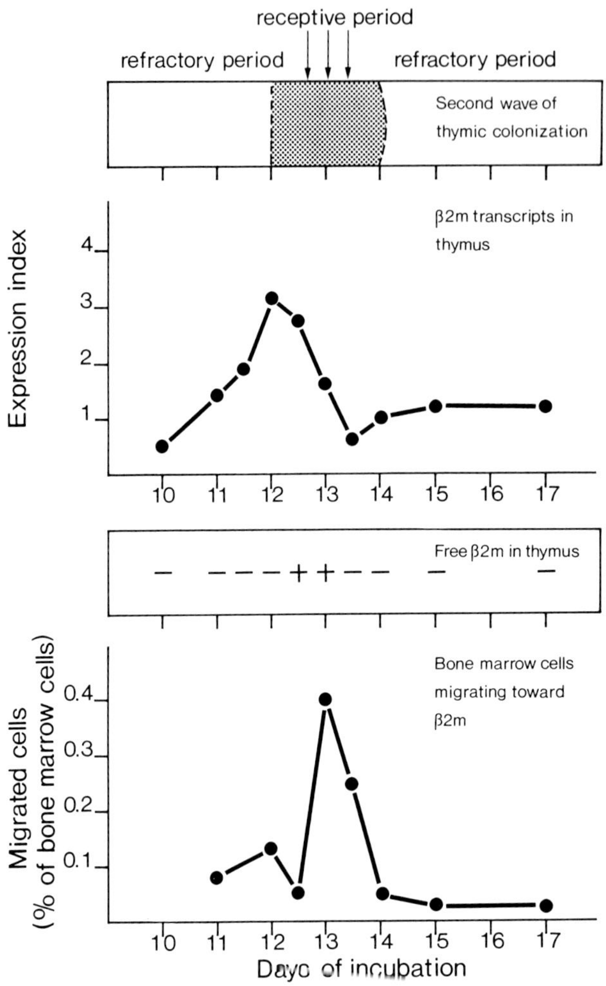

Figure 1 β2m expression and β2m chemotactic activity during the second wave of thymus colonization. Quantification of 1.3-kb β2m transript in the thymus during embryogenesis was performed by scanning of the Northern blot autoradiography after standardization (Dunon et al., 1990a). Detection of free β2m on thymus section was obtained by peroxidase immunostaining using antibody which detects only β2m in its free form. The percentage of bone marrow cells migrating toward β2m at a concentration of around 3 ± 10^{-11} M in our assay (Imhof et al., 1990) was calculated for each different stage of embryogenesis.

ACKNOWLEDGMENTS

We thank Brigitte Riwar and Barbara Hesse for technical assistance, and Hanspeter Stahlberger for artwork. The Basel Institute for Immunology was founded and is supported by F. Hoffmann–La Roche, Switzerland.

REFERENCES

Ben Slimane, S., Houllier, F., Tucker, G. and Thiery, J.P. In vitro migration of avian hemopoietic cells to the thymus: Characterization of a chemotactic mechanism. Cell Differ. 1983; 13:1–24.

Champion, S., Imhof, B., Savagner, P. and Thiery, J.P. The embryonic thymus produces chemotactic peptides involved in the homing of hemopoietic precursors. Cell 1986; 44:781–90.

Coltey, M., Jotereau, F.V. and Le Douarin, N.M. Evidence for a cyclic renewal of lymphocyte precursor cells in the intraembryonic chick thymus. Cell Differ. 1987; 22:71–82.

Dargemont, C., Dunon, D., Deugnier, M.A., Denoyelle, M., Girault, J.M., Lederer, F., Le, K. H. D., Godeau, F., Thiery, J.P. and Imhof, B.A. Thymotaxin, a chemotactic protein, is identical to β2-microglobulin. Science 1989; 246:803–6.

Deugnier, M.A., Imhof, B.A., Bauvois, B., Dunon, D., Denoyelle, M. and Thiery, J.P. Characterization of rat T cell precursors sorted by chemotactic migration toward thymotaxin. Cell 1989; 56: 1073–83.

Dunon, D., Kaufman, J., Salomonsen, J., Skjoedt, K., Thiery, J.P. and Imhof, B. A. T-cell precursor migration toward β2-microglobulin is involved in thymus colonization of chicken embryos. EMBO J., 1990a; 9:3315–3322.

Dunon, D., Salomonsen, J., Skjødt, K., Kaufman, J. and Imhof, B.A. Ontogenic appearance of MHC class I (B-F) antigens during embryogenesis. Dev. Immunol. 1990b; 1:127–135.

Imhof, B.A., Deugnier, M.A., Girault, J.M., Champion, S., Damais, C., Itoh, T. and Thiery, J.P. Thymotaxin: A thymic epithelial peptide chemotactic for T-cell precursors. Proc. Natl. Acad. Sci. U.S.A. 1988; 85:7699–703.

Imhof, B.A., Deugnier, M.A., Bauvois, B., Dunon, D. and Thiery, J.P. Properties of pre-T cells and their chemotactic migration to the thymus. In: *Thymus Update*. Vol. 1 (Kendall, M.D., and Ritter, M.A., eds.). 1989; pp. 3–19.

Imhof, B.A., Dargemont, C., Deugnier, M.-A. and Dunon, D. A chemotactic assay compatible with the recovery of cells after migration. In: *Immunological Methods IV* (Lefkovits, I., and Pernis, B. eds.). Academic Press, Orlando, Florida, 1990; 235–249.

Jotereau, F.V., Houssaint, E. and Le Douarin, N.M. Lymphoid stem cell homing to the early thymic primordium of the avian embryo. Eur. J. Immunol. 1980; 10:620–7.

Koller, B.H., Marrack, P., Kappler, J.W. and Smithies, O. Normal development of mice deficient in β2m, MHC class I proteins and CD8+ T cells. Science 1990; 248:1227–1230.

Le Douarin, N.M. (1978). Ontogeny of hematopoietic organs studied in avian embryo interspecific chimeras. In: *Differentiation of Normal and Neoplastic Hematopoietic Cells*. Cold Spring Harbor, New York, pp. 5–31.

Le Douarin, N.M., Jotereau, F.V., Houssaint, E. and Thiery, J.P. Primary lymphoid organ ontogeny in birds. In *Chimeras in Developmental Biology*. (Le Douarin N.M., and McLaren A., eds.). Academic Press, New York, 1984, pp. 179–216.

Zijlstra, M., Bix, M., Simister, N.E., Loring, J.M., Raulet, D.H. and Jaenisch, R. β2-Microglobulin deficient mice lack CD4–CD8^{+} cytolytic cells. Nature, 1990; 344:742–746.

165
Kinetics of B-Cell Emigration from the Chicken Bursa of Fabricius

Olli Lassila
Turku University, Turku, Finland

INTRODUCTION

The avian bursa of Fabricius provides a unique model to study different steps in the B-cell development (1). To fulfill its function, i.e., immunoglobulin (Ig) V-gene diversification, it is colonized by committed B-cell precursors from the embryonic mesenchyme between days 8 and 14 of incubation. Antibody variability is generated by somatic gene conversion in the developing bursa (2). Within bursal follicles the B cells proliferate extensively (8–12 hr per generation) (3). Between days 13 and 17 of incubation the time for doubling the cell population corresponds to the cell cycle time indicating that cell death and/or export does not occur. Bursal cell traffic to other sites of the body starts to occur at 18 days of incubation and this export continues during the functional maturation of the avian B-cell compartment in the newly hatched period, decreasing by the time of bursal involution (4).

In the present study emigration of B cells from the chicken bursa of Fabricius was evaluated by local in situ labeling of bursal cells by fluorescein isothiocyanate (FITC). The results demonstrate that only a small fraction of daily turnover of the cells leave the organ. These results indicate that in spite of a very rapid rate of bursal cell birth, relatively few cells are exported to the periphery, the majority dying in situ in the bursa.

MATERIALS AND METHODS

Experimental Design

Inbred chicks of various ages were labeled with FITC via anal route. After 3–18 hr, the chickens were bled and killed, and the number of FITC-positive cells among mononuclear cells of blood, bursa, thymus, and spleen were counted as previously described (5).

RESULTS

Phenotype of Bursal Emigrants

The FITC solution was applied to the anal lips of the chicks. Anal sucking movements were able to transport the dye into the bursal lumen, where it was further transported through the follicle-associated epithelium into the bursal follicles. Within minutes it stained the bursal cells both in the medulla and the cortex. By characterizing these FITC-labeled bursa-derived cells outside of the bursa with various B-cell–specific monoclonal antibodies like anti-μ, anti-λ, anti-Bu-1, anti-γ, or anti-α showed that practically all labeled cells were phenotypically B lymphocytes. In the blood and the spleen, the recent emigrants were exclusively IgM isotype–bearing cells.

Rate of Cell Export

In the peripheral blood, the number of FITC-positive cells doubled between 3 and 6 hr after per bursam labeling. The data in Table 1 show the estimation of the number of bursal emigrants/day of chickens at 2–3 weeks of age. These estimates give the value of 10^7 migrants/100 g of body weight, or 4–5% of all the cells in the bursa at that time. These values are based on an assumption that there is a linear increase of emigrants in the blood and that the migrants observed in other organs, like spleen, are coming via blood circulation. These results demonstrate that only a small proportion of the bursal cells leave the organ.

DISCUSSION

The present study indicates that the majority of the bursal cells die in the bursa after a short lifespan. However, what are the reasons for this kind of overproduction has not yet been established. We assume that during the embryonic colonization, the bursa positively selects precursor cells, which have functionally rearranged and expressed germ line–encoded immunoglobulin molecules on the cell surface (6,7). B cells in the bursa are immature, they proliferate in an antigen-independent manner, and antibody diversity is generated in the bursa within a population of surface Ig-expressing cells by a somatic gene conversion. Because each gene conversion event can lead to multiple amino acid changes in the V region and the process starts already during embryonic development (2), it is most unlikely that exogenous antigens are required for the induction of diversification (8). It has been estimated that the rate of productive gene conversion event may be in the order 1 per

Table 1 Estimation of the Number of Bursal Emigrants

Age (days)	No. of FITC + ve cells/10^6 PBLs	No. of PBLs (10^{-6})	No. of bursal emigrants into PBLs/24 hr (10^{-6})	No. of bursal cells (10^{-6})	% of emigration of bursa cells/day
10	6400	60	3.1	93	3.1
17	9810	180	14.1	254	5.5

Values are obtained after in situ FITC labeling following quantitation of PBLs 3 hr later. Values for 24 hr were obtained by multiplying by 8 and by the total number of PBLs.

10–15 cell divisions (2). The high bursa cell death might be thus due to abortive gene conversion events. This model would indicate that the selection of the bursal cells to maturity and to export represents the overall efficiency to form an Ig antigen receptor that is structurally sound to be able to deal with the antigen outside of the bursa.

Another possibility is that the immature B cells in the bursa are selected negatively by autoantigens. Immature bursal cells may be sensitive to the engagement of a surface Ig (sIg) receptor by autoantigens, which would signal deoxyribonucleic acid (DNA) degradation and cell death through the endogenous pathway of apoptosis (9). Activation of this process in immature bursal cells by the binding of the Ig receptor to self-antigens may, therefore, be the mechanism which produces clonal deletion and consequently self-tolerance in a similar was as in the thymus (10).

REFERENCES

1. Pink JRL, Lassila O. B cell commitment and diversification in the bursa of Fabricius. Curr Topics Microbiol Immunol 1987; 135:54–64.
2. Weill JC, Reynaud CA. The chicken B cell compartment. Science 1987; 238:1094–8.
3. Lydyard PM, Grossi CE, Cooper MD. Ontogeny of B cells in the chicken. I. Sequential development of clonal diversity on the Bursa. J Exp Med 1976; 144:79–87.
4. Woods R, Linna TJ. The transport of cells from the bursa of Fabricius to the spleen and the thymus. Acta Pathol Microbiol Scand 1965; 64:470–6.
5. Lassila O. Emigration of B cells from chicken bursa of Fabricius. Eur J Immunol 1989; 19:955–8.
6. McCormack W, Tjoelker L, Carlson L, Petryniak B, Barth C, Humphries E, Thompson C. Chicken IgL gene rearrangement involves deletion of a circular episome and addition of single nonrandom nucleotides to both coding segments. Cell 1989; 56:785–91.
7. Mansikka A, Sandberg M, Lassila O, Toivanen P. Rearrangement of immunoglobulin light chain genes in the chicken occurs prior to the colonization of the embryonic bursa of Fabricius. Proc Natl Acad Sci USA 1990; 87:9410–20.
8. Lassila O, Lefkovitz I, Alanen A. Immunoglobulin diversification in bursal duct ligated chickens. Eur J Immunol 1989; 19:1343–5.
9. Duvall E, Wyllie AH. Death and the cell. Immunol Today 1986; 7:115–9.
10. Smith CA, Williams GT, Kingston R, Jenkinson EJ, Owen JJT. Antibodies to CD3/T-cell receptor complex induce death by apoptosis in immature T cells in the thymic cultures. Nature 1989; 337:181–3.

166
T-Lymphocyte Precursors Adhere to Thymic Endothelium

Patricia Ruiz, Dominique Dunon, Barbara Hesse, and Beat A. Imhof
Basel Institute for Immunology, Basel, Switzerland

INTRODUCTION

Colonization of the mouse thymus by hemopoietic cells occurs mainly during ontogeny and development. However, influx of such cells may continue during adult life but at a very low level (Scollay et al. 1986; Kyewski, 1987; Savagner et al. 1988). Homing of T-lymphocyte precursors implies complex molecular events including transportation of precursors from their site of emergence via blood circulation to the thymus (Savagner et al., 1986). Ample evidence suggest that extravasation of precursors from the perithymic endothelium to the thymus is guided in part by a chemotactic mechanism exerted by a gradient of free β_2-microglobulin (Imhof et al. 1988; Dunon et al. 1990; Chapter 164). One of the essential steps in this process is the adhesion of precursors, present in the blood vessel, to the perithymic vascular endothelium.

Cell-cell interaction between mature hemopoietic cells and endothelium has been extensively studied and three structural classes of molecules have been found to be involved. Mel-14, ELAM-1, and PADGEM/GMP-140 belong to the group of lectin binding, so-called the selectin family. ICAM-1, ICAM-2, VCAM-1/INCAM-110, and PECAM-1/EndoCAM (Albelda et al., 1990; Osborne, 1990; Springer, 1990) belong to the group designated as cell adhesion molecules (CAMs) and more widely to the Ig superfamily. Most of these molecules can be induced to be expressed on certain endothelium by tissue inflammation in vivo or by cytokine treatment in vitro. The third type of molecules, the integrins, are widely distributed on different issues, mediating cell-cell as well as cell-substrate contacts. They consist of an α and a β subunit with seven β chains characterized to date (Osborne, 1990).

In contrast, interaction of hemopoietic precursors with endothelium during development is still an untapped field and nothing is known about the adhesive molecules involved. In the present study, we focused our interest on the homing molecules involved in the binding of hemopoietic precursors present in the blood stream on the thymus endothelium. In order to carry out biochemical studies, we established an in vitro model using hemopoietic precursors and endothelial cell lines. Various precursor cell lines have been tested for their binding capacity on frozen sections of thymus. The selected cells were used for binding studies on endothelial cell lines of thymic origin, and antibodies against known adhesion molecules have been tested for their blocking activities. Furthermore new functional monoclonal antibodies against endothelium have been produced and antigen expression on the various cell lines studied.

MATERIALS AND METHODS

Cells

The pro–T-cell line FT-F1 obtained from R. Palacios was produced and described in Pelkonen et al. (1987). The cells were grown in culture medium in the presence of interleukin-2 (IL-2). Endothelial cells eEnd.2 (derived from mouse embryo) and tEnd.1 (derived from mouse thymus) are both endothelioma cell lines containing the polyoma middle T oncogene, and have been described in Williams et al. (1989).

FITC Coupling to pro–T Cells

Fluorescein isothiocyanate (FITC) (Sigma, St. Louis, Missouri) was prepared as a 25.7-mM stock solution in dimethylsulfoxide (DMSO) (Fluka, Buchs, Switzerland) and processed as previously described (Imhof et al., 1990). Briefly: 100 μl stock solution was added to 900 μl cell suspension containing 5-40 × 10^6 cells in Dulbecco's modified Eagle's medium (DMEM) and incubated at 4°C for 15 min in the dark. Labeled cells were then centrifuged through a layer of 5 ml 10% bovine serum albumin (BSA) for 15 min at 460 g at room temperature. Cells were washed with DMEM and viability tested using trypan blue.

Adhesion Assays

Endothelial cells were seeded into 96-well Costar microtiter plates (3×10^4 cells/well) and cultured for 24 hr. After removing the medium, FITC-labeled pro–T cells were coincubated (10^5 cells/200 μl) for 2 hr at 20°C. Unbound cells were then removed from the endothelia by washing three times with Dulbecco's phosphate-buffered saline (PBS) (DPBS) containing 1% BSA by flicking the plates. Fluorescence, corresponding to bound cells, was measured by a Titertek Fluoroskan II reader in DPBS only (Imhof et al., 1990).

In situ binding was performed on freshly prepared frozen section from newborn mouse tissue. Organs were embedded and frozen in Tissue-Tek, O.C.T. Compound (Miles Inc., Elkhart, Indiana), sectioned to 5 μm, and then mounted onto glass slides. The sections were outlined by a PapPen (SCI Science Services, Munich, West Germany) and immediately placed into DPBS containing 1% BSA for at least 10 min. Slides were dried around the PapPen marked area and the tissue section then loaded with 10^5 pro–T cells in 200 μl. Binding was allowed to occur for 40 min at 8°C on a mini-shaker Kühner (Basel, Switzerland) at 50 rpm. Slides were then vertically placed into DPBS containing 0.5% glutaraldehyde and 2% formaldehyde. After 20 min of fixation at room temperature, pro–T cells bound to the tissue section were counted under a microscope.

Immunofluorescence

Frozen sections were fixed with acetone and labeled with hybridoma supernatant from the monoclonal antibody EA-1 raised against eEnd.2 cells, followed by an FITC-conjugated goat-antirat IgG antibody (Jackson Immuno Research, West Grove, Pennsylvania).

RESULTS AND DISCUSSION

Hemopoietic T-Cell Precursor Cell Binds to Frozen Sections of Thymus

Hemopoietic precursor cells were studied for their capacity to bind to frozen sections of newborn mouse thymus (Stamper and Woodruff assay; Woodruff et al., 1987). Among tested lines, the pro–T cell, FT-F1, adhered with good efficiency to thymic blood vessels (Fig. 1). The cells bound in groups preferentially to the larger vessels in the region of the thymic corticomedullary junction. Pro–T cells bound also to frozen sections of newborn mouse liver. On all other tested organs pro–T cells did not adhere; i.e., binding seemed to be specific for lymphoid organs. However, statistical analysis revealed that twice as many cells bound to the thymus as to the liver, suggesting a specific homing mechanism for pro–T cells to the thymus.

By testing several established endothelial cell lines as a possible binding partner for FT-F1 cells, we found eEnd.2 (derived from 12-day-old mouse embryos) and tEnd.1 (derived from the thymus of newborn mice) to be most efficient. Attempts to induce a higher binding capacity by treatment of the endothelium with cytokines failed. By contrast, endothelial cells cocultured with thymic epithelia doubled their capacity for pro–T cell binding (Fig. 2a). Thymic epithelial cells alone did not bind pro–T cells.

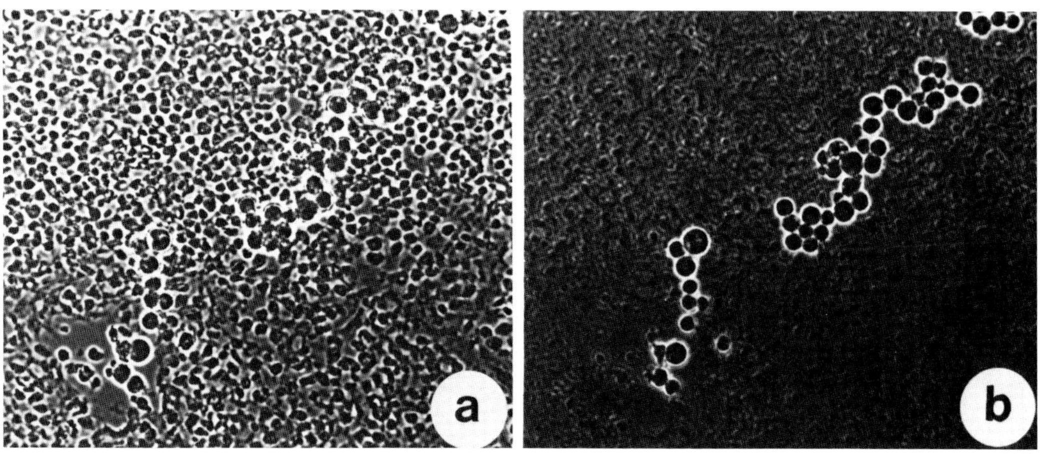

Figure 1 Binding of FT-F1 pro–T cells to frozen sections of newborn thymic tissue using phase contrast microscopy. (a) Level of focus is on thymic tissue; (b) level of focus is on pro–T cells. Note that pro–T cells bound in the region of a thymic capillary.

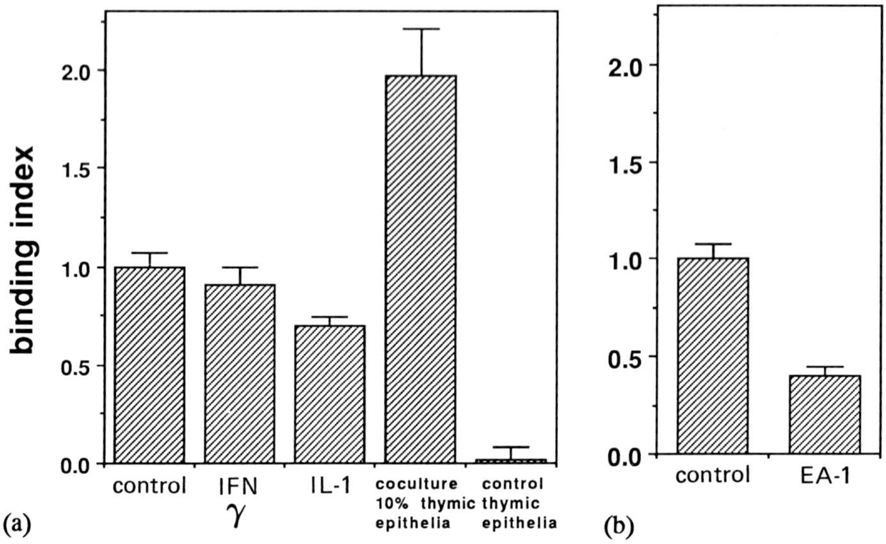

Figure 2 Binding of FT-F1 cells on endothelial monolayer. (a) Influence of culturing in the presence of IFN-γ, IL-1 or thymic epithelial cells on binding capacity. (b) Effect of adding antibody EA-1.

These results suggest that homing to the thymus may use molecular mechanisms different from those extensively described for lymphocyte adhesion to endothelia mediated by inflammation.

Monoclonal Antibody Inhibiting Pro–T-Cell Adhesion to Endothelium

To try to identify molecules involved in homing to the thymus, we prepared monoclonal antibodies in rats against the two endothelial cell lines (embryonic and thymic) and tested them for functional activity. Antibody EA-1 blocked binding of FT-F1 cells to tEnd.1 endothelial cells (Fig. 2b). Experiments are presently underway to determine the exact nature of this blocking activity. The results from these studies may lead to the understanding of embryonic homing mechanisms involved in pattern formation. Whether adhesion molecules which participate in cell-cell adhesion of mature hemopoietic cells with endothelium play a role during embryogenesis remains to be determined.

ACKNOWLEDGMENTS

We thank Dr. Marie Kosco for help with the production of monoclonal antibodies and for critical reading of the manuscript. Dr. Ron Palcacios for giving FT-F1 cells, and Dr. Erwin Wagner for the endothelial cells. The Basel Institute for Immunology was founded and is supported by Hoffmann–La Roche & Co. Ltd., Switzerland.

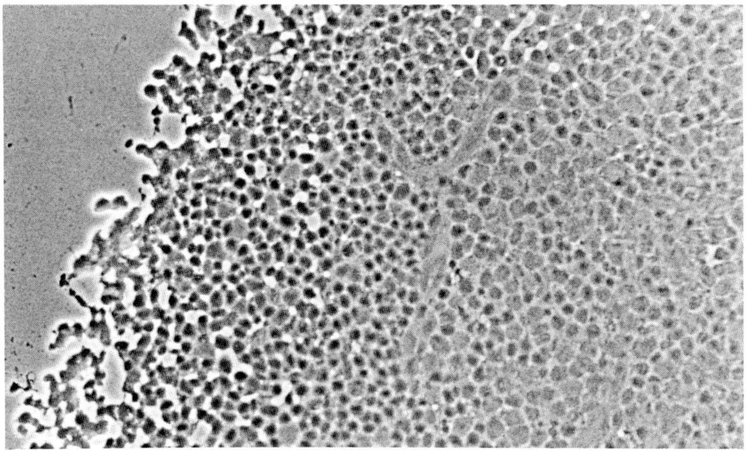

(a)

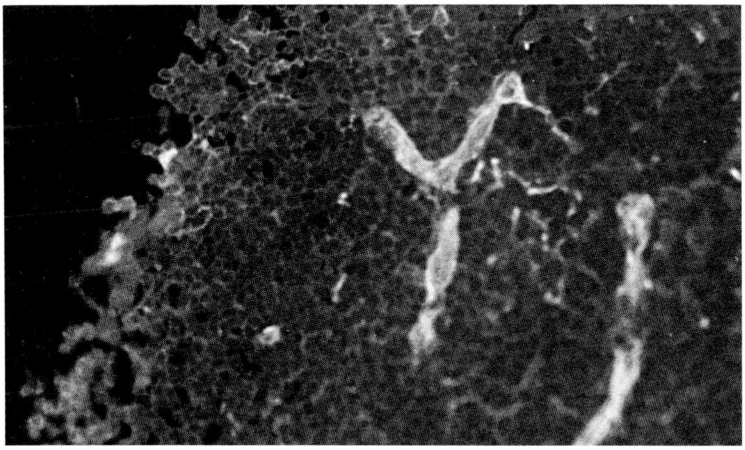

(b)

Figure 3 Immunofluorescence of antibody EA-1 on newborn thymus. (a) Phase contrast microscopy; (b) corresponding immunofluorescence. Intrathymic endothelial cells are stained.

REFERENCES

Albelda, S.M., Oliver, P.D., Romer, L.H., and Buck, C.A. EndoCAM: A novel endothelial cell-cell adhesion molecule. J. Cell. Biol. 1990; 110:1227–1237.

Dunon, D., Kaufman, J., Salomonsen, J., Skjoedt, K., Thiery, J.P. and Imhof, B. A. T-cell precursor migration toward β_2-microglobulin is involved in thymus colonization of chicken embryos. EMBO J. 1990; 9:3315–3322.

Imhof, B.A., Deugnier, M.A., Girault, J.M., Champion, S., Damais, C., Itoh, T. and Thiery, J.P. Thymotaxin: a thymic epithelial peptide chemotactic for T-cell precursors. Proc. Natl. Acad. Sci. U.S.A. 1988; 85:7699–703.

Imhof, B.A., Schlienger, C., Handloser, K., Hesse, B., and Gisler, R. Assay for quantitation of cell-cell adhesion using fluorescent dyes. In: Levkovits, I., and Pernis, B., eds., *Immunological Methods IV*. Academic Press, New York, 1990, pp. 251–263.

Pelkonen, J., Sideras, P., Rammensee, H.G., Karjalainen, K., and Palacios, R. Thymocyte clones from 14 day mouse embryos. J. Exp. Med. 1987; 166:1245–1258.

Kyewski, B.A. Seeding of thymic microenvironments defined by distinct thymocyte-stromal interactions is developmentally controlled. J. Exp. Med. 1987; 166:520–538.

Osborne, L. Leukocyte adhesion to endothelium in inflammation. Cell 1990; 62:3–6.

Savagner, P., Imhof, B.A., Yamada, K.M., and Thiery, J.P. Homing of hemopoietic precursor cells to the embryonic thymus: Characterization of an invasive mechanism induced by chemotactic peptides. J. Cell Biol. 1986, 103:2715–1727.

Savagner, P., Bauvois, B., Deugnier, M.A., Imhof, B.A., and Thiery, J.P. Aspects of haemopoietic cell dynamics: Ontogeny and targeted migration. Ann. Inst. Pasteur/Immunol. 1988; 139:409–431.

Scollay, R., Smith, J., and Stauffer, V. Dynamics of early T cells: Pro thymocyte migration and proliferation in the adult mouse thymus. Immunol. Rev. 1986, 91:129–157.

Springer, T.A. Adhesion receptors of the immune system. Nature 1990; 346, 425–434.

Williams, T.A., Risau, W., Zerwes, H.G., Drexler, H., Aguzzi, A., Wagner, E.F. Endothelioma cells expressing the polyoma middle T oncogene induce hemangiomas by host cell recruitment. Cell 1989; 57:1053–1063.

Woodruff, J.J., Clarke, L.M., and Chin, Y.H. Specific cell-adhesion mechanisms determining migration pathways of recirculating lymphocytes. Ann. Rev. Immunol. 1987; 5:201–222.

167
Germinal Centers: Yesterday, Today, and Tomorrow
A Matter of Life and Death

Paul Nieuwenhuis
University of Groningen, Groningen, The Netherlands

INTRODUCTION

When Beat Imhof asked me to give the final presentation at this meeting, words once spoken by Dr J. Klein (Max Planck Institut, Tübingen, West Germany) crossed my mind, and I quote (1):

> One of the signs of growing old is when you are invited to deliver general lectures. Such an invitation means either that you are not expected to have much specific to say or that you are thought of as being around long enough to acquire old age wisdom. Either way, the invitation is not very flattering.

Nevertheless, I accepted gracefully. These closing remarks will not be a summary of all the exciting data that have been presented these last few days. What I will do, however, is to try and summarize ±150 years of germinal centre research, eventually to take a brief glimpse at the future.

GERMINAL CENTERS YESTERDAY

Birth of a Lymphocyte: A Role for Germinal Centers?

At the beginning of the nineteenth century, some scientists still believed that life could originate from lifeless matter (generatio spontanea). So it was believed, e.g., that lymphocytes (*Lymphkörperchen, Lymphzellen*), especially in intestinal lymph, could originate by aggregation of small fat droplets in the chyle (Fig. 1a) (for discussion, see Ref. 2). One of the main arguments against this hypothesis came from observations by Brücke (3) on the lymphocyte content of afferent and efferent lymph of mesenteric nodes. Even in animals fed on a low-fat diet, the efferent lymph contained high numbers of lymphocytes in sharp

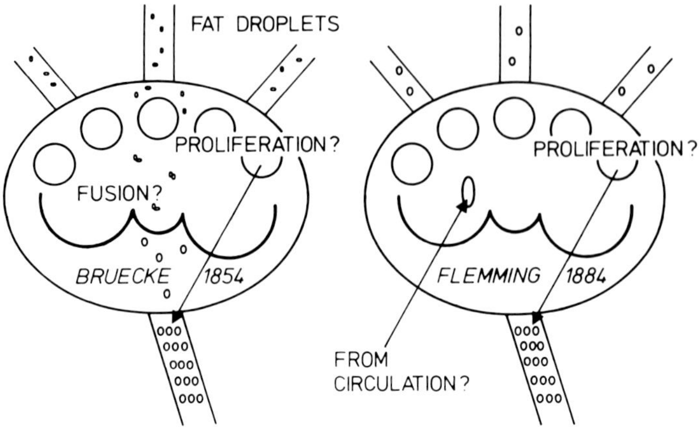

Figure 1 Schematic representation of questions asked respectively by Brücke (2) and Flemming (1884) (see Ref. 4) on the origin of lymphocytes.

contrast to the very few present in the afferent lymph. Consequently, he concluded that lymphocytes (*Lymphkörperchen*) would have their origin within the lymph nodes:

> Es ist gewiss und unzweifelhaft, dass die Lymphkörperchen in den Lymphdrüsen gebildet werden, und zwar nicht aus Keimen, welche der Chylusstrom in dieselben hineinbringt, sondern aus solchen, welche sich auf dem Drüsengewebe, als auf ihren mütterlichen Boden entwickeln (Ref. 2, p. 131).

Some 30 years later, Flemming, in his studies on tissue regeneration, also studied the question why efferent lymph contains many more lymphocytes than afferent lymph. He envisaged two possibilities:

> Entweder sie erfolgt durch Theilungen der Zellen, die in den Maschen des Reticulums der Knoten und Strängen lagern; oder sie geschieht in der Art, dass aus den Blutgefässen dieser Knoten und Strängen fortdauernd oder schubweise Leukozyten auswandern, so dass also einer Art kontinuierlichen Kreislaufs dieser Elemente aus dem Blut in die Lymphe und mit dieser wieder ins Blut statt finden würde (4) [Fig. 1b].

As he observed high mitotic activity in the lightly staining central parts of secondary nodules (*Sekundär-knötchen*) in the cortex of the lymph nodes studied (Fig. 2a), he concluded: "Die Lymphknoten und die 'Darmfollikel' sind Brutstätten der Neubildung von Lymphozyten auf dem Wege indirecten Theilungs" (Ref. 4, p. 57). Subsequently Flemming referred to these areas of high mitotic activity as *Keimzentren*, or germinal centers (Ref. 4, e.g., p. 55, and Ref. 5, e.g., p. 361).

Death of a Germinal Center

It took not long before objections against Flemming's hypothesis of germinal centers being the only source of lymphocytes were raised. In 1912, Downey and Weidenreich (6) observed that large lymphocytes, which they considered to be the "*Mutterform der kleine Elemente*," not only could be found within germinal centers, but throughout the lymphoid tissues and even in the thoracic duct. So the whole of the lymphoid tissue would seem to serve as a continuous source for its own inhabitants and they concluded: "So ist damit die

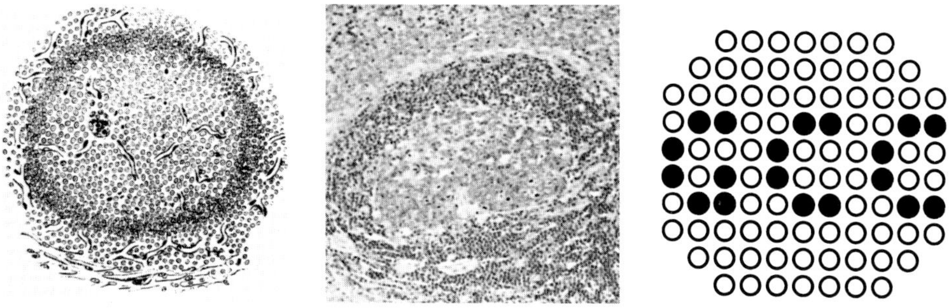

a b c

Figure 2 Three different views on a germinal center: (a) from Flemming (4), fig. 5, indicating mitotic activity in a secondary nodule (Sekundär-knötchen); (b) germinal center in rat spleen, 4 days after i.v. injection of sheep red blood cells (methylgreen-pyronin stain); (c) logo of Germinal Centre Conferences (as from 1981) with closed circles (GCC, red) indicating centroblasts and open circles (remainder, blue) indicating mantle zone lymphocytes. Typical methylgreen-pyronin stain.

Frage nach der Herkunft der kleinen Lymphozyten gelöst." Objections against Flemming's hypothesis of germinal centers being at all a possible source of lymphocytes were presented by Hellman in a large series of papers (e.g., see Ref. 7). His two major arguments were:

1. As one might expect the production of lymphocytes to be a continuous process, the *Keimzentren* of Flemming seemed to be a rather unlikely source, as these structures were found to be subject to considerable changes in size and activity (as, by the way, had already been noticed by Flemming himself). Mitotic activity within these structures could be increased by the injection of all kinds of toxins, which was the reason why Hellman preferred the name *Reaktionszentren* over *Keimzentren*, and consequently ascribed to them a role "im Dienste der Ausbildung der Immunität."
2. Along with an increase of the mitotic activity of a germinal center, the mantle zone of small lymphocytes does not grow from the germinal center. In contrast, germinal centers not seldom were found completely lacking a small rim of darkly staining lymphocytes.

Support for Hellman's objections against Flemming's hypothesis came from the work of Sjøvall (8), who, after subjecting rabbits to repeated bleedings, which resulted in a 25% drop in lymphocyte count in the blood, was unable to find any changes in germinal center activity. She concluded: "die Reaktionszentren (haben) nichts mit den Lymphozyten-production zu tun."

Also from the work of Glimstedt (9) it seemed rather unlikely that germinal centers contributed to the normal population of the lymphoid tissue. In his studies on germ-free guinea pigs, these animals were found to be completely lacking any germinal center, but nevertheless contained an otherwise normally developed lymphoid tissue, a finding which has since been repeatedly confirmed. So by the middle of this century, Flemming's hypothesis on the role of germinal centers had died an untimely death.

The Thymus

In the late 1950s and early 1960s, many exciting things happened in immunology, among which a major one was the discovery of the recirculation of lymphocytes by Gowans (10) (cf. "kontinuierlichen Kreislaufs", Ref. 4). By now, available data could explain how efferent lymph contains more lymphocytes than afferent lymph, and how the continuous delivery of large numbers of lymphocytes into the blood stream could be reconciled with a constant level of lymphocytes in the blood. Still, these data could not answer questions related to the *origin* of the (recirculating) lymphocytes.

Although the *true* function of the thymus had been described early in 1900 by Beard (11), in 1921, Hammar (12), in a paper ominously enough published in the journal *Endocrinology*, stated: "All these facts thus contain as many confirmations . . . of the fact . . . that the thymus is not or does not consist of lymphoid tissue," and . . . : "The thymus is an epithelial organ, infiltrated with lymphocytes."

Until 1961, little if any experimental evidence was available to indicate that the thymus played a major role in the development of the immune system. In that year, Miller (13), who was kind enough to allow me to paraphrase the title of his 1967 paper in the journal *Lancet*, "The Thymus: Yesterday, Today and Tomorrow" (14), published data showing that thymectomy of newborn mice was associated with a deficiency in the lymphocyte population of the blood and lymphoid tissues, an inability to reject foreign skin grafts, and premature death attributed to infection (wasting disease). This was the beginning of the golden age of thymology, of which we have not seen the end yet.

Serendipity in Immunology

Apart from the obvious reason for introducing the thymus in this summary of germinal center research, i.e., as a source of lymphocytes, there is another reason, namely, the "accidental" (with apologies to Dr. Miller) nature of the discovery of the role of the thymus in the immune system. Four years before Miller's 1961 publication (13), MacLean et al. (15), who had performed neonatal thymectomy in rabbits, had (re)confirmed that the thymus should not be considered as a source of lymphocytes. Owing to the fact that mice are neonatally less mature than rabbits, Miller succeeded where MacLean et al. failed, as "luck" would have it.

This luck has played a major role in many discoveries in medical science, including immunology. In recent years the role of luck has gained more attention and the term has now been replaced by serendipity, which was defined by Humphrey (16) as "the unexpected observation seized upon and turned to advantage by the prepared mind." In two papers on serendipity in immunology, Humphrey (16,17) extensively describes various examples related to his own work and that of others. Here I would like to add another serendipitous finding, especially as it brings me back to germinal centers, at least to B cells.

The Bursa of Fabricius

In the chicken, a small round pear-shaped diverticulum extending from the dorsal side of the cloaca for the first time was described in 1604 by Fabricius, and later was called the bursa of Fabricius in his honor. Fabricius considered it to be a storage place for spermatozoa to be used for fertilization during the egg-laying process. Later, however, it was found that this bursa never contains any spermatozoa, and, moreover, disappears at sexual maturity. Up to the summer of 1954, bursectomy experiments had failed to reveal any specific function for the bursa. It then happened that in a class demonstration involving the injection of chickens with *Salmonella typhi* O antigen, some chickens immediately died after the injection, whereas three others failed to produce the expected agglutinin antibodies. When the wing-band numbers of these animals were checked, it appeared that they had been bursectomized early after hatching (18,19). From this chance observation and subsequent systematic research, the significance of the bursa of Fabricius as the major source of B cells (i.e., bursa-derived cells) and its role in the development of antibody potential became established.

As mammals do not have a bursa of Fabricius, a bursa-equivalent was postulated (20), and for a while the mammalian gut-associated lymphoid tissue (GALT) was considered to have a central lymphoid role, like the bursa in chicken (21). In our own experiments we showed (22) that it was essentially the richness in germinal centers (which we had shown to be a source of antibody-forming cell precursors (AFCPs) (23) of structures like GALT that allowed the erroneous interpretation of GALT as a central lymphoid organ.

Revival of Germinal Centers

At the time when the central roles of the thymus and the bursa of Fabricius were being established, germinal centers also gained new interest. Thus, members of the Biology Division, Oak Ridge National Laboratory, Oak Ridge, Tennessee, and of the Institute of Pathology, University of Bern, Switzerland, guided by C. C. Congdon and H. Cottier, decided to bring together workers interested in the field. The result was an International Conference on "Germinal Centres of Lymphatic Tissue" (the first Germinal Centre Conference [GCC]) held in Bern, June 1966. In his closing remarks Cottier stated: "Many participants expressed an interest in meeting again in a few years to reexamine our understanding of the relationship of germinal centres and immune responses" (Ref. 24, p. 466). And so a series of international conferences was started dedicated to in vivo immunology.

Until the eighth meeting held in Cambridge, 1984, the driving force behind these meetings, apart from everchanging local organizing committees, was Dr. M. G. Hanna, Jr., Frederick Cancer Center, Frederick, Maryland, originally of Oak Ridge, Tennessee, who's highly valuable contributions should especially be gratefully acknowledged here. The fact that germinal centers were now a regular focus of interest at subsequent meetings—at least nominally dedicated to these structures—did not imply that the veil of mystery was lifted from these structures (see Fig. 2b). This led Humphrey (25) to entitle his invited lecture at the fifth GCC, held in Tiberias, Israel, in 1975: "The Still Unsolved Germinal Centre Mystery." At the seventh GCC, held in Groningen, The Netherlands, 1981, Humphrey (26) delivered another lecture on germinal centers, which was entitled: "The Still Unsolved Mystery of the Germinal Centre (Continued)." Later still, at the occasion of the centennial anniversary of Flemming's first description of *Keimzentren*, I referred to germinal centers as "structures, which have yet to reveal their last secret" (27). In 1981, Humphrey, rather succinctly summarized germinal center knowledge by saying:

> The evidence is now good that the production of B-memory cells (i.e. cells capable of responding to further antigenic stimulation, with T cell help, by antibody production) is stimulated by antigen-antibody complexes retained via C_3 on follicular dendritic cells (FDC) in germinal centres, at least for T dependent antigens in the mouse (Ref. 26, p. 739)

GERMINAL CENTERS TODAY

Now, nine years later, at the tenth GCC, where do we stand? Has "the mystery" been solved? (see Fig. 3.) Despite the many excellent contributions at this meeting, still some question marks remain related to the precise role of the various factors involved in the life history of a germinal center. In his summing up as cochairman of the session on B-cell development, Rajewski mentioned three decisions a B cell had to make, which are a matter of life or death for this cell. In regard to these decisions, one more question should be added, i.e., how does a B cell "decide" whether it will function as an antibody-forming cell precursor and transform into a plasmablast, giving rise to a clone of plasma cells, or whether it considers itself to be a germinal center precursor cell to clonally expand within a germinal center to give rise to a new generation of B-memory cells.

Are these questions mere semantics or do they constitute real problems, which in my opinion have received too little attention yet? Are there separate lineages/subsets or does the "choice" reflect different maturation stages, or is it influenced by varying local microenvironmental signals either by direct cell-cell interaction (role for adhesion molecules?) or by local messages (interleukins?)? (For a discussion, see Ref. 28.)

Other points of interest that came up at this meeting (i.e., related to germinal centers) are a better understanding of the role of follicular dendritic cells (FDCs) in rescuing germinal center B cells from programmed cell death (also by some designated apoptosis) and substantial evidence for the occurrence of somatic mutation within germinal centers. The size of this volume in itself bears witness to the many other topics discussed at length, which are beyond the scope of this "summary."

GERMINAL CENTERS TOMORROW

At this meeting we have seen a first and reasonably convincing successful attempt to mimic germinal centers in vitro by culturing a mixture of B cells, FDCs, and T cells (Kosco et al., Chap. 118). Kosco concluded: "Collectively these data suggest that the in vitro system described is representative of a germinal center and can be used to identify necessary components interacting in the microenvironment."

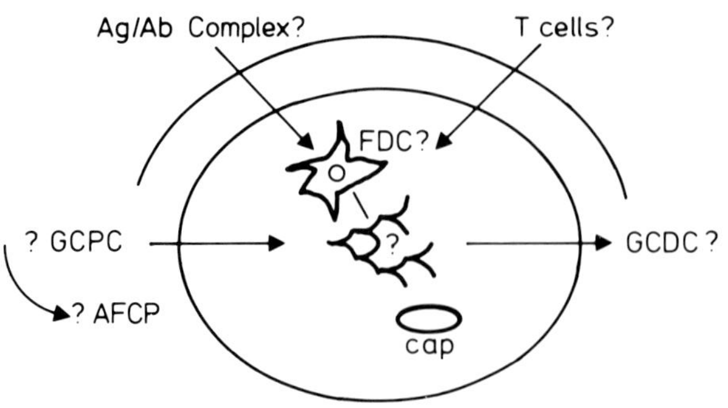

Figure 3 Schematic representation of various factors involved in the formation and function of a germinal center. Question marks indicate areas of ongoing research. Ag/Ab: antigen/antibody; FDC: follicular dendritic cell; GGPC: 8 germinal center precursor cell; GCDC: germinal center derived cell; AFCP: antibody-forming cell precursor; cap: capillary inside germinal center.

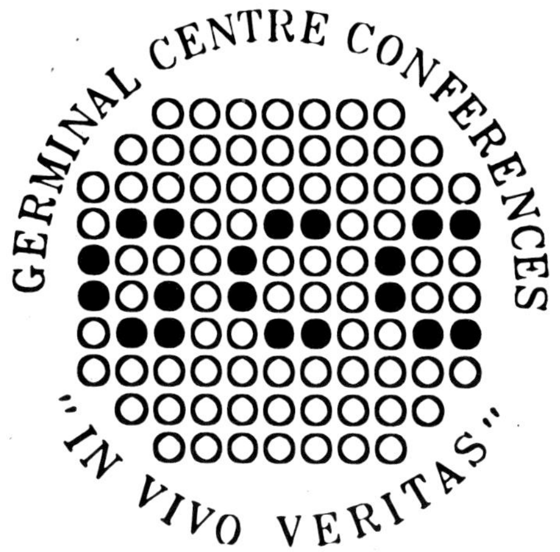

Figure 4 Suggested logo for future Germinal Centre Conferences.

Until presently, germinal centers were "in vivo only" structures par excellence, and as such highly symbolic of the general interest in in vivo immunology, which has been the running theme of these meetings. If future germinal center research indeed would focus on in vitro models, one might perhaps ask: Is there life after 10 GCC? Fortunately enough, in vivo immunology relates to more than germinal centers, as is witnessed by the rather elaborate name of these meetings: "International Conference on Lymphatic Tissues and Germinal Centres in Immune Reactions." Moreover, these meetings per se function as real "germinal centers," constituting a highly creative microenvironment selecting the really bright ideas, and usually leaving one with pleasant memories.

If we stick to the theme that has run through all our previous meetings, i.e., in vivo immunology, guided by the motto *in vivo veritas*, I see a bright future ahead for these kinds of meetings, which—just for short—might be called Germinal Centre Conferences. To support this idea, I would like to present a new logo (see Fig. 4) to accompany us on our road of better understanding the enigmatic pathways of the lymphocyte (*Lymphzelle* or *Lymphkörperchen*) with which it all began.

ACKNOWLEDGMENTS

It is a pleasure to thank Ms. Marga de Wolff for a typing job well done, Mr. Hemmo Meiborg for excellent photography, and Mr. Peter van de Sijde for expert "fiddling" with his computer in producing the new logo.

REFERENCES

1. Klein, J. *Hegemony of Mediocrity in Contemporary Sciences, Particularly in Immunology.* Seminar given in Boston, April 14, 1984.
2. Brücke, E. Ueber die Chylusgefässe und die Resorption der Chylus. Denkschriften der kaiserlichen Akademie der Wissenschaften. Mat. Nat. Wiss. Classe. Wien, 1854, 6:99.

3. Brücke, E. Ueber den Bau und die physiologische Bedeutung der Peyerschen Drüsen. Denkschriften der kaiserlichen Akademie der Wissenschaften. Mat. Nat. Wiss. Classe, Wien, 1851, 2:21.
4. Flemming, W. Studien über Regeneration der Gewebe: I. Die Zellvermehrung in den Lympdrüssen und verwandten Organen, und ihr Einfluss auf deren Bau. Arch. Mikr. Anat. 1885, 24:50.
5. Flemming, W. Studien über Regeneration der Gewebe: VII. Schluss-bemerkungen über die Zellvermehrung in den lymphoiden Drüsen. Arch. Mikr. Anat. 1885, 24:355.
6. Downey, H. and Weidenreich, F. Ueber die Bildung der Lymphozyten in Lymphdrüsen und Milz IX: Fortsetzung der "Studien über das Blut und die Blutbildenden und -zerstörenden Organe" von F. Weidenreich. Arch. Mikr. Anat. 1912, 80:306.
7. Hellman, T. Die Reaktionszentern des lymphatischen Gewebes. Anat. Anz., 1939, 87:132 (Ergänzungsheft zum 87 band)
8. Sjøvall, H. Experimentelle Untersuchungen über das Blut und die Blutbildende Organe—besonders das lympatische Gewebe—des Kaninchens bei wiederholten Aderlässen. Acta Pathol. Microb. Scand. 1936, Suppl. 27.
9. Glimstedt, G., Bacterienfreie Meerschweinchen. Acta Pathol. Microb. Scand. 1936, Suppl. 30.
10. Gowans, J. L. The recirculation of lymphocytes from blood to lymph in the rat. J. Physiol. (Lond.) 1958, 143:84.
11. Beard, J. The source of leukocytes and the true function of the thymus. Anat. Anz. 1900, 18:550.
12. Hammar, J. A., The new views as to the morphology of the thymus gland and their bearing on the problem of the function of the thymus. Endocrinology 1921, 14:731.
13. Miller, J. F. A. P., Immunological function of the thymus. Lancet 1961, 2:748.
14. Miller, J. F. A. P., The thymus: Yesterday, today and tomorrow. Lancet 1967, 2:1299.
15. MacLean, L. D., Zak, S. J., Varco, R. L. and Good, R. A. The role of the thymus in antibody production: an experimental study of the immune response in thymectomized rabbits. Transplant. Bull. 1957, 4:21.
16. Humphrey, J. H. Serendipity in immunology. Ann. Rev. Immunol. 1984, 2:1.
17. Humphrey, J. H. Serendipity and insight in immunology. Br. Med. J. 1986, 293:185.
18. Glick, B., Chang, T. S. and Jaap, R. G. The bursa of Fabricius and antibody production. Poultry Sci. 1956, 35:224.
19. Chang, T. S., Rheins, M. S. and Winter, A. R. The significance of the bursa of Fabricius in antibody production in chickens. 1. Age of chickens. Poultry Sci. 1957, 36:735.
20. Cooper, M. D., Perey, D. Y., McKneally, M. F., Gabrielsen, A. E., Sutherland, D. E. R. and Good, R. A. A mammalian equivalent of the avian bursa of Fabricius. Lancet 1966, 1:1388.
21. Cooper, M. D., Perey, D. Y., Gabrielsen, A. E., Sutherland D. E. R., McKneally, M. F. and Good, R. A. Production of an antibody deficiency syndrome in rabbits by neonatal removal of organized intestinal lymphoid tissues. Int. Arch. Allergy 1968, 33:65.
22. Nieuwenhuis, P. The rabbit appendix: A central or peripheral lymphoid organ? Adv. Exp. Med. Biol. 1971, 12:25.
23. Nieuwenhuis, P. Germinal centers: A microenvironment for the production of antibody forming germinal cell precursors. Adv. Exp. Med. Biol. 1973, 29:95.
24. Cottier, H., Hess, M. W. and Stoner, R. D. Summary and closing remarks In: *Germinal Centers in Immune Responses*, Cottier, H., Odartchenko, N., Schindler, R., and Congdon, C. C., eds.). Springer-Verlag, Berlin, 1967, p. 460.
25. Humphrey, J. H., The still unsolved germinal centre mystery. Adv. Exp. Med. Biol. 1976, 66:711.
26. Humphrey, J. H., The still unsolved mystery of the germinal centre (continued). Adv. Exp. Med. Biol. 1982, 149:739.
27. Nieuwenhuis, P. and Opstelten, D. Functional anatomy of germinal centres. Am. J. of Anat. 1984, 170:421.
28. Kroese, F. G. M., Timens, W. and Nieuwenhuis, P. Germinal center reaction and B lymphocytes: morphology and function. In: *Current Topics in Pathology*, Springer-Verlag, Heidelberg, 1990, 84/1, 118.

Index

About the Editors

BEAT A. IMHOF is a Member of the Basel Institute for Immunology, Switzerland. The author or coauthor of several articles and papers, he is a member of the Swiss Society for Biochemistry. Dr. Imhof received the M.S. (1980) and Ph.D. (1983) degrees from the Swiss Federal Institute of Technology, Zürich, Switzerland.

SONIA BERRIH-AKNIN is a Researcher for the Institut National de la Santé et de la Recherche Médicale at the Centre Chirurgical Marie-Lannelongue, Le Plessis-Robinson, France. The author or coauthor of several articles, she is a member of the New York Academy of Sciences, French Society of Immunology, and Society of Neuroimmunology. Dr. Berrih-Aknin received the M.Sc. (1977) and Ph.D. (1984) degrees from the University of Paris, France

SOPHIE EZINE is a Researcher for the Institut National de la Santé et de la Recherche Médicale at the Hôpital Necker, Paris, France. The author or coauthor of several articles and papers, she is a member of the French Society of Immunology. Dr. Ezine received the M.Sc. (1978) and Ph.D. (1987) degrees from the University of Paris, France.